Principles of
Public Health Practice

Principles of Public Health Practice

Third Edition

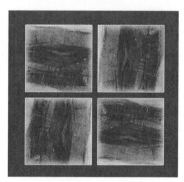

Edited by

F. Douglas Scutchfield, MD

Peter P. Bosomworth Professor of
Health Services Research and Policy
College of Public Health
University of Kentucky
Lexington, KY

C. William Keck, MD, MPH

Professor and Chair Emeritus
Community Health Sciences
Northeastern Ohio Universities Colleges of
Medicine and Pharmacy
Rootstown, OH

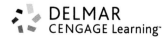

Australia • Brazil • Japan • Korea • Mexico • Singapore • Spain • United Kingdom • United States

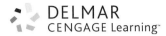
DELMAR
CENGAGE Learning™

Principles of Public Health Practice, Third Edition
F. Douglas Scutchfield and
C. William Keck

Vice President, Career and Professional Editorial: Dave Garza

Director of Learning Solutions: Matthew Kane

Senior Acquisitions Editor: Tari Broderick

Managing Editor: Marah Bellegarde

Product Manager: Natalie Pashoukos

Editorial Assistant: Anthony Souza

Vice President, Career and Professional Marketing: Jennifer McAvey

Marketing Director: Wendy Mapstone

Marketing Manager: Michelle McTighe

Marketing Coordinator: Scott Chrysler

Production Director: Carolyn Miller

Production Manager: Andrew Crouth

Senior Content Project Manager: James Zayicek

Senior Art Director: Jack Pendleton

Library of Congress Control Number: 2008931929

ISBN-13: 978-1-4180-6725-0

ISBN-10: 1-4180-6725-3

Delmar
5 Maxwell Drive
Clifton Park, NY 12065-2919
USA

Cengage Learning products are represented in Canada by Nelson Education, Ltd.

For your lifelong learning solutions, visit **delmar.cengage.com**

Visit our corporate website at **cengage.com**.

Printed in United States of America
2 3 4 5 6 13 12 11 10 09

DEDICATION

This book is dedicated to two groups of individuals. The first is our wives, Phyllis and Ardith, for their patience and support during the preparation of this book. It was from them we stole the nights and weekends to edit and write this text. Without their love and support, this book would not be in your hands.

If we are able to see any distance, it is because we had mentors who allowed and encouraged us to stand on their shoulders. We also dedicate this book to them. They include Abram Benenson, Kurt Deutschel, William Foege, John Hanlon, Alex Langmuir, William McBeath, George Pickett, and William Willard.

CONTENTS

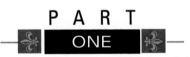

P A R T
ONE
The Basis of Public Health / 1

P A R T

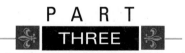

TWO

Settings for Public Health Practice / 149

P A R T

THREE

Tools for Public Health Practice / 233

P A R T
FOUR
The Provision of Public Health Services / 445

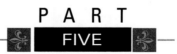

P A R T
FIVE
The Future of Public Health Practice / 735

ACKNOWLEDGMENTS

There are many people who have made important contributions to the successful completion of this book. The contributing authors merit the largest share of our gratitude, of course. The field of public health is broad and ever changing, and we felt the need to call widely on the expertise of many of our colleagues. Their willingness to participate with us in this endeavor is appreciated, as is their positive response to editing suggestions we made.

We especially thank Dr. Lois Nora, President and Dean, Northeastern Ohio Universities Colleges of Medicine and Pharmacy; Melody Hall at the University of Kentucky; Dr. J. Michael Moser, Director of Health for the City of Akron, Ohio; and Matthew A. Stefanak, Health Commissioner, Mahoning County General Health District for their understanding and support of this project. In addition, a special thank you is in order to Emma Lovely and the graduate students in public health at the University of Kentucky. Our editors, Natalie Pashoukos and Tari Broderick, deserve special mention for their help and support in the preparation of this manuscript.

FOREWORD

Public health has never received the recognition it deserves. The late nineteenth and early twentieth centuries have been referred to as the "Age of Modern Medical Miracles," yet it was not "miracles" of high technology that brought this nation to the health status it now enjoys. Instead, it was public health advances that accomplished that: clean water, proper housing, immunization, eradication of smallpox, increased life expectancy, and the understanding of preventive medicine as exemplified by healthy lifestyle choices.

In the past decade, we have seen two separate movements in the national and global worlds of public health. In the United States, we have seen the erosion of the infrastructure of public health, not because the practitioners of public health or its teachers were negligent but because both the Congress and the administrative branch, with their minds on other things, contributed to the present sorry state of affairs. The Republican Party presented the nation with a Contract with the American People, which unlike most contracts was signed only by the government. The administrative branch conceived the idea of "re-inventing" government. Public health was caught in a pincers movement, both sides of which could have more honestly labeled their efforts as "downsizing," a euphemism for activities that frequently undermine institutions and their infrastructures while reducing them in size.

The terrorist effort, mailing anthrax bacilli to prominent individuals, demonstrated our woeful inadequacy of institutions and infrastructure, which we trusted to forge the necessary alliances between health surveillance, health management, and agencies of the law necessary to respond to a bioterrorist attempt at mass destruction. Even the communication was confusing with multiple voices telling different stories. No one seemed to be in charge, in spite of the fact that the threat of bioterrorism cannot honestly be called new.

The other great movement that affects global as well as national public health is the technological advances made in communication. These new capabilities auger well, if properly harnessed, not only for the health of America but also the health of the world. Public health has been improving its ability to use these new tools, particularly the unbelievable explosion of informatics in the form of e-mail and the Internet. They have been of great assistance in the transmission of knowledge about the tremendous growth of science, including the scientific basis for public health problems and interventions, and advances in genetics and vaccines. The mapping of the genome and advances in genetic engineering have provided public health and medicine with knowledge hitherto almost unimaginable. And the development of new vaccines, always a welcomed advancement, comes at the very time when we need all of the expertise we can muster in this field, especially if we are to respond adequately to bioterrorism.

The word "globalization" has become one of our current buzzwords, and although most of the popular writing on the subject has to do with the economics of globalization, it is inextricably tied to the health of those nations to be globalized. We have truly globalized only two things, and we have done them well: we have globalized the spread of infectious disease, and we have seen the exportation of the cigarette into every nook and cranny of the planet. These things being true and both being the fruits, if you will, of the industrialized world, it stands to reason that we have the obligation to globalize health. The benefits of economic globalization aside, economic globalization cannot take place if the health of developing nations is not tremendously improved. These nations are too sick to contribute to economic globalization; only the globalization of good health can change that situation.

I do not view the health status of the world with discouragement, but rather see it as an unprecedented challenge for public health, which comes at a time when we have tools recently undreamed of that can aid us in our quest. In earlier years, I worried how we could ever bring health to the developing world because it lacked a health infrastructure. But science leapfrogged over that issue, and with the cell phone and the Internet, all it takes now is organization.

Just a few years ago, representatives of the almost 150 schools of medicine and osteopathic medicine in the United States, who turn out practitioners to treat injury and illness and return people to a previous state of health without making much effort to take them beyond that, met in dialogue on several occasions with representatives of the field of public health. The early enthusiasm of both sides to better meld medicine and public health has faded to a lackluster substitute for what we started out to do. That situation has to be reversed. I can't think of a professional challenge presented to two interrelated but distinct groups simultaneously that carries such promise if properly guided.

It is obvious, therefore, that there is an important role for a book that synthesizes state-of-the-art information about the problems and challenges of public health for the benefit of both students and current practitioners. I believe that Drs. Scutchfield and Keck have provided such a book. They have brought together the wisdom of many of the most knowledgeable health professionals in North America to provide the best information possible about current public health organizations and practice. For the new student, the book provides an introduction to the field of public health practice. For the current practitioner, it is a unique and vital reference. Those who make public health policy should not do so without understanding the content of this book. Only when there are enough knowledgeable and committed individuals will deplorable human suffering and unaffordable economic costs be prevented. This book is a step in that direction.

C. Everett Koop,
MD, ScD

PREFACE

Recent years have witnessed a quiet, yet dramatic, philosophic renaissance in the field of public health. Largely unnoticed by the general public, in the wake of the dramatic findings catalogued by the Institute of Medicine in their 1988 report, *The Future of Public Health*, the profession has recast itself. The vision, mission, and core functions of public health have been defined and clarified. Competencies for public health workers and performance standards for public health services have been developed and applied. National professional associations have expanded in number and effectiveness. Calls for accreditation of health departments, development of quality improvement activities, and credentialing of public health professionals are receiving attention and action. The structure of local health departments has changed very little, but efforts to better define what a local health department is and discussions of possible agency accreditation procedures and processes suggest that coming years may see serious attention paid to the organization and structure of local health agencies.

The historical underfunding of public health came into sharp focus with the attacks on the World Trade Center and the Pentagon in September 2001, followed by the mailing of anthrax spores to prominent politicians, and, more recently, the catastrophe spawned by Hurricane Katrina. The limited capacity of the United States to respond effectively to man-made or natural disasters led to a new public focus on public health capacity and new funding to improve preparedness for catastrophic event response. This did not translate, however, into broader respect for other public health services. The potential for public health to contribute to improved health status remained underappreciated as funding was shifted from other areas of public health activity to improve preparedness or fell victim to limited budgets and other spending priorities. This has resulted, in most public health jurisdictions, in an overall decrease in available funding.

With increasing complexity and attention to the profession there are new challenges for those who are responsible for public health. The management, administration, and financing of public health requires a new public health worker, one not only with detailed knowledge of the science of their discipline but also knowledge of how public health operates and the role that members of the public health workforce play in the provision of those public health services. They need, as well, additional leadership skills transferred from those developed in the private sector.

Today's public health practitioners find themselves in a changing and somewhat ambiguous environment. Challenging and exciting possibilities abound, but resources are limited. The government's role is paramount, but there is public mistrust of government. Health reform is at the front of the public's mind, but the focus is on illness care rather than health promotion and disease prevention. An expanding public health agenda calls for innovative responses, but the public is divided on priorities for action.

Successful management of health departments and other community health agencies requires enlightened and strong leadership. Public health leaders need to understand the contributions that can be made by the application of public health principles to community health problems, to work with communities to involve them in understanding and addressing the problems that threaten them, and to engineer constructive evolution of their agencies to effectively perform in a changing and uncertain environment.

The special challenges and unique environment of public health practice requires a large and competent workforce. Very few of the approximately 500,000 individuals employed as public health workers at all levels of government in the United States have formal public health training or even share a common academic base. The steady growth of public health training programs in the United States suggests appropriately trained individuals will continue to increase in number, but the fact remains that wide variation continues in the capacity of local health departments across the country to meet the needs of the populations they serve. Nonetheless, improvement of the public's health will require that the core functions of public health be competently executed. The cadre of public health leaders and workers must continue to expand, armed with both a clear vision of the role of public health in maintaining and improving health, and the skills required to make that vision a reality. This combination of challenges and opportunities suggests to us the need for *Principles of Public Health Practice, 3rd Edition.*

This book's third edition is intended for two main audiences. The first is students of the public health professions who would benefit from access to a broad text describing the organization, administration, and practice of public health in the unique and changing environment of the United States. The second is the public health professional who may be working in the field without the benefit of formal exposure to course work in public health practice, or who wishes to have on hand a review of recent developments in the field.

ORGANIZATION

This new edition is organized into five major parts with three appendices. The first part describes the current public health environment by introducing the basic concepts and development of public health practice, determinants of health status, the legal aspects on which public health practice is based, and recent changes in public health practice. This section also includes two new chapters that describe the making of public health policy and public health ethics.

Part two addresses the contributions made to public health at the federal, state, and local levels. Part three contains chapters that describe and discuss available tools to effectively manage a typical health department. Part four of this new edition describes public health practice in a number of substantive environments, including a new chapter on public health preparedness. Part five focuses on the role of the public health department in an evolving health system and suggests a vision of the ideal health department of the future. The appendices contain a new entry on evidence-based public health practice.

NEW TO THIS EDITION

A new table has been added to the front of the text which outlines how the core competencies for public health practice map to each chapter. Learning objectives and key terms are listed at the beginning of each chapter and there is a comprehensive glossary in the back of the book. Review questions appear at the end of each chapter.

Additionally, an online companion including the instructor's manual, PowerPoint presentations, and test banks, was created to accompany this text. The instructor's manual provides the instructor with talking points for case studies and policy issues, suggested group and individual activities and assignments, and answers to the review questions.

CONTRIBUTOR LIST

Myron Allukian, DDS, MPH
Oral Health Consultant
Massachusetts League of Community Health
    Centers and Lutheran Medical Center
Boston, MA

Susan P. Baker, MPH, ScD
Adjunct Associate Professor
Department of Health Policy and Management
Bloomberg School of Public Health
Johns Hopkins University
Baltimore, MD

Ronald Cada, DrPH
Retired, State of Colorado
Lincoln, NE

Zhuo Chen, PhD, MS
Economist & Prevention Effectiveness Fellow
Office of Workforce & Career Development
    and Office of Strategy and Innovation
    Centers for Disease Control & Prevention
Atlanta, GA

Janet L. Collins, PhD
Director, National Center for Chronic Disease
    Prevention and Health Promotion
Centers for Disease Control
Atlanta, GA

Julia F. Costich, JD, PhD
Chair, Department of Health Services
    Management
College of Public Health
University of Kentucky
Lexington, KY

Noe C. Crespo, MPH, MS
Doctoral Student
Graduate School of Public Health
San Diego, CA

Laura Hall Downey, DrPH
Assistant Professor
Department of Community Health Sciences
The University of Southern Mississippi
Hattiesburg, MS

Diane Downing, RN, MSN
Public Health Program Specialist/Nurse Manager
Department of Human Services
Arlington, VA

John P. Elder, PhD, MPH
Professor
Division of Health Promotion
Graduate School of Public Health
San Diego State University
San Diego, CA

Michael Eriksen, ScD
Professor and Director
Institute of Public Health
Georgia State University
Atlanta, GA

Linnea Evans, MPH
General Health Scientist
Office of the Director, Global Health
Promotion
National Center for Chronic Disease
Prevention and Health Promotion
Atlanta, GA

Elizabeth Fee, PhD
Chief of the History of Medicine Division
National Library of Medicine
Bethesda, MD

Kristine Gebbie, DrPH, RN
Dean, Hunter Bellevue School of Nursing
Hunter College,
New York, NY

Grace Gorenflo, MPH, RN
National Association of County and City
Health Officials
Washington, DC

Lawrence W. Green, DrPH
Adjunct Professor
Cancer Center
University of California
San Francisco, CA

Anne Haddix, MS, PhD
Chief Policy Officer
Office of Strategy and Innovation-Office of the
Director
Centers for Disease Control and Prevention
Atlanta, GA

Paul K. Halverson, MHSA, DrPH
Director
Arkansas Department of Health
Little Rock, AR

Alan Hinman, MD, MPH
Sr. Public Health Scientist Public Health
Informatics Institute
Task Force for Child Survival and Development
Decatur, GA

Carol J. Rowland Hogue, PhD, MPH
Terry Professor of Maternal and Child Health,
Professor of Epidemiology
Rollins School of Public Health
Emory University
Atlanta, GA

Alan M. Jacobs, PhD
Chair, Department of Geological and
Environmental Sciences
Youngstown State University
Youngstown, OH

C. William Keck, MD, MPH
Professor and Chair Emeritus
Community Health Sciences
Northeastern Ohio Universities Colleges of
Medicine and Pharmacy
Rootstown, OH

Michael R. King, MD, MPH
Assistant Professor
Department of Family and Community
Medicine
University of Kentucky
Lexington, KY

Cynthia Lamberth, MPH, CPH
Director, Kentucky Public Health Leadership
Institute and Center for Public Health
Systems and Services Research
College of Public Health
University of Kentucky
Lexington, KY

Linda Landesman, DrPH, MSW
NYC Health and Hospitals Corporation
New York, NY

Carolyn Leep, MS, MPH
  National Association of County and City
    Health Officials
  Washington, DC

Carl Leukefeld, DSW
  Bell Alcohol and Addictions Chair
  Department of Behavioral Science and Center
    on Drug and Alcohol Research
  University of Kentucky
  Lexington, KY

Patrick Libbey, BA
  Former Executive Director
  National Association of City and County
    Health Officials
  Washington, DC

Samuel C. Matheny, MD, MPH
  Professor and Chair
  Family Practice and Community Medicine
  University of Kentucky
  Lexington, KY

David McQueen, ScD
  Associate Director for Global Health
    Promotion
  Centers for Disease Control
  Atlanta, GA

A. Richard Melton, MPH, DrPH
  Director
  Utah Department of Health
  Salt Lake City, UT

Michael Moser, MD, MPH
  Director of Health
  Akron Health Department
  Akron, OH

James F. Mosher, JD
  Senior Policy Advisor
  The CDM Group, Inc.
  Felton, CA

Nancy Myers, PhD, RN
  Associate Professor
  Community Health Sciences
  Northeastern Ohio Universities Colleges of
    Medicine and Pharmacy
  Rootstown, OH

Carrie B. Oser, PhD
  Department of Sociology and Center on Drug
    and Alcohol Research
  University of Kentucky
  Lexington, KY

Kevin A. Pearce, MD, MPH
  Professor and Vice Chair
  Department of Family and Community
    Medicine
  College of Medicine
  University of Kentucky
  Lexington, KY

Robert L. Phillips, Jr., MD, MSPH
  Director, The Robert Graham Center: Policy
    Studies in Family Medicine and Primary Care
  Washington, DC

DuWayne Porter, MPH, RS
  Director of Health
  Portage County Health Department
  Ravenna, OH

Katharine C. Rathbun, MD, MPH
  Concentra Medical Clinic
  Baton Rouge, LA

Edward P. Richards, JD, MPH
  Professor and Director,
  Program in Law, Science, and Public Health
    Louisiana State University Law Center
    Baton Rouge, LA

Thomas Ricketts, PhD
  Professor and Director, North Carolina Rural
    Health Research Program and Program on
    Health Policy Analysis
  University of North Carolina
  Chapel Hill, NC

William L. Roper, MD, MPH
Dean and Vice Chancellor for Medical Affairs
School of Medicine
University of North Carolina
Chapel Hill, NC

Louis Rowitz, MA, PhD
Professor
Community Health Sciences
University of Illinois
School of Public Health
Chicago, IL

Kakoli Roy, PhD
Senior Economist
Office of Workforce and Career Development
Centers for Disease Control and Prevention
Atlanta, GA

F. Douglas Scutchfield, MD
Peter Bosomworth Professor of Health
    Services Research and Policy
Colleges of Public Health and Medicine
University of Kentucky
Lexington, KY

Maria Sequi-Gomez, MD, ScD
Adjunct Associate Professor
Department of Health Policy and
    Management
Bloomberg School of Public Health
Johns Hopkins University
Baltimore, MD

Laverne Snow, MPA PhD(C)
Utah Department of Health
Salt Lake City, UT

Michele Stanton-Tindall, PhD, MSW
College of Social Work and Center on Drug
    and Alcohol Research
University of Kentucky
Lexington, KY

William Stoops, PhD
Department of Behavioral Science
College of Medicine
University of Kentucky
Lexington, KY

Donna Stroup, PhD, MSc
Executive Director
Data for Solutions
Decatur, GA

Patricia M. Sweeney, JD, MPH, RN
Assistant Professor
Department of Health Policy and
    Management
Graduate School of Public Health
University of Pittsburg
Pittsburgh, PA

Stephen Thacker, MD, MSc
Director, Office of Workforce and Career
    Development
Centers for Disease Control and Prevention
Atlanta, GA

James C. Thomas, MPH, PhD
Associate Professor of Epidemiology
Director, Program in Public Health Ethics
Gillings School of Global Public Health
University of North Carolina
Chapel Hill, NC

Hugh Tilson, MD, DrPH
Adjunct Professor
Gillings School of Global Public Health
University of North Carolina
Chapel Hill, NC

Ralph Timperi, MPH
Association of Public Health Laboratories
Silver Spring, MD

Paula M. Usita, PhD
    Associate Professor
    Graduate School of Public Health
    San Diego State University
    San Diego, CA

Alfredo E. Vergara, MS, PhD
    Assistant Professor, Department of Preventive
        Medicine and Deputy Director
    Vanderbilt Institute for Global Health
    Vanderbilt University School of Medicine
    Nashville, TN

Sten H. Vermund, MD, PhD
    Professor, Department of Pediatrics and
        Director, Institute for Global Health
    Vanderbilt University School of Medicine
    Nashville, TN

Susan C. Waltman, JD, MSW
    Greater New York Hospital Association
    New York, NY

Isaac B. Weisfuse, MD, MPH
    NYC Department of Health and Mental Hygiene
    New York, NY

Steven H. Woolf, MD
    Professor of Family Medicine, Epidemiology
        and Community Health
    Virginia Commonwealth University
    Richmond, VA

REVIEWERS

Rachel T. Abraham, MD, MPH
Assistant Professor
Director, Public Health Grand Rounds
Director, Office for Public Health Practice and
Department of Community Medicine
West Virginia University
Morgantown, WV

Gwendolyn F. Foss, DNSc, RN
Associate Professor, School of Nursing
Coordinator, Graduate CHN and School of
Nursing
University of North Carolina
Charlotte, NC

Mary Ann Littleton, PhD
Assistant Professor, Department Public Health
East Tennessee State University
Johnson City, TN

Mary Helen McSweeney-Feld, PhD
Assistant Professor, Health Care
Programs
Iona College
New Rochelle, NY

Stacey B. Plichta, ScD
Professor, College of Health Sciences
Old Dominion University
Norfolk, VA

Wayne B. Sorenson, PhD
Associate Professor, Health Administration
Texas State University
San Marcos, TX

PUBLIC HEALTH COMPETENCIES BY CHAPTER

Specific Competencies	Chapter 1	Chapter 2	Chapter 3	Chapter 4	Chapter 5	Chapter 6	Chapter 7	Chapter 8	Chapter 9	Chapter 10	Chapter 11	Chapter 12	Chapter 13	Chapter 14	Chapter 15	Chapter 16	Chapter 17
DOMAIN #1: ANALYTIC ASSESSMENT SKILLS																	
A. Defines a problem.		X		X			X				X		X	X		X	X
B. Determines appropriate uses and limitations of both quantitative and qualitative data.				X							X		X	X		X	X
C. Selects and defines variables relevant to defined public health problems.				X					X		X		X	X		X	
D. Identifies relevant and appropriate data and information sources.		X		X					X	X	X		X	X		X	
E. Evaluates the integrity and comparability of data and identifies gaps in data sources.				X							X		X			X	X
F. Applies ethical principles to the collection, maintenance, use, and dissemination of data and information.					X	X	X				X	X	X			X	
G. Partners with communities to attach meaning to collect quantitative and qualitative data.							X					X				X	
H. Makes relevant inferences from quantitative and qualitative data.				X						X	X		X	X		X	
I. Obtains and interprets information regarding risks and benefits to the community.				X		X					X		X			X	
J. Applies data collection processes, information technology applications, and computer systems storage/retrieval strategies.												X				X	
K. Recognizes how the data illuminates ethical, political, scientific, economic, and overall public health issues.		X	X	X	X		X				X		X	X		X	X

Specific Competencies	Chapter 1	Chapter 2	Chapter 3	Chapter 4	Chapter 5	Chapter 6	Chapter 7	Chapter 8	Chapter 9	Chapter 10	Chapter 11	Chapter 12	Chapter 13	Chapter 14	Chapter 15	Chapter 16	Chapter 17
DOMAIN #2: POLICY DEVELOPMENT/PROGRAM PLANNING SKILLS																	
A. Collects, summarizes, and interprets information relevant to an issue.		X		X		X	X	X	X	X	X		X	X			X
B. States policy options and writes clear and concise policy statements.							X	X	X				X				
C. Identifies, interprets, and implements public health laws, regulations, and policies related to specific programs.							X	X	X	X							
D. Articulates the health, fiscal, administrative, legal, social, and political implications of each policy option.		X		X			X	X	X				X		X		
E. States the feasibility and expected outcomes of each policy option.				X			X	X	X				X				
F. Utilizes current techniques in decision analysis and health planning.							X	X					X			X	
G. Decides on the appropriate course of action.							X	X			X			X	X		
H. Develops a plan to implement policy, including goals, outcome and process objectives, and implementation steps.							X	X							X		
I. Translates policy into organizational plans, structures, and programs.							X	X	X					X	X		
J. Prepares and implements emergency response plans.							X										
K. Develops mechanisms to monitor and evaluate programs for their effectiveness and quality.							X		X					X		X	
DOMAIN #3: COMMUNICATION SKILLS																	
A. Communicates effectively both in writing and orally, or in other ways.							X			X	X						
B. Solicits input from individuals and organizations.							X				X	X	X			X	
C. Advocates for public health programs and resources.		X		X	X	X	X		X		X	X					
D. Leads and participates in groups to address specific issues.						X	X				X	X					
E. Uses the media, advanced technologies, and community networks to communicate information.		X					X		X		X	X		X			
F. Effectively presents accurate demographic, statistical, programmatic, and scientific information for professional and lay audiences.			X	X			X		X	X	X		X	X		X	

Specific Competencies	Chapter 1	Chapter 2	Chapter 3	Chapter 4	Chapter 5	Chapter 6	Chapter 7	Chapter 8	Chapter 9	Chapter 10	Chapter 11	Chapter 12	Chapter 13	Chapter 14	Chapter 15	Chapter 16	Chapter 17
G. Listens to others in an unbiased manner, respects points of view of others, and promotes the expression of diverse opinions and perspectives.							X				X	X					
DOMAIN #4: CULTURAL COMPETENCY SKILLS																	
A. Utilizes appropriate methods for interacting sensitively, effectively, and professionally with persons from diverse cultural, socioeconomic, educational, racial, ethnic, and professional backgrounds, and persons of all ages and lifestyle preferences.						X			X				X				
B. Identifies the role of cultural, social, and behavioral factors in determining the delivery of public health services.		X		X			X									X	
C. Develops and adapts approaches to problems that take into account cultural differences.				X			X										
D. Understands the dynamic forces contributing to cultural diversity.				X			X				X						
E. Understands the importance of a diverse public health workforce.							X		X							X	X
DOMAIN #5: COMMUNITY DIMENSIONS OF PRACTICE SKILLS																	
A. Establishes and maintains linkages with key stakeholders.	X	X	X	X		X	X		X			X		X			
B. Utilizes leadership, teambuilding, negotiation, and conflict-resolution skills to build community partnerships.							X		X			X		X			
C. Collaborates with community partners to promote the health of the population.		X	X	X			X		X			X		X			
D. Identifies how public and private organizations operate within a community.	X	X	X	X	X	X			X			X		X		X	
E. Accomplishes effective community engagements.				X			X		X			X		X		X	
F. Identifies community assets and available resources.	X		X	X					X			X	X	X		X	
G. Develops, implements, and evaluates a community public health assessment.									X		X	X		X		X	
H. Describes the role of government in the delivery of community health services.		X	X	X	X	X	X	X	X	X							X

Specific Competencies	Chapter 1	Chapter 2	Chapter 3	Chapter 4	Chapter 5	Chapter 6	Chapter 7	Chapter 8	Chapter 9	Chapter 10	Chapter 11	Chapter 12	Chapter 13	Chapter 14	Chapter 15	Chapter 16	Chapter 17
DOMAIN #6: BASIC PUBLIC HEALTH SCIENCES SKILLS																	
A. Identifies the individual's and organization's responsibilities within the context of the essential public health services and core functions.	X	X	X			X		X	X	X						X	X
B. Defines, assesses, and understands the health status of populations, determinants of health and illness, factors contributing to health promotion and disease prevention, and factors influencing the use of health services.	X		X	X			X					X	X	X		X	
C. Understands the historical development, structure, and interaction of public health and health care systems.	X	X	X					X	X	X							
D. Identifies and applies basic research methods used in public health.				X									X			X	
E. Applies the basic public health sciences, including behavioral and social sciences, biostatistics, epidemiology, environmental public health, and prevention of chronic and infectious diseases and injuries.		X		X					X		X		X	X			
F. Identifies and retrieves current relevant scientific evidence.				X				X	X				X				
G. Identifies the limitations of research and the importance of observations and interrelationships.		X	X	X				X					X				X
H. Develops a lifelong commitment to rigorous critical thinking.		X	X			X	X						X				X
DOMAIN #7: FINANCIAL PLANNING AND MANAGEMENT SKILLS																	
A. Develops and presents a budget.								X			X						
B. Manages programs within budget constraints.							X	X			X				X		
C. Applies budget processes.								X			X				X		
D. Develops strategies for determining budget priorities.				X							X		X		X	X	
E. Monitors program performance.							X	X			X		X	X		X	
F. Prepares proposals for funding from external sources.								X			X						
G. Applies basic human relations skills to the management of organizations, motivation of personnel, and resolution of conflicts.		X				X		X			X						
H. Manages information systems for collection, retrieval, and use of data for decision making.							X									X	

Specific Competencies	Chapter 1	Chapter 2	Chapter 3	Chapter 4	Chapter 5	Chapter 6	Chapter 7	Chapter 8	Chapter 9	Chapter 10	Chapter 11	Chapter 12	Chapter 13	Chapter 14	Chapter 15	Chapter 16	Chapter 17
I. Negotiates and develops contracts and other documents for the provision of population-based services.						X											
J. Conducts cost-effectiveness, cost-benefit, and cost utility analyses.							X						X				
DOMAIN #8: LEADERSHIP AND SYSTEMS THINKING SKILLS																	
A. Creates a culture of ethical standards within organizations and communities.						X	X		X		X						
B. Helps create key values and shared vision and uses these principles to guide action.		X	X		X		X							X	X		
C. Identifies internal and external issues that may impact delivery of essential public health services (i.e., strategic planning).			X	X		X	X		X	X	X				X		X
D. Facilitates collaboration with internal and external groups to ensure participation of key stakeholders.			X	X		X	X		X			X			X		
E. Promotes team and organizational learning.		X	X			X	X		X								X
F. Contributes to development, implementation, and monitoring of organizational performance standards.			X			X	X		X						X	X	
G. Uses the legal and political systems to effect change.		X	X	X	X	X	X	X	X								
H. Applies theory of organizational structures to professional practice.			X	X											X		

Specific Competencies	Chapter 18	Chapter 19	Chapter 20	Chapter 21	Chapter 22	Chapter 23	Chapter 24	Chapter 25	Chapter 26	Chapter 27	Chapter 28	Chapter 29	Chapter 30	Chapter 31	Appendix A	Appendix B	Appendix C
DOMAIN #1: ANALYTIC ASSESSMENT SKILLS L. Defines a problem.		X	X	X	X	X	X	X	X	X	X	X	X	X			
M. Determines appropriate uses and limitations of both quantitative and qualitative data.				X	X		X			X						X	
N. Selects and defines variables relevant to defined public health problems.		X	X	X	X	X	X	X	X	X							
O. Identifies relevant and appropriate data and information sources.		X	X	X	X	X	X	X	X	X	X	X	X	X		X	

Specific Competencies	Chapter 18	Chapter 19	Chapter 20	Chapter 21	Chapter 22	Chapter 23	Chapter 24	Chapter 25	Chapter 26	Chapter 27	Chapter 28	Chapter 29	Chapter 30	Chapter 31	Appendix A	Appendix B	Appendix C
P. Evaluates the integrity and comparability of data and identifies gaps in data sources.			X	X			X	X	X							X	
Q. Applies ethical principles to the collection, maintenance, use, and dissemination of data and information.				X			X										
R. Partners with communities to attach meaning to collect quantitative and qualitative data.				X			X	X	X		X	X					
S. Makes relevant inferences from quantitative and qualitative data.			X	X	X		X	X	X	X	X	X				X	
T. Obtains and interprets information regarding risks and benefits to the community.			X	X	X	X	X	X	X	X	X		X		X	X	
U. Applies data collection processes, information technology applications, and computer systems storage/retrieval strategies.			X				X										
V. Recognizes how the data illuminates ethical, political, scientific, economic, and overall public health issues.			X	X	X	X	X	X	X	X	X	X	X		X		
DOMAIN #2: POLICY DEVELOPMENT/PROGRAM PLANNING SKILLS																	
L. Collects, summarizes, and interprets information relevant to an issue.			X	X	X	X	X	X	X	X	X				X	X	
M. States policy options and writes clear and concise policy statements.			X	X			X	X	X		X	X	X				
N. Identifies, interprets, and implements public health laws, regulations, and policies related to specific programs.			X	X	X	X	X	X	X		X	X	X				
O. Articulates the health, fiscal, administrative, legal, social, and political implications of each policy option.			X	X			X	X	X		X			X			
P. States the feasibility and expected outcomes of each policy option.			X	X			X	X	X		X						
Q. Utilizes current techniques in decision analysis and health planning.			X	X			X										
R. Decides on the appropriate course of action.			X	X			X				X	X					
S. Develops a plan to implement policy, including goals, outcome and process objectives, and implementation steps.			X				X				X						

Specific Competencies	Chapter 18	Chapter 19	Chapter 20	Chapter 21	Chapter 22	Chapter 23	Chapter 24	Chapter 25	Chapter 26	Chapter 27	Chapter 28	Chapter 29	Chapter 30	Chapter 31	Appendix A	Appendix B	Appendix C
T. Translates policy into organizational plans, structures, and programs.			X	X		X	X	X	X		X	X	X				
U. Prepares and implements emergency response plans.						X	X		X								
V. Develops mechanisms to monitor and evaluate programs for their effectiveness and quality.			X				X	X	X		X	X					
DOMAIN #3: COMMUNICATION SKILLS																	
H. Communicates effectively both in writing and orally, or in other ways.				X	X	X	X	X	X	X							
I. Solicits input from individuals and organizations.			X	X		X	X										
J. Advocates for public health programs and resources.			X	X	X		X	X	X		X	X	X				
K. Leads and participates in groups to address specific issues.				X			X				X						
L. Uses the media, advanced technologies, and community networks to communicate information.			X	X		X	X	X	X								
M. Effectively presents accurate demographic, statistical, programmatic, and scientific information for professional and lay audiences.			X	X	X		X	X	X	X	X	X		X			
N. Listens to others in an unbiased manner, respects points of view of others, and promotes the expression of diverse opinions and perspectives.				X			X					X					
DOMAIN #4: CULTURAL COMPETENCY SKILLS																	
F. Utilizes appropriate methods for interacting sensitively, effectively, and professionally with persons from diverse cultural, socioeconomic, educational, racial, ethnic, and professional backgrounds, and persons of all ages and lifestyle preferences.	X		X			X				X							
G. Identifies the role of cultural, social, and behavioral factors in determining the delivery of public health services.	X	X	X	X	X		X	X	X			X	X				
H. Develops and adapts approaches to problems that take into account cultural differences.			X	X		X		X	X		X	X					
I. Understands the dynamic forces contributing to cultural diversity.			X	X		X		X	X				X				
J. Understands the importance of a diverse public health workforce.			X	X			X	X			X		X				

Specific Competencies	Chapter 18	Chapter 19	Chapter 20	Chapter 21	Chapter 22	Chapter 23	Chapter 24	Chapter 25	Chapter 26	Chapter 27	Chapter 28	Chapter 29	Chapter 30	Chapter 31	Appendix A	Appendix B	Appendix C
DOMAIN #5: COMMUNITY DIMENSIONS OF PRACTICE SKILLS																	
I. Establishes and maintains linkages with key stakeholders.			X	X	X	X				X		X					
J. Utilizes leadership, teambuilding, negotiation, and conflict-resolution skills to build community partnerships.	X			X										X			
K. Collaborates with community partners to promote the health of the population.			X	X	X	X	X				X	X		X			
L. Identifies how public and private organizations operate within a community.			X	X	X	X	X	X	X		X	X		X			
M. Accomplishes effective community engagements.				X			X				X	X					
N. Identifies community assets and available resources.			X	X		X	X	X	X		X	X	X				
O. Develops, implements, and evaluates a community public health assessment.				X			X				X	X		X			
P. Describes the role of government in the delivery of community health services.		X	X	X		X	X	X	X	X	X	X	X	X			
DOMAIN #6: BASIC PUBLIC HEALTH SCIENCES SKILLS																	
I. Identifies the individual's and organization's responsibilities within the context of the essential public health services and core functions.	X		X	X	?	X	X	X	X	X	X	X	X	X			
J. Defines, assesses, and understands the health status of populations, determinants of health and illness, factors contributing to health promotion and disease prevention, and factors influencing the use of health services.		X	X	X		X	X	X	X	X	X	X	X	X			
K. Understands the historical development, structure, and interaction of public health and health care systems.			X	X	X		X	X	X	X	X	X	X			X	
L. Identifies and applies basic research methods used in public health.			X	X			X			X			X			X	
M. Applies the basic public health sciences, including behavioral and social sciences, biostatistics, epidemiology, environmental public health, and prevention of chronic and infectious diseases and injuries.		X	X	X	X	X	X			X			X				
N. Identifies and retrieves current relevant scientific evidence.			X	X	X	X	X	X	X	X	X		X	X		X	
O. Identifies the limitations of research and the importance of observations and interrelationships.				X			X	X	X	X		X		X		X	
P. Develops a lifelong commitment to rigorous critical thinking.				X				X	X	X		X					

Specific Competencies	Chapter 18	Chapter 19	Chapter 20	Chapter 21	Chapter 22	Chapter 23	Chapter 24	Chapter 25	Chapter 26	Chapter 27	Chapter 28	Chapter 29	Chapter 30	Chapter 31	Appendix A	Appendix B	Appendix C
DOMAIN #7: FINANCIAL PLANNING AND MANAGEMENT SKILLS																	
K. Develops and presents a budget.																	
L. Manages programs within budget constraints.												X					
M. Applies budget processes.												X					
N. Develops strategies for determining budget priorities.						X						X					
O. Monitors program performance.			X	X				X	X			X					
P. Prepares proposals for funding from external sources.																	
Q. Applies basic human relations skills to the management of organizations, motivation of personnel, and resolution of conflicts.						X							X				
R. Manages information systems for collection, retrieval, and use of data for decision making.													X				
S. Negotiates and develops contracts and other documents for the provision of population-based services.												X					
T. Conducts cost-effectiveness, cost-benefit, and cost utility analyses.			X								X	X					
DOMAIN #8: LEADERSHIP AND SYSTEMS THINKING SKILLS																	
I. Creates a culture of ethical standards within organizations and communities.	X			X		X		X	X								
J. Helps create key values and shared vision and uses these principles to guide action.	X				X			X	X	X	X	X		X			
K. Identifies internal and external issues that may impact delivery of essential public health services (i.e., strategic planning).	X				X	X					X	X	X	X			
L. Facilitates collaboration with internal and external groups to ensure participation of key stakeholders.	X		X			X		X	X	X		X		X			
M. Promotes team and organizational learning.	X					X											
N. Contributes to development, implementation, and monitoring of organizational performance standards.	X				X			X	X								
O. Uses the legal and political systems to effect change.	X		X								X	X		X			
P. Applies theory of organizational structures to professional practice.	X		X		X	X						X					

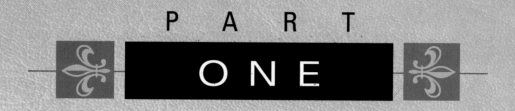

The Basis of Public Health

CHAPTER 1

Concepts and Definitions of Public Health Practice

F. Douglas Scutchfield, MD and C. William Keck, MD, MPH

LEARNING OBJECTIVES

Upon completion of this chapter, the reader will be able to:

1. Identify the individual's and organization's responsibilities within the context of the Essential Public Health Services and core functions.
2. Define, assess, and understand the health status of populations, determinants of health and illness, factors contributing to health promotion and disease prevention, and factors influencing the use of health services.
3. Understand the historical development, structure, and interaction of public health and health care systems.
4. Establish and maintains linkages with key stakeholders.
5. Identify how public and private organizations operate within a community.
6. Identify community assets and available resources.

KEY TERMS

Assessment
Assurance
Biostatistics
Community Medicine
Disease Prevention
Epidemiology
Health
Health Promotion
Health Protection
Policy Development
Prevention
Preventive Medicine
Primary Prevention
Public Health

Public health is defined by John Last as

> An organized activity of society to promote, protect, improve, and, when necessary, restore the health of individuals, specified groups, or the entire population. It is a combination of sciences, skills, and values that function through collective societal activities and involve programs, services, and institutions aimed at protecting and improving the health of all the people. The term "public health" can describe a concept, a social institution, a set of scientific and professional disciplines and technologies, and a form of practice. It encompasses a wide range of services, institutions, professional groups, trades, and unskilled occupations. It is a way of thinking, a set of disciplines, an institution of society, and a manner of practice. It has an increasing number and variety of specialized domains, and it demands of its practitioners an increasing array of skills and expertise. [1(p306)]

The World Health Organization has defined **health** as ". . . a complete state of physical, mental, and social well-being and not merely the absence of disease or infirmity."[2] Societies that approach this ideal state will do so by appropriately balancing services for the diagnosis and treatment of illness with services that promote health and prevent disease.

Unfortunately, our current system of providing health services in the United States is unbalanced because it is tilted strongly toward interacting with people who are ill. This system, focused as it is on illness care, is not prepared to deal with the social issues that affect health. It is likely, for example, that health status is more closely linked to socioeconomic status and its attendant problems than to any other factor. Thus, improvement in our nation's health status will depend more on the effective application of public health techniques than on taking care of people who are ill.

We intend, in this chapter, to make distinctions and definitions that define public health and also differentiate from other related disciplines. This chapter also describes the discipline of public health and introduces concepts, problem areas, and approaches to problem solving that are part of public health practice. These issues and others will be referenced repeatedly and discussed in greater detail in subsequent chapters.

SCIENCE, SKILLS, AND BELIEFS

The scientific basis for public health rests on the study of risks to the health of populations (including risks related to the environment) and on the systems designed to deliver required services. **Epidemiology** and **biostatistics** are the scientific disciplines that underpin inquiry in all of public health. They provide the methods necessary for understanding the risks to the health of populations and individuals and for developing effective risk reduction and health promotion activities.

The skills required for effective public health practice begin with proficiency in applying the techniques required for a particular public health specialization. The most important skill, however, is the capacity to create a vision of the potential for health that exists within a community. With a clear vision comes a sense of direction and a feeling of enthusiasm that are essential if one hopes to engage a population in understanding and reducing risks to its health.

Health departments are the only entities statutorily responsible for the health of their constituent populations. As a result, an underlying belief and responsibility of public health departments is that all members of the community should have access to the health promotion, disease **prevention,** and illness care services they need for good health. Public health is firmly grounded in the concepts of social justice, and its practitioners should be strong proponents of the ethical distribution of resources.

ASSOCIATED DISCIPLINES

Medicine played a substantial role in the development of public health. Many leaders of the public health movement during the mid to late 1800s were physicians. However, at the turn of the twentieth century, the two disciplines, for a variety of reasons, began to drift apart.[3] Recent efforts have been focused on reestablishing the dialogue between public health and medicine to recognize the commonality of interest in the health of the nation's citizens.[4] In addition, recent work has showcased illustrations of effective working relations between medicine and public health.[5]

The public often has difficulty distinguishing between the practice of medicine and the practice of public health. Public health practitioners must be clear about the differences between them. As with medicine, the practice of public health is rooted in science and the scientific method. Medicine applies what we learn from science to the benefit of the individual patient, usually in the pursuit of the diagnosis and treatment of illness. Public health applies the knowledge gained from science to the improvement of the health status of groups of people, usually through health promotion, health protection, and disease prevention activities.

Preventive medicine and **community medicine** are medical disciplines that function, to some degree, as bridges between the practice of medicine and the practice of public health. Preventive medicine physicians work to ensure the primacy and excellence of both individual and community health promotion and disease prevention efforts. Although they may interact primarily with individuals, they also deal with groups seeking to maintain and preserve their health.

Community medicine has developed as a discipline during the past 40 years, and its practitioners concentrate on the preservation of health status in communities rather than individuals. John Last defines community medicine as

. . . the study of health and disease in the population of a specific community. Its goal is to identify the health problems and needs of defined populations, to identify means by which these needs should be met and to evaluate the extent to which health services effectively meet these needs.[1]

Public health clearly includes some elements of medical practice, preventive medicine, and community medicine. It is greater than the sum of these parts, however. It includes many other disciplines, such as nutrition, health education, and environmental health, that contribute to the improvement of the public's health status. Public health also concentrates on **health promotion, health protection,** and **disease prevention.**

Health Protection

Health protection refers to

. . . important activities of public health departments, specifically in food hygiene, water purification, environmental sanitation, drug safety, and other activities in which the emphasis is on actions that can be taken to eliminate as far as possible the risk of adverse consequences for health attributable to environmental hazards, unsafe or impure food, water, drugs, etc.[1(p159)]

Health Promotion

Health promotion refers to

The policies and processes that enable people to increase control over and improve their health. These address the needs of the population as a whole in the context of their daily lives, rather than focusing on people at risk for specific diseases, and are directed toward action on the determinants or causes of health. Health promotion is action oriented and based on public policies, for instance provision of facilities such as bicycle pathways, recreational parks to encourage healthy behavior, and public meeting places to encourage social interaction; and deterring health-harming behavior by promoting smoke-free zones.[1(p159)]

We know that prerequisites for health include a variety of factors such as shelter, food, and education among others. Good health promotion activities may involve educational, organizational, economic, and environmental interventions targeted toward specific lifestyle behaviors and environmental conditions that are harmful to health, with the intention of making health-promoting changes in those conditions.

Disease Prevention

Disease-prevention techniques are usually described in one of three categories: primary prevention, secondary prevention, and tertiary prevention.

Primary Prevention

The first category, **primary prevention,** includes those activities that are intended to prevent the onset of disease in the first place. The classic example of primary prevention is immunization against infectious diseases, but the use of seat belts, the installation of air bags in automobiles, the avoidance of tobacco use, the minimal intake of alcoholic beverages, and the inspection and licensure of restaurants are all examples of common public health activities that exemplify primary prevention.

Secondary Prevention

Secondary prevention refers to techniques that find health problems early in their course so that action can be taken to minimize the risk of progression of the disease in individuals or the risk that communicable illnesses will be transmitted to others. Examples of this principle include the early diagnosis of hypertension with follow-up treatment to minimize the risk of future vascular disease, and the early diagnosis and treatment of sexually transmitted diseases to minimize the transmission potential of those conditions to others.

Tertiary Prevention

Tertiary prevention is focused on rehabilitation in an effort to prevent the worsening of an individual's health in the face of a chronic disease or injury. Learning to walk again after an orthopedic injury or cerebrovascular accident is an example.

Acute Sickness Services

Although public health focuses principally on health promotion and disease prevention, in many circumstances, it has become a provider of acute sickness services to those who cannot obtain these services otherwise. Not surprisingly, sickness services are most often provided by health departments found in inner-city and rural areas of lower socioeconomic status, where access to medical care is limited. This assumption of responsibility for illness care has been controversial. Many insist it is outside the purview of traditional public health functions. Others insist that the assurance of medical services, when they cannot be obtained in any other way, is a clear public health mission, consistent with the responsibility for maintaining the public's health. It is important to recognize that even if the health department provides direct patient care for ill patients, it cannot abrogate its responsibility for population-based services. The health department is one of several organizations in communities that can care for sick patients, but it is the only source of governmental efforts to maintain and improve the health status of the community. That being the case, those who argue that the health department should not be involved in direct patient care services to those unable to access other providers of health care, point out that direct patient care services can and frequently do draw resources away from their unique mission of population-based services.

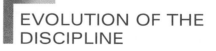

EVOLUTION OF THE DISCIPLINE

Public health departments began to appear in the United States in the middle of the nineteenth century. Since that time, public health methods and programs have evolved to meet the changing needs of the community. Many changes have been driven by scientific contributions to knowledge about risks to health and by improvements in the technology available to respond to public health issues. For more than a century, public health has moved from a period of limited scientific understanding, when infectious diseases were the major cause of death, to a period of significant and growing scientific capacity, as chronic diseases became the major killers. This evolution is discussed in more detail in Chapter 19.

INFECTIOUS DISEASE CONTROL

Scientists came to realize that the major health problems of the day were caused by microorganisms. They also realized that understanding how the microorganisms moved from person to person could lead to strategies to prevent the transmission of disease. This realization was so revolutionary that Milton Terris has called this period the "First Epidemiological Revolution."[6] This allowed communities to develop policies and laws that would protect the public's health and to hire people to enforce them. These governmental *sanitarians* in the nation's first health departments used laws providing for quarantine, safe water, and sewage disposal to significantly reduce the toll taken by communicable disease. The later addition of vaccines and antibiotics increased the effectiveness of infectious disease control efforts. It became increasingly obvious, however, that improved socioeconomic status, decreased crowding, good nutrition, and better education had as much to do with this success story as did the newer medical interventions.[7] This reinforced the lesson that there are *determinants of health* that deserve as much attention as medical interventions when it comes to improving health status.

CHRONIC DISEASE CONTROL

Our struggles with infectious diseases continue in the present day. New organisms appear, such as the human immunodeficiency virus, or HIV, and older organisms, such as the tubercle bacillus that causes tuberculosis, return to fill new niches in our changing environment. The major causes of death and disability in the United States today, however, are chronic illnesses. Our efforts to understand and control them have led to what Terris calls the "Second Epidemiological Revolution."[6]

We are in an era of rapidly increasing understanding of the causes of chronic disease. We have learned that heart disease, cancer, stroke, and many other chronic diseases are caused by multiple factors. A variety of genetic, environmental, and lifestyle factors interact to predispose individuals to chronic illness. In fact, up to 70 percent of premature mortality in the United States is directly related to environmental and lifestyle factors that are potentially controllable by individuals or society.[8] We describe these causes as risk factors, and we realize that such behaviors as the use of tobacco, the excessive use of alcohol, unhealthful nutritional practices, and sedentary lifestyles cannot be altered without the direct, willing participation of the individuals affected in an environment that is supportive of healthful choices.

We are moving beyond an era of professionals doing things for others to one of professionals doing things *with* others to help them minimize risks to their health. It is a time of trying to understand the motivations of human behavior and developing constructive and ethical mechanisms to support healthful behavioral choices. It is also a time of working with governments and communities to create the most healthful living environments possible.

SOCIAL ISSUES

New problems have emerged that have public health implications and that require a new level of understanding to devise effective intervention methods. They include epidemics of violence, drug abuse, teenage pregnancy, and sexually transmitted disease—problems that are not clearly understood but probably due in part to racial and ethnic prejudice, increasing numbers of single-parent families, changing cultural values, and poverty as a social norm.

Scutchfield has termed these new social/public health problems as the "third public health revolution." Understanding these problems requires that we develop new scientific knowledge from disciplines not traditionally associated with public health. We must develop a better understanding of human behavior, communities, their structures, and interaction among them.[9,10] Unfortunately, we are only beginning to understand the epidemiology of these problems and do not yet have robust interventions for most of them.

NEW TOOLS FOR PUBLIC HEALTH PRACTICE

A number of new tools are available to public health professionals to help them carry out public health's core functions. Frequent reference will be made to these tools throughout this textbook because of the important roles they play in the conceptualization, organization, and delivery of public health services. They are just briefly introduced here, but subsequent chapters will deal with these in depth.

Report on the Future of Public Health

The contributions made by public health over the past 100 years have largely been taken for granted. In fact, public health had languished, through inattention, for many decades. Fortunately, the 1988 report titled *The Future of Public Health* by the Institute of Medicine (IOM) focused attention on the discipline.[11] This study details the contributions made by public health while chronicling its current difficulties, and it makes very clear recommendations about how the nation's public health system should be improved to ensure that every citizen in the country has access to needed public health services. This report was a wake up call and initiated many of the activities in public health described in subsequent chapters. Most public health leaders date the renewal of public health to the release of the first IOM Report on the future of public health.

The report defines the mission of public health as "fulfilling society's interest in assuring conditions in which people can be healthy."[11] The Study Committee of the IOM that produced the report recognized that many components of a community must work together for that mission to be successfully accomplished, but they emphasized the unique responsibility of government, at all levels, to ensure success. These governmental responsibilities are usually carried out by health departments, which are the jurisdiction's action arm to accomplish the mission articulated by the IOM. The committee suggested three core public health functions for local and state health departments: **assessment, policy development,** and **assurance.**

By assessment, the committee meant that each public health agency should

> . . . regularly and systematically collect, assemble, analyze, and make available information on the health of the community, including statistics on health status, community health needs, and epidemiologic and other studies of health problems.[11(p7)]

The committee noted that not every agency is large enough to conduct these activities in their entirety, but that each agency bears the responsibility for seeing that the assessment function is fulfilled. In essence, the committee recognized the public health department as the epidemiologic intelligence center for health in the community, providing the information necessary for effective health planning and programming.

By policy development, the committee meant that each public health agency should

> . . . serve the public interest in the development of comprehensive public health policies by promoting use of the scientific knowledge

base in decision-making about public health and by leading in developing public health policy.[11(p8)]

Policy development links science with political, organizational, and community values. It includes information sharing, citizen participation, compromise, and consensus building in a process that nurtures shared ownership of the policy decisions.

By assurance, the committee meant that each public health agency should

> . . . assure their constituents that services necessary to achieve agreed upon goals are provided, either by encouraging actions by other entities (private or public sector), by requiring such action through regulation, or by providing services directly.[11(p8)]

The committee also felt that each public health agency should work with its community to guarantee access to a basic set of health services for each citizen.[11(p8)] This reflects the social justice element of public health. The effective health department will work with other service providers to ensure that good quality, basic services are available to all, even if someone other than the health department provides the services.

The areas of assessment, policy development, and assurance are now considered by most to define the core functions of public health. Unfortunately, most health departments must improve their capacity to carry out the functions and activities associated with these responsibilities. Many health departments are too small to perform them well. They might combine with others or form alliances that allow expertise to be shared. Strong liaisons with academic units, where available, may also provide access to analytical and other skills. The report and subsequent publications drew the distinction between health department activities in assessment, policy development and assurance, and what the community organizations and agencies contribute to those public health functions. It called the larger group of organizations and agencies committed to population-based health activities the *Local Public Health System* (*LPHS*) to draw the distinction

between the health department and all the community resources that contribute to the community's health.

Ten Essential Public Health Services

During the early 1990s, it became apparent that the notion of assessment, policy development, and assurance did not communicate well to policy makers what public health organizations actually do. Although those in public health understood the concept, the layperson had difficulty understanding it. The United States Department of Health and Human Services convened a work group of stakeholders who developed a list of 10 essential health services that should be considered core components of public health practice. These 10 essential services, which were refinements and elaboration of the functions delineated in the IOM report, are:

1. Monitor health status to identify community health problems.
2. Diagnose and investigate health problems and health hazards in the community.
3. Inform, educate, and empower people about health issues.
4. Mobilize community partnerships to identify and solve health problems.
5. Develop policies and plans that support individual and community health efforts.
6. Enforce laws and regulations that protect health and ensure safety.
7. Link people to needed personal health services, and ensure the provision of health care when otherwise unavailable.
8. Ensure a competent public health and personal health care workforce.
9. Evaluate effectiveness, accessibility, and quality of personal and population-based health services.
10. Research for new insights and innovative solutions to health problems.

These ten essential public health services have been used in a variety of ways to facilitate public health activities at the federal, state, and local level. They will be a recurring theme throughout this textbook.[12]

The Future of the Public's Health in the 21st Century

Although there have been a number of IOM reports focusing on public health since the 1988 report, only one deals specifically with public health practice. This follow-up report, *The Future of the Public's Health in the 21st Century*, provides an update from the earlier report. It was begun in 2001 and published in 2003. It recognizes that the initial IOM report dealt with governmental public health, so the latter report focuses on the public health system, organizations other than governmental public health departments that contribute to the public health mission of "assuring conditions in which people can be healthy." Specifically, the report made recommendations for contributions from the community, health care delivery system, employers and business, media, and the academy to achieve the mission of public health. As with the first IOM report on the future of public health, recommendations of this follow-up IOM report will be continually referenced throughout the remainder of this book.

Healthy People 2010

The process of setting national goals and objectives for the nation began in 1979 with the publication of *Healthy People: The Surgeon General's Report on Health Promotion and Disease Prevention*.[8] It was the first such report to emphasize the importance of reducing premature mortality through health promotion and disease prevention programs, and it discussed a series of age-specific goals for the nation to accomplish by 1990. Following that report, the Centers for Disease Control and Prevention (CDC) convened a series of discussions that led to a publication titled *Health Promotion/ Disease Prevention: Objectives for the Nation*.[13]

This document established 226 specific health objectives to be achieved by 1990. These objectives were measurable, specific, and tied to the various priority programs listed under the rubrics of health promotion, health protection, and preventive services.

In 1987, the Public Health Service's Office of Health Promotion and Disease Prevention began a new consultative process with the nation's public health professionals to develop a set of objectives for the year 2000. The resulting *Healthy People 2000: National Health Promotion and Disease Prevention Objectives*,[14] which was published in 1990, articulated three major goals:

1. Increase the span of healthy life for all Americans.
2. Reduce health disparities among Americans.
3. Achieve access to preventive services for all Americans.

More than 300 objectives were listed within 22 priority areas and categorized as Health Status Objectives, Risk Reduction Objectives, and Service and Protection Objectives. *Healthy People 2000* succeeded in establishing a national focus for attainable health status by the year 2000. It has been described by many as creating the destination for health promotion and disease prevention activities.

The success of these efforts led to the creation of the third publication of the series. *Healthy People 2010* was released in 2000. *Healthy People 2010* has two overarching goals: increasing the quality and years of a healthy life and reducing health disparities. The new version includes 467 objectives in 28 focus areas. To focus efforts in *Healthy People 2010*, 10 leading health indicators were chosen for more detailed tracking. These indicators reflect the major public health concerns in the United States and were chosen based on their ability to motivate action, the availability of data to measure their progress, and their relevance as broad public health issues. The 10 indicators are:

1. Physical activity
2. Overweight and obesity
3. Tobacco use

4. Substance abuse
5. Responsible sexual behavior
6. Mental health
7. Injury and violence
8. Environmental quality
9. Immunizations
10. Access to health care

For each of the leading health indicators, specific objectives derived from *Healthy People 2010* will be used to track progress. This small set of measures will provide a snapshot of the health of the nation. The leading health indicators serve as a link to the 467 objectives in *Healthy People 2010* and can become the basic building blocks for community health initiatives.[15]

As is the case with previous *Healthy People* documents listing national health objectives, periodic review of *Healthy People 2010* allows us to refine and examine how we, as a nation, are doing with these objectives. The midcourse review of the *Health People 2010* objectives has recently been completed, and substantial changes have been made in the objectives. We have identified those objectives where we are successful, or likely will be, and where we are falling short (http://www.healthypeople.gov/data). A careful review of *Healthy People 2010* and the midcourse evaluation is "required reading" for those interested in public health practice.

Assessment Protocol for Excellence in Public Health

Before a community can translate its public health problems into objectives for action that are consistent, wherever possible, with national goals, those local public health problems must be identified and prioritized. We have moved beyond the time when significant progress in improved health status is possible by doing things for the community. We now realize that the community must be engaged in the process of identifying and understanding its health problems and determining the remedies to be applied. To this end, the National Association of County and City Health Officials (NACCHO), together with the CDC and other public health professional associations, developed the *Assessment Protocol for Excellence in Public Health (APEX)*.[17] It guides public health agencies in the process of community assessment and public health program planning. APEX helps health departments assess their own internal strengths and weaknesses in terms of their capacity to carry out community needs assessment, to work with the community to understand its health problems and establish priorities for action, and to implement a community plan for reducing public health problems. APEX/PH has proven to be so successful that NACCHO has developed a new, more robust community health planning model called Mobilizing for Action through Planning and Partnership (MAPP). This tool is flexible and is designed to facilitate community-wide health planning efforts. This and other similar programs, such as the Planned Approach to Community Health (PATCH)[18] and the Healthy Cities Project[19] are discussed in Chapter 12.

In the future, growing numbers of local and state health departments will be using APEX, MAPP, PATCH, or Healthy Cities as guides to developing community-based plans for identifying and addressing community health problems. Inherent in that process will be the accurate assessment of risks to health and a growing capacity to communicate those risks to the public at large. Increasingly, these tools will link communities with national efforts to improve health status so that the mission of public health, "fulfilling society's interest in assuring conditions in which people can be healthy," will be realized.

REVIEW QUESTIONS

1. What is the World Health Organization's definition of health?
2. Name and define the three categories of disease prevention.
3. What is the mission of public health?
4. Name the three core governmental public health functions.

5. Define the local public health system.
6. What are the two major goals of *Healthy People 2010*?

REFERENCES

1. Last JM. *A Dictionary of Public Health*. New York, NY: Oxford University Press; 2007.
2. Osamnczk EJ. *Encyclopedia of the United Nations and International Agreements*. Philadelphia, PA: Taylor & Francis; 1985.
3. Starr P. *The Social Transformation of American Medicine*. New York, NY: Basic Books; 1982.
4. Reiser SJ. Topics for our times: The medicine public health initiative. *Am J Public Health*. 1997; 87(7):1098–1099.
5. Lasker R. *Medicine and Public Health: The Power of Collaboration Health*. Chicago, IL: Administration Press; 1997.
6. Terris M. The complex tasks of the second epidemiological revolution: The Joseph W. Mountain lecture. *J Public Health Policy*. March(1) 1983; 8–24.
7. McKinlay JB, McKinlay SM. The questionable contribution of medical measures to the decline of mortality in the United States in the twentieth century. *Milbank Q*. 1977;55(3):405–428.
8. *Healthy People: The Surgeon General's Report on Health Promotion and Disease Prevention*. Washington, DC: U.S. Dept. of Health and Human Services, Public Health Service; 1979.
9. Scutchfield FD, Hartman K. A new preventive medicine for a new millennium. *Aviat Space and Environmental Medicine*. 1996;67(4):369–375.
10. Frumpkin H. Beyond toxicity: Human health and the natural environment. *Am J Preventive Medicine*. 2001;20(3):234–240.
11. Institute of Medicine, Committee for the Study of the Future of Public Health. *The Future of Public Health*. Washington, DC: National Academy Press; 1988.
12. Baker EL, Melton RJ, Strange PV, et al. Health reform and the healing of the public. Forging community health partnerships. *JAMA*. 1994;272(16):1276–1282.
13. *Health Promotion/Disease Prevention: Objectives for the Nation*. Washington, DC: U.S. Dept of Health and Human Services, Public Health Service; 1981.
14. *Healthy People 2000: National Health Promotion and Disease Prevention Objectives*. Washington, DC: U.S. Dept of Health and Human Services, Public Health Service; 1990.
15. *Healthy People 2010*. Washington, DC: U.S. Dept of Health and Human Services, Public Health Service; 2000.
16. *Healthy Communities 2000: Model Standards. Guidelines for Community Attainment of the Year 2000 National Health Objectives*. 3rd ed. Washington, DC: American Public Health Association; 1991.
17. *APEX/PH, Assessment Protocol for Excellence in Public Health*. Washington, DC: National Association of County and City Health Officials; 1991.
18. *Planned Approach to Community Health (PATCH): Program Descriptions*. Washington, DC: U.S. Dept of Health and Human Services; November 1993.
19. *World Health Organizations, Five Year Planning Project*. Fadl, Copenhagen: World Health Organization, Healthy Cities Project; 1988. WHO Healthy Cities Paper, No. 2.

CHAPTER 2

History and Development of Public Health

Elizabeth Fee, PhD

LEARNING OBJECTIVES

Upon completion of this chapter, the reader will be able to:

1. Outline the early development of public health institutions in the United States.
2. Discuss the contribution of social reformers, the United States Army, the Rockefeller philanthropies, and the United States Public Health Service to public health.
3. Explain the significance of bacteriology in the development of public health.
4. Discuss alternate conceptions of public health to the biomedical model.
5. Understand the complex relationships between medicine and public health.
6. Describe the historical impact of war mobilization on public health.
7. Explain the political problems and constraints facing public health officials.
8. Outline the accomplishments of public health over the past 300 years.

KEY TERMS

Bacteriology
Categorical
Chronic Diseases
Communications
Disciplines
Epidemic Diseases
Federal Regulation
Fluoridation
History
Industrial Hygiene
Infrastructure
Mobilization
Patronage
Politics
Poverty
Professional
Quarantine
Research
Sanitation
Social Determinants of Health
Social Medicine

This chapter discusses the **history** and development of public health in the United States and the factors that influenced them. The first section gives an overview of public health in the United States in the eighteenth and nineteenth centuries.

PUBLIC HEALTH IN THE EIGHTEENTH AND NINETEENTH CENTURIES

In the United States, before the twentieth century, there were few formal requirements for public health positions, no established career structures, no job security for health officials, and no formalized ways of producing new knowledge. Public health positions were usually part-time appointments at nominal salary; those who devoted much effort to public health typically did so on a voluntary basis. Until the mid-nineteenth century, public health, like other governmental functions, was usually the responsibility of the social elite. The public health officer was expected to be a statesman acting in the public interest, not a politician answering to a class constituency. Men of property and wealth were believed to be independent of special interests and therefore capable of disinterested judgment.

Charles Rosenberg has eloquently described an earlier conception of both poverty and disease as consequences of moral failure at the individual and social level.[1] Disease attacked the dirty, the improvident, the intemperate, the ignorant; the clean, the pious, and the virtuous, on the other hand, tended to escape. **Epidemic diseases** were the consequence of a failure to obey the laws of nature and God: they were indicators of social and moral dissolution. As cleanliness was linked to godliness, virtue was an essential qualification for managing the state. The conscientious, the respectable, the educated, and the affluent were seen as naturally qualified for public office. Physicians were frequently chosen as public health officers, but lawyers or gentlemen of independent means could also be appointed.

Earliest Public Health Programs and Activities

The first public health organizations were those of the rapidly growing port cities of the eastern seaboard in the late eighteenth century. Here, the American republic intersected with the world of international trade. Local authorities tried to protect the population from the threat of potentially catastrophic epidemic diseases, such as the yellow fever epidemic that had crippled Philadelphia in 1793, while they also tried to maintain the conditions for successful economic activity.[2] Public health programs, when organized at all, were organized locally. As Robert Wiebe has argued, the United States in the nineteenth century was a society of *island communities* with considerable economic and political autonomy.[3]

Public health in this period was also largely a police function. Traditionally, port cities had dealt with epidemics by means of **quarantine** regulations, keeping ships suspected of carrying disease in harbor for up to forty days. However, quarantine regulations clearly interfered with shipping, and they were energetically opposed by those whose economic interests were tied to trade.[4]

Opponents of quarantine argued that diseases were internally generated by the filthy conditions of the docks, streets, and alleys, which provided an ideal environment for *putrefactive fermentation*. City health departments attempted to regulate the worst offenders: graveyards, tallow chandleries, tanneries, sugar boilers, skin dressers, dyers, glue boilers, and slaughterhouses. They also cleaned the privies and alleys and removed dead animals and decaying vegetable matter from the streets and public spaces.[5(p50)]

Influence of Disease

The causes of disease were much in dispute by the mid-nineteenth century. The evidence available was contradictory and suggested no clear resolution to the dispute between those who believed that diseases were brought in from overseas and thus should be fought by quarantine regulations and those who believed that diseases were internally generated and thus should be fought by cleaning up the cities. Health regulations were written and revised more in response to political influence or pressure from merchants than in response to shifts in scientific thinking.

Official health agencies were sporadically moved to action by the threat of great epidemics—the devastating waves of yellow fever and cholera that periodically threatened from Europe, the Caribbean, or Latin America or were detected on ships arriving in New Orleans, Boston, or Philadelphia. These sudden, catastrophic events compelled even politicians and business leaders to devote their attention to sanitary improvements, city cleanliness, quarantines, and hospital construction.

At other times, adults and children were killed continually but in less spectacular numbers by tuberculosis, smallpox, typhus, dysentery, diphtheria, typhoid fever, measles, influenza, malaria, and scarlet fever. These diseases were met with a stolid indifference born of familiarity and a sense of helplessness. It seemed that little could be done beyond attempts to maintain general cleanliness, backed by prayer, fasting, and exhortations to virtue.[5(p87)] When free of the immediate threat of an impending epidemic, politicians tended to ignore the fate of the multitudes of immigrant poor, unless compelled to action by the insistent demands of reform groups or the fear of popular unrest.[6–8]

Early Public Health Reforms

A few cities did have active and energetic reform groups. In New York in 1864, members of the Council of Hygiene and Public Health of the Citizens' Association conducted street-by-street investigations of tenement housing congestion, slaughterhouse and stable conditions, sewage drainage, garbage heaps, and filthy habitations of many sections of the city, and correlated these with outbreaks of infectious disease and premature infant deaths.[9] Dr. Ezra R. Pulling, for example, detailed every case of typhus, typhoid fever, and smallpox found in the notorious Five Points section of Manhattan's Lower East Side. He also carefully mapped all the stables, privies (especially "privies in an extremely offensive condition"), and other *insalubrious locations* in the

area, making obvious the close geographical relationship between disease and its causes.[10]

In other parts of the country, a few farsighted men and women argued for the need to collect vital statistics, register birth and death rates, and keep careful records on the health of the population. The most notable of these was Lemuel Shattuck, a schoolteacher, bookseller, and publisher, who was largely responsible for implementing a system of vital statistics in Massachusetts. Shattuck is especially remembered for his *Report of the Sanitary Commission of Massachusetts*, an extraordinarily comprehensive set of recommendations for public health organization.[11,12]

Shattuck's report advocated a decennial census and collection of data by age, sex, race, occupation, economic status, and locality. It discussed the need for environmental **sanitation,** regulation of food and drugs, and control of communicable disease. Shattuck also recommended attention to well-child care, mental health, health education, smallpox vaccination, alcoholism, town planning, and the teaching of preventive medicine in medical schools.

Shattuck's report was well received by medical reviewers but essentially ignored by the Massachusetts state legislature. Although having little direct impact at the time it was written, the report would become a central reference point for later generations of public health practitioners.

By 1860, public health activities were just beginning to move beyond the confines of local city **politics.** Between 1857 and 1860, quarantine and sanitary conventions were held in Philadelphia, Baltimore, New York, and Boston.[13] Although these conventions gave public health reformers an opportunity to debate the causes of disease and the most appropriate public health responses, the possibility of implementing their ideas was interrupted by the outbreak of the Civil War.

Impact of the Civil War

In its own way, the Civil War helped enforce a national consciousness of epidemic disease: two-thirds of the 360,000 Union soldiers who died were killed by infectious diseases rather than by bullets.[14,15] The ravages of dysentery, spread by inadequate or nonexistent sanitary facilities, were appalling. The United States Sanitary Commission, a voluntary organization inspired by Florence Nightingale's work in the Crimean War, promoted the health of the Union army by inspecting army camps, distributing educational materials, and providing nursing care and supplies for the wounded.

Formation of the American Public Health Association

In 1872, ten health reformers from various parts of the country met in New York City at the home of Stephen Smith and announced the creation of the American Public Health Association (APHA). Its purpose was to advance *sanitary science* and promote the "practical application of public hygiene."[16,17] After a slow start, the new organization grew rapidly. Its members devoted themselves to the reform activities of citizens' sanitary associations and encouraged the formation and development of local and state health agencies. They organized annual meetings and presented papers on infectious diseases and on many of the practical public health issues of the day—from sewage and garbage disposal to occupational injuries and proposals for the medical inspection of prostitutes. The APHA was notable in welcoming physicians, engineers, lawyers, municipal officials, other professional groups, and lay reformers to its membership, and in this respect, it helped mold the specific character of American public health.[18,19]

First State and Local Boards of Health

In the late nineteenth century, state and local boards of health were created in many parts of the country. The first state board of health, formed in Louisiana in 1855, had largely been a paper organization. In the 1870s and 1880s, however, most states instituted their own boards of health. The first working state health board was formed in Massachusetts in 1869, followed by California (1870), the District of Columbia (1871), Virginia and Minnesota (1872), Maryland (1874), and Alabama (1875).[20] The impact of these state boards of health should not be overemphasized. By 1900, only three states (Massachusetts, Rhode Island, and Florida) spent more than two cents per capita for public health services.[21]

The Marine Hospital Service

The origins of a federal organization of public health lie in the provision of medical and hospital care for merchant seamen and sailors. In 1798, the United States Congress had passed the Act for the Relief of Sick and Disabled Seamen to finance the construction and operation of public hospitals in port cities.[22] These hospitals were poorly run and badly managed until 1871, when John Maynard Woodward became Supervising Surgeon of what was now named the Marine Hospital Service.

Woodward and other public health reformers urged the formation of a national system of quarantines and a national health board. In 1879, a disastrous yellow fever epidemic swept up the Mississippi Valley from New Orleans, prompting the United States Congress to create the National Board of Health. This consisted of seven physicians and one representative each from the army, the navy, the Marine Hospital Service, and the United States Department of Justice.

Responsible for formulating quarantine regulations between states, the National Board of Health soon became embroiled in fierce battles over states' rights. Many cities and states had discovered that local quarantine laws could be an excellent source of income as well as a valuable source of political **patronage;** they were naturally reluctant to relinquish these powers to the federal government.[7(pp157–174)] In 1883, after various battles in Congress, the National Board of Health was disbanded, and its quarantine powers reverted to the Marine Hospital Service.

Gradually, the Marine Hospital Service expanded its public health activities into public health research. In 1887, it set aside a single room as a *hygienic laboratory,* which would later be expanded into an important center for the investigation of infectious diseases.[23] In 1912, the Marine Hospital Service became the United States Public Health Service, specifically authorized to investigate the causes and spread of disease and to provide health information to the public.

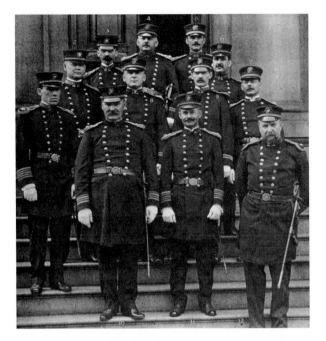

Figure 2.1. Members of the United States Public Health Service in Uniform, Standing for the Examination for Promotion to the Grade of Surgeon.
Courtesy of the National Library of Medicine.

Public Health as Social Reform

The belief that epidemic diseases posed only occasional threats to an otherwise healthy social order had been shaken by the industrial transformation of the late nineteenth century. The burgeoning health problems of the industrial cities could not be ignored; almost all families lost children to diphtheria, smallpox, or other infectious diseases. Poverty and disease could not be treated simply as individual failings but were understood to be consequences of industrialization, urbanization, immigration, and exploitation.

Public Health Responses

The early efforts of city health department officials to deal with health problems were attempts to mitigate the worst effects of unplanned and unregulated growth—a kind of rearguard action against the filth and congestion created by anarchic economic and urban development.[24–29] As cities grew in size, as the flow of immigrants continued, and as public health problems became ever more obvious, pressures mounted for more effective responses to the problems.[30] New York, the largest city and the one with some of the worst health conditions, produced some of the most energetic and progressive public health leaders; Boston and Providence were also noted for their active public health programs; Baltimore and Philadelphia, however, trailed far behind.[25,31–33]

Social Reform

America no longer fit its self-image as a country of independent farmers and craftsmen. Like the countries of Europe, it displayed extremes of wealth and privilege, social misery, and deprivation. Labor and social unrest pushed awareness of the need for social and health reforms. The perceived social anarchy of the large industrial cities mocked the pretensions to social control of the traditional forces of church and state and highlighted the need for new approaches to the multiplicity of problems.[34]

Reformers and Reform Groups

An increasing number of reform groups devoted themselves to social issues and improvements of every variety. Health reformers, physicians, and engineers urged improved sanitary conditions in the industrial cities. Medical men were prominent in reform organizations, but they were not alone.[35] Barbara Rosenkrantz has contrasted public health in the late nineteenth century with the internecine battles within general medicine: ". . . the field of public hygiene exemplified a happy marriage of engineers, physicians and public spirited citizens providing a model of complementary comportment under the banner of sanitary science."[36]

Middle- and upper-class women, seizing an opportunity to escape from the narrow bounds of domestic responsibilities, joined in campaigns for improved housing, the abolition of child labor, maternal and child health, and temperance. They were active in the settlement house movement, the organization of trade unions, the suffrage movement, and municipal sanitary reform. The latter, as municipal housekeeping, was viewed as a natural extension of women's training and experience as the housekeepers of the world.[37] By the early years of the twentieth century, dozens of such voluntary health organizations were established around specific issues, thus providing the impulse and energy behind many public health reforms.[38]

The progressive reform groups in the public health movement advocated immediate change tempered by scientific knowledge and humanitarian concern. Sharing the revolutionaries' perception of the plight of the poor and the injustices of the system, they nonetheless counseled less radical solutions.[39–42] They advocated public health reforms on political, economic, humanitarian, and scientific grounds. Politically, public health reform offered a middle ground between the cutthroat principles of entrepreneurial capitalism and the revolutionary ideas of the socialists, anarchists, and utopian visionaries. As William Henry Welch, a leader of American medicine and public health,

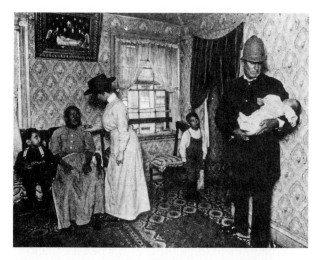

Figure 2.2. Visiting Nurse Comforts Mother as Policeman Takes Baby to the Contagious Disease Hospital, 1916.
Courtesy of the National Library of Medicine.

expressed it to the Charity Organization Society, sanitary improvement offered the best way of improving the lot of the poor, short of the radical restructuring of society.[43(p598)]

Economic Rewards of Reform

Economically, progressive reformers argued that public health should be viewed as a paying investment, giving higher returns than the stock market. In Germany, Max von Pettenkofer had first calculated the financial returns on public health "investments" to prove the value of sanitary improvements in reducing deaths from typhoid.[44] His argument would be repeated many times by American public health leaders. As William Henry Welch explained:

> . . . merely from a mercenary and commercial point of view it is for the interest of the community to take care of the health of the poor. Philanthropy assumes a totally different aspect in the eyes of the world when it is able to demonstrate that it pays to keep people healthy.[43(p596)]

Public health leaders argued that the demand for centralized planning and business efficiency required scientific knowledge rather than the undisciplined enthusiasms of voluntary groups.[45] Public health decisions should be made by an analysis of costs and benefits "as an up-to-date manufacturer would count the cost of a new process." The health officer, like the merchant, should learn "which line of work yields the most for the sum expended."[46]

National and International Health

Public health was quickly becoming a national and even international issue. Although Congress was reluctant to enact federal health legislation, there were mounting pressures for United States attention to public health abroad. As American business was seeking enlarged foreign markets, a vocal group of intellectuals and politicians argued for an assertive foreign policy. The United States began to challenge European dominance in the Far East and

Latin America, seeking trade and political influence more than territory but taking territory where it could. National defense goals included broadening control of trade routes, building a Central American canal, and establishing strategic bases in the Caribbean and Western Pacific.

Cuba and the Panama Canal

In 1898, the United States entered the Spanish-American War, expanded the army from 25,000 to 250,000 men, and sent troops to Cuba. The war showed that the United States could not afford military adventures overseas unless more attention was paid to sanitation and public health: 968 men died in battle, but 5438 died of infectious diseases.[47,48] Nonetheless, the United States defeated Spain and installed an army of occupation in Cuba. When yellow fever threatened the troops in 1900, the response was efficient and effective. An army commission under Walter Reed was sent to Cuba to study the disease and, in a dramatic series of human experiments, it confirmed the hypothesis that yellow fever was spread by mosquitoes. Surgeon Major William Gorgas then eliminated yellow fever from Havana.[49]

This experience confirmed the importance of public health for successful United States efforts overseas. Earlier attempts to dig the Panama Canal had been attended by enormous mortality rates from disease.[50] But in 1904, Gorgas, now promoted to general, took control of a campaign against the malaria and yellow fever that were threatening canal operations. He was finally able to persuade the Canal Commission to institute an intensive campaign against mosquitoes. In one of the great triumphs of practical public health, yellow fever and malaria were brought under control, and the canal was successfully completed in 1914.

Bringing the Lessons Home

United States industrialists brought some of the lessons of Cuba and the Panama Canal home to the southern United States. The South at that time resembled an underdeveloped country within the United States, characterized by poor economic and social conditions. Northern industrialists were already investing heavily in southern education as well as in cotton mills and railroads. John D. Rockefeller had created the General Education Board to support "the general organization of rural communities for economic, social, and educational purposes."[51] Charles Wardell Stiles managed to convince the secretary of the General Education Board that the real cause of misery and lack of productivity in the South was hookworm, the "germ of laziness." In 1909, Rockefeller agreed to provide $1 million to create the Rockefeller Sanitary Commission for the Eradication of Hookworm Disease, with Wickliffe Rose as director.[52] This was to be the first installment in Rockefeller's massive national and international investment in public health.

Rose went beyond the task of attempting to control a single disease and worked to establish an effective and permanent public health organization in the southern states.[53] At the end of five years of intensive effort, the campaign had failed to eradicate hookworm but had greatly expanded the role of public health agencies. Between 1910 and 1914, county appropriations for local public health work increased from a total of $240 to $110,000.[52(pp220-221)]

Public Health at the National Level

In Washington, the Committee of One Hundred on National Health campaigned for the **federal regulation** of public health.[54,55] The committee was composed of such notables as Jane Addams, Andrew Carnegie, William H. Welch, and Booker T. Washington. Its president, the economist Irving Fisher, argued that a public health service would be good policy and good economics, in conserving national vitality.[56]

In 1912, the federal government made its first real commitment to public health when it expanded the responsibilities of the Public Health Service, empowering it to investigate the causes and spread of diseases and the pollution and sanitation of navigable streams and lakes.[57] The responsibilities

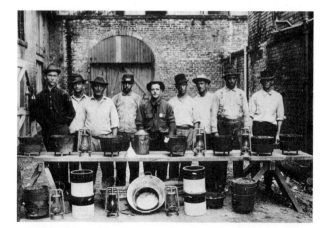

Figure 2.3. **Many Types of Public Health Workers Were Needed During the Plague Epidemic of 1914–1920, Rat Catchers Display the Tools of Their Trade: Kettles, Buckets, and Lanterns.**

Courtesy of the National Library of Medicine.

of the Public Health Service included the medical inspection of immigrants arriving at Ellis Island, field investigations of endemic rural diseases such as trachoma, and groundbreaking research on diseases such as pellagra and Rocky Mountain spotted fever. By 1915, the Public Health Service, the United States Army, and the Rockefeller Foundation were the major agencies involved in public health activities, supplemented on a local level by a network of city and state health departments.

THE PROFESSIONALIZATION OF PUBLIC HEALTH

At the turn of the century, existing health departments were often dominated more by patronage and political considerations than by economic or administrative efficiency. Progressives regretted the evils of politics and wanted to increase the pay and minimum qualifications for health officers to attract personnel on the basis of skill rather than influence. Their attempt to insulate boards of health from local political control was part of a broader movement to make all forms of public administration more rational and efficient by reducing the influence of political bosses and promoting a new group of **professional** administrators.[58] The goal was for a well-trained professional elite to conduct social reform on scientific lines.

These developments led to an increasing demand for people trained in public health to direct the new programs being created at the local, state, and national levels. Those attempting to develop such programs were increasingly critical of the lack of properly trained personnel; part-time public health officers were simply not adequate to staff the ambitious new programs. Public health reformers agreed that full-time practitioners, especially trained for the job, were needed. In 1913, the New York state legislature passed a law requiring public health officers to have specialized training, despite the fact that there was little agreement about what kind of specialized training was needed, much less where it could be obtained.[59,60]

Public health had been defined in terms of its aims and goals—to reduce disease and maintain the health of the population—rather than by any specific body of knowledge. Many different **disciplines** contributed to effective public health work: physicians diagnosed contagious diseases; sanitary engineers built water and sewage systems; epidemiologists traced the sources of disease outbreaks and their modes of transmission; vital statisticians provided quantitative measures of births and deaths; lawyers wrote sanitary codes and regulations; public health nurses provided care and advice to the sick in their homes; sanitary inspectors visited factories and markets to enforce compliance with public health ordinances; and administrators tried to organize everyone within the limits of health department budgets. Public health thus involved economics, sociology, psychology, politics, law, statistics, and engineering, as well as the biological and clinical sciences. However, in the period immediately following the brilliant experimental work of Louis Pasteur and Robert Koch, the bacteriological laboratory became the first and primary symbol of a new, scientific public health.

Bacteriology and Alternative Views of Health and Disease

The rise of **bacteriology** and other scientific advances in the understanding of disease contributed to the professionalization of public health.

The Rise of Bacteriology

The clarity and simplicity of bacteriological methods and discoveries gave them tremendous cultural importance: the agents of particular diseases had been made visible under the microscope. The identification of specific bacteria seemed to have cut through the misty miasmas of disease to define the enemy in unmistakable terms. Bacteriology thus became an ideological marker, sharply differentiating the *old* public health, the province of untrained amateurs, from the *new* public health, which would belong to scientifically trained professionals.

Young Americans who had studied in Germany brought back the new knowledge of laboratory methods in bacteriology and started to teach others. These young scientists were convinced that physicians should stop squabbling over medical ethics and politics and commit themselves to the purer values of laboratory research. Under their influence, the laboratory ideal soon spread throughout progressive public health circles. By the 1880s, Charles Chapin had established a public health laboratory in Providence, Rhode Island, and Victor C. Vaughan had created a state hygienic laboratory in Michigan.

In 1901, William Sedgwick reported on his bacteriological study of water supplies and sewage disposal at the Lawrence Experiment Station in Massachusetts.[61] Sedgwick demonstrated the transmission of typhoid fever by polluted water supplies, and he developed quantitative methods for measuring the presence of bacteria in the air, water, and milk. Describing the impact of bacteriological discoveries, he said, "Before 1880 we knew nothing; after 1890 we knew it all; it was a glorious ten years."[32(p57)]

The powerful new methods of identifying diseases through the microscope drew attention away from the larger and more diffuse problems of water supplies, street cleaning, housing reform, and the living conditions of the poor. The approach of locating, identifying, and isolating bacteria and their human hosts was a more elegant and efficient way of dealing with disease than environmental reform. The public health laboratory demonstrated the scientific and diagnostic power of the new public health. However, by focusing on the diagnosis of infectious diseases, it narrowed the distance between medicine and public health and brought public health into potential conflict with private medical practice. Physicians began increasingly to resent the public health officials' claim to diagnose, and often treat, infectious diseases.

Alternative Models

Although the narrow bacteriological view was dominant, there were several competing models for public health research and practice. It is worth noting the broad and comprehensive definition of public health offered by Charles-Edward A. Winslow, professor of public health at Yale University, in 1920:

> Public health is the science and art of preventing disease, prolonging life, and promoting physical health and efficiency through organized community efforts for the sanitation of the environment, the control of community infections, the education of the individual in principles of personal hygiene, the organization of medical and nursing service for the early diagnosis and preventive treatment of disease, and the development of the social machinery which will ensure to every individual in the community a standard of living adequate for the maintenance of health.[62,63]

Winslow's was not the only broad vision of public health. Alice Hamilton in Illinois conducted a survey of industrial lead poisoning and established the fact that thousands of American workers were being slowly killed by white lead.[64] Unaided by legislation, Hamilton argued, persuaded, shamed, and flattered individual employers into improving working conditions. Almost single-handedly, she created the foundations of **industrial hygiene** in America.

Joseph Goldberger's epidemiological studies of pellagra for the Public Health Service offer another example of a comprehensive approach to public health. In 1914, Goldberger announced that pellagra was due to dietary deficiencies and not to some unknown microorganism. He and his colleagues had cured endemic pellagra in a Mississippi orphanage by feeding the children milk, eggs, beans, and meat. He then teamed up with an economist, Edgar Sydenstricker, to survey the diets of southern wageworkers' families. They showed how the sharecropping system had impoverished tenant farmers, led to dietary deficiencies, and thus produced endemic pellagra.[65]

Alice Hamilton, Joseph Goldberger, and Edgar Sydenstricker were minority voices amid the growing majority focusing exclusively on bacteria. As most bacteriologists and epidemiologists concentrated on specific disease-causing organisms and the individuals who harbored them, only a minority continued to relate the problems of ill health and disease to the larger social environment.[66]

The Relationship Between Public Health and Medicine

Although the broader conceptions of public health required an understanding of economics and politics, the dominant model of public health knowledge was based almost exclusively on the biological sciences. This redefinition of public health in bioscientific terms reinforced the medical profession's claim to preeminence in the field. Physicians felt that because they were the experts in infectious diseases, they were uniquely qualified to become the ultimate authorities in the new, scientific public health.

By the second decade of the twentieth century, nonmedical public health officers were beginning to protest the dominance of public health by medical men. By this time, the sanitary engineers were the only professional group strong enough to challenge the physicians' assumption that the future of public health should be theirs. Civil and sanitary engineers had created clean city water supplies and adequate sewage systems, which were major factors in the declining death rates from infant diarrhea and other infectious diseases.[67–70]

Professional competition between the sanitary engineers and physicians became intense in the early years of the twentieth century as sanitary engineers vociferously complained about the increasing *medical monopoly* of public health. By 1912, 15 states required that all members of their boards of health be physicians, and 23 states required at least 1 physician member; only 10 states had no professional requirement for eligibility.[71]

With the increasing professionalization of public health, physicians came to hold a dominant but not exclusive role in the field. Leadership positions in public health departments and public health agencies were increasingly reserved for physicians. Other scientists, professionals, and nurses might be given subordinate positions. Physicians themselves were increasingly ambivalent about public health. The curious relationships between physicians and nonmedical public health practitioners would shape the subsequent development of public health practice.

PUBLIC HEALTH ORGANIZATION AND PRACTICE

The practical importance of public health was well recognized by the early decades of the twentieth century. The incidence of tuberculosis, diphtheria, and other infectious diseases was falling, apparently in response to energetic public health campaigns. School health clinics and maternal and child health centers were established in many cities with active public support. Registration for the draft in World War I revealed that a substantial proportion of young men were either physically or mentally unfit for combat, and this perception also led to increased political support for public health activities. The influenza epidemic that devastated families and communities from 1916 to 1918 underlined the continuing threat of infectious disease epidemics.

The Waning Influence of Bacteriology

After the first flush of enthusiasm for the achievements of bacteriology, many health departments were now paying more attention to community-based health activities and popular health education. In 1923, Charles-Edward A. Winslow went so far as to announce the ending of the bacteriological age and to describe popular health education as the

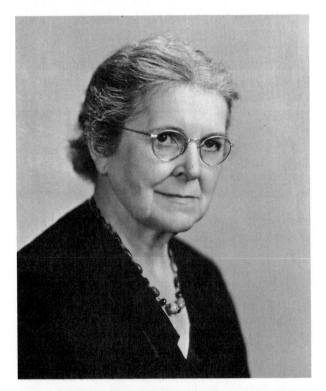

Figure 2.4. Martha May Eliot, Pioneer of Child and Maternal Health. Children's Bureau Photo, Singer, 1954.

Courtesy of the National Library of Medicine.

keynote of the *new public health*, almost as far-reaching in its importance as the germ theory of disease had been some 30 years before.[63(pp53,55),72]

In the 1920s, state and municipal health departments developed new organizational units and increased their hiring of public health personnel, especially public health nurses. Although bacteriological laboratories continued to be important, divisions that were focused on tuberculosis, maternal and child health, venereal diseases, public health administration, and health education played a major role in most state and city health departments, as did divisions of sanitation and vital statistics.

Variation in Public Health Practice

Public health practice varied greatly throughout the states and cities across the country, as shown by an APHA survey of municipal public health department practice in 1923. Although some cities had extensive, progressive, and imaginative programs, others did little beyond offering a few communicable disease clinics and public health inspections.[73]

Continuing Controversy with Medicine

The relationship between the emerging profession of public health and the well-established profession of medicine continued to be problematic and controversial. The increased activity of health departments in the identification and control of infectious diseases brought health officers into conflict with private practitioners. As soon as public health left the confines of sanitary engineering and took on the battle against specific diseases, it challenged the boundaries of medical autonomy. As John Duffy has argued, the medical profession moved from a position of strong support for public health activities to a cautious and sometimes suspicious ambivalence.[74]

Major battles would be fought over the Sheppard-Towner Maternity and Infancy Act of 1921, which provided grants to states to teach prenatal and infant care to mothers.[75] Conservatives denounced the measure as socialistic, and many physicians opposed it as interfering with the proper purview of medicine. These programs were allowed to expire in 1929, showing the difficulties faced by any innovative public health or social welfare legislation in a politically conservative period.

Federal Involvement

The most important federal organization in public health continued to be the United States Public Health Service, an arm of the Federal Security Agency. The Public Health Service aided the development of state health departments by giving grants-in-aid, loaning expert personnel, and providing advice and consultation on specific problems.[76] For example, if a state was facing an unexplained outbreak of typhoid fever or other epidemic disease, the Public Health Service would send epidemiologists to trace the source of the disease and suggest means of preventing its spread.

Influence of the Depression

A major stimulus to the development of public health practice came in response to the Depression, with the New Deal and the Social Security Act of 1935. The Social Security Act represented America's first broad-based social welfare legislation, providing old-age benefits, unemployment insurance, and public health services. Unfortunately, the attempt to include basic medical insurance within the bill was abandoned because of the determined opposition of the medical profession, pharmaceutical companies, and the insurance industry.[77–79] From the public health point of view, however, the Social Security Act was a huge leap forward. Title V of the act established a program of grants to states for maternal and child health services, administered by the Children's Bureau, and provided funds for child welfare and crippled children's programs. Title VI of the act expanded financing of the Public Health Service and allotted federal grants to states to assist them in developing their public health services.

Federal and state expenditures for public health actually doubled in the decade of the Depression, fueling the expansion of local health units. In most parts of the country, efficient provision of public health services to local communities depended on county health organizations, smaller and simpler units than the larger state health departments. In 1934, only 541 counties out of the 3070 counties in the United States had any form of local public health service, but by June 1942, 1828 counties could boast of health units directed by a full-time public health officer.[80] Much of this gain would be lost during the war; by the end of the war, only 1322 counties had an organized health service.[81(p125),82]

Federal Funding and Training

In 1935, for the first time, the federal government provided funds, administered through the states, for public health training. Federal regulations now required states to establish minimum qualifications for public health personnel employed through new federal grants. Thus, it was no longer sufficient for state programs to employ any willing physician; some form of professional public health training was expected.

As a result of the growing demand for public health education, several state universities began new schools or divisions of public health, and existing schools of public health expanded their enrollments. By 1936, 10 schools offered public health degrees or certificates requiring at least one year of attendance.[83] By 1938, more than 4000 individuals, including about 1000 physicians, had received some public health training with funds provided by the federal government through the states.

The economic difficulties of maintaining a private practice during the Depression had pushed some physicians into public health; others were attracted by the new availability of fellowships or by increased social awareness of the plight of the poor. In 1939, the federal government allocated more than $8 million for maternal and child health programs, more than $9 million for general public health work, and more than $4 million for venereal disease control.

Several important trends were stimulated by these federal funds. The first was the development of programs to control specific diseases and of services targeted to specific population groups, the **categorical** approach to public health. Second was the expansion in the number of local health departments. Third was the increased training of personnel, and fourth, the assumption of responsibility for some phases of medical care on the part of health departments.[81](pxii)

Categorical Approach to Public Health

The categorical approach to public health proved politically popular. Members of Congress were willing to allocate funds for specific diseases or for particular groups—health and welfare services for children were especially favored—but they showed less interest in general public health or administrative expenditures. Although state health officers often felt constrained by targeted programs, they rarely refused federal grants-in-aid and thus adapted their programs to the pattern of available funds. Federal grants came in turn for maternal and child health services and crippled children (1935), venereal disease control (1938), tuberculosis (1944), mental health (1947), industrial hygiene (1947), and dental health (1947). The pattern of funding started in the 1930s would thus shape the organization of public health departments through the postwar period. As institutionalized in the National Institutes of Health, it would also shape the future patterns of biomedical research.

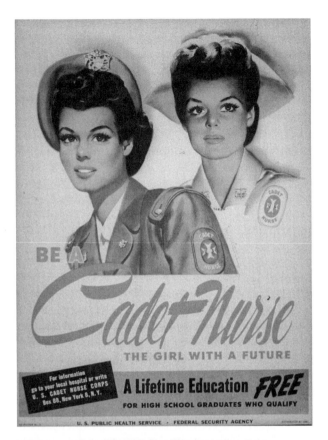

Figure 2.5. Be a Cadet Nurse with a Future. Poster by Jon Whitcomb, United States General Printing Office, United States Public Health Service, Federal Security Agency, Washington, DC.

Courtesy of the National Library of Medicine.

PUBLIC HEALTH AND THE WAR

Mobilization for war acted as another major force in the expansion and development of public health in the United States.[84] Public health was declared a national priority for the armed forces and the civilian population engaged in military production. As James Stevens Simmons, brigadier general and director of the Preventive Medicine Division of the United States Army, announced:

> A civil population that is not healthy cannot be prosperous and will lag behind in the economic competition between nations. This is even more true of a military population, for any army that has its strength sapped by disease is in no condition to withstand the attack of a virile force that has conserved its strength and is enjoying the vigor and exhilaration of health.[85]

The Need for Personnel

Health departments again suffered from a critical shortage of personnel as physicians, nurses, engineers, and other trained and experienced professionals left to join the armed services.[86] In 1940, the United States Public Health Service expanded its program of grants to states and local communities, sending personnel to particularly needy areas. The Community Facilities Act, for instance, provided $300 million to fund health and sanitation facilities in communities with rapidly expanding populations because of military camps and war industries.[87,88]

The Selective Service Exams

The shock of discovering that many of the young men being called into the army were physically unfit for military service provided a powerful impetus for increased national attention to public health. The Selective Service examinations represented the most massive health survey ever undertaken, with more than 16 million young men examined. Fully 40 percent of the young men examined were declared physically or mentally unfit for service, with the leading causes of rejection being defective teeth, vision problems, orthopedic impairments (from polio, for example), diseases of the cardiovascular system, nervous and mental diseases, hernia, tuberculosis, and venereal diseases.[89,90]

Mosquitoes and the Centers for Disease Control

With the war mobilization, hundreds of thousands of workers moved to areas with defense industry plants, and the troops moved to Army camps.[91] Army training camps often had been placed in areas with warm climates, where the Anopheles mosquito bred in profusion, and malaria was endemic. To control malaria in the South, the Public Health Service established the Center for Controlling Malaria in the War Areas. After the war, when substantial funds were made available for malaria eradication efforts, this organization was gradually transformed into the Centers for Disease

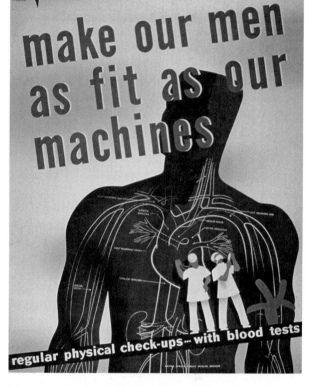

Figure 2.6. Make Our Men as Fit as Our Machines: Regular Physical Check-ups—with Blood Tests. United States Public Health Service poster.
Courtesy of the National Library of Medicine.

Control (now the Centers for Disease Control and Prevention), which would play a major national role in the effort to control both infectious and noninfectious diseases.[92]

POSTWAR REORGANIZATION

In the immediate postwar period, considerable optimism and energy were devoted to the possible reorganization of public health and medical care. Many of the discussions of a future national medical care system posited the potential unification of preventive and curative medicine. Some public health leaders were advocating the direct administration of tax-supported medical care by health departments. Others opposed such a development, feeling that if public health and medical care administration were combined, preventive and educational efforts would be submerged by the demand for costly therapeutic services.[93]

Hospital Construction

While public health officials were debating whether they wanted to take responsibility for medical care services, the Hospital Survey and Construction Act, more popularly known as the Hill-Burton Act, was passed in 1946. Hospital construction, especially in rural areas, promised to bring everyone the benefits of medical science, without disturbing the freedoms of the medical profession or the patterns of paying for their services. The federal government would pay one-third the costs of building hospitals, setting aside $75 million for each of the first five years. No health program had ever been so generous or so popular.

Hill-Burton addressed the national demand for access to medical care without challenging the private organization of medical practice. It thus answered the desire for acute-care services while essentially ignoring preventive care and public health. The United States could have been completely covered by local health departments for a fraction of the cost of Hill-Burton, but there was no strong political constituency for public health that could compete effectively for resources with curative medicine.

Local Health Services

In 1942, the APHA provided a plan for organizing local health services across the nation.[94] Haven Emerson's report, *Local Health Units for the Nation*, found that only two-thirds of the people of the United States were covered by local public health services. It also estimated the cost of providing a modest but adequate basic health service for

each of the 1197 additional local health units proposed. The committee noted that communities of over 50,000 should be able to provide a reasonably adequate local service at the cost of $1.00 per capita or a superior service for only $2.00 per capita.[94(p2)]

A survey of state health departments found that a multitude of agencies, state boards, and commissions were involved in public health activities, as many as 18 different agencies being involved in a single state.[95,96] The money spent for public health work also varied widely, ranging from $0.13 per capita in Ohio to $1.68 in Delaware. In most cases, the states spending the largest sums were spending most of these funds on hospital services rather than on prevention.

Changes in Disease

In the postwar years, the public health community clearly understood that the disease patterns of the country had changed: in 1900, the leading causes of death had been tuberculosis, pneumonia, diarrheal diseases, and enteritis; by 1946, the leading causes of death were heart disease, cancer, and accidents. Recognition of the importance of **chronic diseases** had been temporarily eclipsed by the more urgent demands of infectious disease control during the war. With the return to peace, health departments recognized that they must now come to terms with the problems and prevalence of the chronic diseases.

Social Medicine

In the late 1940s and early 1950s, some American public health officials welcomed the concept of **social medicine** as seeming to offer a fresh perspective on the problems of chronic illness. Iago Galdston, secretary of the New York Academy of Medicine, organized the Institute on Social Medicine in 1947, later publishing its papers as *Social Medicine: Its Derivations and Objectives*.[97] John A. Ryle, professor of social medicine at Oxford University, emphasized the distinctions between the new social medicine and the old public health. Public health, he said, was concerned with environmental improvement, while social medicine extended its view to "the whole of the economic, nutritional, occupational, educational, and psychological opportunity or experience of the individual or of the community."[98] Whereas public health was concerned with communicable diseases, social medicine would be concerned with all health problems—ulcers and rheumatism, heart disease and cancer, neuroses and injuries. Ryle stated that social medicine, in close alliance with clinical practice, posed the exciting challenge of the future.

The Role of Epidemiology

Ernest L. Stebbins, dean of the Johns Hopkins School of Public Health, argued that epidemiology was the essential discipline for dealing with both chronic and infectious diseases.[99] Margaret Merrell and Lowell J. Reed, statisticians from the Hopkins school, made a similar point in a brief paper that would become a classic statement on the *epidemiology of health*. They suggested a graded scale for measuring degrees of health, not simply the absence of illness:

> On such a scale people would be classified from those who are in top-notch condition with abundant energy, through the people who are well, to fairly well, down to people who are feeling rather poorly, and finally to the definitely ill.[100]

The ideas that health could be quantitatively measurable and that it could be advanced in the total absence of disease helped make connections between the new social medicine and the older public health. Epidemiology, broadening its scope to place more emphasis on the social environment, became newly fashionable as "medical ecology."[81] John E. Gordon, professor of preventive medicine and epidemiology at the Harvard School of Public Health and a prominent exponent of the "newer epidemiology," explained how the triad of

"environment, host, and disease" could be applied to noncommunicable organic diseases such as pellagra, cancer, psychosomatic conditions, traumatic injuries, and accidents.[101,102] The notion of a single cause of disease (the agent) was now firmly rejected in favor of multiple causation.[99]

Troubles in Implementation

Social medicine brought considerable optimism about the possibilities for new approaches to the chronic diseases, for the integration of preventive and curative medicine, and for the extension of comprehensive health programs to the whole population.[103] In 1950, Eli Ginzberg introduced a tone of pessimism and caution, however, when he warned optimistic thinkers of an *antigovernment attitude* in the United States and the prevalent assumption that health depended on medical care, with the ever-increasing provision of physicians and hospital beds. He urged public health professionals to do a more effective job of persuading the public that advances in diet, housing, and public health nursing were more important to health than the construction of hospitals. He also noted that while hospitals were being built across the country, local health officer positions stood vacant because communities refused to provide reasonable salaries.[104]

Ginzberg's prognosis proved correct in the political climate of the 1950s. The theoretical innovations of social medicine were not translated into effective health programs; acute-care facilities and biomedical research expanded dramatically in the postwar period, while public health departments struggled to maintain their programs on inadequate budgets with little political support. The postwar construction meant massive expenditures for biomedical research and hospital construction, the partial payment for medical care by expanding private insurance coverage, but the relative neglect of public health services and a complete failure to implement the more radical ideas of social medicine through attention to the **social determinants of health** and disease.

POLITICAL PROBLEMS OF PUBLIC HEALTH

The Committee on Medicine and the Changing Order, supported by the Commonwealth Fund, the Milbank Memorial Fund, and the Josiah Macy Jr. Foundation, recommended the extension of public health services in 1947, but it argued that the quality of public health officers must be improved by better recruitment, training, assured tenure, and adequate salaries.[105] Harry Mustard, on the other hand, protested that the problems of public health were largely political. State health officers were of relatively low rank in the hierarchy of state officials and were limited in their freedom to introduce new proposals. Too often they accepted political constraints and bureaucratic barriers as natural and inevitable.[106] Too seldom were they willing to risk their positions by appealing to a larger constituency.

In retrospect, it also seems clear that public health failed to claim sufficient credit for controlling infectious diseases. The major scientific achievements of the war in relation to health, such as the discovery of penicillin and the use of DDT, were especially relevant to public health. In popular perception, however, scientific medicine took credit for both the specific wartime discoveries and the longer history of controlling epidemic disease. Medicine and biomedical research had essentially seized the public glory, the political interest, and the financial support given for further anticipated health improvements in the postwar world.

Public health departments needed to claim some share of the credit for declining infectious diseases and to move quickly to develop programs for the chronic diseases. Most health departments did neither of these things but simply continued running the same programs and clinics within already established bureaucratic structures. The political atmosphere of the 1950s did not support aggressive new programs, and health department budgets were stagnant, without the funding needed to develop broad new health programs.

The Fluoridation Fiasco

Health departments did implement, or try to implement, one important new and very cost-effective public health measure, the **fluoridation** of water supplies to protect children's teeth.[107] Despite virtually unanimous support from scientific authorities and professional organizations, however, fluoridation was denounced as a communist plot and effectively halted in many cities and towns through vocal local opposition. If such a simple and obviously effective measure could be so energetically opposed, health departments must have perceived the difficulty in instituting more adventurous or expensive interventions.

An Exception: Success with Polio

The one great triumph of the 1950s was the successful development of the polio vaccine and its implementation on a mass scale.[108–110] The success of the polio campaign was due in large part to private funding and a massive public relations campaign by the Foundation for Infantile Paralysis, which raised public awareness and developed public support, interest, and enthusiasm. The appeal for crippled children proved extremely popular, and the polio vaccination campaign, aside from some major setbacks, was a remarkable success.

DECLINE OF PUBLIC HEALTH IN THE 1950S

Despite such public success, in the 1950s the real expenditures of public health departments failed to keep pace with the increase in population.[111] Federal grants-in-aid to the states for public health programs steadily declined, falling from $45 million in 1950 to $33 million in 1959. Given inflation, the decline in purchasing power was even more dramatic. At a time when public health officials were facing a whole series of new, poorly understood health problems, they were also underbudgeted and understaffed.

Health officers were frequently limited to routine clinical responsibilities in child health stations, tuberculosis clinics, venereal disease clinics, and immunization programs, and to communicable disease diagnosis and treatment. They had little or no time for community health education, for studying new health problems, or for developing experimental programs. Indeed, in many areas, health officer positions went unfilled, and local medical practitioners, working part time, provided clinical services on an hourly basis.[112]

Some state legislatures were setting up new agencies to build nursing homes, abate water pollution, or promote mental health, and they simply bypassed health departments as not active or interested in these issues. Public health officials were expressing "frustrations, disappointments, dissatisfactions, and discontentments," said John W. Knutson in his Presidential Address to the APHA in 1957.[113] Public health professionals, he said, must develop more imagination, political skills, and knowledge of human motivation and behavior. Public health students needed a better understanding of social and political forces. Instead of simply learning soon-to-be-outdated factual information, they needed an in-depth knowledge of cultural anthropology, human ecology, epidemiology, and biostatistics.[113] Even with the best possible preparation, the bureaucratic controls of state health departments tended to ensure conformity and discourage young professionals from initiating or taking responsibility for new programs or activities.[114]

In 1959, Milton Terris offered a forceful summary statement of the dilemma of public health. The communicable diseases were disappearing; their place had been taken by the noninfectious diseases that the public health profession was ill prepared to prevent or control. The public understood the fact that **research** was crucial, and federal expenditures for medical research had multiplied from $28 million in 1947 to $186 million 10 years later. Most of this money, however, was being spent for clinical and laboratory research; there was little understanding of the importance of epidemiological studies in

addressing these problems. Schools of public health had been slow to deal with chronic illness, as had health departments, with a few notable exceptions as in the cases of New York and California. Even the small sums spent on epidemiological research had produced dramatic successes, including the discovery of the role of fluoride in preventing dental caries, the relation of cigarette smoking to lung cancer, and the suspected relation of serum cholesterol and physical exercise to coronary artery disease.[115]

In the late 1950s, public health leaders recognized and lamented the failure of their profession to assert a strong political presence or even to perceive the importance of politics to practical public health. The APHA devoted its annual meeting in 1958 to The Politics of Public Health.[116] The editor of the *American Journal of Public Health*, George Rosen, wrote that the education of public health workers should begin with teaching them to think politically and to understand the political process.[117] Raymond R. Tucker, mayor of St. Louis, the city hosting the APHA convention, insisted that public health officials must learn not to confuse the opposition of special interest groups with public opinion, for the general public solidly supported public health reform.[118]

THE 1960S AND THE WAR ON POVERTY

The 1960s saw the collapse of the conservative complacency of the 1950s, the growing power of the civil rights movement, riots in urban African-American ghettos, and federal support for the *war on poverty.* The antipoverty effort and other Great Society programs soon became deeply involved with medical care.[119] Growing concern over access to medical care and hospitalization, especially by the elderly population, culminated in Medicare and Medicaid legislation in 1965 to cover medical care costs for those on Social Security and for the poor. Both programs were built on the *politics of accommodation* with private providers of medical care, thus increasing the incomes of physicians and hospitals and leading to spiraling costs for medical services.[120] Other antipoverty programs, such as the neighborhood health centers that were intended to encourage community participation in providing comprehensive care to underserved populations, fared less well because they were seen as competing with the interests of private care providers.[121]

Most of the new health and social programs of the 1960s bypassed the structure of the public health agencies and set up new agencies to mediate between the federal government and local communities. Medicare and Medicaid reflected the usual priorities of the medical care system in favoring highly technical interventions and hospital care, while failing to provide adequately for preventive services. Neighborhood health centers and community-based mental health services were established without reference to public health agencies.

When environmental issues attracted public concern and political attention in the 1960s and 1970s, separate agencies were also created to respond to these concerns. At the federal level, the Environmental Protection Agency (EPA) was created to deal with such issues as solid wastes, pesticides, and radiation. At the state level, environmental agencies were often separate from public health departments and failed to reflect specific health concerns or public health expertise. Similarly, mental health agencies were often separate from public health agencies.

Thus, the broader functions of public health were again divided among numerous agencies. Losing a clear institutional base, public health had also lost visibility and clarity of definition. For a field that depends so heavily on public understanding and support, such a loss was disastrous.

PUBLIC HEALTH IN THE SEVENTIES AND EIGHTIES

In the 1970s, public health departments became providers of last resort for uninsured patients and for Medicaid patients rejected by private practitioners. By 1988, almost three-quarters of all state and local health department expenditures went for personal health services.[122] As Harry Mustard had predicted some 40 years earlier, direct provision of medical care absorbed much of the limited resources—in personnel, money, energy, time, and attention—of public health departments, leading to a slow starvation of public health and preventive activities.[122(p52)] The problem of caring for the uninsured and the indigent loomed so large that it eclipsed the need for a basic public health infrastructure in the minds of many legislators and the general public.

In the Reagan revolution of the 1980s, federal funding for public health programs was cut. Through the mechanism of the block grants, power was returned to state health agencies, but in the context of funding cuts, this was the unpopular power to cut existing programs.[123] In the context of general budget cuts, state health departments were often left the task of managing Medicaid programs and delivering personal health services to uninsured and indigent populations. State health departments also had to deal with the adverse health consequences of reductions in other social programs; with the problems of a growing poverty population, as evidenced in drug abuse, alcoholism, teenage pregnancy, infant mortality, family violence, and homelessness; and with the health and social needs of growing populations of illegal immigrants.

The AIDS epidemic and the resurgence of tuberculosis revealed the structural contradictions and weaknesses of national and federal health policy.[124] For state and local health agencies, AIDS and tuberculosis exacerbated their existing problems but gave a new visibility and urgency to their public health efforts.[125,126] The public health community urged a major national effort in AIDS education and prevention. Much of the new funding, when it did finally come, went into research and medical care; as usual, education and prevention received much less attention. But at the same time, the mobilization of public concern provided renewed attention to public health and increased political support. The report by the Institute of Medicine, titled *The Future of Public Health*, notes:

In a free society public activities ultimately
rest on public understanding and support,

not on the technical judgment of experts. Expertise is made effective only when it is combined with sufficient public support, a connection acted upon effectively by the early leaders of public health.[122(p130)]

PUBLIC HEALTH TODAY

Since the early 1990s, the whole country has been embroiled in debates over health care reform, welfare reform, drugs, violence, environmental health, and women's health issues. These are all issues of public health, yet public health as such is rarely mentioned. This is partly a failure of public health practice; we need a variety of model public health programs to demonstrate to the country what could be achieved with sufficient political will, expertise, and money. It is also in part a failure of **communications.** Public health professionals have not been very effective in presenting their views and accomplishments to the media, the politicians, and the public.

SUMMARY

The growth in the technical knowledge of public health in the past 100 years has been extraordinary—and insufficiently addressed in this brief account—but our ability to implement this knowledge in health and social reform has advanced little. As we have noted, the issues of public health today include and intersect with the great social issues of modern America: health care reform and the coverage of the uninsured; environmental health and safety; welfare reform and child health; drugs and violence in the streets; women's health, reproductive freedom, abortion, and fertility control; family violence and child abuse; AIDS, tuberculosis, and emerging epidemics; the continuing problems of chronic disease; and the need for home health services and long-term care for an aging population.

Public health is a vitally important field for the future well-being of America, its citizens, and its communities. Public health professionals must learn to communicate better the vital importance of their activities, mobilize public support, build a more effective public health **infrastructure,** and demonstrate clearly the benefits of prevention to the public at large by finding innovative ways of responding to endemic social problems and new crises.

REVIEW QUESTIONS

1. Before the germ theory, what were believed to be the causes of epidemic diseases?
2. How did social reformers begin to tackle the tasks of public health?
3. Why was it difficult to create a National Board of Health?
4. What were the earliest responsibilities of the United States Public Health Service?
5. What disciplines contributed to public health work?
6. In the early twentieth century, what were the alternate possible models of public health?
7. When did the federal government begin to increase funding for public health?
8. What has been the impact of war on public health?
9. What are some of the lessons to be learned from the history of public health?

REFERENCES

1. Rosenberg C. *The Cholera Years: The United States in 1832, 1849 and 1866.* Chicago, IL: University of Chicago Press; 1962.
2. Powell JH. *Bring Out Your Dead: The Great Plague of Yellow Fever in Philadelphia in 1793.* Philadelphia: University of Pennsylvania Press; 1949.
3. Wiebe RH. *The Search for Order, 1877–1920.* New York: Hill & Wang; 1967.
4. Ackerknecht EL. Anticontagionism between 1821 and 1867. *Bull Hist Med.* 1948;22:562–593.
5. Baltimore City Ordinance 11, approved April 7, 1797. In: Howard WT. *Public Health Administration and the Natural History of Disease in*

Baltimore, Maryland, 1797–1920. Washington, DC: Carnegie Institution; 1924.

6. Rosen G. *A History of Public Health.* Expanded ed. Baltimore, MD: Johns Hopkins University Press; 1993.

7. Duffy J. The *Sanitarians: A History of American Public Health.* Urbana: University of Illinois Press; 1990.

8. Rosner D, ed. *Epidemic! Public Health Crises in New York.* New Brunswick, NJ: Rutgers University Press; 1994.

9. Citizens' Association of New York. *Report of the Council of Hygiene and Public Health of the Citizens' Association of New York upon the Sanitary Condition of the City.* New York: Arno Press; 1970: xxi–xxxv.

10. Hudson A. The mapping of property and environment in Manhattan since the 1600s. *Biblion.* Spring 1993;1:47–50.

11. Shattuck L. Report of a *General Plan for the Promotion of Public and Personal Health, Devised, Prepared, and Recommended by the Commissioners Appointed under a Resolve of the Legislature of the State.* Cambridge, MA: Harvard University Press; 1948.

12. Rosen G. *A History of Public Health.* Baltimore, MD: Johns Hopkins University Press; 1993:216–219.

13. *Proceedings and Debates of the Third National Quarantine and Sanitary Conference.* New York: Edward Jones; 1859:179–180.

14. Adams GW. *Doctors in Blue.* New York: Henry Schuman; 1952.

15. Woodward JJ. *Chief Camp Diseases of the United States Armies.* Philadelphia, PA: JB Lippencott; 1863.

16. Cavins HM. The national quarantine and sanitary conventions of 1857–1858 and the beginnings of the American Public Health Association. *Bull Hist Med.* 1943;13:419–425.

17. Kramer HD. Agitation for public health reform in the 1870s. *J Hist Med Allied Sci.* 1948;3:473–488.

18. Smith S. The history of public health, 1871–1921. In: Ravenel MP, ed. *A Half Century of Public Health.* New York: American Public Health Association; 1921:1–12.

19. Ravenel MP. The American Public Health Association: Past, present, future. In: Ravenel MP, ed. *A Half Century of Public Health.* New York: American Public Health Association; 1921: 13–55.

20. Patterson RG. *Historical Directory of State Health Departments in the United States of America.* Columbus: Public Health Association; 1939.

21. Abbott SW. *The Past and Present Conditions of Public Hygiene and State Medicine in the United States.* Boston, MA: Wright & Potter; 1900.

22. Mullan F. *Plagues and Politics: The Story of the United States Marine Hospital Service.* New York: Basic Books; 1989.

23. Harden VA. *Inventing the NIH: Federal Biomedical Research Policy, 1887–1937.* Baltimore, MD: Johns Hopkins University Press; 1986.

24. Blake J. *Public Health in the Town of Boston, 1630–1822.* Cambridge, MA: Harvard University Press; 1959.

25. Rosenkrantz B. *Public Health and the State: Changing Views in Massachusetts, 1842–1936.* Cambridge, MA: Harvard University Press; 1972.

26. Duffy J. *A History of Public Health in New York City, 1625–1826.* New York: Russell Sage Foundation; 1968.

27. Duffy J. *A History of Public Health in New York City, 1866–1966.* New York: Russell Sage Foundation; 1974.

28. Galishoff S. *Safeguarding the Public Health: Newark, 1895–1918.* Westport, CT: Greenwood Press; 1975.

29. Leavitt JW. *The Healthiest City: Milwaukee and the Politics of Health Reform.* Princeton, NJ: Princeton University Press; 1982.

30. Kraut AM. *Silent Travelers: Germs, Genes, and the Immigrant Menace.* New York: Basic Books; 1994.

31. Winslow CEA. *The Life of Hermann M. Biggs: Physician and Statesman of the Public Health.* Philadelphia, PA: Lea & Febiger; 1929.

32. Jordan EO, Whipple GC, Winslow CEA. *A Pioneer of Public Health: William Thompson Sedgwick.* New Haven, CT: Yale University Press; 1924.

33. Cassedy JH. *Charles V. Chapin and the Public Health Movement.* Cambridge, MA: Harvard University Press; 1962.

34. Rosenberg CE, Rosenberg CS. Pietism and the origins of the American public health movement. *J Hist Med Allied Sci.* 1968;23:16–35.

35. Shroyck RH. The early American public health movement. *Am J Public Health.* 1937;27:965–971.

36. Rosenkrantz B. Cart before horse: Theory, practice and professional image in American public health. *J Hist Med Allied Sci.* 1974;29:57.

37. Ryan MP. *Womanhood in America: From Colonial Times to the Present.* New York: Franklin Watts; 1975:225–234.

38. Smillie W. *Public Health: Its Promise for the Future.* New York: Macmillan; 1955:450–458.

39. Wiebe RH. *The Search for Order, 1877–1920.* New York: Hill & Wang; 1967.

40. Hayes SP. The politics of reform in municipal government in the progressive era. In: Hayes SP, ed. *American Political History as Social Analysis.* Knoxville: University of Tennessee Press; 1980: 205–232.

41. Hayes SP. *Conservation and the Gospel of Efficiency: The Progressive Conservation Movement, 1890–1918.* Boston, MA: Beacon Press; 1968.

42. Rogers DT. In search of progressivism. *Rev Am Hist.* 1982;10:115–132.

43. Welch WH. Sanitation in relation to the poor. An address to the Charity Organization Society of Baltimore, November 1892. In: *Papers and Addresses by William Henry Welch, Vol. 3.* Baltimore, MD: The Johns Hopkins Press; 1920.

44. von Pettenkofer M., Sigerist HE, trans. *The Value of Health to a City.* Baltimore, MD: Johns Hopkins University Press; 1941:15–52.

45. Rotch TM. The position and work of the American Pediatric Society toward public questions. *Trans Am Pediatr Soc.* 1909:21:12.

46. Chapin C. How shall we spend the health appropriation? In: Chapin CV, Gorham FP, eds. *Papers of Charles V. Chapin, M.D.: A Review of Public Health Realities.* New York: The Commonwealth Fund; 1934:28–35.

47. Sternberg GM. *Sanitary lessons of the war. In: Sternberg GM, ed. Sanitary Lessons of the War and Other Papers.* Washington, DC: Byron S Adams; 1912:2.

48. Cosmas GA. *An Army for Empire: The United States Army in the Spanish-American War.* Columbia: University of Missouri Press; 1971.

49. Kelley HA. *Walter Reed and Yellow Fever.* Baltimore, MD: Medical Standard Book Co; 1906.

50. Sternberg GM. Sanitary problems connected with the construction of the Isthmian Canal. In: Sternberg GM, ed. *Sanitary Lessons of the War and Other Papers.* Washington, DC: Byron S Adams; 1912:39–40.

51. Fosdick RB. *Adventure in Giving: The Story of the General Education Board.* New York: Harper & Row; 1962:57–58.

52. Ettling J. *The Germ of Laziness: Rockefeller Philanthropy and Public Health in the New South.* Cambridge, MA: Harvard University Press; 1981.

53. Rose W. First annual report of the administrative secretary of the Rockefeller Sanitary Commission; 1910:4. In: Fosdick RB, ed. *The Story of the Rockefeller Foundation.* New York: Harper & Brothers; 1952:33.

54. Rosen G. The committee of one hundred on national health and the campaign for a national health department, 1906–1912. *Am J Public Health.* 1972;62:261–263.

55. Marcus AI. Disease prevention in America: from a local to a national outlook, 1880–1910. *Bull Hist Med.* 1979;53:184–203.

56. Fisher I. *A Report on National Vitality, Its Wastes and Conservation.* Washington, DC: Committee of One Hundred on National Health; 1909. US Government Printing Office Bulletin No. 30.

57. Williams RC. *The United States Public Health Service, 1798–1950.* Washington, DC: US Government Printing Office; 1951.

58. Schiesl MJ. *The Politics of Efficiency: Municipal Administration and Reform In America, 1880–1920.* Berkeley: University of California Press; 1980.

59. Fee E. *Disease and Discovery: A History of the Johns Hopkins School of Hygiene and Public Health, 1916–1939.* Baltimore, MD: Johns Hopkins University Press; 1987.

60. Fee E, Acheson RM, eds. *A History of Education in Public Health: Health That Mocks the Doctors' Rules.* New York: Oxford University Press; 1991.

61. Sedgwick WT. The origin, scope and significance of bacteriology. *Science.* 1901;13:121–128.

62. Winslow CEA. The untilled fields of public health. *Science.* 1920;51:23.

63. Winslow CEA. *The Evolution and Significance of the Modern Public Health Campaign.* New Haven, CT: Yale University Press; 1923.

64. Sicherman B. *Alice Hamilton: A Life in Letters.* Cambridge, MA: Harvard University Press; 1984:153–183.

65. Terris M, ed. *Goldberger on Pellagra.* Baton Rouge: Louisiana State University Press; 1964.

66. Kantor B. *The New Scientific Public Health Movement: A Case Study of Tuberculosis in Baltimore,*

Maryland, 1900–1910 [master's thesis]. Baltimore, MD: Johns Hopkins University; 1985.

67. Meeker E. The improving health of the United States, 1850–1915. *Explorations in Economic History.* 1972;9:353–373.

68. Haines RH. The use of model life tables to estimate mortality for the United States in the late nineteenth century. *Demography.* 1979;16:289–312.

69. Hoffman FL. The general death rate of large American cities, 1871–1904. *Publications of the American Statistical Association.* 1906–1907; 10:1–75.

70. Duffy J. Social impact of disease in the late nineteenth century. *Bull NY Acad Med.* 1971;47: 797–811.

71. Knowles M. Public health service not a medical monopoly. *Am J Public Health.* 1913;3:111–122.

72. Winslow CEA. Public health at the crossroads. *Am J Public Health.* 1926;16:1075–1085.

73. *Report of the Committee on Municipal Health Department Practice of the American Public Health Association, in cooperation with the United States Public Health Service.* Washington, DC: US Government Printing Office; 1923. Public Health Bulletin No. 136.

74. Duffy J. The American medical profession and public health: from support to ambivalence. *Bull Hist Med.* 1979;53:1–22.

75. Meckel RA. *Save the Babies: American Public Health Reform and the Prevention of Infant Mortality, 1850–1920.* Baltimore, MD: Johns Hopkins University Press; 1990.

76. Mullan F. *Plagues and Politics: The Story of the United States Public Health Service.* New York: Basic Books; 1989.

77. Committee on the Costs of Medical Care. *Medical Care for the American People.* Chicago, IL: University of Chicago Press; 1932. Final report.

78. Fee E. The pleasures and perils of prophetic advocacy: socialized medicine and the politics of medical reform. In: Fee E, Brown TM, eds. *Making Medical History: The Life and Work of Henry E. Sigerist.* Baltimore, MD: Johns Hopkins University Press; 1996. In press.

79. Berkowitz ED. *America's Welfare State: From Roosevelt to Reagan.* Baltimore, MD: Johns Hopkins University Press; 1991.

80. Kratz FK. Status of full-time local health organizations at the end of the fiscal year 1941–1942. *Public Health Rep.* 1943;58:345–351.

81. Corwin EHL, ed. *Ecology of Health.* New York: The Commonwealth Fund; 1949.

82. Mustard HS. *Government in Public Health.* New York: The Commonwealth Fund; 1945: 190.

83. Leathers WS, et al. Committee on Professional Education of the American Public Health Association. Public health degrees and certificates granted in 1936. *Am J Public Health.* 1937;27: 1267–1272.

84. Mustard HS, ed. Yesterday's school children are examined for the army. *Am J Public Health.* 1941; 31:1207.

85. Simmons JS. The preventive medicine program of the United States Army. *Am J Public Health.* 1943;33:931–940.

86. Mountain JW. Responsibility of local health authorities in the war effort. *Am J Public Health.* 1943;33:35–40.

87. Williams RC. *The United States Public Health Service, 1798–1950.* Washington, DC: Commissioned Officers' Association of the United States Public Health Service; 1951:612–768.

88. Furman B. *A Profile of the Public Health Service, 1798–1948.* Bethesda, MD: National Institutes of Health; 1973:418–458.

89. Perrott GStJ. Findings of selective service examinations. *Milbank Q.* 1944;22:358–366.

90. Perrott GStJ. Selective service rejection statistics and some of their implications. *Am J Public Health.* 1946;36:336–342.

91. Maxcy KF. Epidemiologic implications of wartime population shifts. *Am J Public Health.* 1942;32: 1089–1096.

92. Ethridge EW. *Sentinel for Health: A History of the Centers for Disease Control.* Berkeley: University of California Press; 1992.

93. Stern BJ. *Medical Services by Government: Local, State, and Federal.* New York: The Commonwealth Fund; 1946:31–32.

94. Emerson H. *Local Health Units for the Nation.* New York: The Commonwealth Fund; 1945.

95. Mountain JW, Flook E. Distribution of health services in the structure of state government: the composite pattern of state health services. *Public Health Rep.* 1941;56:1676.

96. Mountain JW, Flook E. Distribution of health services in the structure of state government: State health department organization. *Public Health Rep.* 1943;58:568.

97. Galdston I, ed. *Social Medicine: Its Derivations and Objectives*. New York: The Commonwealth Fund; 1949.

98. Ryle JA. Social pathology. In: Galdston I, ed. *Social Medicine: Its Derivations and Objectives*. New York: The Commonwealth Fund; 1949:64.

99. Stebbins EL. Epidemiology and social medicine. In: Galdston I, ed. *Social Medicine: Its Derivations and Objectives*. New York: The Commonwealth Fund; 1949:101–104.

100. Merrell M, Reed LJ. The epidemiology of health. In: Galdston I, ed. *Social Medicine: Its Derivations and Objectives*. New York: The Commonwealth Fund; 1949:105–110.

101. Gordon JE. The newer epidemiology. In: *Tomorrow's Horizon in Public Health*. Transactions of the 1950 conference of the Public Health Association of New York City. New York: Public Health Association; 1950:18–45.

102. Gordon JE. The world, the flesh and the devil as environment, host and agent of disease. In: Galdston I, ed. *The Epidemiology of Health*. New York: Health Education Council; 1953:60–73.

103. Smillie WG. The responsibility of the state. In: *Tomorrow's Horizon in Public Health*. Transactions of the 1950 conference of the Public Health Association of New York City. New York: Public Health Association; 1950:95–102.

104. Ginzberg E. Public health and the public. In: *Tomorrow's Horizon in Public Health*. Transactions of the 1950 conference of the Public Health Association of New York City. New York: Public Health Association; 1950:101–109.

105. New York Academy of Medicine, Committee on Medicine in the Changing Order. *Medicine in the Changing Order*. New York: The Commonwealth Fund; 1947:109.

106. Mustard HS. *Government in Public Health*. New York: The Commonwealth Fund; 1945:112.

107. McNeil DR. *The Fight for Fluoridation*. New York: Oxford University Press; 1957.

108. Benison S. *Tom Rivers: Reflections on a Life in Medicine and Science*. Cambridge, MA: MIT Press; 1967.

109. Klein AE. *Trial by Fury: The Polio Vaccine Controversy*. New York: Scribner's; 1972.

110. Paul JR. *A History of Poliomyelitis*. New Haven, CT: Yale University Press; 1971.

111. Sanders BS. Local health departments: Growth or illusion. *Public Health Rep*. 1959;74:13–20.

112. Aronson JB. The politics of public health—reactions and summary. *Am J Public Health*. 1959;49:311.

113. Knutson JW. Ferment in public health. *Am J Public Health*. 1957;47:1489–1491.

114. Woodcock L. Where are we going in public health? *Am J Public Health*. 1956;46:278–282.

115. Terris M. The changing face of public health. *Am J Public Health*. 1959;49:1113–1119.

116. American Public Health Association Symposium—1958. The politics of public health. *Am J Public Health*. 1959;49:300–313.

117. Rosen G. The politics of public health. *Am J Public Health*. 1959;49:364–365.

118. Tucker RR. The politics of public health. *Am J Public Health*. 1959;49:300–305.

119. Davis K, Schoen C. *Health and the War on Poverty*. Washington, DC: Brookings Institution; 1978.

120. Starr P. *The Social Transformation of American Medicine*. New York: Basic Books; 1982:374–378.

121. Sardell A. *The U.S. Experiment in Social Medicine: The Community Health Center Program, 1965–1986*. Pittsburgh, PA; University of Pittsburgh Press; 1988.

122. Institute of Medicine, Committee for the Study of the Future of Public Health. *The Future of Public Health*. Washington, DC: National Academy Press; 1988.

123. Omenn GS. What's behind those block grants in health. *New Eng J Med*. 1982;306:1057–1060.

124. Fox DM. AIDS and the American health policy: the history and prospects of a crisis of authority. In: Fee E, Fox DM, eds. *AIDS: The Burdens of History*. Berkeley: University of California Press; 1988:316–343.

125. Fee E, Fox DM, eds. *AIDS: The Making of a Chronic Disease*. Berkeley: University of California Press; 1992.

126. Krieger N, Margo G, eds. *AIDS: The Politics of Survival*. New York: Baywood; 1994.

CHAPTER 3

Emergence of a New Public Health

C. William Keck, MD, MPH and F. Douglas Scutchfield, MD

LEARNING OBJECTIVES

Upon completion of this chapter, the reader will be able to:

1. Describe briefly the findings of the 1988 and 2003 Institute of Medicine Reports on the Future of Public Health.

2. Describe the key developments that have contributed to the evolution of public health during the past 20 years.

3. List the "Ten Essential Services" and describe how they were developed.

4. Describe some of the achievements of the Public Health Practice Program Office at the Centers for Disease Control and Prevention.

5. Discuss how public health relates to the Medicine/Public Health initiative and Managed Care.

6. Describe public health practice weaknesses that remain to be improved in the coming decades.

KEY TERMS

Local Public Health System (LPHS)

Assessment

Policy Development

Assurance

10 Essential Public Health Services

Council on Linkages

Core Competencies

MPH Core Competencies

Credentialing

Medicine/Public Health Initiative

Managed Care

Medicaid Managed Care

Turning Point Initiative

Performance Measures

Healthy People 2010

INTRODUCTION

In Chapter 2, Dr. Elizabeth Fee chronicled the development of public health in the United States until the early 1990's. She concludes on a note of disappointment that significant advances in public health knowledge during the past 100 years were not matched with the development of a public health infrastructure strong enough to deliver public health services in a manner that the full public impact promised by the evolving science could be achieved. In the late 1980s, many recognized that public health was limited in its ability to effectively deal with the onset of new and frightening problems, such as HIV/AIDS and multiple drug-resistant tuberculosis. These concerns led to a contemporary effort to better define public health responsibilities and bolster public health department capacity. The 9/11 tragedy followed by the distribution of anthrax spores by mail prompted even more attention and focus on assuring that local and state health departments were prepared to meet the public's needs.

The most frequently cited genesis of what became a contemporary public health philosophic renaissance was the seminal work by the Institute of Medicine (IOM) in its study of the United States public health system described in its 1988 report, *The Future of Public Health*.[1] The report is cited throughout this book, illustrating that it serves as a departure point for most, if not all, contemporary public health thinking. The institute's conclusion that public health in the United States is a system in disarray acted as a call to action for the public health profession, a call that the public health community responded to enthusiastically.

President Clinton promised comprehensive health care reform at the time of his election in 1992. This was an additional stimulus to better define the role of public health. Early drafts of the Clinton proposed reform didn't mention the public health system. Public health professionals were committed to assure that the new reform proposal included, prominently, the nation's public health system. Both the IOM report and the professional response to Clinton's initiative were largely focused on the role of governmental agencies in the provision of public health services, while recognizing a broader public health system that included others, beyond health departments, who shared the public health mission of creating conditions in which people can be healthy.

The IOM report and the president's health care initiative, coming relatively close together, acted as driving forces for the public health profession to better define its role and increase public understanding of its contributions to health. The resulting activities were far ranging and productive. They were characterized by a strong sense of purpose; high productivity; and unprecedented collaboration between agencies of the federal government, national public health professional organizations, academic institutions, local and state health departments, and many individuals. This collaboration and focus of effort has created a subsequent period of public health philosophic renaissance.

A second IOM committee in their 2003 report, *The Future of the Public's Health in the 21st Century*[2], reviewed recent national health achievements and examined issues that could undercut health gains if not addressed. This report recognized the special role of government in improving health status and the continuing shortcomings in governmental capacity but also noted that for maximum impact, government must be allied with the contributions of other sectors of society that have enormous power to influence health. This consortium of agencies, institutions, and individuals whose work and activities impact community health status has been called the **Local Public Health System (LPHS)** to distinguish it from the Local Public Health Department. This second report supports the findings of the initial study group and contributes to the ongoing renaissance in public health by charting a course for assuring population health by recommending actions by the

Table 3.1. Major Players in the Recent History of Public Health Discussed in This Chapter

Organization	Role	Website
Institute of Medicine (IOM)	The Institute of Medicine provides independent, objective, evidence-based advice to policy makers, health professionals, the private sector, and the public.	http://www.iom.edu/
Centers for Disease Control and Prevention (CDC)	The major agency of the federal government focused on promoting health and quality of life by preventing and controlling disease, injury, and disability.	http://www.cdc.gov/
Federal Department of Health and Human Services (DHHS)	The United States government department responsible for all civilian health services.	http://www.hhs.gov/
Faculty/Agency Forum	Established the first set of competencies for public health workers in 1993.	http://bookstore.phf.org/product_info.php?products_id=119&osCsid=n6iicsnkt47ke5ii8ulnaigu21
Council on Linkages Between Academia and Public Health Practice (COL)	Works to further academic/practice collaboration to assure a well-trained, competent workforce and a strong, evidence-based public health infrastructure.	http://phf.org/link/index.htm
Association of Schools of Public Health (ASPH)	The national professional organization for the 40 Council on Education for Public Health (CEPH)-accredited schools of public health.	http://www.asph.org/
Council on Education for Public Health (CEPH)	The academic accrediting body for educational institutions (schools and programs) offering degrees in public health.	http://www.ceph.org/i4a/pages/index.cfm?pageid=1
National Association of County and City Health Officials (NACCHO)	The national professional organization for officials directing local health departments.	http://www.naccho.org/
National Association of Local Boards of Health (NALBOH)	The national professional organization for members of local boards of health.	http://www.nalboh.org/
American Public Health Association (APHA)	The national professional organization for public health professionals.	http://www.apha.org/
American Medical Association (AMA)	The national professional organization for United States physicians.	http://www.ama-assn.org/

other members of the LPHS in addition to the health department's activities.

This chapter describes many of the major events of the recent past that are continuing to shape the evolution of public health in this country. Table 3.1 lists and briefly describes the roles of the major organizations that have contributed to events detailed in the body of the chapter.

INSTITUTE OF MEDICINE

The first IOM report mentioned previously is not gathering dust on shelves. Its documentation of the inadequate status of local public health services and recommendations for common mission and core functions got the attention of public health professionals. All public health workers should become familiar with that document and the reasons behind its damning conclusion that the United States public health system is a system in disarray. Among the IOM's disturbing findings were:

- There was no clear, universally accepted mission for public health.

- Tension between professional expertise and politics was present throughout the nation's public health system.

- Public health professionals had been slow to develop strategies that demonstrate the worth of their efforts to legislators and the public.

- Relationships between medicine and public health were, at best, uneasy.

- Inadequate research resources had been targeted at identifying and solving public health problems.

- Public health practice, unlike other health professions, was largely decoupled from its academic base(s).[1]

There were initially mixed reviews of these findings from the public health community. Many public health leaders objected to the characterization of their agency as being in disarray. As the report was more fully digested, however, most public health professionals came to accept the accuracy of the report's description of the public health system in the United States and that something had to be done to reverse the reality.

Local health departments (LHDs) and other elements of the public health system have probably never gotten as much attention as they have received since the IOM report was published. Very real progress has been and continues to be made in responding to the various factors critiqued by the IOM. The introspection fostered by the report has resulted in a growing clarity of the challenges that face the profession. This is helpful, but the magnitude of those challenges is also quite daunting. If there is any comfort, it lies to some degree in the growing national awareness of the needs of communities and local public health practitioners.

There is a growing sense that something has to be done to improve the capacity of LHDs to do their work, and significant steps are being taken to address that situation.

An important first step was general agreement on the mission and functions of public health. In the absence of an identifiable universal mission statement, the IOM suggested the following:

> The mission of public health is to fulfill society's interest in assuring conditions in which people can be healthy.[1(p7)]

Because the IOM was unable to identify universally accepted core functions for LHDs, they proposed the following:[1(pp7–8)]

Assessment: Every public health agency should regularly and systematically collect, assemble, analyze, and make available information on the health of the community, including statistics on health status, community health needs, and epidemiologic and other studies of health problems.

Policy Development: Every public health agency should exercise its responsibility to serve the public interest in the development of comprehensive public health policies by promoting the use of the scientific knowledge base in decision making about public health and by leading in developing public health policy.

Assurance: Public health agencies should assure their constituents that services necessary to achieve agreed upon goals are provided by encouraging actions by other entities (private or public sector), by requiring such action through regulation, or by providing services directly.

Each public health agency should involve key policy makers and the general public in determining a set of high-priority personal and community-wide health services that governments will guarantee to every member of the community. This guarantee should include subsidization or direct provision of high-priority personal health services for those unable to afford them. (This point was, and remains, controversial. There are those who suggest that the role of public health is to care for population health problems and not provide direct medical care, whereas others contend that public health must provide government's response to the medical care needs of those unable to pay for these services.)

The public health community, both practice and academic, embraced the suggested mission and the proposed core functions. They were left, then, to deal with the reality that the IOM had found the nation's public health agencies limited in their capacity to fulfill these functions.

DEVELOPMENT OF THE 10 ESSENTIAL PUBLIC HEALTH SERVICES

The election of President Clinton in 1992 heralded the beginning of an attempt to develop health care reform. As it became clear to public health leaders that very comprehensive reform was the intent, they realized how important it would be to ensure that public health was included in a reform proposal. They also realized that public understanding of the role of public health was limited. The terms assessment, policy development, and assurance had become well accepted by the public health practice and academic communities, but they were poorly understood by the public, the medical care industry, and the policy makers who were drafting the president's reform package. The response to this realization marked the entrance of public health into a period of significant change and growth as a profession. Things had already been changing, of course, but many of those changes had been driven by external factors. Now change was being driven from within the profession, often directly responding to the findings of the IOM.

At the time of the president's inauguration, work had already begun on expanding the three core public health functions to a longer related list of activities or practices that more clearly defined the role of public health in the United States. The Centers for Disease Control and Prevention (CDC)[3] used the three core functions to develop an expanded list of 10 basic public health practices. A version of this list, called the "Core Functions of Public Health," appeared in Title III of the Health Security Act forwarded by President Clinton to Congress in October 1993.[4] The eventual defeat of this attempt to reform the United States health delivery system was a bitter blow to the Clinton presidency, but it was also a bitter blow for public health. This was the first time that a national health care reform effort recognized the importance of public health to improved health status and included public health as an important system element. The defeat of the proposed legislation was not related to the inclusion of public health system issues in the bill.

There was value in better defining the role of public health beyond its usefulness for proposed federal legislation, however. A list of 10 "core functions" was subsequently developed by the Washington State Department of Health.[5] It was comparable to a variation of the list developed by the National Association of County Health Officials, the Association of State and Territorial Health Officials, and the federal Office of the Assistant Secretary for Health.[6] A working group on the core functions of public health was put together in the spring of 1994, co-led by the CDC's Public Health Practice Program Office and the Secretary of Department of Health and Human Service's Office of Disease Prevention and Health Promotion, to develop a consensus of the "essential services of public health."

The resulting statement provided a vision for public health in America: "Healthy People in Healthy Communities," and a mission for public health: "Promote physical and mental health and prevent disease, injury, and disability."[7]

It also provided two brief lists. The first was intended as a description of what public health seeks to accomplish by providing essential services to the public:

- Prevent epidemics and the spread of disease.
- Protect against environmental hazards.

- Prevent injuries.
- Promote and encourage healthy behaviors and mental health.
- Respond to disasters and assist communities in recovery.
- Assure the quality and accessibility of health services.

The second list has been accepted as the consensus description of the **10 essential public health services**:

1. Monitor health status to identify community health problems.
2. Diagnose and investigate health problems and health hazards in the community.
3. Inform, educate, and empower people about health issues.
4. Mobilize community partnerships to identify and solve health problems.
5. Develop policies and plans that support individual and community health efforts.
6. Enforce laws and regulations that protect health and ensure safety.
7. Link people to needed personal health services and assure the provision of health care when otherwise unavailable.
8. Assure a competent public health and personal health care workforce.
9. Evaluate effectiveness, accessibility, and quality of personal and population-based health services.
10. Research for new insights and innovative solutions to health problems.

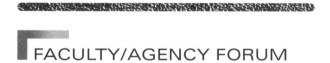

FACULTY/AGENCY FORUM

Funded by the Health Resources and Services Administration (HRSA) and CDC, the Faculty/Agency Forum was established in 1988 to address the educational and academic dimensions of the findings of the IOM. Under the direction of an Advisory Committee consisting of the Executive Directors of the Association of Schools of Public Health (ASPH) and of the American Public Health Association (APHA); and the Presidents of the Association of State and Territorial Health Officials, the National Association of County Health Officials, the United States Conference of Local Health Officers, and the Association of State and Territorial Local Health Liaison Officials, four work groups with broad representation of academics and practitioners were formed. The Forum's major accomplishment in 1993 was the development and publication of a compendium of competencies required for successful public health practice. They listed the skills required under the following headings: analytic, communication, policy development/program planning, cultural, financial planning and management, and basic public health science (epidemiology, biostatistics, environmental health, administration, and behavioral science).[8] The Forum wanted to improve the quality of public health education and establish flourishing, permanent, broad cooperative agreements among schools of public health and major local, regional, and state public health agencies. To that end, the Forum also proposed ways that public agencies and institutions providing graduate education in public health could work together. After completing its work and publishing a report,[8] the Forum went out of existence.

COUNCIL ON LINKAGES BETWEEN ACADEMIA AND PUBLIC HEALTH PRACTICE

The **Council on Linkages** was established in 1991 under a cooperative agreement from HRSA through the ASPH, as a sequel to the Faculty/Agency Forum. It brought representatives from national public health professional organizations and federal agencies together to "improve public

Table 3.2. Council on Linkages Between Academia and Public Health Practice Membership Organizations

American College of Preventive Medicine
American Public Health Association
Association for Prevention Teaching and Research
Association of Schools of Public Health
Association of State and Territorial Health Officials
Association of University Programs in Health Administration
Centers for Disease Control and Prevention
Community-Campus Partnerships for Health
Council of Accredited Master of Public Health Programs
Health Resources and Services Administration
National Association of County and City Health Officials
National Association of Local Boards of Health
National Environmental Health Association
National Library of Medicine
National Network of Public Health Institutes
QUAD Council of Public Health Nursing Organizations
Society for Public Health Education

SOURCE: Council on Linkages Between Academia and Public Health Practice. Available at: http://www.phf.org/link/membership.htm.

health practice and education by refining and implementing recommendations of the Public Health Faculty/Agency Forum, establishing links between academia and the agencies of the public health community, and creating a process for continuing public health education throughout one's career."[9] Membership of the Council on Linkages is listed in Table 3.2.

The council's major contribution is its development of a modernized list of **core competencies** for public health professionals. This list builds on the work of the Faculty/Agency Forum, and it represents almost 10 years of work on this subject by the council and numerous other organizations and individuals in public health academia and practice settings. Their work was compiled and crosswalked with the essential public health services to ensure that the competencies can be used to help

build the skills necessary for providing these services[10] (see Appendix B).

This latest list of core competencies represents a set of skills, knowledge, and attitudes necessary for the broad practice of public health. The competencies are listed under the following eight domains: Analytic Assessment Skills, Basic Public Health Sciences Skills, Cultural Competency Skills, Communication Skills, Community Dimensions of Practice Skills, Financial Planning and Management Skills, Leadership and Systems Thinking Skills, and Policy Development/Program Planning Skills.

Among the council's other accomplishments are:

- Creating and distributing *The Link,* its newsletter, highlighting models of linkages between public health academic and practice settings

- Working through the ASPH (an agency member of the council) to identify practice representatives at each school of public health charged with improving their institution's linkages with practice settings

- Beginning the process of developing Community Public Health Practice Guidelines (such as the Clinical Preventive Service Guidelines), now being carried out by the CDC

- Proposing a public health research agenda based on the 10 essential services

- Promoting and facilitating the development of academic health departments

- Compiling and disseminating tools to foster academic/practice linkages

Unfortunately, federal budget cuts in 2006 resulted in loss of funding for the council. The council's work was facilitated by staff of the Public Health Foundation, and the council was "mothballed" in hopes that future funding could be found to reactivate it.[9] Subsequently, temporary funding was received from the CDC to support the work of the council to modernize the core competencies and to study the so-called workforce pipeline to better understand how individuals make their way into the public health workforce. The council returned to "mothball" status during the summer of 2008, and then received funding into 2009 in the fall of 2008.

MPH CORE COMPETENCY DEVELOPMENT PROJECT

The ASPH launched a project in 2004 to develop a set of competencies that should be evident in graduates with a generalist Master of Public Health (MPH) degree. The initiative began with a review of competencies developed by others for various categories of the public health workforce, including those developed by the Council on Linkages for the general public health workforce. Over the course of several years, a set of competencies reflecting the knowledge, skills, and other attributes that might be expected for emerging public health professionals was developed in the five discipline-specific domains that have been the core of public health training since the mid 1970s: Biostatistics, Epidemiology, Environmental Health Science, Health Policy and Management, and Social and Behavioral Sciences.

During this process, an additional set of seven interdisciplinary, cross-cutting competencies was identified, explored, and incorporated into the final competency set. These new competency areas are listed and defined here:

- **Communication and Informatics:** The ability to collect, manage, and organize data to produce information and meaning that is exchanged by use of signs and symbols; to gather, process, and present information to different audiences in person, through information technologies, or through media channels; and to strategically design the information and knowledge exchange process to achieve specific objectives.

- **Diversity and Culture:** The ability to interact with both diverse individuals and communities to produce or impact an intended public health outcome.

- **Leadership:** The ability to create and communicate a shared vision for a changing future; champion solutions to organizational and community challenges; and energize commitment to goals.

- **Professionalism:** The ability to demonstrate ethical choices, values, and professional practices implicit in public health decisions; consider the effect of choices on community stewardship, equity, social justice, and accountability; and commit to personal and institutional development.

- **Program Planning:** The ability to plan for the design, development, implementation, and evaluation of strategies to improve individual and community health.

- **Public Health Biology:** Public health biology is the biological and molecular context of public health.

- **Systems Thinking:** The ability to recognize system level properties that result from dynamic interactions among human and social systems and how they affect the relationships among individuals, groups, organizations, communities, and environments.

You can find a list of competencies by category at the ASPH website.[11]

PUBLIC HEALTH TRAINING PROGRAMS

When the Council on Education for Public Health (CEPH) took over public health training program accreditation from the APHA in 1974, there were 18 accredited schools of public health. The number had expanded from 10 schools in 1946 to 18 in 1974—an 80-percent increase in close to 30 years. In retrospect, that seems to be a very slow expansion, but at the time, it was viewed as being quite rapid. The growth responded primarily to the infusion of federal funds, including formula or capitation grants, training grants, traineeships for students, greatly expanded biomedical research funding, and even some construction monies. Most of these funds were available only to accredited schools, leaving the independent schools of public health primarily engaged in graduate training as the nation's model of professional public health preparation.[12]

The most notable difference in the public health professional preparation landscape now and 30 years ago is the sheer number of institutions of higher education offering graduate training in public health. Today, CEPH accredits 40 schools and 69 programs, or 109 public health training sites in total.[13]

The most dramatic growth over the past 30 years has occurred in programs outside schools of public health, and much of that growth has occurred in the past 15 years. This is not at all unexpected, given that universities can assemble the resources needed to support a program much more easily than the resources needed to provide the comprehensive offerings required of a school of public health. A program, for example, may offer only a generalist master of public health degree (MPH) or one or two areas of specialization, whereas a school of public health must offer a full range of at least one MPH degree in each of five core required concentration areas, plus at least three doctoral degrees.[14(p13, p21)] Programs, which typically start small but often grow quite large, are the spawning ground for new schools of public health. A number of accredited programs have already made the transition to accredited schools of public health, and it is likely that more will do so.[13]

The growth in the past, however, pales in comparison to the growth that appears to be on the immediate horizon. A change from 18 to 106 institutions in 30 years is an almost six-fold increase. It is likely that number will more than double again in the next 5 to 10 years. In addition to the more than 106 accredited schools and programs, currently 24 institutions are in applicant status and another approximately 50 institutions are on CEPH's "early warning list"—programs and schools that are under development, in early operational stages or just thinking about accreditation. The list grows longer every year, even as many go off this list and on to the accredited list. Public health training is a growth industry and gives every sign of

remaining so in the near future. Also of interest is that among the 106 accredited institutions, there is now one school in Mexico, one program in Canada, and one program in Lebanon.[13]

CREDENTIALING OF PUBLIC HEALTH WORKERS

Among the health workforces in the United States, public health alone has no credentialing process to certify that its workforce has acquired minimal competence. To be sure, most public health workers are licensed or certified in their basic professions—nursing, medicine, environmental health, health education, counseling, laboratory technology, and so on. There is no process, however, to certify competence to practice their profession in a public health setting. This has been a controversial issue in public health for many years, but the development of sets of accepted competencies by such groups as the Council on Linkages (for all public health workers) and, more recently, the ASPH (for MPH degree graduates), sets the stage for a certification process.

The state of Illinois has led the way in this process by forming the Public Health Practitioner Certification Board (PHPCB) in 1998. The PHPCB uses a competency-based **credentialing** process to certify public health administrators and emergency response coordinators and is considering credentialing for other public health occupational categories. In 2001, the Missouri and Kansas departments of health affiliated with the Illinois PHPCB to do the same.[15] Over the past 10 years, an effort at the national level has emerged to certify the competence of public health professionals who hold either the masters or doctorate in public health (MPH or DrPH). In 2002, the ASPH led the way in creating an independent board of public health examiners that was subsequently incorporated in 2005. This board is independent of any of the current public health academic or professional organizations but has representatives of the practice and academic communities as members of its board, along with public representatives. The board examination is under development, using a major national certifying board as a contractor, to develop questions from the five core public health disciplines and the cross-cutting competencies developed recently by ASPH. The National Board of Public Health Examiners administered the first certification examination in the summer of 2008.[16] The value of this examination and certification process will depend in large measure on the extent to which those certified by this board are preferentially hired for jobs or the extent to which public health practice positions require this certification. Experience in the past suggests that public health hiring authorities are more concerned with the salary commanded by individuals than the credentials they hold. The development and experience of this activity should be watched with interest in the public health practice and academic communities.

NATIONAL ASSOCIATION OF COUNTY AND CITY HEALTH OFFICIALS (NACCHO)

The combination in 1994 of the United States Conference of Local Health Officers and the National Association of County Health Officials into a single professional association representing directors of all LHDs, named the National Association of County and City Health Officials (NACCHO), was a very significant occurrence. The organization has grown in strength just as increasing attention has been focused on LHDs, and it has become a very important participant in the many activities related to improving the LPHS.

In the past, the National Association of County Health Officials focused on maintaining its membership, facilitating communication, and continuing education of its members. In its new form, NACCHO is actively involved in developing public policy, its workforce, and leadership; defining and expanding the public health research agenda;

developing tools to assist LHDs with community assessment; and providing technical assistance to public health practitioners. Staff and other resources have grown dramatically, and critical partnerships have been established with other public health professional organizations and key federal agencies, including participation in cooperative agreements with the CDC that provide funding for a number of the organization's expanded activities.

A major ongoing initiative of NACCHO is the development of an operational definition of a functional local health department (LHD).[17] The "definition" consists of a list of activities that every LHD should be able to accomplish. This list is considered to be a set of "standards" that can be used to measure LHD functional capacity. The list can also be used to describe the contributions that should be made to the 10 essential services by LHDs (see Chapter 10), and they can be used as the basis for a proposed national accreditation program for state and local health departments (see Chapter 31).

NATIONAL ASSOCIATION OF LOCAL BOARDS OF HEALTH

The large majority of LHDs are governed by boards of health. They consist of three to 15 members who, depending on the laws affecting the local jurisdiction, serve as advisors or policy makers (see Chapter 10). Boards function as a major link between local public health agencies and the communities they serve, and board members have the potential to wield significant influence on the public health services provided and the resources made available to deliver them. Board members may be health professionals, but the majority of the members are not; few have any training or experience in public health.

Orientation and training of local board of health members has traditionally been left to the LHD they represent, sometimes with assistance from their state health department. Additionally, boards typically focused on their local jurisdiction's needs and interacted minimally, if at all, with other boards in their own geographic area, let alone with boards from other parts of their state or other states.

It was not until the 1980s that boards of health in some states formed their own state local board of health associations. These groups sought to provide training for new board members and organize the influence of board members to address public health issues and the resources needed to deal with them. In November 1992, representatives of states with these kinds of organizations (Georgia, Illinois, North Carolina, Ohio, and Washington) came together and formed the National Association of Local Boards of Health (NALBOH). Since its founding, NALBOH has grown rapidly. It operates offices in Bowling Green, Ohio, and Washington, DC, and is effectively involved in a growing number of activities, including training for board of health members through an annual national education and training conference and a "train the trainer" program, legislative advocacy, emergency preparedness/terrorism, environmental health, oral health, the development of performance measurement standards, and tobacco control.[18] It is reasonable to expect that as its membership and staff grow, NALBOH will become an increasingly important player on the local, state, and national scenes.

PUBLIC HEALTH PRACTICE PROGRAM OFFICE AT THE CDC

The establishment of the Public Health Practice Program Office at the CDC in 1988 marked a new direction for that agency. For the first time, there would be a locus in the CDC dedicated to strengthening the public health infrastructure in the United States. The Office began its work by concentrating its efforts in four areas:[19]

1. Strengthening the professional competencies of the public health workforce

2. Developing information systems that would increase access to public health knowledge

3. Building the organizational capacity of LHDs

4. Strengthening the science base for infrastructure development

Over the ensuing years, while continuing to work in these areas, the Office added to its agenda the development of science-based performance standards for public health organizations and competency standards for practitioners. It intends to use these standards and the Public Health Infrastructure objectives contained in *Healthy People 2010* as a framework for action. The Office was very productive. Among its products are:[19]

- Health Alert Network
- Information Network for Public Health Officials
- Public Health Training Network
- Public Health Leadership Institute (see Chapter 18)
- National Public Health Performance Standards (see Chapter 16)
- Geographic Information Systems Research Center
- National Inventory of Clinical Laboratory Testing
- Electronic Laboratory Reporting (see Chapter 29)
- Clinical Laboratories Improvement Amendments
- Public Health Image Library

The contribution of the Public Health Practice Programs Office to the evolution of public health was very significant. The Office involved representatives of local and state health departments appropriately and proceeded with skill and sensitivity. The Office was reorganized when the CDC underwent a major reorganization beginning April 21, 2005.[20] The Office functions were assigned to the Office of the Chief of Public Health Practice (OCPHP), which ". . . serves as the advocate, guardian, promoter, and conscience of public health practice throughout the CDC and in the larger public health community; ensures coordination and synergy of CDC's scientific and practice activities; and promotes and protects the public's health through science-based, practice relevant standards, policies, and legal tools. Activities in support of the mission are carried out through programs and offices focused on public health law, public health system standards, agency accreditation, and surveillance for emerging issues in public health practice."[21]

MEDICINE/PUBLIC HEALTH INITIATIVE

A joint effort of the American Medical Association (AMA) and the American Public Health Association (APHA), the **Medicine/Public Health Initiative** (MPHI) is an attempt to bridge the gap and develop stronger working relationships between these two disciplines. An initial National Congress in the spring of 1996, which brought national, state, and local leaders together from each discipline to explore common ground, was followed by a second gathering in 1997 at the New York Academy of Medicine. The Academy had been asked to explore and describe the current "state of the art" of collaboration between medicine and public health. Dr. Roz Lasker and the Academy's Committee on Medicine and Public Health sought out case studies demonstrating collaborative efforts and used the meeting to highlight examples of the more than 400 case studies they collected. The nature of collaborative efforts was described in their report, *Medicine and Public Health: The Power of Collaboration,* published later in 1997.[22] In 1998, the Macy Foundation sponsored and published proceedings from a meeting in Florida titled, "Education for More Synergistic Practice of Medicine and Public Health." This conference explored the most effective way to educate and train physicians and public health professionals to enhance the synergistic practice of medicine and public health. The conference did not produce a recommended approach applicable in all situations, but it did produce agreement that the characteristics of successful

collaborative practices should be extended and developed as teaching/learning centers.[23]

By the beginning of 2001, however, despite continued meaningful activities at the local level to bridge the many gaps between medicine and public health, changes in organizational leadership and shifting association priorities at national, state, and local levels made it difficult to sustain the momentum of the MPHI. The events of September 11 and the ensuing fall of 2001 made it clear that collaboration between medicine and public health was extremely important if the public's health was to be protected in a changing world. In October 2002, the presidents of the AMA and the APHA joined with several other organizations to reiterate their dedication to the purposes of the MPHI. A new, more focused agenda emerged focusing on disaster preparedness, reduction of health disparities, improving patient safety, and promoting health care access for the uninsured. Several states, California, Texas and Florida among them, have demonstrably strengthened medicine and public health collaboration, and there is some international focus on this area, as well.[24]

An interesting example of collaboration between medicine and public health can be seen in the Association of American Medical Colleges (AAMC)/Centers for Disease Control and Prevention (CDC) cooperative agreement focused on the development of regional centers to improve medical students' exposure to public health and population medicine. Applicant medical schools for these grants were required to partner with at least one state or local public health agency to enhance population health/public health education for all of their medical students, not only those with an interest in public health. In 2003, seven schools were funded, and in early 2006, an additional 11 schools were funded.[25]

Tangible evidence of the overlap between medicine and public health exists in both the AMA's medical journal, *Journal of the American Medical Association,* which publishes many articles of public health import, and in the AMA's policy positions on public health issues such as tobacco, substance use and abuse, sports injuries, and so forth. Nonetheless, these partnership efforts do not come easily in a culture where the disciplines have developed separately for so long. It will take the continued rededication of leaders and practitioners in both disciplines to cooperate in the many areas of mission overlap that have been identified.[24]

MANAGED CARE

The swing to managed care after the defeat of the Clinton health care proposal could have acted as a stimulus to bring clinical care and public health into the same fold. After all, the central theme of **managed care** was to approach clinical care from a population perspective—that is, to understand the characteristics, epidemiologically speaking, of the managed care company's "covered lives," and to emphasize the employment of those clinical preventive services that would likely improve the length and quality of life for the enrolled population. Correctly done, this should meld with the broader population health promotion and disease prevention activities of public health services, and decrease disease and disability while helping to control medical care costs.

Unfortunately, managed care evolved into an effort focused more on managing finances than on managing care. Many for-profit managed care companies were formed that began to compete for business by offering limited coverage plans for attractive, low prices. Prices were controlled by cutting reimbursements for providers (physicians, hospitals, etc.) and limiting access by patients to the more expensive services.[26] Patients were moved from one plan to another as employers shopped for the best prices. Many states opted to shift financial responsibility to providers by privatizing Medicaid and providing participating companies with a set amount per patient per year, allowing them to keep whatever was not spent. The trade-off was a relatively fixed and predictable state budget that was less than it previously had been. The combination of a transient "covered" population (if patients were leaving the plan before the benefit of preventive

services would be seen, then money spent on prevention was wasted) and a drive to minimize costs created powerful disincentives to vigorously pursue preventive services.

The impact of managed care on health departments was quite variable—some are affected substantially, others not at all. Certainly, those health departments that had been very involved in providing medical care to Medicaid and other underserved populations often were suddenly exempted from eligibility to receive Medicaid payments in those locations where Medicaid was converted to managed care. Because the number of uninsured continued to grow as this process evolved, there was the perverse effect of diminishing resources available to the health care "safety net" as the need increased. Some health departments were able to become credentialed providers for managed care companies and receive reimbursement for some services delivered to managed care patients.[27] The transition to **Medicaid managed care** is now complete in many states, as are policies designed to move LHDs away from providing direct care with federal dollars into a role of facilitating and enabling population services.[28] In an environment of universal access to care, this might make sense. The reality, however, is that fewer health departments than ever are able to offer direct primary health care at a time when the number of people without the capacity to pay for care in the private system continues to grow.[29]

The 1990s were halcyon years for managed care when many believed the approach could "solve" the continued upward spiral of health care costs. However, the push back from accompanying restrictions placed on provider decision making and tightened control of utilization of specialty services and medical technology, forced managed care plans to loosen restrictions on service utilization. As utilization restrictions diminished, the initial decrease in medical care costs created by those restrictions was reversed, and the rate of inflation of medical care costs returned to patterns of escalation.[30] This resulted in a loss of confidence in the managed care paradigm, and decision makers began to look for other ways to control medical care costs. Resulting changes include the advent of "consumer driven health care," or other terms referencing the creation of "health savings accounts," an insurance program to provide first dollar coverage up to a certain amount (commonly $2,000) with the consumer becoming responsible for subsequent costs up to a higher level (commonly $5,000) where catastrophic insurance coverage becomes available. These savings accounts are tax free and can be carried over from year to year. In similar efforts to shift the burden of costs onto the consumer, insurance plans increased the proportion of the health care bill paid out of the insured's pocket as well as imposing deductible payments, co-payments, and higher premiums. All of these changes provide incentives for individuals to avoid needed preventive services or primary care because the costs would be either "out of pocket" or would be subtracted from the cushion against big medical care costs provided by health savings accounts. In many cases, the increase of premiums has forced patients who can ill afford these increased costs for themselves or their family members, to refuse to purchase health insurance from their employer when that option exists. These realities have created a progressive increase in the number of uninsured individuals and families.

The role of public health in this increasingly difficult health insurance environment has not been a concern of those focusing on developing policies, procedures, and mechanisms of payment for medical care. Public health remains a safety net provider, however, and those health departments providing a limited or full range of primary care services are seeing an increased demand for clinical preventive services, such as immunizations, from a population increasingly falling through the cracks of our health insurance payment schemes.

There is some feeling among those who follow these developments that we may be at a point comparable to the early 1990s when the Clinton health insurance plan was introduced. Growing public concern about these issues have led a number of states to develop plans to provide universal access to care, and access to care is once again part of the national political discourse. Some caution that just

fixing elements of the current health insurance system is too limiting. They suggest that having medical care insurance just provides entry to a poorly designed and functioning health care system, and system redesign is necessary. In any event, it appears likely that the issue of universal access to care will be revisited as a key national policy concern, and it is imperative for public health professionals to assure that proposals for reform at the state or national level include the public health system in their programs and financing mechanisms.

TURNING POINT

The **Turning Point Initiative** was begun in 1997 by the Robert Wood Johnson Foundation and the W.K. Kellogg Foundation with the intention "To transform the public health system in the United States to make the system more effective, more community-based, and more collaborative."[31] The underlying philosophy of the program was that, "public health agencies and their partners can be strengthened by linking other sectors (not just the private health care sector, but education, criminal justice, faith communities, business, and others) because the underlying causes of poor health and quality of life are tied closely to social issues that are too complex to be approached by disease models of intervention."[32]

States were invited to apply for funding support, and eventually a network of 23 funded partners were engaged in bringing health-conscious people and organizations to the table to focus on a variety of ways to improve the public's health through a new group of partnerships. State level partnerships focused on:

- Influencing good public policy
- Expanding information technology so data is available to local communities for addressing health concerns
- Stimulating state agencies and organizations to develop comprehensive state health plans

Turning Point also formed five National Excellence Collaboratives that worked to:

- Modernize public health statutes
- Create accountable systems to measure performance
- Use information technology
- Invest in social marketing
- Develop leadership[32]

Funding for the program has ended, but the program can point to a number of significant contributions because of its existence. A visit to the program's website (http://www.turningpointprogram.org) provides access to a number of tools, resources, guides, and lessons learned that can provide assistance to today's public health practitioners. The program can also claim some significant accomplishments during its tenure, including the revamping of public health legislation in Alaska, helping to expand LHD coverage from 22 to all 93 counties in Nebraska, developing a training program for state and local public health officials in New York, and successfully passing all or part of Turning Point's model public health legislation in more than two dozen states.[32]

PUBLIC HEALTH FUNCTIONS PROJECT

Organized by the federal government, this project included representatives of federal public health agencies, national public health professional organizations, and major foundations interested in health. It had subcommittees and projects that included tracking and characterizing expenditures on public health; developing public health guidelines; training and educating the public health workforce; the public health infrastructure chapter of *Healthy People 2010;* and developing public health data for the twenty-first century, public health communications, and the essential services

of public health. The project was created to help clarify the issues and develop strategies and tools to address the identified fragility of the public health infrastructure in the United States.[33] The project completed its work and went out of existence.

NATIONAL PERFORMANCE STANDARDS

As noted in the thorough discussion of performance measurement in Chapter 16, there was steady movement toward the development of public health **performance measures** during the twentieth century. The reasons for this movement are described there in detail. A recent catalyst for this evolution was the development of, and agreement about, the 10 essential services for public health. After all, if the public health profession is in general agreement about the major services required to have as healthy a population as possible, it makes sense to develop a system to measure how well the services are delivered.

The CDC, through its Public Health Practice Programs Office, launched an effort in the mid-1990s to develop a set of standards keyed to the 10 essential services that would help communities measure their capacity to deliver those services. Representatives from state and local health departments, national public health organizations, schools of public health, and federal agencies were brought together to develop performance standards for each of the 10 services. Separate standards for state and local systems were developed, and a continuum of performance levels was identified for each standard. In addition, NALBOH and CDC developed a Local Public Health Governance Assessment Instrument focusing on the governing body accountable for public health at the local level. These three standard measurement tools were field tested in state and local health departments several times, and refined into workable tools now available from the Office of the Chief of Public

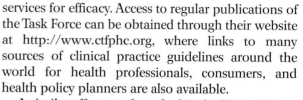

Health Practice at CDC.[34] Many felt that the LPHS performance standards would be a mechanism to measure LHD performance. They may indeed prove helpful in that regard, but it is clear that they really measure the capacity of a community, including all agencies, institutions, and individuals working in the area of health, to deliver those services. It is apparent that communities require a wide variety of services to maintain health, including but not limited to those services provided typically by health departments. The National Performance Standards are now used to assess the LPHS. The standards will be useful in measuring the impact of the consortium of community services required, emphasizing the notion that partnerships remain key to the improvement of health status at the local level.

CLINICAL/COMMUNITY PREVENTIVE SERVICES GUIDELINES

In 1976, the Canadian government convened the Canadian Task Force on the Periodic Health Examination. This expert panel adopted a highly organized approach to evaluating the effectiveness of clinical preventive services. They developed explicit criteria to judge the quality of evidence from published clinical research, and uniform decision rules were used to link the strength of recommendations for or against a given preventive service to the quality of the underlying evidence. The idea was to provide the clinician with a means of selecting those preventive services supported by the strongest evidence of effectiveness. They examined evidence for preventive services for 78 conditions and released recommendations in 1979.[35] Revisions with coverage of new topics were created in 1984, 1986, and 1988. In 2000, the Canadian Task Force on the Periodic Health Examination changed their name to the Canadian Task Force on Preventive Health Care, and the group has continued its work to review clinical preventive

services for efficacy. Access to regular publications of the Task Force can be obtained through their website at http://www.ctfphc.org, where links to many sources of clinical practice guidelines around the world for health professionals, consumers, and health policy planners are also available.

A similar effort was launched in the United States in 1984. The United States Task Force produced its first report in 1989 titled, *Guide to Clinical Preventive Services: An Assessment of the Effectiveness of 169 Interventions.*[36] In 1994, The *Clinician's Handbook of Preventive Services,* the second report of the United States Preventive Services Task Force, as part of the United States Public Health Service's Put Prevention into Practice campaign, was published, followed by a second edition in 1998.[37] Subsequently, there have been periodic updates of its recommendations so that the information remains current and is available to clinicians at http://www.ahrq.gov/clinic/uspstfix.htm. This work has successfully placed clinical preventive services on a strong science base and identified areas of needed research. Moreover, it has provided guidance to health departments that provide many of the scientifically valid services suggested in the *Guide,* such as immunizations or counseling interventions.

The Council on Linkages reasoned in 1993 that the same approach should be used for community-based prevention services. That is, the literature describing effectiveness of community programs and services should be scrutinized to determine which services are effective, which are not, and where the evidence is insufficient to make a judgment. The council decided to seek funding for a demonstration project to determine the value of such an approach and secured funding from the W.J. Kellogg Foundation for a pilot effort. The council set two goals for itself: to assess the desirability and feasibility of developing community preventive service guidelines, and to test the methodology for evaluating existing scientific evidence for the effectiveness of community interventions. It looked at immunization delivery, tuberculosis treatment completion, cardiovascular disease prevention, and lead poisoning prevention. The results indicated the validity of the approach.[38] The CDC was subsequently convinced that the proposal was worthwhile and established a Community Preventive Services Guidelines Project, which is currently ongoing.[39] A variety of community preventive services are currently under review, and interim reports of the project will be found in the literature. The first compendium of project results has been published in a guide entitled, *The Guide to Community Preventive Services.*[40] As with the *Guide to Clinical Preventive Services,* this guide is regularly updated and available at a government-sponsored website—http://www.thecommunityguide.org/.

NATIONAL PUBLIC HEALTH RESEARCH AGENDA

The United States is strongly oriented to medical research and spends more money than any other country in that arena. A very small percentage of resources allocated for health-related research is spent in the domain of public health, however.[41] In a world of limited resources for public health and increasing accountability for positive health status outcomes, it is increasingly important to focus attention on interventions that can be shown to be effective.

The United States Congress increased the budget allocations for research steadily in the early part of the first decade of this new century, however, the National Institutes of Health budget, after doubling in the early part of the last decade, has remained flat for the past several years. The public health community wants to see a larger share of those dollars, or major allocations of new money, targeted to answer questions about community-based services. It is expected that the Community Preventive Services Guidelines Project will, among other things, create a community services research agenda by clarifying the science base for those services and noting where the science base is absent or inadequate.

Others are interested in this issue, as well. Before it was defunded, the Council on Linkages, for example, was working to improve resources available for Public Health Systems Research (PHSR). It had convened annual PHSR Leadership forums to bring those who conduct, fund, and use this type of research together; held "closed door" meetings with PHSR funders; compiled and disseminated research agendas; created a set of "tips" for researchers seeking funding; and assisted in the creation of the PHSR Interest Group at Academy Health. Tools for those interested in PHSR can be found at the organization's website.[42] Academy Health has been funded by the Robert Wood Johnson Foundation to continue the work of building the public health research agenda and has begun the process of building consensus for research priorities. In addition, the Robert Wood Johnson Foundation has funded other PHSR programs to enhance the availability of data for PHSR, create more PHSR researchers, and enhance the dissemination of PHSR results to the practice community.

PUBLIC HEALTH LEADERSHIP INSTITUTES

An important response to the IOM finding in 1988 that suggested leadership in public health was suboptimal was the development of the National Public Health Leadership Institute and the subsequent development of a number of state and regional leadership institutes. These institutes have focused on identifying and training current and future public health leaders. Their development and current statuses are described in Chapter 18.

HEALTHY PEOPLE 2010

Healthy People 2010 is the third iteration of a set of 10-year objectives for improvement in health status in the United States. *Healthy People 2010* contains a section on Public Health Infrastructure (see Chapter 23). The chapter contains 17 objectives: seven in data and information systems, three related to workforce, five addressing public health organizations, and one each for resources and prevention research.[43] The addition of this subject to the document highlights the importance of improving the public health infrastructure and guarantees that progress in this area will be monitored in the best sense of the truism, "What gets measured gets done." Obviously, as the next decade is upon us, there will be a new set of objectives developed. The process of delineating those objectives has already begun. This is an area where those working in public health should follow developments closely, both to provide input for the objective development process and to be aware of the impact that objectives developed for *Healthy People 2020* will have on their work responsibilities.

PUBLIC HEALTH CODE OF ETHICS

Public health, until recently, has been without a formal code of ethics to guide its practice. To be sure, the profession has considered itself to be inherently ethical with its activities based in an ethos of social justice, and has transferred many of the principles of medical ethics to itself. Public health concerns are not equal to those of medicine, however. The discipline focuses more on populations than individuals, and more on prevention than cure. It includes those who are well and for whom the risks and benefits of medical care are not particularly relevant.

The Public Health Leadership Society, an outgrowth of the national Public Health Leadership Institute (see Chapter 18), led a project to create a code of ethics for public health. A group of public health organizations participated in the development of the code. The results of their work are described in Chapter 7 and at the website of the APHA.[44]

TERRORISM AND GENERAL PREPAREDNESS

Chemicals and communicable disease agents have been intentionally employed as weapons in human conflict for many years. Until the 1990s, their use, or contemplated use, focused principally on employment as a battlefield weapon between two opposing armed forces. The attack on the Tokyo subway system with the nerve gas sarin in 1995 brought the danger faced by civilians from chemical and biological attacks to the world's attention. The growth of purposeful attacks on civilian populations around the world created enough concern to stimulate improvement of capacity to prevent and respond to threatened or actual incidents.[30] The terrorist attacks on the World Trade Center in New York City on September 11, 2001, followed by the mailing of letters contaminated with anthrax spores to certain media outlets and national governmental figures in the United States in early October 2001, added new urgency to terrorism preparedness activities.[45]

In the intervening years, substantial attention has been paid to the topic of preparedness in the form of new legislation and funding to help prevent, protect against, and respond to acts of terrorism in this country, as well as natural disasters. State and local health departments, along with many other agencies and institutions, have received significant funding and been included in regional planning and preparedness activities. In general, this combination of resources and enhancement of working partnerships with other health and law enforcement organizations has improved surveillance and response capabilities at the state and local levels. (For a discussion of these issues, see Chapter 23.) However, at the same time that new federal funding for preparedness became available, federal support for many other areas of public health programming diminished. Concomitant revenue shortfalls in many states actually led to reductions in funding for population-based public health services across the country. Instead of building capacity overall, public health agencies have been placed in the position of having to fund their basic services and the new preparedness expectations with what amounts to, in many cases, an overall reduction in funding.

SUMMARY

If a central theme has been emerging as public health reinvents itself, it is the importance of partnerships in practically all phases of that reinvention. Partnerships were essential for the work that led to the development of workforce competencies, and they are essential for the ongoing definition and application of those competencies. The conversion of the IOM's core public health functions into the 10 essential services required partnerships, as did the communication processes used to gain their acceptance by the profession and their inclusion in the Clinton health care reform proposal. The development of several important national public health associations and the evolution of others are examples of people working together as partners. Important work coordinated by federal agencies was and remains characterized by the many different groups and individuals that are brought to the table as meaningful participants. Public health academicians and practitioners are reconnecting, and the relevance of training to practice is improving. Concentrated efforts to bring the separate cultures of medicine and public health more closely together indicate growing awareness that delivery of the 10 essential services and health status improvement are dependent on both sectors working in a coordinated fashion. Indeed, the National Performance Standards, themselves the product of working partnerships, will measure the effectiveness of LPHSs, partnerships by definition.

Public health is in a renaissance period. It has reached new levels of understanding and relevance. Its scientific base is expanding, and its effectiveness is improving. Training programs are growing at an almost exponential rate, and organized efforts are focused on finding and training public health leaders. Resources do not yet match need, and the varying organizational structures at the local level create some barriers to effectiveness and efficiency, but innovation and change have become the norm. It is reasonable to expect this evolution to continue resulting in increasing effectiveness of the profession's organized efforts to protect the public's health.

REVIEW QUESTIONS

1. The 1988 Institute of Medicine report on the *Future of Public Health* was highly critical of public health practice in the United States. List its major criticisms.
2. List at least five key developments that have contributed to the "philosophic renaissance" of public health practice during the past 20 years.
3. The "10 essential public health services" have become a core part of public health thinking and programming in recent years. List three national efforts that are based on their development.
4. Discuss the importance of partnerships to effective modern public health practice at the local level.
5. Describe major areas of public health practice that will need to be improved for future effectiveness of the discipline.

REFERENCES

1. Institute of Medicine, Committee for the Study of the Future of Public Health. *The Future of Public Health.* Washington, DC: National Academy Press; 1988.
2. Institute of Medicine, Committee on Assuring the Health of the Public in the 21st Century. *The Future of the Public's Health in the 21st Century.* Washington, DC: National Academy Press; 2003.
3. Roper WL, Baker EL, Dyal WW, Nicola RM. Strengthening the public health system. *Public Health Rep.* 1993;107(6):609–615.
4. *Health Security Act, Title III-Public Health Initiatives, HR3600.* Washington, DC: 103rd Congress; 1993.

5. Washington State Department of Health. *Public Health Improvement Plan.* Olympia: Washington State Depart of Health; 1994.

6. *Blueprint for a Healthy Community: A Guide for Local Health Departments.* Washington, DC: National Association of County Health Officials; 1994.

7. Public Health in America. Available at: http://www.health.gov/phfunctions/public.htm.

8. Sorensen AA, Bialek RG. *The Public Health Faculty Agency Forum: Linking Graduate Education and Practice, Final Report.* Gainesville: University Press of Florida; 1993.

9. Council on Linkages Between Academia and Public Health Practice. Available at: http://www.phf.org/link/index.htm.

10. Council on Linkages Between Academia and Public Health Practice. *Core Competencies for Public Health Practice.* Washington, DC: Council on Linkages Between Academia and Public Health Practice; 2001. Available at: http://www.phf.org/link/corecompetencies.htm.

11. Association of Schools of Public Health. MPH core competency development project: Introduction to the model. Washington, DC; 2007. Available at: http://www.asph.org/document.cfm?page=851.

12. Evans P. *Council on Education for Public Health.* [personal communication]. Washington, DC; March 2001.

13. Rasar L. *Council on Education for Public Health.* [personal communication]. Washington, DC; November, 2006.

14. Council on Education for Public Health. *Accreditation Criteria: Schools of Public Health.* Washington, DC; 2005. Available at: http://www.ceph.org/i4a/pages/index.cfm?pageid=3352.

15. The Illinois Public Health Practitioner Certification Board, Inc. Chicago, IL; 2007. Available at: http://www.phpcb.org/.

16. National Board of Public Health Examiners. Available at: http://www.nbphe.org.

17. National Association of County and City Health Officials. *Operational Definition of a Functional Local Health Department.* Washington, DC; 2005. Available at: http://www.naccho.org/topics/infrastructure/accreditation/upload/OperationalDefinitionBrochure.pdf.

18. National Association of Local Boards of Health. Available at: http://www.nalboh.org.

19. Public Health Practice Program Office. Available at: http://www.answers.com/topic/public-health-practice-program-office.

20. Notice to Readers: CDC Announces Landmark Reorganization. *MMWR.* 2005;54(15):387.

21. Centers for Disease Control and Prevention. *Office of Chief of Public Health Practice.* Atlanta, GA; 2005. Available at: http://www.cdc.gov/maso/pdf/OCPHPfs.pdf.

22. Lasker RD. *Medicine and Public Health: The Power of Collaboration.* New York: The New York Academy of Medicine; 1997.

23. Hager M. *Education for More Synergistic Practice of Medicine and Public Health.* New York: The Josiah Macy Jr. Foundation; 1999.

24. Beitsch LM, Brooks RG, Glasser JH, Coble YD. The medicine and public health initiative: Ten years later. *AJPM.* 2005;29(2):149–153.

25. Association of American Medical Colleges. *Development of regional centers to improve medical students' exposure to public health and population medicine.* Washington, DC; 2007. Available at: http://www.aamc.org/members/cdc/aamcbased/regionalcenters.htm.

26. Robinson JC. The end of managed care. *JAMA.* 2001;285(20):2622–2628.

27. Scutchfield DS, Harris JR, Koplan JP, et al. Managed care and public health. *J Public Health Manage Pract.* 1998;4(1):1–11.

28. Long SK, Yemane A. Commercial Plans in Medicaid Managed care: Understanding Who Stays and Who Leaves. *Health Affairs.* July/August 2005; 24(4): 1084–1094.

29. Dubay L, Holahan J, Cook A. The Uninsured and the Affordability of Health Insurance Coverage. *Health Affairs.* January/February 2007; 26(1): w22–w30.

30. Holahan J, Ghosh A. Understanding the recent growth in Medicaid spending, 2000–2003. *Health Affairs.* 2005;25(1):52–62.

31. Turning Point. Collaborating for a New Century in Public Health. Available at: http://www.turningpointprogram.org.

32. Lavizzo-Mourey R. Public Health Is for the Public Good. Gene Matthews Public Health Law Lecture. Atlanta, GA: CDC 4th Annual Partnership Conference; 2005.

33. Public Health Functions Project. Available at: http://www.health.gov/phfunctions/project.htm.

34. National Public Health Performance Standards Program Local Public Health System Performance Assessment Instrument. Available at: http://www.cdc.gov/od/ocphp/nphpsp/TheInstruments.htm.

35. Canadian Task Force on the Periodic Health Examination. The Periodic Health Examination. *Can Med Assoc J.* 1979;121:1194–1254.

36. *Guide to Clinical Preventive Services: An Assessment of the Effectiveness of 169 Interventions.* Baltimore, MD: Williams & Wilkens; 1989.

37. *Clinician's Handbook of Preventive Services.* 2nd ed. Washington, DC: Office of Disease Prevention and Health Promotion, US Public Health Service; 1998.

38. Lloyd P, Bialek R, et al. *Practice Guidelines for Public Health: Assessment of Scientific Evidence, Feasibility and Benefits.* Washington, DC: Council on Linkages Between Academia and Public Health; 1995.

39. McGinnis MJ, Foege W. Guide to community preventive services: Harnessing the science. *Am J Prev Med.* 2000;18(1S):1–2.

40. Zaza S, Briss PA, Harris KW. *The Guide to Community Preventive Services.* New York: Oxford University Press; 2005.

41. Council on Linkages Public Health Research Project. Available at: http://www.phf.org/link/phsr/April99Concept.pdf.

42. Council on Linkages. Public Health Systems Research. Available at: http://www.phf.org.

43. *Healthy People 2010.* 2nd ed. Washington, DC: US Depart of Health and Human Services; 2000.

44. American Public Health Association. *Code of Ethics. 2001.* Available at: http://www.apha.org.

45. *Chemical and Biological Terrorism: Research and Development to Improve Civilian Medical Response.* Institute of Medicine, National Research Council. Washington, DC: National Academy Press; 1999.

CHAPTER 4

Social Determinants of Health: Their Influence on Personal Choice, Environmental Exposures, and Health Care

Steven H. Woolf, MD, MPH* and Robert L. Phillips, Jr., MD, MSPH†

LEARNING OBJECTIVES

Upon completion of this chapter, the reader will be able to:

1. Describe the complexities of the relationship between social conditions and individual, environmental, and clinical determinants of health status.

2. Describe how social determinants affect personal health-related choices (e.g., health habits, seeking clinical attention, self-care of diseases), environmental exposures, and access to quality health care.

3. Describe the social conditions of the United States population with respect to education, income, race, ethnicity, homeless, food insecurity, and access to health care.

4. Compare the relative importance of social conditions and advances in medical care in their relative influence on the health status of the population.

5. Describe the contextual policy circumstances and public attitudes that impede or facilitate progress in ameliorating adverse social conditions.

KEY TERMS

Disparities

Inequality

Social Class

Social Determinants

*Departments of Family Medicine, Epidemiology and Community Health, Virginia Commonwealth University
†The Robert Graham Center: Policy Studies in Family Medicine and Primary Care, Washington, DC

INTRODUCTION

Including the crew, the *Titanic* sailed with 2,223 persons aboard, of whom 1,517 were lost and 706 were saved. It will be noted in this connection that 60 percent of the first-class passengers were saved, 42 percent of the second-class passengers were saved, 25 percent of the third-class passengers were saved, and 24 percent of the crew were saved.[1]

United States Senate Commerce Committee Report Investigation into the Loss of the *S.S. Titanic,* 1912.

The health of individuals and of populations is a product of multiple influences (Figure 4.1). Health status is affected by *individual* characteristics, which include both nonmodifiable host factors (e.g., age, gender, race, genotype) and modifiable behaviors. Modifiable behaviors include choices about using health care services and lifestyle habits that affect health, such as diet, physical activity, smoking, substance abuse, sexual behavior, and injury-reducing practices. The influence of host factors is strong—age being the most powerful determinant of health and disease—but personal choices also play a major role. Fully 38 percent of all deaths in the United States are attributed to three modifiable risk factors: smoking, diet, and physical inactivity.

As noted, personal choices unrelated to lifestyle also influence health status, such as those made in relation to accessing health care. People choose whether and how promptly to obtain screening tests while healthy and how quickly to seek clinical attention when symptoms of illness emerge. Delays in diagnosis and treatment can affect health outcomes, as do patients' choices in how carefully to adhere to treatment and follow-up recommendations.

Health is also affected by *environmental* characteristics that exist apart from individual host factors and personal choices. An individual's health is affected by toxic pollutants in the air, water, and food supply. Such effects arise from exposure to environmental tobacco smoke produced by cigarette smokers, to infectious agents transmitted by humans or animals, to asbestos and lead released by old housing, to intentional injuries inflicted by others, and to workplace hazards. Exposure to stress—at home or work—affects both mental and physical health.[2] Children exposed to family and

Figure 4.1. Determinants of Health
SOURCE: Delmar Cengage Learning

parental dysfunction are also more prone to health and developmental disorders.[3]

Finally, health is influenced by *health care*, which includes personal medical care, preventive services (e.g., immunizations), and public health programs. The degree to which health care improves health status is a function of the efficacy and effectiveness of interventions—e.g., screening, diagnosis, treatment—but these effects are dampened when individuals encounter barriers and delays in accessing care and when the care to which they have access is deficient in quality. The outcomes of health care are therefore mediated by both access and quality. Together, health care interacts with individual and environmental characteristics to influence health status.

THE INFLUENCE OF SOCIAL DETERMINANTS OF HEALTH

In turn, individual, environmental, and medical determinants of health are each mediated by social determinants such as education, income, race, ethnicity, neighborhood, and community. Some researchers suggest that behaviors, environmental factors, and health care are the intermediate or "proximal" pathways by which social determinants affect health.[4]

Other chapters in this book delve more deeply into how population health is affected by lifestyle, the environment, and health care. This chapter focuses on how these determinants are, in turn, influenced by social determinants. Krieger defines **Social determinants** *of health* as "specific features of and pathways by which societal conditions affect health and that potentially can be altered by informed action."[5]

Due to space considerations, this chapter focuses on the relationship between disparities in social conditions and health status, delving less into the social justice of the existence of these disparities, a topic with deep ethical and historical roots that is

examined in detail elsewhere.[6] See the works of Rawls[7] and Sen[8] to learn more about social justice.

Also because of space considerations, this chapter focuses on social determinants in the United States. Health status in developing countries is certainly more deeply influenced by social determinants, but the spectrum of problems extends well beyond the topics raised in this chapter to include more egregious social conditions such as civil wars, refugee displacements, and additional issues that are more characteristic of other regions of the globe. Fully 19 percent of the world's population (more than 1 billion people) live in extreme poverty (income less than $1 per day).[9] The prevalence of problems in the United States discussed in this chapter, such as food insecurity and poverty, is far more profound in the developing world. Several excellent publications examine social determinants of health from an international perspective.[10] Chief among these is the work of the World Health Organization Commission on Social Determinants of Health, the establishment of which in 2005 signaled the vital importance of the topic to health status globally.

Although social determinants affecting health are more profound in the developing world, similar patterns of health inequality also exist in industrialized or "developed" countries.[11–12] Universal access to health care, as in the United Kingdom, and more egalitarian income distributions, as in Scandinavian countries, may ameliorate the effects of social determinants—but they do not change the common pattern of differential health outcomes related to socioeconomic or social class.[11–14]

This chapter cannot properly address the deep cross-cutting effects of social conditions on health without first acknowledging the role of confounding variables—the profound clustering of determinants that make it difficult to tease apart the causal effects.[15] The complex interrelationships between the social conditions of individuals, families, and communities complicate any discussion of social determinants of health.[14] People with limited education are more likely to be poor, and the poor have greater difficulty obtaining a good education. Lahelma et al. estimated, based on Finnish data, that at least one-third of health inequalities by education are mediated by occupational class and income.[16] Health inequalities, often labeled as **disparities,** are prominently associated with race and ethnicity; however, limited education and income are also more prevalent among blacks, Hispanics, and other minorities. Reverse causality further complicates observed associations: poverty can cause inferior health status, but illness can also affect the ability to earn income. Perhaps the most difficult complexities involve intergenerational effects, such as the extent to which individuals' health reflects the conditions of their childhood and the social status of their parents and families.[17]

The clustering and interrelationships of these variables make it exceedingly difficult to discuss income, race, or any other individual social determinant of health in isolation, and render impossible any attempt to quantify with certainty the degree to which that variable affects health outcomes. Research in this field makes regular use of statistical techniques, such as multiple logistic regression analysis, to adjust for confounding variables in an attempt to quantify individual effects. Such methods often yield inconsistent results across studies and are often inadequate to deal with the complex interrelationships between social factors. The anatomy of these interrelationships is not well understood. This uncertainty poses questions about where responsibility for disparities lie and where policy interventions should be directed, but it also offers many potential targets for innovation and experimentation and is the focus of active research among social scientists and health services researchers.

Although the details of the causal pathway linking social conditions to health are therefore subject to some uncertainty at this writing, there is little doubt about the magnitude of their cumulative influence on health and disease. Analyzed by education, income, race, and ethnicity, individuals and families who face adverse social conditions have markedly inferior health outcomes on multiple indices, including lower life expectancies, higher prevalence rates for diseases, more severe complications, and higher morbidity and mortality rates.

The magnitude of the disparities is profound.[18] In the United States, a black newborn is 2.4 times more likely than a white baby to die by age one.[19] Compared to white Americans, blacks lose an excess of 2 million years of life each year.[20] As a population, U.S. blacks rank 69th in the world for male life expectancy and 59th in the world for female life expectancy (Tables 4.1 and 4.2). U.S. whites rank 29th and 31st, respectively.

These disparities are longstanding. Although mortality rates for the entire U.S. population—whites and blacks included—have declined steadily over recent decades, black mortality rates have remained 30 percent higher than those of whites.[21] The mechanisms by which poverty affects health outcomes have changed over time, but the strength of the relationship between poverty and health has not. Longitudinal studies in California from 1965 to 1994 found a strong relationship between cumulative exposure to economic disadvantage (below 200 percent poverty) and decreased life expectancy, physical disability, depression, pessimism, hostility, and cognitive problems.[22]

This chapter gives closer scrutiny to the interface between social determinants and health, demonstrating in particular how social conditions influence the major modifiable health determinants—(1) personal choices, (2) the environment, and (3) health care.

Personal Choices

Social determinants affect health by influencing the choices people make in modifying health habits and other risk factors for disease, in seeking clinical attention, and in self-care of disease.

Health Habits and Modifiable Risk Factors

Tobacco use, the leading cause of death in the United States, is more common among persons with limited education. In 2003, the prevalence of current cigarette smoking among persons age 25 and older was 10 percent for persons with a bachelor's degree or higher, 21 percent for those with

Table 4.1. Male Life Expectancy at Birth and Per Capita Expenditure on Health (U.S. Dollars 2003) for U.S. Whites and Blacks and for Other Nations, 2004

Country	Years Life Expectancy (2004)	Per Capita Health Care Expenditure (US$ 2003)	Country	Years Life Expectancy (2004)	Per Capita Health Care Expenditure (US$ 2003)
Iceland	79.0	3821	Chile	74.0	282
Japan	79.0	2662	Portugal	74.0	1348
San Marino	79.0	2957	Bahrain	73.0	555
Australia	78.0	2519	Czech Republic	73.0	667
Canada	78.0	2669	Panama	73.0	315
Israel	78.0	1514	Republic of Korea	73.0	705
Italy	78.0	2139	Slovenia	73.0	1218
Monaco	78.0	4587	Croatia	72.0	494
Sweden	78.0	3149	Dominica	72.0	212
Switzerland	78.0	5035	Mexico	72.0	372
Andorra	77.0	2039	Venezuela, Bolivarian Republic of	72.0	146
Cyprus	77.0	1038	Argentina	71.0	305
Greece	77.0	1556	Barbados	71.0	691
Netherlands	77.0	3088	Oman	71.0	278
New Zealand	77.0	1618	Poland	71.0	354
Norway	77.0	4976	Saint Lucia	71.0	221
Singapore	77.0	964	Tonga	71.0	102
Spain	77.0	1541	Uruguay	71.0	323
Austria	76.0	2358	Antigua and Barbuda	70.0	426
Brunei Darussalam	76.0	466	Bahamas	70.0	1121
France	76.0	2981	Bosnia and Herzegovina	70.0	168
Germany	76.0	3204	China	70.0	61
Kuwait	76.0	580	Cook Islands	70.0	294
Luxembourg	76.0	4112	Ecuador	70.0	109
Malta	76.0	1104	Georgia	70.0	35
Qatar	76.0	862	Jamaica	70.0	164
United Arab Emirates	76.0	661	Libyan Arab Jamahiriya	70.0	171
United Kingdom	76.0	2428	Paraguay	70.0	75
US Whites	**75.7**	**Not available**	Serbia-Montenegro	70.0	181
Belgium	75.0	2796	Slovakia	70.0	360
Costa Rica	75.0	305	Syrian Arab Republic	70.0	59
Cuba	75.0	211	Tunisia	70.0	137
Denmark	75.0	3534	**US Blacks**	**69.5**	**Not available**
Finland	75.0	2307	Albania	69.0	118
Ireland	75.0	2860	Algeria	69.0	89
United States of America	**75.0**	**5711**	Bulgaria	69.0	191

(continued)

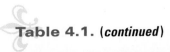**Table 4.1.** (*continued*)

Country	Years Life Expectancy (2004)	Per Capita Health Care Expenditure (US$ 2003)	Country	Years Life Expectancy (2004)	Per Capita Health Care Expenditure (US$ 2003)
Hungary	69.0	684	Samoa	66.0	94
Jordan	69.0	177	Solomon Islands	66.0	28
Malaysia	69.0	163	Armenia	65.0	55
Mauritius	69.0	172	Belize	65.0	174
Morocco	69.0	72	Democratic People's		
Peru	69.0	98	Republic of Korea	65.0	<1
Saint Kitts and Nevis	69.0	467	Guatemala	65.0	112
The former Yugoslav			Honduras	65.0	72
Republic of Macedonia	69.0	161	Indonesia	65.0	30
Turkey	69.0	257	Philippines	65.0	31
Viet Nam	69.0	26	Suriname	65.0	182
Colombia	68.0	138	Dominican Republic	64.0	132
El Salvador	68.0	183	Republic of Moldova	64.0	34
Iran, Islamic Republic of	68.0	131	Azerbaijan	63.0	32
Lebanon	68.0	573	Belarus	63.0	99
Micronesia, Federated			Bolivia	63.0	61
States of	68.0	147	Kiribati	63.0	96
Niue	68.0	655	Uzbekistan	63.0	21
Romania	68.0	159	Bangladesh	62.0	14
Saudi Arabia	68.0	366	Bhutan	62.0	10
Sri Lanka	68.0	31	Comoros	62.0	11
Brazil	67.0	212	Guyana	62.0	53
Cape Verde	67.0	78	Pakistan	62.0	13
Nicaragua	67.0	60	Tajikistan	62.0	11
Palau	67.0	607	Ukraine	62.0	60
Seychelles	67.0	522	India	61.0	27
Thailand	67.0	76	Mongolia	61.0	33
Trinidad and Tobago	67.0	316	Nepal	61.0	12
Vanuatu	67.0	54	Timor-Leste	61.0	39
Egypt	66.0	55	Tuvalu	61.0	142
Estonia	66.0	366	Marshall Islands	60.0	255
Fiji	66.0	104	Kyrgyzstan	59.0	20
Grenada	66.0	289	Russian Federation	59.0	167
Latvia	66.0	301	Eritrea	58.0	8
Lithuania	66.0	351	Lao People's Democratic		
Maldives	66.0	136	Republic	58.0	11
Saint Vincent and the			Nauru	58.0	798
Grenadines	66.0	194	Papua New Guinea	58.0	23

Table 4.1. (*continued*)

Country	Years Life Expectancy (2004)	Per Capita Health Care Expenditure (US$ 2003)	Country	Years Life Expectancy (2004)	Per Capita Health Care Expenditure (US$ 2003)
Sao Tome and Principe	57.0	34	United Republic of Tanzania	47.0	12
Yemen	57.0	32	Chad	45.0	16
Ghana	56.0	16	Guinea-Bissau	45.0	9
Kazakhstan	56.0	73	Nigeria	45.0	22
Myanmar	56.0	394	Mali	44.0	16
Sudan	56.0	21	Mozambique	44.0	12
Turkmenistan	56.0	89	Rwanda	44.0	7
Gabon	55.0	196	Somalia	43.0	n/a
Gambia	55.0	21	Afghanistan	42.0	11
Madagascar	55.0	8	Burundi	42.0	3
Mauritania	55.0	17	Democratic Republic of the Congo	42.0	4
Djibouti	54.0	47	Equatorial Guinea	42.0	96
Senegal	54.0	29	Niger	42.0	9
Congo	53.0	19	Côte d'Ivoire	41.0	28
Haiti	53.0	26	Malawi	41.0	13
Benin	52.0	20	Botswana	40.0	232
Guinea	52.0	22	Central African Republic	40.0	12
Namibia	52.0	145	Zambia	40.0	21
Togo	52.0	16	Lesotho	39.0	31
Cambodia	51.0	33	Liberia	39.0	6
Iraq	51.0	23	Angola	38.0	26
Kenya	51.0	20	Sierra Leone	37.0	7
Cameroon	50.0	37	Zimbabwe	37.0	40
Ethiopia	49.0	5	Swaziland	36.0	107
Uganda	48.0	18			
Burkina Faso	47.0	19			
South Africa	47.0	295			

SOURCE: Data from the *Statistical Annex* of the *World Health Report 2006* and *Health, United States, 2006* (http://www.cdc.gov/nchs/data/hus/hus06.pdf#027) were used for ranking. Mean health expenditures from the *World Health Report 2006* (http://www.who.int/whr/2006/annex/en/index.html). Analysis by the Robert Graham Center.

Table 4.2.   Female Life Expectancy at Birth and Per Capita Expenditure on Health (U.S. Dollars 2003) for U.S. Whites and Blacks and for Other Nations, 2004

Country	Years Life Expectancy (2004)	Per Capita Health Care Expenditure (US$ 2003)	Country	Years Life Expectancy (2004)	Per Capita Health Care Expenditure (US$ 2003)
Japan	86.0	2662	Poland	79.0	354
Monaco	85.0	4587	United Arab Emirates	79.0	661
Italy	84.0	2139	Uruguay	79.0	323
San Marino	84.0	2957	Argentina	78.0	305
Andorra	83.0	2039	Barbados	78.0	691
Australia	83.0	2519	Brunei Darussalam	78.0	466
Canada	83.0	2669	Estonia	78.0	366
France	83.0	2981	Kuwait	78.0	580
Iceland	83.0	3821	Lithuania	78.0	351
Spain	83.0	1541	Panama	78.0	315
Sweden	83.0	3149	Seychelles	78.0	522
Switzerland	83.0	5035	Slovakia	78.0	360
Austria	82.0	2358	Venezuela, Bolivarian Republic of	78.0	146
Cyprus	82.0	1038	Bosnia and Herzegovina	77.0	168
Finland	82.0	2307	Colombia	77.0	138
Germany	82.0	3204	Georgia	77.0	35
Greece	82.0	1556	Hungary	77.0	684
Israel	82.0	1514	Mexico	77.0	372
New Zealand	82.0	1618	Oman	77.0	278
Norway	82.0	4976	Saint Lucia	77.0	221
Singapore	82.0	964	**US Blacks**	**76.3**	**Not available**
Belgium	81.0	2796	Bahamas	76.0	1121
Chile	81.0	282	Bulgaria	76.0	191
Ireland	81.0	2860	Dominica	76.0	212
Luxembourg	81.0	4112	Latvia	76.0	301
Malta	81.0	1104	Romania	76.0	159
Netherlands	81.0	3088	The former Yugoslav Republic of Macedonia	76.0	161
Portugal	81.0	1348	Antigua and Barbuda	75.0	426
Slovenia	81.0	1218	Bahrain	75.0	555
United Kingdom	81.0	2428	Cook Islands	75.0	294
US Whites	**80.8**	**Not available**	Ecuador	75.0	109
Costa Rica	80.0	305	Libyan Arab Jamahiriya	75.0	171
Cuba	80.0	211	Mauritius	75.0	172
Denmark	80.0	3534	Qatar	75.0	862
Republic of Korea	80.0	705	Serbia-Montenegro	75.0	181
United States of America	**80.0**	**5711**	Sri Lanka	75.0	31
Croatia	79.0	494			
Czech Republic	79.0	667			

Table 4.2. (*continued*)

Country	Years Life Expectancy (2004)	Per Capita Health Care Expenditure (US$ 2003)	Country	Years Life Expectancy (2004)	Per Capita Health Care Expenditure (US$ 2003)
Albania	74.0	118	Egypt	70.0	55
Belarus	74.0	99	Honduras	70.0	72
Brazil	74.0	212	Palau	70.0	607
China	74.0	61	Samoa	70.0	94
El Salvador	74.0	183	Solomon Islands	70.0	28
Jamaica	74.0	164	Suriname	70.0	182
Malaysia	74.0	163	Tonga	70.0	102
Niue	74.0	655	Grenada	69.0	289
Paraguay	74.0	75	Mongolia	69.0	33
Saudi Arabia	74.0	366	Uzbekistan	69.0	21
Syrian Arab Republic	74.0	59	Vanuatu	69.0	54
Tunisia	74.0	137	Azerbaijan	68.0	32
Viet Nam	74.0	26	Democratic People's		
Jordan	73.0	177	Republic of Korea	68.0	<1
Morocco	73.0	72	Indonesia	68.0	30
Peru	73.0	98	Maldives	68.0	136
Saint Vincent and			Comoros	67.0	11
the Grenadines	73.0	194	Kazakhstan	67.0	73
Thailand	73.0	76	Kiribati	67.0	96
Trinidad and Tobago	73.0	316	Kyrgyzstan	67.0	20
Turkey	73.0	257	Bolivia	66.0	61
Ukraine	73.0	60	Timor-Leste	66.0	39
Algeria	72.0	89	Bhutan	65.0	10
Armenia	72.0	55	Nauru	65.0	798
Belize	72.0	174	Turkmenistan	65.0	89
Iran, Islamic Republic of	72.0	131	Guyana	64.0	53
Lebanon	72.0	573	Marshall Islands	64.0	255
Philippines	72.0	31	Tajikistan	64.0	11
Russian Federation	72.0	167	Bangladesh	63.0	14
Saint Kitts and Nevis	72.0	467	India	63.0	27
Cape Verde	71.0	78	Myanmar	63.0	394
Fiji	71.0	104	Pakistan	63.0	13
Guatemala	71.0	112	Eritrea	62.0	8
Micronesia, Federated			Tuvalu	62.0	142
States of	71.0	147	Iraq	61.0	23
Nicaragua	71.0	60	Nepal	61.0	12
Republic of Moldova	71.0	34	Papua New Guinea	61.0	23
Dominican Republic	70.0	132	Yemen	61.0	32

(*continued*)

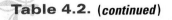

Table 4.2. (*continued*)

Country	Years Life Expectancy (2004)	Per Capita Health Care Expenditure (US$ 2003)	Country	Years Life Expectancy (2004)	Per Capita Health Care Expenditure (US$ 2003)
Lao People's Democratic Republic	60.0	11	Burkina Faso	48.0	19
Mauritania	60.0	17	Chad	48.0	16
Sao Tome and Principe	60.0	34	Guinea-Bissau	48.0	9
Sudan	60.0	21	Burundi	47.0	3
Gabon	59.0	196	Côte d'Ivoire	47.0	28
Gambia	59.0	21	Democratic Republic of the Congo	47.0	4
Madagascar	59.0	8	Mali	47.0	16
Cambodia	58.0	33	Rwanda	47.0	7
Ghana	58.0	16	Mozambique	46.0	12
Djibouti	57.0	47	Nigeria	46.0	22
Senegal	57.0	29	Somalia	45.0	n/a
Haiti	56.0	26	Equatorial Guinea	44.0	96
Togo	56.0	16	Lesotho	44.0	31
Congo	55.0	19	Liberia	44.0	6
Guinea	55.0	22	Afghanistan	42.0	11
Namibia	55.0	145	Angola	42.0	26
Benin	53.0	20	Central African Republic	41.0	12
Cameroon	51.0	37	Malawi	41.0	13
Ethiopia	51.0	5	Niger	41.0	9
Uganda	51.0	18	Botswana	40.0	232
Kenya	50.0	20	Sierra Leone	40.0	7
South Africa	49.0	295	Zambia	40.0	21
United Republic of Tanzania	49.0	12	Swaziland	39.0	107
			Zimbabwe	34.0	40

SOURCE: Data from the *Statistical Annex* of the *World Health Report 2006* and *Health, United States, 2006* (http://www.cdc.gov/nchs/data/hus/hus06.pdf#027) were used for ranking. Mean health expenditures from the *World Health Report 2006* (http://www.who.int/whr/2006/annex/en/index.html). Analysis by the Robert Graham Center.

some college but no bachelor's degree, 28 percent for those with a high school diploma or General Equivalency Developmental (GED) high school equivalency diploma, and 30 percent for those with no high school diploma or GED.[19]

Obesity is more common among the poor, those with limited education, and minorities.[19] Between 1999 and 2002, the prevalence of overweight was 77 percent among black women, compared to 57 percent for non-Hispanic whites.[19] The disparity in overweight by poverty status may be stabilizing in general but has widened among adolescents (Figure 4.2).[23] The major causes of obesity—physical inactivity and unhealthy diets—differ by

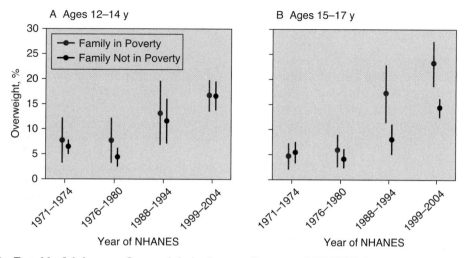

Figure 4.2. **Trend in Adolescent Overweight by Poverty Status and NHANES Surveys, 1971–2004**

socioeconomic status. Between 1999 and 2002, physical inactivity was reported by 31 percent of nonpoor adults and 56 percent of the poor.[19] Physical inactivity was reported by 28 percent of those with some college education and 61 percent of those with no high school diploma or GED.[19] Persons with higher education and income consume more fruits and vegetables.[24–25] Poor adolescents drink larger quantities of sweetened beverages.[23] Black women eat at fast food restaurants at twice the rate of white women.[26]

Other health behaviors also differ by social class. Use of child safety seats is less common among Hispanics and black Americans and among low-income populations.[27] In a 2002 survey, the proportion of women who reported using a contraceptive method at their first sexual encounter was 68 percent for whites, 60 percent for blacks, and 43 percent for Hispanics.[28] A survey of urban children found that those who were disadvantaged were more likely to be sexually active in grades 6, 8, and 10.[29]

The higher prevalence of unhealthy behaviors among disadvantaged populations has multiple explanations,[30–31] but social conditions exert a major influence. Persons with inadequate education, especially those with limited health literacy,

may not appreciate the degree of risk associated with unhealthy behaviors. They may know less about how to reduce risk, such as the effectiveness of pharmacotherapy to help with smoking cessation, the specific foods to avoid or emphasize in a healthy diet, or when contraception is necessary. They also may know less about available resources to help with behavior modification. Illiteracy, language, and cultural barriers may limit the usefulness of information delivered by pamphlets, websites, public health announcements, or advice given by health professionals.

Resources to help with behavior change are often lacking in the communities in which disadvantaged persons reside. The built environment in many urban settings, such as the lack of sidewalks and pedestrian routes from home to shopping, is not conducive to physical activity.[32] High crime rates, few parks, and other factors discourage children and adults from walking or engaging in more vigorous activities outdoors.[33] The consumption of fruits and vegetables is correlated with proximity to supermarkets,[34] but minority and poor communities have fewer supermarkets than do other neighborhoods and live in what some describe as "food deserts."[35–37] The perceived difficulties associated with preparing healthy meals or ordering healthy foods in restaurants increases the predilection to eat at fast-food restaurants.[38]

Minority communities are targets for advertising and marketing that promote unhealthy behaviors. The density of fast food restaurants and advertisements for their products are greater in low-income neighborhoods.[39] Billboards and other media in minority communities promote tobacco products and alcoholic beverages with images and messages that cater to cultural and ethnic backgrounds.[40-42] Cash-strapped schools in low-income school districts are more dependent on other revenue sources, such as vending machines that promote consumption of calorie-dense products.[43-44] Commercials aired on television programming targeted to black viewers include more food and beverage advertisements—for fast food, candy, soda, or meat—than those aired on other television programs.[45-46]

Low-income individuals and families face financial barriers to adopting healthy behaviors. Healthful food options tend to cost more than calorie-dense diets.[24] Disadvantaged individuals often cannot afford the resources that help wealthier individuals to exercise and lose weight. They cannot participate in sports that require expensive equipment, and they can rarely afford membership at fitness centers, commercial weight loss programs, or sports clubs, few of which are located in their communities.[47] Individual counseling sessions with a dietician or trainer are rarely possible.[48] Financial barriers limit options for other forms of behavior modification, such as when out-of-pocket costs limit access to tobacco-cessation medication, contraceptives, car seats, or physician counseling. And such individuals may be "time poor" because their work schedule or other competing demands do not provide the time for exercise, grocery shopping, and the preparation of healthful meals.

Seeking Clinical Attention

The choice to seek health care is influenced by logistical access barriers (as described later in this section), such as lack of providers or health insurance coverage, but social conditions also exert a more subtle influence on the predilection of patients to seek clinical attention, even when access is available. In health systems in which access and insurance coverage are equivalent for blacks and whites, such as the Medicare program and the Veterans Administration, black patients often have higher cancer mortality rates, a disparity attributed in part to delays in detection.[49-51] Influenza vaccination is covered under Medicare, but black beneficiaries, who have lower immunization rates, express less positive attitudes about the vaccine.[52]

Patients with good access but limited education or literacy may be less likely to obtain screening tests (or to follow up on abnormal results) because they do not know about the disease, that screening is recommended, or how to obtain the tests.[53-55] Patients with limited knowledge may also not appreciate the clinical significance of worsening symptoms that require prompt attention, such as the warning signs of a stroke, and may be more likely to harbor misconceptions that cause delays in contacting clinicians. Working class patients often cannot afford to take time off from their jobs or their families.

The choice to seek health care is also influenced by cultural and ethnic factors, such as one's language.[56-57] Efforts to educate patients about the need for care or the logistics of obtaining services are usually unsuccessful when delivered in languages that patients cannot understand. The health beliefs and traditions of certain cultures and ethnic groups may dampen interest in medical care. [58-60] The logic behind preventive care, such as screening for diseases, is countermanded by fatalism and beliefs that disease is spiritually ordained.

Culture, ethnicity, and race influence levels of trust in clinicians and may also contribute to delays in seeking care. Native Americans often prefer traditional healers, such as medicine men, over allopathic physicians.[61] In general, patients exhibit greater reluctance to seek care from individuals of a different ethnic or racial background.[62] Black patients experience well-documented problems with mistrust of white clinicians emanating from their long troubled history with whites, research atrocities such as the Tuskegee experiments, and modern experiences with subtle or overt racism in health care and daily life.[63] Although racial and ethnic concordance between patient and provider is therefore desirable to remove this impediment to care and is known to improve the quality of communication,[64–65] minority communities generally suffer from a shortage of minority clinicians, largely because proportionally few minorities are trained in the health professions.[66–67]

Self Care of Diseases

Among those who obtain care, the same tableau of social conditions influence the choice to follow through on recommendations: to undergo tests, obtain and use medication as instructed, follow treatment instructions, and return for follow-up appointments. Socioeconomic conditions may require patients to forego or delay these steps because they are too expensive or because they give precedence to what they perceive as higher priorities, such as feeding the family, getting to work, and staying safe from violent crime.

Other factors noted previously—educational deficits, literacy and language barriers, cultural and ethnic values—also influence both the ability of patients to understand what they should do and the intensity of their motivation to follow the advice. The effectiveness of treatments for chronic diseases such as diabetes and heart failure depend on self-management by patients, a greater challenge for individuals with less education and resources to draw upon.[68] For patients of all backgrounds, the highly fragmented United States health care system makes it difficult to navigate the logistical complexities of obtaining clinical services, such as getting an appointment, obtaining referrals to specialists, tracking down test results, and negotiating with insurance companies.[69] Individuals with limited education, language difficulties, and scarce resources are at a special disadvantage and highly vulnerable to falling through the cracks in their efforts to navigate the system.

Environmental Exposures

Independent of the personal choices made by individuals, health status is also influenced by the social conditions in which people live, the most obvious being the home itself. For example, aged housing stock and apartment buildings contaminated by lead-based paint or asbestos are more likely to be occupied by disadvantaged residents who cannot afford better housing.[70–71] More destitute conditions force individuals and families to become homeless, where they are exposed to health risks from outdoor threats (e.g., hypothermia, sexual assault) and from the crowded conditions at homeless shelters, such as increased susceptibility to infectious diseases (e.g., tuberculosis).

Factories, waste management facilities, and other sources of air, water, and soil pollution are generally located closer to impoverished residential areas and to minority communities than to more affluent suburbs. This issue, sometimes referred to as *environmental injustice,* has pernicious health consequences.[72] For example, the odds that black urban children will have asthma are 45 percent higher than those for white children living outside of urban settings.[73]

Adults and children living in high-crime areas are at greater risk of violent personal injury from assault or homicide, but more subtle characteristics of communities under stress may also influence the health of their residents.[74–76] For example, the literature suggests that the health of the people in a community is influenced by *social capital* and *social cohesion.* These factors, according to Krieger, "are proposed (and contested) as population level psychosocial assets that potentially can improve population health by influencing norms and strengthening bonds of 'civil society,' with the caveat that membership in certain social formations can potentially harm either members of the group (for example, group norms encourage high risk behaviors) or nongroup members (for example, harm caused to groups subjected to discrimination by groups supporting discrimination)."[5] Just two social determinant constructs, social cohesion and socioeconomic status, explained 89 percent of variance in child health and 93 percent of variance in overall county health in Kansas,[77] and others have reported similar findings.[78–79]

Most disadvantaged individuals and families lack the resources to do the obvious and escape such communities by moving to areas with greater social capital and healthier surroundings. Lacking the job opportunities and income to enable such a move, they remain mired in unhealthy communities where their best efforts at disease prevention can be undermined by frayed social infrastructure.[80] Health outcomes in such areas are affected by languishing, under-funded school systems that compromise educational attainment, inadequate public transportation services that impede access to supermarkets or medical appointments, local work settings that lack the resources for health promotion programs, and insufficient social service agencies, programs, personnel, and resources to help the disadvantaged. Lack of social cohesion has ripple effects, such as lowering participation in political activity (e.g., voting, serving on boards and committees) "which undermines the responsiveness of governments institutions in addressing the needs of the worst off."[81]

Many governments use indices based on multiple social determinants to assess neighborhood risk of poor health outcomes. The Townsend Index, one often used in the United Kingdom, is calculated using four variables: the proportion of people without an automobile, the proportion of households in overcrowded accommodations, the proportion of households that are not owner-occupied, and the proportion of people who are unemployed.[13] A positive Townsend score indicates material deprivation, whereas a negative score signifies comparative affluence. The association between the Townsend Index and unfavorable health outcomes has been widely validated and tends to be most predictive in urban areas. Figure 4.3 shows the distribution of the Townsend Index for New York City (note the high scores in the underprivileged western end of Long Island—the Bronx).

Economic *inequality,* a phenomenon that relates more to relative than to absolute income, is another potential environmental mediator of health. Literature suggests that the adverse health of a population is associated with the steepness of its socioeconomic gradient.[82–86] After adjustment for confounding variables, Lynch et al. found that United States metropolitan areas with high income inequality had higher death rates than communities with more egalitarian distributions. Across 283 Metropolitan Statistical Areas, the combined impact of high levels of income inequality and low per capita income was associated with a burden of mortality equal to the combined total mortality from lung cancer, HIV/AIDS, unintentional injuries, diabetes, suicide, and homicide.[86] Intra-area differences (within regions) in income are more important than those between regions: just as income inequality within countries is more profound than cross-national comparisons, differences within states in the United States are more important than differences between states.[82]

Several famous studies have validated the effects of social class or status on health outcomes. As defined by Krieger, "*social class* refers to social groups arising from interdependent economic relationships among people. These relationships are determined by a society's forms of property, ownership, and labor, and their connections through production, distribution, and consumption of goods, services, and information. Social class is thus premised upon people's structural location within the economy—as employers, employees, self employed, and unemployed (in both the formal and informal sector), and as owners, or not, of capital, land, or other forms of economic investments."[5]

The seminal work on the relationship between social class and health was the Whitehall Study, a 25-year longitudinal study that observed that the position of government employees in the British civil service hierarchy was associated with a gradient of premature mortality.[87] The study heralded a body of research showing that health is influenced by social and geopolitical context. The effects occur in aggregate: although poverty or other single measures are helpful proxies for the collective influence, the combination of factors and their interrelationships contribute most to the relative gradient of social inequality.

The environmental conditions heretofore discussed—violent crime, frayed infrastructure, and social inequality—foster stress and emotional

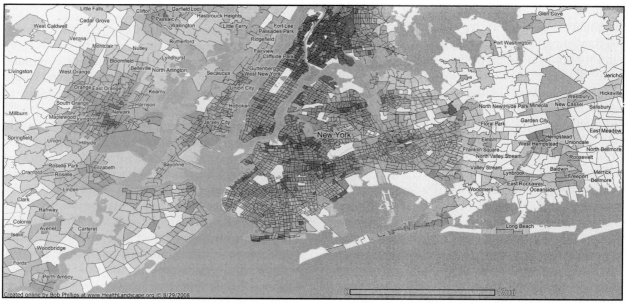

Legend:

Area-Based Socioeconomic Measures, 2000–Townsend Index
- ☐ –5— –2
- ▨ –2—0
- ▨ 0—5

Area-Based Socioeconomic Measures, 2000–Townsend Index (Cont'd)
- ▨ 5—10
- ▨ 10—20
- ▨ 20—30

Figure 4.3. **Townsend Deprivation Index by Census Tract for New York City**

reactions, such as humiliation, resentment, and anger over the experience of deprivation and asymmetric power.[88] Stress and other emotions elicited by these conditions may have direct biological influences on health, physiological functions (e.g., nerve conduction, immunity), and disease progression.[2,89–90] Stress may precipitate depression, posttraumatic stress disorder, and other clinical disorders.[91] It may also foster unhealthy behaviors (e.g., problem drinking, drug abuse, sexual promiscuity, domestic violence) as compensatory mechanisms. In the United States, which has the highest reported incarceration rate in the world, one in eight (12 percent) young black men (age 25–29) is in jail or prison.[92] Living in a neighborhood with increased "psychological hazards" has been shown to have an independent association with obesity.[93]

The influence of environmental conditions on health is perhaps most lasting for children, whose vulnerability to factors outside their control begins in utero. Maternal nutrition, behaviors (e.g., tobacco and substance abuse), and disease states that are brought about by social conditions have established influences on perinatal outcomes, such as infant mortality and low birth weight, but a growing literature suggests that in utero exposures have a more prolonged influence on disease processes manifested later in life. For example, intrauterine growth retardation and low birth weight appear to be risk factors for the development of cardiovascular disease later in life.[94]

Social conditions also shape the home surroundings and experience amid which children are raised. Children's growth and their physical and cognitive health and development are affected by the quality of meals they are served, the opportunities they are given for physical activity, the second-hand tobacco smoke they inhale, and other domestic conditions that, as noted previously, reflect the social conditions of the family. Stresses on parents and families fostered by austere living conditions can affect domestic stability, the quality of parenting, the opportunity to encourage educational advancement and to promote healthy behaviors, and the ability of adults to protect children from injuries. For example, mothers who are psychologically distressed are less likely to fasten children in car safety seats or seat belts.[95] Children in poverty face heightened exposure to emotional and physical trauma from marital discord, family dysfunction, and domestic violence.[96–97] Single-parent households are more common among the poor and minorities.[98] A turbulent community environment can affect children's sense of safety.[99]

The trauma of these childhood exposures can have immediate health consequences—as from child abuse—or can have delayed expression in adolescence, when rebellion, acting out, or other responsive behaviors lead to health problems from sexually transmitted diseases, unwanted pregnancy, tobacco addiction, substance abuse, or violent injuries. Health behaviors learned in childhood and the cumulative disadvantage that arises when one progresses through life stages under conditions of social distress are thought to have lasting consequences on the risks of developing chronic diseases, mental illness, drug abuse, and criminal activity in later years.[100–104] Children raised in poor families are also more likely to experience poverty as adults,[105] which not only affects their personal health status but also creates the conditions in which they, as parents, are at risk of repeating the same cycle with their own children.

Health Care

Social conditions affect the health care that patients receive, both in terms of access (including health insurance coverage) and the quality of care available to those with access.

Access to Health Care

Social conditions create well-known logistical barriers to obtaining health care. Access to care is more limited in disadvantaged and minority communities where health care providers, hospitals, and other clinical facilities are either unavailable or inaccessible due to transportation difficulties.[106–108] Community health centers (CHCs) fill this role in some locales but are unavailable in other needy areas and are often understaffed.[109–110] Growing evidence suggests that having a usual source of care in primary care can ameliorate some of the health disparities wrought by social inequalities.[111] Rates of hospitalization for conditions that should be preventable by receiving robust primary care ("ambulatory care–sensitive conditions") correlate strongly with socioeconomic deprivation, at least in part because vulnerable populations are less likely to have a good source of primary care.[112–113]

Disadvantaged persons and minorities are more likely to be uninsured or underinsured, a major health risk in the market-based health care system of the United States. Fully 31 percent of persons below the poverty threshold are uninsured, and 23 percent report no usual source of care.[19] Middle-class patients are often unable to access or meet eligibility requirements for Medicaid or charity care. With the rapid growth in the costs of health care and prescription drugs, a growing population, including insured as well as uninsured persons, find it difficult to afford co-payments, deductibles, pharmacy bills, and medical supplies. As of 2005, 16–20 percent of adults *with insurance* reported experiencing substantial problems paying their medical bills.[114] Health care spending may be the leading cause of personal bankruptcy.[115]

Quality of Health Care

The quality of care for disadvantaged and minority patients can be compromised if clinicians who care for such patients have deficient training or if the quality of facilities and services to which they have access is limited. Specialists, surgical centers, and other ancillary services are less available to vulnerable populations. Some patients with the same clinical presentation and health insurance coverage receive different care because of their race or ethnicity. Minority patients cared for by clinicians of a different race or ethnicity encounter difficulties with communication and trust and may be more likely to experience inferior outcomes.[64,116] Physicians less readily engage black patients in participatory decision making. A literature review by the Kaiser Family Foundation found 68 studies reporting racial or ethnic deficiencies in cardiac care.[117] In one widely cited study, physicians shown videotapes of simulated patients (actors) with identically scripted complaints were 40 percent less likely to recommend catheterization if the actor was black.[118]

THE MAGNITUDE OF THE PROBLEM

The notion that social conditions can affect health is easily understood, but it is equally easy to dismiss its relative impact on health—in comparison to medical care or biological and genetic determinants—as marginal. It is mistakenly assumed that ameliorating adverse social conditions would improve health on the margins but that more substantial health gains can be anticipated from biomedical research and technological advances in health care.

This assumption is problematic on two grounds. First, the magnitude (effect size) with which social conditions influence health is substantial—in some cases doubling or tripling the risk of death—whereas few biomedical advances affect health outcomes to this degree (see the following section). Second, the prevalence of adverse social conditions is high. Were either untrue—if adverse social conditions were uncommon or if they had minor impacts on health—it would be appropriate to make them less of a priority, but unfortunately the prevalence of societal distress in the United States is quite high despite the nation's overall affluence (Table 4.3).

The substantial prevalence of adverse social conditions, combined with their profound influence on health outcomes, creates the opportunity for social change to influence disease rates on a scale that rivals biomedical advances. As shown in Figure 4.4, age-adjusted mortality rates over the past century have declined at a mean rate of 1 percent per year. Except for the influenza pandemic in 1918, neither the public health advances in the early century nor the technological advances in later decades did much to alter the pace of this decline (Figure 4.4). All the while, however, black mortality rates remained 30 percent higher than those of whites.[21]

Eliminating the black-white mortality gap could save more lives than the year-to-year reductions achieved by biomedical advances. For example, from 1991 to 2000, such advances in medical care averted an estimated 176,633 deaths, but five times as many lives (886,202) would have been saved if blacks experienced the mortality rates of whites.

Addressing the root cause of these disparities could rival medical breakthroughs as a strategy to improve health. For example, if all adults had the lower mortality rate of people who attend college, eight times as many lives would be saved as those saved by medical advances.[127] The ripple effects of such interventions extend beyond health, which makes a business case for social change. Education, for example, yields economic gains not only by improving health—for example, reduced medical spending—but also by enhancing job opportunities, such as health insurance and higher earnings.[128–129] An educated workforce strengthens the economy and global competitiveness.[130] Crime and incarceration rates may be lowered.[131–132] The higher incomes of educated workers boost tax returns to government and reduce demands for welfare assistance and Medicaid.[133] A study that took these broader societal benefits into consideration found that reducing class sizes in grade school would improve the health status of students' lives *and* generate net savings for society ($168,000 per high school graduate).[134] Medical advances cannot produce such sweeping effects, and they rarely save money.[135]

Table 4.3. Prevalence of Societal Influences on Health in the United States

Education

- As of 2005, 15% of U.S. adults age 25 and older had not graduated from high school, and only 28% had graduated from college.[119]
- Compared with other developed countries, U.S. 15-year-old students score below average for proficiency in mathematics, science, and problem solving.[120]
- Approximately 90 million adults in the United States have reading skills that test below high school level. Experts estimate that a similar number lack needed health literacy skills to effectively use the U.S. health system.[53]

Income

- 13% of the U.S. population (18% of children) live in poverty (have incomes below the poverty threshold).[98] The prevalence of severe poverty (incomes of less than half of the poverty threshold) grew by 20% between 2000 and 2004.[121]
- Income inequality has widened steadily in the United States. The Gini index,[5] a key measure of inequality, increased by 3.6% from its most recent low of 0.450 in 1995 to 0.466 in 2004.[98] An analysis for the Brookings Institution found that only the top 10% of the income distribution has experienced growth in real wages and salaries equal to or greater than the rate of growth in the economy.
- U.S. household income, adjusted for inflation, declined by 3.6% between 2000 and 2004, from a median of $46,058 to $44,389.[98]

Race and Ethnicity

- Minorities, the subgroup at elevated risk for adverse health outcomes, represent a growing proportion of the U.S. population.
- Between 2000 and 2050, the proportion of the U.S. population represented by non-Hispanic whites is expected to decrease from 69% to 50%, whereas the Hispanic population is expected to grow from 13% to 24%. Growth is also expected among blacks (from 13% to 15%), Asians (from 4% to 8%), and other races (from 3% to 5%), which include American Indian and Alaskan natives, native Hawaiians, other Pacific Islanders, and those of two or more races.[122] By one estimate, Hispanics and people of color will constitute 47% of the U.S. population by 2050.[123]

Homelessness

- Approximately 3.5 million Americans (1.4 million children) experience homelessness in a given year.[124]

Food Insecurity

- As of 2004, 12% of U.S. households were food insecure (uncertain of having or unable to acquire enough food for all household members because of insufficient money and other resources for food). In 4% of U.S. households, food insecurity reached the point that one or more household members were hungry at some time during the year because they could not afford food.[125]

Access to Health Care

- As of 2003–2004, 18% of U.S. adults and 5% of children had no usual source of health care.
- As of 2005, 16% of the U.S. population (11% of children) lacked health insurance coverage.[98] A survey the same year by the Commonwealth Fund reported that 37% of adults under age 65 were either uninsured or underinsured.[114]
- As of 2003, 49 million Americans (19% of the population) lived in families that spent more than 10% of family income on health care.[126] By the time of the 2005 Commonwealth Fund survey, 16% of adults *with insurance* were reporting substantial problems paying their medical bills.[114]

A strategy to reduce disease in America should emphasize the alleviation of social distress at least as much as medical advances. As stated by Lem Nichols, "it is entirely plausible (but not yet proved) that transferring some money from Medicaid to public housing or education could yield much greater return than would spending the extra dollars within Medicaid or on health care in general."[78] Reverse priorities dominate government policies.[136] Indeed, budget pressures fomented by rising health expenditures, along with political sentiments, have caused Congress and state legislatures to reduce funding for social programs, thereby undercutting an upstream strategy to curtail health spending.[137–138]

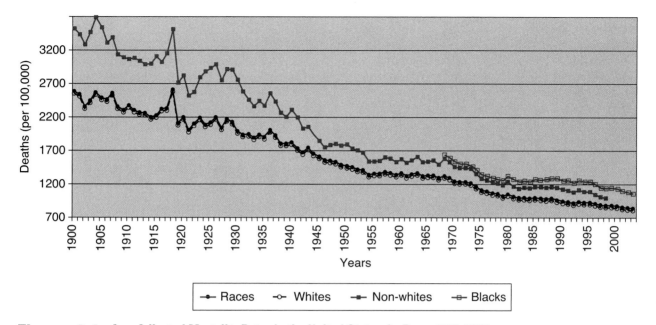

Figure 4.4. Age-Adjusted Mortality Rates in the United States, by Race, 1900–2003

THE CLIMATE FOR SOCIAL CHANGE

The existence of social conditions that compromise health status is as longstanding as civilization itself. Resources have always been concentrated among the aristocracy at the expense of the common man.[139] However, like individual determinants of health, social conditions are often modifiable. Modern countries and cultures differ in their tolerance of social injustice and the willingness of the public and the powerful to sacrifice self-interest to pursue aspirations for social equity. The public in many countries willingly accepts high tax rates to finance social programs and rationing of medical services to ensure universal, equitable access to basic health care.

The American public and its leaders have always found themselves caught in the crosswinds of two prevailing ethics: the utilitarian commitment to the common good and the spirit of individualism and entrepreneurialism on which the nation was founded. The latter fuels the popular sentiment that individuals hold personal responsibility for their success, that the disadvantaged should "pull themselves up by their bootstraps," and that limits exist on the duty of the state or of the affluent to lend assistance to the needy. Reflected in the dominant themes of conservative politics, many Americans are reluctant to expand government and entitlement programs or to pay higher taxes to address social problems.

> The inequality/health policy debate in the United States is caught in a fundamental conflict between the worship of individualism and varying impulses toward egalitarianism . . . Many Americans hold dear a national myth that effort always overcomes bad odds . . . [which] leads quite easily to the conclusion that individuals are responsible

for themselves and that most get the resources they deserve most of the time. My larger point is that this cannot be the cultural myth of a generous society.[78]

Changes in public attitudes and the economic climate that are conspicuous at the time of this writing could foster more concerted efforts in the United States to improve the social conditions discussed in this chapter. For example, poverty and income inequality have resurfaced on the national agenda. Following a period of intense interest in the 1960s—in which the "war on poverty" was the domestic centerpiece of the Johnson administration and garnered visibility from the civil rights movement and outspoken leaders such as Robert F. Kennedy, Jr., Martin Luther King, Jr., and Marian Wright Edelman—the plight of the poor subsequently slipped out of the national consciousness for much of the remainder of the twentieth century. This period was punctuated by blunt reminders of the problem, most notably in 2005 when the nation was horrified by televised images of conditions in Ward 9 of New Orleans in the aftermath of Hurricane Katrina.

Attitudes about the poor were otherwise complacent. A period of relative economic prosperity in the 1990s created favorable conditions in which the vast majority of Americans felt comfortable enough to view the disadvantaged as an isolated sector of the population whose concerns were quite distinct from their own. A downturn in the economy following a recession in 2001 changed circumstances. Corporate earnings fell under more intense global competition and higher operating costs (due in part to rising health care costs), spawning large layoffs by automobile manufacturers and other major employers and an increase in unemployment rates (from 4.0 percent in 2000 to 6.0 percent in 2003).[140]

Problems that had largely been considered the province of the poor—such as lack of health insurance and the inability to afford housing, medical bills, and other daily living expenses—increasingly became the problem of the middle class, a population that existing social safety net and entitlement programs were not designed to serve. As of 2005, 25 percent of adults under age 65 who were unin-

sured for some or all of the prior year reported annual incomes of $40,000 or greater.[114] Nearly half the uninsured were full-time workers. By 2006, the impact from rising medical bills was widespread: a survey by the Employee Benefit Research Institute reported that 28 percent of Americans were having difficulty paying for basic necessities (e.g., food, heat, housing), 33 percent had spent all or most of their savings, and approximately 22 percent had increased their credit card debt or borrowed money.[141] At this writing, the scale of the economic instability is widening.

Public discourse in recent years has paid greater notice to widening income disparities in the United States.[142] News reports chronicle the enormous earnings of corporate executives and how the ratio between management and labor incomes has grown steeply in recent years.[143–144] Real income (adjusted for inflation) for most Americans increased little during this period, if at all, while the government boasted of robust economic growth and productivity. The sense that these gains have accrued mainly to the wealthiest tier of society and that the middle class and the poor face increasing hardship is building interest in new policies to improve income, such as an increase in the minimum wage, enhanced job security, and job training programs.

The desire to improve educational attainment has also increased with greater recognition of the primacy of the "knowledge economy"[130]—competitiveness in the global market depends on employers' and workers' mastery of science, technology, and other disciplines—and of the dismal performance of students in the United States when compared to their counterparts in China, India, and other global competitors. Federal and state officials, along with corporate leaders, see a "business case" in investing in better education from pre-K through college. Politicians now campaign on the issue and are introducing new programs, especially at the state and local level, such as tax deductions for college tuition. Major philanthropies such as the Bill and Melinda Gates Foundation have made a priority of improving America's schools, especially in struggling communities.

Along with heightened interest in addressing income and education, the subject of racial and ethnic disparities remains vibrant.[116] The federal government, private foundations, and nonprofit organizations have launched initiatives to document the ways and the severity with which race and ethnicity influence health status and health care and to explore and formally evaluate potential solutions.[112] The tempo of these efforts is likely to increase as a result of demographic shifts in the United States population that will eventually make non-Hispanic whites a minority group.[122] The marked increase in the number of immigrants entering the United States already exerts profound influence on policy decisions about minorities.

A variety of initiatives seek to intervene at the interface in which social conditions affect health. Following are examples from each of the three nexuses discussed in this chapter: personal choices, environmental exposures, and health care.

Personal Choices

Various national and local initiatives seek to mitigate the conditions that heighten the exposure of disadvantaged adults and children to unhealthy behaviors. Examples include counter-marketing activities in which ad messages are used to undermine the industry's promotion of tobacco products and alcoholic beverages to minorities.[145–146] Other examples include efforts to address lunch menus and vending machine offerings at low-income schools and the work of some urban planners and developers to modify the built environment to encourage physical activity and to develop community gardens and farmers' markets to improve inner-city access to healthy food choices.

Developers of health educational materials, websites, and public health campaigns are giving greater attention to targeted outreach by focusing on language barriers and the cultural concerns and health literacy of their audience.[147] Faith-based organizations and lay health workers are proving effective, especially in black and Latino communities, in disseminating health information and providing social support in seeking care.[148] The most innovative public schools organize classes for adults, offer parenting skill courses, screen children for abuse and neglect, involve parents in the classroom, and host community events.

To make the health care setting more inviting to minorities, and to thereby facilitate prompt clinical attention for screening or the evaluation of abnormal symptoms, health systems are devoting greater attention to cultural sensitivity and to expanding the size of the minority health care workforce. "Patient navigator" programs and chronic disease management services are being developed and tested for disadvantaged patients.[149]

Employers, who increasingly recognize the connection between worksite health promotion and business productivity, offer programs and benefits such as exercise breaks, fitness facilities, heart-healthy cafeterias, occupational medicine clinics, and insurance coverage for preventive services. Although the typical blue-collar worker is not employed by businesses that offer such benefits, that stereotype is beginning to change.

Environmental Exposures

Civil rights organizations have brought greater attention to environmental justice issues, and the public health community has continued its long-standing efforts to implement policies and regulations to reduce exposure to environmental and occupational toxins. For example, policies enacted in past years to eliminate lead from household paint and gasoline continue to yield benefits today, while current efforts focus on other initiatives, such as banning indoor use of tobacco.[150] The ability to move out of unsafe housing conditions and to avoid homelessness is facilitated by programs that offer rent support and foster home ownership.

A variety of public- and private-sector initiatives build infrastructure and social cohesion in disadvantaged communities. They range from the most practical—such as free or discounted bus services to enable residents to shop at supermarkets or visit a physician—to more elaborate programs to improve the home environment for children. Social cohesion can be strengthened by programs to reduce crime, care for the homeless, build community social and health centers, and enhance job opportunities.

More imaginative efforts are envisioned for the future. For example, programs can actively intervene at key times in peoples' lives or when they are most vulnerable. The implementation in Britain of a universal program of home visits by community nurses after childbirth has enhanced childhood development scores and reduced child abuse. These programs are designed to support new parents during the first year of a child's life, offering parents a sense of control over their lives and tools for better parenting.[151] Later in life, opportunities exist to help young people avoid criminal activity and to avoid incarceration.

The public health system in the United States is frequently overburdened by providing personal health care and ensuring preparedness for bioterrorism and other emergencies. Ideally, it should turn its attention to community-level interventions and programs to help resolve the effects of social disparities. Examples might include bringing farmer's markets to impoverished neighborhoods and sponsoring safe exercise activities in high-crime areas. Public health departments can offer leadership and seed capital for the establishment of high-functioning community health centers (CHCs), where teams of health care providers can work together with social services. This model enables the public health department to exit its role in providing personal health care rather than behaving as a "co-predator" to CHCs in the same community. Similarly, public health functions and women, infant, and children nutritional services can be co-located for the ease of patients and integration of care. Successful local models might ultimately be propagated as a federal initiative.

Health Care

As the growing number of uninsured Americans recaptures visibility in headlines, policy makers are facing mounting pressure to adopt health reforms to improve coverage. At this writing, a variety of options are under consideration. They include incremental efforts to expand coverage for children and to lower the age of eligibility for Medicare, and more sweeping reforms such as the adoption of universal health coverage or a single-payer system. Other measures to improve access to health care for vulnerable populations are also in play, notably the expansion of CHCs. Strong mental health programs, particularly when coupled with primary care, can help individuals escape conditions of social deprivation.

The national effort to improve quality and reduce medical errors includes targeted efforts directed at problems that occur disproportionately among minority patients. Blue-ribbon panels and major studies have documented that patients with the same clinical presentation and insurance coverage often receive different care due to the mispereptions or subconscious biases of clinicians.[116] Centers of excellence have been established to study the causes and solutions of such disparities so that patients can count on receiving a consistent standard of care regardless of their race or ethnicity.

Although these developments are hopeful signs that progress in reducing social distress and health disparities can be achieved, several challenges dim the prospects for dramatic reforms. Perhaps the most formidable constraint is the lack of resolve (political will) within society itself. Disquiet about social injustice may not be sufficiently acute in the United States to motivate the public or its leaders to accept large sacrifices for equity, such as reordering the priorities of government or paying higher taxes. Competing values in American culture reflect the tension between altruism and a longstanding aversion to policies that bear too close a resemblance to socialism. Power centers and special interests that stand to lose exert considerable influence in resisting such changes. Politicians are reluctant to take positions that seem likely to disappoint constituents and potential campaign donors.

A second obstacle to dramatic social change is cost. Although, as discussed earlier, optimistic economic analyses forecast long-term net savings to society if it invests in improving education and other social determinants of health, the upfront costs remain problematic at this writing,[152] when the federal government is experiencing enormous budget deficits from housing and other crises and when state and local governments are struggling to make ends meet. For example, most school districts rely on property taxes for revenue, and impoverished communities have few resources to draw upon to finance transformational changes in their school systems. Small businesses, the predominant employer for most of the middle class, cannot afford to offer health promotion benefits, such as membership in fitness clubs or weight loss counseling.

The third major challenge is the inherent complexity of the social tapestry itself, which renders unsuccessful many well-meaning attempts at social change, especially those that rely too much on simplistic expectations. Critics of anti-poverty programs frequently cite their lack of success in alleviating poverty. Only a few strategies to improve educational attainment have been evaluated or proven effective in well-designed, controlled studies.[153] Successful efforts at social change are likely to require multi-pronged interventions across sectors. Apart from the sizable costs and the difficulties of stove-piping that such ambitious endeavors encounter, the ideal blueprint for such efforts remains speculative until social scientists acquire a better understanding of the interrelationships between social determinants of health.

Advocates for social justice find encouragement in the belief that all three of these major obstacles are surmountable with perseverance, and until then, progress in improving social conditions continues to occur at the local level and in a steady sequence of incremental national initiatives. Winston Churchill, Harry Truman, and Hubert Humphrey each quoted the maxim that nations are judged by how they treat the most vulnerable and disadvantaged segments of society. The alleviation of social distress therefore stands not only as a means for improving public health but also as an expression of civilized society.

REVIEW QUESTIONS

1. What is the causal relationship between social conditions and health status?
2. How do social determinants affect personal health-related choices, environmental exposures, and access to quality health care?
3. What is the prevalence of adverse social conditions in the United States?
4. What are the principal arguments for the contention that ameliorating social conditions can be more influential than advances in medical care?
5. What aspects of the current policy climate might foster interest in addressing social determinants of health, and what factors remain impediments?

REFERENCES

1. Report of the Committee on Commerce, United States Senate. *Investigation into Loss of* S.S. Titanic. Report No. 86, 62nd Congress. Washington, DC: Government Printing Office; 1912:5. Available at: http://www.senate.gov/artandhistory/history/resources/pdf/TitanicReport.pdf. Accessed January 1, 2007.
2. Tosevski DL, Milovancevic MP. Stressful life events and physical health. *Curr Opin Psychiatry.* 2006;19:184–9.
3. Taylor SE, Lerner JS, Sage RM, Lehman BJ, Seeman TE. Early environment, emotions, responses to stress, and health. *J Pers.* 2004;72:1365–93.
4. Henderson G. Introduction to Part II: The influences of social factors on health and illness. In: *The Social Medicine Reader.* Henderson GE, King NMP, Strauss RP, Estroff SE, Churchill LR, eds. 1997. Durham, NC: Duke University Press; 1997:103.
5. Krieger N. A glossary for social epidemiology. *Epidemiol Bull.* 2002;23:7–11.
6. Doyal L, Gough I. *A Theory of Human Need.* London: Macmillan Press; 1991.
7. Rawls J. *A Theory of Justice,* rev ed. Cambridge: Harvard University Press; 1999.
8. Sen A. *Inequality Reexamined.* Oxford: Clarendon Press, New York: Russell Sage Foundation, and Cambridge. MA: Harvard University Press; 1992.
9. United Nations. *The Millenium Development Goals Report.* 2006. Available at: http://unstats.un.org/unsd/mdg/Resources/Static/Products/Progress2006/MDGReport2006.pdf.
10. Irwin A, et al. The commission on social determinants of health: Tackling the social roots of health inequities. *PLoS Med.* 2006;3:e106.

11. *Social Determinants of Health*. Marmot M, Wilkinson RG, eds. Oxford: Oxford University Press, 1999.

12. Adler NE, Boyce WT, Chesney MA, Folkman S, Syme SL. Socioeconomic inequalities in health: No easy solution. *JAMA*. 1993;269:3140–5.

13. Townsend P, Phillimore P., Beattie A. *Health and Deprivation: Inequality and the North*. London: Croom Helm Ltd; 1988.

14. Goldman N. Social inequalities in health disentangling the underlying mechanisms. *Ann NY Acad Sci*. 2001;954:118–39.

15. Kilbourne AM, Switzer G, Hyman K, Crowley-Matoka M, Fine MJ. Advancing health disparities research within the health care system: A conceptual framework. *Am J Public Health*. 2006;96: 2113–21.

16. Lahelma E, Martikainen P, Laaksonen M, Aittomaki A. Pathways between socioeconomic determinants of health. *J Epidemiol Community Health*. 2004;58:327–32.

17. Lawlor DA, Ebrahim S, Davey Smith G. Adverse socioeconomic position across the lifecourse increases coronary heart disease risk cumulatively: Findings from the British women's heart and health study. *J Epidemiol Community Health*. 2005;59:785–93.

18. Murray CJ, et al. Eight Americas: Investigating mortality disparities across races, counties, and race-counties in the United States. *PLoS Med*. 2006;3 [Epub ahead of print].

19. National Center for Health Statistics. *Health, United States, 2005 with Chartbook on Trends in the Health of Americans*. Hyattsville, MD: National Center for Health Statistics; 2005. Available at: http://www.cdc.gov/nchs/data/hus/hus05.pdf#summary. Accessed November 4, 2006.

20. Franks P, Muennig P, Lubetkin E, Jia H. The burden of disease associated with being African-American in the United States and the contribution of socio-economic status. *Soc Sci Med*. 2006; 62:2469–78.

21. Satcher D, Fryer GE Jr, McCann J, Troutman A, Woolf SH, Rust G. What if we were equal? A comparison of the black-white mortality gap in 1960 and 2000. *Health Aff*. 2005;24:459–64.

22. Lynch JW, Kaplan GA, Shema SJ. Cumulative impact of sustained economic hardship on physical, cognitive, psychological, and social

functioning. *N Engl J Med*. 1997;337: 1889–1895.

23. Miech RA, Kumanyika SK, Stettler N, Link BG, Phelan JC, Chang VW. Trends in the association of poverty with overweight among US adolescents, 1971–2004. *JAMA*. 2006;295:2385–93.

24. Drewnowski A. Obesity and the food environment: Dietary energy density and diet costs. *Am J Prev Med*. 2004;27(3 Suppl):154–62.

25. Popkin BM, Zizza C, Siega-Riz AM. Who is leading the change? U.S. dietary quality comparison between 1965 and 1996. *Am J Prev Med*. 2003;25:1–8.

26. Pereira MA, et al. Fast-food habits, weight gain, and insulin resistance (the CARDIA study): 15-year prospective analysis. *Lancet*. 2005;365:36–42.

27. Agran PF, Anderson CL, Winn DG. Violators of a child passenger safety law. *Pediatrics*. 2004;114: 109–15.

28. Frost JJ, Driscoll AK. Sexual and Reproductive Health of U.S. Latinas: A Literature Review. Report No. 19. Guttmacher Institute, 2006. Available at: http://www.guttmacher.org/pubs/2006/02/07/or19.pdf.

29. Barone C, Ickovics JR, Ayers TS, Katz SM, Voyce CK, Weissberg RP. High-risk sexual behavior among young urban students. *Fam Plann Perspect*. 1996;28:69–74.

30. Lynch JW, Kaplan GA, Salonen JT. Why do poor people behave poorly? Variation in adult health behaviours and psychosocial characteristics by stages of the socioeconomic lifecourse. *Soc Sci Med*. 1997;44:809–19.

31. Droomers M, Schrijvers CT, Mackenbach JP. Educational level and decreases in leisure time physical activity: Predictors from the longitudinal GLOBE study. *J Epidemiol Community Health*. 2001;55:562–8.

32. Humpel N, Owen N, Leslie E. Environmental factors associated with adults' participation in physical activity: A review. *Am J Prev Med*. 2002;22: 188–99.

33. Schweitzer JH, Kim JW, Mackin JR. The impact of the built environment on crime and fear of crime in urban neighborhoods. *J Urban Technol*. 1999; 6:59–73.

34. Morland K, Wing S, Diez Roux A. The contextual effect of the local food environment on residents' diets: The atherosclerosis risk in communities study. *Am J Public Health*. 2002;92:1761–7.

35. Moore LV, Diez Roux AV. Associations of neighborhood characteristics with the location and type of food stores. *Am J Public Health*. 2006;96:325–31.

36. Baker EA, Schootman M, Barnidge E, Kelly C. The role of race and poverty in access to foods that enable individuals to adhere to dietary guidelines. *Prev Chronic Dis*. 2006;3:A76. Epub June 15, 2006.

37. Briggs JE. "In 'food deserts' of city, healthy eating a mirage." *Chicago Tribune*, July 18, 2006.

38. Satia JA, Galanko JA, Siega-Riz AM. Eating at fast-food restaurants is associated with dietary intake, demographic, psychosocial and behavioural factors among African Americans in North Carolina. *Public Health Nutr*. 2004;7:1089–96.

39. Block JP, Scribner RA, DeSalvo KB. Fast food, race/ethnicity, and income: A geographic analysis. *Am J Prev Med*. 2004;27:211–7.

40. Altman DG, Schooler C, Basil MD. Alcohol and cigarette advertising on billboards. *Health Educ Res*. 1991;6:487–90.

41. Gardiner PS. The African Americanization of menthol cigarette use in the United States. *Nicotine Tob Res*. 2004;6(suppl 1):S55–65.

42. Alaniz ML, Wilkes C. Pro-drinking messages and message environments for young adults: The case of alcohol industry advertising in African American, Latino, and Native American communities. *J Public Health Policy*. 1998;19:447–72.

43. Wechsler H, Brener ND, Kuester S, Miller C. Food service and foods and beverages available at school: Results from the School Health Policies and Programs Study 2000. *J Sch Health*. 2001;71:313–324.

44. Government Accountability Office. *School Meal Programs: Competitive Foods are Widely Available and Generate Substantial Revenues for Schools*. GAO-05–563. Available at: http://www.gao.gov/cgi-bin/getrpt?GAO-05–563. Accessed January 1, 2007.

45. Henderson VR, Kelly B. Food advertising in the age of obesity: Content analysis of food advertising on general market and African American television. *J Nutr Educ Behav*. 2005;37:191–6.

46. Outley CW, Taddese A. A content analysis of health and physical activity messages marketed to African American children during after-school television programming. *Arch Pediatr Adolesc Med*. 2006;160:432–5.

47. Powell LM, Slater S, Chaloupka FJ, Harper D. Availability of physical activity-related facilities and neighborhood demographic and socioeconomic characteristics: A national study. *Am J Public Health*. 2006;96:1676–80.

48. Gettleman L, Winkleby MA. Using focus groups to develop a heart disease prevention program for ethnically diverse, low-income women. *J Community Health*. 2000;25:439–53.

49. L.A. Ries, et al. The annual report to the nation on the status of cancer, 1973–1997, with a special section on colorectal cancer. *Cancer*. 2000;88:2398–2424.

50. Etzioni DA, Yano EM, Rubenstein LV, et al. Measuring the quality of colorectal cancer screening: The importance of follow-up. *Dis Colon Rectum*. 2006;49:1002–10.

51. Lantz PM, et al. The influence of race, ethnicity, and individual socioeconomic factors on breast cancer stage at diagnosis. *Am J Public Health*. 2006;96:2173–8.

52. Lindley MC, Wortley PM, Winston CA, Bardenheier BH. The role of attitudes in understanding disparities in adult influenza vaccination. *Am J Prev Med*. 2006;31:281–5.

53. Nielsen-Bohlman L, Panzer AM, Kindig DA, eds. *Health Literacy: A Prescription to End Confusion*. Committee on Health Literacy, Institute of Medicine. Washington: National Academy Press; 2004.

54. Gullatte MM, Phillips JM, Gibson LM. Factors associated with delays in screening of self-detected breast changes in African-American women. *J Natl Black Nurses Assoc*. 2006;17:45–50.

55. Deskins S, et al. Preventive care in Appalachia: Use of the theory of planned behavior to identify barriers to participation in cholesterol screenings among West Virginians. *J Rural Health*. 2006;22:367–74.

56. Luquis RR, Villanueva Cruz IJ. Knowledge, attitudes, and perceptions about breast cancer and breast cancer screening among Hispanic women residing in South Central Pennsylvania. *J Community Health*. 2006;31:25–42.

57. Fiscella K, Franks P, Doescher MP, Saver BG. Disparities in health care by race, ethnicity, and language among the insured: findings from a national sample. *Med Care*. 2002;40:52–9.

58. Simon CE. Breast cancer screening: Cultural beliefs and diverse populations. *Health Soc Work*. 2006;31:36–43.

59. Whittle J, et al. Do patient preferences contribute to racial differences in cardiovascular procedure use? *J Gen Intern Med.* 1997;12:267–73.

60. Cykert S, Phifer N. Surgical decisions for early stage, non-small cell lung cancer: Which racially sensitive perceptions of cancer are likely to explain racial variation in surgery? *Med Decis Making.* 2003;23:167–76.

61. Novins DK, Beals J, Moore LA, Spicer P, Manson SM, AI-SUPERPFP Team. Use of biomedical services and traditional healing options among American Indians: Sociodemographic correlates, spirituality, and ethnic identity. *Med Care.* 2004;42:670–9.

62. Chen FM, Fryer GE, Phillips RL, Wilson E, Pathman DE. Patients' beliefs about racism, preferences for physician race, and satisfaction with care. *Ann Fam Med.* 2005; 3:138–143.

63. Smith DB. *Health Care Divided: Race and Healing a Nation.* Ann Arbor: University of Michigan Press; 2002.

64. Cooper-Patrick L, et al. Race, gender, and partnership in the patient-physician relationship. *JAMA.* 1999;282:583–9.

65. Saha S, Komaromy M, Koepsell TD, Bindman AB. Patient-physician racial concordance and the perceived quality and use of health care. *Arch Intern Med.* 1999;159:997–1004.

66. *Missing Persons: Minorities in the Health Professions.* Washington, DC: Sullivan Commission; 2004.

67. *In the Nation's Compelling Interest: Ensuring Diversity in the Health Care Workforce.* Washington, DC: National Academy Press; 2004.

68. Bodenheimer T, Lorig K, Holman H, Grumbach K. Patient self-management of chronic disease in primary care. *JAMA.* 2002;288:2469–75.

69. President's Cancer Panel. Voices of a broken system: Real people, real problems. 2001 Available at: http://156.40.135.142:8080/webisodes/pcpvideo/voices_files/index.html. Accessed May 28, 2006.

70. Jacobs DE, et al. The prevalence of lead-based paint hazards in U.S. housing. *Environ Health Perspect.* 2002;110:A599–606.

71. Hood E. Dwelling disparities: How poor housing leads to poor health. *Environ Health Perspect.* 2005;113:A310–7.

72. Morello-Frosch R, Lopez R. The riskscape and the color line: Examining the role of segregation in environmental health disparities. *Environ Res.* 2006;102:181–96.

73. Aligne CA, Auinger P, Byrd RS, Weitzman M. Risk factors for pediatric asthma. Contributions of poverty, race, and urban residence. *Am J Respir Crit Care Med.* 2000;162(3 Pt 1):873–7.

74. Mackenbach JP, Kunst AE, Cavelaars AE, Groenhof F, Geurts JJ. Socioeconomic inequalities in morbidity and mortality in Western Europe. The EU Working Group on Socioeconomic Inequalities in Health. *Lancet.* 1997;349:1655–9.

75. Diez Roux AV, et al. Neighborhood of residence and incidence of coronary heart disease. *N Engl J Med.* 2001;345:99–106.

76. Kaplan GA. What is the role of the social environment in understanding inequalities in health? *Ann NY Acad Sci.* 1999;896:116–9.

77. Singh GK. Socioeconomic and behavioral differences in health, morbidity, and mortality in Kansas: Empirical data, models, and analysis. In: Tarlov AR, St Peter RF, eds *The Society and Population Health Reader. Vol II: A State and Community Perspective.* New York: The New Press; 2000.

78. Nichols LM. The case for additional research on the relationship between socioeconomic status and health. In: Auerbach JA, Krimgold BK, eds.*Income, socioeconomic status, and health: Exploring the relationships.* Washington, DC: National Policy Association; 2001:132–136.

79. Kaplan GA. Economic policy is health policy: Findings from the study of income, socioeconomic status, and health. In: Auerbach JA, Krimgold BK, eds. *Income, Socioeconomic Status, and Health: Exploring the Relationships.* Washington, DC: National Policy Association; 2001:137–149.

80. Lynch JW, Smith GD, Kaplan GA, House JS. Income inequality and mortality: importance to health of individual income, psychosocial environment, or material conditions. *BMJ.* 2000;320:1200–4.

81. Daniels N, Kennedy B, Kawachi I. Justice is good for our health. In: Daniels N, Kennedy B, Kawachi I. *Is Inequality Bad for Our Health?* Boston: Beacon Press; 2000:14.

82. Wilkinson RG. Putting the picture together: Prosperity, redistribution, health, and welfare. In: Marmot M, Wilkinson RG, eds. *Social Determinants of Health.* Oxford: Oxford University Press; 1999:256–274.

83. Wilkinson RG. Income distribution and life expectancy. *Br Med J.* 1992;304:165–8.

84. Kaplan GA, Pamuk ER, Lynch JW, Cohen RD, Balfour JL. Inequality in income and mortality in the United States: Analysis of mortality and potential pathways. *Br Med J.* 1996;312:999–1003.

85. Stronks K, van de Mheen HD, Mackenbach JP. A higher prevalence of health problems in low income groups: Does it reflect relative deprivation? *J Epidemiol Community Health.* 1998;52:548–57.

86. Lynch JW, et al. Income inequality and mortality in metropolitan areas of the United States. *Am J Public Health.* 1998;88:1074–80.

87. Marmot MG, et al. Health inequalities among British civil servants: The Whitehall II study. *Lancet.* 1991:337:1387–93.

88. Leventhal T, Brooks-Gunn J. Moving to opportunity: An experimental study of neighborhood effects on mental health. *Am J Public Health.* 2003;93:1576–82.

89. Cassel J. The contribution of the social environment to host resistance. *Am J Epidemiol.* 1976; 104:107–23.

90. Taylor SE, Repetti RL, Seeman T. What is an unhealthy environment and how does it get under the skin? *Annu Rev Psychol.* 1997;48:411–47.

91. Schulz AJ, et al. Psychosocial stress and social support as mediators of relationships between income, length of residence and depressive symptoms among African American women on Detroit's eastside. *Soc Sci Med.* 2006;62:510–22.

92. *Facts about Prisons and Prisoners.* Washington, DC: The Sentencing Project, 2006. Available at: http://www.sentencingproject.org/pdfs/1035.pdf. Accessed January 1, 2007.

93. Glass TA, Rasmussen MD, Schwartz BS. Neighborhoods and obesity in older adults: The Baltimore memory study. *Am J Prev Med.* 2006; 31:455–63.

94. Baum M, Ortiz L, Quan A. Fetal origins of cardiovascular disease. *Curr Opin Pediatr.* 2003;15:166–70.

95. Witt WP, et al. Children's use of motor vehicle restraints: Maternal psychological distress, maternal motor vehicle restraint practices, and sociodemographics. *Ambul Pediatr.* 2006;6:145–51.

96. Rutter M. Poverty and child mental health: Natural experiments and social causation. *JAMA.* 2003;290:2063–4.

97. Freisthler B, Merritt DH, LaScala EA. Understanding the ecology of child maltreatment: A review of the literature and directions for future research. *Child Maltreat.* 2006;11:263–80.

98. DeNavas-Walt C, Proctor BD, Lee CH. U.S. Census Bureau, Current Population Reports, P60–231, *Income, Poverty, and Health Insurance Coverage in the United States: 2005.* U.S. Government Printing Office, Washington, DC; 2006.

99. Mijanovich T, Weitzman BC. Which "broken windows" matter? School, neighborhood, and family characteristics associated with youths' feelings of unsafety. *J Urban Health.* 2003;80:400–15.

100. Case A, Fertig A, Paxson C. The lasting impact of childhood health and circumstance. *J Health Econ.* 2005;24:365–89.

101. Graham H, Power C. Childhood disadvantage and health inequalities: A framework for policy based on lifecourse research. *Child Care Health Dev.* 2004;30:671–8.

102. Wadsworthx ME. Changing social factors and their long-term implications for health. *Br Med Bull.* 1997;53:198–209.

103. Kuh DL, Ben Shlomo Y, eds. *A Life Course Approach to Chronic Disease Epidemiology. Tracing the Origins of Ill Health from Early to Adult Life.* Oxford: Oxford University Press, 1997.

104. Kahn RS, Wilson K, Wise PH. Intergenerational health disparities: Socioeconomic status, women's health conditions, and child behavior problems. *Public Health Rep.* 2005;120:399–408.

105. Hertz T. *Understanding Mobility in America.* Washington, DC: Center for American Progress; 2006. Available at: http://www.americanprogress. org/kf/hertz_mobility_analysis.pdf. Accessed May 12, 2006.

106. Field K, Briggs D. Socio-economic and locational determinants of accessibility and utilization of primary health-care. *Health and Social Care in the Community.* 2001;9:294–308.

107. Zuvekas SH, Weinick RM. Changes in access to care, 1977–1996: The role of health insurance. *Health Serv Res.* 1999;34:271–9.

108. Hendryx MS, Ahern MM, Lovrich NP, McCurdy AH. Access to health care and community social capital. *Health Serv Res.* 2002;37:87–103.

109. Forrest CB, Whelan EM. Primary care safety-net delivery sites in the United States: A comparison of community health centers, hospital outpatient

departments, and physicians' offices. *JAMA.* 2000;284:2077–83.

110. Rosenblatt RA, Andrilla CH, Curtin T, Hart LG. Shortages of medical personnel at community health centers: Implications for planned expansion. *JAMA.* 2006;295:1042–9.

111. Starfield B, Shi L, Macinko J. Contribution of primary care to health systems and health. *Milbank Q.* 2005;83:457–502.

112. Agency for Healthcare Research and Quality. *2004 National Healthcare Disparities Report.* AHRQ Publication no. 05-0014. Rockville, MD: US Department of Health and Human Services; 2004.

113. Shi L, Stevens GD. Disparities in access to care and satisfaction among U.S. children: The roles of race/ethnicity and poverty status. *Public Health Rep.* 2005;120:431–41.

114. Commonwealth Fund. *2005 Biennial Health Insurance Survey.* Available at: http://www.cmwf .org/surveys/surveys_show.htm?doc_id=367929.

115. Himmelstein DU, Warren E, Thorne D, Woolhandler S. Illness and injury as contributors to bankruptcy. *Health Aff.* 2005 January–June;Suppl Web Exclusives:W5-63–W5-73.

116. Smedley BD, Stith AY, Nelson AR, eds. *Unequal Treatment: Confronting Racial and Ethnic Disparities in Health Care.* Committee on Understanding and Eliminating Racial and Ethnic Disparities in Health Care, Board on Health Sciences Policy, Institute of Medicine. Washington, DC: National Academy Press; 2003.

117. Lillie-Blanton M, Rushing OE, Ruiz S, Mayberry R, Boone L. *Racial/Ethnic Differences in Cardiac Care: The Weight of the Evidence.* Publication No. 6041. Menlo Park, CA: The Henry J. Kaiser Family Foundation; 2002.

118. Schulman KA, et al. The effect of race and sex on physicians' recommendations for cardiac catheterization. *N Engl J Med.* 1999;340:618–26.

119. U.S. Census Bureau. Table 1a. Percent of High School and College Graduates of the Population 15 Years and Over, by Age, Sex, Race, and Hispanic Origin: 2005. Available at: http://www. census.gov/population/socdemo/education/cps20 05/tab01a-01.xls. Accessed January 1, 2007.

120. National Center for Education Statistics. Table 399. Average reading literacy, mathematics literacy, science literacy, and problem-solving scores of 15-year-olds, by sex and country: 2003. Available at: http://nces.ed.gov/programs/digest/

d04/tables/dt04_399.asp. Accessed January 1, 2007.

121. Woolf SH, Johnson RE, Geiger HJ. The rising prevalence of severe poverty in America: A growing threat to public health. *Am J Prev Med.* 2006;31:332–341.

122. U.S. Census Bureau. U.S. interim projections by age, sex, race, and Hispanic origin. 2004. Available at: http://www.census.gov/ipc/www/usinterimproj/.

123. Kaiser Family Foundation. *Key Facts: Race, Ethnicity, and Medical Care.* Menlo Park, CA; 2003.

124. The National Law Center on Homelessness and Poverty. Homelessness in the United States and the human right to housing. January, 2004. Available at: http://www.nlchp.org/content/pubs/HomelessnessintheUSandRightstoHousing.pdf.

125. *Household Food Security in the United States, 2004/ERR-1.* Economic Research Service/USDA. Available at: http://www.ers.usda.gov/publications/err11/err11fm.pdf.

126. Commonwealth Fund. *2005 Biennial Health Insurance Survey.* Available at: http://www.cmwf. org/surveys/surveys_show.htm?doc_id=367929.

127. Woolf SH, Johnson RE, Fryer GE Jr, Rust G, Satcher D. The health impact of resolving racial disparities: An analysis of U.S. mortality data. *Am J Public Health.* 2004;94:2078–81.

128. Woolf SH, Johnson RE, Phillips RL Jr, Philipsen M. Giving everyone the health of the educated: Would social change save more lives than medical advances? *Am J Public Health.* In press.

129. Muennig P, Fahs M. The cost-effectiveness of public postsecondary education subsidies. *Prev Med.* 2001;32:156–62.

130. Muennig P. Health returns to education interventions. Available at: http://devweb.tc.columbia. edu/manager/symposium/Files/81_Muennig_paper.ed.pdf. Accessed November 4, 2006.

131. Graham PA, Stacey NG, eds. *The Knowledge Economy and Postsecondary Education: Report of a Workshop.* Committee on the Impact of the Changing Economy on the Education System, National Research Council. Washington, DC: National Academy Press; 2002. Available at: http://www.nap.edu/catalog/10239.html. Accessed November 4, 2006.

132. Lochner L, Moretti E. The effect of education on crime: Evidence from prison inmates, arrests, and self-reports. *American Econ Rev.* 2004;94:155–89.

133. Belfield C. The promise of early childhood education. Available at: http://devweb.tc.columbia.edu/

manager/symposium/Files/72_Belfield_paper.ed. pdf. Accessed November 4, 2006.

134. Rouse CE. The labor market consequences of an inadequate education. Available at: http://devweb. tc.columbia.edu/manager/symposium/Files/77_ Rouse_paper.pdf. Accessed November 4, 2006.

135. Muennig P, Woolf SH. The cost-effectiveness of education as a health intervention: An analysis of the health and economic benefits of reducing the size of classes. *Am J Public Health*. Submitted.

136. The CEA Registry. Available at: https://research. tufts-nemc.org/cear/default.aspx. Accessed November 4, 2006.

137. Woolf SH. Society's choice: The tradeoff between efficacy and equity and the lives at stake. *Am J Prev Med*. 2004;27:49–56.

138. National Head Start Association. *Special Report: Funding and Enrollment Cuts in Fiscal Year 2006*. Washington, DC: National Head Start Association Research and Evaluation Department; 2004. Available at: http://www.nhsa.org/download/ research/FY2006_Budget_Cuts.pdf. Accessed October 21, 2005.

139. Tanner R. Governors wrestle with Medicaid changes. Associated Press. August 7, 2006. http://www.examiner.com/a-206747~Gover- nors_Wrestle_With_Medicaid_Changes.html. Accessed September 6, 2006.

140. Phillips K. *Wealth and Democracy: A Political History of the American Rich*. New York: Broadway Books; 2002.

141. U.S. Department of Labor, Bureau of Labors Statistics. Where can I find the unemployment rate for previous years? Available at: http://www.bls. gov/cps/prev_yrs.htm. Accessed January 1, 2007.

142. Employee Benefit Research Institute. *2006 Health Confidence Survey*. EBRI Notes, November 2006, Vol. 27, No. 11. Available at: http://www.ebri. org/pdf/notespdf/EBRI_Notes_11-20061.pdf. Accessed December 27, 2006.

143. Seize the chance. The politics of inequality have shifted: Now policy must follow. *Washington Post*. December 24, 2006:B6.

144. Fonda D. If this is a boom why does it feel like a squeeze? *Time*. November 10, 2003;162(19):62, 64, 66.

145. The top takes off: That rhetoric about giveaways for multimillionaires? It's accurate. *Washington Post*. May 7, 2006:B6.

146. Siegel M, Biener L. The impact of an antismoking media campaign on progression to established smoking: Results of a longitudinal youth study. *Am J Public Health*. 2000;90:380–386.

147. Niederdeppe J, Farrelly MC, Haviland ML. Confirming "truth": More evidence of a successful tobacco countermarketing campaign in Florida. *Am J Public Health*. 2004;94:255–7.

148. Brown SA, Garcia AA, Winchell M. Reaching underserved populations and cultural competence in diabetes education. *Curr Diab Rep*. 2002;2: 166–76.

149. Elder JP, et al. Interpersonal and print nutrition communication for a Spanish-dominant Latino population: Secretos de la Buena Vida. *Health Psychol*. 2005;24:49–57.

150. Fowler T, Steakley C, Garcia AR, Kwok J, Bennett LM. Reducing disparities in the burden of cancer: The role of patient navigators. *PLoS Med*. July 2006;3(7):e193.

151. CDC. State-specific prevalence of current cigarette smoking among adults and secondhand smoke rules and policies in homes and workplaces— United States, 2005. *MMWR*. 2006;55:1148–51.

152. Wadsworth M. Early life. In: *Social Determinants of Health*. Marmot M, Wilkinson RG, eds. Oxford: Oxford University Press; 1999: 44–63.

153. Finn JD, Gerber SB, Boyd-Zaharias J. Small classes in the early grades, academic achievement, and graduating from high school. *J Educ Psychol*. 2005;97:214–223.

CHAPTER 5

Public Health Policy and the Policy-Making Process

Thomas C. Ricketts, PhD

LEARNING OBJECTIVES

Upon completion of this chapter, the reader will be able to:

1. Understand the policy-making process in public health in the United States as a form of story telling.
2. Recognize the major frameworks for understanding policy making in the United States.
3. Understand key terms and interpretive structures in public health policy making, including the role of numbers, facts, symbols, and timing.
4. Comprehend the major theories that motivate policy making and politics in public health.
5. Describe the basic structure of public health policymaking and the institutions where this takes place.

KEY TERMS

Academics
Agenda
Bureaucracies
Bureaucrats
Community
Elites
Great People
Liberal Traditions
Media
Policy
Policy Entrepreneurs
Politics
Professionals
Scientists
Special Interests
Window of Opportunity

Public health can be viewed as a fusion of classical American themes. Its politics fit well into the thread of the American political story. This chapter describes public health policy making and politics using a familiar structure of story telling. Public health touches practically all of the elements of American society because it deals with the quality of the lives of the people who inhabit the United States. Forces beyond our borders also affect the public's health, and the policy making in public health easily stretches into international affairs. Even the physical structure of the land and buildings we inhabit has an effect on our health, which allows the policies for public health to intersect with the politics and policy making of engineering, infrastructure, and the environment. Given this breadth, it might appear to the casual observer that the politics of public health may be either too broad to be usefully characterized or made up of a shifting set of special political rules and structures that are impossible to coherently describe.

In a sense this is true; for example, in public health the "special" politics of farm subsidies and agriculture combines with the politics of international chemical manufacturing to affect population exposure to hazardous chemicals for farmworkers.[1] Governmental public health agencies are then charged with dealing with the resulting harm. At any given time, national agricultural or trade policy may "trump" the policies of formal public health agencies. But the way in which one dominates the other usually follows rules and theories common to all three domains in American politics and policy making. Public health is just one of many political and policy streams in the American context that can be interpreted and "explained" using general political theory and policy frameworks.

In this chapter, the description of public health politics unfolds as a story much like you might describe an event in a newspaper. A good journalist knows that the story must answer the who, what, when, where, how, and why questions. This story telling approach doesn't deviate very much from the guidance given by a well-accepted definition of politics. Harold Lasswell described **politics** as "who gets what, when (and) how" and titled his influential analysis of American politics with those words.[2] That definition is repeated to this day because it explains so well what politics is all about. But to complete the description, the additional questions of when and why are justifiably added.

John Kingdon uses much the same taxonomy in describing how **policy** is generated.[3] He describes a wide range of elements important to policy creation that fall into the journalist's categorical questions, but he places more or less emphasis on some elements than others. His book, *Agendas, Alternatives and Public Policies,* is one of the most widely used texts in courses that focus on health and public health policy although it is intended for a general audience of people seeking to understand policy. There are political scientists and policy experts who have viewed the public health and health policy worlds as a more or less coherent whole[4,5] with public health seen as a special subset of health politics[6,7] or as a coherent subject in and of itself.[8]

Others have seen the health policy process as fitting into a model with recognizable phases. Beaufort Longest promotes this form of structured conceptualization to guide managers in the health system.[9] He identifies a policy formulation phase, drawing from Kingdon, and then a policy implementation phase that provides feedback via a policy modification stage. His emphasis is on formal legislation because that form of policy direction fits better with the management of formal institutions. Others see the policy process as something that can be better understood through the lesson on case studies and the history of specific issues. Harrington and Estes continue a series of volumes that cover a range of issues in the fourth edition of their book,[10] and McLaughlin and McLaughlin make use of many specific policy examples within a general structure of policy analysis to give a sense of how health policy works.[11] The use of anecdotes and histories of how past policy has emerged and the application of a generalized model or the combination of the two approaches have been the standard way to present health policy making and elaborate the processes of health policy. The approach used in this chapter is intended to sensitize the individual who is in a situation where policy and politics are operating to the forces that are in play.

WHO CONTROLS POLITICS AND WHO MAKES POLICY?

It is fitting to start with a description of the people who take the lead in politics and policy because while we can speak easily about a decision being subject to "politics," we know that politicians drive this process. The same can be said for policy making: it is a people process. There are, however, special classifications of people who dominate politics and policy, and they are called by names such as elites, professionals, entrepreneurs, and even "great" people. Understanding the people involved goes a long way toward understanding politics and policy.

Elites

It may come as no surprise to most Americans that a relatively small group of **elites** make most political decisions. It is widely recognized that there are identifiable people whose economic or social position give them more "weight" in politics than their role as a single voter or individual claimant on government. Most Americans easily accept that some "types" of people are more politically influential. Theories that describe the dominance of elites go beyond that simple observation and posit that practically all decisions are made by the same small set of elite actors, and the elites can be identified by their social, economic, or occupational characteristics. The background to elitist theories of political dominance is that the elites are consistently in charge and that little gets done without their blessing or stimulation. In public health, it is hard to see the field run by a select few other than as a result of general governmental control of most of the formal structure. Public health may be viewed as insulated from elites because of its general population focus and broad applicability of its benefits. Nevertheless, policies and laws that favor industry over people or protect some groups and not others are often the result of the "normal" politics where elites hold sway over decision making.

Even in public health, local boards and commissions are often controlled by the more powerful sectors of society and the economy. These people, who are charged with representing the community as a whole, often are chosen from the well-educated and financially successful elements of their communities. The decision-making process in local public health has been described as a process whereby "The result is that elites discuss the problem and work through solutions with other elites, not citizens."[12]

The fascination with the quality of natural leaders and ruling classes goes back to antiquity, but the modern study of elites can be traced back to Vilfredo Pareto (1848–1923). Pareto was opposed to the emerging big political idea of his time, the spread of the voting franchise; "universal suffrage," he said, "matters but little whether the ruling class is an oligarchy, a plutocracy, or a democracy." However, he was squarely in favor of the dominance of elites.

Two American commentators on elites, Robert Dahl and C. Wright Mills, were more accommodating of the concept of elite dominance coexisting with democracy. Dahl saw elites as those who were willing to function to control politics, and that there was a voluntary and informal structure that actually "ran things." This system of elitism was actually open to all. This follows the belief among Americans that, with luck and hard work, anyone can become rich or powerful. This theme is repeated in the autobiographies of Benjamin Franklin, Malcolm X, and the stories of Horatio Alger.

C. Wright Mills is a little more definite in his identification of the people who run America: business people, politicians, and the military. These people run the show because they have found common cause with each other and managed to create central structures for control and stability. These institutions, such as corporations, universities, and even big churches, are where the influence of Wall Street or of the banks can be felt. Their elite dominance will be even more pervasive if the idea of privatization of health care edges over into public health.

More recently the elites have been charged with abandoning their natural responsibility and separating themselves from society. Christopher Lasch titled his social criticism "The Revolt of the Elites" and described how the rich and influential can hide within gated communities and separate themselves from the normal risks of life by dint of their economic and social power. Public health has been viewed as outside the province of the elites because it is part of the dirty work of governing: "The public at large views public health as dirty and unpleasant work, removed from the concerns of the broad spectrum of society, especially the world of the power elites."[13]

Although we may feel that public health is an activity that is antithetical to elite dominance, we find many instances of elites either leading reform in public health or exerting great influence on the direction of public health policy through foundations and corporate boards. The Robert Wood Johnson Foundation, the Commonwealth Fund, the Milbank Memorial Fund, the W.K. Kellogg Foundation, and the Kaiser Family Foundation are but a few of the many philanthropic organizations that take an active role in influencing the direction of public health policy, either through direct funding of experimental and model programs or through training and socialization of leaders. The W.K. Kellogg foundation and the Robert Wood Johnson Foundation have programs whose goals are to develop individuals who will make up the elite of public health. These programs orient emerging experts and practitioners to the world of power and government with goals of bettering the nation's health by creating leadership capital.

Professionals

For health care and public health, there is tradition of interpreting the emergence of policies from a viewpoint that considers **professionals** and professional roles as dominating the process. This might be a form of the distributed "**great people**" theory of change, but health care and public health professionals have special social and economic roles that they play that are not replicated in other policy domains.

Paul Starr in his excellent review of the history of medicine in America, *The Social Transformation of American Medicine,* pointed out the special role that professionals play in our society. By professional, we mean any group that is given some power or degree of influence that rests with their social or economic role. Priests and ministers are given "special" powers, as are lawyers, accountants, military men, police, and even brokers by dint of their training and expected behavior for the benefit of society rather than themselves. A useful definition of a professional is one who is expected to act in behalf of another or of society rather than themselves in certain spheres. Their behavior is guided as much by ethical standards as by legal or political norms, but their recognition depends upon a highly political process.

The states have retained the power to license and regulate the healing professions through their "police power" to protect the health, safety, and welfare of the public. This provides a complementary legal justification for the professional role of physicians that is tied to the protective power of the state governments expressed through public health. Starr's work traces this process, and he uses the image of medicine as a "sovereign" profession that acts as a controlling force in the emergence of professional public health.

Health professionals have been expected to behave "benevolently," and this may extend to a sense of public responsibility that often translates into a "public" health role. Recently they have discovered that "the benevolence of their work world is eroding in the face of growing concern over their responsiveness to public needs."[14] This clash of the professional tendency to benevolent (often paternalistic) activity and of market responsiveness is not new, but it is creating new problems for medical professionals who were once comfortable with their dominant role in society.

Trends

Health care has become more and more labor intensive, but the labor intensification has not necessarily transformed the traditional clinical roles of physician and nurse. The explosion of "new health professions" includes expansion of roles and responsibilities for professionals who complement and extend more traditional health professional disciplines. This has benefited public health to some degree by allowing for more cost-efficient direct care in some systems as physician assistants and nurse practitioners assume leadership or coordinating roles where once medical physicians were exclusively in charge.

Health professions will grow rapidly in the near future, but growth will be most rapid among the support professions: technicians, aides, therapists, and assistants who provide low-wage or low-salary services provided under the direction of physicians, within organized systems, or in the open market for personal services. Health professionals are more and more employees rather than independent entrepreneurs. This trend creates a sense of instability for the sovereign professions, but the trend can support organized public health as a viable option for professionals used to working in bureaucratic structures. The pressure on human resources in the general health care field affects public health disproportionately due to the relatively low wages in the public sector and the general inability of government agencies to respond to labor market changes. In public health, the pace of professional development has been slower than in medical care, and there are concerns that a public health workforce shortage is emerging.[15]

The politics of the national public health workforce are played out at the federal level as advocates vie for funds to support training programs and incentive systems to attract individuals into the field. At the state level, there are debates over how much support to provide universities and community colleges to prepare practitioners in the health professions as well as for prevention and public health careers. To date, these politics have been separated into silos that reflect the professional "division of labor."

Bureaucrats and Bureaucracies

This is an example of the "whos" getting mixed with the "what" of government. The bureaucracy is a necessary part of the system, but **bureaucrats** behave in ways that transcend and, in many ways, defy organizations and their missions. Some might say that studying bureaucracy has more of a place in administration than politics, but the nature and structure of bureaucracy either makes many policy options infeasible or facilitates their implementation. Understanding how **bureaucracies** work and how much power they can wield in the implementation of policies is a necessary political skill. Any policy analysis that is considering options and alternatives for future action must include an assessment of the capacity of the bureaucracy to achieve the stated goals for policy.

Since the release of the 1988 Institute of Medicine (IOM) report on the *Future of Public Health* there has been a series of reorganizations of public health at the federal and state levels.[16] Public health agencies, especially at the national level, were reoriented toward what were termed "core" services. The IOM committee recommended a more unified and conceptually coherent mission for public health calling for reorganization that unified the assurance, assessment, policy development, and evaluation activities of public health.

This generalized mission did not give specific structural guidance to public health agencies, but over the next decade, a process of reorganization occurred, especially in the federal government, using these rubrics. The identification of core services or concepts allowed the Public Health Functions Steering Committee organized in response to the federal initiatives to identify areas where communications could be tightened, lines of control shortened, and a general process of accountability added to the overall public health mission (see Exhibit 5.1). This process was mirrored by the states as they also reorganized along these lines, seeking streamlined structures and more clarity in goals and tasks.

The fact that such a coordinating committee could have this kind of administrative success is

---

EXHIBIT 5.1 Membership of the Public Health Functions Steering Committee

The Public Health Functions Steering Committee was created in 1994 by a consortium of key players in public health and operated through 2000. It was chaired by the Assistant Secretary for Health of the U.S. Department of Health and Human Services and the Surgeon General with coordination within DHHS. The consortium was made up of the following:

- American Public Health Association
- Association of Schools of Public Health
- Association of State and Territorial Health Officials
- Environmental Council of the States
- National Association of County and City Health Officials

- National Association of State Alcohol and Drug Abuse Directors
- National Association of State Mental Health Program Directors
- Public Health Foundation
- The U.S. Agency for Health Care Policy and Research
- Centers for Disease Control and Prevention
- Food and Drug Administration
- Health Resources and Services Administration
- Indian Health Service
- National Institutes of Health
- Office of the Assistant Secretary for Health
- Substance Abuse and Mental Health Services Administration

---

relatively unique to public sectors but not unknown in other sectors of government, especially when there is a need to set industry-wide or cross-industry standards for measurement, communication, and regulation of conflicting regulatory standards. Such coordinating committees are active in the electronics and communications industries to assure interoperability and to allow computer systems to "talk" to each other.

California attempted a reform in 2004 issuing a report that called for a general restructuring of the public health authority and a formal reorganization of the public health system in that state (http://www.lhc.ca.gov/lhcdir/170/report170.pdf). The major recommendations from that report were for bureaucratic restructuring and a focus on getting the right scale and mechanisms for accountability in place. Any enterprise whose constituency is the entire population requires careful and close attention to the demands and needs of bureaucracy to make any meaningful change in individual or collective behavior beyond what occurs as a result of natural competition for money and power.

Scientists/Academics

The role of scientists and academics in policy making and politics differs to some degree from that of professionals in public health and is reflected in a delineation between the academic, or "ivory tower," world of research and teaching and the practical day-to-day work of delivering services. **Academics** have influence in policy making where there is a high degree of complexity, and technical language is the norm. This is somewhat parallel to the power derived from mastery of knowledge on the part of medical professionals, but, in the case of public health, the knowledge base is much wider to encompass issues of pollution, water quality management, disease propagation, risk factors, and the relative effectiveness of prevention versus control measures.

Academics have been criticized for holding themselves aloof from the worlds of practical policy making and politics[17] and often see themselves as clearly separate and untainted by the quotidian. In fact, the research and academic worlds have long been enmeshed in political battles, and their influence and participation remains substantial. This is particularly so in public health where the academic homes of the field grew from practical needs to understand the nature of vectors and diseases and how to organize and manage a relatively uniform public service structure. A contemporary program such as the Community-Campus Partnerships for Health highlights the practical involvement of the academy in local policy making and governance (http://depts.washington.edu/ccph/index.html).

The National Institute of Health (NIH) recognized the need to connect the work of "bench" **scientists** more closely to the delivery of health care and the application of public health policy at the community level. To that end, the organization has created the Clinical and Translational Science Awards (CTSA) funding mechanism to organize what was previously a relatively unconnected set of independent research projects. (http://www.ncrr.nih.gov/clinical_research_resources/clinical_and_translational_science_awards/). The focus is on the translation of discoveries into treatment for patients, but there are also very strong community-level components in many of the projects that have been funded as of early 2008. This attempt to use funding mechanisms to push scientists to work more closely with community-focused programs represents a "brute force" approach to linking two kinds of special "whos": laboratory-based scientists and community actors who come from a social science tradition. How well this connection works will depend upon the relative control of the policies that shape NIH funding by the two groups as well as other key actors.

Media

The **media** serve a unique function in modern democracies. Some have called it a separate branch of government that provides another check to power in the tradition of the "fourth estate."[18] Others see it as a political player on its own, functioning as form of special interest group.[19] In public health policy, the media are important in the dissemination of information from central and professional sources and are often seen are functioning more like messengers rather than shapers of policy. However, the media may not recognize important "news" that the public needs until it fits into their expectations of what is newsworthy or interesting to the public. For example, in the coverage of AIDS, the disease and its threat were an isolated and technical issue until a major film star and other personalities were revealed to be infected or died from the disease. The media could then focus the issue with the drama of the struggle of recognizable "personalities."[20]

One use of the media to promote public health has been the rise of conscious "social marketing."[21] This is the use of the media to foster social change and promote behaviors and beliefs that either experts or elites consider beneficial for society as a whole. The process of social marketing has the potential for influence in policy making as well because the messages flow "down" to the public as well as "up" to policy makers. Social marketing may be somewhat akin to a political "campaign" intended to generate policy change or to elect someone to office. The same principles apply of clarity and simplicity of message, repetition, and the use of persuasive symbols. For example, the anti-tobacco advertising program was intended not only to change individual behavior but also to foster political changes.[22]

The People, the Public

Alan Wolfe argues that Americans have adequate access to democratic mechanisms but that the quality of democracy has degraded, in that participation is both uninformed and heavily influenced by **special interests**.[23] Public health is a beneficiary of all the avenues of participation in the democratic process with a range of national interest groups and coalitions engaged at all levels of government; these include groups such as the American Public Health Association (APHA) and the American Cancer Society (ACS). Local interests are reflected by organizations such as the Healthy Ansonians, which are grass-roots groups whose organizations are concerned with health in a broad sense but focus their work on a local system or government structure.

The public has an independent voice in policy making but that is often filtered through institutions and organizations. The media and interest groups often offer more direct connections between the public and policy makers, especially in the case of elections and in recall or referendums. Whether the public is more or less engaged in public health policy making is open to debate. Policy making does ebb and flow with the public mood, and the public has been able to express preferences for complex problems in health care and public health.[24,25] The American public is aware of public health issues, and there is formal participation at the local level through membership on boards and commissions, but more often the public's involvement is viewed through the lens of **community.**[26] Much of the democratic engagement of Americans in public health is through these community groups who are concerned with the general health of their fellow citizens or of a specific group of people at risk or suffering from a disease. These groups cross over political boundaries in the sense of voting districts and representation in general government. This may weaken the formal political power of the public's involvement in policy making for public health at some levels, such as in localities or at the state level for groups focused on a specific disease, but allow it to function more effectively at others.

Public opinion is more often measured through polling, and health and public health are often included in broad scale assessments of public priorities. Research America conducted a national sample survey in 2004 to gauge Americans' support for and knowledge of public health. They found widespread awareness of public health, 56 percent of respondents reported personally knowing someone working in the field of public health.[27] Public health is often conflated with "health" in surveys and opinion polls, and the general issue of "health" is usually a relatively high priority of Americans. However, this is usually expressed in terms of insurance coverage, the costs of pharmaceuticals, or some aspect of health financing. The Kaiser Family Foundation has funded a program of surveys whose topics cover almost all aspects of health, including public health. They have, for example, issued focus studies of the role of public health agencies in the treatment and prevention of sexually transmitted disease.[28] However, they do not

include "public health" as a main search topic on their "Health Poll" page, including bioterrorism, environmental health, smoking, violence and sexual health, among others, as the search terms. This is a reflection of the general indifference to public health as an issue in and of itself.

Policy Entrepreneurs

Policy making in the United States has become its own industry. The emergence of multiple "think-tanks" and advocacy groups has created a well-developed "market of policy ideas." Many of these entities have been created around single ideas that were promoted by individuals. Medical savings accounts, for example, were developed by John C. Goodman, who then created the National Center for Policy Analysis (NCPA) as an organizational vehicle to promote this idea. In turn, the NCPA expanded to advocate for a range of conservative and libertarian ideas. Tom Oliver pointed out the significant role that policy entrepreneurs played in the politics of health reform as well as in broader public health policy making.[29] Most of the important leaders in public health can be viewed as **policy entrepreneurs** of some form as they seek to promote their vision of change through formal policy making or in the political arena.

In public health, there are individuals who are closely identified with specific policy solutions. For those policies that are successfully implemented, the recognition of those individuals places them more in the "great people" category. While they are struggling to attract policy attention to their ideas, they are viewed more as entrepreneurs trying to build support for a policy or an approach. *Moments in Leadership: Case Studies in Public Health Policy* highlights the struggle of some of these policy entrepreneurs who were eventually successful in bringing policies into being. The policy innovations they promote do not necessarily have a unique and inevitable pathway toward implementation. The development of the *Guide to Clinical Preventive Services* promoted by Michael McGinnis, for example, led to adoption by both public agencies and private groups. The policy innovation in this instance was a more general policy solution to a broad scale problem. The downstream policies are yet to be realized, but the promotion of evidence-based guidance for clinical prevention is now a well-established idea.

Great People

In the nineteenth and early twentieth century, the driving forces of history and societal progress were often embodied in the lives of "great men." The American polity and its economy were the result of efforts of the greats: the founding fathers of Washington, Franklin, Jefferson, and later Lincoln, and the Roosevelts. Our industry thrived given the vision and energy of Carnegie, Rockefeller, and Edison. Public health had its own great men and women: Lemuel Shattuck, William Gorgas, William Sedgewick, Dorothea Dix, and Clara Barton are often invoked to help explain why certain decisions were made and the course of events changed to allow for progress. The role of great people in making policy and influencing politics is an important consideration is understanding politics, but it is also a way by which certain political positions and policy platforms are promoted by invoking an important historical figure as being somehow connected to the decisions of the present. Great people do make important differences in their time, but they may have even greater influence as symbols used by their successors.

Luther Terry, Joseph Califano, and C. Everett Koop are often regarded as "great people" in the history of public health for their individual contributions to the political dialogue and the policies that emerged while they served as Surgeon General. They gave voice to positions that were unpopular in government because the policy decisions that had to flow from their words would cost entrenched interests heavily. They used their place of power to "speak truth to power." The post they held survives, but in name only; reorganization in the Dept. of HHS has left the Public Health Service as a largely ceremonial title and role as titular head of the U.S. Public Health Service Commissioned Corps. The "bully pulpit" of the Surgeon General has been largely torn down by recent administra-

tions that see the role of the Surgeon General as more of a symbol than as an actor.[30]

Interest Groups

The power of interest groups in American politics and policy making is perhaps the dominant interpretive lens for understanding how policy emerges. Interest groups are embedded deeply in our political systems because their explicit support by the founding fathers (e.g., Madison's factions) and their implicit recognition in the Constitution (the right to petition government) combined with the ease with which we allow groups to coalesce and receive formal recognition. The United States tax code recognizes several types of voluntary organizations that can influence the political process. So called 501(c)(3) organizations are "absolutely prohibited from directly or indirectly participating in, or intervening in, any political campaign on behalf of (or in opposition to) any candidate for elective public office." However, these organizations can participate in "voter education" activities, which is a very gray area. Those not-for profit, tax-exempt associations can, however, participate in lobbying activities that attempt to influence legislation as long as it is not the majority of their activity. Other more political organizations can be recognized as 501(c)(4), but donations to those organizations are not tax-exempt, and their participation in politics is permitted. Examples of these organizations include the American Association of Retired Persons (AARP), the National Rifle Association (NRA), MoveOn.org, and the Christian Coalition. So-called "527" organizations have recently emerged as another vehicle for financing political activities. They are formed to influence issues, not candidates, and are not regulated by the Federal Elections Commission (FEC). They are influential in conservative and liberal movements and include groups such as Emily's List, Swift Boat Veterans for Truth, and the Sierra Club.

The current role of interest groups in health policy is found to be most effective when they function in coalitions,[4] or as advocacy coalitions.[31] Interest groups are not always successful in achieving their goals. For example, there has long been a recognition that rural economic interests have not been powerful,[32] but the interest group coalition surrounding rural health care has been especially effective in getting attention and favorable policies in Congress.[33]

In public health, interest group activity has a very fluid structure. The many factions and stakeholders in the public health field see their claim to policy attention as paramount. The APHA itself can be viewed as more of a federation of groups working under a "big tent" of progressive interests. The Association includes many sections, caucuses, and Special Primary Interest Groups (SPIGS) that are as varied as podiatric health, disability, homelessness, laboratory, food and nutrition, and chiropractic. These groupings allow individuals who may identify professionally more with a specific discipline (e.g., epidemiology) or profession (e.g., chiropractic) to combine for common advocacy and programs support. The Association has attracted criticism by conservatives as too much concerned with a "social justice agenda" and not focused on practical public health policy issues.[34] This "drift" in focus and message can impair an advocacy group in its ability to provide a clear and cogent message. However, when there is a need for a broad-based coalition to motivate a large number of supporters in a coherent campaign, these larger associations can provide the breadth of support necessary to motivate politicians. These broad scale movements in support of policy change are often called "grassroots" because they rise from the ground up.

In recent years, movements that appear to be generated from grass-roots activity have been shown to be manipulated by interests operating more or less centrally. This charge has been leveled at the Christian Right and their involvement in national elections as centralized advocacy groups mobilized conservative ministers and churches. These campaigns, called "astro-turf," emphasizing their artificiality, are controversial and, on the one hand, do reflect broad involvement or voice from voters and citizens, but their original motivation is clearly from political centers and professional operatives. This tendency toward "professionalization"

of membership groups has happened on the left and right as the recruitment of the media and the use of sophisticated communications technologies requires substantial technical knowledge and experience.[35]

WHAT ARE PUBLIC HEALTH POLITICS AND POLICY MAKING ALL ABOUT?

The "whats" of policy making in public health are the topics and issues that are being considered and for which policy is being made. These are intangible things in a system that is largely devoted to the distribution of resources, favor, or restraint. What we are debating or considering on any given day will certainly change, but there are issues that tend to rise and fall in the degree of attention they receive in the policy-making process. Describing an **agenda** for policy making has been one of several useful interpretive structures that help outside observers as well as policy makers themselves understand what is going on.

Agendas and Plans

At any time in the political life of the nation, some issues seem to dominate the news and the attention of the public. This is also true for public health. Whether it the issue is smoking cessation or preparedness for bioterror, only a few topics tend to rise to the top of the political agenda in any given year. Only so much time is available to legislators and administrators to make policy changes. The most important issues that these individuals and institutions confront at any given time are collectively called the policy agenda. The idea of an "agenda" with a limited set of issues is an established idea in political analysis. Anthony Downs described an "issue-attention cycle" that tracked how the attention of politicians and policy makers was dominated at times by specific issues that then faded away over time.[36] John Kingdon emphasizes the importance of the somewhat restricted policy agenda and described how specific topics came onto or dropped off of the national policy agenda.[3] Baumgardner and Jones argued that the narrow focus that the agenda-setting process brings to a few issues tends to hide the overall continuity that underlies the system where there is a relatively constant process of policy building more or less behind the scenes.[37] Their public health-oriented example of tobacco and pesticide legislation traced a pattern of relatively constant and incremental policy formation that allowed more distributed benefits of regulation to trump the concentrated costs to specific industries. This notion of the balance of benefits and costs was posited originally by James Q. Wilson, who suggested that there were paradoxical situations where the concentration of costs on a particular industry or social sector would negate the ability of policy advocates to pass legislation that had diffuse benefits. One example of this is emissions abatement in electrical production to clean the air of pollutants.[38] However, there are multiple examples of how these "imbalanced" policies have been enacted to benefit the public's health[29] (see Table 5.1).

Patient politics are the "normal" redistribution of resources that benefit a well-organized interest group, for example, in health care, the use of Medicare funds for graduates medical education. The "entrepreneurial politics" quadrant is where public health politics are most often played out. For example, pollution abatement, seat belt laws, vaccine requirements, and other policies that burden individuals or small groups but distribute the benefits widely across populations are entrepreneurial in nature. They require aggressive, creative arguments for policy makers to grasp the benefits of their passage, and widespread acceptance on the part of the political community and the public.

Laws, Rules, Regulations

The "laws of the land" are distributed across the constitution of the United States, the separate constitutions of the several states, and the enacted codes of the nation and the states. These form only a part of the formal legal structure for the nation, as there are many other sets of rules, codes, regulations, statutes, and policies that either guarantee certain rights, set obligations, or guide or restrict action in some way. Public health law is often described as having its primary basis in the common law "police powers" reserved to the states. In reality, in the twenty-first century, a robust mix of statutes and legal structures affect the public's

Table 5.1. Wilson's Framework for Policy Analysis

		BENEFITS	
		Concentrated	**Diffuse**
COSTS	**Diffuse**	**Patient politics** *Politically attractive*	**Majoritarian politics**
	Concentrated	**Interest Group politics**	**Entrepreneurial politics** *Politically Unattractive*

Concentrated Effects
- Large magnitude
- Occur immediately
- Direct traceable impact
- Identifiable group of geography

Diffuse Effects
- Small in magnitude
- Occur over time
- Indirect less traceable impacts
- Broad, less identifiable population

SOURCES: Adapted from Oliver TR. The politics of public health policy. Annu Rev Public Health. 2006;27:195–233.[29] and Wilson JQ. American Government: Institutions and Policies. Lexington, MA: D.C. Health and Company; 1992.[39]

health or the public health structure and draw on a broad range of legal sources. The stability of this mixed set of legal authorities was jolted by the terrorist attacks of 2001 where multiple jurisdictions and conflicting authorities were revealed to be threats to the protection of the public.[40]

The process of "modernizing" public health law was underway before the terrorist attacks, and the attacks served to some degree as focusing events that opened a window of opportunity for sweeping change in public health law. The Turning Point Initiative of the W.K. Kellogg Foundation and the IOM's 1988 report, *The Future of Public Health* called for widespread rewriting of the nation's public health statutes. Following the attacks of 9/11, efforts were set in motion to modernize state public health and emergency powers acts, and model statutes were disseminated and distributed. This was met with some resistance as debates erupted over how much additional "coercive" power should be given to government. The politics of this debate brought left-wing civil libertarians together with right-wing traditional libertarians, both concerned with erosion of individual right and freedoms. This resistance blunted some of the most aggressive efforts, and the changes that were made in the following years tended to be incremental and clarifying rather than broadly reforming.

Political struggles sometimes emerge as 1 or more of the 50 states or other jurisdictions contend with the federal government over the applicability or the intensity of some specific law or regulation. This federal-state-local tension is apparent in public health law as localities often react to strong concentrated pressure from groups to restrain behavior (anti-smoking ordinances) or industry (abatement rules) that may exceed their statutory powers or conflict with interests whose abilities to sway legislatures is much greater than their ability to move local councils.

Institutions

In speaking of institutions in politics and policy, we are referring to the major elements of the political structure, such as the legislative branch or the executive branch, but also include informal institutions

such as the media or "big business." In referring to the institutional power of government, we are referring to how the structures and traditions of that branch have become powerful in and of themselves.[41] Steinmo described institutions and "simple rules" that serve as the "foundation for political behavior," and these institutions are very powerful in defining the policy agenda and the outcomes of policy debates.[42] Some who emphasize institutions go so far as to say that the rules are in fact laws that guide political behavior, and that all people function according to their rational self-interest. In health policy, Paul Feldstein presents this argument for the development of health policy.[43]

In public health politics, it is accepted that certain institutional players operate more or less consistently toward the development of public health policy. Big business is seen as predictably opposing adding restrictions on emissions or tightening workplace rules, whereas organized labor may regularly take the opposite stance. These generalizations, themselves, signal the recognition of an institutional player identified by some symbolic collective term.

Some institutions are somewhat special to public health. In the field, we often speak of "public-private partnerships" as being a special mechanism to bridge the gaps between institutional interests. The same holds when the "community" is invoked as a unitary element to either be considered or consulted.[44,45]

Symbols

Politics is played out with many symbols being invoked to promote policies or to rally support for programs.[2,46] Public health, itself, can be used in a symbolic sense by politicians when they call for "more funding for public health" or for programs that "protect the public's health." Those two uses convey very different meanings depending on the context. The rhetoric of politics requires the use of symbols to both define concepts as well as align related groups and policies.[47] The ability to manipulate symbols is now considered a key attribute of the successful politician or political movement. The careful crafting of political messages brought Newt Gingrich to power, and his method of "capturing the rhetorical high ground" is a lesson learned by both the left and right.[48]

Public health has been viewed as the expression of "social justice" by some and as a pragmatic mechanism to ensure national productivity by others.[49,50] The use of metaphors is as important to the conduct of debate as it is to the development of policy. Structuring a public health debate around a notion of a healthy "ecology" would generate substantially different outcomes than a debate where the dominant theme was the creation of healthy individuals or a healthy economy. In recent years, public health improvement has focused on the role of "place" and neighborhood in creating the opportunities and conditions in which people can live healthier lives.[51] This use of place-based metaphors and identifiers has shifted policy discussions away from "personal behavior" toward more general mechanisms to intervene to improve health.

Rights and Freedoms

Some argue that the basis for government is the protection of individual rights; John Locke argued that "civil government is the proper remedy for the inconveniences of the state of nature."[52] To Locke, that "state of nature" is freedom, and government's proper role is to preserve that freedom mainly by preserving our fundamental rights of property and autonomy. In public health, the essential rights we often speak of are those that protect us from interferences and harm. These are often called negative rights in contrast to positive rights that entitle us to some benefit, such as health care or privacy. However, the complex relationship between liberty and rights creates a tension that is very apparent in public health. Mill's principle that our liberties, meaning rights to freedom of action, end where we begin to harm others is not sufficient to justify a robust public health approach.[53] Prevention and protection provide a form of extension of our positive rights that allow us freedom to enjoy cleaner air, safe water, and longer lives.

Arguments over rights in public health can pit the collective and the individual in stark terms. The right to smoke cigarettes may be invoked by some who are actually more concerned with noninterference. Likewise, the rights of others to clean air is expressed more effectively when it is cast as a protection rather than a guarantee. Mary Ann Glendon sees these conflicts over contending rights as misplaced and reflective of a society "obsessed with laws."[54] Public health is often more comfortable set in the context of a contractual world where the balance between fungible interests can be resolved. Absolute rights create irresolvable conflicts. Dan Beauchamp sees public health as a social and governmental process that is essentially pragmatic in nature, an expression of democracy itself, not a "thing" guaranteed in a structure of law-based rights.[55]

The relationship between universal human rights and public health was made forcefully by Jonathan Mann who argued that people could not function with dignity without their health and that public health systems were the best means of producing and protecting health.[56] This connection is now recognized as a movement of its own with the *Health and Human Rights* journal founded by Mann, expressing the central arguments that promoting the public's health promotes justice and prosperity and is a moral obligation of governments and individuals.[57] Mann's belief was that ". . . in the modern world, public health officials have, for the first time, two fundamental responsibilities to the public: to protect and promote public health ands to protect and promote human rights."[58]

Governments

Government and public health are joined closely; public health is often thought of exclusively as a government activity, but it is much more especially when you consider the important interaction among personal behavior, corporate decisions, and formal government policy. The United States is blessed (or cursed) with many types and levels of government. The states ceded power to the federal government via the Constitution, but they also had the power to create entities that can tax, control the disposition of property, restrain individual behavior, and issue rules and regulations under the rubric of public health. The United States conducts a "census of governments" every five years. The latest reported that there were 87,576 different government entities in the United States as of June 30, 2002; 38,967 are general-purpose local governments with the balance as special-purpose local government. There are 13,506 school districts and 35,052 special districts.[59] The 3,034 county units as well as many subcounty municipal units operate health departments or cooperate in a multicounty health district. Of the approximately 3000 local public health departments, many are structured by county government, but others are structured by municipalities. This multiplicity of government creates the potential for a chaotic mixture of conflicting roles and standards as each governmental entity seeks to maintain its own power and autonomy; this is not the case for public health because the profession has been able to develop general guidelines, if not enforceable standards, for the field. These standards, combined with federal guidance from the CDC, have given the American public health system a reasonable level of uniformity across the many jurisdictions. The "professional" nature of public health has overcome the potential barriers of separate and multiple government structures to create a relatively uniform "practice" of governmental public health.

This is not to say that there is complete uniformity; indeed, it is the lack of harmonization of standards and procedures that the profession has recognized as the Achilles heel of the American public health system. The IOM committees that have issued reports on the state and future of public health in the United States have been clear in their concern over the lack of effective standards, describing the system as in "disarray" in 1988[60] and "a governmental public health structure that is fragmented, inadequately funded and needs updates" in 2003.[26] The variation among states has been described by the IOM committee as "profound in structure substance and procedures," yet the system has been functional. This, in turn, speaks to the resilience of the American governmental system where the many layers of the structure tend to support a common democratic impulse, creating a form of competitive civic competence.

Communities

Communities are a unique facet in policy making in the United States, and they are especially relevant in public health, which tends to emphasize community.[61] Community is a potent symbol in many issue domains, including politics, economics, demography, geography, public health, and health care delivery itself. However, the value of symbols lies in their defiance of strict definitions; symbols can bring together people for common action by obscuring their specific differences.[47] A progressive person who wants to promote a program that sees health as a collective responsibility can coexist with a conservative person who sees health as an individual responsibility when they both agree that the solution to a health issue lies in changing "community values."

In the process of identifying and addressing social needs, there are "units of analysis" or "denominators" that are more or less suited for use by the policy world for assistance in decision making. Ordinary people also want to understand what is happening in their everyday lives so they can improve their conditions of life or avoid dangers and threats, and the status of their immediate environment is often expressed as a rate or proportion ("one out of every six Chicagoans will suffer from diabetes"). These rates, denominators, and administratively defined populations have been used since the inception of governments to describe populations. They are usually based on geopolitical boundaries, but much effort has recently gone into characterizing areas that were set up to expedite the delivery of mail. Whether these are the right denominators (or areas, or communities) on which measures of health, or lack of it, for communities should be based is open to discussion. Given that the process creates boundaries and groups, one would expect to hear a good deal of such discussion. However, there is less than might be expected given the very crucial importance of denominators in generating any kind of statistical rate for measures of population health. The acceptance of existing geopolitical and postal geography for epidemiology has been almost universal, and the citizenry as well as the politicians have been essentially passive, leaving the process to the experts. That might change when the measures are intended to describe how well prepared a community is to cope with its problems. We are used to have our problems described to us but not so used to having rates and measures that say, in effect, "we're not up to the job." The recent search for measures of social capital and various rankings of counties as high or low in social capital may open the door for a reaction to this kind of characterization.

The identification of communities and boundaries for some form of measurement is familiar to policy makers. When confronted with a need to act on a problem, the policy maker sees the problem tied closely to the boundaries that represent what the policy maker can control, and those boundaries are fixed, often constitutional, and "real" in both their perception and utility for policy.[62] Figure 5.1 depicts the relationship between the normal policy boundaries and the relevant boundaries that enclose problems that relate to water quality and air pollution

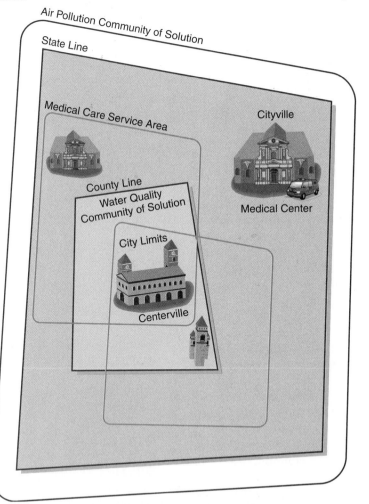

Figure 5.1. Communities of Solution from *Health is a Community Affair*

SOURCE: Reprinted by permission of the publisher from HEALTH IS A COMMUNITY AFFAIR by the National Commission on Community Health Services, p. 3, Cambridge, Mass.: Harvard University Press, Copyright © 1966 by The President and Fellows of Harvard College.[63]

and the "communities of solution" for those problems. The figure is drawn from *Health is a Community Affair*, published in 1966 by the National Commission on Community Health Services.

Note: This chapter draws on the concepts of "communities of solution" and problem-sheds renamed "communities of need" as a way to develop an approach to the measurement of community capacity to improve population health. This chapter also accepts the realities of a relatively fixed policy landscape represented by county and state lines as equally valid to the landscapes of solutions and problems as seen by epidemiologists, public health professionals, medical care practitioners, and the public.

WHEN DOES PUBLIC HEALTH POLICY MAKING HAPPEN?

"Timing is everything in politics" is an oft-repeated nostrum likely to be heard or written in relationship to any specific issue. In public health, the reliance on continuing protections in the infrastructure, water quality, safety, air quality, and responsiveness to immediate and overwhelming threats, such as AIDS, SARS, bioterror, presents political challenges to public health. The field must maintain and regenerate infrastructure as a continuing process that relies on annual budgets and long-term commitments, as well as react swiftly and effectively in uncertain political terrain when new issues arise, often overnight. The combination of long-term predictability and unpredictability creates pressure for public health leaders to assume Janus-like capabilities, which can challenge even experienced political operatives.

Temporal factors in the politics of public health reflect broader political trends and cycles. These are discussed in policy texts as **windows of opportunity** or of specific cycles tied to elections and budgets. However, the force of history looms large in political consideration in many fields but especially in public health where we are often given only the lesson of history to help anticipate what may happen in the future. The contemporary terrain includes a potential massive outbreak of avian influenza, and the lessons of the 1918 outbreak figure heavily as both a template for action as well as a mechanism for stimulating attention.

Windows of Opportunity

Policy windows are those periods in the policy-making process where things can and do change, where ideas emerge "whose time has come," or when a series of "coincident events" create conditions that are favorable to the implementation of a policy that was formerly "premature" of "unacceptable." The brute force of big events, such as a terrorist attack, can create conditions for broad-scale reform in the public health structure, or the force of such an event can be dissipated in endless discussions of changes that need to be made while the real political power, in the form of funding or leadership, is lacking.

An example of a "concentrating" event in public health that opened windows of opportunity was the rise of HIV/AIDS that stimulated changes in research funding, treatment access, laws and rules of privacy, and the perception of the public toward various high-risk groups. The practical political impact is reflected in the rise in influence of pressure groups interested in fast-track research.

Election Cycles

In government, windows of opportunity open often when the people in charge change, and this cycle is somewhat regular due to elections and term limits. The power of elections to change the political landscape has recently been demonstrated. In the words of William Roper, former CDC and HCFGA chief, writing in November of 2006 after the Democrats gained control of the House and Senate:

> There will be a window of opportunity in 2007 to legislate on some key health and health care issues, but by early 2008 that window will have closed, as the presidential campaign will be then be in full swing.

This speaks to the powers of elections past as well as anticipated elections. The national policy process is punctuated by regular congressional and presidential elections that open up windows of opportunity for policy change, especially if there is a sharp change in the power structure. The new leadership in Congress or the White House will sometimes see a "mandate for change" that can reflect public pressure, acquiescence to major changes, or retrenchment in policies.

Funding Cycles

American politics in public health is, in a sense, dominated by our annual budgeting process. Although we do create long-term authorizations, and recurring budgets are relatively stable, we generally pass state and local budgets every year. This puts almost every aspect of governmental public health "at risk" for legislative involvement. The annual crisis-driven budget cycle in the Congress known as "reconciliation" has become well known as the source of ill-considered and often extensive policy making. The Congress has set certain rules for its budget process, but divided government with Democrats in the majority or in office in the Presidency and Republicans holding the other branch created budget stalemates that required extraordinary processes to pass appropriations. These so-called Omnibus bills (OBRA, SOBRA, COBRA, TEFRA, BBA, and BBRA) included many enabling and directive laws that changed public health policy. Some were considered in hearings and the "normal" legislative process and included in final passage; others were the result of rushed compromises as part of huge and often contradictory enactments.

Selected public health issues have become leverage points in this process. Stem cell research and late-term abortions, for example, have been "hot-button" items that are inserted in larger bills with the goal of forcing a vote that will in effect stall passage of appropriations for "normal" government activities. Because these are germane to health, they are often inserted in the appropriations bills for labor, health and human services, and education—the cluster of appropriations that covers much of federal health activities. This often slows or even completely stalls final action on the funding bills. The solution necessary to keep government running is to pass continuing resolutions that essentially set in place funding levels as the level of the previous year's appropriations. In February of 2007, Congress essentially agreed to give up on passing appropriations for many parts of government, including health and human services, by extending the relevant continuing resolution through Fiscal Year 2007. This is an unusual approach even in a process that has apparently no set rules and is an outgrowth of the divided government that has become common early in the twenty-first century.

Agendas as Schedules

The budget cycle is one temporal element of the agenda process. Election cycles and the natural history of policy proposals, the "issue-attention cycle" mentioned earlier, are also important to the timing of policy events. There are also contrived agendas that presidents, agency heads, congressional leaders, or caucuses set that control the ascent of issues into the policy-making process. Presidents are now fond of declaring a 100-day agenda; Newt Gingrich created a "contract with America" that was essentially an agenda for a large voting bloc in Congress; and in the 109th Congress, Speaker Nancy Pelosi declared a 100-hour schedule in the House of Representatives with specific legislative goals. These structured agendas can be derailed; for example, Gingrich's plans were interrupted by a breakdown in Medicare reform when rural hospital interests balked at budget cuts. However, they also can be just as powerful in keeping issues out of the process as they are in promoting policies. Secretary of HHS, Michael Leavitt, entered office with a 500-day plan (http://www.hhs.gov/500DayPlan/500dayplan. html) that essentially signaled to his agency that no substantive work would be done on anything except what was included in the list.

History

George Santayana is famously quoted as saying that "those who cannot learn from history are condemned to repeat it." More recently, the author David McCullough said: "History is a guide to navigation in perilous times. History is who we are and why we are the way we are." These wise admonitions can well be applied to the development of policy in public health or any field, but they are especially true in public health where human history is richly embroidered with the struggle to cope with disease, disability, and threats to life. Certainly, we must imagine new futures and innovative ways to cope with emerging infections, and lives always bounded by the threat of terror; however, that does not take away the value of the lessons of history. The recounting of *The Great Influenza* by John M. Barry drove home the need to change how we were prepared to react to the H51C bird virus. The speed of transmission, the breadth of the pandemic, and the failure of many rationally developed policies are realities that can be learned best by putting them in the context of lived history.

Politicians are inclined to reflect on historical events to give their current policy proposals a place in history as well as allow their constituents to interpret what they are proposing by drawing comparisons. Historical symbology plays an important role in contemporary policy development. Likewise, historical failures often condemn certain ideas to the trash heap. Health planning, for example, was an idea whose time had come, and its apparent failure marked it to this day as a poor way to allocate resources and even worse as a policy option.[64]

WHERE DO PUBLIC HEALTH POLITICS AND POLICY MAKING HAPPEN?

The notion of place in policy making is a subtle concept, but often the geographical context of a policy decision is the most important factor shaping how it evolves and is applied. The United States is a large and largely self-sufficient nation, and its politics reflect a particularism and tradition of independence that often rejects other national models. These conditions hold in public health as well. The nation was built on a tradition of self-reliance and invention that followed necessity. Its social and political structures as well as its public health system emerged from pragmatic local and national accommodations to the realities of a rapidly growing, industrializing nation that had immense natural resources to exploit.

American Values

The development of American values has been traced by historians and contemporary critics of the nation. De Tocqueville's observations remain trenchant and are often repeated to this day. More contemporary writers and observers reflect with some amazement on the continued applicability of reference to values and moral systems in explaining and predicting public health policy. James Morone, a political scientist, suggests that we are a nation with a strong moral streak combined with a national affection of individualism.[65,66] This paradoxical combination of a tendency to impose values as well as celebrate their rejection is used as much to explain policy failure as to anticipate and shape policy decisions.

For public health, the paradox presents very practical problems. The pressure to preserve individual liberties flies directly in the face of the need to protect the commons, to exert restraint on behavior through various proscribed activities.[67] These conflicts are most apparent in issues such as motorcycle helmets and anti-smoking ordinances. Morality is often invoked in ways that may strike the observer as strange. In obesity policy making, for example, it may seem apparent that overweight is a public health problem with a clear solution. However, a "blaming the victim" counterargument can be invoked based on a sense that there is a conflict between personal and collective moral positions.[68]

Border Realities

As you know, the United States is a continental nation with two neighbors: Canada, with a very similar cultural and economic structure, and Mexico, with different languages, differing cultures, and a developing economy. This geography has important implications for public health policy making in that the nation faces a huge array of environments and conditions to either promote or thwart vectors and living conditions. The long contiguous borders allow for populations of people as well as animals and microbes to move easily into and out of the country. These physical conditions have been managed by a quarantine and inspection systems (similar measures have been implemented on the borders between states, namely, medfly control in California).[69] Challenging policy making along the border today is the ebb and flow of humans into and out of the United States. The rapid and sustained rise of immigration, illegal and otherwise, from the south has created population health concerns that confront the public health system.

The influx of Mexican and other South American immigrants into the United States, largely to fill low-wage jobs, has become a major policy issue transcending health care and public health. This situation represents how the politics and policy mechanisms of a more broadly applicable issue can dominate a more specific one; the interesting twist to this policy dominance is that the more specific policies of public health tended to thwart the more "powerful" and more broadly applicable policies of immigration. The politics of immigration caused some states and the federal government to curtail access to safety net programs for individuals who could not show proof of legal residence.[70,71] The border itself has generated a new definition of a population to calculate epidemiological rates.[72,73] The border represents another form of public health threat when considered in the context of terrorism and bioterrorism threats.[74]

Regional Concerns

The geography of the United States reflects historical as well as geological and meteorological realities. The nation was settled or conquered from east to west, and the indigenous peoples were pushed into the sparsely settled and arid western lands, which were then largely ignored. The South embraced slavery and created a disenfranchised population that, when freed, sought to migrate to places where there was more tolerance and opportunity. These realities of place and people created the basis for persisting inequities and disparities in health.[75] The geography of race and ethnicity once saw concentrations of groups in certain places, for example, Hispanics in the western border states and poor blacks in the rural South and central northern cities. Those patterns are quickly breaking down as populations continue to be very mobile, and new immigrants move to places where jobs are available far away from the "traditional" settling places. There remain significant geographic and regional clusters of poverty and lack of development that create regional political pressures. Those areas are also marked by their very poor public health statistics.[76]

The region that includes and immediately borders the Appalachian Mountains were long synonymous with persistent rural poverty. To address poverty in those towns and counties, regional, quasi-political structures were created to build infrastructure and support development. The Tennessee Valley Authority and later the Appalachian Regional Commission were created to focus efforts in paces that were common in their economic and social characteristics but crossed many state boundaries. These regional solutions to common geographic problems are not well accepted in the federal structure; the power base to support them is diffuse and unorganized and often conflicts with claimants and stakeholders in the states and localities who are included in the region.

Other regional "authorities" have been developed with the intent of closing persistent economic gaps. These also include substantial attention to health and public health issues. The Delta Regional Authority and Denali Regional Commissions include direct support for health care delivery and prevention and public health.

Federalism

The federal structure of American government is a unique characteristic of the American polity that is very important to public health policy.[16] Federalism refers to the system of government where the original, sovereign powers of government rested within the several states, and those states ceded specific powers to the federal or central government by ratifying the Constitution. The states retained the common law "policy powers," which reserved to them the responsibility and the power to protect the public's health, safety, and welfare. To exercise this power, the states were free to create other levels of government as they saw fit: counties, towns, municipalities, and authorities. This left the nation with a very complex structure of state, local, and national government with the principal responsibility for public health held by the states.

This complexity, as it relates to public health, is viewed as both a weakness and a strength.[60] Federalism, to Oliver, allows us to experiment to some degree with policy formation where the states operate as the "laboratories of democracy"; however, that can create bewildering variation in policies in some sectors.[29]

Although the legal basis for public health laws rests in the states and common law, the federal government assumed a leadership role in protecting the public using other clauses in the Constitution, most notable the "Commerce Clause" to justify the Food and Drug Act and other protections for workers or for clean air and water. For much of the twentieth century, it could be said that the notable advances in public health were the result of federal legislation that were the result of federal political structures and process. Toward the end of the century, the federal government, the Congress, and the executive branch, backed away from active promotion of public health issues, and the states were left to either act or to remain passive as the "new federalism" devolved the initiative for further public activity to the states.[16] There remain substantial forces alive for further public health regulation and policy making in Congress and the national executive branch, but the states have been very active in

recent years as they recognize the opportunity to regulate behavior to protect lives (e.g., smoking restrictions), and the need to restructure and modernize bureaucracies to prepare for major threats (e.g., pandemic flu or a bioterrorism attack).

Although this balance of power between the states and the central government may seem ripe for conflict, the tenor of the politics have been cooperative and supportive; the federal government, through grants-in-aid, has sought to foster uniformity and support technical capacity within the states. The states, for their part, have accepted this technical interference in their roles and often identify with the federal agencies, the CDC and the Dept. of HHS, as a unified "public health community." This cooperation often takes the form of technical collaboration with tight links being constructed between specific agencies at the state level and their federal counterparts. These connections may run counter to prevailing state-federal relations between other parts of the executive branches and reflect to some degree the independent power of bureaucracies to find common ground. However, when there are significant disputes between a state or states and the federal government over issues in public health, policy making and policy maintenance can be thwarted (e.g., medical marijuana laws).

WHY PUBLIC HEALTH POLICY? WHY PUBLIC HEALTH POLITICS?

Politics and policy making in the Untied States may seem to be driven by our collective desires to achieve the goals set out in the Preamble to the Constitution. Public health as promoting the general welfare may seem most relevant to some, whereas others may see the establishment of justice as what guides our collective decision making. However, as the debates in the 13 original state assemblies that led to the adoption of the Constitution revealed, there was as much concern about the maintenance of trade and the economy as there was concern with fundamental, philosophical liberties and rights. The practical evolution of public health agencies emerged from practical collective decisions made by local authorities under their interpretation of the reserved police powers. This dependence on pragmatics and local authority complicates any attempt to identify a central answer to the question of "why?" in public health policy making. Over time, we have developed some main themes that can be used to categorize the justifications for public health policy.

Liberal Traditions

The heart of our legal as well as philosophical traditions have focused on the idea that all persons enjoy individual and inviolable rights that the government is bound to protect. The **liberal traditions** of American politics are at the core of the public health policy paradox: how collective action can occur in a nation that values individual liberty. The United States has a long history of balancing the powers of government and the prerogatives and freedoms of the individual. Many of the central conflicts of the republic have come over issues surrounding public health that saw individual rights in conflict with the collective powers and needs of the nation or state.

Liberal justice emphasizes individual responsibility, minimal collective action, and freedom from collective obligations except to respect the fundamental rights of others. John Stuart Mill's essay "On Liberty" remains a much-read guide to the limits of government and the responsibilities of individuals.[77] Liberal justice historically has sought to limit the range of interests people can claim in conditions conducive to well being, but in recent years, a more libertarian model of justice has surfaced that stresses traditional values. F.A. Hayek, a libertarian much admired by the new conservatives, sees the social structures, uniformities, and regularities by which public health advances the common health as merely "spontaneous orders" produced by individuals and organizations, and the dream of social justice as a "mirage."[78]

The alternative to the libertarian theme is one of social justice where the underlying problems of inequality and injustice are taken as a problem and not a condition. This recognition of inequality, or in modern public health parlance, disparity, as a problem subject to policy interventions fits well into Kingdon's structure of how issues move on to an agenda and find a match with policy solutions.

Economics

The United States is a free-market democracy with a strong tradition and a political structure that favors commerce and trade. This economic orientation was explicitly included in the discussions that led to the adoption of the Constitution. The framers were as worried about the effects on commerce as they were on the individual liberties of the new citizens.[79] From the founding of the republic there has been a tension between the demand of commerce and the health of the people; Nancy Milio posed the contrast starkly by asking "Is a healthy profit compatible with a healthy population?"[80]

Conflicts between economic interests and public health are often very public and dramatic. The pressures for profits drive corporations to pollute water and air, which in turn creates measurable health consequences. The Love Canal example is one of many.[81] The role of business is often seen as naturally oppositional to public health interests. Charles Lindblom described the "market prison" that forces elected officials and bureaucrats to favor market expansion over health or public protection.[82] However, there have been significant constraints placed on the freedom of business to ignore the health of the public and equally significant restraints on personal behavior, such as smoking, that have important effects on the viability of business.

The surprising ability of the United States to control the negative health effects of market activity is seen as somewhat surprising by some who see the regulatory advances of the 1960s as somewhat out of step with American traditions.[83] However, aggressive agencies that confront business often "have their wings clipped" as did the Environmental

Protection Agency (EPA) and the Occupational Safety and Health Administration (OSHA) when their enthusiastic enforcement of the laws in the 1970s was met with administrative and Congressional opposition in the 1980s.[84] However, the important thing is that those agencies persisted beyond the 1980s into the twenty-first century, their mechanisms to control pollution or occupational hazards remain in place, and their effects have created an overall better environment and workplace than would have occurred without their work.[55,85]

Values in Public Health: Justice and Utility

Amartya Sen, the Nobel Laureate in economics, speaks of democracy's values as *intrinsic*, (one vote, one person, etc.), *instrumental* (giving voice to the hitherto powerless), and *constructive* (forging new interests and needs in the conditions for social justice through conflict and democratic discussion). These may be seen as values more aligned with notions of justice than with the general welfare.[86] Dan Beauchamp wrote an important essay that equated pubic health with social justice.[50] That juxtaposition has helped structure arguments for expanded government activity in public health as well as greater personal responsibility for health. The notion of public health as social justice brings together the components of Sen's democratic values, serving as an example of how democracy should work, balancing the needs of individuals with the pressures and compulsions of the commons. Indeed, Beauchamp points to the resurgence of democracy as the stimulus for public health progress:

> Surely that 10-year increase in life expectancy since 1950 is mostly due to societal sea changes like the sharp decline in smoking from public health campaigns, causing a big drop in heart disease and lung cancer, or to safer highways, less poverty, less discrimination, and cleaner air. For all that, and for Medicare and Medicaid, we can thank resurgent democracy during the Great Society era and the coming to the fore of public health agencies and activism.[87]

A contending value to justice in public health is utility. Historians of public health often trace the origins of the field to the pragmatic and utilitarian calculations of the Victorians who were concerned with the productivity of the Irish peasants, or the Prussian statesman who were concerned with the strength of their emerging nation and its army.[88] Early promoters of public health reforms saw these as investments in productive human capital and saw modest measures to ensure clean air and water as useful "from a commercial point of view. Much remains in public health as a vestige of the view that the population should be made as productive as possible to enrich the state; modern cost-benefit analysis of preventive measures draws on the theories of welfare economics that sees trade-offs in health and lives as subject to valuation and calculation.[26]

The contrast of utilitarian ideals with those of justice does not present an either/or choice. Each presents a schema to help guide practical policy choices. The elaboration of the utilitarian idea into careful cost-benefit studies that consider the widest possible set of externalities can be matched with a careful assessment of the degree to which principles of justice can be applied. This is accomplished through democratic structures and processes that give voice to both sides.

HOW ARE PUBLIC HEALTH POLICY AND POLITICS ACCOMPLISHED?

Policy making is the creation of laws, rules, and regulations, as well as the structured codes created by the state and the federal government. It is the "stuff" that politics creates, but how? Most of the guidance a student gets in introductory politics and policy classes focuses on the formal structure of lawmaking, which is covered extensively in books and guides. "How a Bill Becomes Law" is a classic title of a description of the steps legislation takes before final passage (see, for example, http://thomas.loc.gov/home/holam.txt for a description). Unfortunately, that process is more the exception than the rule in the U.S. Congress and most state assemblies. Public health lawmaking is like any other legislative process, and it enjoys no special stature as, for example, budgeting might. The entire policy-making process in public health extends well beyond the passage of laws because there are public health policy decisions that control the lives and actions of people and institutions that are made by even the sanitation inspector by applying local ordinances.

Lawmaking

"The law is firmly established as a powerful instrument of public health."[89] That close relationship of law and public health created a sense that we can, with the wise use of legal means, improve the health and well being of Americans by tackling the recognizable threats to health. However, this creates in some minds an over-reliance on legal mechanisms. The current controversies over how to deal with rising rates of obesity, exemplifies the attraction of legal remedies for public health problems as we try to make certain products and practices "illegal." This dependence on formal regulation and lawmaking puts public health in a position as a constant participant in the formal governmental process, where legal language and adherence to procedures becomes paramount.

Public health policy to protect the population is characterized by Turshen as falling into three major realms: cleansing the environment, eradicating disease, and containing disease.[90] These options are contrasted with the preferred option of prevention, which, in Turshen's view, is less often available to public health policy makers. Public health law and policy is more often reactive and structured to clean up after hazards are produced (as in Super Fund legislation), to eradicate vectors after they have spread (as polio vaccines), or to contain them when that is the only option (as in pandemic influenza preparedness). Cleansing the environment can be more progressive if it anticipates the impact of emerging threats. However, the process of cleansing often entails transporting and storing hazardous materials that no one wants. The resistance

to siting landfills and hazardous waste containment facilities can be intense and generates a "NIMBY—Not In My Backyard" response as communities are targeted for these uses.

The lawmaking process is a function of the institutions of Congress and the administration and bureaucracy but replicated across the 50 states. The staggering of terms, the varieties of rules and customs, and the natural tensions of one branch against the other multiplied by the federal structure makes lawmaking a complex and inherently conservative process. In public health, this is especially so due to the relative place of the states in terms of their public health responsibilities.

Intergovernmental Processes

The federal system is an important defining element of the public health structure in the United States. State governments are often said to have the original jurisdiction in public health matters by virtue of their police powers, but the proximity of interest groups and stakeholders often makes it difficult for states to enact tightly restrictive policies and laws that affect producers and communities. Where an industry is an important local contributor to the economy, state legislators are loathe to require controls and set standards that would affect profits.[91] By the same token, state localities have been able to pass laws that set stringent air quality levels, restrict smoking, and change the fat content of cooking oils. This is due as much to their responsiveness to public pressure as their sensitivity to organized business pressures. On the other hand, the federal government has the power and ability to control interstate commerce as well as to set national standards for air and water quality or passenger vehicle safety, as well as the deep pockets to support programs to provide vaccinations. However, many programs and initiatives that form the core of public health are actually state-based with significant but minority federal input. Vital statistics and monitoring, for example, are collaborative efforts where state agencies adopt shared standards and grant-in-aid funds are provided by the federal government to supplement state funds. Maternal and child health programs in the states function with substantial federal block grants, with some states far exceeding the federal commitment, while others barely supplement it.

Oliver argues that, in public health, federalism has produced an unhealthy variation in policies to address common problems;[29] this was recognized in public health, and a "public health statute modernization collaborative" was created with the support of the Robert Wood Johnson and W. K. Kellogg Foundations to align the laws and procedures of the states to allow them to better meet the challenges of public health needs and external threats (http://www.turningpointprogram.org). This process has generated initiatives to compare and assess the performance of state public health agencies.[92] That development threatens to weaken the traditional independence and autonomy of the states.

Local governments often bear the greatest burden of enforcing public health laws and making policy that restricts individual and business behaviors. The National Association of County and State Health Officials estimates that there are 2864 local health departments in the United States.[93] These are often overseen by elected or appointed boards with executive powers and authority, and they contend with state laws set by statewide agencies as well as federal standards and rules, and occasionally have direct responsibility to report to federal officials. This very complex system might seem chaotic in one sense, but it is drawn together by a common notion of the unique profession of public health as well as a broad agreement on the core functions and responsibilities of public health.

Markets for Policy

The economist Paul Feldstein sees policy making and politics subject to market rules, where policy makers are merely balancing their demands with those of other stakeholders, and exchanges of values are accomplished by legislative or administrative "markets."[94] This notion of "trading" in policy is described by Feldstein as an "economic version of interest group theory of legislation" where the special interests are the primary demanders of legislation rather than the people legislators represent.

The suppliers of legislation are the legislators, who redistribute resources, taxes, and power, and the administrative branch that enforces those decisions. The applicability of this framework to public health is more difficult than for other health policy domains. In Feldstein's model, legislation to combat AIDS was not forthcoming until established and recognizable interest groups demanded support for drug research. The evolution of environmental policies that cleaned the air and water are even harder to fit into this theory. Feldstein found that the policies were enacted largely due to a stalemate between contending industrial interests. In the end, he says that the solutions that were put in place were economically inefficient largely because the Congress did not want to cede its power to the market; thus supporting his notion of legislators as suppliers of policy.

Politics of People and Stories

One school of thought sees policy making as structured and subject to scientific rules and patterns, if not fundamental laws. The study of policy analysis has moved itself away from politics, which is seen as emotional and chaotic and manipulated by the unscrupulous or the driven. However, it is the chaos and the struggle that creates the effective stories of politics and is the real theme that supports policy making, even in a professionally dominated, complex world such as public health.

"Organizations, government or private, when they reach a certain size, become 'organized anarchies.'" The anarchic nature of large government is recognizable in the United States in public health policy making. The system is very complex, structurally and conceptually; the stakeholders varied; and, at any given time, any group can dominate. This makes it difficult to apply a "formula" to any description of the process and tends to make it possible to just "tell the story" as it happens. This is where the idea of pure politics comes into play, that is, the point where it is the combination of the personalities, the place, and the time that conspires to make a thing happen or not. In the United States, the tendency is toward less rather than more change given the conscious and unconscious complexity. However the dominance of people and ideas is evident in the politics. In their book describing the failure of President Clinton's health reform plan, David Broder and Haynes Johnson emphasize how flesh-and-blood people with their personal stories make politics run.[95] They emphasize how the people involved in policy making could stand up to institutions and waves of popular sentiment to bring an "idea whose time had come" to a halt. They also made the point that people's stories change people's minds as they gave examples of real stories from the emergency rooms of Los Angeles to the manufactured story of Harry and Louise. The power of story telling was the power behind policy making. In public health, the stories are a bit different but almost always personal, whether coming from the Love Canal or the family of Ryan White; these stories are the heart of the politics as described by major heads and subheads in Table 5.2.

Table 5.2. The Journalistic Approach to Policy Assessment: A Review

Sets	Subsets	Brief Description
Who	Elites	The people who run things; they sometimes get elected but more often are found running the primary institutions.
	Professionals	Physicians, dentists, lawyers. In public health, there is an emerging trend toward more professionalization.
	Bureaucrats	In and out of government, they have enormous negative power and less often recognized positive power, including the ability to manage and complete very complex tasks.
	Scientists/Academics	People with a "code" of science who are respected by the public. Their sustenance comes from a mix of public and private sources, and their values underpin some aspects of public health: the primacy of data and inquiry.
	Media	Once this was restricted to journalists, but the role of media is now becoming much more diffuse.
	"The People," the public	Voters; they appear in public opinion polls, and they function as communities with specific demands.
	Policy Entrepreneurs	They push solutions by generating ideas and then trying to make them policy.
	Great People	Public health has strong historical figures, but the field is not seen as a place where individual power can be exercised. Great people emerge as role models
What	Agendas and Plans	The political agenda for parties; groups form the starting framework for political debates and controversies.
	Laws, Rules, Regulations	They guide human behavior.
	Customs	These aren't written down, but they also guide behavior.
	Institutions	Banks, hospitals, the Congress, the Administration, and interest group systems.
	Symbols	The flag, equality, efficiency, "15% of the GNP," access, and health.
	Rights	The few guaranteed versus the many claimed.
	Governments	The 7000 jurisdictions, boards, commissions, and authorities that tax and distribute benefits.
	Communities	The innumerable ways people get together and relate to each other. Politics is often practiced most intensively at this level.

Table 5.2. (*continued*)

Sets	Subsets	Brief Description
When	Windows of Opportunity	Kingdon's classic "idea whose time has come." Usually either by the confluence of forces or an unexpected event (death, war, election).
	Election Cycles	They influence behavior and what can be done.
	Funding Cycles	The creation of budgets in the United States is a regular cycle in legislation and opens opportunities to change substantive laws at the same time appropriations are set.
	Agendas and Schedules	The legislative and policy making process has limits to the volume of issues. Timing and priority are very important.
	History	It looms large in policy, as we look to past decisions to guide future decisions.
Where	American Values	We have a manifest destiny, we lead the world, we are a melting pot, and we are dominated by Judeo-Christian ideas.
	Border Realities	In reality, we are a continental nation that has two very different borders, Canada (like us) Mexico (unlike us).
	Regional Concerns	"We don't care how you did it up north" is seen on license plates in the South and there's no denying that there are regional values and health realities for the Appalachians or the upper Midwest.
	Federalism	The states do have power in health; policies can change dramatically as you cross a state border.
Why	Liberal Traditions	We are individuals, with individual freedoms, and science and knowledge lead the way (with a dose of Judeo-Christian authority).
	Economics	Adam Smith said we all seek our own satisfaction and that benefits the masses. Likewise, the complexity of the system reflects the efficiencies gained by the division of labor. However, people often do not seek to optimize health, nor is health a compartmentalized process.
	Values	Christian, humanistic. Either take care of the next person directly or let the market do it while maintaining autonomy. Americans embody a paradox where strong individuals conform to common patterns of consumption and belief.
	Justice	A super-value in that all systems and theories claim to create or promote justice.
How	Lawmaking	The "classic" process of passing legislation, but it has rules, and almost all laws take their own special and unique routes to passage.
	Intergovernmental Processes	America is a federal republic with a unique balance of powers between the central government and the states. Power and politics are often devolved to localities; counties, cities, and so on all have influence over public health.
	Market for Policy	Policies compete for attention and acceptance, just as ideas do. Some are "superior" and accepted; others are rejected.
	Politics	The exercise of power, for its own sake, is a real factor in what policies are adopted.
	Making Deals	"How things really get done," the interaction of people and policies, within the constraints of institutions and time.

REVIEW QUESTIONS

1. What are working definitions of *politics* and *policy*, and how do they differ from formal definitions?
2. In what two principal ways do physicians function in the political process?
3. Describe how academics contribute to policy making.
4. What kinds of people promote a policy "solution" for multiple problems? Describe how they fit into the policy process.
5. How do you know if a specific issue is on the national policy agenda?
6. Using the broad definition of "institutions," identify the leading institutions that are most often involved in public health policy making?
7. Discuss how community has been treated in public health policy, and suggest how to improve our understanding of community.
8. Give examples of statistics that are used as symbols in public health policy making in the United States.
9. What are the most important policy cycles that affect public health policy making? Are there ways in which public health policy transcends those temporal cycles?
10. What are the major places where American public health policy making occurs? What place or level is most important and why?

REFERENCES

1. Homedes N, Ugalde A. Globalization and health at the United States-Mexico border. *Am J Public Health*. December 2003;93(12):2016–2022.
2. Lasswell HD. *Politics: Who Gets What, When, How*. 11th ed. New York: The World Publishing Company; 1971.
3. Kingdon JW. *Agendas, Alternatives and Public Policies*. 2nd ed. New York: HarperCollins; 1995.
4. Heaney MT. Brokering health policy: Coalitions, parties and interest group influence. *Journal of Health Politics, Policy and Law*. October 2006;31(5):887–944.
5. Oliver TK, Jr., Tunnessen WW, Jr., Butzin D, Guerin R, Stockman JA, III. Pediatric work force: Data from the American Board of Pediatrics. *Pediatrics*. 1997;99(2):241–244.
6. Litman TJ, Robins LS, eds. *Health Politics and Policy*. 3rd ed. Albany, NY: Delmar Publishers; 1997.
7. Morone JA, Litman TJ, Robins LS, eds. *Health Politics and Policy*. 4th ed. Clifton Park, NY: Delmar Cengage Learning; 2008.
8. Patel K, Rushevsky ME. *The Politics of Public Health in the United States*. New York: M. E. Sharpe; 2005.
9. Longest BB. *Health Policymaking in the United States*. 4th ed. Chicago: Health Administration Press; 2004.
10. Harrington C, Estes CL, eds. *Health Policy*. 4th ed. Boston: Jones and Bartlett; 2004.
11. McLaughlin CP, McLaughlin CD. *Health Policy Analysis an Interdisciplinary Approach*. Boston: Jones and Bartlett; 2008.
12. Scutchfield FD, Ireson C, Hall L. The voice of the public in public health policy and planning: The role of public judgment. *Journal of Public Health Policy*. 2004;25(2).
13. Coye MJ, Foege WH, Roper WL. *Leadership in Public Health*. New York: Milbank Memorial Fund; 1994.
14. Begun and Lippencott: *Strategic Adaptation in the Health Professions*. Jossey Bass; 1993.
15. Robinson TP. Spatial statistics and geographical information systems in epidemiology and public health. *Adv Parasitol*. 2000;47:81–128.
16. Turnock BJ, Atchison C. Governmental public health in the United States: The implications of federalism. *Health Affairs*. 2002;21(6):68–78.
17. Jacobson N, Butterill D, Goering P. Consulting as a strategy for knowledge transfer. *Milbank Quarterly*. 2005;82(2):299–321.
18. Schultz J. *Reviving the Fourth Estate: Democracy, Accountability & the Media*. Cambridge: Cambridge University Press; 1998.
19. Fallows J. *Breaking the News: How the Media Undermine American Democracy*. New York: Pantheon Books; 1996.
20. Singhal A, Rogers EM. *Combating AIDS: Communication Strategies in Action*. Thousand Oaks, CA: Sage; 2003.
21. Grier S, Bryant CA. Social marketing in public health. *Annu Rev Public Health*. 2005;26:319–339.

22. Siegel M. Mass media antismoking campaigns: A powerful tool for health promotion. *Ann Intern Med.* July 15, 1998;129(2):128–132.

23. Wolfe A. *Does American Democracy Still Work?* New Haven, CT: Yale University Press; 2006.

24. Soroka SN, Lim ET. Issue definition and the opinion-policy link: Public preferences and health care spending in the US and UK. *British Journal of Politics and International Relations.* November 2003(5):4.

25. Blendon RJ, Altman DE. Voters and health care in the 2006 election. *N Engl J Med.* November 2, 2006;355(18):1928–1933.

26. Institute of Medicine. *The Future of the Public's Health in the 21st Century.* Washington, DC: National Academy Press; 2003.

27. Research America. APHA National Poll on American's Attitude Toward Public Health. *American Public Health Association 132nd Annual Meeting.* Washington, DC; 2004.

28. Rosenbaum S, Mauery DR, Blake S, Wehr E. *Public Health in a Changing Health Care System: Linkages between public health agencies and managed care organizations in the treatment and prevention of sexually transmitted diseases.* Washington, DC: Kaiser Family Foundation; 2000.

29. Oliver TR. The politics of public health policy. *Annu Rev Public Health.* 2006;27:195–233.

30. Harris G. Surgeon General sees four-year term as compromised. *New York Times.* July 11, 2007.

31. Sabatier PA, Jenkins-Smith HC. The advocacy coalition framework, an assessment. In: Sabatier PA, ed. *Theories of the Policy Process.* Boulder, CO: Westview Press; 1999.

32. Browne WP. Rural failure: The linkage between policy and lobbies. *Policy Studies Journal.* 2001;29(1):108–117.

33. Lambrew JM. The heartland's heartstrings: The power, challenges and opportunities of rural health advocacy in Washington. *North Carolina Medical Journal.* 2006;67(1):55–57.

34. Satel S. Public Health? Forget It; Cosmic Issues Beckon. *The Wall Street Journal.* December 13, 2001.

35. Skocpol T. Voice and inequality: The transformation of American civic democracy. *Perspectives on Politics.* 2004;2(1):3–20.

36. Downs A. Up and down with ecology: The issue attention cycle. *Public Interest.* 1972;28(1):38–50.

37. Baumgadner FR, Jones BD. *Agendas and Instability in American Politics.* Chicago: University of Chicago Press; 1993.

38. Wilson JQ, Dilulio JJ. *American Government: Institutions and Policies.* 9th ed. New York: Houghton Mifflin; 2004.

39. Wilson JQ. *American Government: Institutions and Policies.* Lexington, MA: D.C. Health and Company; 1992.

40. Gostin LO. Public health and civil liberties in an era of bioterrorism. *Crim Justice Ethics.* Summer 2002;21(2):2,74–76.

41. March J, Olsen J. The new institutionalism: Organizational factors in political life. *American Political Science Review.* 1984;78:734–749.

42. Steinmo S, Watts. J. It's the institutions, stupid. Why comprehensive national health insurance always fails in America. *Journal of Health Politics, Policy and Law.* 1995;20(2):329–372.

43. Feldstein PJ. *The Politics of Health Legislation.* 2nd ed. Chicago: Health Administration Press; 1996.

44. Alexander JA, Weiner BJ, Metzger ME, et al. Sustainability of collaborative capacity in community health partnerships. *Med Care Res Rev.* December 2003;60(4 Suppl):130–160.

45. Weiner BJ, Alexander JA, Shortell SM. Management and governance processes in community health coalitions: A procedural justice perspective. *Health Educ Behav.* December 2002;29(6):737–754.

46. Stone D. *Policy Paradox: The Art of Political Decision Making.* 2nd ed. New York: W. W. Norton & Company; 1997.

47. Stone D. Symbols. *Policy Paradox: The Art of Political Decision Making.* 2nd ed. New York: W. W. Norton & Company; 1997a:137–162.

48. Lemann N. Conservative opportunity society. *The Atlantic.* May 1985:22–36.

49. Beauchamp D. Public health, privatization, and market populism: A time for reflection. *Qual Manag Health Care.* 1997;5(2):73–79.

50. Beauchamp DE. Public health as social justice. *Inquiry.* 1976;13(1):3–14.

51. Kawachi I, Berkman LF. *Neighborhoods and Health.* New York: Oxford University Press; 2003.

52. Locke J. *Second Treatise of Civil Government.* New York: Liberal Arts; 1951.

53. Beauchamp DE. *The Health of the Republic. Epidemics, Medicine, and Moralism as Challenges*

to Democracy. Philadelphia, PA: Temple University Press; 1988.

54. Glendon MA. *Rights Talk: The Impoverishment of Political Discourse*. New York: Free Press; 1991.

55. Beauchamp D. *Health, Social Justice and the Other Great Society*. Chapel Hill: University of North Carolina at Chapel Hill; 2007.

56. Gostin LO. Public health, ethics and human rights: A tribute to the late Jonathan Mann. *Journal of Law Medicine & Ethics*. 2001;29:121–130.

57. Tarantola D, Gruskin S, Brown TM, Fee E. Jonathan Mann: Founder of the health and human rights movement. *Am J Public Health*. Nov 2006;96(11):1942–1943.

58. Mann JM. Medicine and public health, ethics and human rights. In: Beauchamp DE, Steinbock B, eds. *New Ethics for the Public's Health*. New York: Oxford; 1999:83–93.

59. U.S. Census Bureau. *2002 Census of Governments, Volume 1, Number 2, Individual State Descriptions*. Washington, DC: U.S. Government Printing Office; 2002.

60. Institute of Medicine. Committee for the Study of the Future of Public Health. *The Future of Public Health*. Washington, DC: National Academy Press; 1988.

61. Ricketts TC. *Community Capacity to Improve Population Health: Defining Community*. Research Triangle Park: Research Triangle Institute; August 2001. Draft report to the Robert Wood Johnson Foundation.

62. Thomas WI, Znanieki F. *The Polish Peasant in Europe and America*. Eli Zaretsky ed. Urbana: University of Illinois Press; 1996.

63. National Commission on Community Health Services. *Health is a Community Affair Report*. Cambridge, MA: Harvard University Press; 1966.

64. Morone JA. *The Democratic Wish, Popular Participation and the Limits of American Government*. New York: Basic Books; 1990.

65. Morone JA. Enemies of the people: The moral dimension to public health. *Journal of Health Politics, Policy and Law*. 1997;22(4): 993–1020.

66. Morone J. *Hellfire Nation, the Politics of Sin in American History*. New Haven, CT: Yale University Press; 2003.

67. Baron JH. Medical police and the nanny state: Public health versus private autonomy. *Mt Sinai J Med*. July 2006;73(4):708–715.

68. Saguy AC, Riley KW. Weighing both sides: Morality, mortality, and framing contests over obesity. *J Health Polit Policy Law*. October 2005;30(5):869–921.

69. Roe E. *Narrative Policy Analysis, Theory and Practice*. Durham, NC: Duke University Press; 1994.

70. Jaklevic MC. This side of the ethical border. Hospitals feel duty of keeping immigrants healthy despite federal limits. *Mod Healthc*. September 3 2001;31(36):52–54.

71. Ku L, Matani S. Left out: Immigrants' access to health care and insurance. *Health Aff (Millwood)*. January–February 2001;20(1):247–256.

72. Mireles LR. Occupational safety and health on the U.S.-Mexico border. *New Solut*. 2003;13(1): 115–120.

73. Olson T. Trauma, policy, and public health on the U.S.-Mexico border. *Public Health Nurs*. January–February 2007;24(1):2–5.

74. Olson D, Leitheiser A, Atchison C, Larson S, Homzik C. Public health and terrorism preparedness: Cross-border issues. *Public Health Rep*. 2005;120 Suppl 1:76–83.

75. Swift EK, ed. *Guidance for the National Healthcare Disparities Report*. Washington, DC: Institute of Medicine; 2002.

76. Pickle LW, Mungiole M, Jones GK, White AA. *Atlas of United States Mortality*. Hyattsville, MD: U.S. Department of Health and Human Services; 1996.

77. Mill JS. On liberty. http://bartleby.com/130/: accessed October 22, 2008.

78. Hayek FAV. *The Mirage of Social Justice*. London: Routledge and Kegan Paul; 1976.

79. Hofstadter R. From the American Political Tradition. In: Serow AG, Shannon WW, Ladd EC, eds. *The American Polity Reader*. New York: W. W. Norton & Company; 1993:42–47.

80. Milio N. *Public Health in the Market*. Ann Arbor, MI: University of Michigan Press; 2000.

81. Wolff S. Love Canal revisited. *Jama*. March 16, 1984;251(11):1464.

82. Lindblom C. The market as prison. *The Journal of Politics*. 1982;44:324–336.

83. Beauchamp D. The law, the market, and the health of the body politic. *Hastings Cent Rep*. July–August 2002;32(4):44–46.

84. Dryzek JS. The good society versus the state: Freedom and necessity in political innovation. *The Journal of Politics*. 1992;54(2):518–540.

85. Milikis SM, Mileur JM, eds. *The Great Society and the High Tide of Liberalism*. Amherst, MA: The University of Massachusetts Press; 2005.

86. Sen A. Democracy as a universal value. *Journal of Democracy*. 1999;10(3):3–17.

87. Beauchamp DE. Health care spending: The democracy connection; September 28, 2006. Available at: http://www.talesofcoppercity.com/talesofcoppercity/public_health/index.html. Accessed March 23, 2007.

88. Porter D. *Health, Civilization and the State. A History of Public Health from Ancient to Modern Times*. London: Routledge; 1999.

89. Mello MM, Studdert DM, Brennan TA. Obesity—The new frontier of public health law. *N Engl J Med*. June 15 2006;354(24):2601–2610.

90. Turshen M. *The Politics of Public Health*. New Brunscwick, NJ: Rutgers University Press; 1989.

91. Freudenberg N, Galea S. The impact of corporate practices on health: Implications for health policy. *Journal of Public Health Policy*. 2008;29(1):86–104.

92. Mays GP, Halverson PK. Conceptual and methodological issues in public health performance measurement: Results from a computer-assisted expert panel process. *Journal of Public Health Management and Practice*. 2000;6(5):59–65.

93. Leep CJ. *National Profile of Local Health Departments*. Washington, DC: National Association of County & City Health Officials; 2006.

94. Feldstein PJ. *The Politics of Health Legislation an Economic Perspective*. 2nd ed. Chicago: Health Administration Press; 1996.

95. Johnson H, Broder D. *The System, the American Way of Politics at the Breaking Point*. Boston: Little, Brown and Company; 1995.

CHAPTER 6

The Legal Basis for Public Health Practice

Edward P. Richards III, JD, MPH
and Katharine C. Rathbun, MD, MPH

LEARNING OBJECTIVES

Upon completion of this chapter, the reader will be able to:

1. Identify the police powers under the United States Constitution and understand how they relate to public health.
2. Describe the concept of an administrative agency and how health departments are created.
3. Recognize the differences among criminal, civil, and administrative law and how each relates to public health.
4. Describe the limits on public health law from the United States Constitution and from state law, particularly due process and *habeas corpus*.
5. Identify sources of legal liability for a public health official and understand the effects of federal and state tort claims acts on this liability.
6. Describe the legal status of public health reporting.
7. Describe the parallels between emergency power laws and routine public health actions.

KEY TERMS

Area Warrant

Color of State Law

Due Process

Governmental Functions

Habeas Corpus

Health Officer

Mitigate the Hazard

Official Capacity

Parens Patria Power

Personal Capacity

Police Power

Proprietary Functions

Public Nuisance

Reportable Disease or Injury

Sovereign Immunity

Public health has become a broad and flexible concept that encompasses both the traditional definition of practices that benefit the health of the community and personal health services, such as hypertension treatment. Legally, however, the basis for traditional public health and personal health services are very different. For example, although the state has broad powers to order vaccination to prevent the spread of a dangerous communicable disease, the state has limited power to require competent adults to undergo medical treatment for personal illness such as hypertension. This chapter focuses on the legal basis for public health practices that are directed at the health of the community.

The core of public health law is coercive action under state authority, the **police power.** In the best of circumstances, this authority may be needed only to encourage educational efforts. At other times, however, public health authorities must seize property, close businesses, destroy animals, or involuntarily treat or even lock away individuals. Such powers are rooted in earlier times, when the fear of pestilential disease was both powerful and well founded. As communicable diseases such as smallpox, tuberculosis, and polio were brought under control in the 1960s, the public and even some public health experts began to believe that there was no longer a need for coercive public health measures.

The terrorist attack on the United States on September 11, 2001, followed shortly by anthrax-laden letters sent to public figures, brought bioterrorism to the public's consciousness, reviving ancient fears of pestilence. The sequella of Hurricane Katrina and growing fears of pandemic flu have raised questions about the capabilities of the public health infrastructure and the potential reach of public health laws in an emergency. These fears have forced a rethinking of public health law authority.

This chapter has three objectives: (1) to place public health law in its historical context and to show why this matters in understanding contemporary public health practice and public health emergency powers; (2) to show how public health law

fits into the general rules for administrative agency law; and (3) to outline core areas of public health law practice.

HISTORICAL PERSPECTIVE

In the United States, law is shaped by the past through the accretion of cases that provide precedent to guide contemporary judges. Although precedent can be changed by legislation or later legal decision, until these old cases are overruled, they remain the law. More fundamentally, the breadth of public health authority can only be understood in the context of the history of epidemic disease and its impact on social order.

Pestilence is one of the *Four Horsemen of the Apocalypse* in the Book of Revelation, reflecting its position as a primal fear of society. Despite recent fears of bioterrorism and pandemic flu, it is difficult for individuals born after the ready availability of antimicrobial drugs and immunizations to appreciate the historic dread of deadly epidemics. Civilizations have fallen because of communicable diseases, and pestilence has done more to eradicate indigenous cultures than has force of arms or religion.[1] At the time of the drafting of the United States Constitution, epidemic disease was seen as a national security risk as great as that of a foreign invasion. When the courts, including the United States Supreme Court, first outlined the reach of public health authority, they held that state authority was nearly unlimited because the consequences of failing to control an epidemic could be the destruction of the state itself. This assumption was based on the traditional laws of nations that recognize that the preservation of the state is of primary importance.

This concern with public health authority was driven by real events. The major colonial cities were on rivers in coastal marsh areas and were subject to both mosquito-borne illnesses, such as yellow fever, and the illnesses of contaminated water, such as cholera and typhoid. Smallpox also made a regular appearance. Soon after the Constitution was ratified, an epidemic of yellow fever raged in New York and Philadelphia. The flavor of that period was later captured in an argument before the Supreme Court:

> For ten years prior, the yellow-fever had raged almost annually in the city, and annual laws were passed to resist it. The wit of man was exhausted, but in vain. Never did the pestilence rage more violently than in the summer of 1798. The State was in despair. The rising hopes of the metropolis began to fade. The opinion was gaining ground, that the cause of this annual disease was indigenous, and that all precautions against its importation were useless. But the leading spirits of that day were unwilling to give up the city without a final desperate effort. The havoc in the summer of 1798 is represented as terrific. The whole country was roused. A cordon sanitaire was thrown around the city. Governor Mifflin of Pennsylvania proclaimed a nonintercourse between New York and Philadelphia.[2]

The extreme nature of the actions, including isolating the federal government, which was sitting in Philadelphia at the time, was considered an appropriate response to the threat of yellow fever. The terrifying nature of these early epidemics predisposed the courts to grant public health authorities a free hand in their attempts to prevent the spread of disease, as the following quote from United States Supreme Court illustrates:

> Every state has acknowledged power to pass, and enforce quarantine, health, and inspection laws, to prevent the introduction of disease, pestilence, or unwholesome provisions; such laws interfere with no powers of Congress or treaty stipulations; they relate to internal police, and are subjects of domestic regulation within each state, over which no authority can be exercised by any power under the Constitution, save by requiring the consent of Congress to the imposition of duties on exports and imports, and their payment into the treasury of the United States.[3]

These powers, called police powers, resided in the states during the period between the Declaration of Independence and the ratification of the Constitution. Under the Constitution, the police power was left to the states, whereas the new federal government was given the power to regulate trade between the states, and regulate all aspects of foreign trade and policy, including the war powers. It was assumed that the federal government would have a limited role and that most governmental functions would be carried out by the states. Over the next 200 years, the federal government assumed the primary role in many areas of government, but most public health services are still provided by state and local government. Traditionally, the federal government directed these actions by providing funding and expert assistance. As part of the strengthening of national security and surveillance laws after the terrorist attacks on 9/11, Congress has given the federal government more powers to direct and even commandeer state and local resources, as well as to use the military in public health and national security emergencies.[4]

PUBLIC HEALTH DEPARTMENTS AS ADMINISTRATIVE AGENCIES

Other chapters in this book outline the different public health functions and the different organizational structures for public health agencies. There are thousands of public health agencies, ranging in size from state agencies, to big city public health departments that rival the size of many state health departments, to small city and county departments that may have only a handful of employees. Because the majority of public health departments are small and have limited resources, public health law must accommodate both big city and state health departments and small city and county departments.

Governmental Organization

State and local governments are divided into three branches: the legislative branch, executive branch (the president or governor), and judicial branch. The legislature is the primary branch, in that it shapes and funds the branches. Public health departments are government agencies, created by statutes—called enabling statutes—passed by the state legislatures. The state legislature determines how much of the very broad state police power is given to the health department, the organizational structure of the health department, and its funding. The state legislature or state constitution can also give the cities and counties the power to establish and fund local health departments and to use the state's police powers to enforce local public health ordinances. The process is the same for all governmental agencies, including those in the federal government: agencies are created by the legislature, the legislature gives them their powers and mandates, and the legislature provides their funding.

While the legislature shapes the judicial and executive branches through enabling statutes and through funding, the other branches of government have independent authority, referred to as the doctrine of separation of powers, which acts to check the power of the legislature and each other. After the legislature establishes an agency such as a public health department, the legislature cannot run the agency. Any agency that enforces laws must be part of the executive branch. In the federal government, agencies such as the Centers for Disease Control and Prevention (CDC) are under the control of the president. At the state level, public health agencies are under the control of the governor, mayor, or other local official—not the state legislature. There can be legislative agencies, such as the Congressional Budget Office, but the agencies can only do studies and publish reports; they cannot enforce laws.

If the legislature wants to protect an agency from politically driven decisions by the executive branch, it can create an independent agency. At the federal level, the director of an independent agency is appointed by a board or commission, rather than the president. The members of the board are appointed by the president, but they will serve fixed terms that overlap, so that a president can only appoint new members as vacancies occur on the board. This buffers the agency head from day-to-day political interference by the executive branch. The IRS and the Consumer Product Safety Commission are examples of independent federal agencies.

In some states and localities, the public health department is organized as an independent agency, with the director reporting to a board of health. The board may be appointed by the governor or mayor, or several elected officials may each appoint a member. These boards can protect the independence of the health director, but many do not take this responsibility seriously.

Agency Organization and Access to Legal Services

Public health agencies operate at both the state and the local level. They may be controlled at the local level, with the state health department administering federal grants and providing services such as data aggregation and expert advice. The primary decision making and the provision of legal services is local, with larger departments having their own lawyers and smaller departments using the city or county legal department. In the state-controlled model, the state health department runs and controls the local departments. Depending on the state, legal services will be provided by the State Attorney General's office, or the health department will have its own lawyers. Many states have hybrid models with varying levels of state control of local departments, and, like the state-controlled departments, may have their own counsel, or depend on other agencies for legal services.

There are potential conflicts when the legal services are delivered by attorneys whose primary

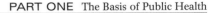

allegiance is not to the health department. For example, the State Attorney General is an independent elected official, who may have different enforcement priorities than the governor or the health director. City and county legal departments may not have the necessary expertise, and they often see public health enforcement actions as less important than their primary work of criminal prosecutions, land use regulation, consumer protection, and the other activities that have a higher public profile than septic tank permits and enforcing dog laws. In smaller communities, legal services are often provided by private attorneys with limited public health law skills, and departmental funding seldom allows the purchase of adequate legal services. Limited access to expert public health law services complicates public health practice, especially when the **health officer** must act quickly.

THE LEGAL STANDARDS FOR PUBLIC HEALTH LAW

The popular perception is that there are two types of laws: criminal laws, enforced by the government and leading to fines and imprisonment; and civil laws, which are privately enforced in actions such as medical malpractice or private business litigation. Agencies such as health departments sometimes rely on criminal laws, but most public health enforcement actions are governmental civil actions. Governmental civil actions can lead to fines, loss of business permits or licenses, destruction of dangerous property, and even personal restrictions such as quarantine, but they cannot be used to imprison individuals as a punishment.

Criminal Law Standards

Understanding the distinction between civil and criminal laws is key to understanding the difference in legal standards for public health actions and government criminal prosecutions. The Bill of Rights provides specific rights to persons who are arrested and prosecuted for crimes. The accused has the right to remain silent, which means that individuals cannot be forced to testify against themselves. The government cannot search an individual's home for evidence of a crime without a warrant approved by a judge. The judge must determine that credible evidence exists that the person was involved in a crime and that specific evidence of the crime is in the house. This is called a probable cause warrant. Accused persons have a right to confront their accusers; to present witnesses to support their case; to have a trial by a jury; and, perhaps most importantly for indigent defendants, the right to have an attorney and the requirement that the government pay for the lawyers if the defendant is indigent. If the defendant is brought to trial, the government must prove the case against the defendant beyond a reasonable doubt. This bundle of rights is called criminal law **due process** because it refers to the process that the state must go through to prosecute an individual for a crime.

Because the consequences of a criminal prosecution are so grave, the United States Supreme Court requires that criminal laws clearly specify what behavior is forbidden. Criminal laws and regulations must be passed by the legislature, they must be specific, and they cannot be modified by the law enforcement agency or other executive branch agencies. These rights are intended to protect individuals from the power of the state. Although they make criminal prosecutions slow and expensive, and sometimes result in guilty persons going free, it is generally accepted that it is more important to protect the rights of the innocent than to assure that every criminal is jailed.

Civil Law Standards

The United States Supreme Court has always recognized a bright line between the standards for criminal prosecution and the standards that apply to governmental actions that are intended to protect the public health and welfare. The government has much broader authority to act and can do so in much more flexible ways when the goal is to protect the public and to prevent future harm. Some scholars asserted that certain decisions of the Warren Court in the 1960s and early 1970s limited traditional public health authority.[5] The Rehnquist court overruled these cases.[6] Subsequent cases by the Rehnquist and Robert's courts have shown great deference to government power when it is preventing future harm.

Administrative agencies are given broad authority to use their expertise to develop the most effective strategies for protecting the public, and they may change these strategies as conditions change or as they get better information about their effectiveness. For example, state health departments are charged with protecting individuals and the community from communicable diseases. Rather than the legislature deciding which diseases pose a threat to the public health, the health department is given the authority to establish the list of communicable diseases that must be reported and to perform other public health regulations. These regulations have the same force as a statute passed by the legislature. When individuals or businesses sue the health department to challenge these regulations, the courts generally defer to the agency's expertise and support the regulations even if there is controversy over the best way to solve a particular problem. As one court held, in a case contesting the right of the health department to close gay bathhouses to prevent the spread of HIV:

> . . . defendants and the intervening patrons challenge the soundness of the scientific judgments upon which the Health Council regulation is based. . . . They go further and argue that facilities such as St. Mark's, which attempts to educate its patrons with written materials, signed pledges, and posted notices as to the advisability of safe sexual practices, provide a positive force in combating AIDS, and a valuable communication link between public health authorities and the homosexual community. While these arguments and proposals may have varying degrees of merit, they overlook a fundamental principle of applicable law: "It is not for the courts to

determine which scientific view is correct in ruling upon whether the police power has been properly exercised. The judicial function is exhausted with the discovery that the relation between means and end is not wholly vain and fanciful, an illusory pretense."[7]

The courts justify this deference to a broad agency power on the basis of cost and risk benefit calculations. The courts recognize that due process protections come at a cost to the agency, both in time and in money. The time costs can mean that innocent individuals are exposed to risk for longer, and the monetary costs can mean that the agency does not have the money to carry out its mission. Thus, in a landmark case concerning the due process rights of persons claiming federal disability benefits, *Mathews v. Eldridge*, the court explained that increasing the due process protections for individuals who were denied benefits would come at the cost of those properly entitled to benefits.[8] Although the court did require some due process for benefit denials, it said that the government should consider how much the protections cost and whether they significantly improved the accuracy of the decisions.

More than 30 years later, the *Mathews* decision remains the core precedent for public health due process requirements under the United States Constitution. Although the court has decided few pure public health cases, it has upheld the use of this flexible standard in much more controversial areas, such as the detention of suspected terrorists.

Constitutional Limits on Public Health Law

The government cannot use public health laws to circumvent criminal law protections. For example, in *Ferguson v. City of Charleston*,[9] the court found that the secret screening of pregnant women to detect illegal drug use was unconstitutional because the evidence was used to threaten the women with criminal prosecution. The opinion indicated that the decision would have been different had the state intended to use the information for a legitimate public health purpose. The government cannot use public health quarantine and isolation powers as a substitute for a criminal prosecution, so locking up a suspected murderer to protect the public, without a criminal conviction, would not be allowed as a public health measure. However, if the government can prove that a criminal poses a threat to society if he is released, he may be held as a public safety measure after his prison term has been served.[10] The police power can also be used to incarcerate dangerous persons without full criminal due process protections.[11] Mental health commitments based on the patient being dangerous to others is a police power action, but commitments done to protect the individual from himself are part of the states *parens patria* **power,** the power to protect individuals from harm.[12]

The court has also rejected claims that holding persons in prison who have not been accused or convicted of crimes violates their constitutional rights. Public health detentions have been legally carried out in prisons and jails. In one case, disease carriers were quarantined in a prison. They petitioned the court for release, claiming that they were being punished by being put in prison and treated as prisoners. The court rejected their claim and concluded the following:

> While it is true that physical facilities constituting part of the penitentiary equipment are utilized, interned persons are in no sense confined in the penitentiary, and are not subject to the peculiar obloquy which attends such confinement.[13]

This decision was ratified by the Rehnquist court in a case that rejected claims by pretrial detainees that holding them in prison when they had not been found guilty of a crime, or, in some cases, even charged with a crime, violated their constitutional rights.[14]

Public health laws must be applied fairly. They cannot, for example, be a subterfuge for discrimination against racial or ethnic groups, in violation of the Equal Protection provisions of the United States Constitution. For example, the courts have rejected laws that subjected the Chinese community to special health regulations without providing evidence that Chinese people were at any greater risk of contracting or spreading disease.[15] However, if a public health law's purpose and enforcement is rationally related to protecting the public's health, it will be constitutional even if it has a differential impact on different groups. Laws for controlling the spread of gonorrhea are constitutional, even if the disease is more prevalent in a specific racial or ethnic group, or if they target prostitutes who are mostly women.[16]

Public health laws cannot violate the Interstate Commerce Clause of the United States Constitution, by treating out-of-state businesses differently from in-state businesses. For example, courts have struck down several laws that imposed different sanitary restrictions on out-of-state milk processors. Even if the restrictions are the same for in-state and out-of-state businesses, the courts will strike down laws that unnecessarily discriminate against out-of-state businesses. For example, a requirement that milk must be processed and delivered within 24 hours would put out-of-state dairies out of business. This law would be improper if there was no evidence that the 24-hour rule was necessary to maintain the purity of the milk.

Basic Public Health Due Process

Whenever the state enforces a law or regulation against an individual or business, the individual or business has the right to be heard. This includes the right to know the legal basis for the state action, the charges made by the agency, the chance to examine the evidence supporting the action, and a chance to state a defense. For the regulated party to take advantage of these rights, the agency must provide notice of the time and location of the hearing, or the chance to request a hearing, to the regulated party.

The right to be heard is not a right to a court hearing before a judge. It may be a hearing before a hearing officer who is an employee of the agency, and the regulated party may be required to file all responses in writing, rather than speaking directly to the hearing officer. There is usually no constitutional right to a hearing before the enforcement action, as long as there is a chance to be heard in a reasonable time after the action.[17] For example, when a power failure in a freezer plant created a large quantity of spoiled food, the court allowed the public health authorities to seize and destroy the food before there was a hearing. The court found that defendants would not be prejudiced by making their case later because the state could pay for the value of the food if the judge determined that the state had acted illegally.[18]

If the public health department isolates or quarantines an individual without a hearing, the individual is entitled to a **habeas corpus** proceeding, which the United States Constitution guarantees to every imprisoned or confined person. *Habeas corpus*, roughly translated, means "bring me the body." It requires that a judge review the legality of a person's confinement, usually including a personal statement by the confined person. Because a *habeas corpus* proceeding is held *after* the person has been confined, it does not interfere with the health department's ability to take quick action. Unlike routine court hearings, *habeas corpus* is used only when requested by the confined person. Many, perhaps most, people restricted by public health orders do not want to contest the restriction. In the vast majority of cases, confinement is temporary—for a medical examination, initial treatment of a disease, or some other similarly minor inconvenience. By contrast, requiring hearings before enforcing routine or uncontested public health orders diverts limited resources from other public health agency functions.

State Law Limits on Public Health Actions

The Constitution provides the minimum standards that all states must meet, but individual states may provide more protection for individual and business rights. In some cases, the state constitution provides more protection. For example, there is a New York case raising the question of whether the state could inspect automobile junk yards without a criminal law probable cause warrant and then use evidence from the search in a criminal prosecution. The United States Supreme Court found that the junk yard owner had given up his right to privacy when he applied for a permit to operate the yard, and because a primary purpose for licensing junk yards was to prevent the sale of stolen parts, the owner was on notice that he might be searched for such parts as a condition of running the junk yard.[19] On the same facts, the New York state court did not allow the evidence to be used in a state prosecution because the New York state constitution provided more protection of privacy than the United States Constitution.[20]

Most limits on state public health authority come from laws passed by the legislatures. The two groups pushing for these restrictions are the civil libertarians and business groups. Although their objectives are very different, the resulting legislation has the same effect. Civil libertarian groups may want the state to enforce public health laws and provide social services, but they want the state to provide extensive due process protections when these restrictions affect individual's rights. Business lobby groups, especially small business groups, generally do not want the state to enforce regulations of any kind that affect their members, so they push for laws that provide due process protections and limit enforcement powers.

Many state legislatures have responded to these political pressures by passing laws that impose extensive procedural restrictions on state administrative agency enforcement, including health department enforcement. These restrictions include elaborate court hearing requirements before enforcement; limits on agency rulemaking, taking decision-making powers away from the agency; and generous judicial appeal rights for regulated parties. Given the organized opposition to public health powers, many state public health law practitioners have argued against the federal push to pass model public health statutes. Any attempt to revise state law runs the risk of being hijacked by special interests opposed to regulation, with the result that the final law may reduce agency powers, rather than increasing them.

Laws that encourage judicial review of public health actions encourage state judges to substitute their judgment for the expert decisions of the agency. There is no reason to have a hearing if the judge must always defer to the agency. For example, while there has been pressure in all states to require a live court hearing before individuals are ordered into quarantine or isolation, there is nothing that the judge can evaluate in the hearing that could not be done on written documents. The only issues are whether the health department has the correct person, whether there is legal authority, and the interpretation of the medical tests. The result is that the state wins all the cases, but at a cost in time and effort; in some cases, the public is exposed to significant risk while the person is at large.[21]

While there has been some public controversy over the growing legal restrictions on public health actions because they could potentially limit quarantine and isolation in emergencies, the real cost has been to routine public health enforcement actions such as locating septic tanks, enforcing sanitary regulations, and seizing and destroying dangerous animals. More importantly, at the same time that legal restrictions increase the cost of enforcement, most public health agencies have lost staff and resources over the past decade. This loss of expert staff in the face of expanding responsibilities, combined with the reluctance of public health directors to take politically controversial actions, is the most important limitation on public health authority.

LEGAL LIABILITY

Public health departments and public health officials are frequent targets of litigation. Historically, the federal and state governments had **sovereign immunity,** which was the common law concept that no one could sue the king (government). If the state injured a person, the only way for the individual to get compensation under sovereign immunity was to persuade the legislature to pass a special law authorizing such compensation. After the Civil

War, Congress passed federal laws, including the Civil Rights Acts,[22] which allowed individuals to sue state officials who used state authority to violate the individual's civil rights. Starting in the 1940s, the states and the federal government, responding to the huge legislative burden of private compensation bills and the potential for corruption in private compensation legislation, passed Tort Claims Acts. These provided a legal remedy for negligence claims against the government and its employees.

These laws attempt to balance the rights of injured individuals against the need to deliver cost-effective public services and the need to protect public officials and employees from individual liability for doing their job. Public health officials have to make many unpopular decisions to protect the public health, and they cannot make these decisions if they are worried about liability for themselves or for their jurisdictions. For example, the Mayor of New Orleans reported that fears of liability for declaring an unnecessary evacuation contributed to delaying the call for an evacuation of New Orleans before Hurricane Katrina. The courts have also recognized that because the states have limited duties to provide social services, subjecting the state to costly litigation over the quality of those social services may have the perverse result of having the state limit or eliminate the service.[23]

Individual Liability

Public health officials can be sued in three ways under state law: in their **official capacity,** as a private individual for wrongdoing that is part of their official duties, or as private individuals for wrongdoing that is outside their professional duties. Official capacity means the public health official is a surrogate for the government and is not personally liable if damages are awarded to the plaintiff. These lawsuits are usually brought to stop enforcement of an unconstitutional law or to stop unconstitutional or otherwise illegal behavior by the health agency, and they are governed by the principle of sovereign immunity. Personal lawsuits related to workplace activities can include medical malpractice for clinical work, automobile accidents while on duty, and other ordinary negligence cases that are covered by torts claims acts as discussed later. In both situations, because the wrongdoing is related to the individual's government employment, the state is substituted as the defendant, and the employee is not personally liable for the costs of defense or any settlements or judgments.

If the individual lawsuits assert wrongdoing outside the individual's job, such as criminal activity or knowingly exceeding the legal authority of the job, governmental immunity will not apply. The individual is responsible for the costs of defense and for any settlements or judgments. In some cases, such allegations are added to claims that are based on official conduct to increase the pressure on the official and to persuade the state to settle the case to avoid any chance that the official will be held personally liable. Individuals working as independent contractors rather than employees, such as public health clinic physicians or individuals working for private companies doing public health work for the state, are generally not covered by state immunity and should make sure that their employer provides adequate insurance, or they should acquire personal coverage.

State Law Liability

Liability under state law for job-related wrongdoing by state employees is controlled by the state's Tort Claims Act (TCA). There is also a Federal TCA. TCAs provide a limited waiver of sovereign immunity that allows for recovery of damages for negligence actions for covered activities. State TCAs have differing caps on recovery, ranging from $100,000 to more than $1,000,000, and they generally prevent the recovery of punitive damages and claims based on strict liability theories such as product liability. The claimant must submit a claim to the state before filing a lawsuit, and the state will decide on an appropriate level of compensation. If the claimant is dissatisfied with the offer, or if the state does not make an offer, the claimant can then go to court. Cities do not have sovereign immunity and the coverage for counties depends on the

individual state constitution. Unless the legislature has extended state immunity to its cities, cities are subject to ordinary tort lawsuits with no damage limits. Although cities generally provide the same protections for their employees as states, this can vary. City public health officials should determine if they need additional personal insurance.

TCAs are structured to protect the ability of the state to make policy choices without being second-guessed by tort lawsuits. This is done by dividing state activities into two different classes: governmental functions and **proprietary functions.** Proprietary functions are those that are not unique to government, that is, the government is not doing anything different from private business. For example, paving roads is often done by private contractors. If the state negligently paves a road, and a car is damaged by flaws in the surface, the car's owner could file a TCA claim.

Governmental functions are those that are only done by government or that are part of governmental policy making. There is no clear dividing line between governmental and proprietary functions, and the definitions vary greatly between states. Some states hold that almost all public health functions are governmental, whereas other states find that a substantial group of these functions are proprietary. Traditional public health services, such as restaurant inspection, animal control, health and safety permits and licenses, sanitation, vital statistics, and related functions, are considered governmental in almost all states. Many states do not consider personal medical services, such as prenatal care clinics and general indigent health care clinics, to be governmental functions and apply ordinary medical malpractice law to them, although some states do include these under governmental immunity. However, if the medical service is related to protecting the public, rather than just helping the individual, it should be governmental. Thus, treatment and testing for tuberculosis would be a governmental function.

If the activity is governmental, it is protected from TCA claims if it involves discretionary decision making. If no discretion is allowed, it is called a ministerial act, and the TCA applies. Ministerial tasks do not allow discretion because they either follow a predetermined plan and cannot be changed, such as following a health department checklist regulation, or they do not involve any special expertise related to public health, such as driving a car. For example, plaintiffs were allowed to recover when the government failed to follow its own regulations for approving a polio vaccine.[24]

TCAs do not allow liability for bad policy choices. Unless the claimant can convince the court that the government violated a law, violated its own regulation, or was negligent in carrying out a governmental function, the court will dismiss the claim regardless of the harm. In a classic case, persons exposed to radioactive fallout from above ground atomic bomb testing sued the federal government, claiming it was negligent in conducting tests where the radiation could drift over the community. The government asserted that it had considered the risks of accidental radiation exposure and had decided to go ahead with the test, that is, it made a decision to risk the exposure. The court found that there was no law prohibiting this, and because the claimants could not show that the harm was due to a mistake, rather than a bad policy choice, the court dismissed their claims.[25]

Section 1983 Liability

Section 1983 of the Civil Rights Act of 1871 allows citizens to sue persons who, under **"color" of state law,** deprive them of their constitutional rights. The statute uses the term "color" of law to include actions that, while not directly authorized by state law, are made possible by the power derived from the state law. For example, if the sheriff participated in a Ku Klux Klan lynching, the plaintiff could argue that the lynching was under color of state law because it was facilitated by the legal power of the sheriff. Section 1983 actions can be brought against state officials in their **personal capacity,** but not in their official capacity. Under this law, claims against individuals can be for money damages, but claims against the state can only be for injunctive relief to stop the state from continuing its illegal actions. Section 1983 does

not allow damage claims against the state itself because these are barred by the 11th Amendment to the United States Constitution. City, county, and other nonstate officials can be sued in their official capacity, which allows damages to be obtained from the governmental entity, and in their personal capacity, which can subject them to personal liability. In 1971, the United States Supreme Court allowed claims against federal officials who violate an individual's constitutional rights in *Bivens v. Six Unknown Named Agents of Federal Bureau of Narcotics*, 403 U.S. 388 (1971). A Bivens action is the federal equivalent of a 1983 action and applies to employees of the Public Health Service, the CDC, and other federal agencies. Bivens actions, 1983 actions, and related actions against public health officials have similar requirements.

Section 1983 applies to anyone who acts under state or local legal authority. It reaches everyone working under the authority of the health department, irrespective of their employment status, and can even be applied to volunteers. It does not provide for vicarious liability, so the state or local government is not liable for an individual's actions unless those actions represent governmental policy. Thus, in police brutality cases, the police department will be liable only if the court finds that the officers were acting under a department policy that encouraged or tolerated brutality.

Section 1983 actions must allege that the defendant violated the plaintiff's rights under the Constitution or certain federal laws. Most public health cases allege violations of the constitutional rights of equal protection or due process. Equal protection claims arise from differential treatment that is motivated by improper discrimination, especially discrimination based on race, ethnicity, or religion. Refusing to issue a license or permit because of personal animus against the applicant could also be an equal protection violation, unless there were other rational grounds for the refusal.

To prevail in a case asking for money damages, the plaintiff must prove that the official's conduct violates clearly established statutory or constitutional rights that a reasonable official should have known about. If the official is mistaken about the law but had no reason to know that the actions were improper, or the official is acting under a law later declared unconstitutional, there is no liability. The courts also require that persons bringing Section 1983 actions show significant harm as well as improper conduct, so that small injuries will not support Section 1983 claims. The plaintiff can get injunctive relief to stop the illegal action even if the official cannot be held liable for money damages.[26]

BASIC AREAS OF PUBLIC HEALTH LAW

The legal core of public health is disease control through environmental health, the collection of epidemiologic data, and the enforcement of disease control measures.

Environmental Health

Food sanitation, drinking-water treatment, wastewater disposal, and animal and vermin control have been mainstays of public health since the earliest times. Most public health orders are directed at environmental health problems. Because they affect property, not persons, they do not pose the difficult issues of personal freedom that arise with communicable disease control orders. Environmental health programs also deal with **public nuisances.** A public nuisance can be dangerous property, such as an abandoned mine shaft or a vicious dog, or it can be an activity, such as burning old tires.

Public health authorities can bring legal actions to seize property or to force the owner to **mitigate the hazard.** Private individuals can also bring nuisance suits to force the owners of the property to mitigate the problem. This is a longstanding right, and at least one state court has rejected legislative efforts to limit the right of individuals to bring private nuisance claims against commercial hog farms.[27]

Environmental health regulations pose two central legal questions: whether the government owes compensation to the owners of regulated property, and under what circumstances health officers can enter private premises to look for public health law violations. Both questions arise from the United States Constitution, which requires that property owners be paid a fair price for property taken for public purposes and prohibits *unreasonable* searches and seizures. The difficult problem is deciding if the government has searched the property unreasonably or has taken valuable property for which the owner must be compensated.

If a city condemns a house to widen a street, the city has clearly taken the property and must pay its owner. In contrast, if property is destroyed because it poses a threat to the public health, the owner is not entitled to compensation because the property is not considered to have any value. For example, an early case involved a compensation claim for property that had been demolished to prevent the spread of a fire in San Francisco.[28] The court found that the police power included the right to destroy property if this was necessary to protect the public safety. This destruction was not taking the property for public purpose and thus no compensation need be paid because the fire would have destroyed the house. The court rejected the claim that the authorities should have allowed the owners time to remove their property from the house because such a delay would have increased the danger to the public. The courts have also found that the owners of dangerous animals are not entitled to compensation if the animals are destroyed.[29]

The second legal issue in environmental health is the right of the health department to enter private property to assess environmental health risks. With certain exceptions, the police may not enter private property to search for evidence of criminal activity without a search warrant approved by a judge. Such warrants are difficult and expensive to get and will be granted only when there is evidence of wrongdoing. In contrast, most environmental health inspections are done to ensure that the owner is in compliance with the law, not because the inspector believes that the owner is violating the law.

The courts do not require specific warrants for environmental health inspections. The courts do require that searches be related to a public health purpose and not be a subterfuge for a criminal search. This can be satisfied by having a general plan for the inspections (called an **area warrant**) that describes which buildings will be searched and why.[30] Access by health inspectors can be made a condition of licensure, so that any establishment with a food handling or other public license has to admit inspectors without a warrant.

Disease and Injury Reporting and Investigation

Basic to all public health is the collection of information about cases of communicable diseases, hazardous conditions, and injuries that are significant to public health. This information forms the epidemiological basis for scientific public health. Collecting this information depends on legally mandated reporting by health care providers, employers, and even laymen. It also requires the investigation of disease outbreaks and individual exposures, even the investigation of individual sexual contacts. Reporting duties transcend the patient's right to privacy and the health care provider's obligation to protect the patient's confidential information. Even the stringent privacy requirements of the Health Insurance Portability and Accountability Act of 1996 (HIPAA) have an exception for public health reporting and investigation.[31]

Communicable Disease Reporting

The constitutionality of reporting laws has been upheld in several recent United States Supreme Court decisions. In a case involving the reporting of controlled substance prescriptions, the Court addressed many of the concerns about public health reporting. The Court first noted that common law did not recognize the right to withhold medical information from the state. Such a right of physician-patient confidentiality arises from state or federal law and is subject to limitations such as public health reporting. The Court then held:

> Unquestionably, some individuals' concern for their own privacy may lead them to avoid or to postpone needed medical attention.

Nevertheless, disclosures of private medical information to doctors, hospital personnel, insurance companies, and public health agencies are often an essential part of modern medical practice, even when the disclosure may reflect unfavorably on the character of the patient. Requiring such disclosures to representatives of the State having responsibility for the health of the community, does not automatically amount to an impermissible invasion of privacy.[32]

Every state has laws that require physicians to report certain diseases and injuries to a local or state health officer.[33] Many include reporting requirements for nurses, dentists, veterinarians, laboratories, school officials, administrators of institutions, and police officials. For some diseases, health care providers are required to report only the number of cases they see. Other diseases and conditions require health care providers to give identifying information, such as name, address, occupation, and birth date, as well as information on the disease and how it might have been acquired.

Although states vary somewhat in which diseases must be reported, about 60 diseases are commonly reportable in all jurisdictions. The state health department can provide information on which diseases to report and to whom the reports should be directed. Most health departments accept reports for diseases that are not on the state list of **reportable diseases,** although they may choose not to act on them. Health care providers have no legal liability for making a report, even if it is not required.

Legally required disease control reporting is not subject to informed consent. Health care providers do not need medical records releases for disease reporting because neither they nor their patients have the right to refuse the release of the information. Although patients have no right to be informed that they are being reported to the health department, it is good practice to do so for diseases for which the health department will contact them for additional information. Although many states passed laws in the 1980s and 1990s that discouraged reporting the names of persons with HIV infection, these are being repealed because the CDC is now requiring named reporting as a condition for federal funding of HIV programs.

Law Enforcement Reporting

Every jurisdiction requires health care providers to report certain types of injuries to law enforcement officials or social service agencies. Reportable injuries generally include child abuse, assaults, family violence, and criminal activity. Although the victim may have a plausible explanation of the injury and be anxious to avoid reporting, proper reports should be made despite the victim's wishes. It is not up to the health care provider to investigate the incident before reporting it; that is the job of the agency that receives the report.

Traditional disease reporting and law enforcement reporting merge in new requirements to report potential bioterrorism events and exposures. This includes the occurrence of any suspicious, unidentified conditions and any cases of communicable diseases that may be used as bioterrorism agents, such as tularemia. These reports will be jointly investigated by public health officials, the CDC, and law enforcement agencies.

Disease Investigations

When a case of communicable disease is identified, the contacts of the person who is infected are traced to find the source of the disease and other people who might be infected.[34] Many persons object to contact tracing as an invasion of privacy. Contact-tracing interviews are always voluntary; there is no legal coercion to divulge the names of contacts.[35] A more serious objection, especially with venereal diseases, is the risk of breaches of confidentiality. As a matter of law, the courts do not consider the risk of such breaches of confidentiality to be sufficient reason to restrict contact tracing. As a matter of public health practice, there have been no significant breaches of the confidentiality of public health records.[36] When suspected breaches of confidentiality have been investigated, they are usually traced back to the patient's own disclosures.

It has also been argued that contact tracing is not legally justified because it is too expensive or because it is ineffective. The courts have rejected these arguments because contact tracing is highly efficient in finding infected persons.[37] This was best demonstrated in the campaign to eradicate smallpox, which was not controlled by universal immunization but by extensive contact tracing to find infected individuals.[38] Fellow villagers and tribe members were encouraged to identify any one who might be infected. When people with smallpox were identified, they were isolated, and everyone in the surrounding community or village was vaccinated. In this way, smallpox was eventually reduced to isolated outbreaks and then eradicated.

Testing and Treatment

Disease control measures include involuntary testing for diseases such as tuberculosis, mandatory treatment for communicable diseases, and mandatory vaccination. In the only immunization case ever decided by the United States Supreme Court, the Court held that it was constitutionally permissible to force an individual to be vaccinated for smallpox:

> We are not prepared to hold that a minority, residing or remaining in any city or town where smallpox is prevalent, and enjoying the general protection afforded by an organized local government, may thus defy the will of its constituted authorities, acting in good faith for all, under the legislative sanction of the state. If such be the privilege of a minority, then a like privilege would belong to each individual of the community, and the spectacle would be presented of the welfare and safety of an entire population being subordinated to the notions of a single individual who chooses to remain a part of that population.[39]

Most mandatory immunization laws contain exemptions for individuals who have a high probability of being injured by the immunization. Although the Constitution allows mandatory immunization of religious objectors, most states do not take advantage of this power. Many states now allow parents to opt their children out of vaccinations just because the parents do not like vaccinations. This has been driven by political opposition to vaccinations, and not the rejection of mandatory vaccination laws by the courts. Attempts to reduce the opposition to vaccinations by establishing a national compensation fund for childhood vaccine injuries have done little to reduce the public distrust of vaccinations.

Personal Restrictions

The most intrusive public health measures are ongoing restrictions of an individual's liberty. A classic example is the case of *Typhoid Mary*, a typhoid carrier who was imprisoned after repeatedly violating orders to stop working as a cook. She infected more than a hundred people, and several of them died of the disease. A 1941 case, also involving a typhoid carrier, is a good example of the court's view of the appropriateness of personal restrictions to control disease. The case concerned the issue of whether the identity of typhoid carriers could be disclosed if necessary to prevent them from handling food and thus exposing others to disease. It was argued:

> The Sanitary Code which has the force of law . . . requires local health officers to keep the state department of health informed of the names, ages and addresses of known or suspected typhoid carriers, to furnish to the state health department necessary specimens for laboratory examination in such cases, to inform the carrier and members of his household of the situation and to exercise certain controls over the activities of the carriers, including a prohibition against any handling by the carrier of food which is to be consumed by persons other than members of his own household. . . . Why should the record of compliance by the county health officer with these salutary requirements be kept confidential? Hidden in the files of the health offices, it serves no public purpose except a bare statistical one. Made available

to those with a legitimate ground for inquiry, it is effective to check the spread of the dread disease. It would be worse than useless to keep secret an order by a public officer that a certain typhoid carrier must not handle foods which are served to the public.[40]

The most extreme public health restrictions are quarantine and isolation. (Only in recent years have *quarantine* and *isolation* been separated as legal terms. All historical cases treat them as the same concept.) Quarantine was widely used until the 1950s. For self-limited diseases such as measles, the infected person was required to stay home without visitors. For chronic diseases, such as infectious tuberculosis before anti-tubercular agents were available, the infected person might be required to stay at a sanitarium with other infected patients. With the advent of antibiotics and effective immunizations, quarantine was seldom necessary to prevent the spread of communicable disease. Tuberculosis control programs still use quarantines when dealing with tuberculosis carriers who do not cooperate with treatment and control measures, and for outbreaks of diseases such as measles.

Vital Statistics and Disease Registries

Vital statistics, or birth and death records, are critical to public health and are required in all states. They provide the baseline information on the population and one of the few public health records that are meant to be a complete set, rather than sample. This requires careful enforcement of birth and death reporting laws.

Disease registries are a special class of reporting laws. Most disease registries are statewide and are used to track cancer, chronic diseases, or occupational illness. The CDC aggregates some state registry data into national registries. In general, registry reporting is like disease and injury reporting in that it is mandated, and the patient does not have the right to block it. However, there have been efforts in some states to allow patients to opt out of having their condition reported to the registry. There have also been legal challenges to the confidentiality of registry data, which undermines public support for registries.[41]

PUBLIC HEALTH EMERGENCY LAW

The terrorist attacks on the United States in September 2001 and the subsequent anthrax letters dramatically changed the legal climate in the United States. The president and congress, through laws such as the Homeland Security Act, moved to centralize control of law enforcement and public health emergency preparedness, including bioterrorism response, in the federal government. The states were urged to pass federally sponsored model laws, such as the Model State Emergency Health Powers Act (MSEHPA), which were intended to provide a legal framework for dealing with emergencies.

Ironically, the state and federal governments have dealt with emergencies throughout the history of this country without the need for elaborate emergency powers laws. These new laws are driven by two factors. First, as discussed earlier, state legislatures have weakened many state enforcement powers. Second, the new laws attempt to federalize and militarize public health emergency efforts, which have traditionally been a state and local responsibility.

Many of these laws, including the MSEHPA, ignore the realities of state and local public health infrastructure and resources. They attempt to mandate how state and local agencies will respond in an emergency such as a bioterrorism attack or flu pandemic, potentially locking agencies into wasteful or counterproductive actions, rather than allowing the flexibility to tailor their responses to the situation. In a real emergency, it is expected that the governors of the affected states will override the authority of the health departments through executive orders and run the emergency response from their own office.

More importantly, the rush to pass emergency laws ignores the fundamental problem of public health emergency response: most health departments in the United States are inadequately funded and staffed. They are unable to carry out their existing missions adequately. Passing new laws giving them more powers and more responsibilities, without dramatically increasing their staffing and resources, does not improve emergency preparedness. It does give legislators and the public a false sense of security. The complete failure of the state and federal response to Hurricane Katrina demonstrates the weakness of emergency preparedness based on laws and plans, without the people and resources to implement the plans.

SUMMARY

The state constitutions and the United States Constitution allow broad public health legal powers. The real constraints on public health actions are political and financial, not legal. Public health professionals need to understand the legal framework for their actions. They should work closely with their lawyers and encourage their lawyers to be creative in using the laws that are available to carry out necessary public health actions. In most cases, there will be a way to legally do what is necessary, if the department has the necessary political and financial support.

REVIEW QUESTIONS

1. What is the police power, and which governmental level is generally responsible for police power regulation?
2. Public health departments are administrative agencies. How are they established. and how do they get their powers?
3. What are the three main types of law, and which is the most important for a public health agency?
4. How does *habeas corpus* provide protection against inappropriate public health restrictions?

5. How are due process standards in public health different from those in criminal law?

6. How does Section 1983 of the Civil Rights Act apply to public health officials?

7. Whose permission is required for public health reporting of diseases or injuries?

8. What is the difference between emergency public health actions and the routine public health powers?

REFERENCES

1. McNeil WH. *Plagues and Peoples*. New York: Random House; 1976.

2. *Smith v Turner*, 48 U.S. 283, 340–341 (1849).

3. *Holmes v Jennison*, 39 U.S. 540, 616 (1840).

4. Pandemic and All-Hazards Preparedness Act, Pub. L. No. 109–417, 120 Stat. 3678 (2006).

5. *In re Gault*, 387 U.S. 1 (1967); and *In re Winship*, 397 U.S. 358 (1970).

6. Richards EP. The jurisprudence of prevention: Society's right of self-defense against dangerous individuals. *Hastings Const Law Q.* 1989;329:16.

7. *City of New York v New St. Mark's Baths*, 497 NYS 2d 979, 983 (1986).

8. *Mathews v Eldridge*, 424 U.S. 319 (1976).

9. *Ferguson v City of Charleston*, 532 U.S. 67 (2001).

10. *Kansas v Hendricks*, 521 U.S. 346 (1997).

11. *Allen v Illinois*, 478 U.S. 364 (1986).

12. *Addington v Texas*, 441 U. S. 418 (1979).

13. *Ex Parte McGee*, 185 P 14,16 (Kan 1919).

14. *Bell v Wolfish*, 441 U.S. 520 (1979).

15. *Yick Wo v Hopkins*, 118 U.S. 356, (1886).

16. *Reynolds v McNichols*, 488 F.2d 1378 (10th Cir. 1973).

17. *Camuglia v The City of Albuquerque*, 448 F.3d 1214 (10th Cir. 2006).

18. *North American Cold Storage Co. v City of Chicago*, 211 U.S. 306 (1908).

19. *New York v Burger*, 482 U.S. 691 (1987).

20. *People v Scott*, 79 N.Y.2d 474, 593 N.E.2d 1328, 583 N.Y.S.2d 920 (N.Y. 1992).

21. CDC. Outbreak of Multidrug-Resistant Tuberculosis—Texas, California, and Pennsylvania. *MMWR.* June 8 1990;39(22):369–372.

22. 42 USC 1981, et seq.

23. *DeShaney v Winnebago Cty. Dep't of Soc. Servs.*, 489 U.S. 189 (1989).

24. *Berkovitz by Berkovitz v US*, 486 US531 (1988).

25. *Allen v United States*, 816 F.2d 1417 (10th Cir. 1987).

26. *Ex parte Young*, 209 U.S. 123 (1908).

27. *Gacke v Pork Xtra, L.L.C.*, 684 N.W.2d 168 (Iowa 2004).

28. *Surocco v Geary*, 3 Cal 69 (1853).

29. *Raynor v Maryland Department of Health and Mental Hygiene*, 676 A.2d 978, 110 Md.App. 165 (Md.Sp.App. 1996); and *Altman v City of High Point, N.C.*, 330 F.3d 194 (4th Cir. 2003).

30. *Camara v Municipal Court of City and County of San Francisco*, 387 U.S. 523 (1967).

31. CDC. HIPAA Privacy Rule and Public Health: Guidance from CDC and the U.S. Department of Health and Human Services. *MMWR Supplement.* May 2 2003;52.

32. *Whalen v Roe*, 429 U.S. 589, 602 (1977).

33. Chorba TL, Berkelman RL, Safford SK, Gibbs NP, Hull HE. Mandatory reporting of infectious diseases by clinicians. *JAMA.* 1989;262:3018–3026.

34. Hethcote HW, Yorke JA. *Gonorrhea Transmission Dynamics and Control*. New York: Springer-Verlag; 1984.

35. Woodhouse DE, Muth JB, Potterat JJ, Riffe LD. Restricting personal behaviour: Case studies on legal measures to prevent the spread of HIV. *Int J STD AIDS.* March/April 1993;4(2):114–117.

36. *Guide to Public Heath Practice: Principles to Protect HIV Related Confidentiality and Prevent Discrimination*. Washington, DC: Association of State and Territorial Health Officers; 1988.

37. Potterat JJ, Spencer NE, Woodhouse DE, Muth JB. Partner notification in the control of human immunodeficiency virus infection. *Am J Public Health.* 1989;79(7):874(3).

38. Carrell S, Zoler ML. Defiant diseases: Hard-won gains erode. *Med World News.* 1990;31(12): 20(7).

39. *Jacobson v Massachusetts*, 197 U.S. 11358, 363 (1905).

40. *Thomas v Morris*, 36 NE2d 141, 142 (NY 1941).

41. *Southern Illinoisan v Department of Public Health*, 349 Ill.App.3d 431, 812 N.E.2d 27 (Ill.App. Dist.5 2004).

CHAPTER 7

Public Health Ethics

James C. Thomas, MPH, PhD

CHAPTER OBJECTIVES

Upon completion of this chapter, the reader will be able to:

1. Distinguish public health ethics from medical ethics.
2. Provide an orientation to ethical foundations in public health research.
3. Describe the contributions of utilitarianism and human rights to the ethics of public health practice.
4. Identify core values underlying public health ethics.
5. Describe the steps in ethical decision making.
6. Identify resources for encouraging the ethical practice of public health.

KEY TERMS

45 CFR 46
Applied Ethics
Belmont Report
Bioethics
Common Rule
Human Rights
Informed Consent
Institutional Review Board (IRB)
Medical Ethics
Morally Defensible Decision
Public Health Ethics
Public Health Practice
Research
Siracusa Principles
Tyranny of the Majority
Universal Declaration of Human Rights
Utilitarianism
Vulnerable Individuals

ETHICAL QUESTIONS

The governor of Texas ordered that all middle-school-aged girls be immunized for infection with human papilloma virus, a common sexually transmitted disease linked to cervical cancer. Some parents feel the immunization will make them more likely to have extramarital sex and are thus objecting to the new law. Others point out that the governor's former chief of staff is a lobbyist for the pharmaceutical company that makes the vaccine. Do the lives saved by preventing cervical cancer justify the constraint of some parents' civil liberties? By what other means might the governor bring about an immunization program without appearing to collude with the pharmaceutical industry and thereby undermine the public's trust?

Counties in North Carolina experienced an ice storm in which precipitation that was wetter than snow fell and froze. Power lines collapsed under the weight of the accumulated ice. Families relying on electricity for heat and cooking were left in the cold. Radio stations warned people not to use charcoal grills or kerosene heaters inside the house because of the risk of fires and the generation of carbon monoxide. However, the warnings were not broadcast in Spanish for the Latino immigrant population. In one affected city with a university campus, there were people of still other languages who didn't speak English. What steps should state and county health departments take to ensure the safety of the entire population?

Researchers are studying the challenges, needs, and health outcomes of men recently released from prison. Men on parole are at risk of being sent back to prison if they violate their parole requirements. The requirements can include, for example, not spending time with old friends. During an interview with a parolee, he mentions something he did that was a parole violation. Are the researchers required to report it to the parole officer?

These examples illustrate how ethical issues pervade the practice of public health. To identify ethical issues and then address them requires some familiarity with ethics in general and some practical skills. This chapter will orient you to both the theory and practice of public health ethics.

THE ETHICS LANDSCAPE

A basic question to start with is whether ethics is another word for morality. Are they the same thing? The short answer is, basically, yes. The longer answer is that some people think of morality as being more practical and based in action, and ethics as being more theoretical. More narrowly, the term morality has been used frequently in religious contexts, often around issues of sex and sexuality. To philosophers, however, the term "moral philosophy" is virtually synonymous with "ethics." In this chapter, the term "ethics" refers to both theory and practice.

At a university, the philosophy department will primarily teach ethical theory whereas professional schools, such as medicine, engineering, business, law, journalism, and public health, will teach **applied ethics.** Ethical theory includes concepts such as deontology (ethics based on a sense of duty) and consequentialism (ethics based on fairness of outcomes), and schools of thought such as utilitarianism, virtue ethics, and human rights. Applied ethics is concerned with prescribed actions or policies in ethical situations commonly encountered in a particular profession. Of course, applied ethics is rooted in ethical theory, and ethical theories arise from practical situations. So, the differences are in terms of emphasis and what people spend most of their time thinking about.

Research Versus Practice

Applied ethics can be further divided into research and practice. In the case of public health, **research** is defined as the intent to obtain knowledge that can be generalized to settings and populations other than the ones from which the data were collected.[1]

For example, an epidemiological study of factors affecting the transmission of HIV may be published in a scientific journal because the findings are thought to clarify the infection and epidemic in ways that will benefit populations around the country or even the world. In contrast, **public health practice** is concerned with a particular population. Thus, data collected by a city health department on the occurrence of HIV infections is not considered research as long as the disease surveillance is intended only to facilitate the planning and evaluation of programs to control the transmission of HIV in that city. If the surveillance data are later used to understand transmission in a way that is applicable to other cities, the use of the data becomes research, and additional ethical guidelines, discussed later, are brought to bear.

Distinctions between Medical and Public Health Ethics

Among the health-related professions, the articulation of ethics in public health is a very recent development.[2] Although the American Medical Association (AMA) adopted a code of ethics in 1847, a code of ethics for public health wasn't adopted until 2002. A reason for this 150-year lag may be that for centuries, physicians were considered the experts to turn to for all things related to health. Moreover, public health leadership positions were often filled by physicians. They would naturally refer to the ethical guidelines either received in their training or adopted by the professional (medical) societies to which they belonged. In the past few decades, however, nonmedical professionals, such as health administrators and epidemiologists, have assumed more leadership in public health and have not reflexively turned to the medical community for guidance in ethics.

A key reason that nonmedical ethical guidance is needed for public health is that the field of public health presents ethical dilemmas different from those in medicine. The professional situation most commonly giving rise to ethical dilemmas in medicine is the patient–provider interaction. In the clinic room, the physician is in his or her own setting with symbols of status and power such as diplomas on the wall, a white coat, and stethoscope, and knowledge of things that can heal the patient. In contrast, the patient is often undressed or scantily covered, in need of healing, and mystified by the pharmaceuticals and tools used by the physician. This setting in which the patient is dependent upon and vulnerable to the physician gives rise to most of the ethical dilemmas faced by physicians. Thus, medical ethics concerns itself with preserving the autonomy of the patient and forbidding the physician from knowingly causing any harm.

The principal setting giving rise to the most common ethical dilemmas in public health is not a one-on-one interaction but a many-on-many, that is, the interaction between a health department and the population it serves. Therefore, interactions entail group discussion and democratic processes. Also, public health is often concerned with prevention rather than cure of disease. Thus, it has an extra burden of proof to justify intervening in the life of a person who is already healthy.

A fundamental reality of populations is that one person's actions affect others. This is particularly evident with some infectious diseases. For example, a person with influenza can transmit the infection to others and make them sick. Conversely, by staying isolated, the infected person can prevent transmission to others. Out of concern for those who are well, a health department may infringe on the autonomy of individuals, at times through imposed isolation, but also through required vaccination or regulation of industries. The tension between preserving the health of the community and respecting the rights of individuals is the most common ethical dilemma arising in public health (see Figure 7.1).

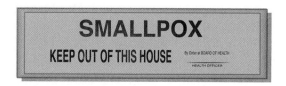

Figure 7.1. Sign Used in Quarantine Against Smallpox

SOURCE: Delmar Cengage Learning.

Bioethics and Public Health Ethics

Although medical and public health ethics arise from different situations, you might think that these two categories of applied ethics would reside together under the big tent of **bioethics.** Along with them would be nursing ethics, environmental ethics, and any other ethics pertaining to living things. In practice, however, centers, books, and courses on bioethics most often address applications of technology affecting the beginning and end of human life. Common concerns are contraception, abortion, gene therapy, termination of life-support, and the right to health care. All of these topics also dominate medical ethics. Thus, although **medical ethics** is logically a subcategory of bioethics, in reality the two are nearly synonymous. Some centers for bioethics are branching out to include **public health ethics** (e.g., the University of Toronto Joint Centre for Bioethics; http://www.utoronto. ca/jcb), but many view ethics through a medical lens and thus overlook public health. Some schools of public health are therefore developing ethics centers or programs that focus on public health concerns (e.g., The University of North Carolina; http://www.sph.unc. edu/general/program_in_public_health_ethics_4011_4045.html).

ETHICS IN PUBLIC HEALTH RESEARCH

Research ethics is the component of public health ethics that bears the closest relationship to medical ethics, in part because many public health studies include interactions between a researcher and a respondent, resembling the interactions between a clinician and a patient. The current guidelines for research ethics have their origins in responses to medical experiments conducted on German concentration camp internees during the Second World War. Following the war, the Nuremberg War Crime Trials led to the creation of the Nuremberg Code in 1947, articulating basic principles for ethical research involving human subjects. The key underlying principle was ensuring that research participation is truly voluntary (addressing the medical ethics concern for the autonomy of the patient). Ensuring voluntary participation requires that potential participants be fully aware of what the research entails, including all the likely risks and benefits. The process by which voluntary participation is ensured came to be known as **informed consent.**

While the principle of informed consent was being articulated in Nuremburg, a study in the United States that did not adhere to this principle was more than 10 years under way. Although conducted by the national Public Health Service, it came to be known as the Tuskegee Study because the Tuskegee Institute, located near the site of the study, was a collaborating institution. The study aimed to assess the health outcomes of untreated syphilis. The participants were not informed of the true purpose of the study. Instead, they were told they would receive treatments for the infection. However, the "treatments" they received were actually procedures for monitoring the progress of the infection. This deception was possible, in part, because the study subjects were low-income, uneducated men from rural Alabama. Much of the medical world was a mystery to them; they simply trusted the word of the highly educated physicians conducting the study.[3]

The deception became even more egregious with the discovery of penicillin in the early 1940s. This cure for syphilis was withheld from the men in the study so the researchers could learn what would happen if syphilis were allowed to follow its natural course. Race relations compounded the ethical lapses of the Tuskegee study. Most of the researchers were white, and the study subjects were black. One might argue that racial attitudes blinded the researchers to the ethical lapses of the study; that is, they held a lower standard for the treatment of poor and uneducated black men. A corollary of this argument would be that the Western world recoiled from the medical experiments of the Holocaust in part because many of the study subjects were white Westerners themselves. The Tuskegee study of untreated syphilis ended in scandal in 1974.

Initially, international bodies articulated research ethics. The United States government had not fully owned the need for research ethics, a realization that would have been demonstrated by developing its own guidelines. This situation was remedied a few years after the end of the Tuskegee Study. The first United States report on research ethics was published in 1979 by the National Commission for the Protection of Human Subjects of Biomedical and Behavioral Research. Known as the **Belmont Report,** it reinforced and elaborated on the principles of the Nuremberg Code.[4] Three key ethical principles were identified: respect for persons, beneficence, and justice. The three principles were then manifested in the practices of informed consent, weighing the risks and benefits to study subjects, and protecting **vulnerable individuals** such as minors, pregnant women, and prisoners.

The practices were codified into federal regulations in 1981. A publication (or "Title") of the Code of Federal Regulations (CFR) addressing human welfare concerns of the Department of Health and Human Services included a section on protection of human subjects. Because it was the 46th section of Title 45, the regulations are referred to as **45 CFR 46.**[5] Also referred to as **the Common Rule,** they establish the role of **institutional review boards (IRBs)** for research on human subjects. Institutions that receive government funds for research are required to have their research approved by a registered IRB. Large institutions, such as universities where much research is conducted, typically have several IRBs. Moreover, researchers receiving government funds are now required to receive training in research ethics. This is often done online through a site such as the Collaborative Institutional Training Initiative (CITI; http://www.citiprogram.org). The training modules teach the viewer about the origins of IRBs, the values that guide them, and the processes they follow. Viewers are taught the elements of informed consent and the concerns for vulnerable populations.

ETHICS IN PUBLIC HEALTH PRACTICE

Ethical principles in public health practice have not been developed along such a well-defined path. And rather than having their origins in the deliberations of international bodies, practice ethics have been country-specific. The following sections describe the ethical schools of thought relevant to public health practice and the values and beliefs inherent to a public health perspective.

Schools of Ethical Thought Relevant to Public Health Practice

The ethical principles in public health, as well as the values and beliefs, do not come from one particular philosophy or ethical school of thought. Rather, several philosophies are prominent in public health ethics.[6] The two most dominant are **utilitarianism** and **human rights.**

Writing in England at the turn of the nineteenth century, Jeremy Bentham articulated the principle of "the greatest happiness of the greatest number,"[7] typically understood today as "the greatest good for the greatest number." With public health's orientation to populations, the utilitarian principle was a natural fit for its ethical deliberations, and it is manifested today in such policy-making tools as the ranking of diseases by incidence and the prioritization of programs by cost-benefit analyses.

Utilitarian thinking was influential among the philosophic radicals in Great Britain in the early nineteenth century.[8] This group included early epidemiologists, biostatisticians, and one of the most prominent of the public health reformers, Edwin Chadwick. An intellectual and great admirer of Bentham, Chadwick was appointed as secretary of the Royal Commission to inquire into the Poor Laws of England. Through work on this commission, Chadwick and others brought attention to the dire health conditions of the new majority in the population, the urban working class, with the publication in 1842 of the pivotal public health document called the "Report . . . on an inquiry into the Sanitary Condition of the Labouring Population of Great Britain".[8] Using the emerging sciences of epidemiology and statistics, this report identified conditions such as polluted water supplies and filthy living conditions that were associated with epidemic diseases observed in Great Britain at the time.[9] Thus, a public health approach that identified the conditions associated with the most prevalent diseases found a natural ally in a utilitarian perspective that also argued for those actions that would benefit the majority of the population.

One of the limitations of utilitarianism is the need for data to enable decisions. In a cost-benefit analysis, for example, important information is often missing on either the costs or the benefits. Conversely, in some situations, the amount of data available can be overwhelming. In either situation, too little or too much information, the result can be inaction.

Another limitation is that, although its egalitarianism and principle of maximization place the majority in the spotlight, bringing attention to the problems of the "masses," a simple utilitarian outlook, risks pushing out of the spotlight those not in the majority. In a utilitarian calculus, each individual becomes a unit and his or her concerns are folded in with those of others, yielding a sum or average that lacks a human face. In this way, the experience of one individual can get swept aside by the momentum of larger numbers. When state laws sanction this **"tyranny of the majority,"** it can have devastating consequences; examples include slavery and eugenics (attempts to rid a race or ethnic group of impurities, often by killing or sterilization).

It was in reaction to the eugenic atrocities of the Third Reich's Holocaust that the **Universal Declaration of Human Rights** was drafted in 1948 as a statement of the minimum protection and benefits due to each human being (http://www.un.org/ Overview/rights.html). Half a decade after the Holocaust, the inadequacy of a utilitarian perspective is evident again in the AIDS pandemic. The overwhelming suffering caused by AIDS has disproportionately affected those in resource-poor areas of the world[10] and groups that have been traditionally marginalized and disenfranchised in resource-rich countries[11]. In neither situation are those with AIDS the people who control the distribution of goods in resource-rich countries. Nor are people living with AIDS around the world likely to figure prominently in a utilitarian calculation of maximizing happiness among the populations in resource-rich nations. It was in this context that Dr. Jonathan Mann of the United Nations Global Program on AIDS invoked human rights as an ethical guiding force in public health.[12]

A human rights perspective is important in public health because of the equal dignity and worth it places in each human being.[13] Equal dignity demands a minimum standard of treatment and respect for each person, providing a needed correction to utilitarianism, in which the dignity and worth of a minority can get lost in the desires of the majority. Modern human rights also bring global attention to the determinants of an individual's health and well-being; including liberty, security, self-determination, access to basic health care, education, nutrition, and a clean environment. Their general acceptance around the world also makes rights a functionally powerful ethical paradigm.

The social, political, and legal natures of human rights, however, are arguably more important than their ability to stand alone as the only ethical paradigm in public health. In some respects, a narrow human rights interpretation is at odds with some public health values. Notably modern human rights are principally individualistic, whereas public health is community-oriented. Although humans are individualistic to some extent, they are also inherently social. Some of the most rewarding and meaningful moments in life are when we care for or nurture another person, and when we receive that care. The word *community* is rooted in the idea of communing, or sharing things in common. Interdependence and community, rather than independence and individualism, are more central to the values of public health.

Article 25 of the Universal Declaration of Human Rights

Everyone has the right to a standard of living adequate for the health and well-being of himself and of his family, including food, clothing, housing and medical care and necessary social services, and the right to security in the event of unemployment, sickness, disability, widowhood, old age or other lack of livelihood in circumstances beyond his control.

Human rights have traditionally been invoked following political and civil abuses by a state against its citizens. Even though one purpose of a government is to enable healthy human interaction, there remains the possibility that it will fail in this function to the point of harming its citizens. Protections and recourse for individuals are undoubtedly needed in this event. However, governments also serve functions that enable, or perhaps even ennoble, people to care for one another. This is seen in part through the redistribution of income and services in the form of taxes, and the creation of public spaces that encourage social interaction. This latter role of government is more akin to public health values.

In addition to interpretations of modern human rights that are not consonant with a public health perspective, a human rights ethic is a tool that is inadequately refined for charting an ethical course for public health. Rights have a binary quality; either they exist or they don't, without gradations. Even among those rights that people agree upon, there is no agreement on the relative weight of one right against another when two rights come into conflict. When two rights are not in conflict, there is no guidance as to which should be pursued first or most aggressively. In these situations, a utilitarian or data-based approach can be helpful.

Other ethical schools of thought relevant to public health are virtue ethics, focusing on individual character (e.g., the character of a public health professional), and care ethics, with its principal attention to the interdependence of people and obligations to care for each other. Religiously motivated ethics have also had their influence on public health. For example, the Civil Rights movement, based largely in African American churches, addressed the inequities of segregation, many of which were manifested in racial health disparities.

Values and Beliefs Underlying a Public Health Perspective

In practical ethics, principles are born from common situations in which the practitioners find themselves. They are also rooted in the core beliefs and values of the profession. A *belief* is something held to be true, and a *value* is something given priority in decision making. Public health is a diverse field, composed of professionals with a wide range of skills, so unanimity in values and beliefs is seldom realized. Nonetheless, there are discernible, dominant shared beliefs and values. They are enumerated in the supporting documents for the Public Health Code of Ethics developed by the Public Health Leadership Society and endorsed by national public health organizations. The values and beliefs are grouped in three topics: health, community, and the bases for action, extracted from the Code documents (http://www.phls.org/home/section/3-26/) and presented next.

Health

1. *Humans have a right to the resources necessary for health.* The Public Health Code of Ethics affirms Article 25 of the Universal Declaration of Human Rights, which states in part "Everyone has the right to a standard of living adequate for the health and well-being of himself and his family. . . ."

Community

2. *Humans are inherently social and interdependent.* Humans look to each other for companionship in friendships, families, and community; and rely upon one another for safety and survival. Positive relationships among individuals and positive collaborations among institutions are signs of a healthy community. The rightful concern for the physical individuality of humans and one's right to make decisions for oneself must be balanced against the fact that each person's actions affect other people.

3. *The effectiveness of institutions depends heavily on the public's trust.* Factors that contribute to trust in an institution include the following actions on the part of the institution: communication; truth telling; transparency (i.e., not concealing information); accountability; reliability; and reciprocity. One critical form of reciprocity and communication is listening to as well as speaking with the community.

4. *Collaboration is a key element to public health.* The public health infrastructure of a society is composed of a wide variety of agencies and professional disciplines. To be effective, they must work together well. Moreover, new collaborations will be needed to rise to new public health challenges.

5. *People and their physical environment are interdependent.* People depend upon the resources of their natural and constructed environments for life itself. A damaged or unbalanced natural environment, and a constructed environment of poor design or in poor condition, will have an adverse affect on the health of people. Conversely, people can have a profound effect on their natural environment through consumption of resources and generation of waste.

6. *Each person in a community should have an opportunity to contribute to public discourse.* Contributions to discourse may occur through a direct or a representative system of government. In the process of developing and evaluating policy, it is important to discern whether all who would like to contribute to the discussion have an opportunity to do so, even though expressing a concern does not mean that it will necessarily be addressed in the final policy.

7. *Identifying and promoting the fundamental requirements for health in a community are a primary concern to public health.* The way in which a society is structured is reflected in the health of a community. The primary concern of public health is with these underlying structural aspects. While some important public health programs are curative in nature, the field as a whole must never lose sight of underlying causes and prevention. Because fundamental social structures affect many aspects of health, addressing the fundamental causes rather than more proximal causes, is more truly preventive.

Bases for Action

8. *Knowledge is important and powerful.* We are to seek to improve our understanding of health and the means of protecting it through research and the accumulation of knowledge. Once obtained, there is a moral obligation in some instances to share what is known. For example, active and informed participation in policy-making processes requires access to relevant information. In other instances, such as information provided in confidence, there is an obligation to protect information.

9. *Science is the basis for much of our public health knowledge.* The scientific method provides a relatively objective means of identifying the factors necessary for health in a population, and for evaluating policies and programs to protect and promote health. The full range of scientific tools, including both quantitative and qualitative methods, and collaboration among the sciences is needed.

10. *People are responsible to act on the basis of what they know.* Knowledge is not morally neutral and often demands action. Moreover, information is not to be gathered for idle interest. Public health should seek to translate available information into timely action. Often, the action required is research to fill in the gaps of what we *don't* know.

11. *Action is not based on information alone.* In many instances, action is required in the absence of all the information one would like. In other instances, policies are demanded by the fundamental value and dignity of each human being, even if implementing them is not calculated to be optimally efficient or cost-beneficial. In both of these situations, values inform the application of information or the action in the absence of information.

Principles in the Ethical Practice of Public Health

The values and beliefs inherent to a public health perspective underlie the 12 principles of the public health code of ethics presented in the text box on the next page. Each principle also relates to one or more of the 10 essential public health services articulated by Public Health Functions Steering Committee. You can view the correspondence between the principles and the services by downloading the code of ethics materials from the Public Health Leadership Society website (http://www.phls.org/home/section/3-26/).

The code of ethics is not the only place that ethical principles in public health have been articulated. Following the international epidemic of sudden acute respiratory syndrome (SARS) in 2002, and in anticipation of a pandemic of influenza, a number of groups have identified ethical principles for the distribution of scarce resources, for social distancing to limit transmission, for keeping the public informed, for the obligations and rights of health care staff who care for the ill, and more. The World Health Organization Project on Addressing Ethical Issues in Pandemic Influenza Planning identified four principles for public health measures:[14]

1. *Public health necessity.* A government should exercise its public health police powers on an individual or group only if the person or group poses a threat to the community such as the likelihood of spreading an infection.

2. *Reasonable and effective means.* The methods by which a threat is addressed should have a reasonable chance of being effective.

3. *Proportionality.* The human burden imposed by a public health regulation should be proportionate to the expected public health benefit.

4. *Distributive justice.* The risks, benefits, and burdens of public health action should be fairly distributed, thereby precluding the unjustified targeting of an already socially vulnerable population.

Speaking to the tension in public health between the rights of individuals and the good of the community, this group noted *The Siracusa Principles,* a set of principles regarding internationally recognized limitations on human rights, established at a meeting in Siracusa, Italy.[15] The four principles for restricting rights for the benefit of the community are as follows: (1) the restriction is provided for and carried out in accordance with the law, (2) the restriction is in the interest of a legitimate objective of general interest, (3) the restriction is strictly necessary in a democratic society to achieve the objective, and (4) there are no less intrusive and restrictive means available to reach the same objective.

The Relation between Ethics and Law

The first of the **Siracusa Principles** says that restrictions of individual rights should only be done in accordance with the law. This begs the question of the ethical nature of the law. Utilitarianism tells us that, in a democratic society, the majority can enact legislation that systematically oppresses or neglects the minority. Intuitively, we might think that laws are the way a society codifies its ethics. Although that is the case with murder, for example, in other situations, a law may have little to do with ethics; and in many instances, ethics are not encoded in the law. An example of a law that is largely unrelated to ethics is the requirement that the President of the United States be at least 35 years old. The rationale behind setting the age at 35 was, in all likelihood, an approximation of an age at which one would be mature enough to fulfill the obligations of the office (this was perhaps a reaction to child kings and queens in history). Experience tells us, however, that there are some people over 35 who do not have the maturity

---

The Public Health Code of Ethics

1. Public health should address principally the fundamental causes of disease and requirements for health, aiming to prevent adverse health outcomes.

2. Public health should achieve community health in a way that respects the rights of individuals in the community.

3. Public health policies, programs, and priorities should be developed and evaluated through processes that ensure an opportunity for input from community members.

4. Public health should advocate and work for the empowerment of disenfranchised community members, aiming to ensure that the basic resources and conditions necessary for health are accessible to all.

5. Public health should seek the information needed to implement effective policies and programs that protect and promote health.

6. Public health institutions should provide communities with the information they have that is needed for decisions on policies or programs and should obtain the community's consent for their implementation.

7. Public health institutions should act in a timely manner on the information they have within the resources and the mandate given to them by the public.

8. Public health programs and policies should incorporate a variety of approaches that anticipate and respect diverse values, beliefs, and cultures in the community.

9. Public health programs and policies should be implemented in a manner that most enhances the physical and social environment.

10. Public health institutions should protect the confidentiality of information that can bring harm to an individual or community if made public. Exceptions must be justified on the basis of the high likelihood of significant harm to the individual or others.

11. Public health institutions should ensure the professional competence of their employees.

12. Public health institutions and their employees should engage in collaborations and affiliations in ways that build the public's trust and the institution's effectiveness.

---

needed for the presidency, and we might well imagine a 34-year-old who is wise and experienced enough to do well in the office. In this and other instances, the law is more about politics and pragmatic issues than about right and wrong.

The "right to a standard of living adequate for health and well-being" mentioned in the Universal Declaration of Human Rights is an example of an ethical tenet not encoded in law. It is not illegal in the United States to be homeless or to lack the means to pay for health care.

From these examples, we see that the door into ethics is not necessarily law (Figure 7.2). In fact, making our public health systems more ethical may entail changing existing laws or enacting laws that do not exist.

ETHICAL DECISION MAKING

If the law does not necessarily tell us what is ethical in public health, how do we make decisions and enact policies that are ethical? There are procedures and steps to aid us in this process, but before describing them, it is worth clarifying what we can reasonably expect from them. We cannot expect to identify a particular answer that is indisputably ethical or, in other words, *the* right answer. We can seldom, if ever, be sure that all relevant considerations have been taken into account for a particular decision. And not everyone gives the same weight

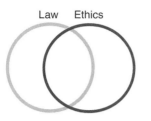

Law   Ethics

Figure 7.2. **The Overlap between Law and Ethics**
SOURCE: Delmar Cengage Learning.

or importance to each consideration. One person or group will favor civil liberties for individuals, and another will favor restriction of some liberties to benefit the health of the whole community.

What we *can* expect is to arrive at a **morally defensible decision,** one that was determined by a fair process and that took into consideration factors that are commonly regarded as important. With different groups of people, a variety of decisions may be made with a similar process and information, but in each case, the group can account for an ethical process of decision making.

Because public health policy is carried out by an agency, usually part of the government, and it affects a population, decision making is a group process. Not only does it entail several people within an agency or at various levels of government, but the Public Health Code of Ethics dictates that representatives from the public be included in the process. Thus, the foundation of ethical decision making in public health is a fair process of deliberation, which is generally considered to have five characteristics:

1. **Transparency:** The process by which decisions are made should be evident to all who are interested (otherwise known as stakeholders), and the decisions made should be publicized.

2. **Inclusiveness:** The interests of all stakeholders should be considered, and stakeholders or their representatives should have an opportunity to contribute to the decision-making process.

3. **Reasonableness:** Decisions should be made on the basis of the best evidence available, and to

the degree possible, should reflect values shared among the stakeholders.

4. **Responsiveness:** Deliberations should address the concerns that led to the deliberations, and there should be opportunities to evaluate decisions and outcomes as new information becomes available.

5. **Accountability:** There should be a means to hold the decision makers accountable for their decisions.

A group that is deliberating in this manner should then follow a several step process. Although they are listed here in a particular order, often in reality the order of the steps gets jumbled, or a group may return to an earlier step after more information is obtained. Examples for each will be applied to the ice storm scenario described at the beginning of the chapter. The principal concern was communication with non-English-speaking populations in North Carolina counties affected by the storm.

1. **Clarify the facts of the situation:** If the ethical question involves a health outcome, what is the occurrence of the disease? What are the risk factors? How do rates compare between males and females, or between different ethnicities? What is the history of the situation? What led to the ethical question arising? What are the financial costs involved?

The list of relevant facts can be quite extensive and seldom are all the desired facts available. Discussion of the remaining steps sometimes refines the question and allows a group to narrow in on particular concerns or to reorient entirely the facts considered relevant. Inevitably, however, the group will have to make a decision with incomplete information.

In the case of the ice storm, who are the non-English-speaking populations? What languages do they speak? Do they have some English speakers among them? Where do they live? How many were affected by the ice storms? Are there cultural factors other than language that may cause them to be at risk during a cold period without electricity?

2. Identify the ethical questions: The process of ethical decision making often begins with an individual or a group identifying an ethical dilemma. The group that deliberates over a response to the dilemma may identify additional ethical questions that were previously unrecognized. They may even conclude that the original question brought to them is not the most important one. Keeping in mind that responsiveness to the original concern is a component of a fair process, the deliberators should confer with the ones who brought the initial concern to either persuade them that their question needs to be reframed or to inform them of the priority of their question among the others identified. In any case, the group should continue the process for only one well-defined ethical question at a time.

An obvious ethical question related to the non-English-speaking populations affected by the ice storm is whether the government of an English-speaking state has an obligation to translate its safety messages into other languages. If so, how many other languages? And how many resources (e.g., finances) should be devoted to this effort? Related questions could pertain to the reasons these populations do not speak English or receive warning messages. For example, have affordable means for learning English been made available to them?

3. Identify the stakeholders and what each stands to lose or gain: The principal intent of this step is to look at the ethical question through the eyes of each group that will be most affected by the decision. The more narrowly stakeholders can be described, the more helpful this step will be. For example, if a question concerns Latino immigrants, the deliberating group may want to consider separately single men, mothers, and dependent children; or those who can speak English and those who can't. This step will be greatly aided if the fair process principle of inclusion is followed and representatives of the various stakeholder groups are among the deliberators.

Another ethnically defined group of stakeholders was the Hmong people who were refugees from war and political strife in Laos. Their needs would be different from those of Latino immigrants because they immigrated legally (many Latinos are undocumented aliens) and thus do not fear contact with government authorities. Moreover, they often immigrate as whole families, whereas Latino immigrants are most likely to be young men. Those addressing the ethical issues need to consider how these factors will affect the actions of the public health officials and other government employees trying to ensure the safety of the population.

4. What do the various schools of ethical thought highlight?: In the previous step, the deliberating group looked at the ethical question through the eyes of various stakeholders. In this step, the group considers the question through the lens of various ethical schools of thought. What does a human rights perspective bring to light? Is it different from what someone would concentrate on with a utilitarian perspective? One or more of the stakeholder groups may adhere to a particular religion. What would be the principal concerns, prescriptions, and proscriptions of those faith perspectives?

A strict utilitarian approach to the ice storm might devalue the safety of a minority of people in favor of efforts to care for the English-speaking majority. Some might suggest that protection from harm in the midst of a public health emergency is a human right. However, if that protection is not written into law, it is hard to make that argument. In contrast, a number of religious traditions insist on an extra effort devoted specifically to any marginalized or vulnerable individuals.

5. What do professional ethical principles, standards of practice, and law suggest?: Here the process turns to resources such as the codes of ethics in public health and other relevant professions. Perhaps there are established "best practices" or even laws to consider. Hopefully, these professional guidelines and laws will move the group toward ethical courses of action. However, it is also possible that flaws in the guidelines or laws may be identified in this process. Then the group of deliberators have to decide whether to let their recommended actions be constrained by existing policies and law or to override them with what they consider to be a truly ethical course of action. In the latter case, they must be willing to deal with a legal challenge or punishment.

The Public Health Code of Ethics states that "Public health should advocate and work for the empowerment of disenfranchised community members, aiming to ensure that the basic resources and conditions necessary for health are accessible to all" (Principle 4), and "Public health programs and policies should incorporate a variety of approaches that anticipate and respect diverse values, beliefs, and cultures in the community" (Principle 8). These two principles point clearly to the obligation of a health department to take particular actions to ensure the well being of non-English-speaking populations in the midst of a public health emergency such as an ice storm.

6. Identify possible alternative courses of action: The options available to a group are seldom as narrow or constrained as they initially appear. In many instances, there is room for nuanced actions in which the pain of the most offensive implications of a decision is blunted with exceptions or modifications for certain stakeholders or in certain situations.

To communicate with non-English-speaking populations in an ice storm, a health department could dispatch an employee to identify and visit every household at risk, or identify a number of bilingual members of the community who could help write a flyer to deliver to each non-English-speaking household. The health department could weigh the effectiveness and cost of each option.

7. Choose the alternative best supported by the preceding analysis: At this point, the time has come for the group to make a decision. As stated earlier, decisions are inevitably made with inadequate information. But by the time the group has reached this step, they have followed a process that has been fair, and they have systematically considered the most important facets. They should make their decision by a process agreed upon in the beginning, whether by a simple majority vote, consensus (in which some of the group may not agree

with the others, but not so strongly that they prevent a decision), or unanimity.

Recalling the elements of fair process, members of the affected communities should contribute to the decision. Different approaches to communication in an ice storm may be most effective with Latinos and the Hmong, for example.

8. Evaluate the actions taken and their eventual outcomes: This step is perhaps the hardest, principally because after a decision has been made, people generally want to move on to other concerns. It takes a high level of commitment to track the effects of a decision and then, in spite of other pressing issues, to consider the quality of a decision made in the past. Yet, in a fully ethical process, those who make a decision truly care about the outcome, not only for those affected by the decision but also to inform future ethical decisions.

Follow-up with the Latino and Hmong populations after the ice storm would help the health department know the elements of a good response to future public health emergencies affecting these populations.

RESOURCES FOR ENCOURAGING ETHICS IN PUBLIC HEALTH

The process just described is rarely implemented. Not many in public health are trained to recognize ethical dilemmas and address them. But ethics is increasingly regarded as an important component of public health, and resources for imparting ethical skills are becoming available. The Public Health Code of Ethics is one such resource. In addition, a list of competencies and skills in public health ethics has been made available online (http://www.phls.org/home/section/3-26/) to inform the development of courses and training materials.

Ready-made materials for teaching or learning ethics are also available free of charge online, including a model curriculum[16] and a series of modules presented through slides and voiceover (http://www2.sph.unc.edu/oce/phethics/). McKeown and Weed have published a helpful lexicon of ethics terms related to public health.[17] A number of textbooks on public health ethics are a good source for information on ethical theory and ethics in public health history.[18–21] There remains a need, however, for materials that impart skills in ethical decision making. The number of academic centers for bioethics is too long to list. However, the websites of a number of international and national institutions addressing public health ethics are listed in the textbox.

The regulated policies of research ethics have helped establish an ethical work environment in research settings. They have brought ethics to the front and center of the minds of researchers. Unfortunately, some researches view the required processes as burdensome, consuming time and creating delays in the research. In some instances, the policies are followed mechanically and resentfully. In this way, they can deaden a person's ethical sensitivity rather than sharpen it. As ethics in public health practice (i.e., apart from research) becomes more institutionalized, one challenge will be to avoid mechanical routinization of tasks and to stimulate ethical sensitivity and skills.

NEEDED FOR THE FUTURE

To move into a future where public health practitioners are energized rather than frustrated by ethical deliberation, it helps to envision processes that encourage and enable individuals to raise ethical concerns; processes that are so highly regarded and rewarding that people want to participate in them and seek out the skills necessary to do so. Those engaged in such a process will benefit from reading case studies reporting how other ethical issues in

> ### International and National Institutions Addressing Public Health Ethics
>
> World Health Organization
>   www.who.int/ethics/en/
> Centers for Disease Control and Prevention (United States)
>   www.cdc.gov/od/science/phec/
> The Provincial Health Ethics Network (Canada)
>   www.phen.ab.ca/
> National Ethics Advisory Committee (New Zealand)
>   www.neac.health.govt.nz/
> Ethics and Health: An International and Comparative Arena (Norway)
>   www.hf.uib.no/i/Filosofisk/ethica/default.html

public health have been identified and addressed. A few case studies are available in a book of epidemiologic examples[22] and the model curriculum in public health ethics mentioned earlier.[16] The field would benefit from many more.

No population has ever been fully isolated from others. Advances in international travel have only heightened the international potential of epidemics and the relevance of the health of one country to the well being of another. As researchers conduct studies outside of their country, and agencies such as the CDC collaborate with other countries, it is important to have an understanding of the ethical perspectives of different countries and cultures, to anticipate differences, and to establish means of working together while also demonstrating mutual respect. Few countries have articulated an ethic related to public health.

The ongoing development of ethics in American public health is limited to the conduct of agencies charged with protecting the health of the public. There are also private companies that affect the health of the public, but they are not seen as having a mandate to protect the health of the public. They include automobile manufacturers and food industries. And of course a healthy work environment is important to employees of all companies. Presently, the practices of companies that affect the health of the public can be regulated by the government. However, regulation is a "stick" rather than a "carrot" approach. Many companies resent regulation and lobby against it. Sorely needed are creative "carrot" approaches that tap into economic incentives while also protecting or improving public health. At the time of this writing, there is an awakening to global climate change. It is becoming fashionable for companies to become more "green," that is, to have less of a negative impact on the environment. This instance may provide insights that will allow us to extend concern for the health of the public, and thus public health ethics, into other facets of our economy and society.

REVIEW QUESTIONS

1. The autonomy of the patient is a prominent ethical principle in medical ethics. In contrast, interdependence between people in a population, and thus the need to sometimes restrict individuals' rights, is more prominent in public health ethics. Why is this?
2. Name one strength and one weakness of utilitarian ethics.
3. Name one strength and one weakness of human rights ethics.
4. What are the Siracusa Principles, and how do they relate to human rights?
5. What are the elements of a fair process of decision making?

REFERENCES

1. MacQueen KM, Buehler JW. Ethics, practice, and research in public health. *Am J Public Health.* 2004;94:928–31.
2. Kass NE. An ethics framework for public health. *Am J Public Health.* 2001;91:1776–82.
3. Jones JH. *Bad Blood: The Tuskegee Syphilis Experiment.* New York: Free Press; 1993.
4. National Commission for the Protection of Human Subjects of Biomedical and Behavioral Research. *The Belmont Report: Ethical Principles and Guidelines for the Protection of Human Subjects of Research.* Washington, DC: US Government Printing Office; 1979.
5. Code of Federal Regulations. Title 45, Part 46, *Protection of Human Subjects*; revised June 23, 2005. Available at: http://www.hhs.gov/ohrp/humansubjects/guidance/45cfr46.htm. Accessed May 23, 2007.
6. Roberts MJ, Reich MR. Ethical analysis in public health. *Lancet.* 2002;359:1055–9.
7. Bentham J. *A Fragment on Government and An Introduction to the Principles of Morals and Legislation.* Oxford: Blackwell Publishers; 1948.
8. Rosen G. *A History of Public Health (expanded ed).* Baltimore, MD: The Johns Hopkins University Press; 1993.
9. Lewis RA. *Edwin Chadwick and the Public Health Movement, 1832–1854.* London: Longmans & Green; 1952.
10. Joint United Nations Program on HIV/AIDS (UNAIDS). *Report on the Global HIV/AIDS Epidemic.* Geneva: Joint United Nations Program on HIV/AIDS; 2000.
11. Centers for Disease Control and Prevention. *HIV/AIDS Surveillance Report.* Atlanta, GA: Centers for Disease Control and Prevention; 1999.
12. Mann JM. Human rights and AIDS: The future of the pandemic. In: Mann JM, Gruskin S, Grodin MA, Annas GJ (Eds). *Health and Human Rights: A Reader.* New York: Routledge; 1999: 216–226.
13. Mann JM, Gostin L, Gruskin S, Brennan T, Lazzarini Z, Fineberg H. Health and human rights. In: Mann JM, Grsuskin S, Grodin MA, Annas GJ (Eds). *Health and Human Rights: A Reader.* New York: Routledge; 1999:7–20.
14. World Health Organization, Project on Addressing Ethical Issues in Pandemic Influenza Planning. Draft paper for working group two: *Ethics of public health measures in response to pandemic influenza.* October 2006. Available at: http://www.who.int/entity/eth/ethics/PI_Ethics_draft_paper_WG2_6_Oct_06.pdf. Accessed May 21, 2007.
15. United Nations, Economic and Social Council. *Siracusa Principles on the Limitation and Derogation Provisions in the International Covenant on Civil and Political Rights,* U.N. Doc. E/CN.4/1985/4, Annex (1985). Available at: http://www1.umn.edu/humanrts/instree/siracusaprinciples.html. Accessed May 23, 2007.
16. Jennings B, Kahn J, Mastroianni A, Parker LS (Eds.). *Ethics and Public Health: Model Curriculum.* Association of Schools of Public Health,

2003. Available at: http://www.asph.org/
document.cfm?page=782. Accessed May 23, 2007.

17. McKeown RE, Weed DL. Ethics in epidemiology
and public health II. Applied terms. *J Epidemiol
Community Health*. 2002;56:739–41.

18. Beauchamp DE, Steinbock B (Eds.). *New Ethics
for the Public's Health*. New York: Oxford
University Press; 1999.

19. Bayer R, Gostin LO, Jennings B, Steinbock B
(Eds.). *Public Health Ethics: Theory, Policy, and
Practice*. New York: Oxford University Press; 2006.

20. Powers M, Faden R. *Social Justice: The Moral
Foundations of Public Health and Health Policy
(Issues in Biomedical Ethics)*. New York: Oxford
University Press; 2006.

21. Anand S, Peter F, Sen A (Eds.). *Public Health,
Ethics, and Equity*. New York: Oxford University
Press; 2006.

22. Soskolne CL, Goodman KW, Coughlin SS.
Case Studies in Public Health Ethics. Washington,
DC: American Public Health Association;
1998.

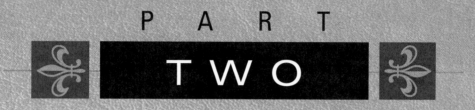

P A R T

TWO

Settings for Public Health Practice

CHAPTER 8

The Federal Contribution to Public Health

William L. Roper, MD, MPH

LEARNING OBJECTIVES

Upon completion of this chapter, the reader will be able to:

1. Describe the evolution of federal government powers and responsibilities in public health.

2. Contrast federal public health powers with those of state and local governments.

3. Assess the sources of federal government influence over public health issues from legal, political, and institutional perspectives.

4. Examine the distribution of public health powers and responsibilities across the executive, legislative, and judicial branches of the federal government.

5. Identify the federal agencies and offices responsible for addressing health issues.

6. Analyze current developments in public health practice that are likely to shape future federal roles in public health.

KEY TERMS

Appropriations Legislation

Authorization Legislation

Efficacy

Enabling Legislation

Medically Underserved Areas

Political Action Committees

Public Health Emergency

Telemedicine

Public health activities in the United States are carried out through the collective actions of governmental agencies and private-sector organizations working at local, state, regional, and national levels. Governmental agencies play leading roles in organizing and coordinating these activities because of their statutorily defined powers and responsibilities and the unique resources and organizational capacities they bring to public health practice. The division of authority and responsibility among federal, state, and local governmental agencies in public health reflects the federalist system of government in the United States and the constitutionally defined powers ascribed to each level of government. The federal government has a profound influence on the structure and content of population-based efforts to protect and improve health within the United States. Tracking the federal influence on public health policy and practice can be difficult, however, because this influence is achieved through numerous policy and regulatory instruments, and it is shaped by a complex array of legal, political, financial, and institutional structures. Nonetheless, a complete understanding of the practice of public health in the United States requires a critical examination of the federal government's many roles and responsibilities. This chapter reviews the legal and political basis for the federal government's contributions to public health activities and examines the primary institutional and policy instruments through which it makes these contributions.

The federal government's roles in public health are carried out through all three branches of government. The legislative branch occupied by the United States Congress holds constitutional authority for creating federal programs, policies, and regulations that influence public health, and for appropriating the federal funds that allow them to be implemented. The executive branch holds the authority for implementing public health programs and enforcing health-related policies and regulations through its many administrative agencies. The executive office also has responsibility for informing the budgetary and legislative processes of Congress. The judicial branch occupied by the federal courts carries out the critical responsibility of interpreting and adjudicating the federal government's public health authority in view of constitutional law, legislative action, and legal precedent.

HISTORY OF FEDERAL INVOLVEMENT IN PUBLIC HEALTH

Federal roles and responsibilities in public health have evolved considerably over time in response to political, economic, legal, and social developments in the nation's history. The federal government played relatively minor roles in protecting and promoting public health throughout much of this history. As scientific knowledge about the causes of disease expanded during the eighteenth and nineteenth centuries, individual cities and states within the United States were the first to respond with public facilities, programs, and regulatory provisions designed to prevent and control diseases within the population.[1] Governmental institutions devoted to health and disease existed almost exclusively at the local and state levels. Meanwhile, federal involvement was limited to the Marine Hospital Service, a system of public hospitals established in 1798 to care for merchant seamen. The federal government's role in health began to expand slowly during the early twentieth century when the Marine Hospital Service was transformed into the United States Public Health Service, and the position of surgeon general was created to lead the institution.[2] By 1918, this institution had received the authority to administer medical examinations to aliens, to experiment with projects to expand health care in rural areas, and to implement programs that prevent and control sexually transmitted diseases.[1] Also during this period, the United States Congress began to explore the use of federal regulatory powers in preventing and controlling diseases. The 1906 passage of the Food and Drug Act created the nation's first federal regulations covering the manufacture, labeling, and sale of food products.

Federal health activities expanded dramatically during the 1920s and 1930s through the creation of numerous governmental programs designed to increase access to personal health services. The Sheppard-Towner Act of 1922 established the first federal grant-in-aid program supporting the delivery of personal health services. This act created the Federal Board of Maternal and Infant Hygiene and authorized it to administer funding to states for maternal and child health services such as home nursing and obstetrical care.[1] The program soon became a widely replicated model for other federal health programs, wherein the federal government provides funding and oversight to state agencies, which in turn design and implement the programs.[3] Similar programs were created to fund the development of local public health clinics (1935), the training of public health workers (1935), the prevention and control of sexually transmitted diseases (1938), and the creation of community mental health centers (1946).

The federal government's involvement in biomedical research and disease control also expanded dramatically during this period. The National Institutes of Health (NIH) was created in 1930 from a former laboratory within the Marine Hospital Service and soon developed the capacity to investigate a broad range of diseases and treatments. Specialized research institutes were soon added to NIH to investigate topics such as cancer, neurological diseases, environmental health issues, and mental health disorders. The federal Center for Disease Control (CDC) was established in 1946, initially to control malaria and other vector-borne diseases during World War II. The CDC's scope of activity grew steadily over the years to cover all communicable disease control efforts and, eventually, a broad range of prevention activities involving chronic diseases, injuries, and environmental health risks.[4] The agency was renamed the Centers for Disease Control and Prevention to reflect this larger scope of activity.

The federal government's dominant role in health care financing was solidified in 1965 with the passage of legislation creating the Medicare and Medicaid programs. The federally administered Medicare program financed medical care for the nation's elderly and, eventually, the nation's permanently disabled populations along with those with end-stage renal disease. Medicaid, by contrast, was created as a federal program jointly funded and administered by the states that financed health services for a variety of low-income populations. Numerous other federal grant-in-aid programs were established during the 1960s and 1970s to fund specific types of health services and programs, including community health centers, family planning services, dental services, tuberculosis diagnosis and treatment, home health care, childhood developmental and screening services, and health professions training programs.[3]

The financial consequences of an expanding federal role in health care and public health became apparent in the 1970s with spiraling national health care expenditures. In response, the federal government assumed another important role within the nation's health system—that of health resources management and planning.[5] Prominent congressional action during the 1970s included the Health Maintenance Organization Act of 1973, which created incentives for the development of health care delivery and financing systems that would later become known as managed care; and the National Health Planning and Resources Development Act of 1974, which established review and certification requirements for the development of new health facilities and services.

A number of federal health initiatives were reorganized and, in some cases, scaled back during the 1980s as overall federal health expenditures continued to escalate. Clusters of related federal grant-in-aid programs supporting health and social services were combined into large block grants that gave states more flexibility over how federal funds could be spent. This federal strategy was used in part to stimulate efforts by states and local governments to develop further their health and social service systems.[6] Critics, however, charged that block grants were also used to mask overall reductions in federal funding for these services.[7] Block grants established specifically for public health activities included the Maternal and Child Health Block Grant, the Family Planning Block Grant, and the Preventive Health and Health Services Block Grant.[8] Also during this period, the federal Health Care Financing Administration (HCFA), now known as the Centers for Medicare & Medicaid Services (CMS), implemented bold changes in health care payment policies within the Medicare program to encourage greater efficiency in health care delivery, including a prospective payment system for hospital care in 1984 and a resource-based payment scale for physician services in 1992. HCFA also began large-scale experiments with managed care plans in both the Medicare and Medicaid programs.

Another notable expansion in federal health activity occurred during the 1990s as public concerns turned toward issues of health care quality, patient protection, and health care choice. Historically, individual states had wielded the authority to regulate the practices of health professionals and health insurance plans.[9] Federal involvement in these issues had been limited to the providers and plans that participate in federal health programs such as Medicare, Medicaid, and the Federal Employee Health Benefits Program (FEHBP). The rapid growth of managed care during the 1990s, however, stimulated public concerns about health care quality and choice within private health insurance plans. The legislative response to these concerns was an unprecedented expansion of federal regulatory authority over issues related to clinical practice and health insurance practices.[10–12] Examples include the 1996 congressional legislation establishing a mandatory 48-hour minimum hospital stay for patients after childbirth; and regulations established as part of the Health Insurance Portability and Accountability Act (HIPPA) of 1996 requiring health plans to provide guaranteed renewable insurance coverage to patients with pre-existing medical conditions.

The federal government's roles in preparing for and responding to **public health emergencies** have dramatically expanded in recent years in the wake of the post-9/11 anthrax attacks, outbreaks of emerging infectious diseases such as SARS and

Monkeypox, and the widely criticized responses to the 2005 Gulf Coast hurricanes. Public health emergencies include both natural and man-made events that have the potential to overwhelm routine public health capabilities due to their scale, timing, or unpredictability. Since 2002, more than $5 billion in federal dollars have been invested in initiatives to strengthen state and local emergency preparedness capacities, including enhanced planning, staffing, training, equipment, and surveillance systems. These initiatives represent a significant expansion in federal responsibility for organizing and financing public health activities.

In addition to these regulatory activities, the federal government has increasingly turned toward informal and indirect ways of influencing clinical practice and quality of care at the population level.[12] One strategy has been to establish standards and systems for measuring quality within federal health care programs such as Medicare and Medicaid. Because large numbers of health care providers and health plans are involved in these programs, these standards and measures influence the care delivered not only to Medicare and Medicaid participants but also to the larger population of health care patients and consumers.[13] The federal government's influence as a dominant payer for health services has increased in recent years with further expansions in federal health care programs, including creation of the State Children's Health Insurance Program (SCHIP) for low-income children and families in 1997 and creation of an outpatient prescription drug benefit for Medicare beneficiaries beginning in 2006.

Another important source of influence has been the federal government's convening power to bring together health plans, providers, and other health care stakeholders to reach voluntary, collective agreements on strategies for improving health care accessibility and quality. Examples include the federal government's involvement in efforts to develop and expand the Health Plan Employer Data and Information Set (HEDIS) system for monitoring the performance of health plans, and more recently the federal government's roles in developing measures of health care quality as part of the collaborative National Forum for Health Care Quality Measurement and Reporting.[14]

As yet another strategy for addressing public concerns about health care quality, the federal government has steadily strengthened its support for health services research, outcomes research, and prevention research during the 1990s. Spearheaded by federal agencies such as the Agency for Healthcare Research and Quality, or AHRQ (formerly the Agency for Health Care Policy and Research, or AHCPR), along with CMS and CDC, these federally sponsored research initiatives have sought to uncover ways of applying existing health knowledge, resources, and technologies to realize improvements in health care quality and outcomes.[15] Increasingly, these initiatives have also focused on disseminating such evidence broadly among health professionals to improve the practice of health care and public health on a population-wide basis. In the contemporary era of health care and public health, the federal government's purchasing power, convening power, and research power have proven to be powerful instruments in shaping the nation's public health and medical care systems.

POWERS AND ACTIONS OF THE FEDERAL GOVERNMENT IN PUBLIC HEALTH

The federal government's authority in the realm of public health originates with the United States Constitution, which divides governmental power between the state and federal levels. The strongest and most visible sources of federal power in public health flow from the constitutional authority to tax, spend, and regulate interstate commerce.[16] The most direct way in which the federal government uses its taxation and spending powers to benefit public health is through the allocation of federal resources to public health programs and services. Federal taxing and spending authority enables the federal government to exist as the nation's single

largest purchaser of health services. Similarly, this authority allows the federal government to fund a broad array of categorical grant programs and block grant programs that support public health programs and services delivered at state and local levels. Total federal health spending has increased dramatically over the past 35 years, from $4.8 billion in 1965 to nearly $644 billion in 2005 (see Figure 8.1).[17] Correspondingly, the federal share of all health expenditures in the United States has risen from 12 percent in 1965 to 32 percent in 2005. By comparison, state and local government spending on health has remained relatively stable at 13 to 14 percent of all United States health expenditures. Federal health expenditures are projected to climb to $713 billion by 2008, continuing to account for more than one-fifth of all health spending.

Personal health services account for the vast majority of federal spending in health. In 2005, 88 percent of the $400 billion in federal health expenditures was dedicated to federal programs that finance the delivery of personal health services.[17] These programs include Medicare, Medicaid, FEHBP, the Department of Defense and Department of Veteran's Affairs' health care systems that provide health care to active-duty military personnel and veterans, the Civilian Health and Medical Program for the Uniformed Services (CHAMPUS) that covers health care for family members of military personnel, and the State Children's Health Insurance Program (SCHIP) that covers health care for low-income uninsured children. Because state governments participate in funding both Medicaid and SCHIP, federal expenditures account for only part of the program costs associated with these programs. Overall, the federal government accounted for 22 percent of the nation's total expenditures for health services and supplies in 2005, with another 18 percent contributed by state and local governments.[17]

Approximately $10.7 billion in federal funds were allocated to public health programs in 2005, such as the Maternal and Child Health Block Grant and the Preventive Health and Health Services Block Grant (see Table 8.1).[17] Consequently, federal public health spending comprised only 1.7 percent

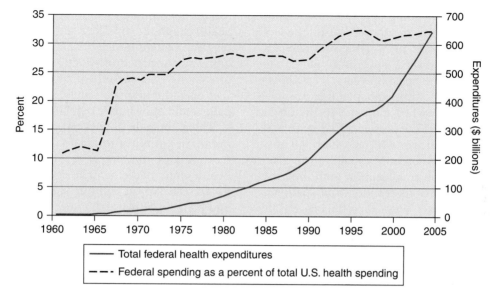

Figure 8.1. **Trends in Federal Health Spending: 1960 to 2005**

SOURCE: Data from U.S. Centers for Medicare and Medicaid Services. National Health Expenditure Data. http://www.cms.hhs.gov/NationalHealthExpendData/02_NationalHealthAccountsHistorical.asp.

Table 8.1. **Federal Health Spending in 2005**

	Federal Health Expenditures ($ Billions)	Percent of Total Federal Health Expenditures	Percent of Total Governmental Health Expenditures
Medicare	342,047	53.1	100.0
Medicaid (Title XIX)	178,797	27.8	57.1
SCHIP (Title XXI)	3,846	0.6	69.3
Workers' Compensation	759	0.1	2.3
Department of Defense	26,088	4.1	100.0
Maternal/Child Health	628	0.1	23.7
Veterans' Administration	30,202	4.7	100.0
Vocational Rehabilitation	391	0.1	77.0
General Hospital/Medical	6,191	1.0	24.4
Substance Abuse/Mental Health	3,226	0.5	–
Indian Health Services	2,212	0.3	100.0
Public Health Activity	10,719	1.7	19.0
Research	31,305	4.9	86.3
Structures & Equipment	7,272	1.1	38.2
Total	643,681	100.0	71.3

SOURCE: Data from U.S. Centers for Medicare and Medicaid Services. National Health Expenditure Data 2005. http://www.cms.hhs.gov/NationalHealthExpendData/02_NationalHealthAccountsHistorical.asp.

of all federal health spending in 1999, down from 4.4 percent in 1965. This trend results from the fact that federal spending on personal health services has dramatically outpaced spending on public health programs over the past 35 years. By comparison, state and local government spending on public health programs reached almost $46 billion in 2005, accounting for 17.7 percent of all state and local health expenditures and 81 percent of all governmental expenditures on public health programs.

In addition to resource allocation authority, the federal government uses its taxation and spending powers in several other ways to influence public health. First, the federal taxation power is often used to discourage private activities and behaviors that threaten the public's health, and to encourage activities that enhance public health and well-being.[16] For example, the federal government imposes excise taxes on cigarettes and alcohol that help to discourage consumption of these harmful products by raising the total prices that consumers must pay. Similarly, federal fuel taxes can be viewed as instruments for discouraging excessive fuel consumption that is harmful to air quality. The use of governmental taxation powers for purposes of behavior modification raises some important ethical issues because this strategy could be perceived as governmental endorsement of harmful activities, and because this strategy could lead government to become financially dependent on the tax revenue generated by harmful activities. Such ethical issues are less apparent when federal taxation powers are used to encourage behaviors that benefit public health. For example, the federal government provides tax exemptions to employers that provide health insurance coverage for their workers.[18]

Second, the federal government uses its spending authority to influence the actions of state governments that receive federal funds.[16] The federal government may establish a variety of conditions that states must meet to receive funds through various federal grant-in-aid programs. For example, the federal government requires state Medicaid programs to establish a minimum set of program benefits and to conform with federal program eligibility criteria to receive federal Medicaid funds. The federal government also uses its spending on non-health programs to induce states to undertake activities that benefit public health. For example, federal highway construction programs frequently include provisions that encourage states to adopt policies that promote highway safety, such as seatbelt campaigns and speed-limit regulations.

Third, the federal government frequently uses its spending authority to create new information and technologies that improve the practice of public health and medicine. The federal government is by far the largest funding agency for biomedical and behavioral research concerning health. By supporting the work of federal researchers as well as university-based scientists, the federal government engages in the discovery of new health interventions and new ways of organizing, delivering, and financing these interventions. These discoveries shape the scope and content of work carried out by health professionals and health care facilities across the nation as well as globally. Frequently, federally funded research provides the scientific foundation for the development and marketing of new drugs, devices, and other technologies produced by the pharmaceutical and health technology industries. In many cases, these discoveries also inform the design and implementation of health policies and regulations carried out by federal, state, and local governments. In 2005, the federal government spent $31.3 billion for health-related research through agencies such as NIH, CDC, CMS, and AHRQ.[17] Most of these resources are devoted to the biomedical research sponsored by NIH, with relatively modest resources supporting the more applied public health and health services research sponsored by other agencies.

Although the power to tax and spend is substantial, the federal government's authority to regulate interstate commerce is often regarded as its most important instrument for influencing public health.[16] This authority provides the legal basis for federal involvement in public health issues that historically have fallen within the exclusive domain of state and local governments, including water and air quality, food and drug safety, occupational health, and health care quality and patient protection.

Under this authority, Congress has passed legislation regulating industrial and commercial activities that introduce toxins into the air, water, and soil; the manufacture, labeling, and sale of pharmaceuticals and food products; the working conditions that employers maintain for their personnel; and most recently the practices of health insurance plans and their affiliated health care providers. The constitutional provisions protecting state sovereignty, however, impose strict limits on the federal government's commerce power. The United States Supreme Court has ruled against a variety of federal legislative and executive actions that were perceived to interfere in purely intrastate issues, including federal restrictions on the possession of handguns and the disposal of hazardous waste. The federal government's public health authority related to interstate commerce is therefore heavily dependent upon judicial interpretations of constitutional law. These interpretations evolve over time as case law develops and as legal, social, and political values change.

In addition to its official constitutional powers, the federal government also uses a variety of informal mechanisms for influencing public health. Both elected and appointed officials within the federal government frequently use the visibility and stature of their federal offices to advance public health causes and address public health issues.[19] These mechanisms may include raising public awareness about important public health topics through speeches, conferences, publications, and public education campaigns; convening major stakeholders in public health to identify important public health problems and potential solutions; and communicating and negotiating with relevant organizations or governments to achieve voluntary participation in and compliance with public health initiatives. In some cases, these activities may be undertaken to create broad-based political support for specific legislation under consideration by Congress. In other cases, these activities are undertaken exclusively to influence the behavior of individuals and organizations through informal mechanisms and are therefore unrelated to legislative agendas within the federal government. As an example, the National Cancer Institute recently launched a campaign to encourage employers to provide comprehensive health insurance coverage for all evidence-based cancer-screening services for age-appropriate employees. Employers that do so are recognized with a federal award known as the CEO Cancer Gold Standard. The U.S. surgeon general often leads federal government efforts to inform and influence health-related decision making among individuals, health professionals, health care organizations, and other stakeholders. A variety of other government officials may also provide federal leadership on specific health policy issues, including administrators of key federal agencies within the United States Department of Health and Human Services (Dept. of HHS), and individual members of Congress that have a strong knowledge of and interest in public health issues.

ORGANIZATION OF FEDERAL PUBLIC HEALTH RESPONSIBILITIES

The Legislative Branch

Most legislative action involving federal health programs and policies can originate in either house of Congress. Constitutional provisions, however, require that legislation involving the levying of taxes begin in the House of Representatives. Two basic forms of legislative action are undertaken by Congress: (1) **authorization legislation** is used to create or modify federal programs and policies; and (2) **appropriations legislation** is used to allocate federal funding to authorized programs. Authorization legislation begins when a member of Congress submits a bill that proposes to create or alter the structure and operation of a federal program, policy, or agency. Often this bill includes specifications for the program's maximum expenditure amount and duration.

The process through which an authorization bill becomes a law includes the familiar steps of

(1) assignment to a legislative committee for review and consideration; (2) committee hearings to facilitate legislative deliberation on the bill; (3) committee markups during which committee members offer amendments; (4) committee reporting of the bill to the full legislative body (House or Senate) for further amendments and approval; (5) House and Senate joint conferencing on the bill after versions are approved by each house of Congress; (6) final approval of the conference bill in both houses; and (7) approval (or veto) by the president. Voting majorities of two-thirds in each house are required to overturn a presidential veto.

Health-related authorization bills are reviewed and considered by numerous legislative committees within the House and Senate, but four committees process the majority of such legislation.[7] In the Senate, the Finance Committee holds jurisdiction over all proposals involving Medicare and Medicaid, whereas the Health, Education, Labor, and Pensions Committee considers legislation involving public health programs, health workforce and medical education issues, health regulatory issues (e.g., food and drug regulations or medical privacy regulations), and health research initiatives (e.g., NIH programs). In the House, Medicare legislation falls under the jurisdiction of the Ways and Means Committee; however, bills involving Medicare Part B (physician services and ancillary services) also fall under the purview of the Commerce Committee. Additionally, the House Commerce Committee considers most legislation involving Medicaid, public health programs, health workforce issues, health regulatory issues, and health research initiatives.

Appropriations bills are handled as part of the congressional budget process. This process makes a key distinction between entitlement programs and discretionary programs. Entitlement programs are those for which the authorizing legislation requires the federal government to pay benefits to all individuals, governments, or other entities that meet program eligibility criteria. Spending on entitlement programs currently makes up more than half of all federal spending.[7] The largest health-related federal entitlement programs include Medicare and

Medicaid. For these programs, federal expenditures are determined largely by the number of individuals that meet the eligibility criteria, rather than by explicit legislative action. By contrast, discretionary programs are subject to Congress' annual appropriations process. This process involves congressional consideration of 13 different bills that fund discretionary programs. Each body of Congress has an appropriations committee to oversee this process, with subcommittees providing the detailed review and consideration of individual appropriations bills. Appropriations for most public health programs are included in a bill that funds the departments of Labor, HHS, and Education. Appropriations for Department of Veterans Affairs health programs are included in a separate bill considered by the Subcommittee on Veterans' Affairs in each house of Congress.

Congress maintains several established mechanisms for obtaining information about the health issues, policies, and programs under its consideration.[20] The Government Accountability Office (GAO), often considered the watchdog arm of Congress, is charged with monitoring the financial and operational performance of federal agencies and programs, and with investigating policy issues of significant congressional interest. The GAO maintains an analytical division devoted to issues of public health and health services delivery, which wields substantial influence over federal public health policy by informing Congress about the performance of federal public health programs and about the need for policy and programmatic changes. Much of the GAO's work is undertaken in response to requests from individual members of Congress. Another legislative institution, the Congressional Budget Office (CBO), provides the legislature with information about the current and potential cost of federal programs and policies. In the domain of federal health policy, the CBO is active in producing estimates of future federal health care expenditures resulting from current and proposed health programs, as well as estimates of the costs incurred by health care purchasers and providers in complying with current and proposed health care regulations. These estimates are often profoundly influential, and occasionally controversial, in congressional policy debates. A third congressional institution that is active in the federal health policy arena is the Congressional Research Service (CRS), which analyzes and syntheses information from a variety of sources to inform legislative decision making. The CRS produces systematic reviews of the scientific literature that are relevant to federal health policy decisions, as well as descriptive analyses of existing federal and state laws that may inform these decisions.

The Executive Branch

The executive branch of federal government comprises the executive office of the president, the cabinet-level departments, and several independent agencies. The majority of health-related programs and policies are administered by the Dept. of HHS; however, a number of other executive departments administer such programs, including the Departments of Education, Labor, Veterans Affairs, Defense, Agriculture, Transportation, and Homeland Security. Additionally, several administrative units within the executive office of the president play important roles in the development, coordination, and management of public health policies and programs. These governmental agencies and their contributions to public health are detailed next.

Department of Health and Human Services

When most think of the federal role in health, they think of the Department of Health and Human Services (DHHS). In fact, the majority of the health-related activities of the federal government are in this department. An examination of the organizational chart in Figure 8.2 gives a quick look at the various programs of the department. Of the units in the department, eight comprise the United States Public Health Services. The following sections contain descriptions of those eight units.

Centers for Disease Control and Prevention

The Centers for Disease Control and Prevention (CDC) is the agency of the federal government that

comes to mind when public health issues or concerns are discussed. The CDC is the agency of the federal government that focuses on prevention, disease control and surveillance, and epidemiologic and laboratory investigations associated with disease. It also focuses on infectious diseases; chronic disease control and prevention; and environmental, occupational, and injury-prevention concerns. An examination of the CDC's organizational chart (Figure 8.3) illustrates that these efforts are accomplished through a variety of centers, offices, and institutes. The CDC is the nation's public health agency. In addition, it also has an international mission, a mission that was responsible for the eradication of smallpox, arguably the greatest public health accomplishment of the century. These efforts are the result of a large and talented pool of intramural scientists who focus on the public's health and a close working relationship with research centers around the United States, frequently funded by the CDC.

The CDC began out of efforts in the 1940s to control malaria in the southeastern United States, so that troops training for WWII were not exposed to the disease. From this arose its initial charter that focused on infectious disease epidemiology and laboratory services. To reflect this mission it was named the Communicable Disease Center. Subsequently, it then took on a larger mission where its epidemiologic and laboratory capacity could have an impact and it was renamed the Center for Disease Control. Further development and reorganization over the years led to the Centers for Disease Control, with several centers of activity, and most recently, a change to the Centers for Disease Control and Prevention. The latter reflects the fact that the CDC is the nation's prevention agency, and Congress specifically allowed the CDC acronym to continue to be used, as the result of its identification with an organization that is renowned both here and abroad.

Of the federal agencies, the CDC has the closest relationship with state and local health departments. The organization has long provided support in a variety of ways. They have assigned federal epidemiologists, using the elite Epidemic Intelligence Service (EIS), and public health advisors who worked with state and local health departments on disease

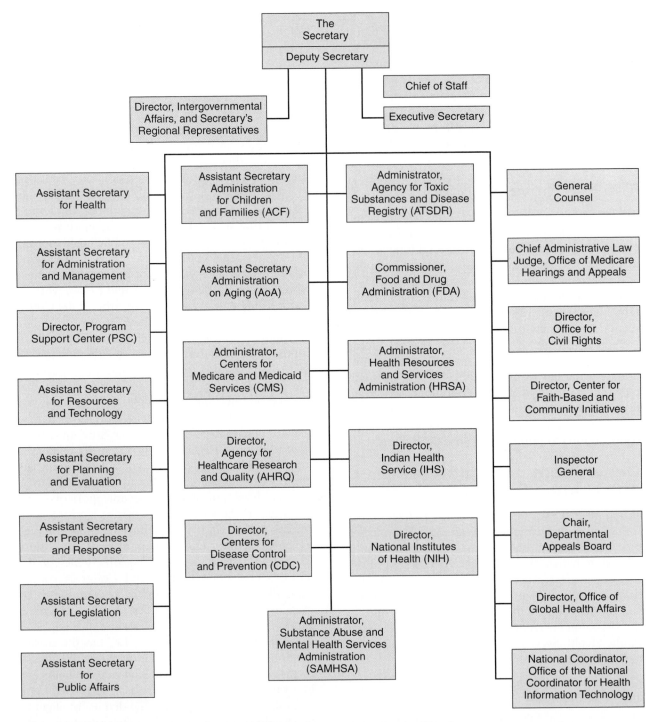

Figure 8.2. **Organization of the U.S. Department of Health and Human Services**

SOURCE: U.S. Department of Health and Human Services http://www.hhs.gov/about/orgchart.html.

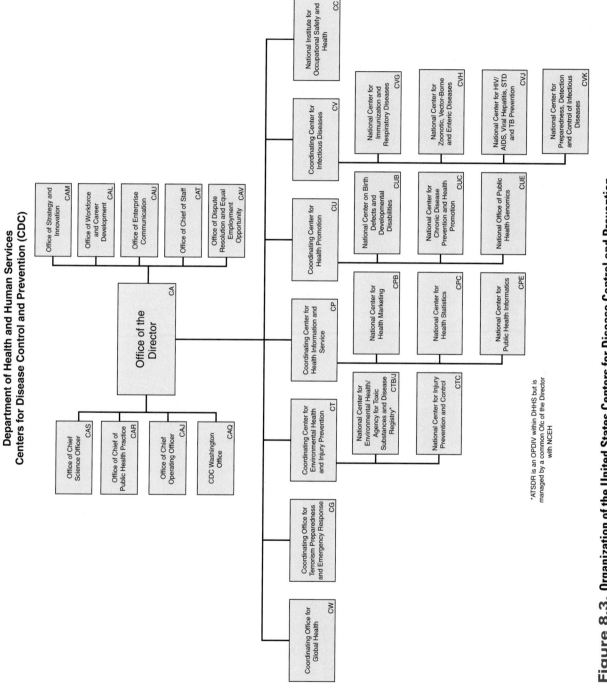

Department of Health and Human Services
Centers for Disease Control and Prevention (CDC)

Figure 8.3. Organization of the United States Centers for Disease Control and Prevention

SOURCE: U.S. Department of Health and Human Services http://www.cdc.gov/about/organization/pdf/cdcOrgChart061008.pdf.

control activities.[4] The CDC also provides the backbone for infectious disease surveillance and responses to epidemics that are identified by those surveillance systems. By working with new and novel infectious disease agents and assisting state labs in their efforts to implement clinical laboratory improvement across the United States, the laboratories of the CDC have been a valuable resource to state public health labs. The CDC has, since its inception, provided training to state and local public health agency employees to help upgrade the public health workforce.

Other Agencies of the U.S. Public Health Service

A number of other agencies, in addition to the CDC, provide important support and leadership for public health activities. A quick examination of those and their public health relationships and activities help understand the broad support for public health in the DHHS.

Health Resources and Services Administration (HRSA)

The operating branches of HRSA contain many programs that directly relate to public health. The Maternal and Child Health Branch is perhaps the most prominent. With the passage of the Social Security Act of 1935 (SSA), funds were made available from the federal government to state health departments to fund maternal and child health activities. This federal grant program, Title V of the SSA, has provided, since that time, a steady source of state support for programs designed to improve health care to mothers and infants. The program activities range from prenatal care to care for children with special needs. This program also merits special attention, since this is the first foray into federal funds transfers to state health departments and has been the model for other federal grant-in-aid programs. The requirement for a state plan for both maternal and child health and maintenance-of-effort requirements, where the state cannot replace existing state funding for federal dollars, has become a part of many other federal state initiatives. More detail about Maternal and Child Health programs is provided in Chapter 26, written by Dr. Carol Hogue.

The second program with significant public health impact that HRSA administers is the HIV/AIDS program. While there are options for funding of not-for-profit agencies and organizations, this branch provides support to state and local health departments to deal with the HIV/AIDS cases in their jurisdiction. The HIV/AIDS program is the home of the Ryan White Program, designed to facilitate direct patient care and supportive services for individuals with HIV infection or AIDS.

The largest single program in HRSA is the Bureau of Primary Health Care. This program is designed to provide support for community health centers across the United States. It has a major grant program to assist these centers with care for indigent patients and/or other hard-to-reach groups such as the homeless. While it may not seem necessarily important to public health, there are many partnerships between those community health centers and the local health department. These partnerships are important to major program efforts that both public health and primary health care share, such as immunizations or the treatment of STDs.

The Bureau of Health Professions has seen substantial decline in its mission and resources over the last several years, as the federal government has chosen not to aggressively pursue efforts to redress workforce shortages in several important areas, notably primary care and nursing. The bureau has little to do with public health, other than their support of the Public Health Training Centers scattered strategically around the country in schools of public health. These centers were designed to address the pressing need for educating the new public health workforce.

There are a number of other components of HRSA, including the remnants of the Hill-Burton Program, designed in the 40s to increase the number of hospitals and now committed to assuring that hospitals supported by federal Hill-Burton funds continue their commitment to indigent care in those facilities. In addition, the Federal Office of Rural Health Policy is a part of HRSA. The opportunity for that office to focus on issues of rural public health has been limited by the amount of funding it has had over the last several years.

The largest and most prestigious of the components of the U.S. Public Health Services is the National Institutes of Health. The budget of the NIH surpasses any other branch of the Public Health Service. Congress recently doubled the NIH budget and is likely to continue to increase the funding for basic research on diseases. The NIH is composed of a series of institutes focused on individual diseases or conditions. The largest are the National Cancer Institute and the National Heart Lung and Blood Institute. These institutes operate to accomplish major scientific research efforts focused on understanding diseases, their etiology, and treatment. They do this through intramural and extramural research funding. The former is the research programs of those who are employees of the NIH, many senior scientists, and scholars, and the latter is focused on the research of basic scientists in physiology and cell biology in the nation's medical schools. While few of the institutes are concerned with public health and its practice, many do contribute to the work of public health departments, such as the work of the National Cancer Institute, The National Institute of Allergy and Infectious Disease, and the National Institute of Environmental Health Sciences. Recently, the NIH has begun to concern itself with the translation into community practice of the research it funds. This new initiative may have the potential for an impact on public health because public health schools, in many cases, represent the largest interaction between the academic medical center and the community, a key to obtaining funding for translation research. This development should be watched closely by those in practice as it provides an opportunity for public health to become more involved with essential public health service,[10] focused on finding and using new information in public health.

Agency for Healthcare Research and Quality (AHRQ)

This federal agency is one that might have potential for its impact on public health, but unfortunately has not moved in that direction. AHRQ focuses on issues surrounding the quality, financing, and delivery of medical care services. It has been the source of most of the research on the electronic health record, the use of information technology in delivering medical care services, and quality issues in medical care. Its budget is small by comparison with other agencies of the U.S. Public Health Service and its research mission is sharply circumscribed by its congressional appropriation. The major contribution it has made to public health is its work on preparedness, where it has had a mandate to address the issues related to the capacity of the medical care system to deal with a major disaster. The hope for the public health research community is that AHRQ will have the opportunity to grow, and to begin to recognize and work with the public health community in addressing the new public health systems and services research agenda.

Food and Drug Administration (FDA)

The FDA is concerned with a variety of domaines that it regulates. It has jurisdiction over human and veterinary drugs, biological, radiation, health devices, food, and cosmetics. The most visible and largest role that FDA plays is in the approval of new drugs. Currently, the FDA is in a dilemma. Both pharmaceutical firms and patient advocates are anxious to assure that new drugs for patients are rapidly approved and made available for the market. The FDA is vulnerable to criticism if it too quickly moves drugs on to the market that subsequently are shown to cause human harm. While this is the most visible role of the FDA, it is not the focus of its relationship to public health. The public health's primary concern with the FDA's role is in the food safety program. Public health has long had a role to play in assuring food safety, for example with inspections of restaurants. The National Food Safety Program of the FDA is a vital part of the effort to assure that safe food reaches the marketplace. The FDA, of course, does not have all of the federal government's activities in food safety, the U.S. Department of Agriculture, the CDC, and a number of other agencies in the federal establishment share responsibility for food safety. Another area of common concern with the FDA is their role in production of biologics, notable in the case of public health, as in the licensing of new vaccines for use. There continues to be a steady increase in the production of new vaccines such as those against the Human Papilloma Virus and the Rotaviruses. The continued production and licensing of these vaccines benefits the public's health by providing more primary prevention possibilities for addressing significant human illnesses. The development of vaccine schedules and the activities of public health immunization programs are altered as these new vaccines come on line and public health departments must continue to follow the vaccine approval process to assure that they are current with their vaccine knowledge.

Indian Health Service (IHS)

This unit of the public health service provides medical care to the nation's American Indian and Alaska Native populations. Treaty obligations with American Indian populations included, in many cases, responsibility to provide medical care to those tribal reservations. The IHS currently provides health services to approximately 1.5 million American Indians and Alaska Natives who belong to more than 557 federally recognized tribes in 35 states. The IHS is unique in another way, as it provides all the health care for American Indian Reservations and in many cases that includes all the components of a health care system, including public health responsibility, as well as direct medical care responsibility. Thus it represents one of a few total health care system under the jurisdiction of one organization in the United States.

Substance Abuse and Mental Health Services Administration (SAMHSA)

This unit of the public health services provides mental health services, substance abuse prevention, and treatment services. It provides grants to states to achieve its mission of preventing and treating both mental illness and substance abuse. The current epidemic of drug abuse has strained the capacity of most local programs to deal with the numbers requiring drug treatment and rehabilitation. Providing treatment appears to be a much better approach to this drug problem than incarceration of those who are addicted to drugs. The lack of resources to provide that treatment has slowed the nation's attack on drug abuse.

Other Agencies of the USDHHS

The Centers for Medicare and Medicaid Services (CMS) has the largest budget of any of DHHS's agencies. CMS's primary mission is administering

three large medical care payment systems. These include Medicare (Title 18 of the Social Security Act), a federal program that provides funding for medical services to the nation's over 65 population, those who are permanently disabled, and those who suffer from End Stage Renal Disease. Second, Medicaid (Title 19 of the Social Security Act), a federal and state cooperative program designed to provide needed medical care to those families who meet certain eligibility criteria and live in poverty. And third, the State Children's Health Insurance Program (SCHIP), (Title 21 of the Social Security Act), a state-federal partnership program, similar to Medicaid, designed to provide medical care for children who live in poverty.

The SCHIP and Medicaid programs are of substantial interest to those in public health. These programs, as they focus on the poor, provide at least some support for a number of health departments who serve in many communities as the primary care provider of last resort. In addition, many services provided by the local health department, without compensation, prior to the passage of these funding methods are now receiving at least some funds to support programs, such as the immunizations, or home health services. In some cases, the availability of funding for these activities and traditional patrons of the health department have changed the way that health departments function. As reimbursement developed, many health departments moved away from providing population-based services and became another community medical care provider, as they were reimbursed for the latter and not for the former. In many states, however, Medicaid and SCHIP have moved to managed care models of delivery, emulating the private sector's efforts to control costs. When that occurred, in many situations, the financial base that the health department depended on disappeared as those patients moved to regular primary care providers who offered services that the health department in the past had provided.

CMS has the largest budget of DHHS, and is the single source of much of the funding of medical care. As such, it has the potential to influence the delivery of medical care services in the United States. By emphasizing quality, for example, it increases the quality of care provided to its beneficiaries, but by setting the baseline for how providers are reimbursed for quality care, that can change the way care is provided to everyone. Close attention to developments in a state's Medicaid and SCHIP programs are vital to assuring that if funding is available for services provided by the health department, those services are billed. As spokespeople for the health of the poor and underserved, public health officials should always be monitoring the development of their state Medicaid and SCHIP program, not only to assure that local public health has been considered in decisions about reimbursement but also in providing the best possible care to their community's indigent population.

Many staff offices exist at the level of the Secretary of the Department of Health and Human Services. Two are particularly important to public health. The first is the Office of the Surgeon General of the U.S. Public Health Service (USPHS). The USPHS has existed since the late 1700s, and is a uniformed service of the DHHS. The assumption is commonly made that the Surgeon General (SG) has command responsibility for the USPHS, however, that is in not the case, as the SG has staff but not line responsibility. The Surgeon General does have a "bully pulpit" to serve as the nation's family doctor. Some have been more successful with that role than others; Dr. C. Everett Koop became a household name as the result of his efforts in dealing with the public's understanding of the dangers of tobacco and his role in providing information about HIV/AIDS. The visibility of the office has made it a key part of the effort to control disease both here and abroad.

The Second is the Office of Health Promotion and Disease Prevention. This office has had responsibility for a number of initiatives of DHHS in health, some of which it continues to administer. One of the most visible is the responsibility for the series of health objectives for the nation. Since 1990, there has been a set of 10-year objectives for health improvement. The notion of Management by Objectives led to the initial set of objectives in 1990 and the new set created ever 10 years. The number of focus areas and objectives has continued to grow, and this effort has been key to the focusing

necessary to establish direction for a number of agencies and organizations, some only tangentially related to health.

There are also a number of staff offices, several of which have relevance to public health. These include the Office of Global Health, the office of Minority Affairs, HIV, population, and women's health.

Other Federal Agencies with Public Health Responsibilities

A number of other federal agencies are not part of HHS but nonetheless contribute substantially to federal public health activities. Many of these agencies carry out their public health activities in close collaboration with administrative units of HHS. Key among these agencies is the United States Department of Agriculture (USDA), which sponsors an array of health-related programs involving nutritional support, food safety, and farm-worker and rural health. Among the best-known public health programs administered by this department is the Special Supplemental Food Program for Women, Infants, and Children, commonly known as WIC, which provides food assistance and nutritional education for pregnant women, postpartum and breastfeeding women, infants, and young children in low-income households. Another large nutrition program administered by the department is the Food Stamp Program, which provides low-income individuals and families with assistance in purchasing food products to reduce hunger and improve diet among disadvantaged populations. The USDA also contributes to public health activities through a broad range of rural development programs, including initiatives to improve access to health care in rural areas through **telemedicine** projects that deliver health interventions through telephone and video technologies, and through efforts to attract and retain health professionals in **medically underserved areas** that lack adequate numbers of physicians and other health personnel.

The USDA administers several other nutritional programs for low-income populations, including a food commodity distribution program and the

National School Lunch and School Breakfast Programs. The USDA's Food Safety and Inspection Service works to ensure the safety of meat and poultry products through the routine inspection and evaluation of product production, content, and labeling. The department's Office of Public Health and Science works closely with the FDA and CDC to evaluate food-borne disease risks within the population and to develop policies, plans, and regulations to prevent and control these risks. The department also operates a consumer education program on food-borne illnesses jointly with the FDA, which strives to expand the use of safe food handling and preparation practices among consumers.

The Environmental Protection Agency (EPA) makes substantial contributions to federal public health activities through its role in developing and enforcing a wide array of environmental health and safety regulations. The EPA's regulatory authority extends to air quality, water quality, radiation exposure, solid waste disposal, pesticides and toxic substances, and issues of environmental justice. In addition to enforcing federal environmental laws and developing regulations authorized by these laws, the EPA maintains an array of partnerships with businesses and community organizations designed to foster voluntary efforts to improve environmental health conditions. These partnerships include efforts to reduce the production of greenhouse gasses, to promote energy conservation within businesses and communities, and to prevent environmental pollution associated with pesticide use. The EPA also administers a variety of public education and information dissemination programs designed to encourage environmentally sound practices among consumers and businesses.

The United States Department of Housing and Urban Development (HUD) engages in public health issues through programs to address the health risks associated with housing and homelessness, and to address the health needs of populations residing in public housing facilities and shelters. HUD maintains a large program to reduce lead poisoning risks in housing units that are supported through federal housing assistance programs, and to educate citizens about lead hazards

and optimal prevention and abatement practices. The department also administers the federal Lead-Based Paint Hazard Control Program, which funds state and local governments to implement initiatives that control and abate lead hazards in privately owned low-income housing units and in areas near Superfund cleanup sites. Similarly, HUD administers programs to promote safety and prevent injuries in low-income housing facilities, and it cooperates with HRSA in administering federal grant programs to support the provision of health education and primary health care services to homeless populations (through the Health Care for the Homeless Program and the Outreach and Primary Health Services for Homeless Children Program) and to residents of public housing facilities (through the Public Housing Primary Health Care Program). HUD also maintains several programs that promote access to quality health care facilities by offering low-cost mortgage insurance to hospitals, nursing homes, assisted-living facilities, and nonprofit group medical practices for use in construction or rehabilitation of these facilities. The largest federal programs administered by HUD—such as the Operating Subsidy for Public Housing Program, the Section 8 Rental Certificate and Voucher Program, the Federal Housing Administration mortgage insurance programs, and the Community Development Block Grant Program—do not address health issues directly, but they nonetheless endeavor to impact socioeconomic determinants of health through efforts to reduce homelessness, improve housing quality and affordability for low- and moderate-income populations, and enhance community facilities and services.

The United States Department of Education plays an important role in federal public health activities through its programs to address the health education and health services needs of students. The department administers the Safe and Drug-Free Schools Program, which is the federal government's primary instrument for preventing and reducing violence and drug, alcohol, and tobacco use in and around the nation's schools through education and outreach interventions. This program funds state and local education agencies and state governor's offices to implement a variety of education and prevention programs, and involves close collaboration with other federal agencies within the CDC, the NIH, the Administration on Children and Families, and the Office of National Drug Control Policy. Similarly, the department provides administrative assistance and support for the Healthy Schools Healthy Communities Initiative, a federal program administered by HRSA to fund the development of school-based health centers that provide comprehensive primary care, health promotion, and disease prevention services to at-risk children. The department also assists state, local, and private educational institutions in developing health education and health promotion curricula for students through its Office of Educational Research and Improvement. This office funds the development, evaluation, and dissemination of a wide range of educational initiatives, including those devoted to educating students about health issues and practices for disease prevention and health promotion.

The United States Department of Labor contributes to the federal government's public health agenda through its programs and policies to promote health and safety in the workplace. The department's Occupational Safety and Health Administration (OSHA) develops and enforces federal regulations regarding workplace safety and health conditions, as authorized under the federal Occupational Safety and Health Act. These regulations include those related to indoor air quality, noise exposure, hazardous materials exposure, protection from hazardous equipment and facilities, and employee training regarding safety practices. OSHA also develops partnerships with employers to encourage voluntary compliance with beneficial health and safety practices.

Other health-related programs administered by the department include the Safe Work/Safe Kids Initiative, which involves efforts to educate employers, parents, and schools about the health and safety issues faced by youth workers, and efforts to enforce state and federal child labor laws. The Labor Department is also charged with enforcing and adjudicating provisions of the federal Family

and Medical Leave Act (FMLA), which allows eligible employees to take unpaid leave from jobs to care for family members. The department's Pension and Welfare Benefits Administration is actively involved in enforcing federal regulations covering employer-provided health insurance benefits. These regulations include provisions of the Newborns' and Mothers' Health Protection Act of 1996, which mandates minimum hospital stay benefits for women after childbirth; provisions of HIPAA 1996, which requires employer-provided health insurance benefits to be more portable and renewable for employees; and provisions of the Employee Retirement and Income Security Act of 1974 (ERISA) which, among other things, creates standards for employer-provided health insurance plans. The Department of Labor also oversees worker compensation benefits provided to federal employees and workers covered under the federal Black Lung Benefits Program (for mine workers) and the federal Longshore and Harbor Workers Compensation Program (for workers employed on or near United States navigable waters).

The United States Department of Transportation (DOT) maintains an array of federal public health programs involving the safety of public and private transportation systems. The department's Federal Highway Administration operates programs to improve pedestrian and bicycle safety, encourage safe driving practices, and enhance highway construction and maintenance to prevent roadway-related injuries and fatalities. These programs include both infrastructure improvements and educational initiatives, such as the Federal Safe Routes to School Program, which promotes walking and bicycling to school with a focus on both injury prevention and physical activity promotion strategies. Another division within the department, the National Highway Traffic Safety Administration (NHTSA), is charged with developing and enforcing safety standards for motor vehicles, and with providing discretionary grants to state and local governments for local highway safety initiatives. This agency also contains an active research unit that investigates trends in driving behavior and in motor vehicle crashes, and that evaluates the effectiveness of traffic safety programs. Other divisions within DOT administer safety policies and regulations for commercial motor vehicles, aviation, railroads, public transit agencies, and maritime transportation.

Two cabinet-level departments contribute substantially to federal public health efforts primarily through the large health care systems that they operate. The United States Department of Defense (DOD) operates a health care system for the nation's military personnel and their family members that includes nearly 100 hospitals and more than 500 ambulatory clinics that serve more than 8.2 million individuals worldwide.[22] The department is also actively engaged in research and development activities to identify more effective and efficient ways of delivering health care to its populations. Findings from these activities often inform the design and operation of other public and private health care systems.

Similarly, the United States Department of Veterans Affairs (VA) operates a health care system for the nation's military veterans, consisting of 173 medical centers, 391 outpatient centers, and 131 nursing facilities organized within 23 regional networks. The department's Veterans Health Administration oversees this system, which focuses its services on a priority population of low-income veterans with service-connected health problems. The VA health system includes Veteran Outreach Centers that provide readjustment counseling services for veterans of armed hostilities, including and following the Vietnam War. The VA also maintains a variety of outreach programs for homeless veterans and for those with alcohol and drug abuse problems. A substantial biomedical and health services research program also exists within the VA system, which makes valuable contributions to the existing body of scientific knowledge about health, disease, and health services delivery.

Many other federal agencies maintain targeted contributions to public health activities. For example, the United States Department of Justice (DOJ) and the and Federal Trade Commission (FTC) work to protect health care consumers by enforcing federal antitrust policy against health care institutions. Likewise, the United States Department of

Commerce (DOC) sponsors a variety of research and development projects that focus on the use of telemedicine applications for enhancing health care accessibility, efficiency, and quality. The federal government's newest cabinet-level department, the Department of Homeland Security, oversees federal activities in preparing for and responding to both natural and human-made disasters.

Several administrative units within the executive office of the president play important roles in the development, coordination, and management of federal public health policies and programs. Key among these units is the Office of Management and Budget (OMB), which is responsible for preparation of the president's budget proposal to Congress and for the overall financial management of federal programs and services. The OMB is also responsible for implementing provisions of the 1993 Government Performance and Results Act, which requires federal agencies to develop and measure specific performance objectives for the programs and policies they administer.[23] Under this initiative, public health organizations that receive federal funding are developing outcome objectives and performance measures in an effort to demonstrate accountability for these federal funds.[24] Another unit within the executive office, the Domestic Policy Council, is charged with developing coordinated federal policies to address broad-based health and social issues. Created in 1989, the council consists of the administrators of major health and social services agencies within the federal government, and has developed policies in areas such as tobacco control, children's health insurance, gun safety, patient's rights, and Medicare policies. The executive office also includes offices that conduct policy development and coordination activities on important public health issues such as environmental quality, AIDS policy, science and technology policy, and drug prevention and control.

The Judicial Branch

Federal courts also play important roles in shaping public health policy and practice, primarily through their authority to interpret federal public health powers in view of constitutional provisions and federal laws passed by Congress. Federal courts have jurisdiction over issues that involve federal laws, such as when citizens, corporations, or governments dispute federal public health regulations and programs on the constitutional grounds of state sovereignty. Federal courts also have jurisdiction over disputes that arise between citizens, corporations, or governments of different states. Thus, interstate conflicts involving environmental issues such as water quality, air pollution, or hazardous waste disposal fall within the domain of federal courts.

The federal judiciary is organized in a three-tier structure, with United States district courts serving as the trial courts where most federal cases begin. There are 94 federal court districts in the United States, with at least 1 district existing within each state. The second tier of the federal judiciary comprises the 12 United States courts of appeals. These courts hear cases that are appealed from the district court level, as well as cases that are appealed from decisions made by federal regulatory agencies. The United States Supreme Court is the third tier of the judiciary, consisting of the chief justice and eight associate justices. The Supreme Court hears a limited number of cases that involve the Constitution or federal law. These cases may originate either in lower federal courts or in state courts.

The Supreme Court has been profoundly influential in clarifying the division between federal and state public health authority in recent years. An increasingly prevalent interpretation of constitutional law, often referred to as the concept of new federalism, holds that governmental police powers are largely reserved for the states under constitutional law, and are therefore restricted at the federal level.[16,25] In keeping with this concept, the Supreme Court has overturned a number of federal public health laws that sought to assert federal regulatory authority over that of the states. Recent examples include the 1997 court decision to overturn provisions of the Brady Handgun Violence Prevention Act requiring background checks on handgun purchasers[26] and the 2000 decision to overturn civil rights provisions of the Violence Against Women Act of 1994.[27]

THE FEDERAL POLICY-MAKING PROCESS

The process of federal policy making in public health derives not only from the established congressional committee structure and system of legislative rules described earlier but also from the complex and changing array of individuals and organizations outside the legislative branch of government that engage in the federal political process. These entities contribute information, advice, and, in some cases, campaign funds in an effort to inform and influence congressional decision making on public health issues.[19,28] Such contributions may be made informally through communication and interaction with individual members of Congress and their staffs, or formally through testimony given at congressional hearings, study commissions, and task forces. Some of these entities also attempt to influence congressional decision making by appealing directly to members of the public, including the constituents of key members of Congress, through public education efforts and mass media campaigns.

The nonfederal entities involved in informing and influencing federal legislative decisions in health policy are many and varied, and have grown over time in tandem with the federal government's expanding involvement in health-related programs and regulations. These entities fall into one of six general categories: professional and trade associations, issue-oriented interest groups, political action committees, individual corporations and labor unions, policy think tanks, and nonpartisan research firms.[29] The latter two types of organizations generally contribute information, research and policy recommendations only, and do not engage directly in lobbying members of Congress nor in contributing to congressional campaign funds (federal law prohibits tax-exempt nonprofit organizations from engaging in these activities). **Political action committees,** by contrast, are formed primarily to participate in electoral politics through campaigning and contributing to campaign funds.

In addition to these nongovernmental groups, federal health agencies in the executive branch of government play important roles in informing and influencing congressional decision making, often in tandem with groups outside the federal government. These agencies wield considerable influence in the legislative policy-making process because members of Congress often rely on them as key sources of information about federal health programs and policy needs, and because these agencies are often directly involved in the annual process of preparing the president's budget proposal to Congress. As a consequence, interest groups in public health often attempt to inform and shape congressional decision making indirectly through their relationships with federal health agencies.

The federal legislative process is informed not only by organized interest groups, advocacy associations, and executive-branch federal agencies, but also by recognized nonpartisan experts in science and policy. Congress uses a number of mechanisms for obtaining outside expertise relevant to policy deliberations, and these mechanisms are particularly important when complex issues of public health and biomedical science are involved. One formal mechanism for obtaining this advice is to invite testimony from leading experts as part of congressional hearings and study commissions. These experts are often drawn from academic institutions and independent research institutes. Another important mechanism is the creation of a standing federal advisory commission by congressional legislation. An example of such a commission is the Medicare Payment Advisory Commission (MedPAC) established by the Balanced Budget Act of 1997 to advise Congress on policy issues affecting the Medicare program. Like its predecessors, the Prospective Payment Assessment Commission and the Physician Payment Review Commission, MedPAC consists of a panel of experts from academia, the health professions, and government that produces regular reports and briefings on the performance of the Medicare program for Congress, and recommends policies and regulations for legislative consideration.

Another institution that serves as a nonpartisan source of information and advice for the Congress is the Institute of Medicine (IOM) of the National Academies. The IOM and the National Academies conduct their work by forming committees of leading volunteer scientists from around the world. The IOM provides unbiased, vital, and authoritative advice on health policy. It examines important issues in public health and medicine in response to requests from Congress and other federal agencies.[31] Though organizationally independent from Congress and the federal government, the IOM plays critical roles in informing legislative decision making. It has produced a large number of influential studies and reports on public health issues. Every report produced by the IOM goes through an extensive review by external experts. Since 1970, when the IOM was added to the academy, policy-makers, professionals, and society leaders have relied on this authoritative information ranging from infectious disease control and prevention, to bioterrorism, medical errors, and health care quality.

The numerous nonfederal experts and interest groups active in federal public health policy are far from unified in their policy interests and advocacy strategies. Nonetheless, their collective impact on the federal policy-making process is substantial, both as sources of information and as agents of political influence. Some elements of the contemporary policy-making process remain controversial and subject to change, particularly in view of concerns that existing campaign financing laws allow political contributions to play a growing role in this process.[32] Despite such concerns, the federal legislative process remains a pluralistic approach to governmental decision making in the allocation of public health resources and in the regulation of personal and commercial actions influencing health.

THE FEDERAL REGULATORY PROCESS

The federal government's influence on public health derives not only from legislative activity but also from the actions of executive-branch federal agencies in developing and enforcing regulations on personal, professional, and commercial behavior. A federal agency's authority to develop and enforce regulations originates from one or more sources: the **enabling legislation** that defines or modifies an agency's scope of authority, and the authorizing legislation that defines the purpose and activities of programs and policies administered by the agency.[7,33] Most agencies develop regulations using the notice-and-comment procedure established by the federal Administrative Procedure Act. Under this procedure, agencies develop regulations pursuant to the relevant legislative directives, publish drafts of these regulations in the Federal Register, solicit and consider comments from interested individuals and organizations, and modify regulations in response to these comments. Final regulations are codified by publication in the Code of Federal Regulations. Additionally, some federal agencies are required to use formal adjudication mechanisms as part of their regulation development process, including the use of cross-examination and rebuttal witnesses. These agencies include the Federal Trade Commission (FTC), the Consumer Product Safety Commission (CPSC), and the Occupational Safety and Health Administration (OSHA).

In many cases, the legislative authority to promulgate regulations is distributed across multiple federal agencies. For example, authority over health insurance benefits regulation is distributed across the United States DOL (for employer-provided insurance), CMS (for Medicare, Medicaid, and SCHIP), the United States DOD (for military personnel and families), and the United States Office of Personnel Management (OPM) (for federal employees and families). For this reason, effective regulatory development and enforcement at the federal level often requires interagency coordination. In some cases, presidential executive orders are used to ensure coordination and consistency in the regulatory policies developed by multiple federal agencies. President Clinton used this approach in 1998 to implement regulatory provisions of the Patient's Bill of Rights initiative uniformly across all health plans participating in federal programs. In other cases, federal agency coordination is achieved through informal interaction among relevant agencies during the regulatory development process.

The notice-and-comment procedure used for federal regulation development provides interest groups with an important avenue for influencing federal public health policy outside the federal legislative process. Groups that represent the institutions and individuals affected by federal regulations are typically the most active participants in this procedure. When regulations are finalized and encoded, the federal judicial system becomes the primary venue for affected entities to pursue claims about federal regulatory authority and enforcement. The federal courts adjudicate three primary types of claims regarding federal regulations: claims that a regulation exceeds the authority granted to the federal government under the Constitution; claims that a regulation exceeds the authority granted to the federal agency by congressional legislation; and claims that a regulation is enforced improperly or inequitably by the federal agency.[34] Claims of the latter type typically begin with adjudication by the federal agency involved and can be appealed directly to the United States appellate courts. Other types of claims most often originate in United States district courts.

Just as Congress uses outside advisory groups to inform legislative decision making, many federal agencies rely on advisory groups to propose and review regulatory decision making. For example, MedPAC, which was established by congressional legislation in 1997, frequently provides comments and feedback to HHS concerning proposed and current regulations developed for the Medicare program by CMS. In other cases, presidential executive orders are used to empanel advisory commissions that assist federal agencies developing health-related regulations. For example, the National Bioethics Advisory Commission was established by executive order in 1995 to advise executive agencies regarding the development and enforcement of federal policies and regulations governing research involving human subjects. In other cases, regulatory advisory bodies are created through the initiatives of federal agencies themselves, such as the EPA's Common Sense Initiative, which involves representatives from industry, environmental justice organizations, labor organizations, and state and local governments in a consensus-based regulatory development process.[35]

INTERGOVERNMENTAL RELATIONSHIPS

Federal public health activities achieve their impact on population health largely by influencing the activities undertaken by public health institutions at other levels of government and the private sector. Federal public health grant-in-aid programs shape the types of activities carried out by state health agencies and their counterparts operating at the local level. Federal regulatory actions also exert a strong influence on state and local public health activities because public health agencies operating at these levels are often responsible for monitoring and enforcing compliance with federal regulations. Clearly, this strong federal influence enables state and local public health agencies to undertake a much broader scope and scale of activity than would be possible otherwise. This influence may also pose challenges for states and localities. One frequent criticism is that federal spending policies induce state and local government agencies to develop policies and programs in response to federal revenue streams rather than in response to community needs and priorities.[36] Another criticism is that the federal government's regulatory authority often creates unfunded mandates, which oblige state and local governments to undertake activities without providing the federal funds to cover the costs of these activities.[37] For these reasons, determining the desirability and appropriateness of federal action in public health is not always straightforward. Federal actions can have unintended effects on public health practice at state and local levels.

Federal agencies shape state and local public health activities in ways other than through spending and regulatory authority. These agencies frequently lend technical assistance and scientific expertise to states, counties, and municipalities seeking to implement public health programs and policies within their jurisdictions. The CDC is perhaps the best-known federal agency for undertaking such activities, which include regular consultation with state and local health officials regarding disease prevention, detection, and control strategies; development of information and communication systems to facilitate state and local interaction with CDC officials; development of model programs and standards for implementation at state and local levels; and assignment of CDC officials to work in state and local public health agencies to facilitate the exchange of knowledge and expertise. Most other federal health agencies are involved to some extent in efforts to support state and local public health activities through information dissemination and technical assistance.

Federal agencies are involved to a lesser extent in the direct provision of public health services at the state and local level. Federal agencies engage in direct service provision most often in response to emergencies and disasters that have the potential to exceed state and local public health capacities.[38] Examples include outbreaks of unusual or particularly harmful infectious diseases, and natural disasters such as floods, earthquakes, and hurricanes. In relatively rare cases, federal agencies may engage in direct service provision to respond to large-scale health threats such as a major infectious disease outbreak or a natural disaster. A 2006 study of public health activities performed in the nation's largest local public health jurisdictions (at least 100,000 residents) found that direct federal involvement in performing public health activities occurred in less than half of these jurisdictions.[20] Where such involvement did occur, the activities most commonly performed by federal agencies included investigating adverse health events, providing access to laboratory services needed for public health surveillance and investigation, and developing support and communication systems among health-related organizations (see Table 8.2).

The federal government also plays important roles in shaping global public health policy and practice through relationships with public health institutions in other countries. Many of these activities are carried out through participation in the World Health Organization (WHO), a specialized unit of the United Nations founded in 1948 to

Table 8.2. Federal Agency Involvement in Local Public Health Activities: 1997 and 2006

Public Health Activities	Proportion of Communities Reporting Federal Involvement	
	1997	2006
Any activity	44.2%	61.2%
Assessment activities		
Assessment of community health needs	6.8%	7.6%
Survey of behavioral risk factors	4.6%	11.9%
Investigation of adverse health events	21.9%	28.5%
Use of public health laboratory testing	15.7%	21.3%
Analysis of health determinants	5.2%	9.4%
Analysis of preventive services use	2.6%	3.0%
Policy development activities		
Communication networks among agencies	10.6%	17.9%
Health briefings for elected officials	3.4%	13.3%
Prioritization of community health needs	5.7%	6.9%
Implementation of priority health initiatives	9.7%	11.2%
Community participation in health planning	4.6%	5.2%
Resource allocation planning	2.3%	5.6%
Resource deployment consistent with plan	5.7%	12.0%
Assurance activities		
Assessment of local public health agency	0.6%	3.9%
Provision/linkage to needed health services	8.3%	10.3%
Evaluation of public health services	4.3%	3.9%
Program monitoring and improvement	4.0%	9.9%
Health information provision to the public	10.0%	22.8%
Health information provision to the media	5.4%	21.0%

SOURCE: Authors' analysis of data from: Mays GP. Complex and adaptive systems: Changes in the organizations contributing to local public health activities. Paper presented at the 2007 Academy Health Annual Research Meeting. Orlando, FL: June 2007.

foster international cooperation in addressing public health issues and in strengthening national health systems. Through its participation in WHO, the federal government helps establish international standards and policies on issues such as disease detection, surveillance and reporting; health technology purchasing and dissemination; vaccine and pharmaceutical products use; environmental health conditions; and the accessibility and quality of health care services. The CDC is often the federal government's lead agency for carrying out WHO-sponsored initia-

tives in global disease prevention, control, and eradication. The CDC also maintains an array of related activities in global public health surveillance and capacity-building, including training programs for public health workers from foreign countries. Another federal agency that frequently engages in international cooperative efforts around health issues is the United States Agency for International Development. This agency helps impoverished and recovering foreign countries develop programs for family planning and reproductive health, infectious disease prevention and control (particularly HIV/AIDS), child survival, and maternal health. These types of international initiatives strengthen the nation's defenses against global health risks while simultaneously helping to achieve global improvements in health and well-being.

THE FUTURE OF FEDERAL CONTRIBUTIONS TO PUBLIC HEALTH

Heightened public concerns about bioterrorism and emergency preparedness have ushered in an era of stronger direct federal involvement in public health infrastructure development and capacity building. Still, the federal government's efforts to protect and promote health at the population level derive principally from its authority to allocate resources to public health programs and to regulate activities that have important effects on health. Undoubtedly, these federal roles will remain powerfully influential forces in the public health system of the future, even as shifts in political power and public priorities alter the specific forms and functions of federal public health initiatives. Emerging trends within the nation's public health system, however, suggest that the federal government may rely more heavily than previously on its ability to shape public health policy and practice through informal leadership, particularly its power to convene major stakeholders in public health and mobilize collaborative, multi-institutional responses to public health issues.

Among the new developments that are placing increased emphasis on federal public health leadership is the expanding collection of stakeholders that contribute to population health. A growing number of institutions and professionals outside the realm of governmental public health are using population-based approaches for identifying health needs and risks, preventing disease and injury, preparing for natural and man-made disasters, and improving

the effectiveness and efficiency of health services delivery.[39–42] Consequently, public health professionals face unprecedented opportunities to align the interests and actions of these diverse stakeholders to improve population health. Federal health agencies are uniquely positioned to bring together these entities on a national level for purposes such as reaching consensus about priority health needs and risks, pooling resources and expertise, identifying optimal intervention strategies, coordinating programs and services, and negotiating organizational roles and responsibilities in public health.

Public health's expanding array of stakeholders includes the many public safety and emergency response organizations that play key roles in public health preparedness planning. These stakeholders also include health care providers, insurers, and businesses, which are increasingly exploring population-based approaches for disease prevention and disease management to meet market demands for lower health care costs and improved health outcomes.[42–47] Community-based organizations such as churches, civic groups, human service providers, educational institutions, and philanthropies are also assuming larger roles in public health activities, particularly as these institutions gain an enhanced understanding of the relationships between population health status and social and economic determinants of health.[43,48,49] In the private sector, pharmaceutical companies and health information technology firms are expanding their involvement in population-based disease management interventions and health education campaigns, particularly as they recognize the social and economic gains to be realized from more appropriate use of preventive and therapeutic interventions.[50,51] Given this expanding array of stakeholders, a key federal leadership challenge lies in using its visibility and influence within the health system to mobilize multi-institutional responses to national public health priorities.[52,53]

A second, related development in the nation's public health system is the growing recognition that many of the nation's most pressing public health problems cannot be addressed through governmental action alone nor through public health action alone. The growing epidemic of obesity presents a prime example of such a problem that requires coordinated responses from public health agencies, clinicians, schools, businesses, food manufacturers and regulatory agencies, and the transportation and land use planning sectors, among others. Another example exists in the persistent disparities in health experienced by population groups defined by race and ethnicity, gender, education and income, disability, geographic area, and sexual orientation.[54] Although the nation as a whole has realized substantial gains in population health in recent decades, the nation's minority and disadvantaged populations bear a disproportionate burden of disease, injury, and mortality—particularly African Americans, Hispanics, Native Americans, and Pacific Islanders.[55,56] Addressing the unmet health needs of minority and disadvantaged populations will require concerted, sustained action from the full complement of health, social, economic, and cultural institutions that influence these populations. Such action will require strong, and perhaps unprecedented, leadership at the national level to mobilize and coordinate responses to persistent population-based disparities in health.

Another emerging development in the nation's public health system involves the complex and evolving dynamics of disease transmission. The resurgence of well-known diseases such as tuberculosis and pneumonia, combined with the emergence of new diseases caused by agents as varied as SARS and hantavirus, has demonstrated the continuing threats to population health posed by infectious agents and environmental toxins.[57–59] New scientific evidence suggests that infectious agents and environmental toxins may be important contributors to many common chronic diseases, including peptic ulcer disease, atherosclerosis, heart disease, cancer, and arthritis.[60–62] The emergence of drug-resistant strains of infectious diseases such as tuberculosis and *Staphylococcus aureus* raises concerns that the nation's armamentarium of antimicrobial interventions may be losing its effectiveness due to overuse and inappropriate use in clinical applications.[63] The nation's public health organizations are

further challenged by the variety of mechanisms through which new and previously unobserved diseases are introduced within populations. Increasingly, disease transmission is a global process facilitated by the ease and speed with which humans, animals, agricultural products, and pollutants move between countries and regions of the world.[57,59] Moreover, the environmental and climatic changes occurring in many regions of the world potentially create opportunities for disease transmission cycles to extend into previously unaffected areas (e.g., the 1999 West Nile Virus outbreak in New York City). These multiple, global transmission routes make it impossible for health professionals practicing at the community level to keep apprised of all possible disease risks facing a population of interest. Moreover, disease outbreaks due to acts of bioterrorism remain a constant threat to population health in the modern geopolitical environment.[57]

In view of the complex and changing patterns of disease epidemiology, the federal government faces new imperatives to mobilize international partnerships for disease control and public health preparedness. At the same time, the federal government faces imperatives to strengthen communication and information-sharing mechanisms among the variety of domestic health care providers and public health institutions involved in disease prevention, identification, monitoring, and control. Ensuring the full cooperation of international and domestic stakeholders in disease control efforts is unlikely to be achieved through federal regulatory and financing initiatives alone. Consequently, the federal government's informal powers in public agenda setting, consensus development, and coalition building are likely to become increasingly important in addressing the nation's emerging disease risks.

These emerging developments in the nation's public health system demand that the federal government continue to exert a major influence on public health practice and policy in the years to come. This influence is essential for addressing health issues and disease risks that are too broad in scope and scale for individual states and localities to resolve effectively on their own. The federal government's formal authority to influence public health is necessarily restrained by the constitutionally guaranteed powers of states to construct their own public health programs and policies in response to local priorities and needs. This formal authority is also subject to the federal political processes that shape congressional legislation in public health. The federal government's informal mechanisms for influencing public health policy and practice, which collectively can be described as public health leadership strategies, are less dependent on legal and political structures. Strong leadership is an increasingly important power in the contemporary public health environment comprised of diverse institutional stakeholders, persistent health disparities, and global disease processes.

REVIEW QUESTIONS

1. Describe four sources of federal governmental power within the public health system, and provide an example of how these sources of power are used to influence public health.
2. How does the federal government's role in financing personal health services compare with its role in financing public health services? What reasons may explain any similarities or differences in these roles? What reasons may explain any changes in these roles over time?
3. What factors or conditions place limits on the scope of federal authority over health issues?
4. Identify three cabinet-level departments other than the Department of Health and Human Services that exercise significant authority and influence over health issues. Describe a health-related program or responsibility within each of these departments.
5. Identify four mechanisms through which the federal government influences the public health activities undertaken by state or local governments.
6. Describe three mechanisms through which Congress obtains information and expertise on health issues.
7. Identify three different types of health issues upon which the federal courts have responsibility to act, and provide an example of each.
8. What developments are likely to explain the substantial increase in federal government involvement in local public health activities as suggested in Table 8.2?

REFERENCES

1. Hanlon G, Pickett J. *Public Health Administration and Practice*. New York: Mosby; 1984.
2. Institute of Medicine, National Academy of Sciences. *The Future of Public Health*. Washington, DC: National Academy Press; 1988.
3. Shonick W. *Government and Health Services: Government's Role in the Development of the US Health Services 1930–1980*. New York: Oxford University Press; 1995.
4. Centers for Disease Control and Prevention. History of CDC. *MMWR*. 1996;45:526–528.
5. Anderson OW. *Health Services in the United States: A Growth Enterprise Since 1875*. Ann Arbor, MI: Health Administration Press; 1985.
6. Omenn GS. What's behind those block grants in health? *N Engl J Med*. 1982;306(17):1057–1060.
7. Kennan SA. Legislative relations in public health. In: Novick LF, Mays GP, eds. *Public Health Administration: Principles for Population-Based Management*. Gaithersburg, MD: Aspen Publishers; 2000;539–566.
8. Leviss PS. Financing the public's health. In: Novick LF, Mays GP, eds. *Public Health Administration: Principles for Population-Based Management*. Gaithersburg, MD: Aspen Publishers; 2000:413–430.
9. Brennan TA, Berwick DM. *New Rules: Regulation, Markets, and the Quality of American Health Care*. San Francisco, CA: Jossey-Bass; 1996.
10. Moran DW. Federal regulation of managed care: An impulse in search of a theory. *Health Aff*. 1997;16(6):7–33.
11. Fuchs BC. *Managed Health Care: Federal and State Regulation*. Washington, DC: Congressional Research Service; 1997.
12. Roper WL. Regulating quality and clinical practice. In: Altman SH, Reinhardt UE, and Shactman D, eds. *Regulating Managed Care: Theory, Practice,*

and Future Options. San Francisco, CA: Jossey-Bass; 1999:145–159.

13. Scheffler RM, Clement DG, Sullivan SD, Hu TW, Sung HY. The hospital response to Medicare's Prospective Payment System: An econometric model of Blue Cross and Blue Shield plans. *Med Care*. 1994;32(5):471–485.

14. Miller T, Leatherman S. The National Quality Forum: A "me-too" or a breakthrough in quality measurement and reporting? *Health Aff*. 1999; 18(6):233–237.

15. Eisenberg JM. Health services research in a market-oriented health care system. *Health Aff*. 1998;17(1):98–108.

16. Gostin LO. Public health law in a new century: Part II, public health powers and limits. *JAMA*. 2000;283(22):2979–2984.

17. Centers for Medicare and Medicaid Services. Health expenditures by sponsors: Business, household, and government. http://www.cms. hhs.gov/NationalHealthExpendData/06_ NationalHealthAccountsBusinessHousehold Government.asp#TopOfPage. March 1, 2006. Accessed October 25, 2006.

18. Pauly MV. *Health Benefits at Work: An Economic and Political Analysis of Employment-Based Health Insurance*. Ann Arbor: University of Michigan Press; 1999.

19. Litman TJ. The politics of health: Establishing policies and setting priorities. In: Lee PR and Estes CL, eds. *The Nation's Health*. 4th ed. Boston, MA: Jones and Bartlett; 1994: 107–120.

20. Mays GP. Organization of the public health delivery system. In: Novick LF, Mays GP, eds. *Public Health Administration: Principles for Population-Based Management,* 2nd ed. Gaithersburg, MD: Aspen Publishers; 2008:69–126.

21. Kahn CN III, Ault T, Isenstein H, Potetz L, Van Gelder S. Snapshot of hospital quality reporting and pay-for-performance under Medicare. *Health Aff* (Millwood). January–February 2006;25(1): 148–62.

22. De Leon R, Bailey S. *Military Health System: A Joint Overview Statement*. Washington, DC: US House of Representatives, Committee on Appropriations, Defense Subcommittee; 2000.

23. Government Accountability Office. *Performance Budgeting: Past Initiatives Offer Insights for GPRA*. Washington, DC: GAO; March 1997.

24. National Research Council, Panel on Performance Measures and Data for Public Health Performance Partnership Grants. *Assessment of Performance Measures for Public Health, Substance Abuse, and Mental Health*. Washington, DC: National Academy Press; 1997.

25. Ferejohn JA, Weingast BR. *The New Federalism: Can the States Be Trusted?* Palo Alto, CA: Hoover Institution Press, Stanford University; 1997.

26. Wing KR. *The Law and the Public's Health*. Ann Arbor, MI: Health Administration Press; 1999.

27. Gostin LO. *Public Health Law: Power, Duty, Restraint*. San Francisco: University of California Press; 2001.

28. Rochefort DA, Cobb RW. *The Politics of Problem Definition: Shaping the Policy Agenda.* Lawrence: University of Kansas Press; 1997.

29. Berry JM. *The Interest Group Society*. New York: Little Brown & Co; 1984.

30. Kahn CN III, Kuttner H. Budget bills and Medicare policy: The politics of the BBA. *Health Aff (Millwood)*. 1999;18(1):37–47.

31. Berkowitz ED. *A History of the Institute of Medicine: To Improve Human Health*. Washington, DC: National Academies Press; 1999.

32. Gais T. *Improper Influence: Campaign Finance Law, Political Interest Groups, and the Problem of Equality*. Ann Arbor: University of Michigan Press; 1996.

33. Schick A. *The Federal Budget: Politics, Policy, Process.* 2nd ed. Washington, DC: Brookings Institute; 2000.

34. Federal Judicial Center. *The Federal Courts and What They Do*. Washington, DC: Government Printing Office; 1997.

35. Environmental Protection Agency. Consensus Decision-Making Principles and Applications in the EPA Common Sense Initiative. Washington, DC: Government Printing Office; 1997.

36. Conlan TJ. *From New Federalism to Devolution: Twenty-five Years of Intergovernmental Reform*. Washington, DC: Brookings Institute; 1998.

37. Posner PL. *The Politics of Unfunded Mandates: Whither Federalism?* Washington, DC: Georgetown University Press; 1998.

38. Turnock BJ. *Public Health: What It Is and How It Works*. Gaithersburg, MD: Aspen Publishers; 2000.

39. Roper WL, Koplan JP, Stinnet AA. 1994. Public health in the new American health system. *Frontiers of Health Serv Manage*. 1994;10(4):32–36.

40. Baker EL, Melton RJ, Stange PV, et al. Health reform and the health of the public. *JAMA.* 1994;272:1276–1282.

41. Showstack J, Lurie N, Leatherman S, Fisher E, Inui T. Health of the public: The private-sector challenge. *JAMA.* 1996;276(13):1071–1074.

42. Roper WL, Mays GP. The changing managed care—public health interface. *JAMA.* 1998; 280(20):1739–1740.

43. Lasker, RD. *Medicine and Public Health: The Power of Collaboration.* New York: Academy of Medicine; 1997.

44. Halverson PK, Mays GP, Kaluzny AD, Richards TB. Not-so-strange bedfellows: Models of interaction between managed care plans and public health agencies. *Milbank Quarterly.* 1997;75: 113–138.

45. Christianson JB. The role of employers in community health care systems. *Health Aff.* 1998;17(4): 158–164.

46. Lee D, Lopez L. An invitational workshop on collaboration between quality improvement organizations and business coalitions. *Joint Commission J on Quality Improvement in Health Care.* 1997; 23(6):334–341.

47. McLaughlin CP. Balancing collaboration and competition: The Kingsport, Tennessee experience. *Joint Commission J on Quality Improvement.* 1995;21(11):646–655.

48. Bruce TA, McKane SU. The community-based public health initiative: Lessons learned. In: Mays GP, Miller CA, and Halverson PK, eds. *Local Public Health Practice: Trends and Models.* Washington, DC: American Public Health Association; 2000.

49. Mays GP, Miller CA, Halverson PK. *Local Public Health Practice: Trends and Models.* Washington, DC: American Public Health Association; 2000.

50. Keys IR. Take it to heart: A national health screening and education project in African-American communities. A joint project of the NMA and Bayer Corporation. *J of the Nat Med Assoc.* 1999; 91(12):649–652.

51. Hirano D. Partnering to improve infant immunizations: The Arizona Partnership for Infant Immunization (TAPII). *Am J Prev Med.* 1998; 14(3 suppl):22–25.

52. Marcus L. *Renegotiating Health Care: Resolving Conflict to Build Collaboration.* San Francisco, CA: Jossey-Bass; 1999.

53. Hatcher MT, Niccola RM. Building constituencies for public health. In: Novick LF, Mays GP, eds. *Public Health Administration: Principles for Population-Based Management.* Gaithersburg, MD: Aspen Publishers; 2000;510–520.

54. US Department of Health and Human Services. *Healthy People 2010: Understanding and Improving Health.* Washington, DC: Government Printing Office; 2000.

55. Smith DB. *Health Care Divided: Race and a Healing Nation.* Ann Arbor: University of Michigan Press; 1999.

56. Hogue CJR, Hargrave MA. *Minority Health in America: Findings and Policy Implications from the Commonwealth Fund Minority Health Survey.* Baltimore, MD: Johns Hopkins University Press; 2000.

57. Centers for Disease Control and Prevention. *Preventing Emerging Infectious Diseases: A Strategy for the 21st Century.* Atlanta, GA: CDC; 1998.

58. Binder S, Levitt AM, Sacks JJ, Hughes JM. Emerging infectious diseases: Public health issues for the 21st century. *Science.* 1999;284(5418): 1311–1313.

59. Mayer JD. Geography, ecology and emerging infectious diseases. *Soc Sci & Med.* 2000;50(7–8): 937–952.

60. Gupta S, et al. Elevated Chlamydia pneumoniae antibodies, cardiovascular events, and azithromycin in male survivors of myocardial infarction. *Circulation.* 1997;96:404–407.

61. Baseman JB, Tully JG. Mycoplasmas: Sophisticated, reemerging, and burdened by their notoriety. *Emerging Infect Dis.* 1997;3:21–32.

62. Muhlestein JB, Anderson JL, Hammond EH, et al. Infection with Chlamydia pneumoniae accelerates the development of atherosclerosis and treatment with azithromycin prevents it in a rabbit model. *Circulation.* 1998;97:633–636.

63. Vermund SH, Fawal H. Emerging infectious diseases and professional integrity: Thoughts for the new millennium. *Am J Infect Control.* 1999;27(6): 497–499.

CHAPTER 9

The State Public Health Agencies

A. Richard Melton, MPH, DrPH and Laverne Alves Snow, MPA, PhD(C)

LEARNING OBJECTIVES

Upon completion of this chapter, the reader will be able to:

1. Develop knowledge of the history and roles of state health agencies.

2. Describe the Institute of Medicine's reports on public health and describe how implementing recommendations could affect public health policy and structure.

3. Recognize the challenges associated with funding state and local public health programs with federal, state, local, and private funds.

4. Develop insight into the processes and challenges of formulating state-level public health priorities and policies and building consensus to support them.

5. Describe the variation in leadership structure among state health agencies and comprehend the benefits and disadvantages associated with each.

6. Apply the information and resources provided in this chapter to foster further learning about state health agencies and track changes in state health agency roles, programs, and health concerns.

7. Describe the importance of identifying and assessing emerging public health problems and the role of state health agencies in implementing activities to meet these needs.

8. Describe the consequences of an aging public health workforce, and identify and evaluate potential approaches to address these concerns.

9. Comprehend the importance of public health informatics in helping a state health agency meet its core functions of assessment, policy development, and assurance.

10. Recognize the leadership role of state health agencies in helping create health information exchange networks.

11. Identify and apply tools for evaluating the effectiveness of public health programs.

KEY TERMS

Disease Registry

Enumeration

Informatics

Interoperability

(Special Thanks to Sara Ellis Simonsen, RN, MSPH, Research Associate, University of Utah Public Health Program, for her work on researching statistics and preparing the figures and to Allen Korhonen, Deputy Director, Utah Department for his help in preparing this chapter.)

Medicaid

Medicare

Public Health Competencies

Public Health Informatics

Sick Building Syndrome (SBS)

Super-Agency

Toxic Mold

Umbrella Agency

Vital Records

Vital Statistics

INTRODUCTION

Public health has widely embraced its core functions to be assessment, policy development, and assurance as described in the landmark 1988 Institute of Medicine (IOM Committee) report, *The Future of Public Health*.[1] The report pointed out that public health was in disarray and the roles and responsibilities of various levels of governmental public health agencies were not clearly defined. Adopting this challenge has been a quest for public health leaders for nearly two decades. The appropriate questions for leaders at the state level include:

- What should be the roles and responsibilities of state health agencies (SHAs)?

- How should public health roles, responsibilities, and resources be assigned among other state agencies and between state and local governmental entities?

In this chapter, the roles, responsibilities, and structures of SHAs will be discussed. These include public health functions and services that have significant influence on the public's health, some of which are frequently found within the SHA and some are often found outside the SHA. Issues related to the purpose and activities of state-level boards of health are presented as well as qualifications and appointments of SHA directors. In addition, recommendations from the 1988 IOM Committee are provided to facilitate comparing current and past choices to recommended structures and processes. Internet links to resource documents are included to enhance a deeper understanding of the materials covered. At the end of the chapter, you will find questions that provide a review of topics covered as well as a challenge to think about and apply concepts and issues relevant to the environment in which SHAs operate.

HISTORY

Massachusetts was the first state to take responsibility for the health of its people by creating a board of health in 1869. By 1909, all states had health departments whose tasks focused primarily on the recording of births and deaths (**vital records**) and the control of communicable diseases. Today, state health departments have expanded their activities to include improving the health of children and pregnant women, controlling chronic diseases, preventing injuries, regulating health care facilities, developing emergency medical services and other health care resources, and protecting the environment.

The 1988 IOM Committee noted that states are close enough to the people to maintain a sense of their needs and preferences, yet large enough, in most cases, to command the resources necessary to get the important jobs done.[1] In fact, because state health departments were created to meet the differing needs and preferences of the people in each state, their functions and activities show wide variation. They also vary in organizational structure, per capita expenditures, staffing patterns, political influence, responsibilities for local health services, and relationships with other federal, state, and local agencies. Because some state health agencies are not organized at the cabinet level and therefore are not truly "departments" of state government, the Association of State and Territorial Health Officials (ASTHO) adopted the term *state health agency* to signify that the agency of state government is vested with primary responsibility for public health within the state.[2] A listing of these agencies and their directors can be found at StatePublicHealth.org,[3] and many of the organization charts can be found on the ASTHO website.[4]

In the 2002 report, *The Future of the Public's Health in the 21st Century*, the IOM Committee reviewed the achievements of public health in recent years and projected challenges that face public health in the new century using the guiding principles of *Healthy People 2010*.[5,6] They also examined in some detail the continuing variation in organizational structure and responsibilities of state and local public health agencies. Recommendations from the 1988 and 2002 IOM Committee reports are included as yardsticks for comparison with actual conditions.

ROLES OF STATE HEALTH AGENCIES

The core public health functions of assessment, policy development, and assurance together imply an agenda-setting role, especially at the state level. Each SHA must identify goals and strategies to improve the health of its citizens. To set and implement this agenda, the agency assesses the health status and needs of the population; plans strategies and health programs to address unmet needs; obtains financial assistance to support these plans; sets and enforces standards; provides technical assistance to local health departments and other governmental and nongovernmental agencies; and,

in limited circumstances, delivers direct health services. In most states, local health departments are the primary government entity providing public health services directly to local communities.

Expert guidance for defining state agency roles and responsibilities comes from many sources. In 1994, the Public Health Functions Working Group, a committee convened by the United States Department of Health and Human Services (HHS) with representatives from all major public health constituencies, agreed on a list of the essential services of public health.[7] This list of services translates the three core functions into a more concrete set of activities, called the 10 Essential Public Health Services. In addition to this definition of services, The National Public Health Performance Standards Program (NPHPSP), a collaborative effort of seven national public health organizations, establishes and implements national performance standards for state and local public health systems and for governance bodies such as local boards of health.[8,9] The vision for the NPHPSP is "excellence in public health practice," and the mission is "to improve the quality of public health practice and performance of public health systems." These standards identify the optimal level of performance for state public health agencies. In 2001, the Council on Linkages between Academia and Public Health Practice published a document describing required **public health competencies** (see Appendix C).[10]

Traditional Roles for State Health Agencies

Until the 1940s, SHAs focused almost solely on six basic public health services: collection of vital records and statistics, control of communicable diseases, environmental sanitation, laboratory services, public health education, and maternal and child health. As antibiotics and vaccines became available to control the spread of communicable diseases, citizens voiced their desire for state government to give attention to other health problems. In the late 1950s, the United States Congress began offering states federal funds to support new categories of services for certain groups of people or for specific diseases. These categorical programs addressed areas in which SHAs traditionally had not been involved, including heart disease, diabetes, mental retardation, migrant labor, ethnic and racial minorities, and the construction of new health facilities such as hospitals and clinics.

This expansion of SHA activities has continued, stimulated by the availability of federal funds, the necessity of meeting federally enacted mandates, and the growth of state health laws. For example, in the past decade, SHAs have expanded activities that target reducing tobacco use, responding to possible acts of bioterrorism, and addressing asthma as a public health problem.

In 1997, 33 states reported substantial use of the Healthy People 2000 national objectives in setting state objectives and program priorities.[11] The availability of baseline data often determined the selection of health objectives. As part of their state health planning process, many states have developed new and complex data systems to track progress toward meeting current objectives and setting new ones based on the national health objectives for 2010. Nationally, work has begun on a new set of national objectives for 2020.

Typical Responsibilities

Typical responsibilities performed by nearly all SHAs are presented in Table 9.1. Many of these activities are expansions and variations on the original six basic functions, particularly health information (vital records and statistics), disease and disability prevention (communicable disease control and laboratory services), health protection (environmental sanitation), health promotion (public health education), and maternal and child health services.

Table 9.1. Typical Responsibilities of a State Health Agency

Health Information
- Recording and issuing certified copies of birth and death certificates
- Publishing health statistics
- Birth defects registry
- Cancer registry

Disease and Disability Prevention
- Screening newborns for inborn errors of metabolism
- Immunization programs
- AIDS screening, counseling, and partner notification
- Tuberculosis control
- Screening children for lead
- Investigating disease outbreaks
- Laboratory testing for infectious diseases
- Medical care for children with handicapping conditions
- Education on use of occupant restraints in vehicles
- Laboratory testing for weapons of mass destruction (biological, chemical, and radiological)

Health Protection
- Testing waters in which shellfish are grown
- Issuing permits for sewage disposal systems
- Monitoring drinking water systems
- Inspecting dairies
- License hospitals, nursing homes, and home health agencies
- Examining and certifying emergency medical personnel
- Inspecting clinical laboratories

Health Promotion
- Food vouchers for pregnant women, infants, and children (WIC)
- Prenatal care for low-income women
- Dental care for low-income children and adults
- School health education
- Family planning services
- Cholesterol and high blood pressure education programs
- Tobacco use cessation programs

Improving the Health Care Delivery System
- Scholarships for medical and nursing students
- Certificates of need for construction of health facilities
- Development of rural health policies and services
- Collecting and analyzing data on health care costs

Health Information

The collection and preservation of vital records and the analysis and use of information from such records are major functions of SHAs. SHAs are the legal repositories for birth and death records in most states. They may also keep records of marriages, divorces, and terminations of pregnancy. More recently, states have begun to gather and analyze data on the health of the population and the characteristics of the medical care delivery system.

Data from these vital records, along with data from **disease registries,** surveys of populations and of health care providers and facilities, disease case reports, screening programs, and laboratory analyses, are used for several purposes such as influencing the creation, continuation, or modification of programs; identifying disease patterns or outbreaks; identifying racial and ethnic health disparities; determining priorities for resource allocation; and planning health care delivery sites and facilities.

Disease and Disability Prevention

Preventing disease and disability, particularly infectious disease, is a unique function of SHAs in every state. No other state agency is given the lead responsibility for these functions. As measles and other communicable diseases have been brought under control, SHA attention and resources have shifted to other health problems such as AIDS, hepatitis, breast cancer, injuries, and cardiovascular disease. State activities in these areas include screening programs, laboratory testing, health education, technical advice, issuance of isolation and quarantine orders, immunizations, public information, and chemotherapy.

Health Promotion

Going beyond educating the population on how to avoid infectious diseases, health promotion efforts in SHAs now focus on lifestyle issues, maintenance of health, and prevention of injury. Health education programs at schools and workplaces address diet, exercise, tobacco use, and stress reduction, with emphasis on reducing risk factors for cancer

and cardiovascular diseases. The latest focus of health promotion is in the area of obesity. Worldwide, obesity has increased in epidemic proportion. We are facing an unprecedented public health epidemic of overweight and obesity that may lead to the first generations in our nation's history that will live shorter lives than their parents, with many of those years being in poor health. The projected long-term health care costs of this epidemic are staggering. All ages and races and both genders are affected directly or indirectly. SHAs are beginning to lead all sectors of public health to work together to develop a focused, consistent, and coordinated approach to create a culture and environment that make a healthy choice the easy choice.

Health Care Delivery

The involvement of SHAs in direct delivery of care began with clinics for pregnant women and children. As federal and state funds have become available, direct services have expanded to include family planning, cancer screening, dental health, treatment for tuberculosis and sexually transmitted diseases, and, most recently, primary medical care. In each of these undertakings, the state's role centers on program planning, setting and enforcing standards, developing procedures, and providing technical assistance and funding, whereas the clinical care is usually delivered at the local level, through either the private or public health delivery system.

Areas of Significant Variation in Health Agency Roles

Before 1960, almost all public health functions provided by states were located in SHAs. As programs became more complex and as demands for new types of services increased, many public health activities were assigned to other state agencies. Based on a 2005 survey by the Association of State and Territorial State Health Officials (ASTHO), Table 9.2 shows the great variation in responsibilities assigned to the SHA in the states, and Table 9.3 shows other agencies that share responsibility for

Table 9.2. Diversity in State Health Agency Programs and Functions

Public Health Function or Program	Agencies Reporting Full Authority	Agencies Reporting Partial Authority
Drinking Water Regulation	21	21
Environmental Health	25	23
Environmental Regulation and Management	11	28
Food Safety	31	17
Health Facility Regulation and Inspection	40	7
Health Professional Licensing	18	19
Medicaid	10	9
Medical Errors Reporting	17	11
Medical Examiner	12	4
Mental Health	9	10
Public Health Laboratories	47	3
Tobacco Prevention and Control	42	9
Substance Abuse Prevention	16	12
Vital Statistics Administration	49	2
WIC	47	3

SOURCE: Association of State and Territorial Public Health Officials, 2005 Salary and Agency Infrastructure Survey.

Table 9.3. Health Responsibilities Often in State Agencies Other Than the State Health Agency

Department of Agriculture
- Inspects grocery stores
- Inspects food processing plants

Department of Education
- Supervises health teaching in schools
- Supervises delivery of health services in schools

Department of Environmental Quality
- Controls air pollution
- Controls water pollution
- Oversees solid and hazardous waste disposal

Department of Health Professions
- Licenses 12 categories of health professionals

Department of Labor and Industry
- Regulates occupational health and safety

Department of Medical Assistance Services (Medicaid)
- Finances medical care to the indigent and categorically needy
- Funds a health status screening program for children
- Provides case management services for newborns

Department of Mental Health, Mental Retardation, and Substance Abuse Services
- Operates mental hospitals
- Directs community mental health and substance abuse services

Department of Motor Vehicles
- Educates the public on occupant safety and seatbelt use

Joint Commission on Health Care
- Develops legislative proposals for improving access to medical care

some public health activities.[12] New problems often generate new programs that are assigned to new agencies rather than generating changes in existing SHAs. Public health leaders may be perceived as having no interest in new ideas or as not having the political skills needed to lead and direct a particular program. Often, special interest groups want separate administration for their particular programs so they can exert more control over operations. Sometimes, governors want to put their "stamp" on a new program to become, for example, the "environmental" or the "education" governor by creating new agencies to address their special issues.

IOM Committee Recommendations

In 1988 and again in 2002, The IOM Committee analyzed this fragmentation of public health functions and made specific recommendations regarding closer linkages between programs that now exist in separate agencies.[1,5]

Areas where variation and fragmentation can be observed include mental health; health care financing, including placement of the **Medicaid** program; and environmental protection.

Mental Health

As reflected in the ASTHO 2005 survey, the SHAs are also the state mental health authority in only 9 states, and only 10 SHAs indicate they have any responsibility for mental health issues at all.[12] This division of leadership at the state level results in separate service delivery systems at the local level, with little coordinated planning around patient needs.

IOM Committee Recommendations

The 2002 IOM Committee continues to recommend that public health and mental health leaders devote efforts to strengthening the linkages between the two fields, particularly to integrating these functions at the service delivery level.[5]

Yet, little has been done to implement this recommendation. Mental health agencies have strong advocacy groups interested in separate systems that lobby state legislatures for money and facilities, sometimes at the expense of public health programs.

Financing Medical Care

The state's participation in financing medical care usually resides outside the SHA. When the federal Medicaid program started in 1965, states had to select a single state agency to manage the program. Initially, some states assigned this role to health departments. As the Medicaid program grew, both in dollars and in numbers of people receiving care, responsibility for operating the program shifted either to a separate state agency or to the social services/welfare agency. Only 10 SHAs manage their state's Medicaid program.[12]

Coordination and Control of Medicaid Services. When the SHA retains responsibility for the Medicaid program, there is greater integration of Medicaid-financed services with other public health services, using the same delivery system. Thus, both federal Medicaid and state public health funds are coordinated to provide services to eligible patients. When public health and Medicaid are administered separately, on the other hand, the SHA loses some of its control, particularly over programs for pregnant women and children, the largest constituency served by Medicaid.

As Congress continues to expand Medicaid eligibility and states try to address falling rates of insurance coverage for their citizens by covering more pregnant women, children, and adolescents, the Medicaid budgets often far exceed the public health budgets. State funds allocated to Medicaid bring federal dollars to each state, on a matching basis, whereas state funds appropriated for public health often stand alone. Because Medicaid is an entitlement, many of the services it provides must be funded each year. Figure 9.1 shows the national annual and cumulative growth of Medicaid enrollment from 1999 through 2005. Because the cost of this growth must be funded each year, many SHAs feel that Medicaid and public health compete for

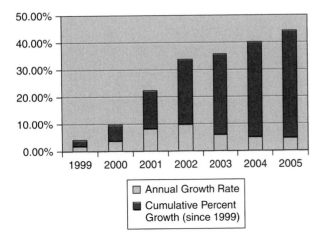

Figure 9.1. Percent Change in United States Medicaid Enrollment

SOURCE: Trends and Indicators in the Changing Health Care Marketplace (#7031), The Henry J. Kaiser Family Foundation, February 2005.

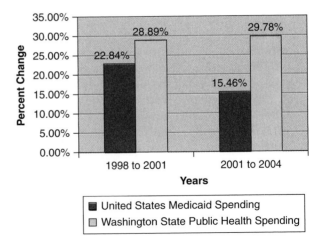

Figure 9.2. Changes in Medicaid Spending and Public Health Spending

SOURCE: **Medicaid Data:** Kaiser Family Foundation and Sonderegger Research Center 2006, Trends and Indicators in the Changing Health Care Marketplace http://www.kff.org/insurance/7031/print-sec1.cfm.

Washington State Data: Public Health Financing Trends, Presentation to the Joint Select Committee on Public Health Finance, Legislative Fiscal Committee Staff, 2005 http://www.leg.wa.gov/NR/rdonlyres/ 23EB8885-0B43-4143-8F64-C47AAEAA8CBC/ 22981/PHFinancingTrends999991.pdf.

state funds, with public health usually losing the battle. As a result, SHAs have resisted being in the same organization or being responsible for this function. Figure 9.2 shows the percent growth for Medicaid nationally for two three-year periods, 1998 to 2001 and 2001 to 2004, compared to the growth of state spending for the same period for public health in Washington state. It is also true, however, that wherever public health programs are located in state government, they are in competition for scarce state funds with Medicaid, education, transportation, law enforcement, and all other large state programs.

IOM Committee Recommendations

Although the 1988 IOM Committee report recommended that each state health agency include responsibility for Medicaid, most state health officers continue to oppose any attempt to take back this function.[1] They believed it would detract from, rather than enhance, their public health activities, by linking them too closely to welfare programs.

Although the 2002 IOM report recognizes the advantages of the state health agency having responsibility for Medicaid, there is no direct recommendation to make this change.[5]

Environmental Protection

The removal of environmental health programs from SHAs has been viewed as a significant loss to public health, unlike mental health, which has never been a significant part of SHAs, and medical care financing, which moved to separate agencies without much protest from state health officials. Many environmental monitoring and control activities previously handled by SHAs, in areas such as air pollution, groundwater contamination, and solid and hazardous waste disposal, have been transferred to separate environmental protection agencies.

These programs grew from health departments' original work in sanitation but became increasingly complex as technology advanced and more potential pollutants were identified. Citizens demanded more protection of and from the environment, businesses became concerned about the costs of compliance with environmental health standards, and regulatory decisions became more complicated. Directors of SHAs frequently had no expertise in new environmental issues. Governors and legislators, wanting to give greater visibility to environmental issues, created new environmental agencies, following the example of the federal Environmental Protection Agency (EPA).

IOM Committee Recommendations

The 1988 IOM Committee noted that this separation of environmental health functions has led to a lack of coordination of efforts and an inadequate analysis of the health effects of environmental problems. Environmental protection agencies are more likely to focus on regulatory requirements and engineering technology than on risk to human health. Therefore, they recommended that state and local health agencies strengthen their capacities for identifying, understanding, and controlling environmental problems as health hazards. In some states, even after environmental programs were transferred, expertise in environmental health risk assessment has been retained within the state health agency as a resource for the environmental agency.[1]

The number of SHAs that are the lead environmental agencies has shown a steady decrease, from 19 in 1978 to 11 as reported in the 2005 ASTHO survey.[12] However, most SHAs have responsibility for some environmental health functions, usually food protection, safe drinking water, radiation control, health risk assessment, or toxic substance investigation. Recently, the federal government has provided funding to SHAs to improve states' capacity for surveillance, laboratory, and response

functions especially for biological and chemical agents used in bioterrorism.

New Roles

The responsibilities of SHAs are changed by the addition of new activities as well as the transfer of some programs to other entities. Some examples of important new areas of involvement for SHAs are suicide prevention, outdoor environmental cleanup, public health informatics and the environmental public health tracking network.

Suicide Prevention

Suicide prevention has traditionally been seen as the responsibility of the mental health agency in the state, which may or may not be located in the SHA. However, because the potential for youth suicide attempts is affected by so many factors, prevention efforts can be addressed by a variety of agencies, including SHAs, state and local education agencies, mental health entities, juvenile justice agencies; and emergency services, and law enforcement entities at the state and local level.[13]

State prevention plans or suicide prevention councils have been established in 49 states. However, unclear authority and accountability, resource constraints, and collaboration challenges are common factors limiting the implementation of these plans.

As with many health issues of concern to communities, SHAs are often the conveners and provide leadership for such planning efforts. Public health expertise in data collection and analysis, public education, and population-based programs make SHAs a crucial player within state governments to address suicide prevention and effectively lead multi-agency and multi-sector approaches.

Indoor Environmental Cleanup

Emerging environmental issues such as chemicals, mold, and drugs within buildings have created new roles for SHAs. In recent years, the new drug of choice for abuse is methamphetamine. "Meth" producers often use apartments and old homes as manufacturing laboratories. The "cooking" procedures result in toxic byproducts that contaminate these residences or "laboratories." The public, through legislative action, has demanded that SHAs define standards for the cleanup of these facilities before they may be re-inhabited. More recently, the demand is for SHAs to define a level of cleanup that must be attained after there is only suspected methamphetamine use in a residence but where no cooking is suspected. In neither situation is the science sufficient to set reliable standards, yet legislatures are mandating action by the SHA. Similar challenges exist with **"toxic mold"** and **"sick building syndrome."** In all of these situations, there is a perception of and possible real health risk, yet the science is still insufficient to support definitive action.

Public Health Informatics

Another emerging issue faced by SHAs is their role in internal and community-wide public health and health services **informatics** activities. Data collection and analysis is a critical function for SHAs. These activities help identify changing needs for health programs as well as emerging threats to the public's health. As information systems have evolved, the field of **public health informatics** helped research and test new methods and tools for using technology to enhance SHAs' ability to identify and assess current and future priorities for legislation, funding, and program activities. Nearly all activities of public health are now supported by some form of information technology.

Embracing technology brings to mind the words of Johann Wolfgang Van Goethe, "The heights charm us, but the steps do not; with the mountain in our view we love to walk the plains." If a challenge is "a test of one's abilities or resources in a demanding but stimulating undertaking," technology in itself presents a new set of tests for public health. These tests or steps for state public health leaders include the following:

- Providing a vision for a systemwide approach to innovation and technology adoption
- Competing with other enterprises for recruiting, retaining, and supervising qualified technical

staff; securing funds for and selecting or developing new systems

- Adopting and implementing standards to support integration of old systems with new systems within the organization as well as with public and private health care partners outside the organization
- Funding ongoing system maintenance and enhancements

As with all administrative support functions, securing time and money for these activities competes head on with the demand for resources for providing direct public health services.

Technology, while riddled with significant hurdles, provides opportunities to improve the effectiveness, timeliness, and efficiency of public health services. Public health has long understood the value of computer-based registries for individual health events such as births and deaths, cancer, birth defects, injury, and trauma. Many of these, however, by necessity, were developed as silos or standalone systems. If they were integrated for data sharing, they were only done so on a vertical basis, and even then, often in only one direction, from local to state to federal programs. The Internet has provided opportunities to think about doing public health business in new ways, which is both good news and bad news for program administrators. While creating demand for new options never dreamed about in the early history of state health responsibilities, these options come with a steep curve for keeping pace with innovations, infrastructure, and training modeled by the private health care and business sectors.

There are many good examples of early technology adopters. **Vital statistics** programs have implemented electronic birth certificate systems, and electronic death certificate systems are now following. Not only does this facilitate the assessment function of public health, but it also enables public health agencies at the state and local levels to provide certificates to citizens faster and in more convenient locations. Immunization information systems are another example of the use of technology to improve data collection and analysis. In addition to enhancing reporting activities, information systems can provide an important decision support tool for public and private health care providers to deliver services in a more timely and appropriate way.

Creating **interoperability** among public health data systems is a current challenge. Many states are developing integrated systems for managing child health services as well as communicable disease surveillance and outbreak management. The Environmental and Public Health Tracking System program, discussed in the next section, is another good example of the use of technology to collect, integrate, and analyze disparate sources of data.[14] This program provides SHAs and others interested in environmental health new information for assessing environmental impacts on health.

Over the next decade, SHAs will be expected to assume greater leadership roles in the creation of longitudinal or "life time" electronic medical records through communitywide administrative and clinical data sharing networks. As part of the effort to create a nationwide **health information exchange** system, SHA leaders will be called on to facilitate these advances both inside their agencies and among community partners throughout their states even when these activities push and threaten the current way of doing business. The contributions to improving quality of care, patient safety, and access to services must be demonstrated to outweigh costs and challenges. In addition to securing resources, technical knowledge and skilled staff, creation and adoption of vocabularies and standards are required for efficient data exchange and effective decision support tools. Policies and laws as well as ethical concerns to address appropriate data sharing, assuring protection of privacy and confidentiality, security and integrity of data, and rules for advancing interoperability must be tackled while not creating new road blocks for desirable exchanges. Public health programs will need to understand how the data they collect could be considered "clinical data" and therefore part of the information to be exchanged. Public health systems must be configured to both send and receive data from health care agencies, including hospitals, emergency departments, clinics, pharmacies, laboratories, home health and long-term care facilities, in addition to traditional national and local data exchange partners. SHAs will benefit from ongoing efforts to support public health informatics. Both training in public health informatics and continued investment in health information systems are needed to meet the challenges of evolving computer technology and changing health information needs.

Environmental Public Health Tracking Network

The 2000 Pew Environmental Health Commission report, *America's Environmental Health Gap*,[15] identified an increasing influence of the environment and environmental contaminates on public health. This influence was evidenced by the sharp increase in numbers of noninfectious illnesses and deaths associated with environmental factors during the previous 20 years. For example, Americans reporting asthma in 1995 was 75 percent higher than the rate in 1980. Americans are increasingly aware and concerned about the impact the environment has on their health. These and other considerations led to federal funding for a national Environmental Public Health Tracking Network (EPHTN).

The EPHTN aims to provide public health officials, researchers, and others ready access to data related to environmental hazards, monitoring, exposure, and health effects to facilitate better understanding of the interactions between the environment and health. To accomplish that aim, the Centers for Disease Control and Prevention (CDC), working with selected federal, state, local, academic, and professional partners, decided to construct an environmental network. This network was to provide data in a standardized and linkable format, along with some innovative analytical tools and expertise to assist users in understanding the environmental and public health interactions. CDC and partners are in the first year of a five-year implementation phase to develop the data, tools, and expertise for the network.[16]

Construction of the network has met some unique challenges. Data identified for inclusion in the network were often collected for regulatory or other purposes. For example, the hospital discharge databases being used as a source for asthma data was collected to monitor patient safety and other quality of care measures. Information such as the address and identity of patients, although not as important in quality of care assessment, is very important for epidemiological studies of environmental exposure and risk. In addition, environmental data are collected primarily for enforcement purposes, not to determine exposure levels. Hence, the location of monitoring tends to focus on enforcement problems and not on potentially exposed populations. Through the implementation of EPHTN, federal, state, and local public health and environmental quality agencies have worked closely with each other to ensure both perspectives accurately understand the data, and mutually useful methods are being developed to link health and environmental data.[17] Through an iterative process, the EPHTN is anticipated to grow both in content and in national coverage. The first phase of the project became available for public use in September 2008, with additions and enhancements expected to occur each year through the five-year implementation cycle.

Health Protection

Citizens' concern with the general cleanliness of the environment has expanded, requiring state oversight of public drinking water, ambient air, food service facilities, sewage systems, and sources of radiation. SHAs have also been asked to regulate the medical care delivery system. Initially, this was to ensure the hygiene, proper staffing, and safety of health facilities. However, anxiety over the increasing costs of health care led policy makers to give SHAs responsibility for regulating facility charges, bed capacity, service enhancement, and gathering data on health care costs. For more information, see the reference on State Health Planning and Development Agencies.[18] More recently, SHAs have been assigned responsibility for monitoring the availability and quality of medical care provided to the population.

Access to Care and Patient Safety

To improve access to care, health departments recruit physicians for medically underserved areas and provide scholarships and loans for medical and nursing students.[19] Thus, SHAs have been charged with protecting not only the health status of communities but also the public's access to quality medical care. More recently, studies have identified medical error as a major cause of death and disability.[20] SHAs are beginning to lead efforts to guard patient safety in hospital settings, including encouraging adoption of best practices and system modifications to reduce the probability of errors during medical procedures and in prescribing practices.

Specific examples of patient safety activities at the state level range from a fully funded nonprofit agency for conducting patient safety analysis and improvement managed outside the SHA to incremental activities funded with existing SHA budgets. The state of Pennsylvania has a Patient Safety Authority and patient safety reporting system.[21] The program is funded by a bed tax that generates approximately $5 million a year used to support this separate nonprofit agency. It is charged with analyzing patient safety events and developing statewide interventions. This program analyzed 196,000 reports of adverse events or near misses in 2006. Oregon has established an Oregon Patient Safety Commission as a standalone organization.[22] Minnesota, Massachusetts, and Vermont have incorporated patient safety activities into other existing state governmental agencies.[23] The Utah Department of Health has funded a half-time position for patient safety located in the Division of Health Systems Improvement.[24] The focus of Utah's program is to apply a public health surveillance perspective in conjunction with an ongoing community-based steering committee and industry-based users group.

ORGANIZATION OF STATE HEALTH DEPARTMENTS

In the United States, there are 57 SHAs (1 in each of the 50 states, the District of Columbia, American Samoa, Guam, Puerto Rico, the Federated States of Micronesia, Northern Mariana Islands, and the U.S.

Virgin Islands), each of which may be a freestanding, independent department or a component of a larger state agency.

Super-agencies and Umbrella Agencies

Beginning in the 1960s, SHAs were merged with other departments, usually social services or welfare departments, to form super-agencies, or they were placed under a cabinet secretary in an umbrella agency, following the pattern of the federal Department of Health and Human Services (HHS). The main difference between these two types of consolidation is that a SHA usually retains more autonomy under the umbrella arrangement.

In 1952, only Maine and Missouri had state public health functions in an umbrella or super-agency. By 1969, there were 8 states with such arrangements; by 1972, there were 16 states; and by 1980, 22 states.[25,26] SHAs in 20 states plus the District of Columbia were part of such agencies in 2000, indicating that some states had reversed this consolidation.[27] The continuing trend to restructure or consider restructuring is an ongoing issue. The National Governors Association (NGA) studied this trend in 1996 and again in 2004. Figure 9.3 shows

the results of the 2003 study as reported in their 2004 report.[28] In these studies, the NGA also defined four categories for SHAs. The definitions for these are provided in Table 9.4 and shown graphically in Figure 9.4. The results of the survey are shown in Figure 9.5. In its 2005 survey, ASTHO reported that 26 of the 50 state agencies were "freestanding," whereas 24 are a part of an umbrella agency of some kind.[12]

The stated purpose of bringing together several separate departments under one roof was to increase coordination between programs serving the same population groups and to provide more political control over policy decisions. These super-agencies most often bring together health and social services for the aged, children and adolescents, families, the developmentally disabled, those needing income assistance, and those with substance abuse

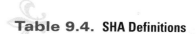

Table 9.4. SHA Definitions

Traditional public health agency: A type of state health agency that oversees public health and primary care only. Although it may also administer one other health-related program (i.e., environmental health, alcohol and drug abuse, etc.), its responsibilities are usually limited to improving or protecting the overall health status of the public.

Super public health agency: A type of state health agency that oversees both (a) public health and primary care and (b) substance abuse and mental health. This would likely include administering services supported by the federal Substance Abuse Prevention and Treatment (SAPT), Block Grant and the Community Mental Health Services (CMHS), and block grant programs.

Super health agency: A type of state health agency that oversees (a) public health and primary care and (b) the state Medicaid program.

Umbrella agency: A type of state health agency oversees (a) public health and primary care, (b) substance abuse and mental health, and (c) the Medicaid program, as well as (d) other human services programs.

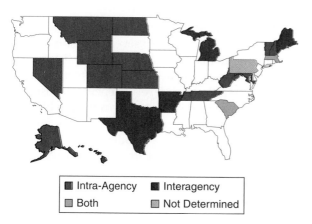

Figure 9.3. State Health Agency Restructuring Initiatives, January 1–December 31, 2003

SOURCE: National Governors Association, *Transforming State Health Agencies to Meet Current and Future Challenges*, 2003.

SOURCE: National Governors Association (NGA), *Transforming State Health Agencies to Meet Current and Future Needs*.

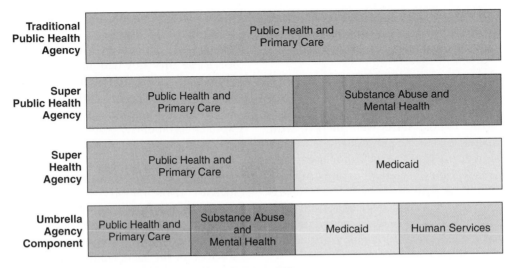

Figure 9.4. Common State Health Agency Organizational Structures

SOURCE: National Governors Association, *Transforming State Health Agencies to Meet Current and Future Challenges*, 1996.

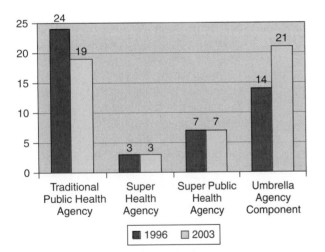

Figure 9.5. Comparison of State Health Agency Structures, January 1, 1996 and January 1, 2003

SOURCE: National Governors Association, *Transforming State Health Agencies to Meet Current and Future Challenges*, 1996 and 2003.

problems. The director or secretary of such an agency is usually a political appointee, frequently with little or no health expertise.

Public Health Opposition

Public health leaders have generally opposed mergers to super-agencies for several reasons. Super-agencies and umbrella agencies may be seen as more efficient and better at creating focused policy agendas, but cabinet-level agencies focused on health may be more responsive to the health needs of the state. Super-agencies tend to focus more on services for the poor or families with problems, rather than on protecting or improving the health of the total population. Unless service delivery at the local level has also been merged or co-located, there may be little benefit to patients from such mergers of agencies at the state level. One of the main reasons for the separation was the perception that the SHA had difficulty obtaining funds from the legislature because the welfare services represented such a large portion of the budget.

IOM Committee Recommendations

The 1988 IOM Committee recommended that each state have a department of health that groups all primarily health-related functions under professional direction and separate from income maintenance (welfare) functions of state government.[1]

Name of the SHA

If it is an independent entity, part of an umbrella agency, or a secretariat, the SHA is often titled the Department of Health, Department of Public Health, or Department of Health Services. If combined with another agency, the public health unit is usually called a Division of Health or Public Health.

When public health functions have been combined with environmental functions, health is more likely to appear in the agency title, for example, Department of Health and Environment, than when public health is combined with social services agencies. The latter type agencies are frequently named the Department of Human Resources or Human Services, supporting the assertion that public health's visibility is lost when such mergers occur.

State Boards of Health

In the late 1800s, state governments created boards of health even before state departments of health to make rules to prevent the spread of diseases and improve general sanitary conditions in the states. As these boards hired employees to enforce the rules, departments of health were organized. In 1972, all but four states had a state board of health in some form.[29] In its 2005 survey, ASTHO reported that 23 of the 50 states have a board of health in some form. This shift has accompanied the continued trend to politicize public health organizations, moving from citizen oversight of boards to oversight by the governor or appointee.

Role of Boards of Health

In 1972, 37 (80 percent) of the 46 boards were policy making, that is, responsible for making, adopting, promulgating, and enforcing rules and

regulations pursuant to state health codes. The remaining 9 boards were advisory only and usually located in states where public health functions had been consolidated into a **super-agency** or an **umbrella agency.**

From 1971 to present, major changes continued to take place in SHAs. By 2000, only 21 states had boards still making policy, and 14 others just had advisory boards or committees at the department level. Whereas 80 percent of states with freestanding departments of health retained a board of health, only half of the states in which public health was located in a super-agency or an umbrella agency had a board. From 1972 to the 2005 survey, the number of boards of health responsible for hiring the state health director also decreased to 4.[5]

The executive branches of state governments assumed the functions previously assigned to boards of health, with policy decisions being made by political appointees instead of citizens' groups. As governors seek more control over health policy, they want the authority to select health directors who will carry out political platforms.

Specialized Boards and Committees

Replacing or supplementing the board of health in many states are specialized boards or committees established by state statute or rule to oversee particular programs. Many of these boards are technical, bringing to the SHA particular expertise not found in the staff, for example, in genetics or rural health. Other special boards are established to make decisions on a particular function in the SHA, such as rules regarding the practice of emergency medical technicians, licensure of hearing aid dispensers, or expansion of health facilities. Special interest groups have lobbied state legislatures to establish these committees, establishing defined memberships representing the regulated community and the public, in preference to having policies made by a board of health or the state health director.

IOM Committee Recommendation

The 1988 IOM Committee recommended that each state have a health council that reports regularly on the health of the state's residents, makes health policy recommendations to the governor and legislature, promulgates public health regulations, reviews the work of the state health agency, and recommends candidates for director of the department. The committee proposed that the purpose of the council should not be the control of health matters by health professionals but the making of policy judgments on public health by lay citizens.[1] In reality, however, most states appear headed in a different direction, with less power given to such a representative group and more control residing in the elected and appointed officials of the executive branch of state government.

State Health Directors

The title of the chief executive of the SHA is usually director or commissioner; in a few states, the position is called state health officer or secretary. A more important factor is not the title but who makes the appointment. Whether the director of the department is appointed by the governor, a board, or the head of an umbrella agency or super-agency is a critical factor in determining the health director's level of authority, access to state policy makers, and participation in health policy decisions.

The 2005 ASTHO survey found that the director of the SHA is appointed by the governor to a cabinet-level position in 26 states, by the head of a super-agency in 20 states, and by the state board of health in 4 states.[12] Where there is direct access to the governor, the health director has a greater opportunity to influence health policy in both the executive and legislative branches.

Qualifications of State Health Directors

Traditionally, a physician held the position of state health officer, with medical requirements being part of state law. At first, most of these physicians had no training in public health. As schools of public health were created, however, physicians who were trained specifically for positions in public health administration directed most SHAs. In 1977, all but 6 states had physician health directors.[30] Twenty-three of the 44 physicians were specialists in public health and preventive medicine, and 30 had a public health degree. In the 2005 survey, ASTHO reported that statutes in 21 states required the health officer to be a physician while 8 required either a Master of Public Health (MPH) or experience in public health. One other state required either a medical degree or another doctoral degree. The report also pointed out that 15 states had no statutory requirements for the qualifications of the health officer. The remaining 14 states required either public health experience or some other unreported requirement. Figure 9.6 demonstrates the wide variation in the qualifications of the state health officials at the time of the survey.

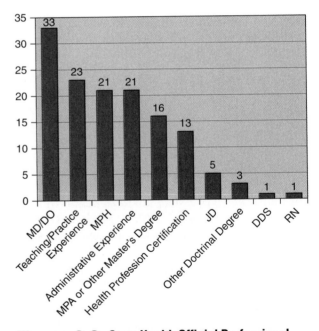

Figure 9.6. State Health Official Professional Education

SOURCE: Courtesy of the Association of State and Territorial Health Officials.

Tenure of State Health Directors

Increased turnover in state health directors and changes in required qualifications have occurred as the positions have become more political. In the first half of this century, many state health officers served from 20 to 35 years. They were respected leaders in health affairs in their communities and also were frequently leaders in state medical societies. For example, the terms of the first two state health officers in Virginia covered a total period of 48 years, from 1908 to 1956.

By contrast, the tenure of state health directors has decreased markedly in the past 20 years. In 1997, the average tenure for former state health officials from all 50 states was 4 years.[31] Of the 57 health officials in states and territories in 1989, only 3 remained in those same positions 10 years later.[32] State health directors appointed by boards of health generally had longer tenure in office than those appointed by governors because new governors often want to appoint new department heads who will carry out their policies and initiatives. Thus the largest number of changes in state health officials occurs in election years. According to ASTHO, in 2007, the average tenure of a state health official is now 40 months.[33]

IOM Committee Recommendations

The 1988 IOM Committee recommended that the director of each department of health be a cabinet-level officer, with doctorate-level education as a physician or other health professional, education in public health, and extensive public sector administrative experience.[1] Provisions for tenure in office, such as specific terms of appointment, should be enacted, the committee said, to promote needed continuity of professional leadership. In recent years, only four states have had specific terms of appointment for their state health directors.

The Need for Flexibility

Evolving health needs require flexible organizations. Very little of the SHA structure should be codified in statutes. This increases the SHA's capability to respond to new issues and needs, such as knowledge concerning genetic diseases or changing problems and evolving technology affecting injury prevention. Ideally, the state health director can restructure the agency and adjust resources to address emerging problems.

Staffing

The numbers and kinds of staff needed at the state level depends on many factors. These include the responsibilities assigned to the SHA; distances between population centers; types and numbers of health care facilities to be regulated; density and economic status of populations served; degree of responsibility for direct delivery of services; and the number, size, autonomy, and sophistication of local health departments. Community values and goals can also affect SHA programs and staffing needs.

Public Health Workforce

Identifying staffing requirements and assessing the adequacy of skills of the public health workforce is problematic because of the significant differences in states, research assumptions, and data collection methods of the different organizations that have undertaken the task of **enumeration.** In 1980 and 2000, HRSA enumeration efforts estimated that the number of federal, state, and local public health professionals increased by about 120,000 over the 20-year period.[34] A 2005 HRSA survey of selected states demonstrated the wide range of variability between states in the makeup and diversity of workforce between state and local health agencies as shown in Figures 9.7 and 9.8.[35] Data from the United States Bureau of Census supports the conclusion that the numbers continued to increase through 2006. Although there was an apparent decrease in state staffing in 2004 and in local staffing in 2005, the estimated number of employees at both levels continues to increase.[36] Even though the numbers increase, there is great concern with the number of experienced and trained public

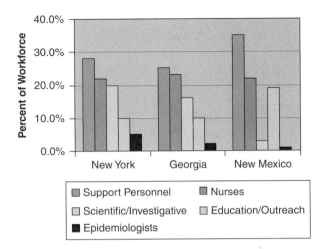

Figure 9.7. Public Health Workforce in New York, Georgia, and New Mexico by Classification

SOURCE: Public Health Workforce Study January 2005 Health Resources and Services Administration http://bhpr.hrsa.gov/healthworkforce/reports/publichealth/default.htm.

health professionals as expressed in a report issued by ASTHO and the Council of State Governments in 2004.[37] The following are key findings from the survey on which the report is based:

- Public health faces a rapidly aging workforce whose average age is 46.6 years.
- Public health will see retirement rates as high as 45 percent over the next five years.
- Current vacancy rates are already up to 20 percent in some states.
- Public health employment turnover rates have reached 14 percent in some parts of the country.

Clearly there are challenges ahead if we hope to maintain an adequate workforce to staff our nation's SHAs.

FUNDING

As with staffing patterns, the expenditures of SHAs are difficult to compare across the nation because the responsibilities of these departments vary so widely. For almost 20 years, the Public Health Foundation collected data on public health expenditures by categorical program. In 1991 (the last year for which data are available), SHAs spent $11.2 billion on public health programs. Three-quarters of these expenditures were for personal

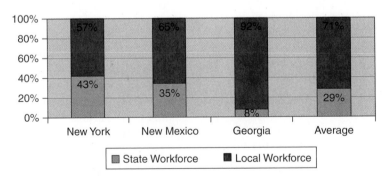

Figure 9.8. State and Local Public Health Workforce in New York, New Mexico, Georgia, and an Average of the Three States

SOURCE: Public Health Workforce Study January 2005 Health Resources and Services Administration http://bhpr.hrsa.gov/healthworkforce/reports/publichealth/default.htm.

health services, including $1.5 billion for the operation of institutions.[38] Most of these personal health funds were used at the local level, either through local health departments, subunits of the SHA, or contracts with other service providers.

In the 1990s, the focus of data collection changed from categorical program expenditures, such as dollars for tuberculosis control, to funds spent on the 10 essential public health services. The Public Health Foundation surveyed 9 states as a sample of nationwide expenditures. These states reported spending $8.8 billion on the essential public health services in 1995.[39] Expenditures were not limited to SHAs but also included local public health and state substance abuse, mental health, and environmental agencies. Sixty-nine percent of the funds were spent on personal health services such as direct care services provided to individuals (under category 7b of the 10 essential services).[40] The remaining 31 percent of expenditures were for population-based services, which are those interventions directed to the entire population. The population-based services averaged $42 per capita across the nine states. Table 9.5 shows which governmental agencies spent the money.

These data emphasize that public health activities are carried out by a variety of state and local agencies, not just state health departments; however, the survey report also concluded that obtaining comparable data across all states for such expenditures would be very difficult.

Sources of Funds

In 1990 (the last year of data specific to all states), SHAs received 50 percent of their funding from state legislatures, 37 percent from federal grants and contracts, 7 percent from fees and third-party reimbursements (excluding Medicaid), 3 percent from local sources, and 3 percent from other sources, such as grants from private foundations. The single largest source of federal funds was the United States Department of Agriculture, which oversees the Supplemental Food Program for Women, Infants, and Children (WIC program). This program accounted for 20 percent of all funds spent by SHAs, with 40 percent of these funds used for vouchers for the direct purchase of food. The CDC and the HRSA were the other major sources of federal funds used by SHAs. Beginning in the late 1980s, the expansion of Medicaid to cover more pregnant women and children provided an additional source of funding for services to these population groups. Figure 9.9 shows the funding sources for Washington state and local public health agencies in 2004.

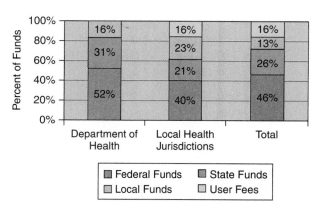

Figure 9.9. Source of Public Health Funding in Washington State, Washington Local Health Jurisdiction, and the Total

SOURCE: Public Health Financing Trends, Presentation to the Joint Select Committee on Public Health Finance, Legislative Fiscal Committee Staff, 2005 http://www.leg.wa.gov/NR/rdonlyres/23EB8885-0B43-4143-8F64-C47AAEAA8CBC/22981/PHFinancingTrends999991.pdf.

Table 9.5. Distribution of Spending for Population-Based Services

Agency	Percent
State health agencies	44%
State environmental agencies	23%
Local health departments	20%
State substance abuse and mental health agencies	13%

SOURCE: Data from Eilbert et al., *J Public Health Manage Prac.* 1997;3(3):1–9.

Categorical and Block Grants

Federal funds come to states both as categorical grants, which focus on a particular health problem or population group, and as block grants, which have a broader public health focus. In general, categorical grant programs are controlled by extensive federal regulations and lengthy reporting requirements. They may lack flexibility to meet variations in state needs.

Block grants were created in the early 1980s to achieve greater flexibility in the use of funds, meaning more efficient use of tax dollars and more cost-effective service to recipients. Initially, the block grants specified no priorities, objectives, or required outcomes. Decisions on how to use the funds were left entirely to state legislatures and governors, who frequently used the grants to fund programs the state was unwilling or unable to support with state revenues. States favored block grants because they provided more opportunities to meet state priorities or fill gaps in state funding. Twenty-one previously separate programs were consolidated into block grant areas. Left as categorical programs were childhood immunization, tuberculosis control, family planning, migrant health centers, and sexually transmitted disease control. The maternal and child health and prevention block grants continue to be major sources of financial support for all SHAs.

Title V—Maternal and Child Health Services Block Grant

The Maternal and Child Health Services Block Grant had its origins in the enactment of the Social Security Act of 1935. It has had 7 major revisions since its inception with the last being the creation of the Maternal and Child Health Bureau and significant amendments made to Title V in 1989. Title V pledged its support of state efforts to extend health and welfare services for mothers and children. Over 70 yeas later, it remains the longest lasting federally funded public health program. In its current form, this block grant suffers from the same problem of continually reduced funding that all block grants are experiencing. Figure 9.10 demonstrates the impact of funding changes to the MCH program by comparing the appropriated fund level with the impact that inflation has had on the ability of states to operate the program.

Prevention Block Grant

The Prevention Block Grant[41] is used by SHAs to support chronic disease prevention, health education and risk reduction, emergency medical services, laboratory testing for communicable diseases and environmental toxins, rodent control, dental health, and a variety of other services. Since its inception, this grant has provided the most flexibility of all funding sources used by SHAs. However, the multiplicity of uses of these grant dollars state by state made it hard for Congress to track exactly which services were being funded with the Prevention Block Grant. As a result, Congress failed to increase funding for this grant at the same rate it did for categorical grants.

In 1992, Congress modified the Prevention Grant, linking it to the National Health Objectives for the year 2000. Beginning in 1993, all expenditures from the grant had to be directed toward specific national objectives, as selected by each state. A state-level advisory group was required to hold public hearings on proposed uses of the grant funds. In turn, the federal government required more accountability from states in the use of these funds and removed these decisions from the legislative process. Over the past few years, there has been a concerted effort by the national executive branch to eliminate this fund source. However, with significant effort by state and local public health leaders and other partners concerned about the public's health, Congress, while reducing the funding each year, has consistently replaced these funds as shown in Figure 9.11. As part of the effort to justify these necessary funds to the administration and Congress, ASTHO has documented many different successes in a compendium of illustrative examples of the impact of the innovative uses to which states have applied block grant funding.[42]

Newer Sources of Funds

State and federal funding for communicable disease control programs increased markedly during

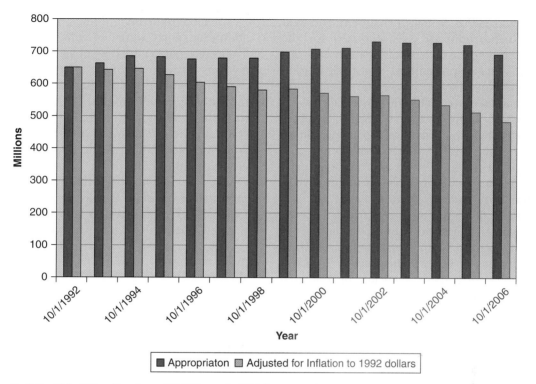

Figure 9.10. Title V Funding from 1992 Through 2006 Compared to the Purchasing Power (Adjusted for Inflation)

SOURCE: Data from MCH Bureau Monograph *Understanding Title V of the Social Security Act* available on the MCH Bureau Web site ftp://ftp.hrsa.gov//mchb/titlevtoday/UnderstandingTitleV.pdf and from Department of Labor Bureau of Statistics *Consumer Price Index for all Urban Consumers and all Items* at ftp://ftp.bls.gov/pub/special.requests/cpi/cpiai.txt.

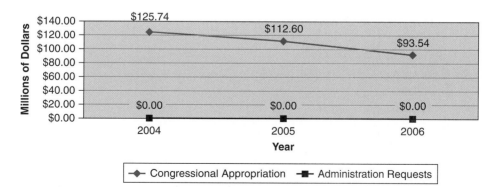

Figure 9.11. Preventive Health and Health Services Block Grant Congressional Funding 2004 Through 2006 Compared to the President's Request

SOURCE: Association of State and Territorial Health Officials Preventive Block funding history 2006.

the 1980s and 1990s, primarily to prevent and treat HIV/AIDS. Expenditures also increased for the control of tuberculosis, sexually transmitted diseases, and vaccine-preventable diseases. During this period, expenditures on chronic disease programs remained stable. This disparity reflects the willingness of appropriating bodies to allocate money to prevent diseases that spread person-to-person, but their relative lack of interest in reducing diseases influenced by lifestyle and behavior, even though the latter are responsible for more morbidity and mortality in the population.

In response to perceived threats from bioterrorism and emerging infectious diseases, the federal government invested funds, beginning in 1999, to improve the public health infrastructure in states aimed at preparing these agencies for potential bioterrorism. Through cooperative agreements with CDC, states received funds to develop better information and communication systems, improve employee skills in surveillance and epidemiology, enhance laboratory capacity for chemical and biological agents, and increase the organizational capacity for response. In reaction to the attack on the World Trade Center on September 11, 2001, funding for preparedness to state and local jurisdictions increased significantly in 2002 and 2003 and has remained relatively stable as shown in Figure 9.12.

Tobacco settlement dollars have provided an additional new source of funding for SHAs. In 1998, 46 states and the tobacco industry settled lawsuits for recovery of the tobacco-related disease costs in Medicaid recipients. State legislatures had the authority to allocate the settlement funds given to each state. By 2000, 15 states had made substantial commitments and others had made lesser commitments to fund tobacco use prevention and cessation programs with these dollars.[43] The tobacco settlement dollars have also been used to fund general public health programs, Medicaid expansion, health research, and a wide variety of nonhealth-related programs in the states.

ACCOUNTABILITY IN THE FORM OF PERFORMANCE STANDARDS

Most SHAs have joined a nationwide effort to focus on performance accountability for the functions assigned or expected of such agencies. In partnership, CDC and the ASTHO have developed a set of performance standards for public health practice in

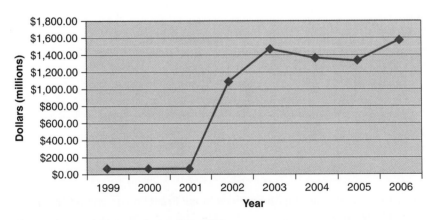

Figure 9.12. Bioterrorism Funding by Year: 1999–2006

SOURCE: Association of State and Territorial Health Officials BT funding history 2006.

SHAs.[44] The standards are organized around the 10 essential public health services. States will collect and analyze data on their achievement of these standards, using a comprehensive performance assessment instrument. The overall goal is to improve the quality and increase the scientific base for public health. In 2006, ASTHO surveyed the states to determine what impact if any the performance standards have had. The survey examined current performance measurement efforts in 40 states.[45] It was designed to contribute to a better understanding of the building blocks of performance improvement in state public health agencies and systems. The survey results also serve to inform efforts to explore the latest push for accountability—public health agency accreditation. Almost 70 percent of respondents (28 of 40) reported performance standards use beyond program and grant requirements. The new direction of the movement for accountability is to have both state and local public health agencies participate in voluntary accreditation. In a 2004 report funded by CDC and the Robert Wood Johnson Foundation, ASTHO and the National Association of County and City Health Officials (NACCHO) agreed to study the feasibility of national accreditation at the state and local level. Although very controversial, both organizations agreed that some form of an accreditation program is feasible.[46] Both organizations are now studying the logistics of developing a national accrediting body.

STATE HEALTH AGENCY RELATIONSHIPS

When President Ronald Reagan moved to distribute funding to the states through block grants instead of categorical grants, he indicated that the strength of the federal government was in collecting and distributing money. It is also true that the federal government is best able to shape public health policy through its ability to direct funds. The Constitution gives legal authority for public health to the states. Local government ends up with most of the responsibility for protecting the health of the people. To protect the health of citizens, SHAs must have a mechanism for delivering services to people where they live and work. The relationship between state and local health departments reflects the geography, politics, and funding patterns of each state.

State/Local Organizational Relationships

A 1998 research brief produced by NACCHO examined this issue and identified four key public health delivery methods at the local level:

- **Centralized:** The local health department is operated by the SHA or board of health, and the local health department functions directly under the state agency's authority.

- **Decentralized:** Local governments have direct authority over local health departments, with or without a board of health.

- **Shared Authority:** The local health department operates under the shared authority of the SHA, local government, and the board of health.

- **Mixed Authority:** Services are provided by a combination of the state agency, local government, boards of health, or health departments in other jurisdictions.[47]

A 2005 ASTHO survey found that although this distribution of "delivery methods"—the number of states in each of these categories—was relatively stable with one state changing from centralized to shared, the actual public health services delivered at the local level continue to vary by state.

Figure 9.13 shows the distribution of these delivery methods among the 50 states.

Whatever the state-local organizational relationship, SHAs are responsible for establishing standards for local public health functions and holding local agencies accountable to those standards. States may develop requirements for specific services to be offered locally, data to be collected and reported, and minimum staffing requirements to be met. Services inappropriate for smaller units, such as the provision of reference laboratories, or for which there must be statewide consistency, such as

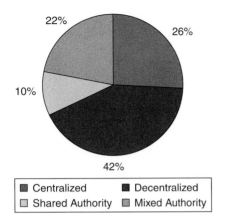

22%
26%
10%
42%

- ■ Centralized　■ Decentralized
- □ Shared Authority　■ Mixed Authority

Figure 9.13. Types of Organizational Structures in Local Public Health Services
SOURCE: Courtesy of the Association of State and Territorial Health Officials.

often sat on boards of health and served as state health officers. As SHAs have become increasingly involved in the direct delivery of care to persons who cannot afford care in the private sector, however, the relationship between the SHA and the state medical society has deteriorated in some states. Whereas earlier physician health officers were invited to participate in medical society meetings, today's nonphysician health officers are viewed with suspicion by the medical community, and they often do not have the same access to medical colleagues that their physician predecessors did. Nonphysician administrators are also frequently criticized for not seeking medical advice or not informing the medical society of their plans.

SHAs need the support of the medical profession to help pass key legislation through state legislatures and to provide medical expertise on many public health issues. Strengthening their relationship with state medical organizations is therefore an important challenge for today's SHAs.

the inspection of health care facilities, are usually organized at the state level. A SHA has the additional responsibility of representing the needs of local health units with other state agencies, within both executive and legislative branches of government. In developing policy and allocating resources, state and local public health officials must communicate and collaborate.[48] Although state-local relationships have often been viewed as a "we/they" situation, state and local public health leaders are working as collaborative partners to foster the view that state and local health agencies are considered part of a total public health system that requires cooperation to succeed. Calling for responsible and responsive state-local public health agencies, Hugh Tilson and Bobbie Berkowitz, point out the imperative for all public health partners to work together to create a competent, all-hazards prepared, highly functioning system that is not in disarray.[49]

Medical Professions

In the early years of this century, the medical profession was strongly supportive of the creation of SHAs, and members of the medical community

SUMMARY

Although SHAs retain ultimate responsibility for protecting the health of their citizens, their roles, significance, and visibility are frequently overlooked. More attention is focused on national and local health agencies. The federal government supplies the majority of government funds for health services through the Medicaid and **Medicare** programs and through categorical and block grants. Local health departments are where citizens generally seek public health services. The SHA may be viewed as just a "pass-through" agency, passing funds and regulations from the federal and state to the local level, but not contributing significantly to the planning, development, and implementation of health services. To obtain or maintain the legal authority and fiscal resources necessary to carry out its mission, a SHA must work with the governor and the state legislature. As noted earlier, the nature of this relationship depends on where health functions are located in the executive branch and how accessible policy makers are to the state health director. The IOM Committee found that many SHAs did not have the influence necessary to acquire needed resources. Without strong state boards of health or other public health advocacy groups such as state public health associations,[50] SHAs frequently have been left powerless and impoverished in the competition over state assets.

The roles and functions of SHAs will continue to evolve as they have in the past. The public depends on state agencies to identify new and emerging threats to their health, and increasingly, needs protection from new causes of morbidity and mortality, such as violence, drugs, emerging infectious diseases, and toxic substances in the environment. At the same time, the need to attend to old challenges, including health disparities among ethnic groups such as excess infant mortality, remain a SHA responsibility as well. The public also expects regulation over health facilities and services to assure effective treatment and protect patient safety. SHAs of tomorrow will be required to meet these expectations with new policies and innovative and cost-effective approaches.

REVIEW QUESTIONS

1. Why is it important to have certain public health functions managed within the jurisdiction of the SHA while others can be effectively managed by other state, local, or nongovernmental agencies? What is the ideal composition of a state health department?

2. What activities are most important for identifying emerging public health concerns? What kind of staff and what qualifications and skills are required to do this effectively?

3. Is it better for the director of the SHA to advance the health policy agenda of the governor, or should the health director be creating the health policy agenda and recommend it to the governor and the state legislature?

4. What are some of the challenging issues related to creating a coordinated and collaborative public health system at the local, state, and national levels? What is a state health director's role in helping create this system?

5. What are the primary sources of funding for state-level public health services? How should these funds be allocated among competing programs? What processes should be used by SHA directors and other community leaders to assure these decisions are fair and responsive to individual state's needs?

6. Historically, what criteria have been used for the selection of SHA directors? What should be considered as the most important qualifications, skills, knowledge, and experience that a SHA director should posses? Why are these important?

7. What role does ASTHO play in supporting SHAs and helping create the public health policy agendas for individual states?

8. At an operational level, what state-level activities support the performance of the three core functions of public health: assessment, policy development, and assurance? How might the changes in organizational structure of SHAs impact resources and agency effectiveness at meeting their responsibilities to perform these three core functions?

9. How can the effectiveness of SHAs be evaluated? What tools and programs are in place to assist in this kind of evaluation? What are the benefits and challenges associated with each?

10. What role should SHAs have in assuring access to quality health services?

11. How can administrative data and clinical data be used to help improve quality of care? How are SHAs currently involved in collecting, analyzing, and disseminating these data? What should they be doing to participate in exchanges of clinical data among health care service providers?

REFERENCES

1. Institute of Medicine, Committee for the Study of the Future of Public Health. The Future of Public Health. Washington, DC: National Academy Press; 1988. Available at: http://books.nap.edu/catalog.php?record_id=1091#toc. Accessed June 1, 2007.

2. Association of State and Territorial Health Officials. By-laws. Washington, DC. Available at: http://www.astho.org/pubs/ASTHOConstitutionandBylaws.pdf. Accessed June 1, 2007.

3. See State Public Health.org. Available at: http://www.statepublichealth.org/index.php?template=sho.php&PHPSESSID=4c5a528094ddab68ce0e6c5732f6325e. Accessed June 1, 2007.

4. Association of State and Territorial Health Officials. Summary of the Organization of Public Health Services within the States and Territories of the United States; 2003. Available at: http://www.astho.org/templates/display_pub.php?u=JnB1Yl9pZD05OTTc=. Accessed June 1, 2007.

5. *Healthy People 2010: Understanding and Improving Health.* 2nd ed. Washington, DC: US Department of Health and Human Services; 2000. US Government Publication No. 017-001-00550-9. Available at: http://www.healthypeople.gov/. Accessed June 1, 2007.

6. Institute of Medicine. *The Future of Public Health in the 21st Century.* Washington, DC: National Academies Press; 2003. Available at: http://www.nap.edu/catalog/10548.html#toc. Accessed June 1, 2007.

7. Public Health Functions Steering Committee Report, *Public Health In America.* Washington, DC; 1994. Available at: http://www.health.gov/phfunctions/public.htm. Accessed June 1, 2007.

8. These seven agencies are: the American Public Health Association (APHA), the Association of State and Territorial Health Officials (ASTHO), the Centers for Disease Control and Prevention (CDC), the National Association of County and City Health Officials (NACCHO), the National Association of Local Boards of Health (NALBOH), the National Network of Public Health Institutes (NNPHI), and the Public Health Foundation (PHF).

9. Centers for Disease Control. National Public Health Performance Standards Program. Atlanta, GA. Available at: http://www.cdc.gov/od/ocphp/nphpsp/. Accessed June 1, 2007.

10. Council on Linkages between Academia and Public Health Practice. Core competencies for public health professionals. April 11, 2001. Available at: http://www.trainingfinder.org/competencies. Accessed June 1, 2007.

11. Measuring Health Objectives and Indicators: 1997 State and Local Capacity Survey. Washington, DC: Public Health Foundation; 1998.

12. Association of State and Territorial Health Official Report: 2005 SHO Salary And Agency Infrastructure Survey. Washington, DC; 2006. Available at: http://www.astho.org/pubs/2005SalarySurveyFinal.pdf. Accessed June 1, 2007.

13. Association of State and Territorial Health Officials Issue Brief: State Efforts to Prevent Youth Suicide. Washington, DC; 2004. Available at: http://www.astho.org/pubs/Suicide—Litts.ppt#385,25,High-risk Approach. Accessed October 14, 2008.

14. Centers for Disease Control and Prevention National Environmental Public Health Tracking Program. Available at: http://www.cdc.gov/nceh/tracking/network.htm. Accessed September 10, 2007.

15. Pew Charitable Trusts. America's environmental health gap: Why the country needs a nationwide health tracking network. Baltimore, MD.; 2000. Available at: http://healthyamericans.org/reports/files/healthgap.pdf. Accessed June 1, 2007.

16. Centers for Disease Control. Environmental public health indicators. Atlanta, GA; 2004. Available at: http://www.cdc.gov/nceh/indicators/. Accessed June 1, 2007.

17. National Association of County and City Health Officials. Local public health perspectives on environmental public health tracking. Washington, DC; 2005 Available at: http://www.complianceconsortium.org/Events/MEI_Forum_June_05_Chicago/ChukMEI05.ppt. Accessed June 1, 2007.

18. A good example of the history of State Health Planning and Development Agencies (SHPDA) can be seen on the Alabama website. Available at: http://shpda.state.al.us. Accessed October 14, 2008.

19. For example, see California's Health Profession Education Foundation website. Available at: http://www.healthprofessions.ca.gov/progfacts.htm.

Accessed June 6, 2007. Information on the national Health Resources and Services Administration (HRSA) program can be seen at http://nhsc.bhpr.hrsa.gov/jobs/. Accessed June 6, 2007.

20. For example, see the Institute of Medicine's reports, *To Err is Human: Building A Safer Health System* and *Crossing the Quality Chasm: A New Health System for the 21st Century*. Available at: http://www.iom.edu/?id=12735 and http://www.iom.edu/?id=12736. Also see Aspden, P, Wolcott, J, Bootman, JL, Cronenwett, LR. (Eds.) *Preventing Medication Errors: Quality Chasm Series*. Available at: http://www.nap.edu/catalog/11623.html#toc. Accessed June 6, 2007.

21. Patient Safety Authority, Commonwealth of Pennsylvania. Available at: http://www.psa.state.pa.us/psa/site/default.asp. See also Pennsylvania Patient Safety Reporting System (PA-PSRS). Available at: http://www.psa.state.pa.us/psa/cwp/view.asp?a=1165&q=441808. Accessed June 6, 2007.

22. Oregon Patient Safety Commission website. Available at: http://www.oregon.gov/DHS/ph/pscommission/index.shtml. Accessed June 6, 2007.

23. Minnesota Alliance for Patient Safety, Massachusetts Coalition for the Prevention of Medical Errors, and Vermont's Health Care Reform of 2006 Agency of Administration or Patient Safety Surveillance and Improvement System. Available at: http://www.mnpatientsafety.org/index.php?option=com_content&task=view&id=20&Itemid=37, http://www.macoalition.org/, and http://www.leg.state.vt.us/statutes/fullchapter.cfm?Title=18&Chapter=043A or http://hcr.vermont.gov/improve_quality/promote_quality_improvement. Accessed June 6, 2007.

24. Utah Department of Health, Division of Health System Improvement Patient Safety website. Available at: http://www.health.utah.gov/hsi/patientsafety.htm. Accessed June 6, 2007.

25. Public Health Foundation. SHAs-freestanding agencies v. super-agencies. Public Health Macroview. Washington, DC; 1995;7(1):1.

26. Public Health Foundation. Public Health Agencies 1980. A Report on Their Expenditures and Activities. Washington, DC; 1981.

27. Association of State and Territorial Health Officials. Fact sheets regarding state health information. State Health Agency Profile Database. Washington, DC. Available at:

http://www. statepublichealth.org/. Accessed March 8, 2007 from ASTHO database.

28. National Association of Governors. Transforming State Health Agencies to Meet Current and Future Changes. Washington, DC; 2003. Available at: http://www.nga.org/cda/files/0411HEALTHAGENCIES.pdf. Accessed June 1, 2007.

29. Gossert DJ, Miller CA. State boards of health, their members and commitments. *Am J Public Health.* 1973;63(6): 486–493. Available at: http://www.ajph.org/cgi/reprint/63/6/486. Accessed June 1, 2007.

30. Terris M. Letter to all state health officials on results of questionnaire on training and experience. New York Medical College; December 2, 1977.

31. Shon K. SHO tenure study. Internal memo. Washington, DC: Public Health Foundation; September 17, 1999.

32. Association of State and Territorial Health Officials: Study of State Health Official Turnover. Internal document. Washington, DC; 2000.

33. Association of State and Territorial Health Officials personal communication with author. Washington, DC; 2007.

34. Health Resources and Services Administration. The Public Health Workforce Enumeration. Washington, DC; 2000.

35. Health Resources and Services Administration. Public Health Workforce Study January 2005. Washington, DC; 2005. Available at: http://bhpr.hrsa.gov/healthworkforce/reports/publichealth/default.htm. Accessed June 1, 2007.

36. U.S. Census Bureau. Federal, state, and local governments: Public employment and payroll data. Washington, DC; 2006. Available at: http://www.census.gov/govs/www/apes.html. Accessed June 1, 2007.

37. Association of State and Territorial Health Officials. State public health employee worker shortage report: A Civil service recruitment and retention crisis. Washington, DC; 2004. Available at: http://www.astho.org/pubs/WorkforceShortageReportFinal.pdf. Accessed June 1, 2007.

38. Public Health Agencies. 1991: An inventory of programs and block grant expenditures. Washington, DC: Public Health Foundation; 1991.

39. Eilbert KW, Barry M, Bialek R,et al. Public health expenditures: developing estimates for improved policy making. *J Public Health Manage Prac.* 1997;3(3):1–9. Available at: http://www.ncbi. nlm.nih.gov/entrez/query.fcgi?cmd=Retrieve&db= PubMed&list_uids=10186718&dopt=Abstract. Accessed June 1, 2007.

40. Essential Pubic Health Services, Public Health Foundation Internet site. Available at: http://www. phf.org/infrastructure/resources/Turnock.ppt#321,1, Essential Public Health Services: What They Are and What They Do. Accessed October 14, 2008.

41. Preventive Health and Health Services Block Grant. Available at: http://www.cdc.gov/ nccdphp/blockgrant/. Accessed June 6, 2007.

42. Association of State and Territorial Health Officials. Making a difference, a compendium of illustrative examples of the impact of the innovative uses to which states have applied block grant funding. Washington, DC; 2001. Available at: http://www.astho.org/templates/display_pub. php?pub_id=364. Accessed June 1, 2007.

43. Show us the money: An update on the states' allocation of the tobacco settlement dollars. A report by the Campaign for Tobacco Free Kids. American Cancer Society, American Heart Association, American Lung Association; 2002. Available at: http://tobaccofreekids.org/reports/settlements/ 2002/fullreport.pdf. Accessed June 1, 2007.

44. The Centers for Disease Control and Prevention (CDC). National Public Health Performance Standards Program. Atlanta, GA. Available at: http://www.cdc.gov/od/ocphp/nphpsp/. Accessed June 1, 2007.

45. Association of State and Territorial Public Health Officials. An examination of state use of performance standards. Washington, DC; 2006. Available at: http://www.astho.org/pubs/ AnExaminationofStateUseofPerformance StandardsFINAL.pdf. Accessed June 1, 2007.

46. Robert Wood Johnson Foundation. Exploring public health experience with standards and accreditation. Washington, DC; 2004. Available at: http://www.rwjf.org/files/publications/other/ publichealthaccreditation.pdf. Accessed June 1, 2007.

47. National Association of County and City Health Officials. Research brief: NACCHO survey examines state/local health department relationships. Washington, DC; 1998. Available at: http:// archive.naccho.org/documents/Research_Brief_2. pdf. Accessed June 1, 2007.

48. Joint Council of State and Local Health Officials. Principles of collaboration between state and local public health officials. Washington, DC: Association of State and Territorial Health Officials and National Association of County and City Health Officials; February 2000. Available at: http://archive.naccho.org/documents/ resolutions/Principles-of-Collaboration-Between-state-local.pdf. Accessed June 1, 2007.

49. Tilson, H, Berkowitz, B. The public health enterprise: Examining our twenty-first-century policy challenges. Health Affairs; 2006. NO. 4:900-910; 10.1377/hlthaff.25.4.900. Available at http:// content.healthaffairs.org/cgi/reprint/25/4/900? maxtoshow=&HITS=10&hits= 10&RESULTFORMAT=&author1=tilson& andorexactfulltext=and&searchid= 1&FIRSTINDEX=0&volume=25&resourcetype= HWCIT. Accessed June 12, 2007.

50. Information about state public health associations can be found on the American Public Health Association State Affiliates web page. Available at: http://www.apha.org/membergroups/states/State RegPHA/. Accessed June 10, 2007.

CHAPTER 10

The Local Health Department

Carolyn J. Leep, MS, MPH, Grace Gorenflo, MPH, RN, and Patrick M. Libbey, BA

LEARNING OBJECTIVES

Upon completion of this chapter, the reader will be able to:

1. Describe the factors that affect local governmental public health practice.
2. Distinguish the differing types of local health department governance models.
3. Recognize the large differences in size among local health departments, in terms of population served, budget, and staffing.
4. Describe how local health department operations are financed.
5. Describe the roles of the local health department in carrying out each of the 10 essential public health services.
6. List a number of activities and services frequently provided by local health departments.
7. Identify the occupations typically employed by local health departments of various sizes.

KEY TERMS

Accountability

Accreditation

Governance

Local Health Department

Workforce

The **local health department** (LHD) is "an administrative or service unit of local or state government concerned with health and carrying some responsibility for the health of a jurisdiction smaller than the state."[1] In some parts of the United States, the LHD is an agency or department of the county, city, or town government. In other places, the LHD is a local or regional office of the state health agency. This chapter provides a historical overview and a current survey of LHDs. It then discusses issues that LHDs are likely to face in the future.

OVERVIEW OF LOCAL HEALTH DEPARTMENTS

The mission of LHDs is to protect, promote, and maintain the health of the entire population of their jurisdiction. A common misperception about LHDs is that their sole, or primary, purpose is to provide health care to the poor and uninsured. However, as articulated in the mission, the LHD provides services and engages in activities that safeguard the health of entire populations. These efforts are often "invisible," and frequently it is only during a public health event that many are aware of the critical role that the LHD plays. Specific examples of the more visible and tangible LHD activities include the following:

- Notifying a school and its community when a student is diagnosed with bacterial meningitis, providing information about measures to take as a result of the diagnosis, and contacting and immunizing all those who have been exposed.

- Providing a wide range of immunizations, including influenza vaccines, childhood immunizations (particularly prior to school entry), and tetanus boosters to emergency responders.

- Educating commercial food handlers about safe food handling procedures, inspecting food establishments, and enforcing codes when they are violated (i.e., shutting down food establishments that have failed inspection).

Another way to describe the role of health departments is in a more academic sense. LHDs fulfill the "three core functions of public health: assessment, policy development, and assurance.[2] Assessment refers to collecting, analyzing, and sharing information about the health of the population. Some examples of this are completing community health assessments, collecting and analyzing vital statistics, and monitoring for and controlling outbreaks of communicable disease. Policy development involves developing public health policies based on scientific knowledge. This includes developing local ordinances to protect the health of the jurisdiction served by the LHD. Assurance includes enforcing public health regulations and working to ensure that appropriate personal health care services are available. LHDs enforce public health statutes enacted by federal and state governments, and they work with health care providers to arrange for health care services for people with limited resources.

In 2006, there were nearly 3000 local governmental agencies fulfilling public health responsibilities at some level in most areas of the country. Every state except Rhode Island either has LHDs or units of the state health agency that serve portions of the state. (However, not all localities are served by a governmental local public health presence, and those that are served do not receive a uniform, consistent set of basic public health services.) The three core functions provide a very broad framework to describe the role of LHDs. However, specific functions and services vary widely among LHDs across the country, as do their organization and financing. The range and variation of LHD characteristics will be described in this chapter.

LHDs operate as part of the nation's public health system, which includes governmental public health agencies at the federal, state, and local levels, as well as the health care delivery system, academia, community entities (e.g., schools, religious groups, and nonprofit organizations), the media, and businesses and employers.[3] The collective efforts of all of these sectors—not only LHDs—influence the conditions in which people can be healthy. The governmental public health agencies stand apart because they "serve as the backbone of this system,"[3] with a unique, constitutionally based responsibility to protect and promote health. Moreover, LHDs play an especially important role because public health services actually reach the population in local communities. A 1988 IOM report articulated the critical role of local public health departments, stating:

> . . . no citizen from any community, no matter how small or remote, should be without identifiable and realistic access to the benefits of public health protection, which is possible only through a local component of the public health delivery system.[2]

To understand the role of LHDs and appreciate their potential impact on the nation's health status, it is important to examine their history and the changing context in which they operate, as well as their current responsibilities and activities.

HISTORICAL PERSPECTIVE

The first governmental public health departments were established in urban areas, in response to health issues related to dense populations. By the late 1800s, LHDs were operating in several cities (Baltimore, Charleston, SC; Philadelphia, Providence, Cambridge, New York City, Chicago, Louisville, Indianapolis, and Boston), largely for the purposes of monitoring and addressing contagious diseases, enforcing quarantine and isolation rules, and eliminating environmental hazards through sanitation measures.[4] As advances in the scientific basis of disease causation, treatment, and prevention were made, additional responsibility for the population's health shifted to the public realm. Early in the twentieth century, more LHDs emerged, including the first in rural areas. These also were established to combat infectious disease outbreaks.[4] The responsibilities of LHDs gradually expanded, mostly around specific infectious diseases, to include

providing immunizations, treatment (such as antibiotics), and health education.[2]

Throughout the twentieth century, additional LHDs were established across the country. By 1953, there were a reported 1239 health departments serving local jurisdictions[5], and in 1989, 2888 health departments had been identified.[6] The number and scope of services of LHDs continued (and continue) to change in response to a number of factors: state statues that govern how the responsibilities for health (and other governmental functions) are shared between the state and local levels;[7] scientific progress in the identification, causation, and treatment of diseases; availability of federal and state funding; epidemics; and evolving needs and characteristics particular to the locality in which LHDs were established.

CONTEXT AT THE TURN OF THE CENTURY

The past 20 years have seen a significant increase in the mobility of the world's population, accompanied by an increase in the speed and expansion of the transmission of infectious diseases. Diseases not only cross geopolitical boundaries, but they now also jump continents. Arguably some of the best examples in this century are the emergence and spread of West Nile Virus, avian flu, and Sudden Acute Respiratory Syndrome (SARS). In addition, the public has been amply warned about the likelihood of a pending influenza epidemic, and numerous preparations have been made to that end. Also, the events surrounding September 11, 2001, clearly illustrated the public health implications of terrorist activities. Combined, these issues have heightened public awareness of the need to be prepared to respond effectively to both intentional and natural disasters, and have also brought LHDs into the public's eye.

Moreover, for the first time, a chronic condition, obesity, reached epidemic proportions and was declared a national threat in 1999[8], heralding new perspectives on population-based interventions for chronic disease.

The increasing availability and use of information technology has transformed the way many LHDs approach their responsibilities. In 1990, less than half (47%) of all LHDs had continuous, high-speed Internet access; by 2006, that number had grown to 93 percent.[1] The advent of more readily available electronic communications has dramatically increased expectations around timeliness of information exchange, among all levels of governmental public health and within communities.

Additionally, several large-scale efforts around the turn of the century have sought to strengthen public health. These include efforts to define public health (the three "core functions"[2] and the 10 essential public health services[9]), measure the performance of public health systems (National Public Health Performance Standards Program[10]), set public health goals (Healthy People 2000 and Healthy People 2010[11]), and develop systems of **accountability** that assure the quality and availability of public health services (as recommended by a 2002 IOM report)[3]. (Increased demand for public accountability has been ignited, in part, over concerns about lack of accounting for federal funds appropriated for public health departments through the Public Health Security and Bioterrorism Preparedness Act of 2002.[12])

As a result of the 2002 IOM recommendation, a national steering committee examined the establishment of a voluntary, national **accreditation** program for state and LHDs, ultimately determining in 2006 that such a program would be both feasible and desirable.[13] *Accreditation* refers to a process for external, reliable, and objective validation of agency performance against a specific set of standards, and some form of reward or recognition for agencies meeting those standards. Many prominent public health leaders view accreditation as a promising strategy to hold health departments accountable, verify that a particular level of performance has been achieved and that quality improvement processes are in place, and to promote uniformity among LHDs.[14] The Public Health Accreditation Board, incorporated in 2007, serves as the national body for state and LHD accreditation. By 2007, approximately 10 states had established accreditation or other standards-related programs for their LHDs.[15]

Another noteworthy effort to define public health involved the definition of a LHD. Concerns about lack of accountability unfolded in the absence of a consensus about what constitutes a functional LHD. Local health official leaders, recognizing the importance of developing a shared understanding of "what everyone, regardless of where they live, should reasonably expect from the local governmental public health presence," released the *Operational Definition of a Functional Local Health Department* in 2005.[16] The Operational Definition is a set of standards framed around the 10 essential public health services, as they relate specifically to LHDs:

1. Monitor health status and understand health issues facing the community.
2. Protect people from health problems and health hazards.
3. Give people information they need to make healthy choices.
4. Engage the community to identify and solve health problems.
5. Develop public health policies and plans.
6. Enforce public health laws and regulations.
7. Help people receive health services.
8. Maintain a competent public health workforce.
9. Evaluate and improve programs and interventions.
10. Contribute to and apply the evidence base of public health.

The standards are the basis for LHD standards of the Public Health Accreditation Board and also are a reference point for all LHDs working to improve their quality and performance.

Amid the changing context in which LHDs operate, at least one constant has emerged: the need for them to demonstrate fulfillment of a consistent set of roles and responsibilities, with an emphasis on swift and effective responses to both anticipated and unforeseen public health threats.

LOCAL HEALTH DEPARTMENT ORGANIZATION AND GOVERNANCE

LHDs vary in several organizational characteristics, including jurisdictional type, relationship to their state health department, governance structure, governing bodies, and size.

Jurisdictional Type

LHDs are governmental entities serving jurisdictions of towns, cities, counties, or districts (see Figure 10.1).[1] Seventy-three percent of LHDs serve a county or combined city-county jurisdiction. Ten percent of LHDs serve district or regional jurisdictions, which usually cover multiple counties, although regions consisting of multiple towns or cities are found in some states. In Idaho, for example, 44 counties were organized into 7 district health departments, each comprising 4 to 8 counties. The district structure created a larger population and tax base for the new health departments, which allowed them to expand staff numbers and skills and provide a broader and more consistent range of services throughout the state.

Relationship to the State Health Agency

The **governance** of a LHD refers to where the ultimate authority for, or control of, its activities resides. Typically, LHDs derive their authority from state health agencies and from the county or city government of which they are a part. Three categories are most often used to describe the relationship between state and LHDs according to how the LHDs are governed: centralized (authority rests with the state health department), decentralized (authority rests with a single or combined local government), and mixed (some combination of the centralized and decentralized).

A fourth category, shared governance, is sometimes used but is not clearly defined. Conceptually, "shared" governance means that both the state health agency and local government govern LHDs. Various sources apply these categories of governance differently.[17–20] Maryland is the only state whose LHD governance is consistently described as shared.

Figure 10.2 shows states by governance type and also shows the number of LHDs in each state.[1] Significant variation exists across United States census geographic regions, such that southern states tend to be centralized, and those in the Midwest are more often decentralized.[21]

Decentralized Governance

In decentralized states, LHDs operate independently from their respective state health agencies. In these states, the local governing bodies for the LHDs typically develop and approve their budgets, set priorities, develop local health ordinances, and hire their directors/health officers.

An important advantage of this model is that the priorities of local government and the community can be integrated easily into the health department's services. Disadvantages can include a lack of communication among departments, noninvolvement of LHDs in state planning and decision making, and uneven service delivery across the state.

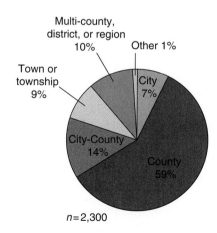

Figure 10.1. Type of Jurisdiction
SOURCE: National Association of County and City Health Officials. (2006) 2005 National profile of local health departments. Washington, DC: NACCHO.

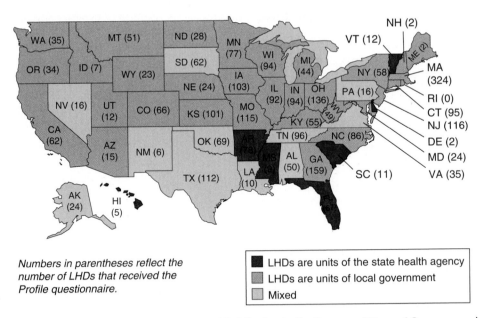

Numbers in parentheses reflect the
number of LHDs that received the
Profile questionnaire.

■ LHDs are units of the state health agency
■ LHDs are units of local government
□ Mixed

Figure 10.2. **LHDs Included in the 2005 National Public Study (by State and Type of Governance)**

SOURCE: National Association of County and City Health Officials. (2006) 2005 National profile of local health departments. Washington, DC: NACCHO.

Centralized Governance

In centralized states, LHDs are units of the state health agencies, and the degree to which they work with local government varies considerably. In Florida, for example, LHDs are entities of state government and also have a direct reporting relationship to county government. The state health department approves the county health department budget, sets priorities, and determines the programmatic emphasis. The county usually contributes tax dollars to the state health department budget and, after developing the county budget, contracts with the state for service. The county makes only limited policy and programmatic decisions. The selection of a county health official is begun by the state health department, with review and appointment made by the county board of commissioners. The county health department staff is also made up of state employees. In some states with centralized governance, however, the LHD may have little interaction with the local government and receive

little or no local tax dollars. LHDs in New Mexico and Delaware are examples at this end of the spectrum. The local offices of the state health department are often organized into regions or districts.

Advantages of this model are more consistency with respect to resource allocation and service provision across the state, interoperable information and communications systems, a more coordinated approach to public health, and the ability to address priorities statewide. Disadvantages include the limited ability of a LHD to focus on locally determined priorities, programs, and policies.

Mixed Governance

Several states include some LHDs that are units of local government and others that are units of the state health agency. In these states, the larger cities and counties typically organize their own independent health department (e.g., Oklahoma City-County and Tulsa City-County Health Departments in Oklahoma), while local or regional offices of the state health department serve the remaining cities or counties in the state. Advantages of this variation include ensuring the availability of state-run public health services in smaller communities that have few resources, while giving broader authority and local control to the health departments serving larger communities. Disadvantages may include inconsistency in policy development and significant variation in services.

Governing Bodies

LHDs may be governed by a local board of health, local elected officials (e.g., county council or commission, city council, mayor), a state health agency, or a combination of these bodies.

Local Boards of Health

Local boards of health are present in most states (Arkansas, Delaware, Hawaii, Louisiana, Mississippi, New Mexico, Rhode Island, and South Dakota are the only states without local boards of health)[22] with varying responsibilities and composition according to state statute. Seventy-seven percent of local boards of health have some governing or policy-making authority, while 13 percent serve in an advisory capacity only.[1] Most often, members of local boards of health are appointed. In some jurisdictions, a local governmental body (e.g., county board of commissioners) serves as the local board of health. In approximately 10 percent of LHD jurisdictions, members are specifically elected to serve on the board of health.[1] Some local boards of health include both elected and appointed members. The size of most local boards of health ranges between three and seven members.[23]

Most local boards of health also serve as a link between LHDs and the community they serve. In this capacity, the board of health represents the community's interest in adopting priorities and establishing needed services, while also communicating with the community about health department goals and services available. Members of boards of health who are not elected officials may also be able to advocate to legislators more directly than is possible for local health officials.

Statistics on local board of health presence and governance are provided in Table 10.1.[1] Nationwide, local boards of health are less likely to be present in larger jurisdictions and also less likely to be the governing body for the LHD in large jurisdictions. Local boards of health are much more common for LHDs that are units of local government than units of the state health agency.

Other Forms of Governance

Approximately 45 percent of all LHDs are not governed by local boards of health.[24] Most of these

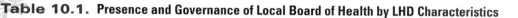

Table 10.1. **Presence and Governance of Local Board of Health by LHD Characteristics**

	Percentage of Jurisdictions with a Local Board of Health	Percentage of LHDs Governed by a Local Board of Health
All LHDs	74%	55%
Jurisdiction population		
<50,000	78%	59%
50,000 to 499,999	72%	50%
500,000+	48%	27%
Governance		
Units of local government	86%	68%
Units of state health agency	32%	5%

LHDs are governed by either state health agencies or local elected officials, such as the county council, county commissioners, board of supervisors, mayor, or city or town council. Some district or regional LHDs, which serve multiple counties, cities, or towns, are governed by separate governing bodies in each jurisdiction, whereas others are governed by a single local board of health or by the state health agency.

Population Served by Local Health Departments

Populations served by LHDs range from very large—approximately 10 million for Los Angeles County and 8 million for New York City—to several communities of fewer than 1000 people.[1]

Figure 10.3 provides statistics on the percentage of LHDs in different size categories and the percentage of the United States population served by LHDs in each size category.[1] Most LHDs serve jurisdictions with relatively small populations. Jurisdictions with fewer than 50,000 residents account for 62 percent of the nation's health departments; 41 percent of all health departments serve jurisdictions with fewer than 25,000 residents. Remarkably, over half (54%) of people in the United States are served by large-jurisdiction health departments (those serving 500,000 or more residents), which comprise only 6 percent of the nation's LHDs. The large number of LHDs with jurisdictions of less than 50,000 serves approxi-

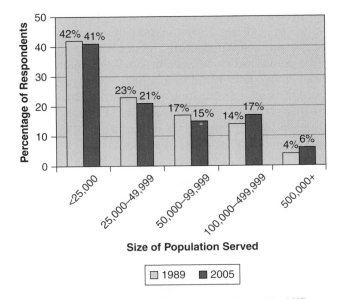

Figure 10.3. Size of Population Served by LHDs: 1989 and 2005 Profile Studies

SOURCE: National Association of County and City Health Officials. (2006) 2005 National profile of local health departments. Washington, DC: NACCHO.

mately 10 percent of the United States population. These numbers illustrate serious issues about resource allocation vis-à-vis smaller health departments, and the implications of perceived return on investment.

As expected, LHD expenditures and number of staff increase as the population served increases (see Table 10.2).[1]

Table 10.2. LHD Expenditures and Staffing by Jurisdiction Population

Population of Jurisdiction	Total Annual Expenditures (Median)	Total Staff FTEs (Median)
<25,000	$340,000	6
25,000–49,999	$890,000	16
50,000–99,999	$2,000,000	33
100,000–499,999	$6,200,000	88
500,000+	$32,000,000	325

LOCAL HEALTH DEPARTMENT FINANCING

LHDs vary widely in budgets (both on total and per capita bases) and in the sources from which they derive their revenue.

Total Annual Expenditures

LHD total annual expenditures range over six orders of magnitude. Some of the smaller jurisdictions in New England have annual expenditures less than $10,000, while the largest metropolitan health departments have annual expenditures on the order of $1 billion. The smallest annual LHD expenditure reported in 2005 was $1,200, whereas the largest was $1.5 billion. Half of LHDs have total annual expenditures of less than $1 million, and 20 percent have total annual expenditures of $5 million or greater (see Figure 10.4).[1]

Per Capita Local Health Department Expenditures

Because LHD annual expenditures are strongly related to the population size of the jurisdiction,

computing per capita expenditures (total expenditures divided by jurisdiction population) is useful for examining differences in governmental local public health investments. Comparisons among spending by LHDs must be made cautiously, however, as the types of services they provide vary greatly. For example, some LHDs provide extensive clinical services, whereas others provide few or none. Some LHDs provide a wide range of environmental health services, while these services are provided by another governmental agency in other jurisdictions (see Figure 10.7 later in this chapter). Table 10.3 provides selected percentiles of per capita annual LHD expenditures.[24] The figures in the first column were computed by subtracting clinical source revenues from total LHD expenditures. This adjustment is intended to remove some of the budget variation that results from differences in the amount of clinical services provided by LHDs.

The mean and median per capita annual LHD expenditures show modest variations with agency characteristics such as jurisdiction population size, type of governance, and degree of urbanization. Much larger variations are seen across states (see Figure 10.5).[1] Median per capita LHD expenditures vary 10-fold across the states, and there is also considerable variation in per capita funding among LHDs within a state.

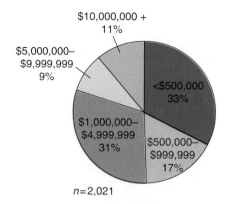

$n=2,021$

Figure 10.4. **Total Annual LHD Expenditures**

SOURCE: National Association of County and City Health Officials. (2006) 2005 National profile of local health departments. Washington, DC: NACCHO.

Table 10.3. **Per Capita Annual Local Health Department Expenditures**

	Nonclinical Revenues[a]	All Revenues
	Median	Median
10th percentile	$8	$9
25th percentile	$14	$17
50th percentile	$23	$29
75th percentile	$36	$50
90th percentile	$59	$84

[a]Excludes Medicaid, Medicare, and other reimbursements for medical care.

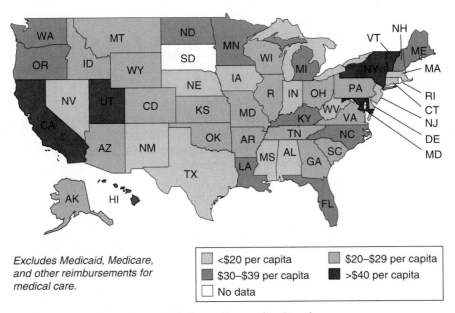

Excludes Medicaid, Medicare, and other reimbursements for medical care.

☐ <$20 per capita   ☐ $20–$29 per capita

■ $30–$39 per capita   ■ >$40 per capita

☐ No data

Figure 10.5. **Median Annual Per Capita LHD Expenditures (by State)**

SOURCE: National Association of County and City Health Officials. (2006) 2005 National profile of local health departments. Washington, DC: NACCHO.

Local Health Department Revenue Sources

LHD revenues come from a variety of sources, including local government; state government; federal funds passed through to LHD by state agencies (federal pass-through); direct funding from federal agencies (e.g., Centers for Disease Control and Prevention, Health Resources and Services Administration, Substance Abuse and Mental Health Services Administration); reimbursement from Medicare, Medicaid, and other insurers; regulatory and patient personal fees; and other sources (e.g., grants from private foundations). Figure 10.6 displays the overall percentage of total LHD revenues by funding sources.[1] Local sources provide the greatest percentage of LHD revenues (29%), followed by state direct sources (23%), and federal pass-through sources (13%).

The amount of funding from these sources varies by governance type. Not surprisingly, local funds contribute to a greater percentage of total LHD revenues on average for agencies that are units of local government than for those that are units of

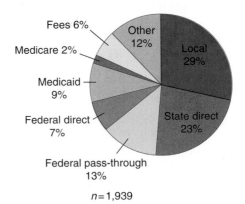

Fees 6%

Medicare 2%

Medicaid 9%

Federal direct 7%

Federal pass-through 13%

Other 12%

Local 29%

State direct 23%

$n = 1,939$

Figure 10.6. **Total LHD Revenues from Various Sources**

SOURCE: National Association of County and City Health Officials. (2006) 2005 National profile of local health departments. Washington, DC: NACCHO.

the state health agency. The latter receive larger percentages of revenues from both state direct and federal pass-through sources. Large differences are also seen across states. Some states' revenues are balanced among local, state, federal, and other

Table 10.4. Variation Among States in Contribution to LHD Revenues from Selected Sources

Revenue Source	State with Highest Contribution	State with Lowest Contribution
Local (city and county)	Missouri (57%)	DE, NM, VT (0%)
State direct	Delaware (79%)	Nevada (4%)
Federal pass through	Vermont (81%)	Maine (2%)
Federal direct	Connecticut (22%)	Many at 0%
Medicare and Medicaid	Alabama (45%)	Many at 0%

sources, whereas others are dominated by one or two sources. Table 10.4 shows the range of contributions to total LHD revenues across states.[1]

LOCAL HEALTH DEPARTMENT FUNCTIONS AND SERVICES

The functions and services of LHDs vary based on the department's authority and resources and by the needs of the community. LHD functions are described in this section organized around the 10 areas of the Operational Definition of a Functional Local Health Department,[16] which mirror the 10 essential public health services. (A description of discrete activities and services is included at the end of this section.)

Monitor Health Status and Understand Health Issues Facing the Community

LHDs must understand the specific health issues confronting their community and how physical, behavioral, environmental, social, and economic conditions affect them. To accomplish this, LHDs both collect community health data and use data collected by other organizations (e.g., other state

Table 10.5. Local Health Departments Conducting Surveillance and Epidemiology

Category	Percentage
Communicable/infectious disease	89%
Environmental health	75%
Chronic disease	41%
Behavioral risk factors	36%
Syndromic	33%
Injury	24%

and local agencies, hospitals, or community-based organizations). Most LHDs conduct surveillance for communicable/infectious diseases and environmental health indicators; some LHDs also conduct surveillance for chronic diseases, behavioral risk factors, and injuries (Table 10.5).[1] Syndromic surveillance is the use of health-related data that precedes diagnosis of disease (e.g., school absence, pharmaceutical use, emergency room visits) to identify potential outbreaks that may warrant a public health response. The utility of syndromic surveillance for identifying bioterrorism-related outbreaks is being explored in some state and LHDs.

Many LHDs work collaboratively with their communities to collect and analyze a wide variety of information related to the community's health in a process known as *community health assessment*. Participation by a wide range of community stakeholders is essential to community health assessment. In 2005, 78 percent of LHDs reported that they had completed a community health assessment in the past three years or intend to complete one in the next three years.[1]

Protect People from Health Problems and Health Hazards

LHDs are responsible for investigating health problems and health threats and for preventing, minimizing, and containing adverse health effects from communicable diseases, disease outbreaks from unsafe food or water, chronic diseases, environmental hazards, injuries, and risky health behaviors. This includes both activities focused on prevention

✿ MONITORING COMMUNITY HEALTH

Alamance County Health Department in Burlington, North Carolina is using GIS (geographic information system) technology to both improve maternal, infant, and environmental health, and to prepare residents (particularly vulnerable populations) and leadership to respond to public health emergencies. Teams collect survey data for a community health assessment using GPS-enabled handheld computers, which link responses to a location, allowing differences in health status to be analyzed and compared across neighborhoods. GIS will be used to create spatial databases of maternal, infant, and environmental health data. Health education and other interventions will be targeted to neighborhoods with the greatest burdens of risk as determined through GIS analysis.

(primary and secondary) and responding to health problems and hazards. Some LHDs provide screening and testing for communicable and chronic diseases (Table 10.6), whereas others provide referrals to such services.[1]

Some LHDs have primary responsibility for many environmental health functions, whereas others have primary responsibility for only a few or none. Figure 10.7 shows the organizations that provide selected environmental health services in LHD jurisdictions across the United States.[1] Environmental health services provided most frequently by LHDs include food safety education and vector control. Regardless of what organization has primary responsibility for these environmental health services, the LHD is responsible for coordinating with that organization and ensuring that the public's health is protected.

✿ Table 10.6. Local Health Department Provision of Testing and Screening Services

Disease or Condition	Percentage Providing
Tuberculosis	85%
High blood pressure	72%
Blood lead	66%
Other STDs	64%
HIV/AIDS	62%
Diabetes	51%
Cancer	46%
Cardiovascular disease	36%

LHDs have a primary responsibility for planning for and responding to public health emergencies, often working with state and federal public health agencies on large-scale events. LHDs also collaborate with other local responders to assist in other emergencies with public health significance, such as natural disasters. Emergency preparedness has received a high degree of attention in recent years, and nearly all LHDs are preparing to respond to a public health emergency by developing and exercising emergency response plans and by training staff to serve in specific capacities (often very different from their everyday jobs) in an emergency. Most LHDs use an "all hazards" approach to emergency planning because responses to any public health emergency (natural or manmade) share many common features. Planning occurs within the context of the National Incident Management System (part of the Federal Emergency Management Agency)[25] because although most emergency situations are handled locally, a major incident often necessitates involvement and assistance from other jurisdictions, the state and the federal government.

Give People Information They Need to Make Healthy Choices

LHDs provide a variety of health education and health promotion activities in their communities, working at both the individual and population levels. Table 10.7 shows the percentage of LHDs with population-based primary prevention programs in selected areas.[1] LHDs work closely with

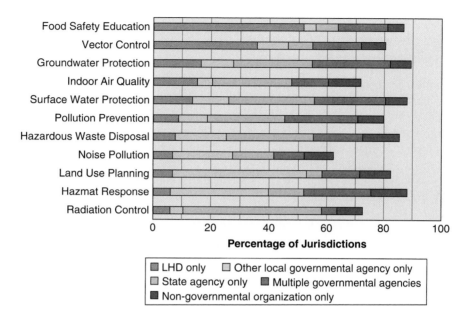

Figure 10.7. Organizations Engaged in Environmental Health Activities

SOURCE: National Association of County and City Health Officials. (2006) 2005 National profile of local health departments. Washington, DC: NACCHO.

members of the population to which a health education or promotion effort is directed to ensure that the program is culturally and linguistically appropriate. LHDs use many different communication channels to reach their target population and frequently work with community partners on health education and promotion efforts. Risk communication is another component of information dissemination. Skillful use of mass media has become increasingly important both for successful health education and promotion programs and for risk communication—a critical facet of providing people with information they need about public health events. Nearly all LHDs partner with their local media.[1]

Engage the Community to Identify and Solve Health Problems

LHDs develop partnerships with public and private health care providers and institutions, community-based organizations, and other government agencies engaged in services that affect health (e.g., housing, criminal justice, education) to collectively identify, alleviate, and act on the sources of public health problems. Over 90 percent of LHDs have a collaborative relationship with schools, emergency responders, the media, physician practices/medical groups, and community-based organizations.[1]

Collective action for public health purposes may be generated through community-wide strategic planning for improving health. MAPP (Mobilizing for Action through Planning and Partnerships[26]) is one tool for such a process, and one community's

Table 10.7. Local Health Department Population-Based Primary Prevention Activities

Condition or Behavior	Percentage Providing
Tobacco use	69%
Obesity	56%
Unintended pregnancy	51%
Injury	40%
Substance abuse	26%
Violence	25%
Mental illness	14%

⚜ BUCKLE UP BOSTON!

Buckle Up Boston! is a child passenger safety program coordinated by the Boston Public Health Commission in collaboration with a host of public and private organizations. Their goal is to increase awareness about child passenger safety and increase usage rates of seats among low-income families in the city of Boston. According to the National Highway Traffic Safety Administration, motor vehicle crashes are the leading cause of unintentional injury-related death to children. Children age four and under who ride unrestrained are at twice the risk of death and injury. Buckle Up Boston! provides car seats to families that might not otherwise have access to them and teaches parents about correct use of child passenger restraints.

⚜ THE WELLNESS CURRICULUM

The Wellness Curriculum, a collaborative project between the Orange County (FL) Health Department and the Orange County Corrections Department, helps to address the health needs of inmates by providing information and education that is useful to them not only while they are in prison but, even more, as they are released into the community. Lack of adequate medical care prior to incarceration, combined with specific prison characteristics, places incarcerated people at higher risk for STDs, HIV, and hepatitis C, and also aggravates chronic conditions such as hypertension and diabetes. This program is targeted to a population that is hard to reach with traditional health education programs and uses surveys of the inmates to identify topics where education is most needed.

experience with MAPP is discussed in the upcoming "Healthy Nashville 2010" boxed feature. Conducting a community health assessment is usually part of this process, and one of the products of strategic planning is a community health improvement plan, which identifies specific action steps to improve community health. Over half of LHDs have developed a community health improvement plan recently, and the vast majority of these plans are based on a community health assessment.[1] Many community health improvement plans are linked to statewide health improvement plans. The identified action steps might be new programs, changes in existing programs at the LHD or another public or private organization, or collaborative efforts to secure funding for needed programs. The community health improvement plan should also include a mechanism to evaluate whether the action steps are achieving the desired goals.

In addition to community-wide processes such as MAPP, LHDs may also work on targeted efforts with a subset of community partners to generate interest in and support for new and emerging public health issues. Raising community awareness of public health needs and soliciting the community's concerns and perspectives about public health issues are important roles of LHD leaders. Most LHD leaders discuss public health issues on local radio and television programs and also have such discussions with local civic groups.[1]

Develop Public Health Policies and Plans

LHDs serve as a primary resource to their governing bodies and policymakers to establish and maintain public health policies, practices, and capacity. Over 80 percent of LHD leaders discuss proposed legislation, regulations, or ordinances with elected officials; participate on local boards or advisory panels responsible for public health policy; and work with the media to inform public health policy.[1] Many

HEALTHY NASHVILLE 2010

MAPP provided the Metropolitan Nashville/ Davidson County Health Department (TN) a way to reconnect with the community and engage them in a sustainable strategic health improvement planning process. Their process, called Healthy Nashville 2010, also offered the Nashville public health community the opportunity to integrate the work of various coalitions into one process, giving overarching direction for all existing health improvement initiatives in the county. Since the Mayor's announcement of the initiative, political support and strong momentum have sparked interest from a broad segment of the Nashville community. Healthy Nashville 2010 has given local public health system partners in Nashville the opportunity to collaborate and to coordinate their programs, decreasing duplication and competition among programs. A significant outcome of MAPP in Nashville has been rebuilding public health policy efforts. For example, Nashville's strategic plan for building sidewalks helped the Leadership Council foster relationships with other governmental agencies.

LHDs also provide technical assistance for drafting proposed legislation, regulations, or ordinances and prepare issue briefs for policymakers. Recent examples include restricted use of tobacco in public places and bans on the use of transfats in restaurants.

Although the modern institution of public health arose as an organized response to the ill effects of industrialization, the focus on broad aspects of social and economic life has been de-emphasized in favor of categorically funded programmatic activities.

SAN FRANCISCO ASTHMA TASK FORCE

In 2002, the San Francisco Department of Public Health facilitated a process to address environmental health disparities in asthma, focusing on indoor air exposures of poor children. Published studies have related poor indoor air quality to the presence of substances frequently found in substandard housing: mites, cockroaches, and mold. The San Francisco Asthma Task Force, which included local public health and social service agencies, nonprofit and community-advocacy organizations, and community members, was formed to investigate the problem and develop recommendations for improving indoor air quality for lower-income tenants. The task force identified several major action strategies:

1. Establishing a cross-agency group to inspect public-housing properties and to create accountability mechanisms that rapidly brought conditions into compliance with the housing code.
2. Establishing standards and guidelines for comprehensive healthy housing, including roles for property owners—requiring government entities to strengthen the relationship between building codes and landlords' legal obligation to tenants to reduce housing-related health risks.
3. Instituting a legal housing-advocacy program for poor patients identified with asthma.

The health department was a key participant, but the project was broadly based in the community and led by community organizations. These recommendations addressed the social context of risk and incorporated nontraditional approaches for providing public health programs and services.

Many local health officials are returning to these public health roots, with more than half of LHDs reporting that they educate officials about health inequities and their causes (i.e., social or economic conditions, and public policy[27]) and support community efforts to change the root causes of health inequities.[1]

Enforce Public Health Laws and Regulations

Various state and local government agencies, including LHDs, are responsible for enforcing public health laws and regulations. Table 10.8 lists the areas of regulation in which LHDs most frequently have responsibility.[1]

A primary role for LHD staff in this arena is to educate regulated individuals and organizations about the meaning, purpose, and benefit of public health laws, ordinances, and regulations, and how to comply. They monitor the compliance of regulated entities and conduct enforcement activities when necessary. LHDs are using creative strategies to increase compliance with public health laws and regulations (see the "Don't Gamble on Food Safety" boxed feature).

Table 10.8. Local Health Department Regulation, Inspection, or Licensing Activities

Area of Regulation, Inspection, or Licensing	% of LHDs
Food service establishments	76%
Public swimming pools	67%
Septic tank installation	66%
Schools/daycare centers	65%
Private drinking water	57%
Lead inspection	53%
Hotels/motels	49%
Campgrounds/RVs	39%
Smoke-free ordinances	38%

DON'T GAMBLE ON FOOD SAFETY

Public Health Seattle-King County developed "Don't Gamble on Food Safety," an inclusive, fast-paced training program for food service workers, to best use valuable training time. The training objectives are to reinforce existing food safety knowledge, teach new safe food practices, and create an experience that will lead to better retention of food safety information. The training is in a game show format with teams of food service workers competing for prestige, points, and prizes. With a food inspector or other food safety expert as host, participants are guided through team selection, competition, and learning about safe food handling principles. Manager and food worker feedback indicates that this training heightens food safety knowledge, changes worker behaviors, and accentuates the importance each individual plays in a safe food service program.

REACH: REAL ESTATE AWARENESS OF THE CONNECTICUT HEALTH CODE

The Ledge Light Health District developed this program to educate and inform local real estate agents of the Connecticut Public Health Code requirements that relate to real estate transactions (water, on-site sewage, lead, and radon). Real estate agents learn about the types of health-related property documents maintained by the Health District, who to contact for information, and how to provide clients with this information in a clear and professional manner.

Table 10.9. Local Health Department Provision of Personal Health Services

Type of health service	Percentage of LHDs Providing	
	2005	1993
Early and periodic screening, diagnosis, and treatment	46%	70%
Prenatal care	42%	63%
Oral health care	31%	44%
Home health care	28%	53%
Obstetrical care	16%	32%
Comprehensive primary care	14%	30%
Behavioral/mental health services	13%	NA
Substance abuse services	11%	NA

Help People Receive Health Services

Access to affordable, appropriate, culturally competent health care is a serious problem in the United States. The federal government estimates that more than 45 million Americans lack health insurance.[28] Although some LHDs provide a variety of personal health services (see Table 10.9)[1], their role is not typically to provide primary health care services. Data on provision of personal health services by LHDs in 1993 and 2005 show a decrease in the number providing personal health services.[1] LHDs work with health care providers and community organizations to identify gaps in personal health services, including preventive and health promotion services, and to develop strategies to close the gaps. LHDs partner with community organizations to increase access to health care and link individuals to personal health care providers in the community.

Maintain a Competent Public Health Workforce

A LHD must employ a competent and diverse staff (i.e., **workforce**) to achieve its goals. Core Competencies for Public Health Professionals define the set of skills, knowledge, and attitudes necessary for the broad practice of public health (see Appendix C).[29] The Core Competencies cover skills in eight domains (analytical/assessment, policy development/program planning, communication, cultural competency, community dimensions of practice, basic public health science, financial planning and management, and leadership and systems thinking) that are defined for three levels of public health professionals (front line staff, senior staff, and supervisory and management staff).

LHDs must evaluate their staff members against these competencies and address deficiencies through continuing education, training, and leadership development activities. A recent survey indicates

BUNCOMBE COUNTY PROJECT ACCESS

The Buncombe County (NC) Health Center is the primary source of medical care for the uninsured in Buncombe County, serving more than 15,000 active patients. The specialty care needs of many of these patients were not being met, however, until a local partnership launched Project Access in 1995. This partnership of county government, local medical society, physicians, service agencies, the hospital, and pharmacists gave health care providers a way to do their "fair share" in providing medical care for the indigent. Through Project Access, 90 percent of practicing physicians in Buncombe County (more than 600) see 10 to 20 individuals referred into their program with no expectation of payment. This program spreads the indigent care burden across the entire medical community so that no single provider is ever required to see more than 20 patients. That represents less than 1 percent of the average practice, a burden that local physicians are willing to bear.

STUDENT OUTREACH AND RESPONSE TEAM (SORT)

The SORT program provides master's level public health students and faculty at Rollins School of Public Health at Emory University with the opportunity to explore public health careers at the local level. It also provides the DeKalb County Board of Health with surge capacity, both in a crisis situation and in everyday work. Not only does the team participate in outbreak investigations, but they also are able to participate in preparedness drills and exercises, mass vaccination clinics, policy meetings, and surveillance activities. Students are able to experience diverse activities and programs in a LHD. As a result, several SORT members have sought and earned positions in LHDs upon graduation.

that most LHDs (72%) are familiar with the core competencies, but less than half are using them to assess competencies or develop training plans.[30]

Maintaining a workforce that reflects the diversity of the community served is critical and becoming more so as the United States population grows increasingly racially and ethnically diverse. Evidence suggests that greater diversity can improve the cultural competence of health professionals and health systems and that such improvement may be associated with better health care outcomes.[31] Yet, over two-thirds of LHD staffs are less racially diverse than the communities they serve.[32] LHDs need to work with community partners, including at educational institutions and job training programs, to address this deficiency.

LHDs' contribution to the public health workforce does not end with their own agency staffs. LHDs can also help to train the future public health workforce in local public health practice by providing educational experiences for students at all levels and by teaching public health curricula. Further, because many others in the community are also engaged in public health interventions, LHDs need to promote the use of effective public health practices by these practitioners.

Evaluate and Improve Programs and Interventions

To maximize their effectiveness, the LHD must have a culture of continuous quality improvement that fosters ongoing, evidence-based evaluation efforts that drive performance improvement activities. They also need to review the effectiveness of public health interventions provided by others in the community. For example, to assess the effectiveness of immunization programs in the community, the LHD needs to evaluate not only its own immunization practices but also those of physicians, clinics, and other health care providers in the community.

Seventy-one percent of LHDs report that they are engaged in quality or performance improvement activities,[33] but little is known about the nature, extent, and focus of these efforts. Clear definitions about quality improvement for LHDs are likely to emerge as the Public Health Accreditation Board evolves and accreditation is launched.

Contribute to and Apply the Evidence Base of Public Health

A number of federal agencies have developed resources to help LHDs identify evidence-based public health practices (see Appendix B). CDC's *Guide to Community Preventive Services* summarizes what is known about the effectiveness, economic efficiency, and feasibility of interventions to promote community health and prevent disease.[34] The Agency for Healthcare Research and Quality publishes the *Guide to Clinical Preventive Services*, which provides recommendations on screening, counseling, and preventive medication topics and includes clinical considerations for each topic.[35] The

National Library of Medicine maintains the Healthy People 2010 Information Access project, which makes information and evidence-based strategies related to the Healthy People 2010 objectives easier to find by providing preformulated PubMed search strategies for selected Healthy People 2010 focus areas.[36] LHDs should apply these resources to practice.

Building an evidence base for public health requires practitioners to share information about effective public health practices and programs. LHD staff members do not have the kinds of incentives for publication that academics do, but their experiences are a critical part of the public health evidence base. At least one state health agency has a program to collect information about exemplary local public health practices and make this information readily available to other LHDs.[37] The National Association of County and City Health Officials (NACCHO) sponsors the Model Practices program, which recognizes effective programs and allows LHD staff to benefit from their colleagues' experiences, to learn what works, and to ensure that resources are used wisely on effective programs that have been implemented with good results. Both model and promising practices are available in a Web-based toolkit.[38]

The idea of LHDs becoming "Academic Health Departments" involved in the academic roles of teaching, service, and research with either formal or informal affiliations with academic institutions is increasingly common.[39–42] In several recent surveys, responding health departments report that a majority are involved in some way with academic institutions.[43,44]

Overview of Specific Programmatic Areas

Another way to consider the work of the LHD is to look at specific program areas. Despite the variation among LHD organization and structure, some specific program areas are nearly universal. Table 10.10 lists the 10 most frequently provided by LHDs.[1]

Table 10.10. Activities and Services Provided Mostly Frequently by LHDs

Activity or Service	Percentage of LHDs
Adult immunization provision	91%
Childhood immunization provision	90%
Communicable/infectious disease surveillance	89%
Tuberculosis screening	85%
Food service inspection or licensing	76%
Environmental health surveillance	75%
Food safety education	75%
Tuberculosis treatment	75%
High blood pressure screening	72%
Tobacco use prevention	69%

THE LOCAL HEALTH DEPARTMENT WORKFORCE

Like most areas of public health, the LHD workforce comprises individuals with a wide variety of academic and professional training. In addition, the number of staff and types of occupations vary according to the size of population served by LHDs and the functions and services provided.

Size and Composition of the Local Health Department Workforce

LHDs in the United States employ a total of approximately 160,000 full-time equivalent (FTE) staff.[1] The United States Census Bureau estimates approximately 246,000 governmental health workers at the local level, which includes not only workers at LHDs but also workers at other local agencies providing health-related services, including emergency medical, mental health, substance abuse, animal control, and environmental health services.[45]

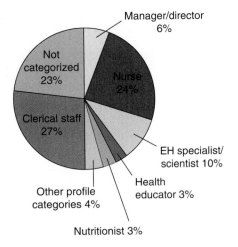

Figure 10.8. Occupations in the LHD Workforce

SOURCE: National Association of County and City Health Officials. (2006) 2005 National profile of local health departments. Washington, DC: NACCHO.

Figure 10.8 illustrates the proportions of the LHD workforce in selected occupations.[1] The occupations that make up the largest percentages of this workforce are clerical staff (27%), nurses (24%), environmental health (EH) specialists and scientists (10%), and managers and directors (6%). The category "other professional occupations" includes physicians, epidemiologists, information

systems (IS) specialists, public information specialists, and emergency preparedness (EP) coordinators (each of which account for less than 1.5% of the LHD workforce). The occupations included in the "not categorized" group are not known, but they likely include mostly nonprofessional or paraprofessional positions. This group also includes some professional occupations (e.g., dentists, attorneys, planners) that are employed in relatively small numbers by LHDs.

Typical Staffing Patterns for Local Health Departments

The types of functions and services LHDs provide also affect their staffing patterns. LHDs that provide environmental health services employ environmental scientists, specialists, or technicians. LHDs that provide a wide range of clinical services employ many types of health professionals. LHDs that provide health promotion programs may employ health educators and community outreach workers.

Despite these differences in employment based on services provided, it is instructive to compare typical staffing patterns for LHDs serving different sizes of jurisdictions. Table 10.11 lists the median numbers of total LHD staff and selected occupations (expressed in FTEs) employed by LHDs serving

Table 10.11. Typical Staffing Patterns for LHDs Serving Jurisdictions within Selected Population Size Categories

Serving <25,000	Serving 50,000–100,000	Serving 100,000–500,000
6FTEs, including:	**33 FTEs, including:**	**88 FTEs, including:**
1 manager/director	1 manager/director	5 managers/directors
2 nurses	10 nurses	20 nurses
1 EH specialist	3 EH specialists	9 EH specialists
2 clerical staff	8 clerical staff	23 clerical staff
	1 nutritionist	3 nutritionists
	1 health educator	2 health educators
	1 EP coordinator	1 EP coordinator
		1 physician
		1 epidemiologist
		1 EH scientist
		1 IS specialist

three different jurisdiction sizes.[1] This analysis shows that LHDs serving small populations typically employ only a few different occupations: a manager or director, nurses, an EH specialist, and clerical staff. In these small LHDs, a single employee may serve in many roles (e.g., a nurse who provides clinical services, conducts disease investigation, and conducts health education and promotion). Certain specialized occupations (nutritionist, health educator, emergency preparedness coordinator) become common in LHDs serving 50,000 or more. Additional specialized occupations (physician, epidemiologist, EH scientist, and IS specialist) become common in LHDs serving 100,000 or more.

Recruitment and Retention of Local Health Department Staff

Like other sectors of public health, LHDs are faced with challenges in recruiting and retaining a competent and diverse workforce. A 2005 survey indicated that approximately 20 percent of LHD workers are eligible to retire within five years.[1] This survey also showed that many LHDs are having problems hiring certain occupations, including nurses, environmental health specialists and scientists, and epidemiologists. The reason for hiring problems cited most frequently was uncompetitive pay and benefits.[30] Difficulty attracting qualified candidates to their geographic area was also a problem for many LHDs, particularly those in rural areas. Efforts to provide public health educational opportunities to a diverse group of students, much as is being done for health care professions, could help alleviate the lack of diversity in many LHD jurisdictions.

PROFILE OF AGENCY TOP EXECUTIVES

The top agency executive of the LHD usually is also the health official, but in some departments, these responsibilities reside in two different individuals. The top agency executive bears responsibility for administrative issues and management of their agencies, and if they lack public health or medical training, they may rely on appropriately trained and licensed health officials or medical advisors to make health or medical decisions.

Selected Characteristics of Agency Top Executive

Most health departments (86%) are served by a full-time agency executive.[1] Not surprisingly, as the population of the jurisdiction served increases, the likelihood that the job of agency executive will be a full-time position also increases, from 80 percent in the smallest agencies to 100 percent in the largest.

Fifty-five percent of local health directors are female, and 92 percent of local health directors are white. Approximately 5 percent are African-American, 3 percent are other races, and 2 percent are of Hispanic ethnicity.[1] Larger LHDs are more likely to have a nonwhite director.[32]

Academic Degrees of Agency Top Executives

Most agency top executives have earned graduate level degrees.[1] Nineteen percent of local health directors have public health graduate degrees (MPH or DrPH), and 17 percent have medical degrees (MD, DVM, or DDS); these degrees are most common for leaders in large jurisdictions. Thirty-four percent of local health directors have nursing degrees (RN, BSN, or MSN), and nursing degrees are most common for leaders in small jurisdictions.

Tenure of Local Health Directors

In contrast to state health officials, many local health directors have been in their positions for many years. The mean tenure of a local health director in 2005 was 8 years, and one-third had held their current position for 10 years or more[1]. Health directors serving large jurisdictions have somewhat shorter tenures on average than those serving small jurisdictions (mean of 6 years for jurisdictions over 500,000 versus 8 years for jurisdictions under 500,000). By contrast, the average tenure of state health department directors in

2000 was 2 years.[46] Many attribute the difference in tenure to a lesser degree of politicization of health officer positions at the local level.

Duties of Local Health Officials

Local health officials have cited leadership, communication, working with elected officials, and financial planning and management as the most important abilities for leading LHDs.[47]

Leadership can be defined as "an activity, not a skill set."[48] Local public health leaders must embrace their role to "mobilize, coordinate and direct broad collaborative actions within the complex public health system,"[3] and take advantage of the many leadership training opportunities that exist.

Communication, with an emphasis on risk communication, is an especially crucial duty in public health. LHDs, as the "backbone" of the local public health system[2], need to have a leader who is skilled in communicating effectively with all entities that influence the public health. Additionally, they need to cultivate trust and credibility with the public they serve, and deliver information about public health threats in an open, honest, and compassionate manner.

Local health officials also need to understand the political environment, and educate decision makers about the return on investments realized through public health practice. Messages must be well-timed and framed within the current political climate. The ability to communicate with these insights, in a concise and compelling fashion, is at the heart of successful relationships with policy makers.

Financial planning and management has become increasingly important over the past several years. A long trend of dwindling federal dollars continues, and many local health officials continually need to do more with less.

FUTURE CONTEXT

Accreditation, attention to the root causes of health inequities, epidemics of chronic disease, and global climate change are anticipated to command the attention of local health officials throughout the beginning of the twenty-first century.

The Public Health Accreditation Board and related state-based accreditation programs provide a means for accountability, quality improvement, and consistency in public health practice. While the existing programs are overwhelmingly voluntary (Michigan and North Carolina are the only two states with mandatory accreditation programs for LHDs), many health departments are either participating or preparing to participate. Documented improvements in public health outcomes and performance offer an increased ability to show positive results of public health resource allocations. Demonstrating accountability in this manner affords visibility among policy makers and the public that public health sorely needs. Additionally, accreditation creates a platform for quality improvement activities that will help LHDs embrace that culture. Moreover, because all LHDs will be held to the same standards, accreditation promotes an unprecedented degree of consistency among local health jurisdictions across the country. Finally, as the number of accredited LHDs grows, it is anticipated that smaller health departments, with limited resources, will turn to regionalization and other means of enhancing capacity to meet the standards and become accredited.

While a wealth of research has demonstrated very disturbing health disparities among racially and ethnically diverse populations, a smaller but increasing body of evidence illustrates the need to address disparities in a broader sense, that is, by answering the question, "Why is there inequality and how can our organizational structure, policies, and practices change to eliminate health inequities?"[27] Health inequities are best addressed through principles of social justice, which include the following:

- Sustained action on the underlying injustice (racism, discrimination, and poverty) rather than treating symptoms or consequences

- Increasing the voice and influence of affected communities

- Convening relevant parties and institutions that can change social conditions

- Support for health equity as a social right[27]

A number of LHDs across the country are transforming public health practice, culture, and structure to address health inequities through these principles.[27] Sharing successes in this arena will facilitate their replication in jurisdictions around the country.

Because obesity is a risk factor for other conditions (e.g., diabetes, cardiovascular disease, and stroke),[49] it is likely that additional epidemics of chronic disease will develop and that advances in health education, behavior change modalities, and public policy will be made. Subsequently, LHDs are apt to find themselves implementing new interventions to combat the epidemics.

Scientists predict that global climate change will result in heat waves, flooding, droughts, air pollution, and intense storms such as hurricanes.[50] Although the health effects of this disturbing trend are not yet fully understood, at the very least, LHDs likely will fulfill many, if not all, of their current responsibilities for natural disasters. Additionally, as scientists learn more and issue additional predictions, and as the effects of global warming are realized, new roles for LHDs probably will emerge.

It is important to remember that unforeseen events also will occur. Regardless of the specific event, a robust government LHD is key to protecting and promoting the community's health. Effective local public health practice will be characterized by demonstrated accountability, heightened visibility, and rapid response to emerging public health threats and emergencies.

REVIEW QUESTIONS

1. What are some of the factors affecting local public health practice?
2. What are the advantages and disadvantages of the various types of governance for LHDs?
3. What are the factors contributing to the variation among services provided by LHDs?
4. Many people regard LHDs as publicly funded health care providers. What is a better description of the role of LHDs?
5. What considerations should drive a recruitment plan for the local public health workforce?

REFERENCES

1. *National Profile of Local Health Departments.* Washington, DC: National Association of County and City Health Officials; 2005.
2. Institute of Medicine, Committee for the Study of the Future of Public Health. *The Future of Public Health.* Washington, DC: National Academy Press; 1988.
3. Institute of Medicine, Committee on Assuring the Health of the Public in the 21st Century. *The Future of the Public's Health.* Washington, DC: National Academy Press; 2002.
4. Pickett G, Hanlon J. *Public Health: Administration and Practice.* St. Louis, MO: Times Mirror/Mosby College Publishing; 1990.
5. Mountin J, Flook E. *Guide to Health Organizations in the United States.* Washington, DC: US Public Health Service; 1953.
6. *National Profile of Local Health Departments.* Washington, DC: National Association of County and City Health Officials; 1990.
7. Turnock, B. *Public Health: What It Is and How It Works.* Gaithersburg, MD: Aspen Publishers, Inc; 1997.
8. Centers for Disease Control and Prevention Press Release, October 26, 1999. Available at: http://www.cdc.gov/OD/OC/MEDIA/pressrel/r991026.htm. Accessed December 15, 2007.
9. *Public Health in America.* Washington, DC: Public Health Functions Steering Committee; Fall 1994.
10. Available at: http://www.cdc.gov/od/ocphp/nphpsp. Accessed December 15, 2007.
11. Available at: http://www.healthypeople.gov. Accessed December 15, 2007.
12. Hebert K, Henderson M, Gursky E. Building preparedness by improving fiscal accountability. *Journal of Public Health Management and Practice.* 2007;13(2):200–201.
13. *Final Recommendations for a Voluntary National Accreditation Program for State and Local Health Departments.* Washington, DC: Exploring Accreditation Steering Committee; September 12, 2006. Available at: http://www.phaboard.org/Documents/finalrec.pdf.

14. Bender K, Benjamin G, Fallon M, Jarris P, Libbey P. Exploring accreditation: Striving for a consensus model. *Journal of Public Health Management and Practice*. 2007;13(4):334–336.

15. National Network of Public Health Institutes. http://www.nnphi.org/home/section/1–15//view/39/. Accessed December 15, 2007.

16. *Operational Definition of a Functional Local Health Department*. Washington, DC: National Association of County and City Health Officials; 2005.

17. Centers for Disease Control. *Profile of State and Territorial Public Health Systems*: US 1990. Washington, DC: US Department of Health and Human Services; 1991.

18. National Association of County and City Health Officials. *Research Brief Number 2: NACCHO Survey Examines State/Local Health Department Relationships*. Washington, DC: NACCHO; 1998.

19. Health Resources and Services Administration. *The Public Health Work Force: Enumeration 2000*. Rockville, MD: US Department of Health and Human Services; 2000.

20. Association of State and Territorial Health Officials. *2005 SHO Salary and Agency Infrastructure Survey*. Washington, DC: ASTHO; 2005.

21. Beitsch L, Brooks R, Menachemi N, Libbey P. Public Health at Center Stage: New Roles, Old Props. *Journal of Health Affairs*. 2006;25(24):12.

22. Unpublished database of local boards of health. Bowling Green, OH: National Association of County and City Health Officials; December 2007.

23. *National Profile of Local Boards of Health*. Washington, DC: National Association of Local Boards of Health; 1997.

24. Unpublished data. 2005 National Profile of Local Health Departments study.

25. FEMA. http://www.fema.gov/emergency/nims/index.shtm. Accessed December 15, 2007.

26. *Mobilizing for Action through Planning and Partnerships*. Washington, DC: National Association of County and City Health Officials; 2000.

27. *Tackling Health Inequities through Public Health Practice: A Handbook for Action*. Washington, DC: National Association of County and City Health Officials; 2007.

28. US Census Bureau. *Income, Poverty, and Health Insurance Coverage in the United States: 2004*. Washington, DC: US Government Printing Office; 2005.

29. Council on Linkages between Academia and Public Health Practice (2001). Core Competencies for Public Health Professionals. Available at: http://www.trainingfinder.org/competencies/list_nolevels.htm. Accessed October 14, 2008.

30. *A Global and National Implementation Plan for Public Health Workforce Development*. Atlanta, GA: Public Health Practice Program Office/Centers for Disease Control and Prevention; 2001.

31. Institute of Medicine, Committee on Institutional and Policy-Level Strategies for Increasing the Diversity of the US Healthcare Workforce. *In the Nation's Compelling Interest: Ensuring Diversity in the Health Care Workforce*. Washington, DC: National Academy Press; 2004.

32. National Association of County and City Health Officials. *Research Brief: Race and Ethnicity of Local Health Department Employees*. Washington, DC: NACCHO; 2007.

33. National Association of County and City Health Officials. Available at: http://www.naccho.org/topics/infrastructure/profile/upload/NACCHO_report_final_000.pdf. Accessed October 14, 2008.

34. CDC. Available at: http://www.thecommunityguide.org/index.html. Accessed December 15, 2007.

35. *Guide to Clinical Preventive Services, 2006*. AHRQ Publication No. 06-0588, June 2006. Agency for Healthcare Research and Quality: Rockville, MD. Available at: http://www.ahrq.gov/clinic/pocketgd.htm.

36. Partners in Information Access. Available at: http://phpartners.org/hp/index.html. Accessed December 15, 2007.

37. Public Health Improvement Project. Available at: http://www.doh.wa.gov/phip/documents/PerfMgmt/05EP/EPreport.pdf. Accessed December 15, 2007.

38. National Association of County and City Health Officials. Available at: http://www.naccho.org/topics/modelpractices/index.cfm. Accessed December 15, 2007.

39. Keck CW. Lessons learned from an academic health department. *J Public Health Management Practice*. 2000;6(1):47–52.

40. Conte C, CS Chang, J Malcolm, PG Russo. Academic health departments: From theory to practice. *J Public Health Management Practice*. 2006;12(1):6–14.

41. Swain GR, N Bennett, P Etkind, J Ransom. News from NACCHO: Local health department and academic partnerships: Education beyond the ivy walls. *J Public Health Management Practice.* 2006;12(1):33–36.

42. Maeshiro R. Health departments and medical schools. *J Public Health Management Practice.* 2006;12(1):31–32.

43. Boex JR, CW Keck, E Piatt, TN Nunthirapikorn, RS Blacklow. Academic health centers and public health departments: Partnership matters. *Am J Prev Med.* 2006;30(1):89–93.

44. Livingood WC, J Goldhagen, WL Little, J Gornto, T Hou. Assessing the status of partnerships between academic institutions and public health agencies. *Am J Pub Health.* 2007;97(4):659–666.

45. US Census Bureau. Federal, *State, and Local Governments Public Employment and Payroll Data.* 2005. Available at: http://www.census.gov/govs/www/apes.html. Accessed December 15, 2007.

46. *Study of State Health Official Turnover.* Washington, DC: Association of State and Territorial Health Officials; 2000.

47. Unpublished data from New Local Health Official Orientation Environmental Scan. Washington, DC: National Association of County and City Health Officials; 2007.

48. National Public Health Institute. Available at: http://www.phli.org/. Accessed December 15, 2007.

49. Centers for Disease Control and Prevention. Available at: http://www.cdc.gov/nccdphp/dnpa/obesity/. Accessed December 15, 2007.

50. Centers for Disease Control and Prevention. Available at: http://www.cdc.gov/Features/ClimateChange/. Accessed December 15, 2007.

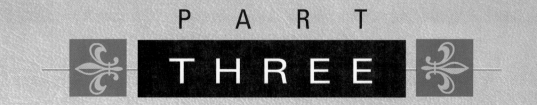

PART
THREE

Tools for Public Health Practice

CHAPTER 11

Epidemiology and Public Health Data

Donna F. Stroup, PhD, MSc and Stephen B. Thacker, MD, MSc

LEARNING OBJECTIVES

Upon completion of this chapter, the reader will be able to:

1. Understand the basic definition and components of public health surveillance as they relate to Essential Service 1: Monitor health status to identify community health problems.

2. Identify and evaluate relevant public health data sources.

3. Recognize and apply ethical principles to the conduct of public health surveillance.

4. Be able to apply basic analytic methods to surveillance data for temporal, personal, and spatial analysis.

5. Understand the basic definition and common study designs for epidemiology as they relate to Essential Service 2: Diagnose and investigate health problems and health hazards in the community.

6. Recognize common forms of bias in the interpretation of epidemiologic data.

7. Be able to compute and interpret measures of risk.

8. Understand effective communication principles and relationships with the media.

9. Recognize culturally appropriate ways of conducting public health surveillance and epidemiologic studies.

10. Recognize how epidemiologic and public health surveillance data can contribute to public health policy decisions.

KEY TERMS

Acceptability

Age Adjustment

Age Standardized

Agent Factors

Alternative Hypothesis

Analytic Epidemiology

Attack Rate

Attributable

Bias

Biologic and Chemical Terrorism

Capture-Recapture Methodology

Case-Control Study

Case Definition

Chance

ACKNOWLEDGEMENTS: Richard C. Dicker is the author of some of the material on epidemiology, which we have retained from an earlier edition. We thank Kaye Smith-Aiken for excellent editing and Jim Walters for assistance with figure preparation.

Chi-Square Test

Cohort Study

Competency Domains

Confidence Interval

Confidentiality

Confounding

Coroner

Cumulative Incidence Rate

Descriptive Epidemiology

Determinant

Disability-Adjusted Life Years (DALYs)

Distribution

Environmental Factors

Epidemic Period

Ethical Standards

Evaluation

Experimental Study

Fisher Exact Test

Health Insurance Portability and Accountability Act (HIPAA)

Health Policy

Health Problem

Health Service

Host Factors

Incidence

Information Bias

Investigator Error

Medical Examiner

Morbidity

Mortality

Natality

National Notifiable Diseases Surveillance System

Null Hypothesis

Observational Study

Odds Ratio

P Value

Pathognomonic

Personal Identifier

Person-Time Rate

Positive Predictive Value

Prevalence

Prevalence Odds Ratio

Prevented Fraction

Privacy

Quality-Adjusted Life Years (QALYs)

Randomized Controlled Trial

Rate

Relative Risk

Representativeness

Risk

Risk Ratio

Secondary Attack Rate

Secular Trend

Security

Selection Bias

Sensitivity

Sentinel Surveillance

Social Determinants

Smoothing Techniques

Standardized Mortality/Morbidity Ratio (SMR)

Statisticians

Timeliness

Time-Series

Two-By-Two Table

Vital Events

Vital Statistics

Years of Potential Life Lost (YPLL)

To address the increasing complexity of public health practice,[1] the Council on Linkages Between Academia and Public Health Practice developed public health competencies linked to 10 essential public health services.[2] In this chapter, we consider how physicians' skills in epidemiology and understanding of public health data can contribute to competencies in Essential Services 1 and 2. Specifically, we use the principles and practice of public health surveillance to address **competency domains** in Essential Service 1, monitoring health status to identify community health problems. We define and discuss epidemiology, the basic science of public health, to address competency domains in Essential Service 2, diagnosing and investigating health problems and health hazards in the community. In this discussion, we indicate where epidemiology and public health data can be used to address selected competencies in the other Essential Services.

The Essential Services contain eight competency domains:

1. Analytic assessment skills
2. Policy development/program planning skills
3. Communication skills
4. Cultural competency skills
5. Community dimensions of practice skills
6. Basic public health science skills
7. Financial planning and management skills
8. Leadership and systems-thinking skills

ESSENTIAL SERVICE 1, MONITORING HEALTH STATUS TO IDENTIFY COMMUNITY HEALTH PROBLEMS

Public health surveillance is the ongoing systematic collection, analysis, and dissemination of health data to those who need to have them. The final link in the surveillance chain is the application of these data to disease prevention and injury control.[3] Surveillance in public health is information for action.

The idea of collecting data, analyzing them, and considering a reasonable public health response to them stems from Hippocrates.[4] Perhaps the first public health action that can be attributed to using surveillance data occurred in the 1300s, when public health authorities in a port near the Republic of Venice prevented passengers from coming ashore during the time of epidemic bubonic plague in Europe.

Domain 1: Analytic Assessment Skills

In the late 1940s, Alexander Langmuir, the first chief epidemiologist of the Communicable Disease Center (now the Centers for Disease Control and Prevention) and the founder of modern concepts of surveillance, broadened the idea of surveillance. Previously, public health surveillance consisted of watching persons at **risk** for specific disease at quarantine stations. Langmuir changed the focus to watching for diseases such as malaria and smallpox. He emphasized rapid collection and analysis of data on a particular disease, as well as quick dissemination of the findings to those who needed the information.[5]

Today, this credo of rapid reporting, analysis, and action applies to approximately 100 infectious diseases and adverse health events of noninfectious etiology at the local, state, and national levels. Ongoing systems of reporting often have resulted from local or national emergencies, such as the discovery of contaminated lots of poliovirus vaccine during the first national vaccination program in 1955, the pandemic Asian influenza in 1957, the outbreak of shellfish-associated hepatitis A in 1961, the appearance of toxic shock syndrome in 1980, the discovery of the hantavirus pulmonary syndrome in the Four Corners area in 1994, the widespread outbreaks of *Escherichia coli* O157:H7 in 1994–1999, an outbreak of West Nile encephalitis in the Northeast in 1999, and the severe acute respiratory syndrome (SARS) pandemic in 2003.

Within days of the investigation of L-tryptophan-associated eosinophilia myalgia syndrome (EMS) in 1990, for example, a national reporting system was implemented for this previously rare and nonreportable condition. And in 2001, in response to anthrax attacks, surveillance for anthrax was quickly implemented[6] to define the problem related to biologic and chemical terrorism (specific competency 1).

Defining a Problem and Other Purposes of Public Health Surveillance

Being able to define a public health problem is, as noted above, the first competency in Domain 1—if a problem cannot be recognized and defined, no surveillance of the problem is possible. And public health surveillance is critical, because it is fundamental to decision making, policy development, program planning (see "Domain 4: Cultural Competency Skills"), and sometimes crisis management. The primary purposes of a surveillance system are:

- describing trends and the natural history of health problems,

- detecting epidemics, providing details about patterns of disease, monitoring changes in disease agents through laboratory testing, planning and setting health program priorities,

- evaluating the effects of control and prevention measures,

- detecting critical changes in health practice,

- evaluating hypotheses about the cause of health problems,

- detecting rare but important cases of disease, such as botulism, and

- generating hypotheses for research.

The Surveillance Cycle

For greatest effectiveness, public health surveillance is conducted in a systematic cycle (Figure 11.1) that has four major steps:

1. collection of data (pertinent, regular, frequent, prompt, timely),

2. consolidation and interpretation of data (orderly, descriptive, evaluative, prompt, timely),

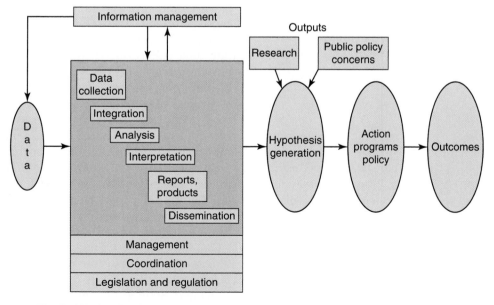

Figure 11.1. The Public Health Surveillance Cycle

3. dissemination of information (prompt, timely; disseminated to all who need to know [e.g., data providers for confirmation and support], policy makers, and action takers), and

4. prompt, targeted action to control existing problems and promptly prevent future ones.

Originally applied only to infectious diseases, the surveillance cycle is now also used in prevention and control programs for injury, cancer, certain cardiovascular diseases, diabetes, and high-risk and unintended pregnancies. Specifically, the surveillance cycle highlights three key points that may be overlooked by for policy makers and program managers (Essential Service 5):

- Promptness is critical at every step of the cycle and is given priority over meticulousness. As a result, changes might occur in surveillance data that do not occur in vital statistics or in the majority of health survey data.

- Reports based on surveillance data are highly descriptive; that is, for the most part, surveillance data provide the numerator for estimated rates of disease occurrence. Surveillance reports generate hypotheses and indicate causes of health problems rather than confirm or establish them.

- Under rare circumstances, surveillance systems are deactivated. For example, when smallpox was eradicated, surveillance was terminated because the smallpox virus was no longer a public health threat.

Case Definition

A **case definition** is a set of standard criteria for determining whether a person should be categorized as having a particular disease or health-related condition. A case definition consists of clinical criteria and sometimes specifies time, place, and person. The clinical criteria usually include confirmatory laboratory tests, if available, or combinations of symptoms, signs, and other findings. For example, the case definition for human rabies requires laboratory confirmation (Figure 11.2a). In contrast, the case definition for Kawasaki syndrome, a febrile rash illness of children with no known cause and no **pathognomonic** laboratory findings, is based on the presence of fever, at least four of five specified clinical findings, and no other explanation for the findings (Figure 11.2b).

Use of a standard case definition increases consistency of surveillance data across time, location, and source of report. For example, the current number of cases of hepatitis A in one area can be compared with the numbers in the same area over time and to the numbers in surrounding areas. When standard case definitions are used, an excess number of observed cases is more likely to represent a true outbreak rather than variation in diagnostic criteria.

Case definitions might vary, depending on purpose and setting. In conducting surveillance for a rare but serious communicable disease, a sensitive case definition, one that is good at identifying true cases (but that may suffer from a high false positive rate), is appropriate. Local health officials need to hear about a patient with clinical findings consistent with plague or foodborne botulism, even if confirmatory laboratory results are still pending, so that they could begin planning the appropriate public health measures that might be required. Similarly, in areas of the world where malaria is endemic but diagnostic tools are rare, the case definition for malaria might be as simple as "fever." In contrast, when conducting epidemiologic research into the cause of disease, the information that the patients have the disease under study is important for accurate data collection. Therefore, the investigator is likely to prefer a specific or "strict" case definition, so that false positives do not bias the analysis.

Critical steps have been taken for standardizing case definitions for both infectious and chronic conditions. In the United States, uniform criteria have been developed for state health department personnel to use when reporting notifiable diseases to the Centers for Disease Control and Prevention (CDC).[7] Based in part on the use of these uniform criteria, as well as the increasing burden of noninfectious conditions throughout the world, the CDC, the Council of State and Territorial Epidemiologists (CSTE), and state chronic disease directors developed the Indicators for Chronic Disease Surveillance.[8] Standard definitions were developed for 73 indicators, selected because of their importance to public health and the availability of state-level

a. Rabies, Human

Clinical Description

Rabies is an acute encephalomyelitis that almost always progresses to coma or death within 10 days after the first symptom.

Laboratory Criteria for Diagnosis

- Detection by direct fluorescent antibody of viral antigens in a clinical specimen (preferably the brain or the nerves surrounding hair follicles in the nape of the neck); or
- Isolation (in cell culture or in a laboratory animal) of rabies virus from saliva, cerebrospinal fluid (CSF), or central nervous system tissue; or
- Identification of a rabies-neutralizing antibody titer greater than or equal to 5 (complete neutralization) in the serum or CSF of an unvaccinated person.

Case Classification

Confirmed: a clinically compatible case that is laboratory confirmed.

Comment

Laboratory confirmation by all of the above methods is strongly recommended.

SOURCE: CDC. Case definitions for infectious conditions under public health surveillance. MMWR. 1997;46:RR10.

b. Kawasaki Syndrome

Clinical Case Definition

A febrile illness of greater than or equal to 5 days' duration, with at least four of the five following physical findings and no other more reasonable explanation for the observed clinical findings:

- Bilateral conjunctival injection; or
- Oral changes (erythema of lips or oropharynx, strawberry tongue, or fissuring of the lips); or
- Peripheral extremity changes (edema, erythema, or generalized or periungual desquamation); or
- Rash; or
- Cervical lymphadenopathy (at least one lymph node greater than or equal to 1.5 cm in diameter).

Laboratory Criteria for Diagnosis

None.

Case Classification

Confirmed: a case that meets the clinical case definition.

Comment

If fever disappears after intravenous gamma globulin therapy is started, fever may be of less than five days' duration, and the clinical case definition may still be met.

SOURCE: CDC. Case definitions for infectious conditions under public health surveillance. MMWR. 1990;39:RR13.

Figure 11.2. Case Definitions for Selected Infectious Conditions

data. Of the indicators, there are 24 for cancer; 15 for cardiovascular disease; 11 for diabetes; 7 for alcohol; 5 each for nutrition and tobacco; 3 each for oral health, physical activity, and renal disease; and 2 each for asthma, osteoporosis, and immunizations. The remaining 10 indicators cover overarching conditions (Figure 11.3).

Attributes of a Surveillance System

To aid in system development and evaluation, defining the attributes of a public health surveillance system is helpful.[9] We cover analytic methods

for assessing these attributes later in this chapter, when discussing Domain 6, basic public health science skills. The eight basic attributes of any surveillance activity are:

- simplicity (elegance of design, limitation of size, ease of operation);
- flexibility (ability of the system to adapt to changing needs, such as the addition of new conditions or data-collection elements);
- **acceptability** (willingness of people and organizations to participate in the surveillance system,

Title	Age (years)	Sex	Data Source*
Poverty	All	Both	CPS
High school completion	18–24	Both	CPS
Life expectancy at birth	All	Both	Vital Statistics
Lack of health insurance	18–64	Both	BRFSS
Self-assessed health status	$\geq = 18$	Both	BRFSS
Recent mental health	$\geq = 18$	Both	BRFSS
Recent activity limitation	$\geq = 18$	Both	BRFSS

Figure 11.3. **Selected Overarching Conditions for Chronic Disease Surveillance**

*BRFSS = Behavioral Risk Factor Surveillance System; CPS = Current Population Survey

SOURCE: CDC, the Council of State and Territorial Epidemiologists, and the Association of State and Territorial Chronic Disease Program Directors. Indicators for Chronic Disease Surveillance. MMWR 2004; 53(RR11);1–6.

including persons involved from outside the sponsoring agency);

- **sensitivity** (completeness of case reporting—the proportion of cases of a disease or health event that are detected by the surveillance system; also used to denote the ability of the surveillance system to detect aberrations or epidemics);

- **positive predictive value** (the proportion of persons identified as case-patients who actually have the condition being monitored);

- **representativeness** (extent to which the data accurately describe the occurrence of a health event over time and its distribution in the population by place and person; includes concepts of case ascertainment bias [discussed in a later section], as well as bias in descriptive information about a reported case [e.g., diagnostic misclassification]);

- **timeliness** (delay between any two or more steps in a surveillance system [e.g., diagnosis and report], best assessed by the ability of the system to provide information for appropriate public health action); and

- cost (resources used to operate the surveillance system, including costs of data collection and analysis as well as costs of analyzing and disseminating information resulting from the system).

These attributes are interdependent in multiple ways. Simplicity is essential if data quality is to be maintained and if consolidation, interpretation, and dissemination are to be implemented promptly. Acceptability is required because voluntary cooperation from both patients and busy public health practitioners is the cornerstone of data collection. Sensitivity and a high positive predictive value are important because surveillance is one approach to screening for the health problems of a community, especially for epidemic diseases and clusters of health events, such as injuries.

Flexibility is critical because surveillance systems often prove to be the only mechanism for detecting new and emerging public health problems. This was the case in detecting West Nile encephalitis and in finding penicillinase-producing Neisseria gonorrhea. Representativeness is necessary if the system is to reflect accurately the occurrence of health problems in all sectors of a geographic area. Finally, timeliness and cost must be an integral part of any surveillance system that is expected to detect health problems and to lead to the institution of effective control and prevention measures.

Evaluation

Evaluation refers to the systematic investigation of the merit, worth, or significance of an object.[10] Since 1970, the practice of evaluation has evolved as a discipline with new definitions, methods, approaches, and applications to diverse subjects and settings.[11] For example, evaluations are generally expected to include a logic model to describe associations among program components and expected and likely outcomes,[12] such as was developed as a strategy for increasing attention to mental health in national surveillance activities.[13]

Evaluation of an operating surveillance system aims to increase the system's utility and efficiency. Evaluation of surveillance systems should address these questions:

1. Is the health event under surveillance of continuing public health importance?

2. Is the surveillance system useful and cost effective? and

3. Are the attributes of the quality of the surveillance system (see the following section) addressed adequately?

In addition, with the continuing advancement of technology and importance of informatics, certain informatics criteria should be reviewed routinely (e.g., hardware/software, interface, data format/coding, and quality checks). The decision to establish, maintain, or de-emphasize a surveillance system should be guided by assessments based on these questions. Ultimately, that decision rests on whether a health event under surveillance is a public health priority, and whether the system is useful and cost-effective.

Relevant Data and Information Sources

Multiple sources of data are useful for monitoring health and identifying problems. These sources include vital statistics, morbidity reporting systems, sentinel providers, risk factor assessment systems, laboratory systems, syndromic surveillance, surveys, registries, and other administrative systems (Table 11.1). We describe selected examples of these systems here. More complete information is available elsewhere.[14]

Vital Statistics. The documentation of **vital events** (births and deaths) is one of the oldest and most complete public sources of health information for the United States and the majority of economically developed countries. The first Bill of Mortality was issued in London in 1532 in response to the fear of a plague epidemic. John Graunt's treatise *Natural and Political Observations on the Bills of Mortality* (1662) is generally recognized as one of the first documents to describe the use of numerical methods for monitoring public health.[15] William Farr, the Superintendent of the Statistical Department of the General Registrar's Office in Great Britain from 1839 to 1879, collected, analyzed, and interpreted vital statistics and disseminated the information in weekly, quarterly, and annual reports.[16] To standardize data on vital statistics, the first international list of causes of death was developed in 1893.[17] In 2006, mortality analysts throughout the world use *International Classification of Diseases* (ICD) 10 codes, which is the tenth revision of the 1893 list.[18]

In the United States, each birth or death certificate contains an individual identifier (e.g., social security number, name), geographic location, date, and personal characteristics (e.g., sex, race, and education for death certificates [see http://www.cdc.gov/nchs]). Data from birth certificates are generally more complete than those of deaths and include length of pregnancy, birth weight, time and place of birth, and selected information on maternal characteristics (e.g., prenatal care and smoking during pregnancy).[19] Linked birth-death files can be used for maternal and infant mortality studies (http://www.cdc.gov/nchs/linked.htm). Data from vital statistics systems have been used for surveillance of mortality associated with acute events (e.g., heat waves[20] and influenza[21]) (Figure 11.4).

Despite these uses, data from vital statistics systems pose certain challenges for public health decision making. First, editing, aggregation, and dissemination might not be done quickly enough for public health intervention. For example, national mortality data are not available for up to 3 years, although a 10 percent sample is available within 12 months of the close of the calendar year.[22] More timely weekly reporting of deaths from 122 United States cities to the CDC has been integral to

Table 11.1. **Selected Public Health Data Sources and Internet Sites**

Data Source	Internet Site
AIDS public use data	http://www.cdc.gov/hiv/software/apids/apidsman.htm
Behavioral Risk Factor Surveillance System	http://www.cdc.gov/brfss
Cancer: Surveillance, Epidemiology and End Results (SEER) data	http://seer.cancer.gov
Consumer Product Safety Commission (CPSC)	http://www.cpsc.gov
Council of State and Territorial Epidemiologists (CSTE)	http://www.cste.org
Food and Drug Administration (FDA)	http://www.fda.gov
Hazardous Substance Release/Health Effects	http://www.atsdr.cdc.gov/hazdat.html
Healthy People 2010 Data	http://www.cdc.gov/nchs/hphome.htm
International Classification of Disease (ICD) Codes	http://www.cdc.gov/nchs/ datawh/nchsdefs/icd.htm
International Vital Statistics (WHO)	http://www.who.int/en/
National Health and Nutrition Examination Survey (NHANES)	http://www.cdc.gov/nchs/nhanes.htm
National Health Care Survey	http://www.cdc.gov/nchs/nhcs.htm
National Health Interview Survey (NHIS)	http://www.cdc.gov/nchs/nhis.htm
National Immunization Survey	http://www.cdc.gov/nchs/nis
National Institute on Drug Abuse (NIDA)	http://www.nida.nih.gov
National Maternal/Infant Health Survey	http://www.cdc.gov/nchs/about/major/nmihs/abnmihs.htm
National Mortality Followback Survey	http://www.cdc.gov/nchs/data/nmfs/nmfsag.pdf
National Notifiable Diseases Surveillance System	http://wonder.cdc.gov/ mmwr/mmwrmorb.asp
National Oral Health Surveillance System	http://www.cdc.gov/nohss
National Survey of Family Growth	http://www.cdc.gov/nchs/nsfg.htm
National Vital Statistics System	http://www.cdc.gov/nchs/nvss.htm
Pediatric and Pregnancy Nutrition Surveillance	http://www.cdc.gov/pednss
PulseNet	http://www.cdc.gov/pulsenet
Sexually transmitted diseases	http://www.cdc.gov/nchstp/dstd/Stats_Trends/Stats_and_Trends.htm
Tuberculosis incidence	http://www.cdc.gov/nchstp/tb/surv/surv.htm
State and Local Area Integrated Telephone Survey (SLAITS)	http://www.cdc.gov/nchs/slaits.htm
U.S. Department of the Interior, Water Quality	http://www.doi.gov
U.S. Department of Transportation, Fatality Analysis Reporting System (FARS)	http://www-fars.nhtsa.dot.gov
U.S. Department of Labor, Employment	http://www.dol.gov
Web-based Injury Statistics Query and Reporting System	http://www.cdc.gov/ncipc/wisqars
Youth Risk Behavior Surveillance System	http://www.cdc.gov/HealthyYouth/yrbs

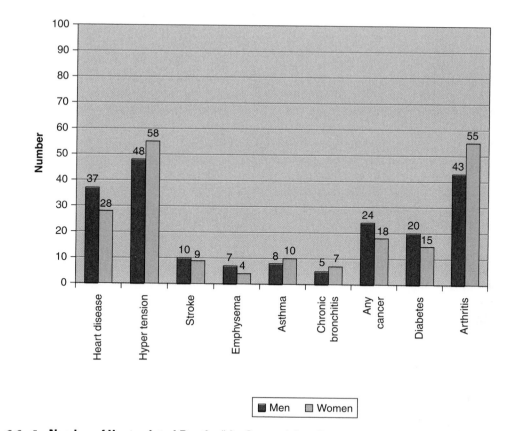

Figure 11.4. Number of Heat-related Deaths,* by Sex and Age Group—United States, 1999–2003

*Exposure to extreme heat is reported as the underlying cause of or a contributing factor to death ($N = 3,442$).

SOURCE: Centers for Disease Control and Prevention. Heat-related deaths United States, 1999–2003. Morb Mortal Wkly Rep MMWR. 2006;55:796–798.

surveillance for influenza epidemics.[23] In addition, automated systems for coding mortality information will move data from clinician to public health practice and should aid in increasing timeliness, both in the United States and internationally (see the section on Informatics).

Second, because the primary purpose of mortality data collection is legal (to aid in burial or criminal investigation), data elements in mortality systems might be limited. For example, the coding of data on external cause (E-code) might not allow investigation of mechanism or manner of injury for prevention and control efforts.[24] For deaths han-

dled by **medical examiners** and **coroners**, more detailed descriptions of circumstances surrounding deaths, including autopsy reports, toxicology studies, and police reports, can be useful.[25]

Third, not all characteristics are reported with full accuracy. Reporting of socioeconomic information related to health (e.g., race, education, and income) is a particular problem because it is reported to bias and may be reported incompletely.[26] Furthermore, information on geographic location should be interpreted with care, because the data might indicate the location where the certificate was completed (e.g., hospital) rather than the place where the vital event occurred (e.g., home or workplace). In addition, using coding schemes developed for underlying cause versus multiple causes of death requires careful statistical examination.[27]

Fourth, mortality statistics might be limited further in developing countries where death registration is inadequate or nonexistent. The use of verbal autopsies, in which a caretaker is interviewed to determine the cause of death, might assist surveillants in following mortality patterns in places without routine death registration.[28] The attributed cause of death might be less accurate in such autopsies for certain acute febrile conditions (e.g., malaria) than for such conditions as maternal causes, injuries, tuberculosis (TB), and acquired immunodeficiency syndrome (AIDS). Also, different techniques in conducting verbal autopsies might affect the accuracy of diagnosis.

Fifth, in all countries, the accuracy and specificity of certain diagnoses is limited as a result of changes in the use of diagnostic categories and codes over time and of the variation in the quality of information. A 1978 study revealed that seven countries in Europe and North America agreed only 53 percent of the time is assigning codes for the underlying cause in a sample of 1,246 deaths.[29] Finally, analysts who use mortality data should consider the impact of using underlying versus multiple cause of death coding.[30]

Despite these limitations, vital statistics are "vital" to surveillance activities. Death certificates have been used to demonstrate progress toward reduction in maternal mortality in association with increased use of prenatal care and other factors. Analyses of death certificates in the United States have highlighted racial differences in mortality rates over time, differences in maternal mortality rates, and preventable premature mortality specific to different populations.

Morbidity Reporting. In 1899, the United Kingdom began compulsory notification of incidence of selected infectious diseases; in 1907, the Office International d'Hygiene Publique, predominantly composed of European member states, was created to collect morbidity data.[31] In the United States, national morbidity data for incidence of

plague, smallpox, and yellow fever was initiated in 1878, and by 1925, all states were reporting weekly to the U.S. Public Health Service on the occurrence of selected diseases. Morbidity surveillance is illustrated by the **National Notifiable Disease Surveillance System**. Physicians, laboratorians, and other health care providers are required by state law to report all cases of health conditions that are notifiable, the majority of which are infectious diseases (http://www.cdc.gov/epo/dphsi/casedef/). Authority to modify the list of notifiable diseases is often granted to the state health officer; in certain states, each change must be newly legislated. Completeness and timeliness of reporting is influenced by the disease severity, availability of public health measures, public concern, ease of reporting, and physician appreciation of public health practice in the community.[32]

Reporting is typically incomplete for the majority of notifiable diseases, and this incompleteness is attributable to multiple causes. Persons who are asymptomatic or having mild symptoms might not seek health care. Patients and physicians might conceal diseases that carry a social stigma or might have adverse consequences in insurability or quality of care. Health care providers might fail to report because they are unaware of regulations or because they might treat the symptoms without a complete laboratory investigation. Completeness of reporting might also be significantly influenced by factors such as medical community interest and publicity; the most important is probably the intensity of surveillance efforts, which is linked to availability of resources. For example, a study of underreporting of acute viral hepatitis in the United States demonstrated that homosexual men with hepatitis B and blood transfusion recipients with non-A non-B hepatitis were less likely to be reported than members of other risk groups.[33]

Still, incomplete data can be useful. Epidemics, as well as general temporal and geographic trends, can be determined as long as the proportion of cases detected remains consistent over time and across geographic areas. A comparison between cases of viral hepatitis reported by practitioners in private practice and cases reported in a population covered by an insurance plan in Israel demonstrated that, although completeness of reporting by the physicians was only 37 percent, the distribution of reported cases by season and age was similar to that recorded among the insured population.[34]

Sentinel Providers. Networks of health care providers have been organized into **sentinel surveillance** systems to gather information on selected health events. The majority of these networks have been organized by practicing physicians on a voluntary basis; in certain European countries, these networks have formed firm associations with public health authorities and academic centers, and often form the basis for morbidity surveillance.[35] In the United States, the CDC maintains a sentinel health event verification system for occupational risk, which is a state-based network of health care providers that focuses on reporting specific occupational conditions.[36]

The strengths of sentinel provider systems include the participants' commitment, the possibility of collecting longitudinal data, the system's flexibility in addressing a changing set of conditions, and the ability to gain information on all patient-provider encounters, regardless of severity of illness. The most severe limitation of this type of system is that the population served by these physicians might not be representative of the general population. In addition, the illness must be fairly common to provide representative incidence data from a limited sample of physician contacts. For example, a voluntary network of general practitioners in Belgium was initiated in 1978,[37] and its selected practitioners were representative of Belgian general practitioners according to age, sex, and geographic location. These practitioners provided weekly reports to the network, and they were sent a summary of results each quarter. The list of health problems included vaccine-preventable diseases, respiratory conditions, and suicide attempts, and selected health problems, such as mumps and measles, reported continuously, while others were reported less frequently. A high level of participation was documented, with the degree of form completion and continuity of reporting as criteria for assessment. The network was evaluated in terms of possible **biases** (e.g., nonparticipation of practitioners and difficulties in estimating the population at risk for the health problems under study); subsequently, methods have been developed to reduce these biases.[38]

Risk Factor Assessment Systems. For certain chronic conditions, morbidity data typically come from population surveys, registries, and health services sources (see later discussion in this chapter) to assess the magnitude and changes in known risk factors, daily living habits, health care, major social and economic features, and morbidity and mortality.[39] The surveillance of risk factors for a condition is a particularly useful approach for chronic diseases, because of both the long latency between exposure and disease, and the multifactor etiology of the majority of chronic conditions. In addition, selected risk factors can be addressed effectively by policy, laws, or comprehensive community approaches.[40]

In the United States, selected risk factors are monitored by the Behavioral Risk Factor Surveillance System (BRFSS), the world's largest, ongoing telephone health survey system, which has tracked health conditions and risk behaviors in the United States yearly since 1984. BRFSS is conducted by the 50 state health departments and those in the District of Columbia, Puerto Rico, Guam, and the U.S. Virgin Islands, with support from the CDC. It provides state-specific information about such health concerns as asthma, diabetes, health care access, alcohol use, hypertension, obesity, cancer screening, nutrition and physical activity, and tobacco use. Federal, state, and local health officials and researchers use this information to track health risks, identify emerging problems, prevent disease, and improve treatment recommendations.[41] Recently, the BRFSS sample size was expanded to allow analysis of data from selected metropolitan and micropolitan areas[42] (Figure 11.5).

Risk-factor surveillance in environmental public health involves hazards and exposures as well as outcomes. An example of a hazard surveillance source is the environmental air-monitoring data from 4,000 state and local monitoring sites in the United States, the collection of which is mandated by the Clean Air Act.[43] Data are collected and

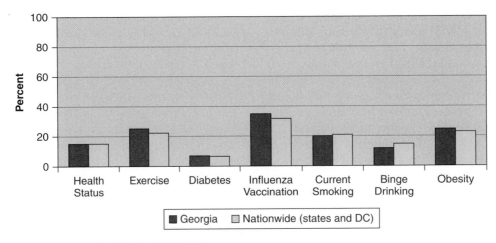

Figure 11.5. SMART* BRFSS, Georgia, 2004

*Selected Metropolitan/Micropolitan Area Risk Trends from the Behavioral Risk Factor Surveillance System.

SOURCE: Centers for Disease Control and Prevention (CDC). Behavior Risk Factor Surveillance System: turning information into health [homepage on the Internet]. Atlanta, GA: US Department of Health and Human Services, CDC; 2006. Available at: http://www.cdc.gov/brfes/. Accessed October 5, 2006.

published routinely for six air pollutants (carbon monoxide, lead, nitrogen dioxide, ozone, particulate matter, and sulfur dioxide) covered by the national air-quality standards.[44] An example of exposure surveillance is the use of the results of blood lead testing among children, used to assess the effectiveness of programs designed to reduce environmental lead hazards.[45]

Laboratory Systems. The data from laboratories are critical in confirming reports of certain infectious conditions and of certain chronic conditions (e.g., chronic viral hepatitis or hemoglobin A1C for diabetes). In the United States, reporting from the majority of public health laboratories is automated.[46] In England, microbiology laboratories report specified infections each week to the Communicable Disease Surveillance Centre.[47] The advantages of a laboratory-reporting system are specificity, flexibility in adding new diseases, timeliness, and the amount of detail that can be provided. Reports can indicate trends or the appearance of

rare infections originating from a common source that could not be identified by a single laboratory. One disadvantage of this type of system is that the number of persons from whom specimens are collected and tested usually is not reported. In addition, the persons tested might not be representative of the population at risk. Further, whereas laboratory reporting provides details about the microorganism, it often lacks key information about the patient (e.g., risk factors or exposures). For certain infections (e.g., toxic shock syndrome) no laboratory test is available, and for certain common illnesses, a patient specimen might not be taken (e.g., influenza).

In hospitals, nosocomial infection surveillance is often based on a review of laboratory records by an infection-control nurse or other designated staff. The National Nosocomial Infection Study was initiated to monitor the frequency and trends of nosocomial infection in United States hospitals. Approximately 160 hospitals participate in a voluntary national surveillance system, with microbiology

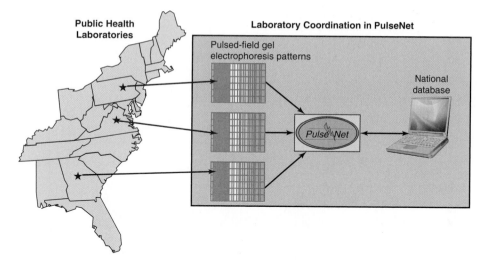

Figure 11.6. **PulseNet: The National Molecular Subtyping Network for Foodborne Disease Surveillance**

SOURCE: Centers for Disease Control and Prevention (CDC). PulseNet [homepage on the Internet]. Atlanta, GA: US Department of Health and Human Services, CDC; 2006. Available at: http://www.cdc.gov/pulsenet/. Accessed October 5, 2006.

studies reported on 90 percent of infected patients.[48] A network of medical center laboratories throughout the world conducts surveillance of antibiotic resistance for different pathogens.[49]

Molecular biology has enhanced surveillance in public health. In the United States, data from public health laboratories that perform DNA "fingerprinting" on bacteria are collected in a network known as PulseNet[50] (Figure 11.6). The network permits rapid comparison of these fingerprint patterns through an electronic database. For example, similar pulsed-field gel electrophoresis patterns of *E. coli* O157:H7 bacteria isolated from ill persons demonstrate that the bacteria come from a common source (e.g., a widely distributed contaminated food product.[51])

Syndromic Surveillance. The need for a strong infrastructure for data and information systems is being reemphasized today, not only as countries face the emergence and reemergence of infectious diseases,[52] but also as a result of the

increasing threat of biologic and chemical terrorism.[53] Plans for detecting terrorist events include strengthening current surveillance systems from clinicians, hospitals, and laboratories, as well as establishing new ones. Recent developments in surveillance for terrorism-related outbreak detection includes surveillance for syndromes, rather than specific diseases; this type of surveillance is called *syndromic surveillance*[54]; these systems can be very timely because the clinical signs and symptoms are available prior to the availability of laboratory testing syndromes rather than laboratory results are used. Additionally, states and local areas have used existing clinical, administrative, pharmacy, and laboratory data, as well as surveillance of emergency calls for medical assistance, admissions of patients to intensive-care units for respiratory conditions, and over-the-counter medication sales[55-57] (Figure 11.7). Although syndromic surveillance is a relatively new methodology, its activities have been evaluated, and their utility has been demonstrated for public health in the twenty-first century.[58] (We

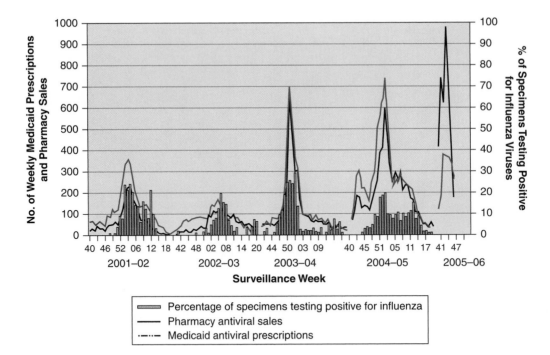

Figure 11.7. Number of Weekly Medicaid Prescriptions and Pharmacy Sales of Antiviral Influenza Medications versus Percentage of Specimens Testing Positive for Influenza Viruses by Surveillance Week—New York City, 2001–02, 2002–03, 2004–05, and 2005–06 Influenza Seasons

SOURCE: Centers for Disease Control and Prevention. Increased antiviral medication sales before the 2005–06 influenza season New York City. Morb Mortal Wkly Rep MMWR. 2006; 55:277–279.

discuss methods for analyzing data from syndromic surveillance systems in the section on basic public health sciences skills in this chapter.)

Surveys. Household surveys of the general population are effective surveillance activities. The National Health Interview Survey conducted in the United States (http://www.cdc.gov/nchs) is an ongoing, nationwide, in-person survey of approximately 40,000 households (approximately 100,000 persons) of the civilian noninstitutionalized population. This survey, conducted in 1982–1996, 1997, 2003, and 2004, includes a set of basic health and demographic questions, as well as one or more sets of supplemental questions on specific health topics. In England and Wales, the General Household Survey provides information on risk behaviors and disparities.[59] In the People's Republic of China, sentinel sites, known as disease surveillance points, are chosen through a statistical sample of provincial areas. Health care professionals at these sites collect mandated information on acute infectious conditions and data on health events and medical encounters for the entire population within their jurisdiction.[60]

Such nationwide surveys efficiently generate national estimates, of the prevalence of diseases, injuries, behaviors, etc., but local programs can benefit from involvement in data collection and the flexibility to adapt the process to their particular needs. Interview surveys such as BRFSS (discussed previously) can obtain self-reported health information with only minor differences from in-person interviews in the reported prevalence of health conditions.[61] In economically developed countries where the majority of residences have telephones, the advantages of telephone interviews are lower cost and the ease of supervising interviewers. To obtain information concerning sexual activity in the United States, states have begun periodic administration of the school-based Youth Risk Behavior Survey (YRBS), a multistage sampling survey of high school students.[62]

Surveys that employ hospital records and other medical care records can provide information on diagnoses, surgical procedures, and patient demographic characteristics. Although computerization of parts of these records has enabled their use for routine surveillance, a major limitation of using such records occurs when unique personal identifiers are not recorded, because repeat admissions and discharges of individual patients usually cannot be identified. Hospital discharge surveys have been useful for surveillance of certain medical care technologies, such as trends in the use of hysterectomies in the United States (particularly by geographical region), in the rate of medical procedures by sex and race, and in the assessment of quality of care.[63]

Other sources of morbidity health information from surveys include the United Nations International Children's Emergency Fund (UNICEF), the World Health Organization (WHO), international conferences, nongovernmental organizations (NGOs), and population laboratories (e.g., the International Center for Diarrheal Disease Research, Bangladesh). Although the health problems in the majority of low-resource settings are similar, it is best for one country to avoid relying on data from other countries, because geographic differences can affect the incidence of a condition. In addition, the health impact associated with certain conditions, such as hepatitis B, rotavirus, or malaria, can vary across regions and countries. For example, in 2000, Ethiopia developed the Ethiopia Demographic and Health Survey, the first comprehensive nationally representative health survey to be implemented as part of the worldwide Demographic and Health Surveys project.[64] Data from this survey have been used to emphasize the particular burden of disease in that country as compared with nearby sub-Saharan regions.

Registries. As suggested in the previous section, health professionals are increasingly recognizing the potential usefulness of medical records in public health practice.[65] At the national level, Medicare data have been adapted for research purposes; locally and regionally, managed care organizations have established research activities based on the records of their patient populations.[66] Specifically, medical records are the source of data for registries, comprehensive longitudinal listings of persons with particular conditions, which can include detailed information about diagnostic classifications, treatments, and outcomes.[67] Registries have also been used to ensure the provision of appropriate care and to evaluate changing patterns of medical care; unlike other disease information systems, registries cut across the different levels of severity of illness and can provide information across time about individual persons. To improve the quality of care for the treatment of other chronic diseases, registries are being developed for stroke[68] and diabetes.[69]

Population-based cancer registries typically have relied on multiple sources of data, most importantly, clinical pathology laboratories and hospital diagnoses (Figure 11.8). Death certification is also critical to these registries, as are other records, such as those from oncology or radiotherapy units, where available. The idea of recording data for all cases of cancer in communities began in the first half of the twentieth century, with the original purpose being to describe patterns and trends.[70] The growth in the number of registries and their use in following patients and analyzing quality of care and survival with comparability across different locations and distinct racial/ethnic groups has led to internationally recognized data collection and reporting standards.[71] In the United States, population-based registries, based on the Surveillance of Epidemiology and End Results (SEER) model, have been developed that conduct surveillance for

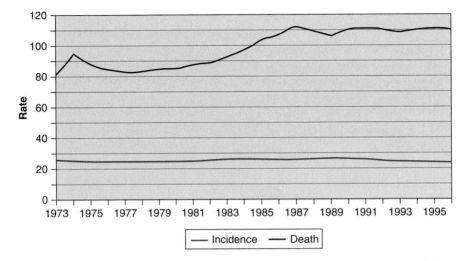

Figure 11.8. Incidence Rate and Death Rate of Invasive Breast Cancer, by Year—United States, 1973–1998
SOURCE: National Cancer Institute. SEER: Surveillance, Epidemiology, and End Results [homepage on the Internet]. Bethesda, MD: US Department of Health and Human Services, National Institutes of Health; 2006. Available at: http://seer.cancer.gov/. Accessed October 5, 2006.

cancer, and the national Coordinating Council for Cancer Surveillance was organized in 1995 to facilitate a collaborative approach among the involved organizations and to ensure maximal efficiency.[72]

Surveillance for birth defects was initiated in certain parts of the world in response to the thalidomide tragedy in the early 1960s; registries were established to provide reliable baseline rates for specific birth defects and to detect increases in the prevalence of birth defects as a means of rapidly identifying human teratogens.[73] The CDC has conducted birth defects surveillance in metropolitan Atlanta since 1967 by using multiple sources of ascertainment of all serious birth defects observed in stillborn and live-born infants or recognized by signs and symptoms apparent during the first year of life.[74] This birth defects registry system has been a valuable resource for monitoring rates of change of specific defects and for conducting numerous genetic and epidemiologic investigations of risk factors for birth defects.[75] In addition to monitoring birth defect rates and serving as the basis for

epidemiologic studies, the data from these state registries are used to evaluate the effectiveness of prevention activities and to refer children for health services and early intervention programs.[76]

Other Administrative Systems. In addition to the CDC, various federal agencies are involved in collecting data that are useful for public health. For example, the Food and Drug Administration (FDA) conducts post-marketing surveillance of adverse reaction to drugs,[77] and the Consumer Product Safety Commission conducts surveillance on product-related injuries.[78] The Hazardous Materials Information System of the Department of Transportation, established in 1971, provides reporting of spills associated with interstate commerce on a voluntary basis.[79]

Insurance records and workers' compensation claims have been useful sources of morbidity data for injuries and illnesses in specific geographic locales (Figure 11.9). For example, in an evaluation of claims for workers' compensation as an adjunct

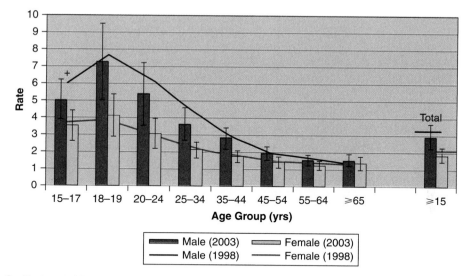

Figure 11.9. Estimated Rates of Nonfatal Occupational Injuries and Illnesses Among Workers Treated in Hospital Emergency Departments, by Age Group and Sex of Worker—United States, 1998 and 2003

SOURCE: Centers for Disease Control and Prevention. Nonfatal occupational injuries and illnesses among workers treated in hospital emergency departments United States, 2003. Morb Mortal Wkly Rep MMWR. 2006; 55: 449–452.

to an occupational lead surveillance system, the usefulness of claims was demonstrated: the likelihood that a company had a case of lead poisoning strongly correlated with the number of claims against the company.[80] In addition, using medical claims data for surveillance can be limited by lack of comparability among data from different jurisdictions (because of varying regulations governing completion of forms) or the accuracy of diagnostic recording.[81]

Ethical Principles for Surveillance

Any data collection that involves collaboration with communities of people must adhere to ethical principles of respect for persons and balance benefit with risk.[82] Well-defined **ethical standards** exist for epidemiologic research[83] and for statistical compilation and data analysis.[84] However, the primary purpose of surveillance is Essential Service 1, to monitor health status to identify community health problems. Thus, public health surveillance

is not research in the sense of data collection for generalizable knowledge.[85]

This distinction is relevant for at least two reasons. First, the ethical standard of respect for persons might be challenged by the benefit to communities that the collection of data may provide.[86] This exception is acknowledged in infectious disease surveillance, as well as the collection of data for disease registries. Second, surveillance data must be disseminated quickly to public health practitioners, including those who originally gathered the data, as well as to decision makers throughout public health organizations and, depending on the character of the information, to other public service agencies and the community. Surveillance data are more often related to identifying a public health problem than to problem solving. The dissemination of surveillance data frequently stimulates the search for additional data that comes from other sources.

This distinction, however, does not exempt the public health practitioner from adhering to ethical practices when conducting surveillance. Preventing inappropriate disclosure of surveillance data is essential both to the privacy of persons with reported cases of disease and to the trust of participants in the surveillance system. As applied to personally identifiable information (as opposed to aggregate data or data about institutions), **confidentiality** refers to a status accorded to information that indicates that it is sensitive for stated reasons, must be protected, and access to it controlled. **Privacy** refers to the claim of individual persons, and the societal value representing that claim, to control the use and disclosure of personal data. **Security** includes the safeguards (administrative, technical, and physical) in an information system that protect it and its information against unauthorized disclosure and that limit access to authorized users in accordance with an established policy.[87]

The protection of confidentiality begins with limiting data collection and transmission to a minimum and includes ensuring the physical security of surveillance records, the discretion of surveillance staff, and legal safeguards. To elicit public health surveillance information from the public and from health care providers, strong laws that ensure a careful procedure for maintaining and reporting data are frequently necessary to ensure the privacy of personal information[88] (see also Chapter 6, The Legal Basis for Public Health Practice).

Privacy regulations in the United States are based on a patchwork of state and local legislation and might not adequately protect electronic health information. Recent laws introduced in the U.S. Congress, such as the Health Insurance Portability and Accountability Act, include definitions of protected information and descriptions of disclosures that can occur with or without consent. Sometimes forgotten in the discussion of health information privacy is the concept that use of electronic information systems can often improve the security of data.[89]

The physical protection of records is governed by rules of conduct for persons involved in the design, development, operation, or maintenance of any surveillance system. For example, confidential records must be kept locked up at any time they are not in use. When confidential records are in use, they must be kept out of the sight of persons not authorized to work with the records. Except as needed for operational purposes, copies of confidential records should not be made. When confidential surveillance records are in the possession of other agencies, provision should be made for protecting those records.

The provision of data containing identifiers of individual persons or establishments should be held to the minimum number of practitioners deemed essential to perform public health functions. Categories of identifiers should be sufficiently broad to avoid inadvertent identification of a person or institution. In particular, the release of information related to limited geographic areas (e.g., a city or county) must be considered carefully to protect confidentiality.[90] Other methods of data security, which involve statistical disclosure techniques, are discussed in the Methods to Preserve Confidentiality of Data section (p.39).

Domain 2: Policy Development/ Program Planning Skills

The surveillance data acquired by the means discussed in the previous sections have important uses for policy development and program planning. First, surveillance can help organizations and government agencies set public health priorities. Missouri, for example, has developed an innovative model that uses surveillance data to rank diseases in order of priority.[91] Specifically, surveillance data can be used to address disparities in health.[92] At the national level, surveillance data have been used to set priorities for allocating limited resources.[93] In addition, a key function of surveillance data is setting policies for research.[94]

Domain 3: Communication Skills

Critical to the usefulness of surveillance systems is the timely dissemination of surveillance data to those who need the information. Data analyses should be regularly published and interpreted. Whatever the publication format, it must be appropriate for the intended audience, because audiences affect data collection and interpretation, as well as dissemination. Regular and timely data dissemination allows for effective control and prevention. Because "those who need to know" include persons with little epidemiologic knowledge or background (i.e., policy makers and administrators), data reports should be simple and easy to understand. For example, data on the percentage of persons in the United States who are overweight or obese has been available since the 1980s (Figure 11.10a); however, not until the data were portrayed in maps across time did this problem receive widespread national attention[95] (Figure 11.10b).

Domain 4: Cultural Competency Skills

Communities around the world face a bewildering array of public policy concerns: poverty, education, housing, safe food and water, employment, social justice, access to health care, and so on. To assist these communities, as public health practitioners, we must work with communities to help them prioritize how to deal with these issues. For surveillance, this means collecting the data that will help us identify problems and effective interventions. A challenge for health providers is the lack of data to measure the association between health and socioeconomic status. The gradient of health with socioeconomic status is a challenge for public health;[96] yet, without data to measure this gradient, we have no way of intervening. Previously, we discussed the problem inherent in reporting race/ethnicity in public health surveillance data.[97,98] Also important is educational background, which for certain conditions creates a greater disparity than that caused by race.[99]

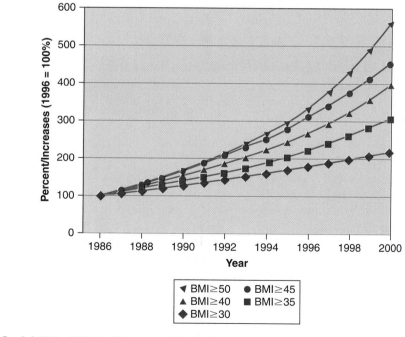

Figure 11.10. (a) 1996–2000. Self-Reported Body Mass Index, United States

SOURCE: Sturm R. Increases in clinically severe obesity in the United States, 1986–2000. Arch Int Med. 2003; 163:2146–2148. Copyright © 2003, American Medical Association. All Rights Reserved.

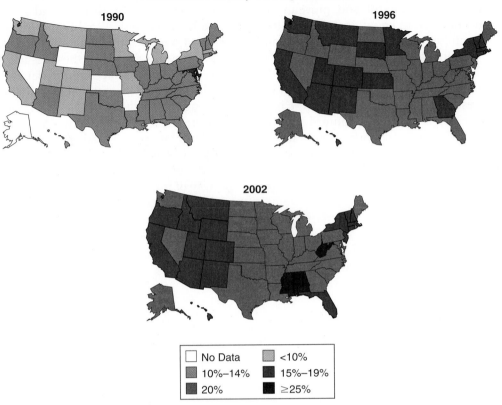

Figure 11.10. **(b) 1990–2002. Self-Reported Body Mass Index, United States**

SOURCE: Centers for Disease Control and Prevention (CDC). Behavior Risk Factor Surveillance System: turning information into health [homepage on the Internet]. Atlanta, GA: US Department of Health and Human Services, CDC; 2006. Available at: http://www.cdc.gov/brfss/. Accessed October 5, 2006.

To navigate the delicate social dynamics of race/ethnicity and educational levels, public health practitioners must acquire skills in cultural competency. The American Medical Association's Liaison Committee on Medical Education (LCME) has defined cultural competency as "an understanding of the manner in which people of diverse cultures and belief systems perceive health and illness."[100] This competency relates to the language used in questionnaires and interviews, an understanding of community values and norms, and the communication of surveillance results. Even if a proposed policy is effective, has minimal risk, and is reasonably priced, community concerns such as perception of risk or acceptability might preclude its adoption. For example, a coalition of agencies in California wanted to address the problem of elevated breast and cervical cancer risk for Vietnamese women as demonstrated by cancer registry data. These agencies evaluated media campaigns versus using lay health workers to educate the affected population, and determined that lay health workers were more effective at encouraging women to actually obtain the appropriate cancer-screening tests because the health workers used their cultural knowledge and social networks to create change.[101]

Domain 5: Community Dimensions of Practice Skills

Establishing a Surveillance System

When a new surveillance program is established, its creators must clearly understand the program's purpose—what data need to be obtained and how and when they are to be used. A particular surveillance system might have more than one goal (e.g., monitoring the occurrence of both fatal and nonfatal disease or injury, evaluating the impact of a public health intervention, or detecting epidemics for control and prevention). A single health event (e.g., influenza or cervical cancer) might require multiple surveillance systems to track morbidity, mortality, laboratory tests, exposures, and risk factors. The key question is, "What action will be taken?" It is critical that practitioners and decision makers have a specific action-oriented commitment to using data effectively for public health action.

To ensure that a surveillance system meets the needs of public health decision makers and their communities, the objectives of the system must be thoroughly detailed. Everyone who might make decisions on the basis of the surveillance data should be involved in the process.

Domain 6: Basic Public Health Sciences Skills

Analysis

Surveillance practitioners should ensure that surveillance data are analyzed appropriately and interpreted in a timely manner. Programmed data analysis packages are the first step in data analysis, but results of analyses should be reviewed, and customized analysis should be done as needed. Surveillance information must be analyzed first in terms of time (temporal analysis), place (spatial analysis), and person (analysis of personal characteristics). More sophisticated methods, such as cluster and **time-series** analyses, methods for evaluation, statistical approaches to confidentiality, data mining, and computer mapping techniques, might be subsequently appropriate. In any analysis of surveillance data, inappropriate inference can produce misleading results. To avoid this pitfall, we recommend three considerations:

1. pattern does not demonstrate causation,
2. association is not causation, and
3. the lack of randomization (fundamental to statistical inference) limits conclusions.

For example, illustrating the first point, an increase in reported cases in a surveillance system may be due to a change in case definition or other reporting artifact rather than a true increase in disease incidence. An example of the second point is that the association of mortality with grey hair clearly does not mean that hair color causes mortality.

Randomization uses chance to assign study participants to a treatment group or a particular exposure. It minimizes the differences among groups by equally distributing people with particular characteristics among all the intervention groups. Thus, researchers do not know which treatment is better; given what is known at the time, any of the treatments chosen could benefit the participant. Clearly, this is impossible in surveillance and impractical in many epidemiologic situations.

Temporal Analysis. Characterizing a health event among a population by time is critical in determining the historical trends, baseline levels and epidemics, and projections for the future of the event. The most effective choice of time pattern varies with the health condition being studied. For the majority of chronic diseases, the most useful time pattern is the **secular trend**, the annual number or rate of disease across multiple years (Figure 11.11). For injuries, the most revealing time pattern might be by day of the week and time of day. For acute infectious diseases, the choice might be seasonal patterns or an **epidemic period** during which the reported number of cases exceeds the usual number of cases (Figure 11.12). Special circumstance can require judgment in choice of study period. For example, at high-profile events that might be related to **biologic or chemical terrorism**, hourly reporting can be critical (see the Syndromic Surveillance section earlier in this chapter).

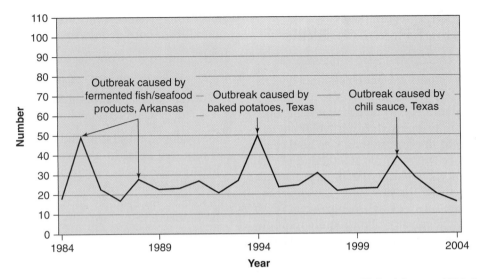

Figure 11.11. Botulism, Foodborne. Number of Reported Cases, by Year—United States, 1984–2004

Home-canned foods and Alaska Native foods consisting of fermented foods of aquatic origin remain the principle sources of foodborne botulism in the United States. No substantial outbreak has occurred since 2001.

SOURCE: Centers for Disease Control and Prevention. Summary of notifiable diseases United States, 2004. Morb Mortal Wkly Rep 2006; 53:179.

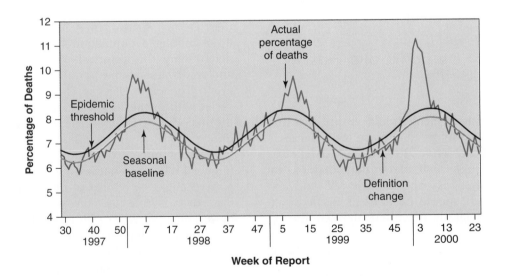

Figure 11.12. Percentage of Deaths Attributed to Pneumonia and Influenza, 122 Cities Mortality Surveillance System, 1997–2000

SOURCE: Centers for Disease Control and Prevention. Surveillance for influenza United States, 1997–98, 1998–99, and 1999–00 seasons. Morb Mortal Wkly Rep MMWR; 51 (No. SS-7): 110.

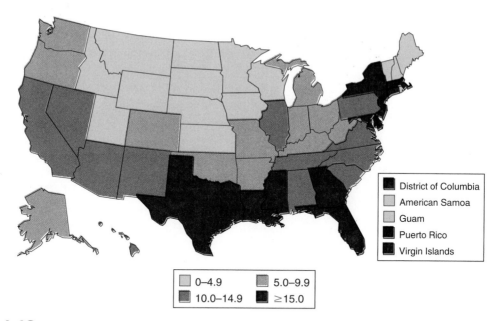

Legend:
- District of Columbia
- American Samoa
- Guam
- Puerto Rico
- Virgin Islands

0–4.9   5.0–9.9
10.0–14.9   ≥15.0

Figure 11.13. Acquired Immunodeficiency Syndrome (AIDS) Incidence—United States and U.S. Territories, 2004

SOURCE: Centers for Disease Control and Prevention. Summary of notifiable diseases United States, 2004. Morb Mortal Wkly Rep 2006; 53:179.

More sophisticated methods (e.g., time-series or smoothing techniques) can be used to model long-term patterns in the data,[102] controlling for the effect of age over time[103] or assessing the effect of the incubation period of infectious conditions.[104]

Spatial Analysis. Characterizing surveillance data from a population by place provides insight into the geographic extent of the problem (Figure 11.13). Characterization by place includes the assessment of occurrence according to place or residence (country, state, county, census tract, street address, map coordinates), birthplace, employment, and school district. Place also considers disease occurrence by categories such as urban or rural, domestic or foreign, and institutional or non-institutional. Analysis of data by place can indicate hypotheses regarding reservoirs, vehicles, manner of spread, and causes. For example, communicable diseases are spread from person to person more rapidly in urban areas than in rural areas, primarily because the greater population density of the urban

area provides more opportunities for susceptible persons to come in contact with a source of infection. On the other hand, diseases that are transmitted from animals to humans often have a greater incidence in rural and suburban areas as a result of greater opportunity for humans to come into contact with disease-carrying animals, insects, and so forth. For example, Lyme disease has become more common as humans have moved to wooded areas where they come into contact with infected ticks. Place as a risk factor for multiple chronic conditions emphasizes the importance of **social determinants** of health.[105]

Spatial analysis includes techniques for quantifying spatial patterns, modeling risk surfaces, and assessing hypothesized relationships between outcomes (e.g., cancer) and specific exposures. The simplest, and perhaps most easily understood, spatial analysis is a geopolitical map (Figure 11.14). An early example of spatial analysis is John Snow's mapping of the addresses of cholera victims in 1854 to assess their proximity to putative pollution

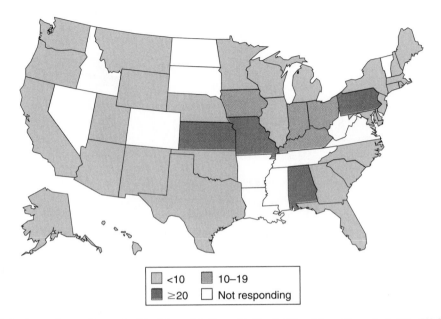

Figure 11.14. Prevalence Rates for Resident Adults with Peak Blood Lead Levels ≥25 g/dL by State—Adult Blood Lead Epidemiology and Surveillance Program, United States, 2003–2004 Annual Average

SOURCE: Centers for Disease Control and Prevention. Adult blood lead epidemiology and surveillance United States, 2003–2004. Morb Mortal Wkly Rep MMWR; 55;876–879.

sources (i.e., water pumps). To address the problem that large land areas appear to have larger disease burden, other mapping methods have been developed to visually portray populations at risk.[106] Other statistical methods for spatial analysis include statistical **smoothing techniques** and algorithms to preserve confidentiality and address limited disease counts,[107] Bayesian methods,[108] and geographic information systems (GIS), which allow manipulation of "layers" of public health data.[109,110] In any spatial analysis, forms of models do not convey any causal relationship; all models have assumptions about the data, and the choice of spatial weights can affect conclusions.[111]

The Analysis of Personal Characteristics. Persons can be described in terms of their inherent characteristics (age, sex, race), acquired characteristics (marital status, vaccination status),

behaviors and activities (occupation, leisure activities, use of medications/tobacco/seat belts), and the circumstances under which they live (socioeconomic status, access to health care). These characteristics, activities, and conditions determine to a considerable degree which persons will be at increased or decreased risk for different diseases and other adverse health events. With the development of sophisticated molecular techniques, descriptive epidemiology can extend to assessing the role of individual genetic risk for disease.[112] More complex methods to assess patterns in personal characteristics include logistic regression, classification and regression tree analysis,[113] and categorical methods.[114]

Aberration Detection. A critical purpose of surveillance is to detect unusual clusters of disease (aberrations in time or space or both) and to implement timely intervention. The first step in establishing an aberration-detection system is to agree on the definition of an *outbreak*. For example, the CDC has defined an outbreak of a foodborne disease as two or more cases of infection by a common agent that are linked epidemiologically.[115] The majority of statistical methods for outbreak detection require a baseline count and a decision mechanism (statistical test) to judge whether current counts significantly exceed the baseline.[116] Terrorism preparedness has generated renewed interest and development in outbreak detection,[117] such as data mining.[118] In evaluating aberration-detection algorithms, attention should be given to sensitivity and specificity of the application.[119,120]

Analytic Methods for Evaluation. In the evaluation of a surveillance system, statistical methods can be used to assess selected attributes of the system (see the previous discussion). Assessments of representativeness, sensitivity, and positive predictive value all require comparison of the data in the surveillance system with another (or standard) source of data for the same condition. One example of such a method is **capture-recapture methodology**.[121,122] In its simplest form, this method requires a second source of data and a matching of cases from the two sources.[123] Thus, the two data sets need to be linked in some way. When **personal identifiers** are lacking (which is the case with the majority of national surveillance systems), probabilistic methods can be used.[124] Record linkage is also useful in updating records or increasing the amount of information in a single surveillance system.[125] However, practitioners must take care to ensure that linking data files does not increase the risk personal disclosure.

Methods to Preserve Confidentiality of Data. Preserving the confidentiality of health records can be approached through two broad classes of methods. The first class consists of controlling access to data, either through legislation (see Chapter 6) or through data aggregation or suppression; for example, tables of counts can suppress cells with fewer than, say, five persons, or records can be aggregated within a geographic area that has a population large enough to protect against disclosure.[126] The second class of methods uses rounding techniques or statistical cell perturbation, so that statistical properties of the data set remain intact, but individual records no longer describe an actual person.[127] Because these data-protection methods can limit the scope of analysis, agencies have explored practices and procedures to prevent public disclosure, but to permit more in-depth analyses of data for public health intervention and policy purposes. These include licensing agreements,[128] data-release policies,[129] and establishing secure remote sites.[130]

Domain 7: Financial Planning and Management Skills

Management of the persons who are needed for conducting surveillance to provide information for control and prevention programs is essential. Because practitioners skilled in working with health data and management problems are often sought for advice, competence in consultation is also important. Proficiency in human relations is required of every public health practitioner who deals with colleagues in implementing tasks related to health data and community health problem management.

Domain 8: Leadership and Systems-Thinking Skills

Relationships with Other Health Practitioners

Health data and its management are important for public health practitioners who have a range of special competencies. In addition to epidemiologists, **statisticians** play a special role in accessing and managing data sources and evaluating and interpreting results. Laboratory staff have a critical role in executing tests that identify the exact cause of a health problem and that confirm the presence of the problem among those persons who present with symptoms and signs of the condition.

Health policy makers need to understand health data if effective strategies are to be designed to control and prevent a community health problem. Similarly, **health service and program managers** need to understand the findings of studies and policy analyses if they are to be persuaded to provide services and to conduct effective programs.

Informatics

Readers might have difficulty envisioning a time when practicing epidemiology and surveillance did not involve computers. By now, public health practitioners fully recognize that information science and computer technology are essential tools for practicing public health. The increase in availability of computers to analyze and transmit data and the decrease in the cost of such technology offers both increased opportunities and challenges for surveillance. On the basis of the Core Competencies for Public Health Professionals, the CDC developed a set of essential skills in public health informatics related to using information for public health practice, using information technology to increase one's individual effectiveness in public health, and managing information technology projects to improve the effectiveness of the public health agency.[131]

For example, the CDC's Epi Info™ is a publicly available computer program designed to assist public health data management and analysis (http://www.cdc.gov/epiinfo/). This tool has been used successfully in both economically developed and developing countries, and the program's information is available in seven languages (English, French, Spanish, Arabic, Russian, Chinese, and Serbo-Croatian). The technical manual or portions of it have been translated into these languages as well as into Italian, Portuguese, German, Norwegian, Hungarian, Czech, Polish, Romanian, Indonesian, and Farsi.

The explosive development of technology includes the development of high-capacity storage devices, expansion of the capabilities of the Internet, use of local- and wide-area networks for entry of surveillance data at multiple computers simultaneously, and development of new programming tools, video and computer integration, and voice and pen input. Interoperability systems, including data standards, are needed to allow maximal use of these advancements.[132] A more integrated approach to data collection is motivated by an interest in data from new syndromic surveillance sources (e.g., pharmacy data or school and workplace absenteeism), access in electronic format, and heightened concerns about security and confidentiality with easily available data on intranet or Internet sites.[133] In 1996, the U.S. Congress passed the **Health Insurance Portability and Accountability Act (HIPAA)** (P.L. 104-191), which mandated development and implementation of standards for exchanging financial and administrative data related to health care[134] and concurrent changes in technology to allow timely and secure data reporting and access to data across governmental and geographic boundaries.[135]

Informatics has also been helpful in transmitting molecular data on isolates of certain pathogens (e.g., the previously discussed pulsed-field gel electrophoresis patterns of *E. coli* 0157:H7 through PulseNet [http://www.cdc.gov/ncidod/dbmd/pulsenet/pulsenet.htm]). In addition, computerization can facilitate and enhance regular and personal contact among public health officials, health care providers, and others who participate in such activities as a closed electronic mail system. The Emerging Infections Network, a national program in which hundreds of infectious diseases practitioners across the United States participate, uses an electronic mail conference for online discussion when new insights into disease occurrence are needed and allows for close communication between public health officials and health care providers.[136] The National Library of Medicine assembles and disseminates bibliographies on new developments in public health informatics.[137]

System Integration

Historically, data systems, as discussed in this chapter, have been developed in regard to the study of specific diseases or health events (e.g., TB, sexually transmitted diseases, or birth defects). Subsequently, independently developed disease-specific computer applications for use at the state and local level for collecting, entering, analyzing, and transmitting data have arisen. These categorical systems result from distinct funding streams, mechanisms for delivering clinical care and health services, and organizational systems. Although these systems have played a key role in standardizing data collection and reporting across the nation for their respective systems, lack of integration among specific diseases or health events hinders usefulness. Variables common to multiple systems, classification and coding schemes, user interfaces, database formats, and methods for data transmission and analysis have not been standardized or reused. Thus, personnel at local and state health departments must use multiple systems that are not linked or merged. This disease-based approach has resulted in lack of utility of data collected, incomplete reporting, and delays and burdens in reporting.

The opportunities created by informatics and the development, implementation, and use of standards for exchanging financial and administrative data related to health care have connected groups that previously did not work together (e.g., the National Library of Medicine's Unified Medical Language System and the U.S. College of American Pathologist's Systematized Nomenclature of Medicine [SNOMED]). Having similar standards and coding for data enables data sharing among agencies interested in population health, privacy protections for medical information, and security of data transmission and storage.[138] To be most effective, public health must take advantage of other information development activities to be able to use data from any source, with rapid and secure dissemination of data to those who need to act to improve communities' health.[139]

ESSENTIAL SERVICE 2, DIAGNOSE AND INVESTIGATE HEALTH PROBLEMS AND HEALTH HAZARDS IN THE COMMUNITY

Alexander Langmuir articulated in simple words what the epidemiologist does: "The basic operation of the epidemiologist is to count cases and measure the population in which they arise," so that rates can be calculated and the occurrence of a health problem can be compared among different groups of people.[140] *The Dictionary of Epidemiology* reflects both dimensions of science and public health practice in its definition of epidemiology "as the study of the distribution and determinants of health-related states or events in specified populations, and the application of this study to the control of health problems."[141]

The phrase **health problem** is used in this definition (in place of the word *disease*) because epidemiologists and public health agencies now find themselves responsible for a range of conditions. As we have seen in the section on Essential Service 1, in addition to infectious diseases (e.g., TB, influenza), noninfectious health problems (e.g., cancer, automobile crash injuries among adolescents, exposure among miners to coal dust, and unintended pregnancies among teenagers) are also high-priority public health problems in countries worldwide.

The term **distribution** in the definition addresses the association of health events to person, places, and time; in other words, the relationship between the health problem and the population among which it exists. The characteristics of the population are usually provided in terms of age, sex, and the places where people live and where the health event occurs.

The word **determinants** refers to both the direct causes of the health problem and the factors that determine the risk for the problem. These factors are often classified into three groups:

- host factors,
- agent factors, and
- environmental factors.

Host factors characterize persons afflicted with the health problem and their susceptibility to it. **Agent factors** are those that characterize the mechanisms that lead to disease or injury. **Environmental factors** are those that determine the exposure of the host group to the agent. In an epidemic of food poisoning, for example, the host group includes the persons who ate the food and became ill. The agent factors are those related to the cause of the problem (e.g., *Salmonella* bacillus) that might contaminate turkey or egg dishes. The environmental factors are those that provide suitable circumstances for the agent to survive (e.g., improper handling of food) and those that determine the exposure of the host group.

Domain 1: Analytic Assessment Skills

As noted previously in this chapter, the practice of epidemiology includes the study of the distribution and determinants of health-related states or events. The study of the distribution—the association of health events to person, place, and time—is called **descriptive epidemiology**. The study of determinants—causes and risk factors—is the domain of **analytic epidemiology**. Both aspects are necessary in providing a complete picture of the health event among the population. Just as a newspaper reporter must describe the what, who, when, where, and why of a story, the epidemiologist must address the health event itself, as well as its person, time, and place characteristics, and finally its causes.

Domain 2: Policy Development/ Program Planning Skills

Epidemiologic data can provide the scientific foundation for policy development and program planning. For example, the *Guide to Community Preventive Services* (Community Guide) provides systematic searches and syntheses of the scientific literature on specific health problems; this is particularly important when the literature is considerable, inconsistent, uneven in quality, or even inaccessible. The Community Guide summarizes what is known about the effectiveness, economic efficiency, and feasibility of interventions to promote community health and prevent disease.[142] In 2000, a Community Guide analysis determined that state laws that establish the legal blood alcohol concentration (BAC) limit for automobile drivers at 0.08 percent reduced alcohol-related fatalities by 7 percent. On the basis, in part, of this finding, the U.S. Congress required that states enact 0.08 percent BAC laws or risk losing federal highway construction funds. Since passage of that requirement, all 50 states have enacted legislation decreasing the legal BAC to 0.08 percent. With all states enacting and enforcing the 0.08 percent BAC laws, experts estimate that 400–600 fewer alcohol-related deaths will occur on our roadways each year.

An international example of the importance of epidemiologic data to policy development is the Data for Decision Making Project.[143] The goals of this project were to strengthen the capacity of decision makers to identify data needs and interpret and use data appropriately; to enhance the capacity of technical advisors to provide valid, essential, and timely data to decision makers; and to strengthen health information systems at local, district, regional, and national levels. The strategy was tested in Bolivia, Cameroon, Mexico, and the Philippines, where decentralization of health services led to a need to strengthen the capacity of policy makers to use information more effectively. An evaluation of the strategy demonstrated that its implementation improved public health; consequently, the strategy has been institutionalized in participating countries. For example, data on tobacco use and health was used to implement a tobacco prevention program in Mexico.

Domain 3: Communication Skills

Communicating the results of field investigations and epidemiologic studies is an essential part of the effective and ethical practice of public health. Information should be shared with:

1. those in a position to intervene in regard to the health problems and to prevent further occurrence,
2. other affected members of the community, and
3. the broader scientific community.

The communication plan for the research results should be developed before the study is initiated.[144]

The first part of the communication plan should be aimed at those in a position to intervene. Recommendations to group patients by cohort during a nosocomial infection outbreak, to vaccinate children in a community, or to close a restaurant, for example, should be communicated with a full understanding of any cost for or barriers to implementation. In this context, principles of risk communication are important.[145]

Second, broader communication messages for the community have at least two purposes. The first is to solicit community support, for example, in the case of mass vaccination.[146] The second is to educate the community to prevent future health problems. The CDC's *Morbidity and Mortality Weekly Report* (*MMWR*) and secure communication tool *Epi-X* are critical resources, because they enable timely dissemination of urgent public health results and recommendations.[147]

The news media can be important partners in public health practice, if they are approached carefully.[148] In some ways, public health is its own worse enemy in media relations: "Some risks we have gotten quite right: tobacco is a serious health hazard. In other areas, our findings are less clear [to us and to others]. Butter is bad, and margarine is good. No—margarine with high levels of trans-fatty acids is actually bad. Eat less red meat, but cook it well to kill potential lurking pathogens. Don't cook it so well that you charbroil it, though—that could create a carcinogenic coating."[149] This difference in culture between the public health community and the media has at least four components:

1. Public health scientists exercise a great deal of control over their manuscripts, but they cannot have the same degree of control over the scientific articles written by journalists, because this goes against the independence of journalism and the decentralized structure of the mass media.

2. The timing of public health investigations, although urgent, allows authors to check their manuscripts and to use the opinions of other scholars, whereas journalists have much less time to produce a story.

3. News stories are shorter, contain less information, are organized in a different manner, and transform scientific language to nontechnical language.

4. News stories are generally intended to report on the answer and thus do not handle scientific uncertainty well.

In part to address the relationship between the field of epidemiology and the media, the CDC developed the Knight Fellowship Program to provide journalists a closer look at the practice of public health, including disease investigation, scientific research, field practice, and interaction with colleagues.[150]

Dissemination of results in the scientific literature documents findings for future research and investigation. Publication in the peer-reviewed scientific literature is an essential activity for public health. First, these publications provide credibility for public health science through the peer-review process. Second, they make overlooking or ignoring research results more difficult for the public and the media. Third, these publications provide information for independent investigators to validate other researchers' results.

Finally, public health practitioners might determine that publication in the peer-reviewed literature is less important that other forms of communication. This might be the result of lack of time or perception that journal editors are not interested in "reports from the field." The CDC's online journal *Preventing Chronic Disease* has addressed this concern for the field of chronic disease prevention and control by encouraging submission of multisectoral approaches and practice reports.40

Domain 4: Cultural Competency Skills

For public health outbreak investigations, the American Medical Association's definition of cultural competency—"an understanding of the manner in which people of diverse cultures and belief systems perceive health and illness"—[translates into respect for and understanding of cultural differences, which involves physicians' self-awareness and sensitivity to patients' culture, as well as adaptation skills. For example, language and culture are important factors in TB outbreak investigations. The ability to understand cultural norms and to bridge the gaps that exist between cultures requires training and experience. Influencing patients to participate in a contact investigation increasingly depends on the cultural competency of the health care worker. For example, using family members as interpreters is not recommended because the majority of family members do not have a medical orientation and because patients might be reluctant to reveal their contacts to a family member. To increase their cultural competency, public health workers should complete training derived from the National Standards for Culturally and Linguistically Appropriate Services in Health Care.[151]

For optimal effectiveness, public health research and practice activities must involve the community.[152] The CDC's network of Prevention Research Centers brings academic researchers, community members, and public health agencies together to collaborate on developing effective strategies. This collaboration illustrates a community-based participatory research paradigm, an orientation to research that focuses on long-term associations among academic, government, and community partners and incorporates community theories, practices, and participation into research activities.[153] Findings are tested and applied in the field so that real-world influences are accounted for, all available resources are accessed, and researchers and communities expand each other's capacity for addressing health problems.[154]

The Community Guide (discussed previously) provided a systematic review of the effectiveness of selected population-based interventions to address social determinants of health disparities focused on interventions within three strategic areas: (1) early childhood development opportunities, (2) affordable family housing in safe neighborhoods, and (3) access to culturally competent health care systems. Recognizing that health is the product of multiple levels of influence (genetic and biologic processes, individual behaviors, and the context within which

people live), public health must address elements in the social environment that affect health. These social determinants that might be amenable to community interventions can, in turn, lead to improved health outcomes. Results from the Community Guide's systematic review provided sufficient evidence to recommend two interventions: center-based programs for children from families with low incomes and rental vouchers that would allow choice of residential location.[155]

In the United States, our cultural diversity is a national treasure. We have population groups that represent countries worldwide. This fact poses both challenges and opportunities, however. Minority populations are often at greater risk for chronic diseases because of living conditions and lifetime exposure to certain risk factors;[153] at the same time, this diversity affords us the ability to hear the voices of others and to begin the process of crafting the solutions for the prevention and control of disease, injury, and disability. It also means that these solutions can be relevant to other countries.[156]

Domain 5: Community Dimensions of Practice Skills

The epidemiologic investigation includes field work and office (or computer) work—following up individual case reports of adverse health events, assessing risk in a community, and conducting epidemiologic studies to identify causal relationships. An epidemiologic investigation might focus on an epidemic (e.g., an outbreak of infection), a cluster of events (e.g., injuries or leukemia), or the presence of risk factors for disease (e.g., tobacco use or an occupational exposure).

Domain 6: Basic Public Health Sciences Skills

Numbers and Rates

Counting the number of events—the number of new cases of hepatitis A reported this week, the number of infants who died this year, the number of new cancers diagnosed this month—is a common and essential activity of a health department. The numbers can be grouped by time, place, and person to provide an informative description of the magnitude and pattern of a health problem or service (see Essential Service 1). The numbers can indicate clusters or outbreaks of disease in the community, or the numbers can be used to guide health policy and resource allocation (Domain 2)—for example, the number of hospital beds needed, the best location of a satellite clinic, or the dollar amount to request for HIV-counseling in the next budget.

Because counts do not involve consideration of population size or demographic changes, they are insufficient for assessing an individual's or a population's risk for adverse health events. To characterize risk, **rates** rather than counts must be used. Calculating rates for different groups by age, sex, geographic location, exposure history, or other characteristics can identify persons at increased risk for disease (Figure 11.14). Identifying these groups at high risk is vital in developing and targeting effective control and prevention strategies (Domain 2). Rates are also preferred over counts for comparing health conditions within a population across time or among different populations, because rates involve consideration of the size of the population and the specific period.

To calculate a rate, the count must be divided by an appropriate denominator, usually an estimate of the population from which the counts in the numerator occurred. (In practice, such rates are usually expressed per 1,000 population or per 100,000 population.) For example, if the numerator is the number of women with diagnosed breast cancer as identified by a statewide cancer registry during the previous year, an appropriate denominator might be the estimated midyear female population of the state, on the basis of census figures. If the numerator is restricted to women of a certain age or higher, the denominator should be restricted similarly. These rates provide an estimate of the 1-year risk for breast cancer among women in that population. Using these standard population units facilitates comparisons of disease or death rates among different groups.

As illustrated by this example, denominators for public health data are often population estimates from the U.S. Bureau of the Census.[157] Based on the census, which is conducted every 10 years, the bureau provides detailed breakdowns of the population by age, race/ethnic group, sex, and census track. Between census years, the bureau provides less detailed estimates. States often develop more detailed estimates for use in their own jurisdictions for the years between the national censuses.

Common Measures

The most common health outcomes measured by public health agencies are those related to **morbidity** (illness, injury, and disability), **mortality** (death), and **natality** (birth). Morbidity measures include disease incidence and prevalence. Mortality measures include crude, specific, and standardized mortality rates as well as years of potential life lost. Selected commonly used measures for morbidity and mortality are described in the following discussion.

Morbidity Measures. Morbidity measures quantify a population's likelihood of developing or having an illness, injury, disability, or other adverse health condition. An **incidence rate,** sometimes referred to simply as **incidence,** is the rate at which new events (e.g., new cases of disease) occur among a population during a stated period. The numerator is the number of persons who experience new cases of illness among a population during a specified period. The denominator is either a sum of the time during which all persons were observed (**person-time rate**) or the average or mid-period size of the population.

An **attack rate** or **cumulative incidence** is a measure of incidence calculated most commonly during the investigation of an acute outbreak of disease. This number is simply the proportion of the population that experienced illness during a specified period. The numerator is the number of new cases. The denominator, however, is the size of the population at the beginning of the observation period. The attack rate is a measure of the probability or risk for experiencing illness.

The **prevalence rate,** often referred to simply as **prevalence,** is the proportion of persons among a population who have a particular disease or attribute at a specific point in time or during a specified period. Prevalence differs from incidence in that prevalence includes all cases, both old and new, among the population during the specified time, whereas incidence is limited to new cases only. Prevalence is most often measured by cross-sectional surveys of a population.

Point prevalence refers to prevalence measured at a particular point in time (i.e., the proportion of persons with a particular disease or attribute on a particular date). Period prevalence refers to prevalence measured over an interval of time (i.e., the proportion of persons who had a particular disease or attribute at any time during the interval).

Mortality Measures. The **mortality** rate, or death rate, quantifies the frequency of occurrence of death among a defined population during a specified period.

The crude death rate (or crude mortality rate) is the number of deaths from all causes for the entire population, divided by the population. In the United States in 2005, a total of 2,448,017 deaths were recorded. The 2005 estimated midyear population was 296,410,404. The crude mortality rate, therefore, was 825.9 deaths/100,000 population.[158]

To assess or compare the mortality experience of different population groups, death rates can be calculated specifically for those groups. An age-specific death rate is a death rate limited to a particular age group. Similarly, a sex-specific or race-specific death rate is limited to one sex or one racial group, respectively.

The infant mortality rate, a type of age-specific death rate, is used by all nations as a key public health indicator. The numerator is the number of deaths among children aged <1 year reported during a specific period, usually a calendar year. The denominator is the number of live births reported during the same period. The infant mortality rate is usually expressed per 1,000 live births. In 2003, the United States infant mortality rate was 6.85 infant deaths/1,000 live births.[159]

A cause-specific death rate is the mortality rate from a specified cause for a population. The numer-ator is the number of deaths attributed to a specific cause. The denominator is the same as the crude death rate (i.e., an estimate of the entire population). Cause-specific death rates are usually expressed per 100,000 population. In the United States, diseases of the heart and malignant neo-plasms have had the two highest cause-specific death rates since at least 1950, but the gap between the two has narrowed considerably.[159]

Often, one wishes to compare the mortality experience of different populations or of the same population across time. However, because death rates increase with age, a higher crude death rate among one population than another might simply reflect that the first population is older, on average, than the second. When the underlying age distribution of two (or more) populations varies, practition-ers can either compare age-specific death rates or compute **age-standardized** (or **age-adjusted**) death (or mortality) rates.

Age-standardized death rates are based on statistical techniques that eliminate the effects of different age distributions among different populations. In effect, an age standardized rate is a "What if?" rate—what would the overall death rate be if the age distributions of the two (or more) populations were the same? This is accomplished by applying the observed age-specific rates from each population to a standard population. For years, the standard population recommended by the CDC's National Center for Health Statistics (NCHS) was the 1940 population of the United States. However, now the 2000 United States population is the standard.

Years of potential life lost (YPLL) is a measure of the impact of premature mortality on a population.[159] For a person who dies "prematurely" (usually defined as either before age 65 years or before the average life expectancy is reached), YPLL is calculated as the difference between that defined end point and the actual age at death. For an entire population, the YPLL is the sum of the individual YPLLs (Figure 11.15). Cause-specific YPLL can be calculated for specific causes of death.

The years-of-potential-life-lost rate represents years of potential life lost per 1,000 population

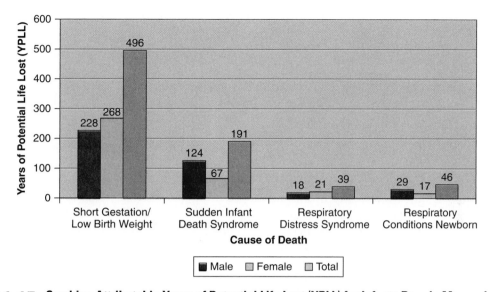

Figure 11.15. Smoking Attributable Years of Potential Life Lost (YPLL) for Infants Born in Massachusetts, 2001

SOURCE: Published in American Journal Of Preventive Medicine, Vol 4, Livengood et al, pp 268–73, Copyright Elsevier (1988).

who are aged less than the specified end point. YPLL rates are used to compare premature mortality among different populations, because YPLL alone does not involve consideration of differences in population size. Furthermore, YPLL rates can be standardized by age to adjust for differences in the underlying age distribution of populations.

Quality-adjusted life years (QALYs) is the standard unit of measure in a cost-utility analysis that reflects the quality of life, or desirability of living, as well as the duration of survival. Quality of life is integrated with length of life by using a multiplicative formula and discounting length of life by quality of life expected.[160] The measures are based on surveys of individual persons, where they are asked to weigh a particular health state against perfect health and against death by using methods such as person trade-off, time trade-off, and standard gamble.[161]

Disability-adjusted life years (DALYs) is a variant of QALYs used by WHO that measures the burden of disease, not only from premature mortality, but also from disability. It is a composite measure (sum) of time lost as a result of premature mortality (YPLL, with life expectancy of 82.5 years for females and 80 years for males), and time lived with a disability, adjusted for the severity of the disability. An expert panel weights the severity of disability by using methods similar to those used for QALYs. Also included in the calculation of DALYs are age weights (different values of life for each age) and discounted future years of life.[162] Critics of using DALYs have examined the heuristic nature of the value judgments and the fact that the components do not allow a distinction between use for measuring burden and allocating resources and the fact that age-weighting and discounting methods minimize the importance of conditions affecting older persons and those living with a disability.[163]

Descriptive Epidemiology

In descriptive epidemiology, data on the health problem among the population are organized and summarized by time, place, and person (see Essential Service 1). A necessary first step, this descriptive step allows the epidemiologist to become familiar with the data and generate hypotheses for further study.[164]

Analytic Epidemiology

Analytic epidemiology is concerned with the search for causes and effects, or the "why" or "how" of an event. The key feature of analytic epidemiology is the use of a comparison group. With a case report or case series, apparently unusual features can be described for one or more persons with disease, but this information cannot answer the question about how unusual those features really are. In an analytic epidemiologic study, the comparison group explicitly provides such information. If persons with a particular characteristic are more likely than those without the characteristic to experience a certain disease, then the characteristic is said to be associated with the disease. The characteristic can be a demographic factor (e.g., age or sex), a constitutional factor (e.g., blood group or immune status), a behavior (e.g., smoking or having eaten potato salad), or a circumstance (e.g., living near a toxic waste site). These factors help to identify populations at increased risk for disease, which can lead to appropriate targeting of public health prevention and control activities (Domain 7), as well as to ideas for future etiologic research.

For example, in an outbreak of hepatitis A, almost all the patients had eaten pastries from a particular bakery and had drunk the city's utility system-supplied water. An epidemiologic study was conducted during which consumption by patients was compared with consumption by a comparable group without hepatitis A. Almost all members of the comparison group had drunk the city-supplied water, but a limited number had eaten pastries. The study therefore implicated the bakery rather than the city's water supply as the source of the outbreak, which would have remained unknown without the comparison group.[165]

Types of Studies. Most epidemiologic studies of public health practice fall into two broad categories: **experimental** and **observational**. In an experimental study, the investigator determines the exposure category for each person (clinical trial) or community (community trial), then follows the participants or communities to identify effects. Experimental studies provide the most compelling evidence for causality (see the following discussion) and are required in certain settings; for example, the FDA requires multiple types of experimental studies before approving a candidate drug or therapeutic agent. However, experimental studies are not often used in public health. Randomization of communities is costly, often impractical, and may be unethical if standard measures are effective even if undocumented or preliminary.

More commonly, epidemiologists conduct observational studies, in which the investigator simply observes the exposure and outcome status of each study participant.[166] The two most common types of observational studies are the cohort study and the case-control study. In a **cohort** study, characteristics of a target group (e.g., their exposure to a carcinogen) are defined at the beginning of the study. Persons in the target group are followed for the subsequent development of the health events under study (e.g., cancer). The difference between a cohort and an experimental study is that, in a cohort study, the epidemiologist observes rather than dictates the exposure status of the participants. It would not be ethical, for example, to allocate humans to exposure to a known carcinogen.

After a follow-up period, the rate of disease occurrence among the exposed group is compared with the rate of disease occurrence among the unexposed group. The length of follow-up depends on characteristics of the health event and its etiology, ranging from days for acute diseases to decades for cancer, cardiovascular disease, and other chronic diseases. The Framingham study is a well-known cohort study in which >5,000 residents of Framingham, Massachusetts, have been followed since the early 1950s to determine the rate of and risk factors for cardiovascular disease.[167] A modification of this design is the retrospective cohort study. In this design, participants with or without a health condition are asked about prior exposures. For example, a group of men identified at a point of time in the past were asked about their lifetime consumption of caffeine; those with high lifetime consumption were compared with those with light lifetime caffeine consumption in the diagnosis of prostate cancer.[168]

The second and, in practicing public health, more common type of observational epidemiologic study is the **case-control study**. In a case-control study, a group of persons with disease ("case-patients") and a comparable group of persons without disease ("control subjects") are enrolled. The exposure or risk factor status of each enrollee is ascertained, and the exposure pattern of cases is compared with the exposure pattern of controls. The purpose of the control group is to provide an estimate of the expected or baseline exposure level or pattern among the population from which the cases arose. An exposure that is more common among case-patients than among control subjects is said to be "associated" with the disease, as in the study of hepatitis A cited previously.[166] The key to

well-designed case-control studies is to select an appropriate control group that provides a valid estimate of the baseline exposure.

The Two-by-Two Table. A **two-by-two table** is a cross-tabulation of the exposure and disease data from a cohort or case-control study. The traditional data layout for a two-by-two table is illustrated in Table 11.2. Each cell contains the number of study subjects with the exposure status as indicated in the row heading to the left and with the disease status indicated in the column heading above. For example, c represents the number of persons in the study who were not exposed, but who became ill (or case subjects) nonetheless.

Data from the investigation of an outbreak of gastroenteritis following an Easter Sunday dinner are presented in Table 11.3 (Cassius Lockett,

Table 11.2. Data Layout and Notation for a Standard Two-by-Two Table

	Ill/Case-patients	Well/Control subjects	Total	Attack rate
Exposed	a	b	a + b	a/(a + c)
Unexposed	c	d	c + d	c /(c + d)
Total	a + c	b + d	a + b + c + d	(a + c)/(a + b + c + d)

Table 11.3. Consumption of Ham and Risk for Gastroenteritis After an Easter Sunday Dinner, State A, April 2000

	Ill	Well	Total	Attack rate
Ate ham	16	11	27	59.3%
Did not eat ham	1	6	7	14.3%
Total	17	17	34	50.0%

California Department of Health Services, personal communication, 2000). The table provides a cross-tabulation of ham consumption (exposure) by presence or absence of gastroenteritis (outcome). Attack rates (59.3 percent for those who ate ham; 14.3 percent for those who did not) are provided to the right of the table.

Measures of Association. A measure of association quantifies the strength or magnitude of the association between the exposure and the health outcome of interest. Measures of association are sometimes called measures of effect because, if the exposure is causally related to the disease, the measures quantify the effect of being exposed on the risk for disease. In cohort studies, the measure of association of choice is the risk ratio or rate ratio. In case-control studies, the measure of choice is the odds ratio.

A **risk ratio** or **relative risk** compares the risk for disease or other health outcome between two groups (e.g., an exposed and unexposed group). It is calculated as the ratio of two risks (attack rates, cumulative incidences), as follows:

$$\text{Risk ratio} = \frac{\text{risk}_{\text{exposed}}}{\text{risk}_{\text{unexposed}}} = \frac{a/h_1}{c/h_0}$$

The risk ratio based on the data presented in Table 11.3 is 59.3/14.3 = 4.1. That is, persons who ate ham were 4.1 times more likely to experience gastroenteritis than those who did not eat ham. Note that the risk ratio will be >1.0 when the risk among the exposed group is greater than the risk among the unexposed group. The risk will be equal to 1.0 if both groups have the same risk for disease (i.e., if exposure is unrelated to risk for disease). The risk will be <1.0 if the risk for disease among the exposed group is less than the risk among the unexposed group, as would be expected when the exposure is a protective one such as vaccination or prophylactic antibiotic use or the use of folic acid to prevent neural tube defects.

In the majority of case-control studies, the sizes of the exposed and unexposed groups are unknown, and the number of controls is decided by the investigator. Without true denominators, attack rates (risks) cannot be calculated; therefore, risk ratios cannot be calculated directly. However, the **odds ratio** can be calculated as its own measure of association, and when the disease is relatively rare, the odds ratio approximates the risk ratio. The odds ratio is calculated as

$$\text{Odds ratio} = \frac{ad}{bc}$$

During an outbreak of Legionnaires' Disease, 13 cases occurred among residents of a small community. Control subjects were selected from local physician logs. Ironically, visiting the local hospital appeared to be associated with illness, as displayed in Table 11.4 (Joel Ackelsberg, New York City Department of Health, personal communication, 2000). The odds ratio, calculated as $12 \times 18/(4 \times 1)$, was 54.0. This odds ratio indicates a

Table 11.4. Legionnaires Disease and Exposure to Hospital A, State B, 1998

	Case-patients	Control subjects	Total
Visited hospital	12	4	16
Did not visit hospital	1	18	19
Total	13	22	35

strong association. Subsequent cultures of the cooling tower atop the hospital grew *Legionella pneumophilia* with patterns indistinguishable from clinical samples from the patients.

Incidence and prevalence among different populations can also be compared. A rate ratio and a prevalence ratio compare two incidence or prevalence rates, respectively, by dividing one by the other. A **prevalence odds ratio** is calculated as the odds ratio described previously, but uses prevalent cases rather than incident cases.

Finally, the **standardized mortality ratio** and the **standardized morbidity ratio** (both abbreviated as **SMR**) are measures of association commonly used in occupational epidemiology, wherein the number of observed deaths (or new cases) are divided by the expected number, taking into account the age distribution of the population.[169]

Measures of Public Health Impact

A measure of public health impact puts the association between exposure and disease into a public health context. It quantifies how much of the disease occurrence among a population can be attributed to the exposure being studied. For example, for an exposure that apparently increases one's risk for disease (e.g., smoking and lung cancer or undercooked hamburgers from Restaurant A and diarrhea), the **attributable risk** quantifies the amount of disease allegedly caused by the exposure. This measure can also be interpreted as the amount of disease that might be (or might have been) avoided if the exposure were removed (or had never existed). For an exposure such as vaccination that reduces one's risk for disease, the **prevented fraction** quantifies the reduction in disease burden attributable to the exposure.[170]

In one of their classic papers on smoking, Doll and Hill reported that the lung cancer mortality rates for smokers and nonsmokers were 1.30 and 0.07/1,000 persons/year, respectively.[170] Because only 0.07 deaths/1,000 is expected in the absence of smoking, the proportion of deaths among smokers attributable to their smoking (attributable risk percentage) was 100 percent $\times$ (1.30 − 0.07)/1.30 = 95 percent. Although smoking also contributed to

an increase in cardiovascular disease deaths, the attributable risk percentage was much smaller, only 23 percent. The prevented fraction can be multiplied by the total number of cases of a specific disease to obtain a "body count"—the absolute number of preventable cases attributable to a specific risk factor, a compelling measure for policy makers.[171]

Tests of Statistical Significance

Not every elevated risk ratio or odds ratio indicates a causal association between exposure and disease. Particularly when the risk ratio or odds ratio is only slightly deviant from 1.0, or when a study has only a limited number of subjects, the apparent association simply might be a chance finding. Tests of statistical significance are tools to evaluate the role of chance in explaining the finding.

The test of an association for statistical significance is an analysis that begins with the assumption that the exposure is *not* related to disease. This assumption is known as the **null hypothesis.** The **alternative hypothesis,** which can be adopted if the data indicate that the null hypothesis is implausible, is that exposure *is* associated with disease. A statistical test appropriate for the data is then selected and applied. For the majority of data in a two-by-two table format, either a **Fisher exact test** (which is best for studies with relatively few subjects) or a **chi-square test** is appropriate. If the data in the table have been matched in some way, then other tests are more appropriate.[172]

The test of significance provides the probability (or chances) of finding an association as strong as, or stronger than, the one observed, if the null hypothesis were in fact true (no relationship actually exits). This probability is called the **P value.** A highly limited P value is produced by data that are substantially inconsistent with the null hypothesis, and thus indicates that one is unlikely to observe such an association if the null hypothesis were true. When the P value is smaller than the cutoff specified in advance (e.g., .05), the null hypothesis is discarded as implausible in favor of the alternative hypothesis. This cutoff point is set by determining what percentage of the time the analyst is willing to reject a true null hypothesis and conclude an erroneous association exists (5 percent in our example). Note that, in practice, the majority of data might be amenable to multiple statistical tests, which occasionally leads to different conclusions.

The statistical test for the data in Table 11.3 yielded a P value of .046. Because this P value is smaller than the specified cutoff of .05, we can reject the null hypothesis and adopt the alternative hypothesis that eating ham was indeed associated with an increased risk for becoming ill. Note that a P value of approximately .05 indicates that 5 percent of the time, we might observe data that supports an association, even if none exists, unlikely but certainly within the realm of possibility. If the ham had come directly from a commercial processor, the investigator might prefer a greater level of statistical assurance that is a smaller P value of $<.01$ or 1 out of 100, before claiming that a company's hams are associated with illness and should be recalled from supermarket shelves and consumers.

The P value for the data in Table 11.4 is .00004. Therefore, the likelihood that the association of visiting the hospital and experiencing legionellosis can be attributed to chance is extremely limited, and the null hypothesis can be rejected.

Confidence Intervals

Another technique for quantifying the statistical likelihood of an observed measure of association is the **confidence interval.** A confidence interval surrounds the observed value and provides an indication of its statistical precision. The confidence interval is a range of values that is computed in such a way that a given proportion of such intervals (most often 95 percent) will contain the true value of the risk estimate. A narrow confidence interval reflects high precision in the observed value, whereas a wide confidence interval reflects more variability and less precision. Investigators often infer that the confidence interval is the range of values consistent with the data in the study. As a result, a confidence interval can also be used as a test of statistical significance—a 95 percent confidence interval that includes the null hypothesis value of 1.0 cannot reject the null hypothesis, whereas a 95 percent confidence interval that does not include 1.0 can

reject the null hypothesis. This use of the confidence interval in place of statistical testing is heuristic and might not always provide the same results.

For example, the 95 percent confidence interval for the data in Table 11.4 (odds ratio = 54.0) is from 5.4 to 544.0. This interval does not include 1.0; therefore, as with the chi-square test, the null hypothesis can be rejected. The interval is wide, indicating that the actual observed value of 54.0 is not precise. Nonetheless, all of the values in the interval, even those at the lower end, indicate a strong association between visiting the hospital and developing legionellosis.

Interpretation and Inference

An elevated risk ratio or odds ratio does not necessarily indicate a causal relationship between the exposure and the health outcome. In fact, other explanations of the apparent association should be assessed first. These possible explanations are chance, selection bias, information bias, confounding, and investigator error.

Randomness, or **chance,** is one possible explanation for an observed association. The role of chance is assessed through using tests of statistical significance. A substantially limited P value indicates that it is unlikely for us to observe these data if the null hypothesis is true, and that chance is an improbable explanation for the observed association. Note that statistical tests and P values only address the role of chance—they do not address problems in how the study was designed, conducted, or analyzed; thus, these measures will not address any bias that might exist.

A second explanation for an observed association is selection bias. **Selection bias** is a systematic flaw in how participants were selected, enrolled, or categorized, which results in an erroneous estimate of the association between exposure and disease. Consider a hypothetical case-control study of toxic shock syndrome at the time when its association with tampon use was suspected but not confirmed. The diagnosis was not well-known at the time, but physicians might have been reminded of the diagnosis if they knew the patient had been using a tampon. If diagnosis-based-on-exposure had been common, the effect on the two-by-two table would have been to load up the *a* cell, resulting in an artificially elevated odds ratio. Bias can also result from other selection, enrollment, and categorization problems such as differences between persons who agree versus those who decline (or are too sick) to participate, from the use of volunteer control subjects, who have their own reasons for participating, and by enrolling persons with asymptomatic disease as control subjects.

A third explanation for an observed association is information bias. **Information bias** is a systematic flaw in the information collected from or about the participants in the study that results in an erroneous estimate of the association between exposure and disease. If patients are more likely to recall an exposure than control subjects, then that exposure will appear to be associated with illness. If interviewers probe more thoroughly when interviewing patients than control subjects, or data abstractors review hospital charts of patients more vigorously than charts of control subjects, the exposure will appear to be associated with illness.

A fourth explanation for an observed association is confounding. **Confounding** is a mixing of two effects, specifically when an unstudied risk factor is associated with both the exposure and outcome under study. Consider a hypothetical, poorly randomized clinical trial in which more cancer patients with early stage disease receive investigational drug A than tried-and-true drug B, and more cancer patients with late-stage disease receive tried-and-true drug B than investigational drug A. Assume that persons with early stage disease survive longer than persons with late-stage disease. Even if investigational drug A is no better than tried-and-true drug B, drug A will appear to be associated with improved survival, compared with drug B, because drug A was preferentially administered to persons with early-stage disease. In this example, the unstudied risk factor is stage of disease, resulting in an apparent association between drug A and improved survival when no such effect truly exists.

A fifth explanation for an observed association is **investigator error**. Investigator error can result from erroneous data entry or manipulation, inappropriate analysis, or misinterpretation. This might be unintentional or intentional.

Assuming that an observed association does not appear to be attributable to chance, selection bias, information bias, confounding, or investigator error, a causal relationship might well be the explanation. Multiple criteria have been proposed for helping an investigator decide whether an association should be considered causal. These criteria include the magnitude of association (the larger the risk ratio or odds ratio, the more plausible), biologic plausibility, consistency with other studies, dose-response effect (increasing exposure associated with increased risk for disease), and exposure preceding disease.[171] These criteria involve judgment, and reasonable people can disagree about whether the available evidence is sufficient to demonstrate causality.

Domain 7: Financial Planning and Management Skills

We have discussed the ways in which epidemiology can support the science and effectiveness of public health activities. Public health agencies increasingly are required to assess quantitatively the quality of their programs. In addition to being effective and of high quality, public health activities must now demonstrate cost-effectiveness. Competency in assessing the effectiveness of prevention[173] includes scientific quantitative policy methods to fundamentally change and improve public health decision making. In this way, public health and health care programs and policies deliver the greatest possible improvement in the health and quality of life of a given population for the expenditure.[174]

Domain 8: Leadership and Systems-Thinking Skills

In the preamble of the 1948 WHO constitution, "health" was defined as "a state of complete physical, mental, and social well-being and not merely the absence of disease or infirmity."[175] This indicates that epidemiologic and public health data contribute to a holistic approach to public health—one that concentrates on the needs, preferences, and assets of the whole community, rather than on individual parts.

Zaza and Briss[176] define multiple benefits to a holistic approach to public health. First, programs can leverage each other's strengths. For example, a program that identifies women at high risk for cancer as a result of lack of preventive screening might also be an opportunity for delivering interventions associated with diet and physical activity aimed at decreasing risk for cardiovascular disease.[177] Second, a holistic approach involving multiple stakeholders has a greater chance of being acceptable to the target population.[178] Third, a holistic approach opens the possibility for earlier identification of the problem and for development of multiple interventions being delivered in a more efficient manner, much more than what might be expected in the activities of a categorical program. For example, the Steps to a Healthier U.S. Program,[179] an integrated chronic disease prevention and health-promotion program, involves a range of sectors (e.g., public health, business, health care, and education), for example, effective approaches to preventing tobacco initiation.[180] Finally, such a holistic approach is more likely to be sustained when categorical programs expire as a result of lack of funding.[181]

In this context, decisions affecting the health of communities are best driven by data that are collected carefully and analyzed rigorously. The term "evidence-based public health" seems to have permeated every conversation about prevention planning, implementation, and evaluation. Certainly, in the majority of medical science branches, the concept of evidence-based medicine seems to be expected. In this regard, the **randomized controlled trial (RCT)** provides the standard of evidence. Yet, to wait for an RCT addressing critical problems of public health seems impracticable, if not unethical. Indeed, the holistic approach described previously, driven by community needs and preferences, might create a tension between community input and the best available science.

The *American Heritage Dictionary* defines *evidence* as "a thing or things helpful in forming a conclusion or judgment."[182] Thus, we recognize a range of evidence in making decisions about public health in communities. A precise definition of evidence and a framework for practice are provided by Brownson et al.[183] Early decisions about whether something should be done about a problem often rely on surveillance data, surveys, or studies that report the burden of disease risk, disease burden, or cost. In deciding what should be done, multiple forms of evidence might be used. For example, the Community Guide[184] provides reviews and recommendations about different public health interventions (educational, policy, environmental, and systems change). However, these evidence-based recommendations might need to be analyzed for individual communities. The intervention of cancer screening among Vietnamese women discussed previously (see Essential Service 1, Domain 4: Cultural Competency Skills) illustrates that even if a proposed policy is effective, has minimal risk, and is priced reasonably, community concerns such as perception of risk or acceptability might preclude its adoption. Our interventions might have unintended consequences related to our progress (e.g., obesity or antibiotic resistance).[185] These unintended effects must be examined in the context within which they occur.

Challenges and Opportunities

Public health data must be communicated clearly to policy makers for effective public health practice. In the early 1990s, public health analysts used the National Health and Nutrition Examination Survey (NHANES) to illustrate an association between the amount of lead in people's blood and the lead in the environment, presumably as a result of the widespread use of leaded gasoline[186] (Figure 11.16). The health risks related to these data were not lost on policy makers who subsequently reduced the allowable levels of lead in gasoline.[187]

Leadership in public health presents multiple challenges. First, we need the science to determine which interventions are efficacious, and then the major challenge is to implement them effectively. For example, the Diabetes Control and Complications Trial, a randomized clinical trial held during

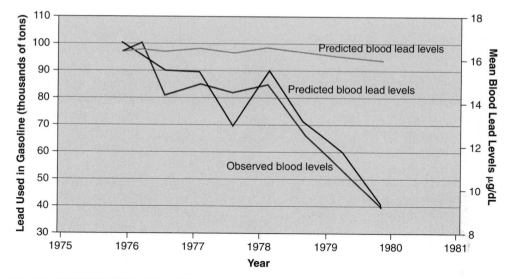

Figure 11.16. NHANES II Blood Lead Measurements, 1975–1981

SOURCE: Pirkle JL, Brody DJ, Gunter EW, et al. The decline in blood lead levels in the United States. The National Health and Nutrition Examination Surveys (NHANES). JAMA 1994; 272:284–291. Copyright © 1994, American Medical Association. All Rights Reserved.

1983–1993, demonstrated that with intensive control (i.e., keeping blood glucose levels as normal as possible), we could reduce microvascular complications of diabetes by 40–70 percent, depending on the type of complication.[188] Yet, as of 1995, a study by the CDC reported that approximately 18 percent of the population of persons with diabetes did not achieve this level of glucose control,[189] especially among populations at greatest risk for complications.[190]

Public health surveillance is the cornerstone of public health practice, and epidemiologic research is the basic science of public health. Both require high-quality data and analysis appropriate to the needs of the population at risk for diseases , injury, and disability. Only then can we ensure that the public's health is served.

REVIEW QUESTIONS

1. Refer to Figure 11.2b for the official case definition for Kawasaki syndrome.
   Discuss the pros and cons of this case definition for the three purposes listed.

   a. Diagnosing and treating individual patients.
   b. Tracking the occurrence of the disease for public health records.
   c. Conducting research to identify the cause of the disease.

2. In one community of 4,399 persons, 115 persons became ill with a disease of unknown etiology. The 115 cases occurred among 77 households. The total number of persons living in these 77 households was 424.

   a. Calculate the overall attack rate in the community.
   b. Calculate the **secondary attack rate** in the affected households, assuming that only one case per household was a primary (community-acquired) case.
   d. Is the disease distributed evenly throughout the population?

3. Assume you are working in a state health department in which none of the following conditions is on the state list of reportable diseases. For each condition, what sources

of data might be available if you wished to conduct surveillance? What factors make one source of data more appropriate than another?

a. *E. coli*

b. Spinal cord injury

c. Lung cancer among nonsmokers

4. In the 1920s, health care workers in Great Britain first began to suspect an association between cigarette smoking and lung cancer, on the basis of the fact that the majority of patients who acquired lung cancer were also smokers. As a result, during 1930–1960, multiple epidemiologic studies were undertaken to try to quantify the association between cigarette smoking and lung cancer. Two of these studies, one in 1947 by Sir Richard Doll and one in 1951 by A. B. Hill, are considered classics. Doll compared the smoking history of a group of hospitalized patients with lung cancer with the smoking history of a similar group without lung cancer. Hill categorized a group of British physicians according to their smoking histories and then analyzed the causes of death among those who died to determine whether cigarette smokers had the highest incidence of lung cancer.

a. What hypotheses are both Doll and Hill attempting to test?

Doll's study: Data for this study were collected from hospitalized patients in London and the surrounding communities during a 4-year period (April 1948–February 1952). Hospital personnel at >20 hospitals were asked to contact investigators whenever a patient was admitted with a new diagnosis of lung cancer. These patients were then interviewed about their prior smoking habits. At the same time, investigators interviewed a random sample of patients from the same hospitals, but with different illnesses, about their smoking habits.

Hill's study: Data for this study were obtained from physicians listed in the British Medical Register who resided in England and Wales as of October 1951. At the beginning of the study, a questionnaire was used to collect information about the physicians' past and present smoking habits. They were then categorized according to their exposure to cigarette smoke. In the ensuing years, investigators gathered information about deaths attributed to lung cancer from death certificates and other mortality data.

b. Name the study design used in Doll's study.

c. In Doll's study, why were investigators interested in interviewing patients who were hospitalized for disorders other than lung cancer? Why was studying patients from the same hospital important? Why do you think Doll chose to conduct his study among hospitalized patients?

Doll's study: Approximately 1,700 persons with lung cancer, all aged <75 years, were eligible for this study. Approximately 15 percent were not interviewed because of death, severity of illness, discharge from the hospital, or inability to speak English. An additional group of patients were interviewed for the study but were later excluded when their initial diagnosis of lung cancer proved to be wrong. The final study group included 1,465 case-subjects (1,357 men and 108 women). Table 11.5 presents data on men who were included in the study.

d. From Table 11.5, calculate the proportion of lung cancer patients and other patients who smoked.

Table 11.5. Incidence of Lung Cancer According to Smoking Status

	Lung Cancer	No Lung Cancer
Cigarette smokers	1,350	1,296
Nonsmokers total	7	61
Total	1,357	1,357

e. What type of study was Hill's study?

Recall that data for Hill's study were obtained from the population of all physicians listed in the British Medical Register who resided in England and Wales as of October 1951. In October 1951, questionnaires were mailed to 59,600 physicians. The questionnaire asked physicians to classify themselves into one of three categories: (1) current smoker, (2) ex-smoker, or (3) nonsmoker. Smokers and ex-smokers were asked how much they smoked, their method of smoking (e.g., whether they inhaled, whether they used a cigarette holder), the age at which they started to smoke, and if they had stopped smoking, how long since they last smoked. Nonsmokers were defined as persons who had never consistently smoked as much as one cigarette per day for as long as one year. Usable responses were received from 40,637 (68 percent) of the physicians (34,445 men and 6,192 women).

f. How do you think the 68 percent response rate might affect the study's results?

Hill and his colleagues focused only on physician respondents aged ≥35 years. The occurrence of lung cancer among respondents was documented for November 1951–October 1961. Over this 10-year period, 4,957 persons in the cohort died, 157 from lung cancer. Four of these 157 deaths were not documented, leaving 153 confirmed deaths from lung cancer. Table 11.6 provides the number of deaths from lung cancer by number of cigarettes smoked per day. (The daily smoking rate was available for only 136 of the 153 decedents). Person-years at risk are displayed for each smoking category.

g. Using data from Table 11.6, calculate lung cancer mortality rates, rate ratios, and rate differences for each smoking category. What is the overall trend concerning lung cancer mortality rates? How would you interpret your findings for the rate ratio and rate difference categories?

Table 11.7 presents information about deaths caused by lung cancer, according to the decedents' cigarette smoking status.

5. What do the data in Table 11.7 indicate regarding smokers, nonsmokers, and ex-smokers? What does this imply from a public health perspective?

Table 11.8 presents results from both Doll's and Hill's studies and the number of cigarettes respondents smoked per day.

6. What are similarities of Doll's study and Hill's study? What are differences? How would you account for the differences?

Table 11.6. Mortality from Lung Cancer by Smoking Status

Daily Number of Cigarettes Smoked	Deaths from Lung Cancer	Person-Years* at Risk	Mortality Rate* per 1000 Person Years	Rate Ratio*	Rate Difference per 1,000 Person-Years
0	3	42,800	0.07	referent	referent
1–14	22	38,600	0.57	8.1	0.50
15–24	54	38,900	1.39	19.8	1.32
25+	57	25,100	2.27	32.4	2.20
All smokers	133	102,600	1.30	18.6	1/23
Total	136	145,400	0.94	Not applicable	

Table 11.7. Mortality from Lung Cancer by Smoking Status

Cigarette Smoking Status	Number of Lung Cancer Deaths	Mortality Rate per 1,000 Person-Years	Rate Ratio
Current smokers	133	1.30	18/6
Ex-smokers: years since quitting			
<5 years	5	0.67	9.6
5–9 years	7	0.49	7.0
10–19 years	3	0.18	2.6
20+ years	2	0.19	2.7
Nonsmokers	3	0.07	1.0 (ref.)

Table 11.8. Risk of Lung Cancer Morbidity and Mortality According to Smoking Status

Number of Cigarettes Smoked Daily	Odds Ratio from Doll's Study	Rate Ratio from Hill's Study
0	1.0 (ref)	1.0 (ref)
1–14	7.0	8.1
15–24	9.5	19.8
≥25	16.3	32.4
All smokers	18.5	9.1

7. What of the following criteria for causality are met by the data from these two studies? (*Answer "yes" or "no" for each*)

- Strength of association?
- Consistency with other studies?
- Exposure precedes disease?
- Dose-response effect?
- Biologic Plausibility?

8. An estimated 18.2 million persons in the United States have diabetes, resulting in increased risk for cardiovascular disease, renal failure, and early death. Diabetes is a condition in which the body cannot use the sugars and starches (carbohydrates) it takes in as food to make energy. Both genetics and lifestyle play a role in who gets diabetes. To investigate whether having a family history of diabetes is related to self-reported diabetes in a substantial representative sample, researchers analyzed data from the National Health and Nutrition Examination Survey (NHANES) during 1999–2002. NHANES is a continuous, population-based survey of noninstitutionalized adults (age ≥20 years) in the United States. Data are collected in two ways: an interview conducted in a person's home and a physical health examination. Diabetes status was assessed by asking whether a person had ever been told by a physician or other health professional that he/she has "diabetes" or "sugar diabetes" other than during pregnancy.

a. What epidemiologic aspect of diabetes is this survey designed to measure?

b. List three limitations presented by this survey design for assessing the true burden of diabetes in the United States?

c. What demographic information would be important to collect regarding the persons surveyed?

9. Participants were asked whether any biological member of their family, living or deceased, had ever been told he/she had

Table 11.9. Frequencies and Percentages of Self-Reported Persons with Diabetes by Demographic and Risk Factors, Adults Aged ≥20 Years in the United States, 1999–2002

	Total (n)	Diabetic (n)	Weighted* Percent (95 Percent CI)
Total	10,283	991	6.5 (5.9–7.1)
Men			
All races	4,802	481	6.7 (5.9–7.5)
Non-Hispanic white	2,396	196	6.2 (5.1–7.3)
Non-Hispanic black	887	108	8.2 (6.5–9.9)
Mexican-American	1,129	130	5.3 (3.9–6.7)
Women			
All races	5,481	510	6.3 (5.5–7.2)
Non-Hispanic white	2,674	170	5.1 (4.4–5.8)
Non-Hispanic black	1,034	140	11.4 (9.2–13.6)
Mexican-American	1,266	148	7.7 (6.2–9.3)
Age (years)			
20–39	3,618	61	1.7 (1.1–2.2)
40–59	2,964	256	6.6 (5.6–7.5)
≥60	3,701	674	15.1 (13.9–16.4)
Poverty income ratio (PIR)			
PIR <1.00 (poverty)	1,743	208	7.9 (6.0–9.8)
PIR 1.00–1.85	2,138	278	8.7 (7.3–10.1)
PIR ≥1.86	5,222	378	5.3 (4.7–6.0)
Education level			
Less than high school	3,559	514	10.9 (9.5–12.3)
High school/GED	2,361	200	6.5 (5.4–7.5)
More than high school	4,321	273	4.7 (3.8–5.5)
Body mass index (BMI)b			
BMI <25	2,752	143	3.1 (2.3–3.9)
BMI 25–29	3,087	298	5.9 (4.8–7.0)
BMI ≥30	2,662	386	11.2 (10.1–12.4)

*For extrapolation of diabetes prevalence to the adult, noninstitutionalized, civilian U.S. population, weighted percentages incorporate NHANES sampling weights to account for unequal selection probabilities and nonrandom sampling design.

diabetes. Family history information was not available from 216 persons. The Disease Detectives defined family history as having a first-degree relative (parent or sibling) with diabetes.

The overall estimated prevalence of diabetes among adults was 6.5 percent. Refer to Table 11.9 to answer questions 9a and b.

a. Describe the pattern of diabetes by sex, race/ethnicity, and age.

Table 11.10. **Frequencies of Self-Reported Persons with Diabetes by Family History of Disease, Adults Aged ≥20 Years in the United States, 1999–2002**

Family History	Total	Diabetic
No	6,895	344
Yes	3,172	618

b. How would you describe the relationship between weight and diabetes?

In this survey, 3,172 adults reported having a family history of diabetes in a first-degree relative within the study population of 10, 283. Table 11.10 displays data on the report of diabetes for these 3,172 adults and the others without family history.

c. Calculate the appropriate risk estimate to assess the association of family history with diabetes in this study. Interpret your answer for a group of your friends.

d. List two reasons other than genetic disposition why persons with family history might have a different pattern of diabetes in these data.

10. Researchers have reported that the B-vitamin, folic acid, can prevent neural tube defects (NTDs) such as anencephaly and spina bifida. As a result, women can do something to prevent many of these birth defects from happening in the future. The percentage of NTDs among a population that is preventable by supplementation with folic acid is known as the preventable fraction. A group of researchers examined use of folic acid among a cohort of 22,776 pregnant women (Milunsky A, Hick H, Hick SS, et al. Multivitamin/folic acid supplementation in early pregnancy reduces the prevalence of neural tube defects. *JAMA.* 1989;262:2847–52). Of the pregnancies, 49 ended in an NTD. Of these 49 pregnancies, 40 (82 percent) did not take folic acid. The

prevalence of NTDs was 3.5/1,000 among women who never used multivitamins before or after conception or who used multivitamins before conception only. The prevalence of NTDs for women who used folic acid-containing multivitamins during the first 6 weeks of pregnancy was substantially lower—0.9/1,000 women.

a. What is the relative risk of NTDs associated with taking folic acid?

b. What is the percentage of NTDs among a population that is preventable by supplementation with folic acid?

REFERENCES

1. Gebbie K, Merrill J, Tilson HH. The public health workforce. *Health Aff.* 2002;21:57–67.
2. Council on Linkages Between Academia and Public Health Practice. *Core Competencies for Public Health Professionals.* Washington, DC: Public Health Foundation [cited Oct 5, 2006]. Available at: http://www.phf.org/competencies.htm.
3. Thacker SB, Stroup DF. Public health surveillance. In: Brownson RC, Pettiti DB, eds. *Applied Epidemiology: Theory to Practice.* 2nd ed. New York: Oxford University Press; 2006.
4. Eylenbosch WJ, Noah ND, eds. *Surveillance in Health and Disease.* London, England: Oxford University Press; 1988.
5. Langmuir AD. The surveillance of communicable diseases of national importance. *N Engl J Med.* 1963;268:182–92.
6. Williams AA, Parashar UD, Stoica A, et al. Bioterrorism anthrax surveillance. *Emerg Infect Dis.* 2002;8 [cited Oct 5, 2006]. http://www.cdc.gov/eid.
7. Centers for Disease Control and Prevention. Case definitions for infectious conditions under public health surveillance. *MMWR.* 1997;46(RR–10) [cited Oct 5, 2006]. http://www.cdc.gov/epo/dphsi/casedef/index.htm.
8. Centers for Disease Control and Prevention. Indicators for chronic disease surveillance. *MMWR.* 2004;53(RR-11).
9. Romaguera RA, German RR, Klaucke DN. Evaluating public health surveillance. In: Teutsch SM, Churchill RE, eds. *Principles and Practice of*

Public Health Surveillance. Vol 2. New York: Oxford University; 2000:176–93.

10. Milstein B, Chapel T, Wetterhall SF, Cotton DA. Building capacity for program evaluation at the Centers for Disease Control and Prevention. *New Directions for Evaluation.* 2002;93: 27–46.

11. Jack L, Mukhtar Q, Martin M, et al. Program evaluation and chronic diseases: methods, approaches, and implications for public health. *Prev Chronic Dis.* 2006;3(1) [cited Oct 5, 2006]. http://www.cdc.gov/pcd.

12. Stevahn L, King JA, Ghere G, Minnema J. Establishing essential competencies for program evaluators. *Am J Eval.* 2005;26:43–59.

13. Lando J, Williams SM, Williams G, Sturgis S. A logic model for the integration of mental health into chronic disease prevention and health promotion. *Prev Chron Dis.* 2006;3 [cited Oct 5, 2006]. http://www.cdc.gov/pcd/issues/2006/apr/pdf/05_0215.pdf.

14. Stroup DF, Brookmeyer R, Kalsbeek W. Public health surveillance in action: a framework. In: Brookmeyer R, Stroup DF, eds. *Monitoring the Health of Populations: Statistical Principles and Methods for Public Health Surveillance.* New York: Oxford University Press; 2003:1–35.

15. Thacker SB. Historical development. In: Teutsch SM, Churchill RE, eds. *Principles and Practice of Public Health Surveillance.* New York: Oxford University Press; 2000:1–16.

16. Langmuir AD. William Farr: founder of modern concepts of surveillance. *Int J Epidemiol.* 1976; 5:13–8.

17. Eylenbosch WJ, Noah ND, eds. *Surveillance in Health and Disease.* London, England: Oxford University Press; 1988.

18. Mather CD, Fat DM, Inoue M, Rao C, Lopez AD. Counting the dead and what they die from. *Bull World Health Organ.* 2005;83:171–7.

19. Schoendorf K, Branum A. The use of United States vital statistics in perinatal and obstetric research. *Am J Obstet Gynecol.* 2005;194:911–5.

20. Luber GE, Sanchez CA, Conklin LM. Heat-related deaths—United States, 1999–2003. *MMWR.* 2006;55: 796–798 [cited Oct 5, 2006]. http://www.cdc.gov/mmwr/preview/mmwrhtml/mm5529a2.htm.

21. Simonsen L, Reichert TA, Viboud C, et al. Impact of influenza vaccination on seasonal mortality in the US elderly population. *Arch Intern Med.* 2005;165:265–72.

22. Kovar MG. *Data Systems of the National Center for Health Statistics.* Hyattsville, MD: National Center for Health Statistics; 1989. *Vital and Health Statistics,* Series 1. DHHS Publication (PHS)89–1325.

23. Choi K, Thacker SB. An evaluation of influenza mortality surveillance, 1962–1979. I. Time series forecasts of expected pneumonia and influenza deaths. *Am J Epidemiol.* 1981;113:215–26.

24. Tilford JM, Aitken ME, Anand KS, et al. Hospitalizations for critically ill children with traumatic brain injuries: A longitudinal analysis. *Crit Care Med.* 2005;33:2074–81.

25. Kung HC, Hanzlick R, Spitler JF. Abstracting data from medical examiner/coroner reports: concordance among abstractors and implications for data reporting. *J Forensic Sci.* 2001;46:1126–31.

26. National Research Council. *Eliminating health disparities: measurement and data needs.* Panel on DHHS Collection of Race and Ethnicity Data, Michele Ver Ploeg and Edward Perrin, eds. Committee on National Statistics, Division of Behavioral and Social Sciences and Education. Washington, DC: The National Academies Press, 2004.

27. Williams DR, Jackson PB. Social sources of racial disparities in health. *Health Aff.* 2005;24:325–34.

28. Setel PW, Sankoh O, Rao C, et al. Sample registration of vital events with verbal autopsy: a renewed commitment to measuring and monitoring vital statistics. *Bull World Health Organ.* 2005; 83:611–7.

29. Percy C, Dolman A. Comparison of the coding of death certificates related to cancer in seven countries. *Public Health Rep.* 1978;93:335–50.

30. Wall MW, Hunag J, Oswald J, McCulle D. Factors associated with reporting multiple causes of death. *BMC Med Res Methodol.* 2005;4:4 [cited Oct 5, 2006]. http://www.pubmedcentral.gov.

31. World Health Organization. *The First Ten Years of the World Health Organization.* Geneva, Switzerland: World Health Organization; 1958.

32. Silk BJ, Berkelman RL. A review of strategies for enhancing the completeness of notifiable disease reporting. *J Public Health Manag Pract.* 2005;11: 191–200.

33. Alter MJ, Mares A, Hadler SC, Maynard, JE. The effect of underreporting on the apparent incidence

and epidemiology of acute viral hepatitis. *Am J Epidemiol*. 1987;125:133–9.

34. Brachott D, Mosley JW. Viral hepatitis in Israel: the effect of canvassing physicians on notifications and the apparent epidemiological pattern. *Bull World Health Organ*. 1972;46:457–64.

35. Surveillance of influenza-like diseases through a national computer network—France, 1984–1989. *MMWR*. 1989;38:855–7.

36. Kyle AD, Balmes JR, Buffler PA, Lee PR. Integrating research, surveillance, and practice in environmental public health tracking. *Environ Health Perspect*. 2006;114:980–4.

37. Stroobant AW, Van Casteren V, Thiers G. Surveillance systems from primary care data: surveillance through a network of sentinel general practitioners. In: Eylenbosch WJ, Noah ND, eds. *Surveillance in Health and Disease*. London, England: Oxford University Press; 1988:62–74.

38. Lobet MP, Stroobant A, Mertens R, et al. Tool for validation of the network of sentinel general practitioners in the Belgian health care system. *Int J Epidemiol*. 1987;16:612–8.

39. Kalsbeek WD. The use of surveys in public health surveillance: monitoring high-risk populations. In: Brookmeyer R, Stroup DF, eds. *Monitoring the Health of Populations: Statistical Principles and Methods for Public Health Surveillance*. New York: Oxford University Press; 2004:37–70.

40. Wilcox LS. Welcome to Preventing Chronic Disease. *Prev Chronic Dis*. [serial online] 2004; 1[cited Oct 5, 2006 5]. http://www.cdc.gov/pcd/issues/2004/jan/03_0023.htm.

41. Yun S, Zhu BP, Black W, Brownson RC. Comparison of national estimates of obesity prevalence from the behavioral risk factor surveillance system and the national health and nutrition examination survey. *Int J Obesity*. 2006;30:164–70.

42. Centers for Disease Control and Prevention (CDC). *SMART: Selected Metropolitan/Micropolitan Area Risk Trends: SMART Technical Documents and survey Data; Annual Survey Data*. Atlanta, GA: US Department of Health and Human Services, CDC; 2006 [cited Oct 5, 2006]. Available at: http://www.cdc.gov/brfss/smart/technical_infodata.htm.

43. Clean Air Act Amendments of 1990. Public Law 101–549.

44. Johns Hopkins Bloomberg School of Public Health. *iHAPSS 2006: Internet-Based Health & Air Pollution Surveillance System*. Baltimore, MD: Johns Hopkins Bloomberg School of Public Health; 2005 [cited Oct 5, 2006]. Available at: http://www.ihapss.jhsph.edu/.

45. Polivka BJ, Salsberry P, Casavant MJ, Chaudry RV, Bush DC. Comparison of parental report of blood lead testing in children enrolled in Medicaid with Medicaid claims data and blood lead surveillance reports. *J Comm Health*. 2006;31:43–55.

46. Centers for Disease Control and Prevention (CDC). PHLIS surveillance data. Salmonella annual summaries. Atlanta, GA: US Department of Health and Human Services, CDC; 2002 [cited Oct 5, 2006]. Available at: http://www.cdc.gov/ncidod/dbmd/phlisdata/salmonella.htm.

47. Gupta SB, Dingley SD, Lamgni TL, et al. The national CD4 surveillance scheme for England and Wales. *Commun Dis Public Health*. 2001; 4:27–32.

48. Centers for Disease Control and Prevention. Monitoring hospital-acquired infections to promote patient safety—United States, 1990–1999. *MMWR*. 2000;49:149–53.

49. Stelling JM, O'Brien TF. Surveillance of antimicrobial resistance: the WHONET program. *Clin Infect Dis*. 1997;24(Suppl 1):S157–68.

50. Gerner Smidt P, Hise K, Kincaid J, et al. PulseNet USA: a five-year update. *Foodborne Pathog Dis*. 2006;3(1):9–19.

51. Cronquist A, Wedel S, Sewell CM, at al. Multistate outbreak of Salmonella Typhimurium infections associated with eating ground beef—United States, 2004. *MMWR*. 2006;55;180–2.

52. Heyman DL, Rodier G. Global surveillance, national surveillance, and SARS. *Emerg Infect Dis* [serial online]. 2003 Feb [cited Oct 5, 2006]. http://www.cdc.gov/ncidod/EID/vol10no2/03-1038.htm.

53. Bravata DM, McDonald KM, Smith WM, et al. Systematic review: surveillance systems for early detection of bioterrorism-related diseases. *Ann Intern Med*. 2004;140:910–22.

54. Centers for Disease Control and Prevention. Framework for evaluating public health surveillance systems for early detection of outbreaks: recommendations from the CDC working group. *MMWR*. 2004;53(RR-5).

55. Henning KJ. What is syndromic surveillance? *MMWR*. 2004;53(Suppl):5–11.

56. Centers for Disease Control and Prevention. Syndromic surveillance: reports from a national conference. *MMWR*. 2005;54(Suppl).

57. Sloane PD, MacFarquhar JK, Sickbert-Bennett E, et al. Syndromic surveillance for emerging infections in office practice using billing data. *Ann Fam Med*. 2006;4:351–8.

58. Centers for Disease Control and Prevention. *Annotated Bibliography for Syndromic Surveillance* [cited Oct 5, 2006]. Available at: http://www.cdc.gov/epo/dphsi/syndromic/abstracts.htm.

59. Richards L, Fox K, Roberts C, Fletcher L, Goddard E. *Living in Britain No. 31: Results from the 2002 General Household Survey*. London, England: Office of National Statistics, Stationery Office; 2002.

60. Yang G, Hu J, Rao KQ, Ma J, Rao C, Lopez AD. Mortality registration and surveillance in China: history, current situation and challenges. *Popul Health Metr*. 2005;3:3.

61. Nelson DE, Powell-Griner E, Town M, Kovar MG. A comparison of national estimates from the National Health Interview Survey and the Behavioral Risk Factor Surveillance System. *Am J Public Health*. 2003;93:1335–41.

62. Eaton DK, Kann L, Kichen S, et al. Youth risk behavior surveillance—United States, 2005. *MMWR*. 2006;55(SS-5).

63. Centers for Disease Control and Prevention. National hospital discharge and ambulatory surgery data 2005 [cited Oct 5, 2006]. Available at: http://www.cdc.gov/nchs/about/major/hdasd/nhds.htm.

64. Central Statistical Authority[Ethiopia] and ORC Macro. *Ethiopia Demographic and Health Survey, 2000*. Addis Ababa, Ethiopia and Calverton, MD, USA: Central Statistical Authority and ORC Macro; 2001 [cited Oct 5, 2006]. Available at: http://www.measuredhs.com.

65. Cherkin DC, Phillips WR, Gillanders WR. Assessing the reliability of data from patient medical records. *J Fam Pract*. 1984;18:937,939–40.

66. Weiner M, Stump TE, Callahan CM, Lewis JN, McDonald CJ. A practical method of linking data from Medicare claims and a comprehensive electronic medical records system. *Int J Med Inform*. 2003;71:57–69.

67. Gladman DD, Menter A. Introduction/overview on clinical registries. *Ann Rheum Dis*. 2005;64:ii101-2.

68. The Paul Coverdell Prototype Registries Writing Group. Acute stroke care in the US: results from 4 pilot prototypes of the Paul Coverdell National Acute Stroke Registry. *Stroke*. 2005;36:1232 [cited Oct 5, 2006]. http://stroke.ahajournals.org/cgi/content/abstract/36/6/1232.

69. Ferrara A, Quesenberry CP, Karter AJ, et al. Current use of unopposed estrogen and estrogen plus progestin and the risk of acute myocardial infarction among women with diabetes. The Northern California Kaiser Permanente Diabetes Registry, 1995–1998. *Circulation*. 2003;107:43–8.

70. Parkin DM. The evolution of the population-based cancer registry. *Cancer*. 2006;6:603–12.

71. Brewster D, Coebergh J, Storm H. Population-based cancer registries: the invisible key to cancer control. *Lancet Oncol*. 2005;6:193–5.

72. Swan J, Wingo P, Clive R, et al. Cancer surveillance in the U.S.: can we have a national system? *Cancer*. 1998;83:9.

73. Holtzman NA, Khoury MJ. Monitoring for congenital malformations. *Annu Rev Public Health*. 1986;7:237–66.

74. Centers for Disease Control and Prevention. *Metropolitan Atlanta Congenital Defects Program*. Atlanta, GA: US Department of Health and Human Services, CDC; 2005 [cited Oct 5, 2006]. Available at: http://www.cdc.gov/ncbddd/bd/macdp.htm.

75. Kirby RS, Seaver LH. Birth defects research: improving surveillance methods and addressing epidemiologic questions and public health issues. *Birth Defects Res A Clin Mol Teratol*. 2005;73:645.

76. Edmonds LD. Birth defects surveillance at the state and local level. *Teratology*. 1997;56:5–7.

77. Vitillo JA. Adverse drug reaction surveillance: practical methods for developing a successful monitoring program. Medscape Pharmacists. 2000 [cited Oct 5, 2006]. Available at: http://www.medscape.com/viewarticle/408575.

78. US Consumer Product Safety Commission. *National Electronic Injury Surveillance System* [cited Oct 5, 2006]. Available at: http://www.cpsc.gov/lib/neiss.

79. Horton DK, Berkowitz Z, Kaye WE. Morbidity and mortality from hazardous materials events in the personal services industry, 1993–2001: a follow-up report from the Hazardous Substances

Emergency Events Surveillance System. *Am J Ind Med*. 2005;47:419–27.

80. Seligman PJ, Halperin WE, Mullan RJ, Frazier TM. Occupational lead poisoning in Ohio: surveillance using worker's compensation data. A*m J Public Health*. 1986;76:1299–302.

81. Rosenman KD, Kalush A, Reilly MJ, et al. How much work-related injury and illness is missed by the current national surveillance system? *J Occup Environ Med*. 2006;48:357–65.

82. Fairchild AL, Bayer R. Ethics and the conduct of public health surveillance. *Science*. 2004;303:631–2.

83. Centers for Disease Control and Prevention (CDC). *Human Subjects Documents*. Atlanta, GA: US Department of Health and Human Services, CDC; 2005 [cited Oct 5, 2006]. Available at: http://www.cdc.gov/od/ads/hsrdocs.htm.

84. American Statistical Association, Committee on Professional Ethics. *Ethical Guidelines for Statistical Practice, 1999* [cited Oct 5, 2006]. Available at: http://www.amstat.org/profession/index.cfm?fuseaction=ethicalstatistics.

85. Fairchild AL, Bayer R. Ethics and the conduct of public health surveillance. *Science*. 2004;30:631–2.

86. Nicoll A. Protecting health and patient confidentiality, ethics and surveillance. *Current Paediatrics*. 2005;15:581–89.

87. O'Brien DG, Yasnoff WA. Privacy, confidentiality, and security in information systems of state health agencies. *Am J Prev Med*. 1999;16:351–8.

88. Gostin LO, Hodge JG. Privacy and security of public health information. Hyattsville, MD: US Department of Health and Human Services, Centers for Disease Control and Prevention, National Center for Health Statistics [cited Oct 5, 2006]. Available at: http://www.critpath.org/msphpa/ncshdoc.htm.

89. Rudolph BA, Shah GH, Love D. Small numbers, disclosure risk, security, and reliability issues in web-based data query systems. *J Public Health Manag Pract*. 2006;12:176–83.

90. Armstrong MP, Rushton G, Zimmerman DL. Geographically masking health data to preserve confidentiality. *Stat Med*. 1999;18:497–525.

91. Simoes EJ, Land G, Metzger R, Mokdad A. Prioritization MICA: a web-based application to prioritize public health resources. *J Public Health Manag Pract*. 2006;12:161–9.

92. Koh HK, Judge CM, Ferrer B, Gershman ST. Using public health data systems to understand and eliminate cancer disparities. *Cancer Causes Control*. 2005;16:15–26.

93. Thacker SB, Stroup DF, Carande-Kulis V, Marks JS, Roy K, Gerberding JL. Measuring the public's health. *Public Health Rep*. 2006;121:14–22.

94. Stillman FA, Wipfli HL, Lando HA, Leischow S, Samet JM. Building capacity for international tobacco control research: the Global Tobacco Research Network. *Am J Public Health*. 2005; 95:965–8.

95. Marks, JS, Stroup, DF. Surveillance and the Tao of leadership. *Soz Präventivmed*. 2005;50(Supp 1);52–58.

96. Syme SL. Social determinants of health: the community as an empowered partner. *Prev Chronic Dis*. 2004;1 [cited Oct 5, 2006]. http://www.cdc.gov/pcd/issues/2004/jan/03_0001.htm.

97. Williams DR, Jackson JS. Race/ethnicity and the 2000 census: recommendations for African American and other black populations in the United States. *Am J Public Health*. 2000;90:1728–11.

98. Mays VM, Ponce NA, Washington DL, Cochran SD. Classification of race and ethnicity: implications for public health. *Annu Rev Public Health*. 2003;24:83–110.

99. Braveman P. Health disparities and health equity: concepts and measurement. *Annu Rev Public Health*. 2006;27:167–94.

100. Liaison Committee on Medical Education. *Functions and Structure of a Medical School: Standards for Accreditation of Medical Education Programs Leading to the MD Degree*. Washington, DC: 2003.

101. Lam TK, McPhee SJ, Mock J, et al. Encouraging Vietnamese-American women to obtain Pap tests through lay health worker outreach ad media education. *J Gen Int Med*. 2003;18:516–24.

102. Devine O. Exploring temporal and spatial patterns in public health surveillance data. In: Brookmeyer R, Stroup DF, eds. *Monitoring the Health of Populations: Statistical Principles and Methods for Public Health Surveillance*. New York: Oxford University Press; 2003:71–98.

103. Holford TR. Temporal factors in public health surveillance: sorting out age, period, and cohort effect. In: Brookmeyer R, Stroup DF, eds. *Monitoring the Health of Populations: Statistical Principles and Methods for Public Health Surveillance*. New York: Oxford University Press; 2003:99–126.

104. Brookmeyer R. Temporal factors in epidemics: the role of the incubation period. In: Brookmeyer R, Stroup DF, eds. *Monitoring the Health of Populations: Statistical Principles and Methods for Public Health Surveillance*. New York: Oxford University Press; 2003:127–45.

105. Graham-Garcia J, Raines TL, Andrews JO, Mensah GA. Race, ethnicity, and geography: disparities in heart disease in women of color. *J Transcul Nurs*. 2001;12:56–7.

106. Hay SI, Noor AM, Nelson A, Tatem AJ. The accuracy of human population maps for public health application. *Tropical Med Int Health*. 2005;10:1073–80.

107. Goovaerts P. Geostatistical analysis of disease data: estimation of cancer mortality risk from empirical frequencies using Poisson kriging. *Int J Health Geogr*. 2005;4:31–74 [cited Oct 5, 2006]. http://www.ij-healthgeographics.com/content/4/1/31.

108. Diggle PJ, Morris SE, Wakefield JCAHO. Point-source modeling using matched case-control data. *Biostatistics*. 2000;1:89–105.

109. Wall PA, Devine OJ. Interactive analysis of the spatial distribution of disease using geographic information systems. *J Geog Syst*. 2000;2:243–56.

110. Mullner RM, Chung K, Croke KG, Mensah EK. Georgraphic information systems in public health and medicine. *J Med Syst*. 2004;28(3):215–21

111. Jacquez GM. Current practices in the spatial analysis of cancer: flies in the ointment. *Int J Health Geogr*. 2004;3:22–32 [cited Oct 5, 2006]. http://www.ij-healthgeographics.com/content/3/1/22.

112. Culler D, Frimes SJ, Acheson LS, et al. Cancer genetics in primary care. *Prim Care*. 2004;31:649–83.

113. Lemon SC, Rogy J, Clark MA, Friedmann PD, Rakowski W. Classification and regression tree analysis in public health: methodological review and comparison with logistic regression. *Ann Behav Med*. 2003;26:172–81.

114. Preisser JS. Categorical data analysis in pubic health. *Annu Rev Public Health*. 1997;18:51–82.

115. Centers for Disease Control and Prevention. Guidelines for confirmation of foodborne disease outbreaks. *MMWR*. 2000;49(No. SS-01):54–62.

116. Farrington P, Andrews N. Outbreak detection: application to infectious disease surveillance. In: Brookmeyer R, Stroup DF, eds. *Monitoring the Health of Populations: Statistical Principles and Methods for Public Health Surveillance*. New York: Oxford University Press; 2003:203–31.

117. Buckeridge DL, Burkon H, Campbell M, Hogan WR, Moore AW, for the Bio ALIRT Project. Algorithms for rapid outbreak detection: a research synthesis. *J Biomed Inform*. 2005;38:99–113.

118. Fayyad UM, Piatetsky-Shairo G, Smyth P. From data mining to knowledge discovery: an overview. In: Fayyad UM, Piatetsky-Shpairo G, Smyth P, Uthurusamy R, eds. *Advances in Knowledge Discovery and Data Mining*. Cambridge, MA: MIT Press; 1996:1–36.

119. Rolka H, Bracy D, Russell C, Fram D, Ball R. Using simulation to assess the sensitivity and specificity of a signal detection tool for multidimensional public health surveillance data. *Stat Med*. 2005;24:551–62.

120. Waller LA, Hill EG, Rudd RA. The geography of power: statistical performance of test of clusters and clustering in heterogeneous populations. *Stat Med*. 2006;25:853–65.

121. Nanan DJ, White F. Capture-recapture: reconnaissance of a demographic technique in epidemiology. *Chronic Dis Can*. 1997;18:144–8.

122. Hook EB, Regal RR. Completeness of reporting: capture-recapture methods in public health. In: Brookmeyer R, Stroup DF, eds. *Monitoring the Health of Populations: Statistical Principles and Methods for Public Health Surveillance*. New York: Oxford University Press; 2003: 341–60.

123. Knowles RL, Smith A, Lynn R, Rahi JS. Using multiple sources to improve and measure case ascertainment in surveillance studies: 20 years of the British Paediatric Surveillance Unit. *J Public Health* (Oxf). 2006;28:157–65.

124. Quantin C, Binquet C, Bourguard K, et al. Which are the best identifiers for record linkage? *Med Inform Internet Med*. 2004;29:221–7.

125. Machado CJ. A literature review of record linkage procedures focusing on infant health outcomes. *Cad Saúde Pública*. 2004;20:362–71.

126. Armstrong MP, Rushton G, Zimmerman DL. Geographically masking health data to preserve confidentiality. *Stat Med*. 1999;18:497–525.

127. Salazar-González JJ. Controlled rounding and cell perturbation: statistical disclosure limitation methods for tabular data. *Mathematical Programming*. 2005;105:583–603.

128. Seastrom MM. Licensing. In: Doyle P, Lane J, Theeuwes JJM, Zayatz L, eds. *Confidentiality, Disclosure and Data Access: Theory and Practical Applications for Statistical Agencies*. Amsterdam, North Holland: Elsevier; 2002:279–96.

129. Centers for Disease Control and Prevention (CDC). *Global Youth Tobacco Survey*. Data Release Policy. Atlanta, GA: US Department of Health and Human Services, CDC [cited Oct 5, 2006]. Available at: http://www.cdc.gov/tobacco/Global/GYTS/datasets/DataRelease.pdf.

130. Dunne T. Issues in the establishment and management of secure research sties. In: Doyle P, Lane J, Theeuwes JJM, Zayatz L, eds. *Confidentiality, Disclosure and Data Access: Theory and Practical Applications for Statistical Agencies*. Amsterdam, North Holland: Elsevier; 2002:297–314.

131. O'Carroll PW and the Public Health Informatics Competency Working Group. *Informatics Competencies for Public Health Professionals*. Seattle, WA: Northwest Center for Public Health Practice; 2002 [cited Oct 5, 2006]. Available at: http://nwcphp.org/resources/phicomps.v1.

132. Brailer DJ. Interoperability: the key to the future health care system. *Health Aff*. 2005;19 [cited Oct 5, 2006]. http://www.calrhio.org/resources/docs/interoperability.pdf.

133 Rudolph B, Shah Gulzar, Love D. Small numbers, disclosure risk, security, and reliability issues in web-based data query systems. *J Public Health Manag Pract*. 2006;12:176–83.

134. Health Insurance Portability and Accountability Act. HIPAA P. L. 104–191

135. Centers for Disease Control and Prevention. HIPAA Privacy Rule and Public Health. *MMWR*. 2003;52(Suppl):1–12.

136. Kimball AM, Horwitch C, O'Carroll P, et al. APEC Emerging Infections Network: prospects for comprehensive information sharing on emerging infections within the Asia Pacific Economic Cooperation. *Emerg Infect Dis*. 1998;4 [cited Oct 5, 2006]. http://www.cdc.gov/ncidod/eid/vol4no3/kimball.htm.

137. Selden CR, Humphreys BL, Yasnoff WA, Ryan ME. *Current Bibliographies in Medicine: Public Health Informatics*. Rockville, MD: US Department of Health and Human Services, National Library of Medicine; 2001 [cited Oct 5, 2006]. Available at: http://www.nlm.nih.gov/pubs/resources.html.

138. Lober WB, Trigg, L, Karras B. Information system architectures for syndromic surveillance. *MMWR*. 2004;53(Suppl):203–8.

139. Hinman AR, Atkinson D, Diehn T, et al. Principles and core functions of integrated child health information systems. *J Public Health Manag Pract*. 2004;10(Suppl):S52–6.

140. Langmuir AD, Andrews JM. Biological warfare defense. 2. The Epidemic Intelligence Service of the Communicable Disease Center. *Am J Public Health*. 1952;42:235–8.

141. Last JM. *A Dictionary of Epidemiology*. 3rd ed. New York: Oxford University Press; 1995.

142. Zaza S, Briss PA, Harris KW. *The Guide to Community Preventive Services: What Works to Promote Health?* New York: Oxford University Press; 2005.

143. Pappaioanou M, Malison M, Wilkins K, et al. Strengthening capacity in developing countries for evidence-based public health: the data for decision-making project. *Soc Sci Med*. 2003;57:1925–37.

144. Collins JJ, Bodner KM, Baase CM, Burns C, Jammer B, Bloemen LJ. Communication of epidemiology study results by industry: the Dow Chemical Company approach. *J Expo Anal Environ Epidemiol*. 2004;14:492–7.

145. Kreuter MW. Dealing with competing and conflicting risk in cancer communication. *J Natl Cancer Inst Monogr*. 1999;25:27–35.

146. Ball LK, Evans G, Bostrom. Risky business: challenges in vaccine risk communication. *Pediatrics*. 1998;101:453–8.

147. Bernhardt J. Improving health through health marketing. *Prev Chronic Dis*. 2006 [cited Oct 5, 2006]. http://www.cdc.gov/pcd/issues/2006/jul/05_0238.htm.

148. Ransohoff DF, Ransohoff DF. Sensationalism in the media: when scientists and journalists may be complicit collaborators. *Eff Clin Pract*. 2001 [cited Oct 5, 2006]. http://www.acponline.org/journals/ecp/julaug01/ransohoff.htm.

149. Koplan JP, Thacker SB, Levin NA. *Epidemiology in the 21st Century: Calculation, Communication, and Intervention*. Washington, DC: American Public Health Association [cited Oct 5, 2006]. Available at: http://www.apha.org/journal/editorials/editkopl.htm.

150. Centers for Disease Control and Prevention. Notice to Readers: Knight Journalism Fellowships offered at CDC. *MMWR*. 2003; 52;112–3.

151. US Department of Health and Human Services. *National Standards for Culturally and Linguistically Appropriate Services in Health Care: Final Report.* Rockville, MD: US Department of Health and Human Services, Office of Minority Health; 2001[cited Oct 5, 2006]. Available at: http://www.omhrc.gov/clas/index.htm.

152. Lythcott N. Changing the research paradigm: community involvement in population-based research. *Cancer.* 2000;88:1214–16.

153. Wallerstien NB, Duran B. Using community-based participatory research to address health disparities. *Health Promot Pract.* 2006;7:312–23.

154. Franks AL, Brownson RC, Baker EA, et al. Prevention Research Centers: contributions to updating the public health workforce through training. *Prev Chronic Dis.* 2005;2 [cited Oct 5, 2006]. http://www.cdc.gov/pcd/issues/2005/apr/04_0139.htm.

155. Task Force on Community Preventive Services. Recommendations to promote healthy social environments. *Am J Prev Med.* 2003:24(Suppl 3): 21–4.

156. Minkler M: Using participatory action research to build healthy communities. *Public Health Rep.* 2000;115:191–7.

157. US Census Bureau. *US Census, 2000.* Washington, DC: US Census Bureau; 2006 [cited Oct 5, 2006]. Available at: http://www.census.gov/main/www/cen2000.html.

158. Kung HC, Hoyert DL, Xu J, Murphy SL. *Deaths: Final Data for 2005. National Vital Statistics Report.* Hyattsville, MD: US Department of Health and Human Services, Centers for Disease Control and Prevention, National Center for Health Statistics; 2008:56.

159. Wise RP, Livengood JR, Berkelman RL, Goodman RA. Methodologic alternatives for measuring premature mortality. *Am J Prev Med.* 1988;4:268–73.

160. Farnham PG, Ackerman SP, Haddix AC. Study design. In: Haddix AC, Teutsch SM, Shaffer PA, Duñet DO, eds. *Prevention Effectiveness: A Guide to Decision Analysis and Economic Evaluation.* New York: Oxford University Press; 1996:12–26.

161. Dasbach E, Teutsch SM. Cost-utility analysis. In: Haddix AC, Teutsch SM, Shaffer PA, Duñet DO, eds. *Prevention Effectiveness: A Guide to Decision Analysis and Economic Evaluation.* New York: Oxford University Press; 1996:130–7.

162. McKenna M, Michaud C, Murray C, Marks J. Assessing the burden of disease in the United States using disability-adjusted life years. *Am J Prev Med.* 2005;28:415–23.

163. Anand S, Hanson K. Disability-adjusted life years: a critical review. *J Health Econ.* 1997;16:685–702.

164. Goodman MT, Howe HH. Descriptive epidemiology of ovarian cancer in the United States, 1992–1997. *Cancer.* 2003;97:2615–30.

165. Schoenbaum SC, Baker O, Jezek Z. Common-source epidemic of hepatitis due to glazed and iced pastries. *Am J Epidemiol.* 1976;104:74–80.

166. Jepson P, Hohnson SP, Gillman MW, et al. Interpretation of observational studies. *Heart.* 2004; 90:956–60.

167. Dawber TR, Kannel WB, Lyell LP. An approach to longitudinal studies in a community: The Framingham Study. In: The challenge of epidemiology: issues and selected readings. *Bull Pan Am Health Organ.* 2004;619–30.

168. Ellison LF. Tea and other beverage consumption and prostate cancer risk. *J Transcult Nurs.* 2001; 12,56–7.

169. Kahn HA, Sempos CT. *Statistical Methods in Epidemiology.* New York: Oxford University Press; 1989.

170. Doll R, Hill AB. Mortality in relation to smoking: ten years' observation of British physicians. *Br Med J.* 1964;1:1399–1410, 1460–1467.

171. Steenland K, Armstrong B. An overview of methods for calculating the burden of disease due to specific risk factors. *Epidemiology.* 2006;17:512–9.

172. Le CT. *Health and Numbers: A Problems-based Introduction to Biostatistics.* New York: Wiley-Liss, 2001.

173. Meltzer M. Introduction to health economics for physicians. *Lancet.* 2001;358:993–8.

174. Haddix AC, Teutsch SM, Corso PS. *Prevention Effectiveness: A Guide to Decision Analysis and Economic Evaluation.* New York: Oxford University Press; 2003.

175. Last JM, ed. *A Dictionary of Epidemiology.* 4th ed. New York: Oxford University Press; 2001.

176. Zaza S, Briss PA. Community health promotion and disease prevention. In: Last JM, Wallace RB, et al. *Public Health and Preventive Medicine.* Oxford University Press (In press, 2006).

177. Besculides M, Zaveri H, Farris R, Will J. Identifying best practices for WISEWOMAN programs using a mixed-methods evaluation. *Prev Chronic*

Dis. 2006;1 [cited Oct 5, 2006]. http://www.cdc .gov/pcd/issues/2006/jan/05_0133.htm.

178. Anderson LA, Gwaltney MK, Sundra DL, et al. Using concept mapping to develop a logic model for the Prevention Research Centers Program. *Prev Chronic Dis.* 2006;1 [cited Oct 5, 2006]. http:// www.cdc.gov/pcd/issues/2006/Jan/05_0153.htm.

179. US Department of Health and Human Services. *Steps to a Healthier US Initiative.* Rockville, MD: US Department of Health and Human Services [cited Oct 5, 2006]. Available at: http://www.healthierUS.gov/steps.

180. Task Force on Community Preventative Services. *Effectiveness of Mass media Campaigns to Reduce Initiation of Tobacco Use and Increase Cessation.* The Community Guide to Preventive Services. Atlanta, GA: Task Force on Community Preventive Services; 2003 [cited Oct 5, 2006]. Available at: http://www.thecommunityguide.org/tobacco/ tobac-int-mass-media.pdf.

181. Audibert M. Fighting poverty and disease in an integrated approach. *Bull World Health Organ.* 2006;84:151–2.

182. *American Heritage Dictionary.* 4th ed. New York: Houghton Mifflin; 2002.

183. Brownson RC, Baker EA, Leet TL, Gillespie KN, eds. *Evidence-based Public Health.* New York: Oxford University Press; 2002.

184. Task Force on Community Preventive Services. *The Guide to Community Preventive Services.* Atlanta, GA: Task Force on Community Preventive Services; 2003 [cited Oct 5, 2006]. Available at: http://www.thecommunityguide.org.

185. Burke JP. Antibiotic resistance: squeezing the balloon? *JAMA.* 1998;290;1770–1.

186. Pirkle JL, Brody DJ, Gunter EW, et al. The decline in blood lead levels in the United States. The National Health and Nutrition Examination Surveys (NHANES). *JAMA.* 1994;272:284–91.

187. Nriagu JO. The rise and fall of leaded gasoline. *Sci Total Environ.* 1990;92:13–28.

188. Diabetes Control and Complication Trial Research Group. The effect of intensive treatment of diabetes on the development and progression of long-term complications in insulin dependent diabetes mellitus. *N Engl J Med.* 1993;329:997–86.

189. Saaddine JB, Engelgau MM, Beckles, G, et al. A diabetes report card for the United States. Quality of care in the 1990s. *Ann Intern Med.* 2002;136: 565–74. (A more recent update will be published soon we will amend at that time.)

190. Satterfield DW, Volansky M, Caspersen C, et al. Community–based lifestyle interventions to prevent Type 2 diabetes. *Diabetes Care.* 2003;26:2643–52.

CHAPTER 12

Community Health Planning and Programming

Laura H. Downey, DrPH and F. Douglas Scutchfield, MD

LEARNING OBJECTIVES

Upon completion of this chapter, the reader will be able to:

1. Express the importance of citizen engagement in public health assessment, improvement, and planning procedures.
2. Identify and explain national models that can be used for community health assessment, improvement, and planning.
3. Understand the role of *Healthy People 2010* in directing national, state, and local health program planning.
4. Recognize that the national focus areas of *Healthy People 2010* are a result of collaboration and prompt for additional partnerships to achieve these benchmarks.
5. Explain how coalitions serve as a particular type of community organizations and describe the essential components for a developing coalition.
6. Describe the evolving role of community-based participation in public health research and the philosophical underpinnings for the increased role of citizens in public health research and practice.

KEY TERMS

Assessment

Coalition

Community

Community-Based Participatory Research (CBPR)

Deliberation

Leading Health Indicators (LHIs)

Public health is practiced in communities and is focused on populations rather than individuals. In the majority of cases, its practice is focused in local health departments and occurs in a political jurisdiction, such as a county or city. There are some variations; public health can be practiced with populations not defined geographically, such as religious groups, occupational groups, or populations especially vulnerable to diseases regardless of where they live. This chapter is about practice of public health in communities, including community engagement, assessment of community resources and community needs, working with communities for planning and implementing public health programs, the emergence of the community as a partner in research (not as a research subject), and the role of the public in public health.

FINDING THE COMMUNITY IN COMMUNITY HEALTH

As described in Chapters 2 and 3, the public health agenda has steadily expanded over time. Clearly progress on much of today's list of public health responsibilities requires a strong working relationship with citizens as community partners.[1] In this chapter, **community** is broadly defined as all who are affected by public health practice and research, including residents, practitioners, service agencies, and policy makers that may or may not share a geographic or specific physical location. A review of the socioecologic determinants of health as described in Chapter 4 quickly reveals the necessity of working in new ways with communities to deal with the underlying etiology of many of the risk factors responsible for disease and disability. In this era, new public health principles such as community participation, citizen engagement, and community empowerment are central philosophies to successful public health practice. The community is not a passive entity but rather the main "engine" in promoting the public's health.[2] The nature of public health practice is continually evolving in ways that allow, and indeed require, more significant participation

by concerned citizens, civic or nongovernmental organizations, and public associations that provide assistance to traditional public health practitioners for promoting and protecting the public's health.

An empowered public has not been at the core of the historical approach to public health. Often, public health authorities have been guilty of gathering and analyzing data, designing programs, and constructing evaluation instruments without input from community members.[3] Although public health continues to use the term "public," the traditional "public health" system, made up of various organizations, has been, and to a great degree remains, a very closed, professional group whose decision-making process is far removed from common citizens.[4] Gittell has argued that community institutions or organizations fail to continually provide opportunities for citizen participation, particularly low-income citizens who lack the resources to join the political process.[5] An analysis of civic participation in health decision making concluded that engagement requires considerable commitment of time and energy to build the necessary trust among academics, practitioners, and community members.[6]

Over the past 50 years, physicians, policy makers, researchers, and community organizers began to question the role of community and community involvement in public health. In the words of Dr. E.G. McGavran, a public health leader in the 1950s, the issue is, "In scientific public health, we no longer treat the individual—the segment of the community—but the total body politic—mental, physical, social, and economic. We no longer treat individuals who have communicable disease, but we prevent, control, or eradicate the disease in the body politic."[7(p723)] This quote suggests recognition at the middle of the past century that communities should be the locus of concern in public health. The idea of the community as a patient created the community medicine movement of the 1950s and 1960s, with the emergence of medical school Departments of Community Medicine or Community Health during that period.[8]

A National Policy Task Force on community-based public health initiatives pointed out that "community lies at the heart of public health . . . interventions work best when they are rooted in the values, knowledge, expertise, and interests of the community itself . . . community members must participate fully in the identification of health issues and the selection, design, implementation and evaluation or programs that address them."[9(p74)] Emerging public health strategies hold promise for making broad community engagement a more common and authentic practice in the discipline.

EXPANDING CITIZEN ENGAGEMENT

Decisions about health problems in communities, the nature of public health programs designed to deal with those problems, and assessment of program effectiveness is a community responsibility. In fact, democratic traditions in America suggest that local citizens should be engaged with experts to make decisions about things that affect their communities, including those activities that relate to the public's health.[10] This recommendation is further reflected in the Institute of Medicine (IOM) report, *The Future of Public Health*, where the following observation is made (emphasis added) in its recommendations regarding the policy development function of public health:

> The committee recommends that every public health agency exercise its responsibility to serve the public interest in the development of comprehensive public health policies by promoting use of the scientific knowledge base in decision-making about public health and by leading in developing public health policy. *Agencies must take a strategic approach, developed on the basis of a positive appreciation for the democratic political process.*[11(p412)]

How to best deal with that fact and the opportunities it provides for communities to identify problems and lead decision making is a source of ongoing discussion. From those discussions, a variety of proposed approaches has emerged. One of the most powerful is public deliberation. **Deliberation** has been defined as, "the process of establishing intent and resolve, where a person or group explores different solutions before settling on a specific course of action."[12] Public deliberation as a mechanism for public health efforts has a sound underlying rationale. Various forms of deliberative practices, including citizen juries, citizen panels, scenario workshops, deliberative forums, and rapid and participatory rural appraisal are used in the health sector to address community health problems. All of these deliberative approaches are characterized by the inclusion of citizens, who do not have any professional role in health care, in decision-making processes by engaging them in deliberative discussions with other citizens. (These methods seemed to have expanded more rapidly in British Commonwealth countries than in the United States.)[13]

Public deliberation among citizens is a fundamental part of achieving a democracy. Democracy rests on the idea that important decisions, including public health problems, are within the capabilities of ordinary citizens. Not only can ordinary people make critical decisions, but they should make the important decisions that affect their community because they understand their own interests better than experts do.[14] Deliberation encourages citizens to use their intelligence, curiosity, reflectivity, and willingness to reason through tough issues for the improvement of society.[15] Deliberation requires a capacity for empathy and a willingness to engage in a dialogue with others about individual beliefs, with the real possibility of revising those beliefs should evidence warrant it.[16]

Despite the continual interest in engaging citizens in conversation about their health, problems with this approach remain. Ensuring that all the necessary voices are present in the deliberative process remains a persistent difficulty. Key questions remain such as:

- Which voices are being used to make community health decisions?
- What can be done if the individuals who need to be there the most are not present in community discussions?

Democratic principles are critical to achieving the notion that health improvement efforts will be most effective if the community takes ownership of local dialogue and feels connected to the decisions being made. Citizens will engage in local discussions when a connection is made between what is most valuable to them and the problems facing their community.[17] Social change of health behaviors is most successful at the community level when individuals who live and work in the areas affected by key health problems are process participants.[18] For example, these citizen-based approaches have been successfully used to address a range of issues from health care reform and emerging infectious diseases such as the pandemic flu, to local concerns that include inactive youth and obesity.[19–21]

The question is no longer whether citizens should be engaged in public health decisions, but what is the best method of encouraging citizen involvement and integration into the public health decision-making process. Decades ago, Dewey concluded that deliberation, in the search for ways to act, leads to providing people (and thus, their communities) with choices.[22] The ultimate goal of deliberation is to make a choice by evaluating conflicting alternatives. Deliberation is an opportunity to think about a complex social situation and make explicit trade-offs that are inherent to grappling with a public problem.

inform service provision, set and assess goals, and determine the direction of local initiatives. Moreover, assessments lay the foundation for policy development and its key processes, including 1) informing, educating, and empowering people about health issues, 2) mobilizing community partnerships to identify and solve health problems, and 3) developing policies and plans that support individual and community health efforts.[1] Directly connected to the core functions of public health, assessments are the preliminary step and concluding activity for public health program planning and program evaluation.[23]

In recent decades, an increasing number of community health models have been used to assess and improve community health. Each of the models discussed in this chapter recognize the need to include multiple and diverse partners in the assessment and planning process. As IOM has documented extensively, medical trained personnel, community planners, educators and academicians, faith-based and community-based organizations, media, local businesses, and numerous other partners are necessary for keeping the public healthy.[11] Most of the models of community health assessment and planning could benefit from additional attention to the engagement of community residents in the processes of community health models.

COMMUNITY HEALTH ASSESSMENT

Conducting community health assessments is critical to fulfilling essential public health services.[23] Public health's core functions encompass policy development, assurance of conditions for individuals to be healthy, and the assessment of health needs and assets. **Assessment** is the regular and systematic collection, analysis, and dissemination of information on the health of a community, including statistics, community health needs, and scientific studies of health problems.[1,11] Assessments can

TOOLS FOR COMMUNITY HEALTH ASSESSMENT AND PLANNING

A number of planning and programming tools have been developed for use when working with communities. The description of these methods, instruments, and tools will be brief, primarily intended to acquaint readers with some of the various models available. The summary presented in this section should be followed with more detailed investigation and exploration of assessment models by the interested reader. References provided in the

Table 12.1. Community Health Assessment and Planning Models

Model	Website
Planned Approach to Community Health (PATCH)	http://www.usmbha.org/images/projects/promovision/patch.pdf
Mobilizing Action through Planning and Partnership	http://www.naccho.org/topics/infrastructure/MAPP.cfm
Assessment Protocol for Excellence in Public Health	
(APEX/PH)	http://www.naccho.org/topics/infrastructure/APEXPH.cfm

descriptions of these models can provide insight into sources for a more detailed description of each. Before a community begins the planning processes discussed in this chapter, a careful review of the methods available and their strengths and weaknesses needs to be done. Table 12.1 lists the official website where more extensive information on community health assessment models described in this chapter can be found.

All the models discussed in this section share certain common attributes. They begin with the creation of a group of citizens empowered to lead a systematic approach to examining the community's health. This assemblage may be a prior constituted group with some responsibility to act on behalf of the community and deal with its health status, such as the local board of health. It may also be an ad hoc group. Frequently, such ad hoc groups represent "stakeholders" who represent other agencies and organizations in the community with a concern about the community's well being, including its health status. Those who have resources and share concerns with public health official agencies are key to solutions that may be crafted in the process. In fact, some have suggested that a formal "stakeholder analysis" is useful to identify those in the community with common interests in problems identified and the resources that will be necessary to address them.[24,25] When such groups are constituted or identified, it is important to recognize that although they may have some credibility embedded in their mission or constitution, rarely do they represent or engage the ordinary citizens of the community in this process. These individuals and agencies are key, but their efforts should not substitute for citizen engagement.

Collecting and analyzing data, that is, statistics or measures of community health, is necessary for assessing the health and well-being of community members. Data can be obtained through primary or secondary data collection. In some cases, primary or newly collected data from surveys, observations, hospital records, or other means will be used to document the health of community members on certain criteria. In other cases, secondary data or previously collected data is available to inform the assessment and planning process. Using secondary data can decrease the time and costs associated with collection procedures. Quantitative data might not capture all of the information needed to assess the health of a community. When this is the case, some of the models obtain qualitative information as well. This information can be obtained a variety of ways, including focus groups, nominal group processes with existing community groups, or other informal mechanisms for tapping the perceptions of the community. Again, this is an appropriate phase in the process for community deliberative forums to be convened so that a broad array of community members is involved in the assessment and planning for the community's health.

Next the group reviews the data to attempt to identify major community health problems that need to be addressed. They may also establish priorities or search for "root causes" of the problems that they have identified. Regardless of the particular steps, a problem list is developed. The next step is to identify specific programs that can address these community needs that were identified. The basis for such programs can and should be scientific evidence of effectiveness. Although public health is a relative newcomer to evidence-based practice, significant strides have been made over the past decade.[26] The *Guide to Community Preventive Services* provides a list of programs that appear to work, those that don't, and where there is no evidence to ascertain the likelihood of a specific program working to solve the problem.[27] This can be a difficult area because many in positions of responsibility will have "pet" programs that they like but have little or no evidence for their success. For example, the DARE program's impact on youth drug and alcohol use has repeatedly not been demonstrated to be effective, in spite of its apparent appeal to those who have positions of authority in most communities.[28]

The planned program should be oriented to specific outcomes that are focused on improving specific health status problems identified in the earlier part of this process. The most logical step in this regard is to link the initiative to objectives for improving health status, such as those contained in *Healthy People 2010*, its state counterpart, or subsequent iterations of that document.[29] Doing so provides program goals that can be used for both formative evaluations to make changes in the program should it be going awry, and summative evaluations to assure the success of the program. As is the case in planning processes, the evaluation phase of this model ultimately returns to the point of the planning process, and the cycle is repeated. This is a generalized discussion of the approach to community health assessment and planning. The specific programs described next are variations on the theme.

Planned Approach to Community Health (PATCH)

The success of early community-based cardiovascular disease prevention programs represented a lesson in how communities can mobilize for and address multiple community factors that influence health status.[30] Based on the experience of this work, along with the work of Green[31] (specifically his PROCEED and PRECEED health behavior models), the Centers for Disease Control and Prevention (CDC) developed the Planned Approach to Community Health (PATCH).[32]

PATCH has a series of steps similar to other assessment procedures, and it follows the generalized approach previously described. First, residents must be mobilized or recognize a need for addressing health issues in the community. Data collection and organization follows community mobilization. After the data has been collected, health priorities must be determined and an intervention designed and implemented. Finally, evaluation of the intervention should be conducted. An important part of PATCH is the partnership required between CDC and state and local health departments. PATCH was designed by CDC to focus on the role of CDC and state health departments as a resource to local health departments, where the specifics of the program will be implemented. The program is based in the local health department, using materials developed by CDC, and assisted by the state health department, which provides technical expertise and training to those in communities undertaking a PATCH program. Although this program was widely accepted and used by communities extensively in the 1990s, other programs have since superseded it.

Assessment Protocol for Excellence in Public Health (APEX/PH)

The Assessment Protocol for Excellence in Public Health (APEX/PH) was created by the National Association of County Health Officials (NACHO) before it merged with the United States Conference of Local Health Officers to form the National Association of City and County Health Officials (NACCHO) (see Chapter 3). The creation of APEX/PH was done in collaboration with the CDC. APEX/PH consists of three parts. The first part is an organizational assessment designed to facilitate an assessment by the local health department of its own capability to address community health needs and problems. This is an inventory of local health department capacity done by senior staff at the agency. It assures that the issues that might prevent the local health department from being successful in its efforts at community health planning and programming are identified and addressed prior to any effort to engage the community. The notion is to make sure the local health department has the capacity to do a community health assessment and develop programs to address health problems identified in the assessment. This gives the local health department an opportunity to improve its internal capacity to support the process before the community is mobilized for action.

The second part of APEX/PH is the community assessment and planning activity, which requires the creation of a representative community group that examines community data indicators. Findings inform the choice of health status improvement objectives, frequently taken from those contained in the *Healthy People* series to apply locally. Phase three of APEX/PH involves linking the organizational capacity of the health department, appropriately configured, to focus on the problems of the community and to work with a group of community representatives to address the problems identified. This process involves the local health department in assessing and addressing its strengths and weaknesses, and then bringing that renewed health department forward to work with the community to improve health.[33,34]

Mobilizing for Action through Planning and Partnership

Mobilizing for Action through Planning and Partnership (MAPP) is the most recently developed method of performing community assessment and planning. It is substantially different and more complex than its predecessors. Its development benefited from the use of APEX/PH and similar models and was intended to correct deficiencies that were identified from the application of preceding models. In addition, new materials were available to assist the local public health system with the planning and programming process, such as the National Public Health Performance Measure Instruments for the local public health system. MAPP was developed by NACCHO, with major help and support from CDC. MAPP involves not only the public health department but also all the components of the public health system. Recollect that the Local Public Health System (LPHS) (see Chapter 3) is all those community organiza-

tions and agencies that contribute to the mission of public health, "assuring conditions in which people can be healthy."[11] Thus, it involves not only the health department but also other community components that contribute to the socioecologic determinants of health. These include, for example, school systems, the justice system, hospitals, community health centers, and not-for-profit organizations, such as the local chapter of the United Way. The decision to undertake a MAPP process should include recognizing the amount of time and energy that is required to do the entire MAPP process. It requires a major investment, not only from the health department but also from others in the community. Figure 12.1 illustrates the key components of MAPP.

The process includes several steps and four separate assessments. MAPP begins by organizing the community—its organizations, agencies, and stakeholders—into a group to proceed with the MAPP process.[35] This, in turn, is followed by a visioning process, which asks the group to describe how the

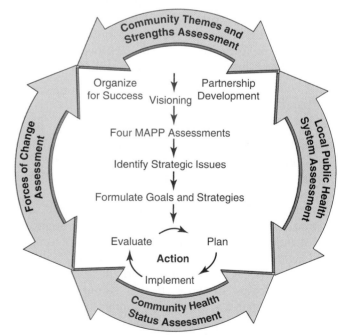

Figure 12.1. Conceptual Model of Mobilization and Action through Planning and Partnership

SOURCE: Delmar Cengage Learning.

community's health should look several years downstream. These steps are places where citizen-deliberative forums can be used to broaden the community's engagement with the process and benefit from their deliberation. This also allows for sharing and agreeing on values and strategic directions.

Next, four separate assessments are undertaken. The four assessments are community themes and strengths assessment, local public health system assessment, community health status assessment, and forces of change assessment. Following those assessments, community members must identify strategic health issues in their community and then formulate goals and strategies to address them. This step can draw heavily on *Healthy People 2010* or its successor in establishing community health objectives consistent with a national set of objectives. This then is followed by an action cycle, involving planning, implementation, and evaluation. Needless to say, the steps are easier to describe briefly, in contrast to actually doing the process. NACCHO provides more descriptions of the process of MAPP and tools that a community undertaking this process can use for leading the work in the correct direction. This process is time intensive but ensures that elements in the community are committed to the process and the outcome of improved community health.[36]

Healthy Cities

The Healthy Cities projects developed from the World Health Organization's (WHO) focus on the "Global Strategy of Health for All by the Year 2000" that were described in the late 1980s.[37] The notion was to mobilize multisectorial approaches to city health problems and issues. This has some natural appeal because it recognizes the socioecological determinants of health (see Chapter 4) and recognizes that many community organizations, public and private, need to collaborate to address underlying etiologies of poor health status. Healthy Cities also had a series of steps similar to the generalized scheme of previously described models. The first step is organizing community relationships already in existence. Unlike other schemes, this community-organizing phase specifically focuses on including community leaders who control

resources in various sectors. The public sector must be involved, but the private sector has much to contribute, as well. The community must complete a community diagnosis or a similar process to identify major health issues in the city. The next step attempts to mobilize all sectors of a community to contribute to the solution of community health issues that have been identified.

An underlying theme is that many health problems have major contributions from outside the health sector, and that the health sector alone may not be successful in solving these problems. Issues such as obesity, for example, would benefit from a multisectorial approach. The parks department could contribute venues and support for physical activity in parks, and the highway and traffic sector could provide bike lanes for individuals to use to go to work and play. The community-planning department could assure that restaurants, grocery stores, and schools are strategically based to allow individuals to walk to those facilities. The grocery stores of the community can cooperate by providing more shelf space for healthier foods and using marketing techniques to facilitate healthy grocery shopping by residents of the community. The strength of this model is in recognizing that the health sector alone cannot create communities that produce healthy people. Finally, the Healthy City model enhances the notion of mutual support and its effect on health. It is understood that the entire city or community mobilizes around health, and each sector will be nurtured by others, creating a community culture committed to health.[38,39]

Community Asset Mapping

Although these models and the generalized approach to community assessment and planning seem powerful and the appropriate tools for public health professionals to use in their efforts to work with the community, a major caveat has been raised about this process: community assets. As McKnight posits, no community was ever built by only defining needs. Instead, he and his colleagues suggest assessments should take a "half-full" as opposed to a "half-empty" approach for true community change. Needs-based surveys insist that residents focus on their emptiness and their insufficiencies. If a culture of deficiency-based assessment becomes the dominant paradigm, then communities could lose the power of wise citizens. Identifying local assets empowers citizens to tap into the capacity that is already available in their community.[40]

Kretzmann and McKnight[41] describe three levels of assets that are available in all communities: individual, associations, and institutions (see Figure 12.2). Each level has resources that are necessary to address a problem, issue, or concern. Individuals living in communities possess significant and diverse gifts, skills, and capacities that can be used to improve community health. All residents have expertise and knowledge that can play an effective role in addressing important local matters. Similarly, when individuals gather as civic associations in pursuit of common goals, another level of collective assets are available to strengthen the community. Whether through formal or informal associations, organized citizens provide additional monetary, service, and educational assets to a community. Local institutions, such as government agencies, school systems, cooperative extension, and hospitals, can increase the level of assets available for developing and sustaining community or neighborhoods improvements.

At its core, asset mapping depends on community members having necessary resources for identifying and solving a community problem or issue, and identifying those assets already available to bring about change.[42] This community-based approach can involve lay citizens as co-creators and co-learners in identifying the desired community outcomes. Moreover, citizens and local organizations and institutions are fundamental to defining the issues to be addressed and creating and implementing the solutions to the issues of concern.[43]

In contrast to traditional needs assessments that focus on mapping deficiencies, asset mapping focuses on the effectiveness of citizens identifying solutions to their own problems and addressing the issues that most affect their community. Community relationships, networks, and individual strengths can be responsive to local needs. Ultimately, asset mapping seeks to empower residents who might traditionally have a limited voice in local processes for addressing local concerns. This more equitable approach can and should be used in conjunction with traditional health assessment methods and tools.[44]

In summary, there are a number of existing models for use by the public health practitioner in attempting to address community health issues. The most sophisticated and time consuming is MAPP. This model developed as an evolution from earlier attempts to provide communities and professionals the tools they need to deal with major community health problems. As we have emphasized, two critical components, deliberative efforts among citizens (not just stakeholders and asset mapping) could enhance the potential for effectiveness in any of the models described in this chapter. Incorporating these two elements into the assessment and planning phase can be a method for ensuring that the broader community is involved and that available community resources are used to address the issue identified in the assessment and planning process. The addition of these two components is likely to increase the power of the process and its success.

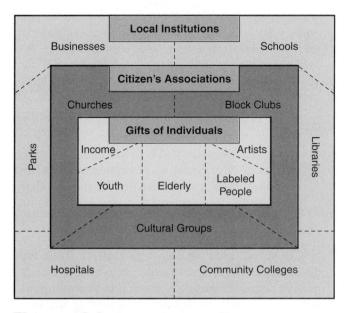

Figure 12.2. Community Assets Map

SOURCE: Kretzmann & McKnight, *Building Communities From the Inside Out.*

HEALTHY PEOPLE 2010

A major issue and concern in any community planning and programming system is the development of programs to address health problems and issues. Programs should be evidence-based, keeping in mind the nature of the democratic process. Additionally, benchmarks should be developed to ascertain where the community conducting an assessment stands in relationship to other communities. For example, is one community's situation better or worse than others similarly situated? A decision could be made to implement a program based on the awareness that a local problem is more severe than it is on average nationally, or is more severe than the situation in a neighboring community. In fact, specific health objectives can indicate the health areas that are out of line with the norm and provide guidance on what a community can aspire to achieve as the result of planning efforts.

Healthy People 2010 is the most ambitious set of health promotion and disease prevention objectives yet developed.[29] *Healthy People 2010* clearly has a role to play in establishing objectives for program planning and evaluation. *Healthy People 2010* is the third iteration of the Healthy People initiative that has progressively identified more comprehensive objectives to achieve better health for all Americans. *Healthy People 2010* is the nation's health plan for the current decade and draws heavily from previous iterations. Over the past three decades, *Healthy People* documents have served as a guiding force in designing and implementing health initiatives for the nation and communities across the United States. This process began with *Healthy People: The Surgeon General's Report on Health Promotion and Disease Prevention* in 1979 and continued with the publication of *Promoting Health/ Preventing Disease: Objectives for the Nation in 1980*.[45,46] In 1990, *Healthy People 2000: National Health Promotion and Disease Prevention Objectives* presented a series of health objectives for the nation to achieve by the turn of the century.[47]

As with the preceding documents, *Healthy People 2010* establishes national health objectives and serves as a framework for developing national, state, and local health promotion and disease prevention plans, with a set of specific health objectives to be achieved by 2010. *Healthy People 2010* represents, as is the case with *Healthy People 2000*, the extensive work that is possible through a concerted effort of diverse agencies, organizations, and individuals working to plan and implement scientific programs for disease prevention. The document's production was coordinated by the Office of Disease Prevention and Health Promotion (ODPHP) of the United States Department of Health and Human Services (Dept. of HHS). Although the federal government provided the leadership necessary to create such an extensive document, input was obtained from private and voluntary organizations, local and state public health departments, mental health agencies, substance abuse prevention and treatment programs, environmental agencies, and individuals resulting in the most comprehensive and current set of national health-related objectives ever presented.[48] The document was not intended to be a plan for government at any level but to be a plan for the nation, with all segments of the nation committed to the objectives and their achievement.

There are two primary goals of *Healthy People 2010* that provide the foundation for other objectives and specific areas of focus:

- **Goal 1:** Increase quality and years of healthy life.
- **Goal 2:** Eliminate health disparities. The concept of health disparities is broadly defined by including health and disease differences that occur by gender, race and ethnicity, education or income, disability, geographic location, or sexual orientation

These two goals inform and provide focus for local, regional, and national health-related efforts for the decade. Plans, programs, and procedures at all levels should be directed at achieving the two overarching goals of *Healthy People 2010*. Objectives in 28 focus areas support the two goals (see Table 12.2). These focus areas range from specific health issues, such as the leading causes of death in the United States, to healthful behaviors, and include other approaches that could be used to improve health outcomes such as enhanced public health infrastructure and health communication. Each focus area is managed by a lead or co-lead agency of the federal government. Lead agencies with recognized expertise in one or more of the focus areas are responsible for supporting and promoting activities directly related to their area of expertise that will ultimately achieve the two primary goals of *Healthy People 2010*.[48]

Healthy People 2010 has evolved through the strengths and lessons learned from previous federal reports while advancing the national approach to improving the health status of all Americans. For example, the 28 objectives in *Healthy People 2010* are similar to the 22 priority areas presented in *Healthy People 2000*. Focus areas ware chosen instead of priority areas so as not to imply prioritization. Similarly, the 467 specific objectives closely align with the 319 specific objectives presented in *Healthy People 2000*, allowing comparison with the preceding set of national health objectives. Each of the *Healthy People 2010* objectives are linked with the 10 **Leading Health Indicators (LHI)** or

primary public health concerns in the United States that were chosen based on their ability to motivate action, the availability of data to measure their progress, and their relevance as broad public health issues.[49] LHI will be used to assess the health of United States residents over the decade and include physical activity, overweight and obesity, tobacco use, substance abuse, responsible sexual behavior, mental health, injury and violence, environmental quality, immunization, and access to health care.

For each focus area, *Healthy People 2010* presents background information about the topic, an overview about disparities, and ideas for future action. A report on the progress of the relevant *Healthy People 2000* objective is also provided. A link is drawn between each objective and other interrelated focus areas, as well as a range of specific objectives that detail the current state of health within each area of focus. Each object has a data-based baseline and targets for outcomes by 2010 that will allow the progress of initiatives to be measured.[48]

Targets are the proposed goal for each health measure for all population groups to reach by the year 2010. This provides the guidance needed for improving quality of life and eliminating health

Table 12.2. *Healthy People 2010* Focus Areas[50]

1. Access to Quality Health Services	15. Injury and Violence Prevention
2. Arthritis, Osteoporosis, and Chronic Back Conditions	16. Maternal, Infant, and Child Health
3. Cancer	17. Medical Product Safety
4. Chronic Kidney Disease	18. Mental Health and Mental Disorders
5. Diabetes	19. Nutrition and Overweight
6. Disability and Secondary Conditions	20. Occupational Safety and Health
7. Educational and Community-Based Programs	21. Oral Health
8. Environmental Health	22. Physical Activity and Fitness
9. Family Planning	23. Public Health Infrastructure
10. Food Safety	24. Respiratory Diseases
11. Health Communication	25. Sexually Transmitted Diseases
12. Heart Disease and Stroke	26. Substance Abuse
13. HIV	27. Tobacco Use
14. Immunization and Infectious Diseases	28. Vision and Hearing

disparities. Data for evaluating the progress of *Healthy People 2010* is updated on a quarterly basis. The National Center for Health Statistics of the CDC maintains *Healthy People 2010* data on a website known as DATA 2010. This website (http://wonder.cdc.gov/data2010/) provides regularly updated information for all the measurable objectives in *Healthy People 2010*. National data is primarily provided on the website, but state-based data are provided where they are available.[48] States such as Delaware, Louisiana, North Carolina, and Virginia, among others, have taken strides to establish strategies for reaching the *Healthy People 2010* objectives.[49]

Healthy People 2010 is more than just a series of national objectives that is far removed from state and local public health practitioners and communities involved in health planning process. *Healthy People 2010* is a touchstone for public health practitioners as they design and evaluate programs. Moreover, it is also a call for the collaboration necessary to achieve such wide-ranging objectives. It is an example of how the participation of nongovernmental organizations and associations, as well as concerned citizens, is necessary to identify areas of mutual interest and to begin or continue collaboration efforts to address these areas.

Although these objectives have been a major force in national health promotion and disease-prevention efforts, there has been criticism of the fact that they contain no definition of responsibility for their achievement and no commitment made in provision of funding to translate these objectives into programs.[50]

COLLABORATIONS TO IMPLEMENT COMMUNITY PUBLIC HEALTH PROGRAMS

The process of development, implementation, and evaluation of public health programs requires community involvement and participation at every step of the process. After the community health needs assessment and asset mapping, establishing a new evidence-based public health program remains a critical issue. Moving from planning, using one of the tools we describe, to action is a key step in the process of improving the public's health. In many cases, if not most, implementation of a new or revamped program requires new or reprogrammed resources. Rarely does the local health department, per se, have those resources, but they are likely to exist in a community, frequently in the hands or under control of other actors in the public health system. In any community, a mechanism for mobilizing partnerships and collaboration for program implementation is imperative if a program is to succeed. This notion is perhaps best expressed in the essential public health service of "mobilize community partnerships to identify and solve health problems."

Public health researchers and practitioners are increasingly exploring alternative methods for linking unique strengths and sharing responsibilities among collaborative partners for improving community health.[51,52] The collective power of diverse individuals and organizations of a community have the capability to tackle public health's most complex problems.[53,54] Coalitions, as a particular type of community organizations, are recognized as a collaborative network in communities that are increasingly used to address leading public health problems, such as those outlined as *Healthy People 2010* focus areas. Coalitions have been successfully used to address issues such as immunization, teen pregnancy, drug/alcohol abuse, and obesity and weight management.[55]

Coalitions are unions of people and organizations working to influence outcomes on a specific problem. Moreover, they involve multiple sectors of the community that come together to address community needs and solve community problems.[56] These groups join to collectively address a broad range of goals that are unattainable by one person or organization. Coalitions promote a critical mass behind social and health issues while conserving resources and reducing duplication of services. These networks cultivate cooperation between diverse sectors of the community that are striving for the same goal.

Although theories relating to community coalitions, community-level initiatives, and their effectiveness in public health practice are still developing, the most comprehensive framework developed to date for forming coalitions is the *Community Coalition Action Theory*.[57] It is important to recognize that coalitions usually form around a specific area of concern in a community, frequently following a community health assessment, where a major issue in the community that needs the communities attention emerges. Coalitions allow for a variety of community resources to focus on the problem, using resources from a variety of community organizations and agencies. Community coalitions are characterized as formal, multipurpose, and long-term alliances. This theory of community coalitions borrows from the philosophies of other collective movements, including community development, citizen participatory action, political science, and group processes. The approach is based upon assumptions that communities can devise solutions to local public health problems; citizens should participate in making, adjusting, or controlling major changes in their community; and changes in the community that are developed by local citizens have longer-lasting implications than imposed changes.

Finally, it is assumed that partnerships will take a holistic approach to solving a problem that will result in greater change than individualistic and fragmented approaches. Through pooled resources, community coalitions can achieve greater outcomes than any single group or agency could achieve independently.[56]

The general focus of coalitions is on "changing systems, rules, social norms, or laws in order to ultimately change the social acceptability of certain behaviors."[55(p161)] As with other participatory approaches, coalitions seek to involve local citizens to ensure that interventions meet the needs of each community and are culturally sensitive. When wide-ranging partners are involved, multiple interventions that focus on the individual and the environment can be carried out simultaneously.

As described by the *Community Coalition Action Theory*, coalitions develop through stages that include *formation, implementation, maintenance,* and *outcomes*. *Formation* begins at the initiation of

funding. After funding is obtained, organizations or individuals interested in joining the partnership are provided with the opportunity to join. As a membership base emerges, with multiple agencies present, the coalition structure must be established. Members are placed on committees as necessary tasks surface. *Implementation* occurs after a needs assessment is conducted. After the needs assessment is complete, programs are developed and implemented. *Maintenance* is an ongoing process that includes monitoring and continuing membership recruitment. Activities outlined in the formation and implementation stage must be fulfilled in the maintenance stage. In the final stage, *outcome*, coalition efforts should result in behavior change. Coalition efforts must continually be evaluated to ensure that education and outreach are beneficial to the community.

A recent critical pathway expands the *Community Coalition Action Theory* by documenting the processes that accompany a community-based coalition development from the formation to implementation stage.[58] This critical pathway presents 12 core components that must be met across each of the developmental stages presented in the *Community Coalition Action Theory*. These 12 core components are essential pieces in the development of coalitions: funding, data, coalition structure, membership, leadership, partnerships, coalition enhancement, community support, education, outreach, publicity, and evaluation. Without each of the key pieces for progress, coalitions could falter and may not succeed in being established. The 12 core components expand as the coalition proceeds through the developmental stages.

As Table 12.3 shows, coalition development is more than simply assembling a group of interested individuals and organizations to achieve a common goal. Certain essential components must exist and certain processes must occur to advance a developing coalition toward sustainability. The pathway provides a practical guide that outlines the milestones that the coalition should meet in the developmental process. Practitioners and community members can use these critical indicators to determine where they are in the process of development and what needs to be done to advance to the next stage.

Table 12.3. Critical Indicators of Progress for a Developing Coalition

Core Components	Phase I Formation	Phase II Implementation	Phase III Maintenance	Phase IV Outcomes
Funding	Collaborate with numerous partners to obtain funding	Sustain funds for coalition continuation		Coalition is financially sustainable to continue projects in the community
Data	Define what data is/is not available	Retrieve, collect and analyze data that would benefit the coalition	Guide coalition efforts with data	Continue to guide coalition efforts with data
Coalition Structure	Define coalition structure	Formalize coalition structure		Attained coalition goals by adhering to coalition structure
Membership	Recruit members by identifying individuals/groups with a similar interest	Empower members to be more involved while seeking new members	Continually seek new members to share work as coalition programs expand	Community groups/individuals are represented by the coalition members
Leadership	Notify the community about the forming coalition	Network with other groups with similar interests	Ensure that tasks get delegated to appropriate people	Core groups of leaders are available to keep the coalition running in case the main leader leaves
Partnerships	Identify potential partners in the community that have similar interests	Assess who is not a partner already but should become a partner	Continue expanding collaboration efforts	All needed partners are at the table for the coalition's success
Coalition Enhancement	Structure and facilitate meetings appropriately	Ensure that active members have a significant role in coalition	Determine future endeavors of the coalition	Coalition is sustainable through active members and extended support
Community Support	Notify community leaders and businesses about the forming coalition	Seek community support to projects	Maintain these relationships by keeping the coalition's agenda at the forefront of supporters' mind	Community recognizes your group's mission and importance
Education	Identify what education is needed in the community	Channel safety messages through the most effective venues	Expand to new channels as the opportunity arises while maintaining those that are effective	Awareness in the community has increased about your public health topic
Outreach	Link with partners already established to get the message/services out	Venture out to new venues that are not currently being used	Identify future opportunities for the coalition to disseminate information	Programs are reaching the targeted groups
Publicity	Build alliances with publicity channels to disseminate information	Keep the coalition efforts or related topics in media messages	Communicate the coalition's agenda in the media	Media/publicity channels are effective in disseminating coalition information to the broader community
Evaluation	Develop an evaluation plan of coalition efforts	Evaluate coalition process, structure, and outcomes regularly	Improve the coalition as needed in accordance with to evaluation	Evaluation is effectively defining and refining coalition efforts

RESEARCH ON COMMUNITY-BASED APPROACHES TO COMMUNITY HEALTH PLANNING, ASSESSMENT, PROGRAM IMPLEMENTATION, AND EVALUATION

Participatory Action Research (PAR) and more specifically **Community-Based Participatory Research (CBPR)** offer a promising approach to public health research and are advancing the practice of community member-academic-practitioner partnerships for community assessment and program planning. Green et al. define PAR as "systematic investigation, with the collaboration of those affected by the issue being studied, for the purpose of education and taking action or effecting social change."[59(p1)] PAR is grounded in the practice of including local citizens in efforts to address social problems, including complex public health problems. PAR is not distinguished by the methods employed, which may be either quantitative or qualitative, but by the active involvement of the people whose lives are affected by the issues under study in every phase of the process.[60]

Philosophical underpinnings of PAR include community empowerment, capacity building, power sharing, process, grassroots control, and negotiation. These underpinnings are well developed and described; PAR is rooted in the notions that people have a right to determine their own development. As an approach, it recognizes the need for local people to participate meaningfully by analyzing their own solutions, over which they have power and control, to lead to sustainable development.[61] These philosophical underpinnings are complemented by the ethical basis of PAR, which includes achieving mutual respect among all parties, being honest about researchers' own objectives, being honest about the benefits to community members, being transparent about how the research finding will be disseminated, and acknowledging

that some of the expected changes that might emerge in the collaborative process are not guaranteed.[61] Central to PAR approaches is the commitment to consciously blurring the lines among the researcher, practitioners, and community members "through processes that accent the wealth of assets that community members bring to the process of knowing and creating knowledge and acting on that knowledge to bring about change."[62(p192)]

CBPR is a direct application of PAR principles. The Agency for Healthcare Research and Quality (AHRQ) defines CBPR as "a collaborative research approach that is designed to ensure and establish structures for participation by communities affected by the issue being studied, representatives of organizations, and researchers in all aspects of the research process to improve health and well-being through taking action, including social change."[63(p3)] CBPR stems from the historical roots of PAR and has emerged as a prime method of applying the PAR philosophy in public health.[64]

The goal of CBPR is to strengthen a community's problem-solving capacity through collective engagement in the research process.[65] Moreover, both approaches, PAR and CBPR, begin with the understanding that the outcome should be action, not just assessment. Community diagnosis is a prime example of these approaches that originate with the intention to act. This action-oriented community diagnosis makes community action the intent of all stages of the assessment.[66]

PAR and particularly CBPR are intertwined with the American philosophy that citizens have a direct and critical role in the democratic process. As Street suggests, PAR can be democratic, equitable, liberating, and life enhancing, enabling the expression of people's full human potential.[67] CBPR requires that students, academics, professionals, and community partners listen to one another, critically discuss common problems and issues, and arrive at solutions and work together to implement those solutions.[68] Although the precise effects and sustainability of CBPR is unknown, experts agree that it benefits community participants, health care practitioners, and researchers alike.[62]

SUMMARY

The contemporary public health professional must work with communities. Communities are the center of public health. Public health professionals must know how to work with their communities to mobilize the community to identify health problems and work with residents to control those health problems. Tools exist to assist with the various stages of working through community health issues and their possible solution. Knowledge and use of these tools will help facilitate their efforts. Although this is perhaps one of the most difficult tasks, it is also one of the most rewarding. It allows for interaction with individuals, often with passionate feelings, to mobilize and use the power of the community to address and solve its problems. The completion of a thorough community health planning and programming process is a source of satisfaction for those leading or involved with the process.

REVIEW QUESTIONS

1. At the beginning of the chapter, the statement is made that the community is the engine in promoting the public's health. In a paragraph, support this statement by explaining the important of community in public health.
2. Explain why a community-based approach is necessary for assessing and addressing current public health conditions.
3. Describe the importance of an asset approach to health assessment and program planning. Give particular attention to how asset mapping can be used in conjunction with more traditional public health assessment models.
4. Describe ways that *Healthy People 2010* encourages collaboration.
5. Identify key characteristics of community-based participatory research and explain how these characteristics could enhance community health initiatives.

REFERENCES

1. Turnock B. *Public Health: What It Is and How It Works*. 3rd ed. Sudbury, MA: Jones and Bartlett Publishing; 2004.
2. Paronen O, Oja P. How to understand a community—Community assessment for the promotion of health-related physical activity. *Patient Educ Couns*. 1998;33:S25-S28.
3. Sharma RK. Putting the community back in community health assessment: A process and outcome approach with a review of some major issues for public health professionals. *J Health Soc Policy*. 2003;16(3):19–33.
4. Heller RF, Heller TD, Pattison S. Putting the public back into public health. Part I. A re-definition of public health. *Public Health*. 2003;117:62–65.
5. Gittell M. *Limits to Citizen Participation: The Decline of Community Organizations*. Beverly Hills, CA: Sage; 1980.
6. Church J, Saunders D, Wanke M, Pong R, Spooner C, Dorgan M. Citizen participation in health decision-making: Past experience and future prospects. *J Public Health Policy*. 2002; 23(1):12–32.
7. McGavran EG. Scientific diagnosis and treatment of the community as a patient. *JAMA*. 1956; 162:723–729.
8. Deuschle KW, Fulmer, HS, McNamara MJ, Tapp, JW. The Kentucky experiment in community medicine. *Milbank Mem Fund Q*. 1966;44(1):9–22.
9. Citrin T. Enhancing public health research and learning through community-academic partnerships: The Michigan experience. *Public Health Rep*. 2001;116(1–2):74–78.
10. Mathews D, McAfee N. *Making Choices Together: The Power of Public Deliberation*. Dayton, OH: Charles F. Kettering Foundation; 2003.
11. Institute of Medicine. *The Future of Public Health*. Washington, DC: National Academy Press; 1988.
12. London S. Thinking together: The art of deliberative dialogue. Available at: http://www.scottlondon.com/reports/dialogue.html.
13. Maxwell J, Rossell S, Forest PG. Giving citizens a voice in healthcare policy in Canada. *BMJ*. 2003; 326(7397):1031–1033.
14. Zinn H. *Declarations of Independence: Cross-examining American Ideology*. New York: HarperCollins; 1990.
15. Fay B. *Critical Social Science*. Ithaca, NY: Cornell University Press; 1987.

16. Mathison S. Deliberation, evaluation, and democracy. *New Directions for Evaluation*. 2000;85:13–26.

17. Scutchfield FD, Ireson C L, Hall LM. Bringing democracy to healthcare: A university-community partnership. *Higher Education Exchange*. 2004;55–63.

18. Green LW, Mercer S. Can public health researchers and agencies reconcile the push from funding bodies and the pull from communities? *American J Public Health*. 2001;91(12):1926–1929.

19. Abelson J, Forest P, Eyles J, Smith P, Martin E, Gauvin F. Deliberations about deliberative methods: Issues in the design and evaluation of public participation processes. *Soc Sci Med*. 2003;57:239–251.

20. Schoch-Spana M, Franco C, Nuzzo JB, Usenza C. Community engagement: Leadership tool for catastrophic health events. *Biosecurity and Bioterrorism: Biodefense Strategy, Practice, and Science*. 2007;5(1):8–25.

21. Scutchfield FD, Ireson CL, Hall LM. The voice of the public in public health policy and planning: The role of public judgment. *J Public Health Policy*. 2004;25(2):197–205.

22. Dewey J, Gouinlock J. *The Moral Writings of John Dewey*. New York: Hafner Press; 1976.

23. Bryne C, Crucetti JB, Medvesky MG, Miller MD, Pirani SJ, Irani PR. The process to develop a meaningful community health assessment in New York state. *J Public Health Manag Pract*. 2002;8(4):45–53.

24. Schmeer K. *Guidelines for Conducting a Stakeholder Analysis*. Bethesda, MD: Partnerships for Health Reform, Abt associates Inc; 1999.

25. Brugha R, Varvasovszky, Z. Stakeholder analysis: A review. *Health Policy and Plan*. 2000;15(3):239–246.

26. Anderson LM, Brownson R, Fullilove MT, et al. Evidence-based public health policy and practice: Promise and limits. *Am J Prev Med*. 2005;28(5S):226–230.

27. Omenn GS, Clark NM. The *Guide to Preventive Services* will be influential in academic health centers: Education, research and links with practice. *Am J Prev Med*. 2000;18(1S):12–14.

28. Perry CL, Komro KA, Veblen-Mortenson S, et al. A randomized controlled trial of the middle and junior high school D.A.R.E. and D.A.R.E. plus programs. *Arch Pediatr Adolesc Med*. 2003;157(2):178–84.

29. US Department of Health and Human Services. *Healthy People 2010*. 2nd ed. Washington, DC: US Government Printing Office; 2000.

30. Fortmann SP, Flora JA, Winkleby MA, Schooler C, Taylor CB, Farquhar JW. Community intervention trials: Reflections on the Stanford five-city project experience. *Am J Epidemiol*. 1995;142(6):576–586.

31. Green LW, Kreuter M. *Health Program Planning: An Educational and Ecological Approach*. 3rd ed. Mountain View, CA: Mayfield Publishing Company; 1999.

32. *Planned Approach to Community Health (PATCH) Program Descriptions*. Washington, DC: US Dept of Health and Human Services; 1993.

33. *APEX/PH, Assessment Protocol for Excellence in Public Health*. Washington, DC: National Association of County and City Health Officials; 1991.

34. Kalos A, Kent L, Gates D. Integrating MAPP, APEXPH, PACE-EH, and other planning initiatives in Northern Kentucky. *J Public Health Manag Pract*. 2005;11(5):401–406.

35. Lenihan P. MAPP and the evolution of planning in public health practice. *J Public Health Manag Pract*. 2005;11(5):381–388.

36. *Mobilizing for Action through Planning and Partnership (MAPP)*. Washington, DC: National Association of County and City Health Officials; 2000.

37. *Global Strategy for Health for All by the Year 2000*. Geneva: World Health Organization; 1981.

38. Norris T, Pittman M. The healthy communities movement and the coalition for healthier cities and communities. *Public Health Rep*. 2000.;115:118–124.

39. *Healthy People in Healthy Communities: A Dialogue Guide*. Chicago, IL: The Coalition for Healthier Cities and Communities; 2000.

40. McKnight J. *The Careless Society: Community and Its Counterfeits*. New York: Basic Books; 1995.

41. Kretzmann JP, McKnight JL. *Building Communities from the Inside Out: A Path Toward Finding and Mobilizing a Community's Assets*. Chicago, IL: ACTA Publications; 1993.

42. McKnight JL. Two tools for well-being: Health systems and communities. *J Perinatol. 1999;*19(6):S12-S16.

43. Missouri Extension Service. FY00-03 Program Development. Available at: http://extension .missouri.edu/about/fy00-03/assetmapping.htm.

44. Williams KJ, Bray PG, Shapiro-Mendoza CK, Reisz I, Peranteau J. Modeling the principles of community-based participatory research in a community health assessment conducted by a health foundation. *Health Promot Pract*. 2007;DOI: 10.1177/15248399062394419.

45. *Healthy People, Surgeon General's Report on Health Promotion and Disease Prevention*. Washington, DC: US Depart of Health and Human Services, Public Health Service; 1979.

46. *Promoting Health/Preventing Disease: Objectives for the Nation*. Washington, DC: US Department of Health and Human Services; 1980.

47. *Healthy People 2000: National Health Promotion and Disease Prevention Objectives*. Washington, DC: US Department of Health and Human Services; 1990. PHS Publication 91-50212.

48. Ochiai E, Blakely C, Wykoff, R. Healthy People: Defining mission, goals, and objectives. In: Keck W, Scutchfield, eds. *Principles of public health*. 2nd ed. Albany, NY: Delmar Thompson Publishers; 2002:161–175.

49. *State Healthy People 2010 Tool Library Archive*. Available at: http://www.phf.org/pmqi/hp2010 .htm.

50. Davis RM. *Healthy People 2010*: Objectives for the United States. *BMJ*. 2000;320:818–819.

51. Israel B, Schulz AJ, Parker E, Becker AB. Review of community-based research: assessing partnership approaches to improve public health. *Annu Rev Public Health*. 1998;19:173–202.

52. Shortell SM, Zukoski AP, Alexander JA, et al. Evaluating partnerships for community health improvement: Tracking the footprints. *J Health Polit Policy Law*. 2002;27(1),49–91.

53. Roussos ST, Fawcett SB. A review of collaborative partnerships as a strategy for improving community health. *Annu Rev Public Health*. 2000; 21:369–402.

54. Weiss ES, Anderson RM, Lasker R. Making the most of collaborations: Exploring the relationship between partnership synergy and partnership functioning. *Health Educ Behav*. 2002;29(6): 683–698.

55. Butterfoss FD, Goodman RM, Wandersman A. Community coalitions for prevention and health promotion. *Health Educ Res*. 1993;8(3):315–330.

56. Berkowitz B, Wolff T. The spirit of the coalition. Washington, DC: American Public Health Association; 2000.

57. Butterfoss FD, Kegler MC. Towards a comprehensive understanding of community coalitions: Moving from practice to theory. In: DiClemente R, Crosby R, Kegler M, eds. *Emerging Theories in Health Promotion Practice and Research: Strategies for Improving Public Health*. San Francisco: Jossey-Bass; 2002:157–193.

58. Downey LH, Ireson CL, Slavova SS, McKee G. Defining elements of success: A critical pathway of coalition development. *Health Promot Pract*. in press.

59. Green LW, George MA, Frankish CJ, Herbert CJ, Bowie WR, O'Neil M. *Study of Participatory Research in Health Promotion: Review and Recommendations for the Development of Participatory Research in Health Promotion of Canada*. Ottawa: Royal Society of Canada; 1995.

60. Cornwell A, Jewkes R. What is participatory research? *Soc Sci Med*. 1995;41:667–676.

61. Gibbons M. Doing a doctorate using a Participatory Action Research framework in the context of community health. *Qual Health Res*. 2002;12(4): 546–558.

62. Minkler M. Using participatory action research to build healthy communities. *Public Health Rep*. 2000;115:191–197.

63. Agency for Healthcare Research and Quality. Community-based participatory research: Assessing the evidence. 2004. Evidence Report/ Technology Assessment. Number 99.

64. White S. *The Art of Facilitating Participation: Releasing the Power of Grassroots Communication*. New Delhi: Sage Publication; 1999.

65. Morone JA, Kilbreth EH. Power to the people? Restoring citizen participation. *J of Health Polit Policy Law*. 2003;28(2–3):271–288.

66. Eng E, Blanchard L. Action-oriented community diagnosis: A health education tool. *Int Q Community Health Educ*. 2006–2007;26(2): 141–158.

67. Street A. *Establishing a Participatory Action Research Group. Nursing Replay: Research Nursing Culture Together*. Melbourne: Churchill Livingstone;1995.

68. Couto R. The promise of a scholarship of engagement. *New England Resource Center for Higher Education*. 2001;Spring:4–7.

CHAPTER 13

Prevention Effectiveness

Kakoli Roy, PhD, Zhuo Chen, MS, PhD, and Anne Haddix, MS, PhD

LEARNING OBJECTIVES

Upon completion of this chapter, the reader will be able to:

1. Describe prevention effectiveness and economic evaluation methods.
2. Distinguish among cost-benefit, cost-effectiveness, and cost-utility analyses.
3. Interpret the results of economic evaluation studies.
4. Recognize challenges and practical issues related to prevention effectiveness studies.
5. Conduct prevention effectiveness studies upon further reading of key references provided in this chapter.

KEY TERMS

Absenteeism
Analytic Horizon
Attributable Fraction
Audience
Cost Analysis
Cost-Benefit Analysis (CBA)
Cost-Effectiveness Analysis (CEA)

Cost-Utility Analysis (CUA)
Direct Cost
Disability-Adjusted Life Year (DALY)
Discounting
Economic Evaluation
Effectiveness
Efficacy
Efficiency
Incremental Cost-Effectiveness Ratio (ICER)
Indirect Cost
Intangible Cost
Morbidity
Mortality
Net Present Value (NPV)
Preventable Fraction
Prevention Effectiveness
Program Costs
Qualify-Adjusted Life Year (QALY)
Randomized Controlled Trials (RCT)
Sensitivity Analysis
Study Perspective
Time Frame
Years of Potential Life Lost (YPLL)

In 2005, the United States spent $1.99 trillion, or 16 percent of gross domestic product (GDP), on health care. The impact of aging, coupled with other demographic and technological changes, is expected to exert continued pressure on health spending, which is projected to reach $4.14 trillion, or 19.6 percent of GDP, by 2016.[1] With over 40 percent of health expenditures financed from the public purse, the ever-increasing share creates challenges for policy makers attempting to balance expenditure on health with spending in other critical sectors, such as education. Although a greater focus on prevention might provide opportunities to further improve health while restraining health care costs, the value of prevention is not obvious. Unlike curative activities, prevention might not have easily identifiable beneficiaries, with the problem further compounded by the differential timing of costs and often delayed benefits, adding challenges in garnering public and political support to fund prevention activities (see Exhibit 13-1).

Public health decision makers, as with other sectors of public expenditure, have to demonstrate the effectiveness and value of health promotion, health protection, and other prevention activities. Convincing policy makers to fund prevention programs requires a comprehensive approach for providing evidence-based information on both costs and effectiveness to assess the return from funds expended for these programs. The term **prevention effectiveness** was coined to describe this body of evidence derived from a systematic assessment of the impact of prevention policies, programs, and practices on health outcomes.

Decision makers in public health are increasingly recognizing the importance of an evidence-based approach as guiding principles for public health practice (see Appendix B). Consequently, prevention effectiveness studies have become a valuable tool in aiding the choice among alternative (often competing) prevention interventions and strategies. For example, the Advisory Committee on Immunization Practices (ACIP) explicitly reviews the evidence on both effectiveness and cost-effectiveness prior to making recommendations on vaccines and immunization practices.[2] A systematic approach frequently adopted in assessing prevention effectiveness requires addressing three critical

EXHIBIT 13-1 Defining Prevention

Prevention is defined as "[O]ne broad-based concept encompassing the reduction of unnecessary suffering, illness and disability and measures health in part as the citizen's sense of well-being."

There are three stages of prevention. *Primary prevention* is the reduction or control of causative factors of potential health problems. It is aimed to reduce the incidence of a disease or injury. *Secondary prevention* is the early detection and treatment of health problems. *Tertiary prevention* involves providing appropriate supportive and rehabilitative services to minimize morbidity and maximize the quality of life, such as the rehabilitation of injuries and the prevention of secondary complications.

Another classification puts prevention activities into three categories: *health promotion, health protection*, and *preventive health services*. Health promotion intends to foster the development of lifestyles to maintain and enhance the state of health and well-being among the general population through promoting health-related information. Health protection is another type of primary prevention, which works by changing the social and physical environment to restrict the access of individuals to pathogens or risk factors usually achieved through legal or regulatory efforts. Preventive health services include counseling, screening, immunization, or chemoprophylactic interventions for individuals in clinical settings.

Source: Public Health Service. *Healthy People 2000: National Health Promotion and Disease Prevention Objectives.* Washington, DC: US Department of Health and Human Services, Public Health Service, 1990; DHHS publication no. (PHS)90-50212.

questions: "What is important?" "What works?" and "What offers best value."[3] In this chapter, we will explain the methods to answer each of these questions, with special emphasis on methods for demonstrating "value" with examples illustrating the practical uses of such information.

WHAT IS IMPORTANT?

Balancing efforts to emphasize the greatest causes of health loss is critical in guiding rational decision-making with limited resources. Consequently, addressing the question "What is important?" starts with an assessment of the relative burden associated with a given disease or health problem. Successful efforts for a systematic assessment of the various dimensions of population health require using valid, accurate, and multiple measures, including mortality, morbidity, and summary measures of burden of disease and quality of life to prioritize conditions for attention[4]. Multiple measures, as opposed to a single measure, are critical because reaching consensus on a single best measure is difficult, with the ranking for conditions by burden varying across these measures, and most importantly, the measures being designed to serve diverse functions (e.g., assess and monitor population health, evaluate effectiveness of health interventions, etc.). This section provides a framework linking the underlying causes with traditional measures of population health (or health outcomes) used for assessing disease burden and the health effects of a prevention strategy.

Mortality

Mortality, or death rate, has been used for centuries to measure burden of diseases and to compare relative burden across diseases.[5] For example, in the United States, chronic diseases—heart disease, cancer, stroke, and chronic lung disease—are the leading causes of death, followed by unintentional injuries and Alzheimer's disease.[6] As a measure of disease burden, mortality has the limitation of being a relatively rare health event, but it remains a critical measure that is simple to define and count with relative ease and accuracy. Relating diseases and risk factors to mortality could help to identify the major causes of death and facilitate priority setting. The top causes of mortality, particularly chronic conditions, are frequently associated with high health care costs.

Although mortality is a good measure for highlighting the causes of death among late life, several other measures have been developed to account for life expectancy at death, or premature mortality, to highlight the causes of death at an early age. A commonly used measure is the **Years of Potential Life Lost (YPLL),** which requires choosing an arbitrary limit of life, with the amount of potential life lost due to death calculated as the difference between age at death and the arbitrary limit. For instance, if the arbitrary limit is set at 75 years, the measure would be reported as YPLL before age 75 (YPLL-75). Chronic diseases, such as cancer and heart disease, are important causes of both mortality and YPLL-75, but injuries, including unintentional injuries, suicide and homicide, and perinatal conditions, which are leading causes of premature death, rank higher as causes of YPLL-75.[6]

In 1993, McGinnis and Foege proposed the concept of "actual causes of death" to emphasize the importance of behavioral (and, usually, modifiable) risk factors that contribute to death in future life stages.[7] They divided the causes of death into genetic and nongenetic factors and demonstrated that half of all deaths are nongenetic and could be prevented, or at least delayed, through behavioral changes. A 2004 update of their analysis reaffirmed that tobacco use, physical inactivity, and poor nutrition were major actual causes of death, followed by other modifiable factors (e.g., alcohol use, sexual practices, and drug use).[8] It is important to highlight that physical inactivity and poor nutrition, which are major contributors to the obesity epidemic, have increased in ranking as actual causes of death. Establishing the importance of behavioral factors as a cause of mortality and morbidity highlights the need for earlier community and policy level interventions that extend beyond the clinical care system.

Morbidity

It is possible for an individual to have a prolonged life but suffer from adverse health conditions. Although mortality does not reflect such suffering, **morbidity** measures the discomfort and psychological stress associated with nonfatal conditions by capturing the incidence or prevalence of acute and chronic conditions, and their consequences. Two such measurements are rate of hospitalization and measurement of disability. Hospitalization rates are relatively easy to collect and useful in some analyses. However, it may be biased or inconsistent over time with the increasing substitution of hospitalization with outpatient treatment.[4] Measurement of disability examines another morbidity dimension (e.g., bone and joint pain, mental health disorders, and hearing and vision disorders). In addition, two commonly used measures of morbidity that are particularly useful in assessing the monetary cost of morbidity are the leading causes of health care expenditures and number of missed workdays. The number of missed workdays, also known as **absenteeism,** measures health-related productivity loss of employees.[9] Employers have increasingly realized the connection between health and employee productivity, resulting in worksite prevention programs. Presenteeism refers to the fact that an employee may be present at work but function with low productivity. Presenteeism can be related to the employee health or health problems associated with the employee's family members. Both absenteeism and presenteesim can be converted to monetary costs by using standard estimates of productivity to measure the impact of morbidity.

Summary Measures

Because mortality and morbidity each have limitations as measures of disease burden, summary measures that combine both dimensions have been employed to measure the overall health status of a population. For the majority of people who do not suffer premature death, it is critical to assess how the conditions they suffer from impact their quality of life or functional status. For any health problem, summary measures combine the quality of life lost to morbidity with the amount of life years lost to mortality. Therefore, in assessing effectiveness of programs and policies, summary measures can capture the impact on both life expectancy and quality of life, the latter capturing both the reduction in severity and length of a condition. Although a number of approaches exist for combining both attributes into a single composite measure, two of the most commonly used are the **disability-adjusted life years (DALYs)** and the **quality-adjusted life years (QALYs).**[10,11]

DALYs combine the life years lost from premature mortality with the health loss experienced by living with a health condition. Although premature mortality is calculated from life tables, the morbidity component is obtained by multiplying years spent living with a condition that results from a particular disease or injury by an associated disability weight rated on a scale ranging from 0 (death) to 1 (perfect health). In contrast, the QALY approach attempts to capture mortality and life in a particular health state with a weighting system that assigns weights ranging from 0 to 1, where 0 corresponds to a health state equivalent to death, and 1 corresponds to optimal health. The QALYs related to a particular health outcome are then expressed as the weight given to a particular health state multiplied by the length of time in that state. Therefore, QALY measures are in terms of gains in health as compared to DALYs, which are in terms of losses in health. Consequently, QALYs are better designed and frequently used to compare the benefits of alternative heath interventions. A ranking of the most common causes of DALYs lost in the United States provides a different perspective than a ranking on the top causes of mortality, with motor vehicle crashes, depression, and alcohol abuse being important causes of lost DALYs but not necessarily of mortality.[12]

Table 13.1 compares the leading causes of health burden by some of the methods of measurement described in this section.

Table 13.1. Leading Causes of Health Burden in the United States

Mortality (2004)[a]	YPLL-75 (2004)[a]	DALY (1996)[b]	Actual Causes of Death (2000)[c]
Diseases of heart	Malignant neoplasms	Ischemic heart disease	Tobacco
Malignant neoplasms	Diseases of heart	Cerebrovascular disease	Poor diet/physical inactivity
Cerebrovascular diseases	Unintentional injuries	Motor vehicle crashes	Alcohol
Chronic obstructive pulmonary diseases	Perinatal Period	Depression	Microbial agents
Unintentional injuries	Suicide	Lung cancer	Toxic Agents
Diabetes Mellitus	Homicide	Chronic lower respiratory disease	Motor vehicle crashes
Alzheimer's Disease	Congenital Anomalies	Alcohol use	Firearms
Influenza and Pneumonia	Cerebrovascular	HIV	Sexual behavior
Nephritis, nephrotic syndrome, and nephrosis	Diabetes mellitus	Diabetes mellitus	Illicit drug use
Septicemia	Chronic liver disease and cirrhosis	Septicemia	

SOURCES: [a]CDC WISQARS website. Available at: http://www.cdc.gov/ncipc/wisqars/. Accessed July 2007.

[b]McKenna MT, Michaud CM, Murray CJL, Marks JS. Assessing the burden of disease in the U.S. using disability-adjusted life years. *Am J Prev Med.* 2005;28:415–23.

[c]Mokdad AH, Marks JS, Stroup DF, Gerberding JL. Actual causes of death in the U.S., 2000 [published erratum appears in *JAMA.* 2005;293:293–4]. *JAMA.* 2004;291:1238–45.

WHAT WORKS?

Assessing the scientific information on the **effectiveness** of an intervention, or addressing "what works?" is critical for public health practitioners attempting to derive the optimal return from limited public resources. For an intervention to eliminate every disease or cure every patient is rare. A related concept is **efficacy,** which refers to the scientific basis for the maximum effectiveness or health improvement obtained from a prevention strategy in expert hands under ideal conditions. Efficacy is often measured in **randomized controlled trials (RCTs)** assessing the impact of a technology on health outcomes. Despite their importance, these studies are expensive in terms of time, effort, and financial resources. However, after

it is known or established that an intervention is efficacious, it is necessary to address how well it works in the real world. Effectiveness measures the impact of an intervention in real-world settings taking into consideration financial and other practical constraints associated with applying an intervention to a target population larger than in the RCTs. Obtaining realistic estimates of effectiveness of intervention in populations, although critical for evidence-based decision making, is a challenge and can, at best, be approximated.

Most of the major causes of disease, injury, and disability are associated with risk factors that might be reduced or eliminated with population-based interventions. After a major health problem has been recognized, public health practitioners must identify the modifiable risk factors associated with the problem to guide the development of appropriate interventions. In assessing an intervention strategy, it is important to know what can be realistically accomplished in terms of reduction in health burden at the population level after the intervention is implemented. The first step is gleaning evidence from research studies on cause-and-effect associations with the health condition. **Attributable fraction** measures the amount of disease or injury that could be eliminated if a risk factor never occurred in a given population. In contrast, the **preventable fraction** measures the proportion of health problem that can actually be avoided by a prevention strategy, and reflects what can be achieved in a real-world setting.

Public health practitioners gather evidence on effectiveness in a variety of ways, including consultation with peer and expert review of the scientific literature.[13–16] Systematic literature reviews, as opposed to expert opinion or narrative reviews, are increasingly recognized as critical for guiding evidence-based public health practice. Such an approach requires the systematic assessment of evidence on effectiveness by a multidisciplinary team of experts using standardized methods to assess the quality, consistency, and strength of evidence,[5–8] followed by a deliberative process for weighing the evidence for setting practice guidelines.[17–20]

The United States Preventive Services Task Force (USPSTF) has been providing comprehensive systematic-review based guidelines for clinical preventive services (and published as the *Guide to Clinical Preventive Services,* or the *Clinical Guide*) since 1989 in the United States.[21] Inspired by the success of the *Clinical Guide,* a sister organization, the Task Force on Community Preventive Services (TFCPS) was convened to develop systematic evidence-based guidelines focused on the clinical system and community based preventive services (and published as the *Guide to Community Preventive Services,* or the *Community Guide*).[22] Both task forces have developed standardized methods for conducting systematic reviews and for translating those into practice guidelines.[13,14] The TFCPS has released several sets of systematic reviews, including a book that compiles these recommendations.[14] The development of evidence-based guidelines might be limited by lack of evidence,

lack of comparable outcomes across studies, and the amount of time and resource it consumes. Despite these potential drawbacks, the success of the *Clinical Guide* and the *Community Guide* highlights the importance of using systematic reviews for developing practice guidelines based on a clear and transparent analytic rationale.

WHAT OFFERS THE BEST VALUE?

In addition to knowing the greatest causes of health loss and identifying preventive interventions that are most effective, public health decision makers need to know which interventions offer the greatest return on investment. **Economic evaluation** provides a systematic approach for assessing and comparing two or more interventions (programs) in terms of their respective costs and benefits. The goal of economic evaluation is to measure the **efficiency,** or the health gain from the funds expended, of one intervention compared to another. Analyses of prevention strategies can only be interpreted in comparison with other reasonable alternatives, for example, compared to doing nothing, using current care, or using other interventions. Evidence from economic evaluations, by identifying programs and activities that provide the greatest benefit per dollar invested, can make useful policy guidance for efficient allocation of limited public health resources.

An economic evaluation study generally adopts one of three approaches: **cost-effectiveness analysis (CEA)**, **cost-utility analysis (CUA)**, or **cost-benefit analysis (CBA)**. Each of these three methods requires a careful cost analysis and an assessment of health effects, both beneficial and adverse events. All three methods measure costs in the same way; the distinguishing feature of each is the way in which health benefits are measured. In addition, economic evaluation studies need to fulfill basic criteria and follow standard methods to ensure that the approaches are comparable.

Framing an Economic Evaluation Study

Before beginning a prevention-effectiveness analysis, researchers must address a number of key methodological issues (see Exhibit 13-2). The *first* methodological issue is the **study perspective,** which determines what costs and benefits should be included, and is dictated in part by the **audience** (i.e., the primary consumers and their informational needs). An economic evaluation study can be performed from a variety of perspectives. The societal perspective takes the broadest view and is preferred for making public health decisions because all costs, benefits, and harms associated are included, regardless of who pays or receives them. Other frequently used perspectives include employer, payer, provider, and patient perspectives. For example, employers might be interested in their health insurance costs, cost of absenteeism, and reduced productivity due to illness. Likewise, patients might weigh their out-of-pocket payments and waiting time with the perceived benefits of care. Each perspective is legitimate in its own right, and sometimes multiple perspectives might be appropriate to address multiple audiences. What is critical is that the study perspec-

tive is clearly stated and that only studies using similar perspectives are compared.

Second, economic evaluation studies should use a **time frame** that includes the time period during which the intervention is implemented. In addition, an appropriate **analytic horizon** should be used to measure all costs, benefits, and harms that accrue from the intervention. The analytic horizon, as shown in Figure 13.1, is generally longer than the time frame because prevention interventions usually have delayed effects lasting beyond the implementation period.

Third, economic evaluation studies should explicitly deal with uncertainty in the model parameters and the effect of varying key model assumptions. **Sensitivity analysis** provides a technique for examining how the results change under different scenarios, assumptions, and with variation in model parameters. Sensitivity analysis assesses the model's robustness, including identifying which variables in the model are "driving" the results and hence warrant more attention.

Fourth, individuals generally prefer receiving (financial and health) benefits as quickly as possible but want to delay adverse events. **Discounting**

EXHIBIT 13-2 Key Issues of Economic Evaluation Studies

1. Define the audience for the evaluation.
2. Define operationally the problem or question to be analyzed.
3. Indicate clearly the prevention strategies being evaluated.
4. Specify the perspective of the analysis.
5. Define the relevant time frame and analytic horizon for the analysis.
6. Determine the analytic method or methods.
7. Determine whether the analysis is to be a marginal or an incremental one.
8. Identify the relevant costs.
9. Identify the health outcome or outcomes of interest.
10. Specify the discount rate or time preference for monetary and nonmonetary costs and outcomes that would occur in the future.
11. Identify the sources of uncertainty and plan sensitivity analyses.
12. Determine the summary measures that will be reported.
13. Evaluate if the distribution of costs and benefits in the population will differ for the alternative prevention-intervention options, including the baseline comparator.

Source: Farnham PG, Haddix AC. Study Design. In: Haddix AC, Teutsch SM, Corso PS eds. *Prevention Effectiveness: A Guide to Decision Analysis and Economic Evaluation*, 2nd ed. Oxford University Press; 2002: 11–12.

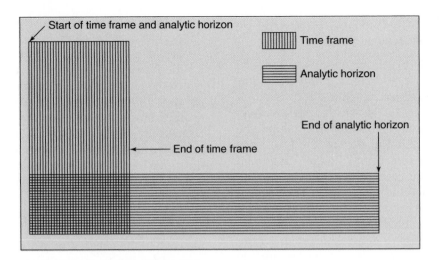

Figure 13.1. Time Frame and Analytical Horizon
SOURCE: Delmar Cengage Learning.

is a technique used to account for differential preferences (or valuation) for events that occur in the future. To reflect this preference for returns that are delivered now, both resources spent and benefits gained in the future are discounted to be comparable to resources spent and benefits gained in the present. The higher the discount rate, the lower the value of events that occur in the future. Hence, a zero discount rate implies that future events have the same value as if they occurred today.

The United States Panel on Cost-Effectiveness in Health and Medicine (PCHM) recommends that both future costs and outcomes be discounted to present values using the 3 percent discount rate in the base-case scenario, with the effect of using different discount rates examined in the sensitivity analysis.[23]

Finally, the scope of an analysis and the intended audience usually determines the choice of an analytic method and the range of costs and benefits to be considered, which not only affect how the analysis is conducted but also the interpretation of results and policy conclusions. A brief description of cost analysis, as well as the three types of economic evaluation methods follows. More detailed descriptions of these methods, including guidelines on conducting such studies, can be found in standard textbooks and online courses.[23–25]

Cost Analysis

Cost analysis involves the systematic collection, categorization, and analysis of intervention (or program) costs, side effects costs, and illness costs. Cost analysis, together with effectiveness assessment, is an important component of all three economic evaluation techniques. Cost analysis can also be used as a standalone evaluation method when only one program is being assessed or when the interventions being assessed and compared are equally effective.

In everyday life, we generally value goods or services by their financial or monetary cost. It is a convenient measure when the good or service has an available "price tag" based on a market transaction. In an economic evaluation study, we think of costs as consequences of choices. Because resources are limited, the decision to implement a particular program will make the resources it consumes unavailable for other alternative uses. Therefore, the true cost of a program requires valuing the benefits that would have been derived had the resources been allocated to their next best use. Economists term it as the **opportunity cost** of a program. The opportunity cost is the value of the benefits forgone by using scarce health care resources for the intervention of interest rather than for alternative purposes. The costing principle in an economic evaluation study involves identifying the opportunity cost associated with a program. Under perfect conditions, the market price of a resource approximates opportunity cost. In reality, assessing the true opportunity cost can be very difficult and requires circumventing challenges using advanced methods. At the minimum, costs can be broken down into **intervention costs, cost of side effects** of the intervention, and **cost of illness** (or disease averted).

The cost of an intervention (or program) includes the costs of all resources expended in management, operation, and implementation of the program or intervention (see Figure 13.2). The cost of side effects includes the incidental hazards and psychological effects associated with the program itself. The cost of illness can be generally categorized into direct, indirect, and intangible costs. **Direct costs** are the cost of medical care associated with diagnosis, management, and treatment had the disease not been prevented. **Indirect costs** refer to the costs incurred or saved due to loss of time in productive pursuits (e.g., absenteeism from work or reduced productivity because of illness) and the value of that time due to changes in the burden of disease or injury. **Intangible costs** are nonmaterial costs such as emotional anxiety, fear, pain, or stigmatization,

which can impose a major burden on a client or a client's family. Quantifying intangible costs is difficult, and although these costs are not included in most studies, their omission must be explicitly stated because they might be a major factor in affecting clients' decisions.

Depending on the perspective of the analysis, costs are often classified into three general categories, (1) program costs, (2) costs to participants, and (3) costs to others affected by the intervention. **Program costs** list the value of all the resources expended on implementation and maintenance of the intervention. **Costs to participants** include out-of-pocket expenses (expenses incurred by participants that are not accounted for in the program costs) and productivity losses. Finally, an intervention might cause adverse events for persons who are not directly participating in the program. Costs to others must be included if the study adopts a societal perspective.

Finally, there are a few critical factors to keep in mind when gleaning data on costs. *First*, in a retrospective study, a researcher attempts to identify costs after the program has begun or been completed. Often it is difficult to collect such data. Data limitations may exist with available datasets because researchers had no control of the data collection process. Hence from time to time, we

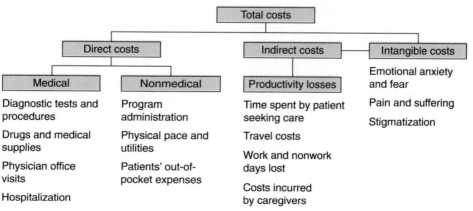

Figure 13.2. Cost Inventory

SOURCE: Prevention Effectiveness Branch, *Centers for Disease Control and Prevention Economic Evaluation Tutorials,* http://www.cdc.gov/owcd/EET/Cost/fixed/PrintAll.html, Prevention Effectiveness Branch, Epidemiology Program Office, Centers for Disease Control and Prevention (CDC), 2001, accessed on April 9, 2008.

have to rely on literature reviews for parameter calibration. In a prospective study, where researchers can design the prevention intervention and collect the data, actual cost data are recorded during the course of the intervention. Therefore cost estimates are more consistent and reliable in prospective studies. *Second*, it is important that the cost data be collected for the same time period in which the intervention was implemented. Selection of the time period is determined by whether seasonality or other time patterns affect either costs or client participation. Both variable costs and startup or fixed costs should be collected and included in the calculation of the total cost of an intervention. *Third*, to summarize results of cost analyses, we must determine a usable form for integration into prevention effectiveness analyses. The cost analyses results need to be expressed as a function of health outcome, for example, cost per unit of intervention.

Cost–Benefit Analysis

Cost-benefit analysis (CBA) is often considered the gold standard for economic evaluation. It is one method in which health outcomes and all costs, including intangible costs, are converted into monetary units based on societal valuation or willingness to pay. CBA generally includes all costs and benefits, discounts them to present value, and then subtracts discounted costs from monetized discounted benefits to estimate the net benefit of an intervention. In effect, CBA compares society's total willingness to pay for the outcomes resulting from a program or policy with the opportunity costs of implementing the program or policy. If total discounted benefits exceed total discounted costs, the intervention is said to have a positive **net present value** (NPV). Although a CBA can be used to estimate the net benefit from a single intervention, when comparing two or more interventions, the logical choice in a CBA is the intervention that yields the highest positive NPV.

CBA is also particularly useful for comparing a wide range of public programs with disparate outcomes, that is, education, housing, defense, and so on. It might be most suitable when the Congress attempts to set priorities and allocate funding across agencies with very different missions and objectives. Although CBA remains the preferred method for regulatory impact analysis in nonhealth sectors (i.e., Environmental Protection Agency), it is less commonly used in the health sector due to concerns about assigning a monetary value to life and health.

Cost–Effectiveness Analysis

Cost-effectiveness analysis (CEA) makes no attempt to assign a monetary value to health outcomes. Instead of monetary units, health outcomes are measured in the most appropriate natural unit. For example, in comparing programs to promote the use of bicycle helmets, the reported health outcome might be "head injuries averted." Other examples of reporting health outcomes in CEA include cases of disease prevented or life years saved. In health and medicine, CEA is the most commonly used economic evaluation method.

The usual question facing the decision maker requires assessing the additional costs and benefits of implementing an intervention compared to status quo. CEA assesses alternative interventions in terms of **incremental cost-effectiveness ratio (ICER),** which calculates the ratio of difference in net costs and net benefits between one scenario and another. The numerator of the ICER is the cost of an intervention, including changes in resource use resulting from the intervention, with the costs of illness and productivity losses averted as a result of the intervention subtracted from intervention costs. The denominator of the ICER is the additional number of health outcomes prevented by the more effective intervention. Thus, the ICER represents the additional cost to achieve one unit of health outcome, such as deaths prevented or life years saved, by implementing one intervention compared to the next most effective intervention.

CEA is most suitable when comparing interventions with similar health outcomes. For example, it might be particularly useful to an STD clinic director in allocating budgets for different programs with a common outcome, for example, cases of STD prevented. The main advantage of CEA is that measuring outcomes in natural units simplifies the analysis and is often more intuitive for users of a study. Some key disadvantages include reduced comparability of efficiency assessments across interventions that produce disparate outcomes (e.g., flu vaccination versus water fluoridation) and the need to focus on a single outcome even when an intervention generates multiple distinct benefits.

Cost-Utility Analysis

Cost-utility analysis (CUA) is a special type of CEA in which health outcomes are composite measures that combine both life years saved and qualify-of-life adjustment for the years lived. The health outcome measure most commonly used for CUA is the quality-adjusted life years (QALYs). The preferred intervention is the one with lowest cost per additional QALY gained compared to the next most effective intervention. However, some international studies prefer the disability-adjusted life years (DALYs). Measuring outcomes in a common metric such as QALYs greatly enhances the comparability of results across programs that produce very different health outcomes (e.g., flu vaccination versus injury prevention), including those that primarily affect quality of life, as well as others that might have a larger impact on premature mortality. CUA might be particularly suitable when the head of a public health agency (i.e., CDC) is trying to set priorities and allocate the budget across different programs within the agency (e.g., cancer control versus immunization programs). It is not surprising that a recently released Institute of Medicine (IOM) report on standardized CEA methods for evaluating economically significant federal regulations affecting health, commissioned by the Office of Management and Budget (OMB) and a consortium of federal agencies, recommended QALY as one of the three outcome measures; the two others being number of deaths averted and life years.

However, a key disadvantage of CUA is the considerable increase over CEA in terms of complexity in health outcome assessment. Both QALYs and DALYs involve subjective assessment of weights that may not be universally accepted. For example, the weights assigned to the 22 health states in DALYs are determined by an expert panel, which works well in practice, but the subjectivity invites doubts and criticisms. The QALYs measure is intuitively more appealing because the weights are preference-based, which is considered more appropriate because it accords with standard welfare economics that suggest resource allocation decisions reflect the preferences of those who will be affected by these decisions. There are well-established methods to elicit individual preference weights (e.g., standard gamble, time trade-off and person trade-off), but controversies remain on many issues, including how the preference weights should be elicited (i.e., from actual clients versus a representative specific group, etc.). Another key difference between DALYs and QALYs is that DALYs weight life according to productivity at different ages, and thus assigning higher weights to working-age individuals. Nonetheless, both measures have wide applicability and are being increasingly used in economic evaluation studies that set public policy priorities.

The three methods of economic evaluation, cost-benefit analysis, cost-effectiveness analysis, and cost-utility analysis, are compared in Table 13.2 in terms of the costs they measure, their units of outcome, and summary measures.

Challenges and Proposed Remedies

The role of economic evaluation, especially CEA, has been increasingly publicized over the past two decades. However, application of economic evaluation in shaping public health policy has been limited, primarily because of methodological and contextual challenges.[31,32] A key problem is that the studies are often not generalizable beyond the specific (local or national) study context. While suggestions[33] for improving generalizability have been proposed, including "generalized CEA" proposed by the World Health Organization,[34] its actual usefulness is yet to be ascertained. A more basic criticism of CEA is the

Table 13.2. **Components of the Three Methods of Economic Evaluation**

| | Costs | | | | Outcome Measure | Summary Measure |
	Direct Medical	Direct Nonmedical	Productivity Losses	Intangible		
CBA	Yes	Yes	Yes	Yes	Monetary unit	Net benefits (benefits–costs)
CEA	Yes	Yes	Yes	No	Natural Unit	Cost-effectiveness ratio (net costs/cases prevented)
CUA	Yes	Yes	Occasionally[a]	No	Health Index	Cost-utility ratio (net costs/quality-adjusted life-years)

[a]The utility measure generally accounts for productivity loss. When it does not account for productivity loss, we need to include it.

EXHIBIT 13-3 An Example of Cost-Benefit Analysis

The smallpox vaccine program was active before 1972, the year smallpox was virtually eliminated in the United States[26] Part of the concern associated with the smallpox vaccine is it uses a "live" vaccinia virus that imposes health risks on those vaccinated and their contacts during the few weeks following vaccination. In 1971, CDC recommended discontinuation of routine smallpox vaccination based on a study that indicated that the total economic costs of vaccination outweighed the benefit, primarily due to the rare natural occurrence of smallpox. Consequently, the cost of side effects (566 per 1 million vaccinated) outweighed the benefit of eliminating the then nearly nonexistent risk of exposure to smallpox for United States civilians, which had not been seen in United States after 1949.

However, the recent threat of bioterrorism after September 11, 2001 led to smallpox vaccination of several high risk groups, including military personnel and public health workers. Costs and unexpected consequences do follow, however, as indicated by a recent incident at The University of Chicago Hospital.[27] The hospital reported that on March 3rd, 2007, a child was transferred into the hospital and later diagnosed with eczema vaccinatum, a complication that resulted from contacts with his father, who was with the military and had been vaccinated three weeks before the contact. Whether the economic benefits of smallpox vaccination would outweigh the costs in today's world and how the relevant protocol should be enforced again falls in the domain of prevention effectiveness research.

---

wide variation in methods across studies, making it difficult to compare results from one analysis to those of another.[35] To improve quality standards and advance comparability across economic evaluation studies, guidelines on standardized methods must be established. The United States Panel on Cost-Effectiveness in Health and Medicine (PCHM), convened by the United States Public Health Service (PHS), took the initiative in establishing guidelines by developing recommendations for "reference case" CEAs.[23]

Although adherence to guidelines in published studies is uneven, with a systematic review of studies published from 1976 to 2001 indicating that only 539 studies had adhered to the PCHM guidelines,[36] standardization of methods appears to be improving over time.[37]

An important challenge in CEA studies is the interpretation of study results in providing recommendations on whether an intervention is a good value for money. One way of organizing the

EXHIBIT 13-4 An Example of Cost-Effectiveness Analysis

Human papillomavirus (HPV) causes cervical intraepithelial neoplasia (CIN); cervical, penile, vaginal, vulvar, and head/neck cancers; and anogenital warts, resulting in serious death and disease among both men and women.[28] Public health authorities recommend routine vaccination of girls aged 11–12 years and catch-up vaccination of girls and women aged 13–26 years with the recently licensed HPV vaccine (Merck & Co., Inc., Whitehouse Station, NJ, USA). The efficacy of the HPV vaccine among men, however, is yet to be established.[29] A recent study indicates that the Incremental Cost-Effectiveness Ratio (ICER) of vaccinating girls before 12 years of age was $4,666 per QALY gained. The ICER of including men and

boys in the program was $45,056 per QALY.[28] Legislators in 24 states have been debating about making the HPV vaccine mandatory. However, Dr. Jo Abramson, the chair of Advisory Committee on Immunization Practices (ACIP), suggested exercising caution because it might be too soon to do so. First, HPV is not contagious; and second, state governments might not have sufficient funding at this time with many other urgent public health priorities consuming a large portion of the public health funding.[30] Aside from information on epidemiologic and economic impact, other factors, including assessment of competing priorities and ethical issues, are also critical when making vaccine policy recommendations.

information is in a "league table" that ranks cost-effectiveness ratios for different interventions, which facilitates comparisons across interventions, including previously published evidence. It is tempting to set a threshold for the ratios, labeling the interventions that have a cost-effectiveness ratio less than a particular threshold as a good buy. It has become common in United States CEA studies to use $50,000 per QALY gained as a threshold for assessing cost-effectiveness of an intervention.[38] The use of the $50,000 benchmark first emerged in 1992 and became more extensively used after 1996. Exploring the history behind this threshold reveals that it is ill defined and not based on solid economic foundations or expert consensus. Rather than arbitrary thresholds, the general recommendation for practitioners of cost-effectiveness studies is to present the cost-effectiveness ratios in a league table and acknowledge the thresholds. Other approaches that are being increasingly used in the literature include estimating the willingness to pay for a QALY and calculating cost-effectiveness acceptability curves that show the probability of an intervention being cost-effective for a range of thresholds.

The **discount rate** used in economic evaluation, including whether to use the same rate for both

costs and benefits, has long been a subject of debate. Researchers have argued that the social value of health is growing over time, and thus a lower discount rate should be used for discounting health effects.[39–41] A recent review on this practice in economic evaluations of health care interventions indicated that whereas the majority of the 147 studies reviewed used either 3 percent or 5 percent as the discount rate, about 28 percent of them did not discount either costs or benefits.[42] The general approach is to use 3 percent as the baseline discount rate, with other rates over a reasonable range (i.e., 0% to 10%) examined in the sensitivity analyses. In addition, the PCHM recommendation is to apply the same rate to discount both costs and health effects.[23]

Another issue that remains unresolved is the treatment of "unrelated" (i.e., indirect or productivity) future costs that result from the lost production due to death and disability. Although many have argued that the future costs should be included,[43] others argue in favor of inclusion.[44] Those who support inclusion believe that health expenditures rise when people live longer. In addition, CEA is consistent with its underlying theory of lifetime utility maximization only if all future medical and nonmedical expenditures are included.[45] For most interventions, these two "diametrically" different approaches produce similar rankings as long as costs are treated consistently.[46] However, if the interventions involve persons with different age groups, this may not be true. The inclusion of future costs can be expected to increase the relative cost-effectiveness of interventions that promote survival among younger adults relative to interventions that promote survival among older adults. An intermediate approach proposes that the difference between future earnings and consumption resulting from mortality prevention be included in CEAs.[41]

However, it must be emphasized that effectiveness and cost-effectiveness are only two of several other factors that must be considered when making choices with limited public resources. Aside from the goal of maximizing population health, it is critical for public health practitioners and decision makers to balance economic efficiency with equity. For example, if two competing interventions are similar in terms of cost-effectiveness, the one that more effectively reduces health disparities by targeting vulnerable groups should be preferred. In practice, rarely are the trade-offs between equity and economic efficiency so simple (e.g., interventions that save lives of older versus younger adults, or high-risk group versus the entire target population). Evidence shows that the fair and equitable distribution of health gains from public resources is preferred over economic considerations.

PRACTICAL APPLICATIONS TO INFORM DECISION MAKING

Including an economic perspective in evaluation of health and health care interventions has become an important and accepted component of health policy and planning. Several countries have been using cost-effectiveness evidence, alongside other types of information, to set priorities and allocate public funds for different (often competing) health interventions. For example, health technology assessments underlie decisions made by the Canadian Coordinating Office of Health Technology Assessment (CCOHTA), the British National Health System (NHS), the Australian Pharmaceutical Benefit Advisory Committee (PBAC), and the United States ACIP. In fact, pharmaceutical companies in Australia[47] and several European countries[48-50] have to prove that their products are cost-effective before they can be reimbursed by the government.

In the United Kingdom, the National Institute for Health and Clinical Excellence (NICE) was established in 1999 to "provide guidance to the NHS on the use of selected new and established technologies."[51] NICE synthesizes evidence on effectiveness and costs of treatment to recommend whether an intervention is a cost-effective use of NHS resources. All appraisals are grounded in a systematic review of the available evidence to assess the safety and efficacy of drugs and devices. In addition, an intervention that is classified as safe and effective may undergo a rigorous assessment to establish its cost-effectiveness, generally expressed in terms of incremental cost per QALY gained.[52]

A review[53] of guidance issued by NICE to the NHS between 1999 and April 2005 identified 86 guidance documents covering 117 technology or client topics. Among the 117 topics, NICE recommendations were "no" for 19 percent, "yes" for 23 percent, "yes with major restrictions" for 32 percent, and "yes with minor restrictions" for 26 percent. Of the negative recommendations, 66 percent were due to insufficient evidence and the rest as a result of unacceptable cost-effectiveness (i.e., below a certain threshold). A valuation issue that has been the subject of intense scrutiny is whether NICE has a threshold above which a technology will not be deemed cost-effective enough to warrant public subsidy via the NHS. Retrospective analysis of published appraisal decisions has identified a general concentration of adopted thresholds in the range of £20,000 ($34,500) to £30,000 ($51,500) per QALY gained in one study,[54] including a suggestion that in practice the threshold may be even more generous, being closer to £45 000 ($77,500).[55] A House of Commons Select Committee inquiry[56] into the matter provided evidence indicating that the NICE threshold may be too generous,[57] raising concern that NICE might have recommended too many new technologies, diverting public resources from other health care technologies that offer a better value for money. More detailed discussion of the threshold and methods for identifying them can be found elsewhere.[58]

NICE continues to play a key role in promoting evidence-based resource allocation decisions in the NHS. Many of the methods used by NICE are transferable to the United States and other countries. For example, a 2003 WHO review[59] of the NICE technology appraisal program noted that NICE appraisals are being widely used as international benchmarks. As of April 2005, the British government announced that NICE would also address matters of public health, providing advice on measures to improve population health, for example, by reducing levels of smoking, alcohol use, and obesity.[52]

In the United States, the National Commission on Prevention Priorities (NCPP) was convened by the Partnership for Prevention in 2003 with the aim of providing decision makers evidence-based information about preventive services that includes health impact and value, guidance about where improving coverage will have the biggest impact, and a resource for building demand for a prevention-focused health care system. In 2006, Partnership for Prevention and Health Partners Research Foundation, under the auspices of NCPP, published a study[60] that ranked 25 evidence-based clinical preventive services recommended by the USPSTF and ACIP based on each service's relative health impact and cost effectiveness. The 2006 ranking is an update of a 2001 ranking of clinical preventive services, and employs a methodology similar to the previous study.[61] Each service received a ranking of 1 to 5 points based on each of two measures—clinically preventable burden and cost-effectiveness—for a total score ranging from 2 to 10. Priorities for

improving delivery rates were obtained by comparing the ranking with what is known about current delivery rates nationally. The three highest-ranking services with a total score of 10 each were discussing aspirin use with high-risk adults, immunizing children, and tobacco-use screening and brief intervention. High-ranking services (with a score of 6 or more) with low use rates include tobacco-use screening and brief intervention, screening adults aged 50 and over for colorectal cancer, immunizing adults aged 65 and older against pneumococcal disease, and screening young women for Chalmydia.[40] The study indicates that that there is significant under-use of preventive services that are very cost effective and have been recommended for years, resulting in unnecessary poor health, lost lives, and inefficient use of health care dollars. In fact, increasing the use of just 5 preventive services to 90 percent has the potential of saving more than 100,000 lives each year in the United States

The majority of cost-effectiveness information currently available in the literature are from high-income countries such as North America, Europe, and Australia.[62] At an international level, the World Bank has employed sectoral CEA to identify disease control priorities in developing countries and essential packages for countries at different levels of economic development.[63,64] However, widespread application of these methods to aid decision making in developing regions such as Asia, Africa, and Latin America, where the majority of the world's poor live, is limited due to several technical shortcomings in generating economic evidence, social preferences, political expediency, and systemic barriers to implementation.[62] The CHOICE (*CHO*osing *I*nterventions that are *C*ost-*E*ffective) project, a WHO initiative developed in 1998, aims to provide policy makers with evidence for allocating scarce resources between a mix of interventions to maximize population health (http://www.who.int/choice/en/). To do so, WHO-CHOICE reports the costs and effectiveness of an extensive range of health interventions for leading causes of, and risk factors for, disease in 14 epidemiological subregions. The results of these CEAs, as well as underlying methodological developments, are assembled in regional databases, which policy makers can adapt to their specific country setting. By using a common set of analytical tools and standardized methods for collecting and analyzing data on costs and effectiveness, WHO-CHOICE circumvents the problem of synthesizing studies that employ different perspectives and measures.

Generalized CEA, a type of sectoral CEA, forms the basis of the WHO-CHOICE approach.[42] This approach overcomes a number of technical barriers, including data unavailability, methodological inconsistencies across studies, and limited generalizability of studies to different settings, to promote the appropriate use of CEA at the regional and country level. To allow meaningful comparisons across regions, costs are expressed in international dollars; effectiveness is measured in terms of DALYs averted; and cost-effectiveness is described in terms of cost per DALY averted.[42] WHO-CHOICE has been using criteria suggested by the Commission on Macroeconomics and Health[65]: interventions that cost less than the average per capita income of a country per DALY averted are considered very cost effective; interventions that cost less than three times the average per capita income per DALY averted are still considered cost effective; and those that exceed this level are not considered cost effective.

It must be emphasized that the availability of aggregate information at the subregional level does not guarantee that findings will actually impact health policy at the national level. Accordingly, WHO-CHOICE recommends the use of a process of "contextualization," whereby the regional estimates can be tailored to the particular demographic, epidemiological and economic situation facing a given country. Condition-specific templates are now available for a number of diseases and risk factors and have been applied to the national context of a number of developed and developing countries. WHO works closely with policy makers on ways of using evidence from WHO-CHOICE in assessing the appropriate mix of interventions to maximize population health for specific settings, while taking into account both health system goals and the broader social goals.

SUMMARY

Countries around the world have demonstrated the need for transparent decision making on what types of health technologies offer good value and can be justifiably funded with finite public funds. Supporting such decisions entails the challenging task of gathering, synthesizing and scrutinizing evidence using appropriate and explicit methods. Prevention effectiveness methods have provided decision makers with an evidence-based approach in determining which health problems to address first, and which policies and interventions to use, and what returns to expect for a given expenditure of resources. Prevention effectiveness information developed systematically using explicit criteria and appropriate data, serves not only clinicians and public health practitioners but also employers, legislators, and communities, with the capability of playing a critical role in transforming and enhancing a prevention-focused health care system.

REVIEW QUESTIONS

1. To whom does the term *audience* refer in a prevention effectiveness study?
2. What is meant by the perspective of a prevention effectiveness study?
3. Which costs should be included when conducting a study from a societal perspective?
4. What is the difference between a study time frame and its analytic horizon?
5. What distinguishes cost-effectiveness analysis (CEA) from cost-benefit analysis (CBA)?
6. Should a highly effective intervention always be supported?
7. Give one example of a final outcome for a needle-exchange program.
8. You have been asked to conduct cost analysis of a nutrition and health education program for middle school students. Your client expects the results to indicate that the program has a substantially low cost because all

of the materials used are donated and the sessions are conducted by students from a nearby university on a volunteer basis. Do you agree?

9. List challenges or issues under debate when performing prevention effectiveness studies?

10. Why do we conduct sensitivity analyses?

REFERENCES

1. Poisal, JA, Truffer C, Smith S., et al. Health Spending Projections through 2016: Modest Changes Obscure Part D's Impact. Health Affairs—Web Exclusive, February, 21, 2007.

2. National Immunization Program, CDC. ACIP: Advisory Committee on Immunization Practices. Available at: http://www.cdc.gov/vaccines/recs/acip/default.htm. Accessed August 8, 2007.

3. Teusch SM. A framework for assessing the effectiveness of disease and injury prevention. *MMWR.* 1992;41(No. RR-3).

4. Thacker SB, Stroup DF, Carande-Kulis V, Marks JS, Roy K, Gerberding JL. Measuring the public's health. *Public Health Rep.* January-February, 2006;121(1):14–22.

5. McKeown T. The direction of medical research. *Lancet.* 1979;2(8155):1281–1284.

6. National Center for Health Statistics. National Vital Statistics System, annual mortality data file, multiple cause-of-death detail, 2004. Hyattsville, MD: U.S. Department of Health and Human Services, Centers for Disease Control and Prevention (CDC), National Center for Health Statistics. Extracted from WISQARS (Web-Based Injury Statistics Query and Reporting System), Office of Statistics and Programming, National Center for Injury Prevention and Control, CDC. Available at: http://www.cdc.gov/ncipc/wisqars/. Accessed July 2007.

7. McGinnis JM, Foege WH. Actual causes of death in the United States. *JAMA.* 1993;217:2207–12.

8. Mokdad AH, Marks JS, Stroup DF, Gerberding JL. Actual causes of death in the United States, 2000 [published erratum appears in *JAMA.* 2005;293: 293–4] *JAMA.* 2004;291:1238–45.

9. Pauly MV, Nicholson S, Xu J, et al. A general model of the impact of absenteeism on employers and employees. *Health Econ.* 2000;11(3): 221–31.

10. Murray C.J.L. Rethinking DALYs. In: C.J.L. Murray and A.D. Lopez, eds. *The Global Burden of Disease.* Cambridge, MA: Harvard University Press; 1996.

11. Torrance GW, Feeny D. Utilities and quality-adjusted life years. *Int J Technol Assess Health Care.* 1989;5:559–575.

12. McKenna MT, Michaud CM, Murray CJL, Marks JS. Assessing the burden of disease in the United States using disability-adjusted life years. *Am J Prev Med.* 2005;28:415–23.

13. Cooper H, Hedges LV, eds. *The Handbook of Research Synthesis.* New York: Russell Sage Foundation; 1994.

14. Mulrow CD, Oxman AD, eds. *Cochrane collaboration handbook.* In: The Cochrane Library [CD-ROM, updated September 1997]. The Cochrane Collaboration. Oxford, England: Update Software;1997:(4).

15. The Cochrane Collaboration. The Cochrane database of systematic reviews, 2005, [database online]. Available at: http://www.mrw .interscience.wiley.com/cochrane/cochrane_clsysrev_articles_fs.html. Accessed August 8, 2007.

16. Stroup DF, Berlin JA, Morton SC, et al. Meta-analysis of observational studies in epidemiology: A proposal for reporting. *JAMA.* April 19, 2000; 283(15):2008–12.

17. Task Force on Community Preventive Services. Introducing the Guide to Community Preventive Services: Methods, first recommendations, and expert commentary. *Am J Prev Med.* 2000a; 19(1S):1–142.

18. Task Force on Community Preventive Services. Recommendations regarding interventions to improve vaccination coverage in children, adolescents, and adults. *Am J Prev Med.* 2000b;18(1S): 92–96.

19. Task Force on Community Preventive Services. Recommendations regarding interventions to reduce tobacco use and exposure to environmental tobacco smoke. *Am J Prev Med.* 2001;20(2S): 10–15.

20. Thacker SB, Ikeda RM, Gieseker KE, et al. The evidence base for public health informing policy at the Centers for Disease Control and Prevention. *Am J Prev Med.* October 2005;29(3):227–33.

21. U.S. Preventive Services Task Force. Guide to Clinical Preventive Services, 2nd ed. Washington, DC: U.S. Department of Health and Human Services; 1996.

22. Zaza S, Briss PA, Harris KW, eds. Task Force on Community Preventive Services. The guide to community preventive services: What works to promote health? New York: Oxford University Press; 2005.

23. Gold MR, Siegel JE, Russell LB, Weinstein MC. *Cost-Effectiveness in Health and Medicine.* New York: Oxford University Press; 1996.

24. Drummond MF, Stoddart GL, Torrance GW. *Methods for the Economic Evaluation of Health Care Programmes.* Oxford, UK: Oxford University Press, 1987.

25. Haddix AC, Teutsch SM, Corso PS, eds. *Prevention Effectiveness: A Guide to Decision Analysis and Economic Evaluation*, 2nd ed. Oxford University Press; 2003.

26. Corso PS, Thacker SB, Koplan JP. The value of prevention: Experiences of a public health agency. *Med Decis Making.* September-October, 2002;22(5 Suppl):S11–6.

27. Vora S, Damon I, Fulginiti V, et al. Severe eczema vaccinatum in a household contact of a smallpox vaccinee. *Clin Infect Dis.* May 15, 2008;46(10): 1555–61.

28. Elbasha EH, Dasbach EJ, Insinga RE. Model for assessing human papillomavirus vaccination strategies. *Emerg Infect Dis.* 2007;13:28–41.

29. Markowitz LE, Dunne EF, Saraiya M, Lawson HW, Chesson H, Unger ER. Quadrivalent Human Papillomavirus Vaccine: Recommendations of the Advisory Committee on Immunization Practices (ACIP). *MMWR Recomm Rep.* March 23, 2007;56(RR-2):1–24.

30. Reinberg, S. Cervical Cancer Vaccine Continues to Spark Debate. *Washington Post*, March 29, 2007, http://www.washingtonpost.com/wp-dyn/content/article/2007/03/29/AR2007032900751.html. Accessed June 7, 2008.

31. Grosse SD, Teutsch SM, Haddix AC. Lessons from cost-effectiveness research for United States public health policy. *Annu. Rev. Public Health.* 2007; 28:19–31

32. Banta DH, Wit GA. Public health services and cost-effectiveness analysis. *Annu. Rev. Public Health.* 2008;29:383–397.

33. Drummond M, Manca A, Sculpher M. Increasing the generalizability of economic evaluations: Recommendations for the design, analysis, and reporting of studies. *Int. J. Technol. Assess. Health Care.* 2000;16:165–71

34. Edejer T, Baltussen R, Adam T, et al. *WHO Guide to Cost-Effectiveness Analysis.* Geneva: WHO; 2003.

35. Drummond M, Pang F. Transferability of economic evaluation results. In: Drummond M, McGuire A, eds. *Economic Evaluation in Health Care: Merging Theory with Practice.* Oxford, UK: Oxford University Press; 2001: 256–76.

36. Sonnad S, Greenberg D, Rosen A, Neumann P. Diffusion of published cost-utility analyses in the field of health policy and practice. *Int. J. Technol. Assess. Health Care.* 2005;21:399–402.

37. Neumann PJ, Greenberg D, Olchanski NV, Stone PW, Rosen AB. Growth and quality of the cost-utility literature, 1976–2001. *Value Health.* 2005; 8:3–9.

38. Grosse SD. Assessing cost-effectiveness in healthcare: History of the $50,000 per QALY threshold. *Expert Review of Pharmacoeconomics & Outcomes Research.* 2008;8(2):165–178.

39. Bos JM, Postma MJ, Annemans L. Discounting health effects in pharmacoeconomic evaluations: Current controversies. *Pharmacoeconomics.* 2005; 23(7):639–4.

40. Gravelle H, Brouwer W, Niessen L, Postma M, Rutten F. Discounting in economic evaluations: Stepping forward towards optimal decision rules. *Health Econ.* March 2007;16(3):307–17.

41. Gravelle H, Smith D. Discounting for health effects in cost-benefit and cost-effectiveness analysis. *Health Econ.* October 2001;10(7):587–99.

42. Smith DH, Gravelle H. The practice of discounting in economic evaluations of healthcare interventions. *Int J Technol Assess Health Care.* Spring 2001;17(2):236–43.

43. Weinstein MC, Stason WB. Foundations of cost-effectiveness analysis for health and medical practices. *New England Journal of Medicine.* 1977; 296:716–21.

44. Russell LB. Is Prevention better than cure? Washington, DC: Brookings Institution; 1986.

45. Meltzer D. Accounting for future costs in medical cost-effectiveness analysis. *J Health Econ.* 1997; 16(1):33–64.

46. Meltzer D. Future costs in medical cost-effectiveness analysis. In: Jones AM, ed. *The Elgar Companion to Health Economics.* Cheltenham, UK: Elgar; 2006: 447–54.

47. Commonwealth of Australia. Guidelines for the pharmaceutical industry on preparations of submissions to the Pharmaceutical Benefits Advisory Committee, including major submissions involving economic analyses. Canberra: Australian Government Publishing Service; 1995.

48. Ministry of Health. Ontario guidelines for economic analysis of pharmaceutical products. Ontario: Ministry of Health; 1994.

49. Elsinga E, Rutten FF. Economic evaluation in support of national health policy: The case of Netherlands. *Soc Sci Med*. 1997;45:605–620.

50. LePen C. Pharmaceutical economics and the economic assessment of drugs in France. *Soc Sci Med*. 1997;45:635–643.

51. National Institute for Clinical Excellence. Appraisal of new and existing technologies: Interim guidance for manufacturers and sponsors. London: NICE; 1999. Available at: http://www.nice.org.uk/guidance/index.jsp. Accessed March 31, 2008.

52. Rawlins MD. NICE Work—Providing Guidance to the British National Health Service. *N Engl J Med*. 2004;351(14):1383–1385.

53. Raftery J. Reviw of NICE's recommendations, 1999–2005. *BMJ*. 2006;332:1266–1268.

54. Editorial. NICE's cost-effectiveness threshold: How high should it be? *BMJ* 2007;335:358–359.

55. Devlin N, Parkin D. Does NICE have a cost effectiveness threshold and what other factors influence its decisions? A binary choice analysis. *Health Econ*. 2004;13:437–52.

56. House of Commons Health Select Committee. Uncorrected transcript of oral evidence 28 June 2007: Q178. (To be published as: HC503 ii.). Available at: http://www.publications.parliament.uk/pa/cm200607/cmselect/cmhealth/uc503-ii/uc50302.htm.

57. Devlin N, Parkin D, Appleby J. Written evidence for the House of Commons Select Committee inquiry on NICE. 2007. Available at: http://www.publications.parliament.uk/pa/cm200708/cmselect/cmhealth/27/2707.htm.

58. Culyer A, McCabe C, Briggs A, et al. Searching for a threshold, not setting one: The role of the National Institute for Health and Clinical Excellence. *J Health Serv Res Policy*. 2007;12,56–58.

59. Hill S, Garattani S, Loenhout JV, O'Brien B, Joncheere KD. *Technology Appraisal Programme of the National Institute of Clinical Excellence: A Review by WHO*. Copenhagen: World Health Organization; 2003.

60. Maciosek MV, Coffield AB, Edwards NM, Flottemesch TJ, Goodman MJ, Solberg LI. Priorities among effective clinical preventive services: Results of a systematic review and analysis. *Am. J. Prev. Med.* 2006;31:52–61.

61. Maciosek MV, Coffield AB, McGinnis JM, et al. Methods for priority setting among clinical preventive services. *Am. J. Prev. Med.* 2001;21:10–19.

62. Hutubessy R, Chisholm D, Edejer TT. WHO-CHOICE. Generalized cost-effectiveness analysis for national level priority-setting in the health sector. *Cost Eff Resour Alloc.* 2003,19;1(1):8,1–13.

63. Jamison DT, Mosley WH, Measham AR, Bobadilla JL. *Disease Control Priorities in Developing Countries*. New York: Oxford University Press; 1993.

64. World Bank. World development report 1993: Investing in health. New York: Oxford University Press; 1993.

65. Commission on Macroeconomics and Health. *Macroeconomics and Health: Investing in Health for Economic Development*. Geneva: WHO; 2001.

CHAPTER 14

Behavioral Community Health Needs Assessment

John Elder, PhD, MPH, Paula M. Usita, PhD, and Noé Crespo, MPH, MS

LEARNING OBJECTIVES[1]

Upon completion of this chapter, the reader will be able to:

1. Describe how to define community health needs and assets.

2. Determine the extent to which human behavior contributes to these needs and assets.

3. List key organizations and individuals you would work with to address health needs in a given area.

4. Briefly describe various health behavior change theories and models, and how they contribute to the "social ecological" framework.

5. Outline a step-by-step approach to changing behavior on a public health scale within the social ecological framework through health communication and social marketing, policy development and enforcement, and skills training.

6. Describe inexpensive and "user-friendly" approaches to monitoring and evaluating the behavior change effort.

7. Apply these skills to a variety of behavior-related health problems.

KEY TERMS

Community

Ecological Models

Formative Research

Key Informants

Models

ONPRIME Model

Outcome Evaluation

Process Evaluation

Self-Efficacy

Social Marketing

Theories

ACKNOWLEDGEMENTS: The authors would especially like to thank Elizabeth ("Katie") Guth Bothwell for her invaluable assistance in editing this chapter.

[1]These core competencies and skills correspond to a variety of sections of the following text. Footnotes are used to designate the parallel components of the ONPRIME model (see Figure 14.1).

THEORIES AND MODELS IN PUBLIC HEALTH BEHAVIOR CHANGE

Current public health promotion and behavior change practices are rooted in diverse **theories** and models. Theories comprise principles devised to explain a group of facts or phenomena, especially a theory that has been repeatedly tested or is widely accepted and can be used to make predictions about social and physical events. Thus, health behavior theories are meant to provide broader understanding of that behavior and its links to the general human condition. Common theories in health promotion derive from the fields of communication, psychology, economics, and more broadly, philosophy. Prominent communication theories guiding this research include McGuire's Communication-Persuasion Model (1989), the Transtheoretical Model (Prochaska & DiClemente, 1983; DiClemente & Prochaska, 1998), and the Elaboration Likelihood Model (Tversky & Kahneman, 1974). Behavior change theories provide strategies for tailoring interventions to individual participants. For example, principles in Behavioral Analysis (Skinner, 1953; Holland & Skinner, 1961; Baer et al., 1968; Miller, 1980) such as goal setting, self-monitoring, and self-reinforcement (Kanfer, 1975) suggest ways of structuring interactive intervention pieces tailored to the individual. The Theory of Reasoned Action (Ajzen & Fishbein, 1980) and Social Learning/Cognitive Theory represent two other commonly referenced psychologically based concepts. Social Cognitive Theory emphasizes the use of observational learning/modeling, as well as targeting a reduction in barriers and enhancing **self-efficacy** (confidence that one can do the behavior) (Bandura, 1986; 1989). Broader theories such as Rogers' Diffusion of Innovations (1983) link communication and behavior change precepts in describing **community** (a group of people defined by one or more common characteristic) and cultural change. Interventions grounded in

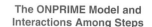

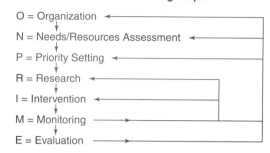

Figure 14.1. The ONPRIME Model (Elder et al., 1994)

theoretical frameworks provide the scientific community with additional evidence on the usefulness of these theories and allow for their refinement.

Models in contrast to theories generally comprise representations of physical structures or processes and the interactions among these structures and processes, meant more to describe and logically link phenomena together than to imply broader meanings underlying these phenomena. The best-known model used in health promotion is Lawrence Green's PRECEDE/PROCEED model (Green & Kreuter, 1999), based in turn on the Health Belief Model (Janz and Becker, 1984). Russell Glasgow's (2002) REAIM (http://www.re-aim.org) also comprises a convenient framework for planning and evaluation. The present article refers specifically to Elder and colleagues' (1994) **ONPRIME model,** which links planning, intervention, and evaluation steps and their specific elements into one staged, recursive process. Based upon the standard approach to community health behavior change (planning, intervention, and evaluation, or "PIE"[2]), the ONPRIME model emphasizes the importance of seven process substeps: *O*rganization, *N*eeds/Resources Assessment, *P*riority Setting, *R*esearch, *I*nterventions, *M*onitoring, and *E*valuation (see Figure 14.1).

Organization refers to whether the program entails working within existing organizations, working through various community gatekeepers

[2]All relevant to Basic Public Health Sciences skills.

or out of the program planner's health office, or sometimes, through grassroots community organizing to develop a sponsoring structure where no apparent candidate exists.[3]

The second element of ONPRIME is *needs and resources assessment*. This phase may include key informant interviews, archival research, race under treatment and surveys, with a special examination of the existing health and related environmental, economic, and social problems of the community.[4] In terms of needs and resources assessment, the community advisors can also point the program planner to types of activities that have been conducted in the past and how the community resources have been, or could be, used to address the existing health problem. Thus, the successful health program looks at the community as one that has many strengths, abilities, and potential resources that can be employed to address a given problem, not as a community that needs outside help.

After data are collected, health officials, community advisory boards, or representative individuals within the community can then examine the health information to help establish health- and disease-related priorities. Generally speaking, communities that have been successful in selecting their own intervention or targeted health *priorities* will be more likely to embrace a program over a longer period of time than those that do not.[5]

Research, in this sense, refers not to epidemiological or survey research to identify health problems (as in the needs/resources assessment phase) but instead to the formative and other qualitative/quantitative research needed to develop health behavior change, intervention concepts, and direct applications. Thus, the qualitative and quantitative research is conducted specifically to develop new techniques or refine old ones. Focus groups and in-depth or brief intercept interviews are the most common examples of qualitative research formats

that can assist the program developer in determining the target audience's perception of a health issue, whether and how they feel something could be done about this issue, and what types of target audiences and target audience segments might exist in the community. Planners can identify individuals (or families, organizations, etc.) who have adopted a practice and compare and contrast them with those who have not. Again, focus group and other types of research with these individuals may be effective in revealing what has influenced some individuals to improve their health or has presented barriers so that others have not. Through such research, program planners can go a long way toward selecting and building on existing practices rather than developing others that might be considered somewhat alien to the target population.

After the aforementioned phases are completed, the planner develops a set of *intervention* activities that address the health issues through the most effective techniques available. Individual level behavior change, skill building, and tailored communication, as well as mass communication, policy change, and changes in the physical environment, can affect the behavior on the small or large scale, respectively. These intervention components derive from the diverse elements of **ecological models,** described in the next section.

Monitoring is the penultimate step in the ONPRIME sequence and a critical element of the planning-implementation-evaluation sequence. Monitoring comprises both the monitoring of the implementation process (e.g., did television spots get aired when they were supposed to?) as well as responses to the intervention (e.g., after a grocery store promotion was undertaken, what sales changes if any were there?). Through regular collection of data sensitive to individual or community response to a program, the implementation team has an excellent feedback tool for themselves and the community. Thus, individuals who may or may not be attuned to statistical analyses and p-values may increase their awareness of how different trends of time series data presented in a graphic format can represent their progress toward an existing health or behavior change criterion. These monitoring data

---

[3]Leadership Skills are essential here, as they are in the Priority Setting stage.
[4]Parallel to the Community Dimensions of Practice Skills.
[5]Communication Skills are essential for the practitioner to develop these priorities in partnership with the community.

may then be used to reinforce individual or community progress or to provide the implementation team with the information needed to alter existing programs to achieve an improved approach.[6]

Finally, *evaluation* is used to determine whether a program was effective or which of its elements were most effective. Evaluation information may be used to determine whether to extend a program and promote its generalization to other communities, or, conversely, whether to terminate the effort.[7]

ECOLOGICAL MODELS OF HEALTH BEHAVIOR[8]

Intervention strategies and other elements of the ONPRIME model are based on the convergence of ecological models of change and validated theories in the fields of community-level health behavior change. The ecological models provide a framework for targeting system and structural changes within the environment, and make it possible to tease out or assess how various levels affect individual and community change. Health communication and behavior change theories will guide the development of micro-environmental interventions.

Ecological Models

Research in socioecology recognizes that individual behavior is often a function of an individual's larger social context (Emmons, 2000). A person's desire to modify his or her own behavior may be impeded by economic, social, and cultural constraints (Stokols, 1996). To engage in health promotion, the social ecological approach involves combining individually focused efforts at change with modifications of the physical and social surroundings.

Emmons (2000) and Cohen, Scribner, and Farley (2000) are among those who have defined the ecological approach. Emmons identified five

levels for intervention development, as well as corresponding targets of change. At the intrapersonal level, the target for change is the individual's behavior through skill development and increasing motivation to change. Improving social support for positive behaviors and targeting social norms occurs at the interpersonal level. Interventions designed in context of school and other organizational environments are examples of organizational-level change. Community- and policy-level change is reflected in attempts to build coalitions and empower the community through social advocacy and subsequent changes in broader social and physical environments (Elder et al., 2006).

Cohen and her colleagues (2000) advocate a similar "structural model" of health behavior change. Four specific factors specified within this model are "availability," "physical structures," "social structures," and "cultural and media messages." *Availability* refers to the accessibility of health-related consumer products (e.g., healthy yet inexpensive foods in local stores). *Physical structures* are those aspects of products or environments that make health-related behavior more or less likely to occur (e.g., bike lanes and clearly designated pedestrian crossings, well-lit and graffiti-free playgrounds, child safety bars over windows). *Social structures* refer both to laws and policies that require or restrict health behaviors and their respective enforcement (e.g., clean indoor air acts and DUI enforcement). Informal social control mechanisms (e.g., parental rule setting about vegetable, soft drink, and dessert consumption) are central to this category as well. Finally, *cultural and media messages* are the messages individuals are exposed to daily that inform them about specific health behaviors and denote social norms underpinning these behaviors. Through its incarnation as "media advocacy" (Wallack & Dorfman, 1996), communication has increasingly been brought to bear on mobilizing public support for policy change, again showing how changes in one structure can result in changes in another (Elder et al., 2006).

Most health promotion theories currently employed by researchers and practitioners address the interconnected nature of individuals within their

---

[6]Relevant to Policy Development/Program Planning Skills.
[7]Also relevant to Policy Development/Program Planning Skills.
[8]See also "Basic Public Health Science Skills."

environments. In addition, the ecological approach holds that any health promotion effort must target behavior change at multiple levels to create a health-promoting climate in the social environment in which people make health-related decisions.

The bulk of this chapter examines existing community health programs within the ONPRIME framework, with special attention on pediatric obesity reduction (Project LEAN [Leaders Encouraging Activity and Nutrition] and the VERB campaign) and arthritis symptom control among seniors (the Arthritis Self Help [ASH] and Arthritis Self Management [ASM] programs). This examination exercise is recommended for health providers and professionals so that they become proficient, sensitive, and dexterous to specific applications of the core concepts described earlier. Although not planned with specific reference to this model, these programs represent the importance of addressing its various components. Thus, those elements that correspond to specific ONPRIME steps are high-

lighted parenthetically with reference to the specific step(s) being addressed.

PEDIATRIC OVERWEIGHT AND OBESITY

The incidence of overweight and obesity has continued to increase in all regions and segments of the United States population. New data from the National Health and Nutrition Examination Survey 2003–2004 (National Center for Health Statistics [NCHS], 2006a) show that around 66 percent of United States adults are either overweight or obese. Even more alarming are the increased rates in the pediatric population, which indicate that 17 percent of children ages 2–19 are overweight, a number up from 11 percent in 1988 (NCHS, 2006b) (see Figure 14.2). As a result, obesity-related

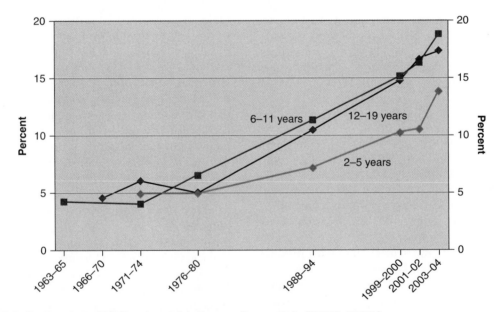

Figure 14.2. Trends in Childhood and Adolescent Overweight (NCHS, 2006b)

SOURCE: National Center for Health Statistics. Health, United States, 2000. Hyattsville, Maryland: Public Health Service. 2004.

NOTE: Overweight is defined as BMI ≥ gender- and weight-specific 95th percentile from the 2000 CDC Growth Charts.

co-morbidities such as type 2 diabetes, hypertension, fatty liver disease, and other diseases are also emerging early in life.

Current information supports the notion that most childhood overweight and obesity is due to unhealthy behaviors and lifestyle choices that are highly shaped and influenced by the environment (Sallis et al., 2000; Sherwood & Jeffery, 2000; Gordon-Larsen et al., 2000). More specifically, poor nutrition (Young & Nestley, 2002), low physical activity (Goran et al., 1999), and increased sedentary behaviors (Crespo et al., 2001) have been identified as the main contributors to these emerging trends in American youth. However the "simple" messages of eating less and moving more have not translated to behavior change. Because apparently simple messages targeting individual change have not resulted in significant changes in these trends, public health efforts are now using intervention models that incorporate various aspects of the human experience such as family, peer groups, schools, community organization, and local and national government. Many strategies have been employed to intervene and reduce pediatric obesity, but results have been mixed (Collins et al., 2006; Flynn et al., 2006; Sharma, 2006). Successful programs have used strategies that target specific and modifiable characteristics at various levels of influence as well as promoting individual and community empowerment to affect change (McKenzie et al., 2003; Nader et al., 1999). This section focuses on two programs that have established a commitment to keeping our children healthy and emphasizes the use of the various steps of the ONPRIME model where appropriate.

Project LEAN

California's Project LEAN (Leaders Encouraging Activity and Nutrition) initially began as one of 10 nationwide programs aimed at promoting low-fat eating (an effort funded by the Henry J. Kaiser Family Foundation in 1987) and has recently extended its mission to increase physical activity and improve bone health. Its activities incorporate the use of nutrition and physical activity programs to promote better nutrition and increased physical activity. Local health departments and community-based organizations are the vehicles for dissemination and implementation of these programs (10 regional offices in California). Project LEAN has uniquely affected health policy in school districts and state legislation and received national recognition through its partnerships with the California Obesity Prevention Initiative and the California Nutrition Network. As a driving force in the fight against pediatric obesity, its programs emphasize the need to create an environment conducive and supportive of positive behavior change.

In its primary stages, LEAN first established objectives based on a *needs assessment* (O*NPRIME*) from available research data, which revealed specific nutritional aspects that would yield favorable health benefits if altered. The data highlighted the role of added sugars, high-fat snacks, and low nutrient rich foods in pediatric obesity. For example, children who eat higher amounts of sugar and sugar-sweetened beverages show signs of poorer heath (Ludwig et al., 2001; Giammattei et al., 2003) and increased risk of diabetes (Schulze et al., 2004; Davis et al., 2005). Similarly, children who consume foods high in saturated fat also show early signs of co-morbid conditions related to obesity such as high blood pressure, hypercholesterolemia, and fatty liver disease (Barton et al., 2006; Marion et al., 2004). Given this evidence, it makes sense to target these food items as a mechanism of intervention.

In 2004, the Successful Students Through Healthy Food Policies (SSTHF) project received recognition for its success in achieving a ban on the sale of sodas and unhealthy snacks in the Los Angeles Unified School district. As such, an *organized* (O*N*PRIME) effort by students, parents, health advocates, teachers, and various community groups took their concerns to the school board and advocated for the removal of sodas and unhealthy snacks in public schools. This effort established specific nutrition-related *priorities* (ONP*R*IME) that would have the most effect on the health behaviors of students (i.e., the removal of sodas and unhealthy snacks). The ban not only addresses the need to educate children and their families about good nutrition but also emphasizes the key roles that the school environment and community officials play in shaping the food choices available to children while they are in school; a position based on previous **formative research** (ONPRIME). Formative research is the first step taken to identify and define the key problems that affect the target population. This step is critical to achieving a comprehensive understanding of the target population and to provide data that informs the development of an intervention or program.

Results of the SSTHF project showed that water and juice sales increased while overall beverage sales declined, salad bars were added where feasible, nutrient and portion size standards were noted for à la carte food items, and at least one vegetarian option was made available. The ban of sodas and unhealthy snacks provides an environment to students that both promotes and nurtures healthier eating. As a social ecological approach (Emmons, 2000; Stokols, 1996; Cohen et al., 2000) to childhood obesity, the SSTHF project implemented *intervention* (ONPRIME) strategies that used organizational-, community-, and policy-level change to address and ensure the availability of healthier food options for children. In the near future, physical education in schools will also be addressed through the establishment of new instructional guidelines for all grade levels as well as the inclusion of fitness centers and pools in new high schools.

Between the years 1998 and 2000, Project LEAN also implemented the Food on the Run (FOR) program through **social marketing.** Social marketing is distinguished from marketing in that the main objective of social marketing is to achieve behavior change for a social good rather than financial gain. FOR used social marketing to strengthen the knowledge and skills of individuals to improve eating and physical activity behaviors and to influence policy change via media advocacy by teens. This approach targeted low-income teens

classified as "early adopters" based on the Diffusion of Innovations theory (Rogers, 1983) to use their leadership capabilities to influence change.

The success of the FOR program can be attributed largely to their initial efforts during their formative *research* phase (ONPRIME). As part of their formative research, FOR used data gathered from various focus groups, commercial marketing, and literature reviews, in addition to the use of **key informants** (individuals that are part of the group of interest) and one-on-one teen interviews. These data helped shape and guide the program objectives and establish the *needs* (ONPRIME) of the target community. Specifically, limited access to healthy foods was identified as one of the major barriers to accomplishing the desired behavioral changes with respect to improving healthy eating habits, and thus became a *priority* (ONPRIME) (Flora & Myrhe, 1998). Consequently, FOR adopted a campaign or *intervention* (ONPRIME) to mobilize teens to advocate for increased accessibility of fruits and vegetables and lower availability of sugary snacks and beverages in their schools.

Teens were first trained and informed about nutrition, physical activity, media advocacy, and policy to provide them with the necessary expertise to be knowledgeable and effective advocates. The California High School Fast Food Survey was released in 2000 as a result of their efforts (Samuels & Associates, 2000). This survey was the first comprehensive survey in California to provide detailed and extensive data on the types of fast foods sold on high school campuses, the factors influencing fast food sales, and the related economic and policy issues surrounding the sale of these foods. This survey provided the data needed to establish an argument toward the role of specific public policies that impede the adoption of healthier practices by adolescents. The survey received state and national recognition and media attention that served as an important tool to disseminate information about the problem and recommendations for future action. *Evaluation* (ONPRIME) data collected after the initial campaign showed that teens improved their nutrition attitudes as well as their related behaviors and knowledge levels (Agron et al., 2002). Similarly, there was increased availability of healthier food and physical activity options in FOR schools (Takada, 2002). Subsequently, advocacy workbooks and a teen website http://www .californiaprojectlean.org were created to promote and reinforce teen advocacy and to *monitor* (ONPRI*ME*) program implementation and effectiveness.

"VERB: It's What You Do."

The VERB campaign, supported and coordinated by the United States Department of Health and Human Services (Dept. of HHS) and the Centers for Diseases Control and Prevention (CDC), is a national social marketing campaign aimed at encouraging daily physically activity in children ages 9–13 (also referred to as "tweens"). VERB uses various aspects of social marketing methods to reach both children and those adults who influence their behavior. The emphasis on daily physical activity is based on the consensus recommendations for at least 30 minutes of moderate intensity physical activity on 5 or more days of the week by the CDC and the American College of Sports Medicine (CDC, 2006 March) (ONPRIME).

The goals of VERB were to 1) increase knowledge and improve attitudes and beliefs about tweens' regular participation in physical activity, 2) increase parental and influencer support and encouragement of tweens' participation in physical activity, 3) heighten awareness of options and opportunities for tween participation in physical activity, 4) facilitate opportunities for tweens to participate in regular physical activity, and 5) increase and maintain the number of tweens who regularly participate in physical activity. To develop and evaluate these goals, VERB planners used a Logic Model for behavior change. In short, the Logic Model uses sequential steps to bring about behavior change. The basic structure of steps is composed of 1) *inputs* (contractors, community infrastructure, and partnerships), 2) *activities* (advertising, promotions, public relations, and national and community outreach), 3) *short-term outcomes* (message delivery and awareness; change in subjective norms, beliefs, self-efficacy, perceived behavioral control, knowledge, and expectations), and 4) *long-term outcomes* (engaging in the desired behavior, maintaining desired behavior, and risk reduction of chronic disease). The "logical" basis therefore was to create a positive "buzz" among the target population (tweens) regarding physical activity and to establish new norms and patterns of physical activity behaviors that meet the health recommendations.

VERB based its campaign on extensive formative research that includes reviews of existing and new research, target audience research, expert consultants, *needs assessments* (O*N*PRIME), and review of other existing campaigns. Formative research also encompassed exploratory research, concept testing, and message testing. These combined efforts have led to the implementation of a media campaign *intervention* (ONPRI*ME*) that is appropriate in content, tone, and execution for the target audience. As a result, VERB has created a media outreach program partnership (O*N*PRIME) with media companies such as ABC Disney, AOL Time Warner, Viacom, Primedia, and other population-specific advertising and marketing entities such as PFI Marketing, G&G Advertising, Telemundo, Univision, *Korean Times, Essence Magazine,* Heart and Soul, Indian Country Today, and American Indian Report. The campaign has used these various communication outlets to disseminate targeted messages such as increase walking (i.e., walking to school or waking the dog), take the stairs instead of the elevator, reduce TV and computer use (to reduce sedentary behaviors), and engage in enjoyable physical activities (dancing, skateboarding, bicycling, and playing outside). The ultimate message of VERB was to encourage tweens to maintain or increase physical activity irrespective of the type of activity. This message was found to be both relevant to the target audience and to have the highest likelihood of success based on data from formative research.

Another important aspect of the VERB campaign was **process evaluation** (ONPRI*ME*). Process evaluation is the assessment of the immediate impact of the program, program implementation, and quality control procedures. The goal of process evaluation is to ascertain whether various aspects of the physical activity campaign were being implemented as planned and whether objectives were being meet. VERB's process evaluation measures reach (how many individuals are being reached), frequency (how often are the messages being delivered), and reactions (qualitative information of attitudes and beliefs concerning the message) provided data that were used to identify problems and weaknesses in the campaign. For example, the continuous tracking survey, a quarterly telephone survey of 300 children aged 9–13, provided data on exposure to the VERB brand, interpretation of the VERB brand and messages, likeability of the message and brand, and product placement. Other process evaluation methods included analysis of campaign advertising, on-site evaluation of VERB-sponsored events, follow-up interviews, interviews with campaign stakeholders, and web tracking.

To determine the impact of the VERB campaign, **outcome evaluation** (ONPRIM*E*) focused on assessing changes in tweens' awareness, knowledge, attitudes, and behaviors with respect to physical activity and how these changes were related to campaign exposures (compared to baseline). The Youth Media Campaign Longitudinal Survey (YMCLS) has been a useful tool in gathering both child and parental outcome data that focused on children's physical activity participation and related attitudes as well as various characteristics of their physical activity behaviors (i.e., type of activity, duration, frequency, and structure). The parental component of the survey ascertained information about perceived strength of parental influence on their child's physical activity level, parental attitudes about their child's physical activity, and basic demographics.

Year 1 results of the VERB campaign indicated that 74 percent of the children surveyed were aware of the VERB campaign. More importantly, data revealed an increase in self-reported levels of free-time physical activity in children aged 9–13, especially among those who were exposed to the VERB campaign. Therefore, as a child's level of awareness of VERB increased, so did their engagement in free-time physical activity sessions (Huhman et al., 2005).

Conclusions

Both Project LEAN and the VERB campaign were effective in promoting and improving the health behaviors of our nation's children. Project LEAN's legislative and political success in improving the environmental availability of healthier food options in public schools has established a model for other programs to follow. The success of LEAN highlights the power of community involvement in affecting change. The VERB campaign has shown that the use of strong media campaign methods also has the potential to change health behavior and increase the physical activity of young children at a national level. As more data are being gathered, we are beginning to build support for further implementation of such community programs. The continuation of LEAN and VERB will increase the likelihood that we may observe a tapering of current trends of childhood obesity in our nation.

CONTROLLING ARTHRITIS

Arthritis is a chronic debilitating disease associated with aging. Efforts designed to improve the quality of life for elderly citizens, including controlling arthritis, is an important health goal.

Population Aging

Population aging in the United States is underway. In 2004, there were 36.3 million older adults, slightly more than 12 percent of the total population. By 2020, there will be 54.6 million older adults, and by 2030, 71.5 million (almost twice the number in 2004). By 2030, people 65 and over will represent 20 percent of the population. The population aged 85 and over is expected to grow

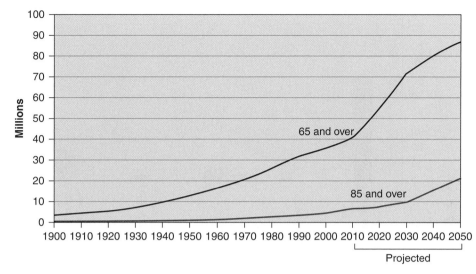

Figure 14.3. Number of People Age 65 and Over (Federal Interagency Forum on Aging-Related Statistics, 2004)

SOURCE: Federal Interagency Forum on Aging-Related Statistics. Older Americans 2004: Key Indicators of Well-Being. Federal Interagency Forum on Aging-Related Statistics, Washington, DC: U.S. Government Printing Office. November 2004.

Reference population: These data refer to the resident population.

NOTE: Data for 2010–2050 of projections of the population.

from 4.2 million in 2000 to 21 million in 2050 (see Figure 14.3).

Racial and ethnic composition of the older population will also change. Whereas non-Hispanic whites represented 83 percent of the older population in 2000, they will represent only 61 percent by 2050. Projections indicate that the aging population will become increasingly diverse by 2050, as the older adult population will be 18 percent Hispanic, 12 percent Black, 8 percent Asian, and 3 percent all other races combined (see Figure 14.4). Projected population growth changes for older Hispanics and Asians are worth noting. While there were 2 million older Hispanics in 2003, there will be 15 million by 2050; among Asians, whereas nearly 1 million were older adults in 2003, 7 million will be by 2050 (Federal Interagency Forum on Aging-Related Statistics, 2004). It is imperative that public health professionals and communities prepare for a growing and aging ethnically diverse society.

Arthritis and Other Chronic Diseases

Chronic diseases are conditions with prolonged illness trajectories, and most are incurable. Although they do not present an immediate threat to life, chronic health conditions impair the health, wealth, and quality of life of individuals, families, communities, and the nation. Common and costly chronic health conditions are heart disease, hypertension, stroke, cancer, diabetes, arthritic symptoms, and respiratory diseases. About 80 percent of older adults have at least one chronic health condition, and 50 percent have at least two (National Center for Chronic Disease Prevention & Health Promotion, 1999). In 2003–2004, an alarming number of older Americans reported having arthritis (55% of women, 43% men) and hypertension (55% of women, 48% of men) (see Figure 14.5) (Federal Interagency Forum on Aging-Related

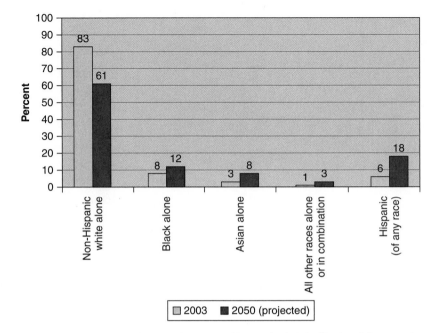

Figure 14.4. Population Age 65 and Over by Race and Hispanic Origin (Federal Interagency Forum on Aging-Related Statistics, 2004)

SOURCE: Federal Interagency Forum on Aging-Related Statistics. Older Americans 2004: Key Indicators of Well-Being. Federal Interagency Forum on Aging-Related Statistics, Washington, DC: U.S. Government Printing Office. November 2004.

Reference population: These data refer to the resident population.

NOTE: The term "non-Hispanic white alone" is used to refer to people who reported being white and no other race and who are not Hispanic. The term "black alone" is used to refer to people who reported being black or African American and not other race, and the term "Asian alone" is used to refer to people who reported only Asian as their race. The use of single-race populations in this report does not imply that this is the preferred method of presenting or analyzing data. The U.S. Census Bureau uses a variety of approaches. The race groups "All other races alone or in combination" includes American Indian and Alaska Native, alone; Native Hawaiian and other Pacific Islander, alone; and all people who reported two or more races.

Statistics, 2006). Interestingly, the percentage of older Americans who reported having arthritis in 2003–2004 was noticeably larger than in 2001–2002 when 39 percent of women and 31 percent of men reported having the condition.

Hence, arthritis specifically comprises a major public health *need* (O*NPRIME*) requiring effective interventions at all levels (Center for the Advancement of Health, 2006).

Arthritis is a term used for a variety of conditions that affect the musculoskeletal system. Problems in the musculoskeletal system occur at the joints, or the meeting place of two or more bones (Arthritis Foundation, 2006). Common symptoms of arthritis include pain, aching, stiffness, and inflammation (Arthritis Foundation, 2006). Some people who have arthritis have difficulty with daily tasks such as walking, climbing stairs, dressing, and

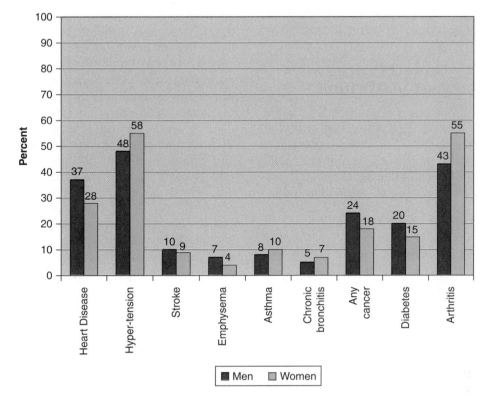

Figure 14.5. Chronic Health Conditions among People 65 and Over (Federal Interagency Forum on Aging-Related Statistics, 2006)

SOURCE: Federal Interagency Forum on Aging-Related Statistics. Older Americans 2004: Key Indicators of Well-Being. Federal Interagency Forum on Aging-Related Statistics, Washington, DC: U.S. Government Printing Office. November 2004.

Reference population: These data refer to the civilian noninstitutionalized population.

NOTE: Data are based on a 2-year average from 2003–2004. The question used to estimate the percentage of people who report having arthritis is "Have you EVER been told by a doctor or other health professional that you have some form of arthritis, rheumatoid arthritis, gout, lupus, or fibromyalgia?" This differs from the questions that were asked to estimate the percentage of people who report having "arthritic symptoms" in *Older Americans 2004*.

brushing teeth. They may also experience psychological problems such as coping with pain and disability, reduction in social well being due to diminished ability to participate in organized groups and school, and financial strain because of the arthritis-related medical costs (Arthritis Foundation, 2006; Center for the Advancement of Health, 2006). Arthritis includes conditions such as osteoarthritis (degenerative joint disease), rheumatoid arthritis

(chronic inflammation of joint lining), gout (condition affecting small joints), juvenile arthritis, and fibromyalgia (pain syndrome involving muscle and muscle attachment areas) (Arthritis Foundation, 1999).

In 1997, nearly 43 million people, or 15 percent of the population, were affected by arthritis, a level that will increase to 60 million by 2020. The CDC estimates that the rate of arthritis will double among adults 65 years and older within the next 25 years (Centers for Disease Control, 2003) (O*NP*RIME).

Community-Based Programs for Persons with Arthritis

Proven strategies for improving older adult health include healthy lifestyles and self-management of chronic disease. Two behavior change programs that are designed to improve the health and well-being of arthritic community members are described next. The sequence of events that led to each program's development was distinct, but both illustrate the value of the ONPRIME model.

Arthritis Self-Help Course

In 1973, Congress passed the National Arthritis Act (PL 93-640). The major objective of the program was to demonstrate, stimulate, and replicate application of available knowledge for the treatment of patients with arthritis and related musculoskeletal diseases (Lorig, 1986). As a result of the legislation, Multipurpose Arthritis Centers (MACs) were developed in the United States, with the Stanford Arthritis Center at Stanford University School of Medicine being among one of the early MACs. A description follows of Stanford's community program efforts from its inception in the 1980s to its ongoing efforts (Lorig, 1986). Thus, community-based arthritis management began with nationally planned funding, which in turn led to the initiation of hospital and community partnerships (O*N*PRIME).

Lorig and colleagues at the Stanford University School of Medicine developed the Arthritis Self-Management (ASM) course to address the arthritis burden (Lorig, 1986). A *needs assessment* (O*N*PRIME) was conducted with persons with arthritis to determine pertinent arthritis issues to better understand patient needs. One hundred patients with arthritis completed a questionnaire, demonstrating the following patient concerns (ONP*R*IME): pain, disability, fear, depression, and deformity (Lorig et al., 1985). Following the gath-

ering of patient reports, researchers conducted a thorough review of the relevant literature and collected information from 50 practicing rheumatologists (Lorig et al., 1985). Based on the needs assessment data, the ASM course was developed. Five values and assumptions underlie the ASM course: 1) patients can learn the principles of arthritis management, including the use of medications; 2) knowledgeable patients can practice self-care and experience health benefits and reduce health care costs; 3) health education should be widely available at a low cost; 4) trained lay persons could deliver structured health education programs; and 5) patients and the professional community would accept lay persons as health educators (Lorig, 1986; Lorig et al., 1985; Lorig & Holman, 1993).

The program was community based (O*NP*R*I*ME) and held at various community locations such as senior centers, churches, libraries, mobile home parks, shopping centers, and hospital conference rooms because most people who have arthritis are not hospitalized (Lorig, 1986). Outreach at various community sites was unique at the time because most arthritis organizations offered programs out of a single community location. During the 12-hour program (taught weekly in 2-hour sessions), participants were presented with and practiced self-management skills such as exercise, relaxation, heat and cold therapies, joint protection, communicating effectively with practitioners, analyzing nontraditional treatments, and problem solving skills (ONPR*I*ME). Participants were encouraged to select and concentrate on the most personally relevant skills (Lorig, 1986). As remains the case today, lay instructors who received 15–18 hours of standardized training taught the majority of the classes. Other teachers included active or retired health care professionals. Lay instructors remain the preferred patient educators because they have been shown to have good outcomes for patients, are cost-effective compared with paid professionals, and thus ensure greater outreach at minimal cost—the latter consistent with the National Arthritis Act passed by Congress. Approximately

15 patients participated in the course at a time (Lorig et al., 1985).

Course materials were purposely kept simple. Each participant in the ASM course receives a copy of *The Arthritis Helpbook* that contains all the course content. No audiovisual materials are used except a 20-page flipchart made by each leader. Deviation from the course materials was discouraged because it would diminish quality control issues. Further, any additional materials would potentially increase costs.

A significant feature of the ASM course that contributed to its early success was that evaluation of the initial course was planned and executed (ONPRIME). Study participants were recruited through newspaper, radio, and television program service announcements. A total of 300 study participants were randomized to begin either the ASM course scheduled immediately thereafter or the one that was to occur 4 months later. Study participants completed self-administered questionnaires at baseline, 4 months, 8 months, and 20 months. Questionnaires covered areas such as demographics, knowledge and frequency of exercise and relaxation, and pain management. Evaluation findings revealed study participants demonstrated increased knowledge and frequency of exercises and relaxation practices, as well as diminished pain compared with controls. Effects diminished over time but remained statistically significant at 20 months (Lorig, 1986).

The success of the ASM course caught the attention of the Arthritis Foundation (AF), which asked to be trained by the Stanford Arthritis Center. At the time, in the 1980s, AF chapters were not offering standardized programs; each chapter developed its own program (Lorig, 1986). Thus, the program was highly attractive to the AF, as consideration of organizational needs and resources is vital to the success of community courses (Lorig, 1986). The ASM course, which began as a controlled community course in Northern California, was soon being offered to persons across the United States in 1981 through pilot demonstration sites. The Stanford team wanted the new courses to develop at a slow pace, so that they could *monitor* and *evaluate* program progress and outcomes (ONPRIME). Additionally, the Stanford team wanted the initial courses to be unaltered and evaluated; the AF agreed (Lorig, 1986). As reported by Lorig (1986), two major problems developed: some trainees were resistant to the course presumably because they had not developed it, and "professional territoriality" issues surfaced wherein some health professionals did not believe laypersons could effectively cover the topics for which they were specifically trained.

Eventually, differences were managed, and the 25 trainees returned to their communities and trained 10 to 20 people who later offered the course. The name of the program was changed from the ASM course to the Arthritis Self-Help (ASH) course under the direction of the AF. The first participants to complete the ASH course completed pretest and posttest evaluations of knowledge, behavior, disability, pain, health care use, and patient satisfaction with medical care. These questionnaires were shortened versions of the ones used in the initial Stanford study. The evaluation data that arrived from the initial trainees was problematic. As reported by Lorig (1986), "When data arrived from the initial trainees, it became obvious that data collection was a low priority. Although each chapter was supplied with questionnaires and written protocol, data collection at best was spotty." (p. 27). The data from the initial trainees showed weaker results than what Stanford had obtained when they offered the course. The Arthritis Foundation Patient Service Committee that was responsible for overseeing the ASH course undertook a second evaluation at a later time. More care was given to data quality control of the pretest and posttest evaluations. The evaluation involved 239 subjects in 12 cities. The evaluation results showed that participants had increased knowledge, exercise, and relaxation, and reduced pain. Demand for the ASH course continued. Soon after, the AF developed its own administrative manual that standardized course content, process, and administration; and more trainers were trained. The ASH course brought positive attention to the AF, which was now reaching people across the United States. The media helped to draw attention to the ASH course; soon the AF was flooded with requests for information on the ASH course.

AF chapters and organizations were growing increasingly uncomfortable with the prospect of having to implement and complete evaluations, however. In 1983, after funding for a 5-site randomized study in 5 states was secured, most AF chapters refused to participate, citing unfairness to persons in the control condition and concern that the AF's positive media image would be compromised by the randomized study. Eventually, 18 months later, 5 sites were enrolled in the study—only 3 were true randomizations, however. Data collection proceeded with greater ease than expected, and subsequently, the AF received funding from the Administration on Aging to disseminate and evaluate the ASH course (Lorig, 1986). Today, ASH courses are still offered by the AF, and the Stanford Arthritis Center also continues to offer the ASM course.

Researchers at Stanford have refined the ASM program over the years based on qualitative and quantitative study results (Lorig et al., 1985). The initial course showed patient improvements in knowledge and self-care behaviors, and reduction in pain, depression, and physical visits. However, later studies showed only a modest relationship between health behavior change and health outcomes (Brady et al., 2003). In later years, Lorig and colleagues incorporated a focus on self-efficacy into the programming. Self-efficacy refers to a person's confidence in his or her belief to achieve a specific desired behavior or state of cognition. Subsequent results showed that the addition of the self-efficacy component led to improved reports of decreased pain and depression (Lorig & Holman, 1993). Additional studies have been conducted, and results continue to show positive outcomes (Lorig et al., 1998). Importantly, the program is now available in other languages; the Spanish Arthritis Self-Management Program has demonstrated

patient improvements in exercise, general health, disability, pain, self-efficacy, and depression at 12 months (Lorig et al., 1999) (ONPRIME). The availability of the program in other languages is critical as the aged population of Americans becomes more ethnically diverse (Federal Interagency Forum on Aging-Related Statistics, 2004).

Arthritis Foundation Education Program

The Arthritis Foundation Education Program (AFEP) is a community-based exercise program for persons with arthritis. AFEP was founded in 1987 by the AF and revised in 1999. AFEP, designed for people with arthritis who were not engaging in regular physical activity, consists of 8 sessions with 2–3 sessions offered per week. The 1-hour sessions are devoted to a combination of 72 exercises (range-of-motion, muscle strengthening, and endurance training), health education, relaxation techniques, and social opportunities. Exercises may be modified to meet individual physical needs. Trained health and fitness professionals who complete a 12-hour training program lead the AFEP programs. Reasons behind the AFEP content include proven benefits of: physical activity on joint mobility, strength, fitness, and range of motion; peer interaction and socialization as counteracting feelings of depression and isolation; and behavior change and educational programs on self-care and mastery of disease symptoms (Brady et al., 2003). Later *evaluations* (ONPRIME) showed reductions in pain and depression, increased self-care behavior and health status, and increased self-efficacy (Brady et al., 2003).

Conclusion

The role of public health in a maturing society cannot be underestimated. The aging of America's population will require greater public health effort to prevent and control chronic health conditions such as arthritis. Ongoing evaluation of existing programs, such as ASH courses, will continue to be important for identifying the best set of educational and behavioral strategies for helping elders to manage their chronic health conditions.

SUMMARY

Community health promotion emphasizing behavior change must be carefully planned, implemented, monitored, and evaluated. A systematic approach to doing so is described in this chapter. Specifically, the ONPRIME (organization, needs/resources assessment, priority setting, formative research, intervention, monitoring and evaluation) model provides a context for ensuring that the necessary elements of an overall approach are addressed. To demonstrate its applicability to a wide variety of target populations and problems, this chapter describes the ONPRIME model in the context of retrospective applications to proven approaches to pediatric obesity and arthritis symptom control among the elderly. ONPRIME integrates many of the public health core competencies within a single phased, recursive model. Specifically, knowledge of and experience with each of the ONPRIME components will contribute toward the development skills in leadership and systems thinking (community *organization*), analysis and assessment (especially *n*eeds assessment and evaluation), policy development and program planning (*prior*ity setting), community dimensions of practice (*n*eeds and *r*esources assessment), communication (*i*ntervention), management (*m*onitoring and *evalu*ation), and cultural competency, as well as basic public health.

REVIEW QUESTIONS

1. List some common public health promotion and behavior change theories.
2. Compare and contrast theories and models used in health promotion. What are the primary components and subcomponents of models?
3. Define and describe socioecological models of health behavior.

For questions 4 and 5: Consider a health promotion intervention with which you are familiar or have read about in detail.

4. What elements of the ONPRIME or other model were addressed in this project and which ones were not? What was the ultimate impact of the program? How might program success or shortcomings have been attributed to observance of these elements of the planning-intervention-evaluation sequence?
5. Was the intervention based on a particular theory or model? Describe how it may have benefited or been hampered by attention or inattention to theory.

NOTES

Agron, P., Takada, E., & Purcell, A. (2002). California Project LEAN's Food on the Run Program: An evaluation of a high school-based student advocacy nutrition and physical activity program. *Journal of the American Dietetic Association*, Adolescent Nutrition Supplement, *102*(3), 103–105.

Arthritis Foundation, Association of State and Territorial Health Officials, Centers for Disease Control and Prevention. (1999). *National Arthritis Action Plan: A Public Health Strategy*. Retrieved September 13, 2006 from http://www.arthritis.org.

Arthritis Foundation. *The Facts about Arthritis*. Retrieved September 13, 2006 from http://www.arthritis.org/resources/gettingstarted/default.asp.

Ajzen, I., & Fishbein, M.(1980). *Understanding Attitudes and Predicting Social Behavior*. Englewood Cliffs, NJ: Prentice-Hall, Inc.

Baer, D., Wolf, M., & Risley, T. (1968). Some dimensions of applied behavioral analysis. *Journal of Applied Behavior Analysis, 1*, pp. 1–24.

Bandura A. (1986). *Social Foundations of Thought and Action: A Social Cognitive Theory*. Englewood Cliffs, NJ: Prentice Hall.

Bandura, A. (1989). *Social learning theory.* Englewood Cliffs, NJ: Prentice Hall.

Barton, A.J.; Gilbert, L., Baramee, J., & Granger, T. (2006). Cardiovascular risk in Hispanic and non-Hispanic preschoolers. *Nursing Research, 55*(3), 172–179.

Brady, T.J., Kruger, J., Helmick, C.G., Callahan, L.F., & Boutaugh, M.L. (2003). Intervention programs for arthritis and other rheumatic diseases. *Health Education & Behavior, 30*(1), 44–63.

Centers for Disease Control and Prevention. (2003). Public health and aging: Projected prevalence of self-reported arthritis or chronic joint symptoms among persons aged >65 years—United States, 2005–2030. *MMWR, 52*(21), 489–491.

Centers for Disease Control and Prevention. (2006 March). *Physical activity for everyone: recommendations.* Retrieved September 13, 2006 from http://www.cdc.gov/nccdphp/dnpa/physical/recommendations/index.htm.

Center for the Advancement of Health. (2006, March). *A new vision of aging: Helping older adults make healthier choices.* Issue Briefing No. 2. Washington, DC.

Cohen, D.A., Scribner, R.A., & Farley, T.A. (2000). A structural model of health behavior: A pragmatic approach to explain and influence health behaviors at the population level. *Preventive Medicine, 30*(2), 146–154.

Collins, C.E. Warren, J., Neve, M., McCoy, P., & Stokes, B.J. (2006). Measuring effectiveness of dietetic interventions in child obesity: A systematic review of randomized trials. *Archives of Pediatric and Adolescent Medicine, 160*(9), 906–922.

Crespo, C.J., Smit, E., Troiano, R.P., Bartlett, S.J., Macera, C.A., & Andersen, R.E. (2001). Television watching, energy intake, and obesity in U.S. children: Results from the Third National Health and Nutrition Examination Survey, 1988–1994. *Archives of Pediatric and Adolescent Medicine, 155*(3), 360–5.

Davis, J.N., Ventura, E.E., Weigensberg, M.J., Ball, G.D.C., Cruz, M.L., Shaibi, G.Q., & Goran, M.I. (2005). The relation of sugar intake to beta-cell function in overweight Latino children. *American Journal of Clinical Nutrition, 82*, 1004–1010.

DiClemente, C., & Prochaska, J. (1998). Towards a comprehensive, trans-theoretical model of change. In Miller, W., & Heather, N. (Eds.), *Treating Addictive Behaviors* (2nd ed.). New York: Plenum Press.

Elder, J., Hovell, M., Mayer, J., & Geller, G. (1994). *Motivating Health Behavior.* New York: Delmar.

Elder JP, Lytle L, Sallis J, Young D, Steckler A, Simons-Morton D, Stone E, Jobe J, Stevens J, Lohman T, Webber L, Pate R, Saksvig B, Ribisl K (in press). A description of the social-ecological framework used in the Trial of Activity for Adolescent Girls (TAAG). *Health Education Research.*

Emmons, K.M. (2000). Health behaviors in social context. In L.F. Berkman & I. Kawachi (Eds.), *Social Epidemiology* (pp. 242–266). New York: Oxford University Press.

Federal Interagency Forum on Aging-Related Statistics. (2004). *Older Americans 2004: Key Indicators of Well-Being.* Washington, DC: U.S. Government Printing Office.

Federal Interagency Forum on Aging-Related Statistics. (2006 October). *Older Americans 2006: Key Indicators of Well-Being.* Federal Interagency Forum on Aging-Related Statistics. Washington, DC: U.S. Government Printing Office.

Flora, J., & Myhre, S. (1998). Key informant interviews with students, experts and LEAN regional coordinators about healthy eating, physical activity and multicultural youth. Sacramento, CA: Public Health Institute, California Project LEAN. Retrieved September 13, 2006 from http://www.californiaprojectlean.org.

Flynn, M.A.T., McNeil, D.A., Maloff, B., Mutasingwa, D., Wu, M., Ford, C., & Tough, S.C. (2006). Reducing obesity and related chronic disease risk in children and youth: A synthesis of evidence with "best practice" recommendations. *Obesity Reviews, 7*(S1), 7–66.

Giammattei, J., Blix, G., Marshak, H.H., Wollitzer, A.O., & Pettitt, D.J. (2003). Television watching and soft drink consumption: Associations with obesity in 11- to 13-year-old school children. *Archives of Pediatric and Adolescent Medicine, 157*, 882–886.

Glasgow, R.E. (2002). Evaluation Models for Theory-Based Interventions: The RE-AIM model. In Glanz, K., Rimer, B.K., & Lewis, F.M. (Eds.), *Health Behavior and Health Education* (3rd ed., pp 531–544). San Francisco: Jossey-Bass.

Goran, M.I., Reynolds, K.D., & Lindquist, C.H. (1999). Role of physical activity in the prevention of obesity in children. *International Journal of Obesity, 23*(S3), S18-S33.

Gordon-Larsen, P., McMurray, R.G., & Popkin, B.M. (2000). Determinants of adolescent physical activity and inactivity patterns. *Pediatrics, 105*(6), 83.

Green, L.W., and Kreuter, M.W. (1999) *Health Promotion Planning: An Educational and Ecological Approach* (3rd edition). Mountain View, CA: Mayfield.

Holland, J., & Skinner, B.F. (1961). *The Analysis of Behavior.* New York: McGraw-Hill.

Huhman, M., Potter, L.D., Wong, F.L., Banspach, S.W., Duke, J.C., and Heitzler, C.D. (2005). Effects of a mass media campaign to increase physical activity Among Children: Year-1 Results of the VERB Campaign. *Pediatrics, 116,* 277–284.

Janz, N.K., & Becker, M.H. (1984). The Health Belief Model: A decade later. *Health Education Quarterly, 11,* 1–47.

Kanfer, F.H. (1975). Self-management methods. In Kanfer, F.H., & Goldstein, A.P. (Eds.), *Helping People Change* (pp. 309–316). New York: Pergamon.

Lorig, K., Lubeck, D., Kraines, R. G., Seleznick, M., & Holman, H.R. (1985). Outcomes of self-help education for patients with arthritis. *Arthritis & Rheumatism, 28*(6), 680–685.

Lorig, K. (1986). Development and dissemination of an arthritis patient education course. *Family & Community Health, 9*(1), 23–32.

Lorig, K., & Holman, H. (1993). Arthritis self-management studies: A twelve-year review. *Health Education Quarterly, 20*(1), 17–28.

Lorig, K., Gonzalez, V.M., Laurent, D. D., Morgan, L., & Laris, B.A. (1998). Arthritis self-management program variations: Three studies. *Arthritis Care Research, 11,* 448–454.

Lorig, K., Gonzalez, V.M., & Ritter, P. (1999). Community-based Spanish language arthritis education program: A randomized trial. *Medical Care, 37*(9), 957–963.

Ludwig, D.S., Peterson, K.E., & Gortmaker, S.L. (2001). Relation between consumption of sugar-sweetened drinks and childhood obesity: A prospective, observational analysis. *Lancet, 357,* 505–8.

Marion, A.W., Baker, A J., & Dhawan, A. (2004). Fatty liver disease in children. *Archives of Disease in Childhood, 89*(7), 648–652.

McGuire, W.J. (1989). Theoretical foundations of campaigns. In R.E. Rice, & C. K. Atkin (Eds.), *Public Communication Campaigns* (pp. 43–66). Newbury Park, CA: Sage.

McKenzie, T.L., Li, D., Derby, C.A., Webber, L.S., Luepker, R.V., & Cribb, P. (2003). Maintenance of effects of the CATCH physical education program: Results from the CATCH-ON study. *Health Education & Behavior, 30*(4), 447–462.

Miller, K.L (1980). *Principles of Everyday Behavior Analysis,* (2nd ed.). Montgomery, CA: Brooks/Cole Publishing Company.

Nader, P.R., Stone, E.J., Lytle, L.A., Perry, C.L., Osganian, S.K., Kelder, S., Webber, L.S., Elder, J.P., Montgomery, D., Feldman, H.A., Wu, M., Johnson, C., Parcel, G., & Luepker, R.V. (1999). Three-year maintenance of improved diet and physical activity: The CATCH Cohort. *Archives of Pediatric and Adolescent Medicine, 153*(7), 695–704.

National Center for Chronic Disease Prevention and Health Promotion, CDC. (1999). Special topic: Healthy aging. *Chronic disease notes and reports, 12*(3). Retrieved September 13, 2006 from http://www.cdc.gov/nccdphp/publications/cdnr/.

National Center for Health Statistics. (2006a). *Prevalence of overweight and obesity among adults: United States, 2003–2004.* Retrieved September 15, 2006 from http://www.cdc.gov/nchs.

National Center for Health Statistics (2006b). Trends in child and adolescent overweight. *Prevalence of overweight among children and adolescents: United States, 2003–2004.* Retrieved September 15, 2006 from http://www.cdc.gov/nchs.

Prochaska, J.O., & DiClemente, C.C. (1983). Stages and processes of self-change of smoking: Toward an integrative model of change. *Journal of Consulting and Clinical Psychology, 51*(3), 390–395.

Rogers, E. 1983. *Diffusion of innovations* (3rdrd ed.). New York: The Free Press.

Sallis, J.F., Prochaska, J.J., & Taylor, W.C. (2000). A review of correlates of physical activity of children and adolescents. *Medicine and Science in Sports and Exercise, 32*(5), 963–975.

Samuels & Associates. (2000). California High School Fast Food Survey: Findings and recommendations. Sacramento, CA: Public Health Institute, California Project LEAN. Retrieved September 13, 2006 from http://www.californiaprojectlean.org.

Schulze, M.B., Manson, J.E., Ludwig, D.S., Colditz, G.A., Stampfer, M.J., Willett, W.C., & Hu, F.B. (2004). Sugar-sweetened beverages, weight gain, and incidence of type 2 diabetes in young and middle-aged women. *Journal of the American Medical Association, 292*(8), 927–934.

Sharma, M. School-based interventions for childhood and adolescent obesity (2006). *Obesity Reviews, 7*(3), 261–269.

Sherwood, N.E., & Jeffery, R.W. (2000). The behavioral determinants of exercise: Implications for physical activity interventions. *Annual Reviews of Nutrition*, *20*, 21–44.

Skinner, B.F (1953). *Science and Human Behavior*. New York: Macmillan.

Stokols, D. (1996). Translating social ecological theory into guidelines for community health promotion. *American Journal of Health Promotion*, *10*(4), 282–298.

Takada, E. (2002). Food on the Run 1998–1999: Environment Evaluation II. Sacramento, CA: Public Health Institute, California Project LEAN. Retrieved September 13, 2006 from http://www.californiaprojectlean.org.

Tversky, A., & Kahneman, D. (1974). Judgment under uncertainty: heuristics and biases. In Kahneman D, Slovic P, Tversky A, eds. *Judgment under uncertainty*. New York: Cambridge University Press; 3–20.

Wallack, L., & Dorfman, L. (1996). Improving health promotion: Media advocacy: a strategy for advancing policy and promoting health. *Health Education Quarterly*, *23*, 293–317.

Young, L.R., & Nestley, M. (2002). The contribution of expanding portion sizes to the U.S. obesity epidemic. *American Journal of Public Health*, *92*(2), 246–249.

CHAPTER 15

The Management of Public Health Organizations

Julia F. Costich, JD, PhD and J. Michael Moser, MD, MPH

LEARNING OBJECTIVES

Upon completion of this chapter, the reader will be able to:

1. Describe general concepts of management theory as they apply to the public health sector.
2. Describe the strategic planning process.
3. Describe the need for and role of partnerships in public health management.
4. List the types of constraints placed on public health managers by the government sectors in which they operate.
5. Describe key aspects of organizational structure in public health agencies.
6. Identify financial management skills and activities commonly found in public health management.
7. List characteristics of human resources management specific to public health practice.
8. Describe tools and approaches used in the control function of public health management

KEY TERMS

Accounting
Budgeting
Categorical Funding
Civil Service System
Controlling
Employee Recruitment, Retention
Financial Management
Fixed Costs
Government Accounting Standards Board (GASB)
Human Resources
Job Description
Leadership
Managerial Accounting
Merit System
Operational Plans
Organizational Structure
Partnerships
Personnel Management
Plan-Do-Study-Act (PDSA)
Public Policy
Span of Control
Strategic Planning
SWOT Analysis
Variable Costs

INTRODUCTION

Management is the discipline that addresses the optimal coordination of human, capital, and material resources to achieve an organization's goals. Whereas important management components of public health agencies such as structure, processes, funding, and evaluation may be governed by external factors, all public health organizations require effective management. The manager is responsible for deploying personnel and other available resources to obtain optimal achievement of agency goals and objectives.

The responsibilities of public health practice are broad and complex, and require a correspondingly broad array of management skills. For example, **personnel management** is an important component of management; personnel management in public health is typically complex because the work of public health requires a wide spectrum of staff education, skills, and personalities. Likewise, planning and finance are critical management components that take on unusual complexity in a public health organization. Planning for a public health organization is complicated by the need to take into account differing priorities derived from agency mission, funding agencies, political agendas, and the wishes of community interest groups. Public health **financial management** often requires simultaneous skill in public sector **budgeting,** grants management, medical insurance billing, and the administration of fee-based programs. Moreover, effective management of a public health organization requires skill in managing external relationships. To a degree unparalleled in other management settings, public health agencies must ensure effective collaboration with other organizations and with the community (or communities) at large to effectively fulfill their mission.

Despite its critical importance, management is often an undervalued skill in public health agencies. Many public health personnel with management responsibilities receive their basic professional education in functional areas such as nursing, medicine, health education, or environmental science, and not in management. These specialists-turned-managers may continue to self-identify with their original specialty, even when most of their day-to-day activity is more properly classified as management. Their professional culture often views "management" as, at best, a necessary evil, and sometimes as an impediment to the achievement of their professional self-realization. New public health managers often assume their managerial roles with limited or no formal training in management. Recognized gaps in management skill are typically addressed with on-the-job training. Managers who lack a firm educational foundation in management are hampered in their efforts by a lack of knowledge of what management science can offer to help them carry out their managerial role. In addition, they may not know about valuable management resources that are available to them or may simply not know how to access these resources.

The need for appropriate training and lifelong professional development among public health practitioners has been more fully discussed elsewhere.[1] However, the need for specific management training for public health managers deserves emphasis here. Too often management training is viewed as a low priority. It may not be included at all in agency training plans. This is unfortunate because fostering management skills is no less important for the success of the public health organization than support of ongoing training in other critical public health skill domains, such as epidemiology, nursing, and environmental health. Management skills are not simply something you grow into. Every well-run public health organization should have a plan to assess and address the needs of senior and middle managers for ongoing development of management skills. In some jurisdictions where the public health organization is part of a larger public entity (e.g., city or state government), there may be general management training programs in which health department personnel can be enrolled. These can be very helpful, but supplemental management education is often needed to prepare for the particular challenges of public health management. Alternatively, opportunities for management training are widely available through institutions of higher education. Although helpful in fostering generic management skills, such programs typically do not address the particular challenges of the public administration environment and the unique demands of managing a public health organization.

Educational programs specifically designed for public health managers are becoming more widely available, although unfortunately still not as readily available as generic management courses. Special management institutes offer high-quality management training often at a premium price. Because not all management techniques and skills can be effectively applied in the public health agency context (a theme to which we will return at several points in this chapter), public health managers seeking training are well advised to consult with colleagues in other jurisdictions and departments before signing up for a course or program. Most public health organizations fall within the service area of one or more academic institutions with public health degree programs, and public health management and administration faculty from these institutions can also serve as valuable resources with whom to discuss the suitability of a management course or program for the public health manager. The take-home message is that a plan to assure suitable management training for public health managers is itself an essential management component for every public health organization.

The Organizational Context of Public Health Management

Public health agencies typically function with some degree of direction from one or more larger governmental entity at the federal, state or municipal level, as described in Chapters 8–10. Aspects of the agency's management may be predetermined by the policies of the larger entity. For example, hiring practices, pay grades, and employee benefits for public health organizations are often determined through a broader **civil service system,** rather than by agency managers. Budget and finance policies typically must follow the dictates of external funding entities. Virtually all public health agencies receive some state and federal grant funding, and these grants are typically accompanied by myriad prescriptions regarding the use of funds and how to account for them. Because state and federal funding for public health organizations is generally granted with the explicit proviso that such funding cannot be counted upon in future years, strategic planning involving use of these funds is challenging.

Another dimension of external influence that must be successfully incorporated by public health managers is the **public policy** dictates of elected public officials and of legislative bodies. In the conventional wisdom, health may be characterized as an area that should not be sullied by the give and take of the political process. Realistically, when public health is a publicly funded activity carried out by public agencies, it is inevitable that the social process that we call politics is a feature. In the first half of the twentieth century, local public health agencies often operated in quiet backwaters under the benign and nominal authority of independent or quasi-independent boards of health. The increases in funding for public health activity over the past century, coupled with modern standards of public accountability, have made that sort of arrangement an anachronism. Today, most public health agencies operate under some form of supervision by elected officials. There is variation in the degree to which public health agencies come under the command and control authority of elected officials, but melding the public health vision and mission with the needs and agendas of elected officials is an important factor in crafting successful management strategies. One of the threshold challenges for a public health manager is to learn and keep abreast of the ways in which those needs and agendas define the parameters of his or her managerial role.

As a general rule, the discretionary authority of senior agency management tends to increase as the size of a public health agency and the population it serves becomes larger. However, like most influences and relationships discussed in this chapter, this one is not absolute. Some small agency managers exercise broad managerial authority and are accountable only to a local board or municipal officials. Conversely, some very large public health organizations have to deal with periods of external micromanagement. All public health organizations must adjust to shifting requirements of state and federal governmental policies and procedures. For example, fiscal procedures in public health agencies must conform to current **Government Accounting Standards Board (GASB)** standards. The range of independent authority in public health management does not diminish the importance of managing a public health organization with skill; rather, it reinforces the need for attention to the specific managerial challenges faced by public health managers and dissemination of successful models for effective management in this challenging environment.

Additional Resources for Public Health Managers

The student or practicing public health professional who is looking for information resources to help acquire new insights and skills in management has a huge literature to draw upon. This literature is very broad and sufficiently uneven that the beginning student or novice manager is ill advised to attempt to navigate it without assistance. Within the general management literature, there is a more focused but still substantial literature on public management. More focused still, books and other resources specializing in public health management have steadily increased in recent decades. In a single short chapter, it is impossible to cover or even summarize all of the key points from the literature of public health management. This chapter is designed as a basic orientation to key management functions as they arise in the context of managing a public health organization. More detailed general reference sources that you can consult include Griffith,[2] Longest et al.,[3] and Novick and Mays.[4] Those seeking the most recent articles in the field or discussions of specialized topics may productively look to peer-reviewed publications such as the *Journal of Public Health*

Management and Practice, Public Health Reports, and the *American Journal of Public Health.*

The fundamental management functions are often categorized as planning, organizing, and **controlling.** We have used these functional categories as the organizing framework for the remainder of this chapter. In addition to a general overview of these broad areas, this chapter provides the reader with an introduction to the areas of financial and human resources management in public health agencies, and provides a discussion on the development of strategic partnerships as a management function for public health. **Leadership** is an important component both of public health management and public health programming. As a cross-cutting topic, this dimension of management is addressed in Chapter 18.

PLANNING

The planning function is intended to prepare an organization for the future and facilitate informed decisions regarding the organization's approach to the achievement of desired outcomes. Planning activities in public health may be categorized as tactical or strategic. Tactical, sometimes called operational, planning is temporally focused in the short term, is relatively narrow in scope, and is linked to specific organizational objectives. In contrast, strategic planning has a longer term focus and is broader in scope. Strategic planning involves a systematic formulation of organizational goals. The longer the effect of a plan and the more difficult it is to reverse once implemented, the more strategic the nature of the plan.

Strategic and **operational plans** should operate concurrently for optimal value because they are complementary. Operational plans can be arrayed under headings derived from strategic plans to structure the implementation of organizational strategy. Concurrent operation of strategic and tactical planning activities can facilitate recognition and exploitation of potential opportunities for synergy.[5]

EXHIBIT 15-1 Examples of Strategic and Tactical Goals

An example of a strategic goal is to reduce preventable mortality among adults living in a community by 10 percent over the next 20 years. A strategic objective related to that goal could be to reduce tobacco-associated deaths in the community. A tactical plan to achieve the strategic goal and objective might involve development of enhanced tobacco cessation programming, including a plan to identify funding sources to support such activities. Another tactical plan related to the strategic goal could be to increase physical activity and reduce obesity and overweight among adults in the community.

Strategic Planning

Strategic planning may be viewed as an activity that seeks to define the organization and its future. A generalized concept for planning can be illustrated by a model that divides the strategic planning process into 10 steps (see Figure 15.1):[6]

1. **Agree upon a process and identify external partners:** Process-related issues include the commitment of key participants to being personally involved (rather than sending a

representative), the use of a facilitator, record-keeping, decision rules such as consensus or majority vote, issues to be addressed, process duration, and time demands. If the process has changed from previous planning cycles or there are new participants, some form of orientation is necessary regarding the order of events, likely time commitment, specific assignments for input and analysis, and goals for the process. The need for partnerships is discussed elsewhere in this chapter, but it is

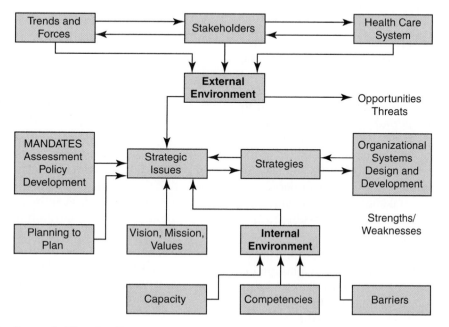

Figure 15.1. Strategic Planning Process

SOURCE: Adapted from Bryson JM. *Strategic Planning for Public and Nonprofit Organizations,* 3d ed, San Francisco: Jossey-Bass, 2004.

important to emphasize that inclusion of key external stakeholders in public health organization planning from the outset can be a critical success factor because their resources and support are particularly crucial for success of the public health mission.

2. **Identify organizational requirements:** Examples of such requirements include resources that the agency needs to provide its essential or mandated services and needs associated with forthcoming or new programs, as well as less tangible needs such as staff professional development, leadership enhancement, improved inter-organizational relationships, and communication with policy makers. Organizational requirements often serve as important criteria in decisions involving choices among possible strategies.

3. **State organizational mission and values:** This stage of the planning process is not normally the time to reexamine mission and values, but restatement of established principles does serve as a framing mechanism that reminds participants of their commitment.

4. **Assess internal and external environments:** Typically, this assessment takes the form of a **SWOT** (strengths/weaknesses/opportunities/threats) **analysis.** Strengths and weaknesses are considered in relation to the agency's internal capacities, competencies, and barriers to goal achievement. Opportunities and threats are identified in the external environment, including trends and forces coming to bear on agency operations, relationships to stakeholders, and characteristics of the health care system within which public health operates locally or statewide.

5. **Ascertain issues to be addressed:** One of the hallmarks of well-led strategic planning is avoiding distracting side issues that can sabotage efficient use of meeting time. Strategic planning sessions should not be the forum for longstanding grievances and rivalries, and an astute manager will identify potential side-tracks in advance and take steps to forestall

unproductive discussions. Because details may be needed to support productive discussion on some agenda items, identifying such items in advance of the actual planning sessions will give responsible staff and other contributors the opportunity to generate the necessary supporting information. Issues can also be characterized in relation to the organizational level at which they arise so that concerns that are limited to the internal operation of a single unit, for example, do not derail a discussion of broader agency-wide issues.

6. **Formulate alternative strategies:** Bryson summarizes four levels of strategy:

   - Grand strategy for the organization as a whole
   - Subunit strategies for parts of larger organizations
   - Program, service, or business process strategies
   - Functional strategies (e.g., information technology or staffing)[6]

   In the public health context, focusing on the system in which the agency functions as well as internal organizational matters fosters a higher level of engagement and cooperation by external partners.

7. **Select specific strategies:** The strategy selection process is facilitated by an agreement in advance regarding selection criteria, particularly where resources must be identified in association with chosen strategies. In concert with assessment of potential new strategies, existing strategies can be examined regarding their ongoing contribution to the agency's mission and goals. It should be noted when adoption of a plan will require consent or confirmation by a policy-making body.

   The last three steps in this model for strategic planning take place after the planning sessions themselves have concluded:

8. **Develop implementation process:** Elements in this step include the identification of timelines, critical success factors, potential

obstacles and tactics to overcome them, and key players, as well as the development of flow charts and other project management tools. Elements of the implementation process that have emerged from earlier phases of the planning process need to be combined and augmented. With a coherent implementation process, progress toward the strategic plan's objectives can be tracked and communicated to staff, external stakeholders, and governing bodies.

9. **Implement strategies:** The initiation of a new strategic focus can provide an opportunity for organizational celebration, press releases, and related events. After the intense and sometimes tedious planning process, this is a time when vision and reality are finally coming into clearer focus. Of course, the hard work of implementation remains to be accomplished, and the milestones identified in the implementation process development phase can provide a sense of achievement when morale wanes.

10. **Evaluate strategies and planning processes:**[6] The lapse of time between strategy formulation and full implementation may be sufficiently long that the original rationale for the strategy can be lost or forgotten. For this and other reasons, a retrospective review of the planning process, including both positive and negative lessons learned, should be part of the plan that emerges from the strategic planning process. Conscientious evaluation is an important step to maximize the value of strategic planning to the public health agency for which it is conducted.

The planning process should be continuous, and upon completion, the model is repeated from the beginning, using the evaluation data as input for the next situational analysis and further refinement of the strategic planning process. Budget cycles, political appointments, and public health-related events can trigger fresh attention to the planning process that managers use to overcome the negative response of staff to the very term "strategic

planning." If planning deteriorates into drudgery over time, a creative approach can energize the process by, for example, engaging more junior staff, rewarding visionary input, or importing officials from other branches of government.

A common critique of strategic planning is its focus on predictable events that have arisen in the past to the exclusion of highly unusual and disruptive threats. For health system managers, this tendency may be accentuated by a longstanding culture of stretching scarce resources. This problem was illustrated when, after the terrorist attacks of 2001, public health agencies were called upon to implement emergency preparedness and response plans with expanded CDC funding. Although a substantial proportion of the new funding could be used to make badly needed improvements to public health infrastructure, agencies were also required to introduce redundancies into communication systems and to acquire emergency stockpiles. Some public health officials interviewed during an assessment of the CDC initiative demonstrated discomfort with the need to allocate resources for events that might never arise, such as "go-kits" that would only be used during response to a terrorist attack.[7] Likewise, hospitals have repeatedly indicated that the exigencies of institutional survival made the concept of surge capacity anomalous. "Managing the unexpected" requires mindfulness, in contrast with mindless adherence to planned modes of action.[8] Public health, with its characteristic mix of routine and crisis, is challenged to combine day-to-day penny pinching with effective planning for novel threats.

Partnerships

One of the most important steps in public health planning is the identification and recruitment of partners who share core values, duties, and constituencies. Examples include representatives of community governance, partners in the provision of public health services, and regional or state health systems, depending on the **organizational structure** within which the agency functions. The fundamental need for inter-agency cooperation has recently been a critical feature of planning for public health emergency preparedness and response, but the need for inter-agency cooperation is not solely a feature of public health emergency planning. The axiom of emergency preparedness that the time to exchange business cards is not in the middle of a crisis can be productively extended to all aspects of public health practice. Cultivation of partnerships in times of relative calm, before they are critically needed, is a vital foundation for response to emergencies and too many other fundamental public health needs.

Public health agencies operate in the sphere of public administration as well as in the broad arena of health care, and their partnerships should range across both dimensions. Local law enforcement and judicial system representatives can be very useful partners when, for example, court orders are required to hospitalize individuals with multiply resistant infections who refuse to comply with medication regimens. Coordination between public health and local hospitals and health care organizations has repeatedly uncovered opportunities to enhance the services provided by public health agencies and the partner organizations. Close coordination with local emergency management authorities can reinforce the ability of a public health agency to respond to the public health needs created by an emergency, whether natural or man-made. Although partnerships make the planning process more complex, they also situate public health as a key element of a community's social capital as it responds to both ordinary and extraordinary challenges.

ORGANIZING

The organization of a public health agency is likely to reflect the cumulative impact of decades of political, economic, demographic, and epidemiological influences. A manager who is new to the agency will be well-served by becoming acquainted with its historical development. Understanding the background to current organizational arrangements can provide valuable insight; an arrangement that might not seem optimal at first acquaintance may become eminently reasonable with the benefit of a historical perspective. Conversely, this approach can help the manager identify areas that are ripe for change because the circumstances that originally shaped the organizational structure are no longer present.

Organizational Structures

Public health agencies are commonly organized by programmatic function with centralized support services such as information technology and financial management. Organizational theory and research has identified practical limits that are useful in structuring managerial roles. The **span of control** concept, for example, helps managers analyze the optimal number of individuals reporting directly to a single manager. For a front-line manager, the direct reports are the unit staff members. At higher levels in the organizational structure, direct reports are managers of smaller units. There is no canonical span of control ratio that is applicable to every situation. Recommendations for optimal span of control often call for manager-to-direct-report ratios between 1:3 and 1:7, but there is no magic formula. Determining the best span of control solution for a particular situation requires thoughtful consideration of a number of factors.

As a general matter, the broader the span of control, the greater the competition for higher management's attention. This experience is shared by staff of public health agencies that are merged with other health and social service functions into omnibus human services departments as units of state or municipal government. They risk loss of organizational identity and status when senior management's span of control becomes extremely broad. It is almost inevitable that some units will attract more favorable attention than others. Conversely, if spans of control are excessively narrow, an organization develops so many hierarchical levels that its ability to respond efficiently to community needs is impaired.

Applying the logic of the span of control model to organization of a local public health agency may be complicated by a number of factors. The city or county government of which a public health agency is a part may have standards for span of control that were designed for other governmental functions, such as public works or public safety. Alternatively, the specialized knowledge required for individual public health program functions can narrow the effective span of control of a public health unit manager. Public health agencies that are part of larger civil service systems may have limited capability to tailor generic supervisor job specifications to their needs. Span of control is a useful concept but as is the case with most "best practice" management concepts, the prudent public health agency manager will take local factors into account when adopting management principles developed from other organizational settings.

Structuring Principles

On an organizational chart, it is often useful to categorize personnel by line or staff functions. *Line* is the term used to define supervisory authority within the organization, and roles such as director, associate director, and department head. The organizational chart demonstrates the hierarchy of managers and subordinates they supervise. *Staff* is the term used to identify personnel with specialized and technical skills who provide support to the supervisory line personnel but who do not have supervisory authority over others. Such categorization has proven utility for quality improvement activities such as training and performance evaluation.

In recent years, many private-sector organizations and some public agencies have explored alternative organizational structures in search of improved efficiency and effectiveness. Under the heading of alternative organizational structures, we include matrix organization models in which employees are categorized by function, by cost or revenue center, or in some other relationship relevant to the organization in question. In the most complex form of matrix management, employees move seamlessly from one category to another as the needs of the organization and the match of their abilities to those needs dictate.

Some alternative organization models deployed in the private sector have featured broad and extensive decentralization of management authority, empowerment of individual employees to explore different approaches to the organization's work, and clouding of the distinction between line and staff. These approaches have found limited acceptance in public health agencies. The public sector in general, and regulatory agencies especially, attach great importance to a consistent approach precisely in accordance with legal and policy authorities. Clear distinctions between staff and line, as well as a command-and-control style, have traditionally been more consistent with this value. Audit requirements for grant funding, particularly with regard to funded positions, introduce other inhibitions on free and easy movement of employees from project to project. Where public health agencies are involved with collective bargaining agreements with unions, an absolute distinction between supervisory employees and bargaining unit employees is often a core contractual feature.

Although it is tempting to try to import the latest management styles to capture the putative advantages of efficiency and effectiveness that are always advertised to accompany these innovations, public health managers are advised to weigh such changes carefully. Public agencies are often criticized for out-of-date management policies. Political pundits often call for government to be "run like a business." In our experience, many public agency managers would cheerfully embrace the private business model if it meant they had access to the same management tools as private-sector managers. But public health agencies are not in the private sector, and the implications of that fundamental reality must always be taken into account by public health managers.

Challenges in Public Health Organization

Periodic re-assessment of an agency's programs and organizational structure falls under the organizing function of management. Programs and services should be offered by a public health agency because a community public health need exists that cannot be better served through another mechanism. A formal community health needs assessment is the textbook starting point for identifying and prioritizing the needs to be met by a public health agency. Of course, the formal data-driven needs assessment must coexist with environmental and political considerations, such as the priorities of influential external entities (e.g., the state health department). It falls to the public health manager to reconcile these sometimes competing forces so that the core mission of the agency is effectively addressed.

An example of the organizing challenges faced by a public health manager is the situation typically referred to as an unfunded mandate. A new activity, service, or program is required by an external entity (federal government, state government, etc.), no additional funding is provided to carry it out, and it is the responsibility of the public health manager to implement. Whatever the merits of the newly mandated function, the manager who becomes responsible for implementing it must make some difficult decisions. In the usual management situation, before a new function is added, there is a business case analysis to determine if resources are available or will be generated to support the new function. With unfunded mandates, this logical approach is bypassed. The manager's choices are (1) cut an existing program, however valuable, to make implementing resources available; (2) find new resources; or (3) squeeze existing resources to make them go further. Choice (1) may have strategic implications relative to agency mission and external relationships. Choice (2) requires action by an external agency to make it a reality and is therefore an external relations challenge. Choice (3) raises challenges in terms of budget, organizational structure, and personnel management. Clearly, there is no textbook answer to such situations. The public health manager who has developed skills in the planning, organizing, and controlling functions can call upon a variety of tools to assess the options, weigh their pros and cons, and make choices with a clear understanding of the likely implications, both in the short term and the long term.

Ideally, when the need for a service or program is no longer as great as the need for other services or programs, the manager shifts resources to an activity in greater demand. In reality, it may take as much or more marketing, selling, and convincing to terminate a program or service that has its own constituency as it does to get a new program or service off the ground. Strategic planning will help a manager recognize the different components of such situations and develop a plan for action that takes them into account. One way of characterizing the difference between management and administration is to say that administration is involved in making sure that individual tasks are done properly, whereas management assures an effective and integrated approach to the organizational needs.

Some public health functions are carried out as part of large, centralized agencies; others are distributed across a larger number of small organizations. For example, in some states, the state health agency or a similar centralized entity is the delivery mechanism for public health services that in other states are delivered by county, city, or township public health agencies. While centralized delivery mechanisms are associated with a risk of insensitivity to local needs and conditions, excessive decentralization can dissipate scarce resources to the extent that none of the small delivery units can provide quality service in a cost-effective manner. Mays and colleagues, assessing data from 315 local public health systems, found that larger entities exhibited higher levels of self-rated performance on a CDC-sponsored survey tool, and that local per-capita spending was a strong predictor of performance level.[9] However, performance did not vary with size across all indicators: multicounty jurisdictions scored lower than single-county entities in 6 of the 10 essential public health services, and performance scores did not improve above a population threshold of 500,000.

FINANCIAL MANAGEMENT

The discipline of public-sector financial management is the subject of many scholarly journals and has the support of several professional organizations.[10] A general list of relevant knowledge and skills includes the following:

- Basic financial and business processes
- **Accounting,** including generally accepted accounting principles, governmental accounting standards, OMB cost principles, indirect cost rates
- Financial data development, analysis, and communication of results to diverse audiences
- Budget development and submission with documentation following prescribed formats and specifications
- Development of cost allocation plans
- Contract negotiation, implementation, and monitoring
- Management and evaluation systems using performance measurement and cost accounting
- Applicable state and federal regulations
- Economic evaluation and analysis (e.g., cost-benefit analysis [CBA], cost-effectiveness analysis [CEA])
- Financial auditing
- Compliance analysis

Funding Sources

A survey of local health departments conducted in 2005 by the National Association of County and City Health Officers (NACCHO) (see Chapter 10) found a wide range of funding sources and an even wider range in the proportion of funding from each source.[11] Local (29%), state (23%), and federal (20%) funding accounted for the large majority across all respondent departments, with the balance made up of Medicaid, Medicare, fees, and miscellaneous sources such as grants and foundation funding. The diversity in funding mix is exemplified by the proportion of local funding, ranging from 0 percent in Delaware, New Mexico, and Vermont to 60 percent in New Jersey.

Another indicator of funding diversity is the role of Medicaid and Medicare revenues, ranging from 45 percent of all local health department revenues in Alabama and 35 percent in Georgia to 0 percent in New Hampshire, New Mexico, Nevada, and Vermont. Revenue per capita also varies widely by state and type of jurisdiction, with Maryland, New York, California, and Utah local health departments spending over $40 per capita and seven other states spending less than $20.

Despite the range of local health department funding configurations across states and localities, a large proportion of agencies fall into a few general categories. Agencies that directly provide a high proportion of the essential public health services (see Chapter 10) have a broader range of funding sources for reasons that include the **categorical funding** for specific types of population-based services as well as the predominance of government funding for clinical services. Conversely, some local health departments provide very limited services themselves and are funded almost exclusively by state pass-through dollars or local levies, while the state public health agency contracts with other providers for the broader range of essential services.

Budgeting

A budget is a detailed accounting of anticipated or actual revenues and expenses. As government agencies, public health departments must comply with many budgetary directives, including statutory and regulatory requirements, as well as policies and procedures set by larger entities of which the agency is a part. These requirements address both revenues and expenditures, forbidding or mandating specific fund acquisition and disbursement. For example, the ability of an agency to raise fees or offer new services may require the approval of a local or state government entity. Another common (and vexing) example is the requirement that funds not expended by the end of the state fiscal year be returned to the state by the local agency.

Financial managers generally distinguish between operating budgets, which address anticipated revenues and expenses for items used in a single year, and capital budgets, which address larger purchases that have longer useful lives. The GASB's summary of the differences between governmental and private-sector accounting notes that government financial statements are prepared "using the *current financial resource flows* measurement focus . . . and a *modified accrual basis* of accounting."[12] Both of the terms in italics deserve closer attention.

Current financial resource flows are the income and expenses that arise when resources actually become available and when liabilities must be paid. In this sense, current financial resource flows are like traditional cash basis accounting practices, or balancing your household checkbook. However, the public health financial manager must also understand and report on the effect of obligations and revenues that fall due at some future point within the reporting period. This approach is closer to the accrual basis of accounting, as might be used to make investments with longer-range financial implications. The combination of these two approaches yields the modified accrual basis described by GASB: "modifications include the fact that expenditures are recognized in the period in which they are expected to require the use of current financial resources, revenue is not recognized until it is available to pay current obligations, and certain long-term liabilities [which would be carried on the books as such under pure accrual accounting] are not recognized until due and payable."

The development of a public health agency budget is typically an open, public process that addresses such factors as resource needs, demand for services by policy makers or the public, changes in the regulatory environment, and unmet or duplicative community needs. Public health agencies have a wide variety of funding streams, including tax receipts, inspection fees, fines and penalties, grants, and reimbursement for specific services delivered to individuals. Some awards come with matching requirements addressing specific fiscal allocations or in-kind provision of staff time, space, and so on.

Financial Statements

Financial statements are important resources for agency management, but they also convey useful information to other audiences. In public health agencies, some financial statements are subject to public disclosure either as a routine matter or through inquiries under open records laws. State reporting guidelines are set by the GASB, and a number of GASB standards are applicable to municipalities, counties, and other government entities.[10] Municipal agencies, including health departments, may be subject to review by the state auditor, in addition to other requirements for external audit.

For daily financial management, the balance sheet is essential as an assessment of the agency's financial position at a given point in time. It provides ready access to an organization's asset base (such as investments, cash on hand, and saleable goods), income streams, and types of expenses, but only for the point in time at which the computation is made. A balance sheet may not be representative of an entire year's transactions because many types of revenue and expense occur less frequently. A common example in public health agencies is contract income that may be disbursed monthly, quarterly, or even annually.

The staff member who is responsible for preparation of balance sheets should have access to all relevant financial information and the combination of experience and expertise necessary to translate the range of background data into a coherent overview of agency financial status.

A complete statement of revenues and expenses, similar to the income statement in the private sector, is a more comprehensive instrument that typically captures an entire year of financial activity. A statement of cash flow is a tool for financial managers who are responsible for assuring that their organization has the cash on hand to meet both routine expenses and, to the degree possible, demands on the budget that arise unexpectedly. A common example in recent years has been steep increases in utility costs, which are typically covered by cutting other expenses or shifting expenditures forward. Although such unplanned increases in operational expenses can be problematic, they are small in comparison with the issues raised by situations that produce major unexpected funding needs. A single case of multi-drug resistant (MDR)

EXHIBIT 15-2 Sample Chief Financial Officer Position Description

Primary Activity: Serves as Chief Financial Officer and manages the administrative support services for the County Health Department. Areas of supervision include finance and accounting, **human resources,** budget, and general services. Responsibilities include those defined, related to, and governed by federal, state, and county laws, statutes, administrative rules, and ordinances. In the fiscal arena, the position is responsible for administering an annual trust fund budget of $X million, involving multiple funding sources from county, state, and federal governments.

Responsibilities:

1. Interprets and ensures implementation of high-level administrative and financial policies established by local, state, and federal entities as related to all levels of health department funding.
2. Oversees health department budget, finance, and accounting operations, including those of special programs and grants.
3. Manages administrative services departmental operations, among which are those of the physical plan management for multiple facilities.
4. Develops the state/county contract, monitors and provides required reports, and recommends contract changes.
5. Administers and manages health department procurement functions.
6. Supervises the management of the personnel department.

Detailed Description:
This is a managerial position responsible for the agency's financial standing as well as direction and supervision of administrative services (human resources, general services, finance and accounting, and budget) within a large county health department. The incumbent serves as the department's Chief Financial Officer (annual budget in excess of $X million) and is required to exercise independent judgment in maintaining internal controls and ensuring the financial viability of the health department. The incumbent participates in local, state, and federal meetings and conferences pertinent to county health department administration and with internal program activities and special projects.

This position coordinates the development of the annual budget request and approved operating budget. It is responsible for overseeing the integrity of the agency's trust funds, maintaining fund balances in accordance with statutory requirements, directing corrective actions, and effecting budget amendments to the approved operating budget. In addition, this position oversees the operations of agency financial and accounting functions in accordance with appropriate regulatory procedures, including all agency trust fund accounts, accounts payable and receivable, travel, fee collections, and third-party billing. This position is responsible for developing the agency's annual state–county contract, monitoring and providing reports required by the contract, and assessing and recommending changes to the contract. This position oversees the agency's purchasing functions, approaching $X million annually, and ensures compliance with appropriate regulatory policies, including approval of purchase orders and contracts in accordance with funding levels in the approved annual operating budget.

In addition to the financial responsibilities, this position oversees the agency's general services functions, including annual building leases, control of property and physical inventory, routine maintenance and safe operation of agency vehicles, and ongoing building repairs and renovations to ensure safe, clean, and functional working environments for staff and clients. This position also oversees agency personnel functions governing employee benefits, classification, recruitment, termination, retirement, payroll, leave and attendance, and insurance claims.

tuberculosis can generate care costs in six figures. Although relatively few local health departments encounter such a case, it is imperative to deal with it when it occurs. When the community is affected by a natural emergency such as a flood or major weather event, it is clearly the duty of the public health agency to attend to the community's public health needs, even if the response exceeds the agency's budget. However, reconciling the unanticipated costs of such necessary responses is an after-action management challenge that may be as difficult in its own way as managing the emergency response. Because public health agencies are often barred by state or local fiscal policies from building reserve or rainy day funds, they do not have access to a common management tool to plan for unusual events. Nonetheless, the high probability that every public health organization will have to deal with unbudgeted major expenses at some point justifies advance management exploration of available options to deal with the fiscal impact of such expenses when and if they are incurred.

Managerial Accounting. In recent years, cost containment and fiscal accountability have become higher priorities for public agencies. Accordingly, it is important for managers to have a detailed understanding of their costs and revenues, in other words, to engage in **managerial accounting.** Private-sector managers have historically found it valuable to distinguish between fixed and variable costs. **Fixed costs** do not change with the level of activity in associated areas. If an entire office suite is rented, for example, the cost will be the same whether one office or all offices are occupied.

When a fixed cost is associated with the production of a specific service, the total unit cost of the output is reduced as the number of units increases because the per-unit cost is spread across a larger number of units. Thus, very small agencies may have higher unit costs than larger ones because there are minimum levels of infrastructure for which they must incur fixed costs. In public health agencies that serve small jurisdictions, traditional public health functions such as tuberculosis and STD screenings may be examples of this phenomenon because the

agency must bear the expense of maintaining capacity that is infrequently used.

Variable costs are those associated with each unit of output, such as the costs of single-use supplies and medications associated with patient visits. Unlike fixed costs, variable costs are not incurred if the relevant service or production does not take place. However, public health services generally require fixed cost inputs such as rent and utilities, so variable costs are typically calculated as additions to fixed costs. For example, a school-based health promotion program could anticipate lower variable costs during the weeks when schools are not in session and program activities do not take place.

Capital budgets can be a major challenge for agencies that are normally funded on a year-to-year basis. Capital acquisitions include facilities and equipment that will have relatively long operating periods, although the precise duration varies by jurisdiction. Because the amount of the expenditure is likely to exceed the capacity of the operating budget, some special appropriation, bonding authority, or levy may be necessary. Bonds are offered on the financial market to facilitate the acquisition of capital by units of government. Those who buy the bonds acquire both the value of the bond itself and a fixed or variable amount of interest. Special tax levies are sometimes mandated by legislative bodies but are more commonly the subject of ballot initiatives that authorize a specific strategy to collect funds, for example, a special tax on hotel rooms or nonresident commuters.

HUMAN RESOURCES

Public health agencies employ professional staff such as physicians, nurses, data analysts, and epidemiologists who may be able to command significantly higher levels of compensation in the private sector than the public health agency can offer. Recruiting and retaining qualified staff are among the most daunting challenges faced by the public health manager.

Job Descriptions

Effective management of staff requires development of **job descriptions** for all employees. A typical job description includes a position title and detailed qualifications for the position, including education, registration or licensure, technical skills, and prior experience. In addition, the position description addresses general and specific responsibilities, performance standards, criteria for performance appraisal, and the salary range. Staffing analysis also addresses the management responsibilities of personnel, identifying front-line, mid-level, and senior managers who are directly responsible for the activities of the organization, and staff who support the work of managers.

Merit Systems

Most United States governmental personnel systems were established during the twentieth century with a focus on protecting public-sector employees from undue political influence on the performance of their duties and their decisions. Government personnel systems are also intended to promote a hiring process that is equitable and professionally administered. In such systems, policy-making positions such as agency heads and their personal staff often serve at the pleasure of the appointing authority, but other employees are hired and hold their positions under some form of merit system.

Merit systems have several characteristics in common. The hiring process is more rigid and much slower than in the private sector and is often based on some form of written examination. The very length of the hiring process often places public agencies in an uncompetitive situation when attractive job candidates are snapped up by more flexible organizations. The individual who will supervise the new employee typically has less input into the hiring decision than is customary in the private sector because the system is structured to minimize the role of personal influence or favoritism. After an individual is hired and completes a probationary period successfully, dismissal for poor performance can be very difficult. Protections against arbitrary or politically motivated dismissal, while well-intended, create a burden of

proof on the public agency manager that is significantly in excess of that faced by a private-sector manager dealing with a similar performance problem.

Public merit systems are a fact of life for public health managers. However challenging, the managerial responsibility in this context is to make the system work to support the agency mission. Agencies with well-developed **human resources** support can reduce the technical burden on managers, but detailed knowledge of personnel and merit system rules remains essential if the public health manager is to be optimally effective. As a corollary, managers must learn to motivate staff performance through means other than discipline to motivate high-quality staff performance.

Public health agency managers have the benefit of a mission that most employees value highly. The commitment and dedication of public health employees to the public health mission is widespread and sincere. Public health managers who respect and understand this motivation can use this understanding to support quality performance within their agency.

Personnel Management Theory

Two points of reference in management theory are the classical and behavioral models. The classical approach advocates that structure be kept simple, with clear-cut authority and responsibility for each position. Each employee is confined to a single specialized function. Supervision is characterized by unity of command and a clear chain of authority, with a single superior directing an employee, and staff communication taking place exclusively through managers, each supervisor having a limited number of subordinates.

Classical managers assume that their employees are solely motivated by financial reward and that they do not value their contribution to the organization's work. Consequently, classical theory-based managers believe subordinates must be constantly supervised and that they will not do their jobs well if they are not. Such managers also believe this approach is the best and the only way to effectively manage an organization.

The behavioral approach assumes that people can enjoy work, and if conditions are favorable, they can exercise control over their own performance. The behavioral model of management contends that the classical theory makes demands on individuals that are incongruent with their needs and questions the classical aggressive supervision and motivation-related assumptions. Behavioral managers believe that people are motivated by the desire to do a good job and by the opportunity to interact with peers. Adoption of this approach results in decentralization of the organization, enlarged and unspecialized responsibilities for staff, employee participation in decision making, and upward and lateral communication among personnel. Just as the advocates of classical management advocate one best way to manage, the advocates of human relations management substitute an alternative universal best way to manage in all situations.

A third and more contemporary approach to management describes a contingency or situational approach to management. In the contingency model, planning, organizing, directing, and controlling are dependent upon the organizational environment and tasks. Contingency managers propose a situational approach, where managers may supervise some personnel and activity using the classical approach, and others using the behavioral approach.

Contingency management shifts from universal principles or methods of management and recognizes that each organization and management problem will have distinctive features. As a result, management strategies must be developed differently for each situation. Rather than select a single best way to manage, contingency managers evaluate a situation and select an appropriate management strategy.

Employee Recruitment and Retention

Due to a cohort effect in earlier hiring for public health, a large turnover of public health staff is expected over the next decade.[13] In recent years, young people have responded to survey questions by assigning a higher ranking to the social meaning and value of work in making job choices. The interest of young people in work that is valued (as opposed to work that generates monetary value) may place public health organizations in a good position to replace these departing employees with well-motivated replacements. We have found that the public health mission has a positive resonance with most people.

Public health agencies that are able to incorporate the public health mission into their recruiting may find it helpful. However, public health managers who want to mine the vein of commitment among young people should be aware that this generation's interest in socially valuable work is accompanied by different attitudes to work and the workplace environment than their predecessors. The younger generation appears to attach less value to promises of pensions and job security and more to work that maintains their interest. They also attach more value to employment that builds marketable skills and workplaces that accommodate the scheduling of family responsibilities and personal interests. Flexibility and understanding will be important attributes for the public health managers who want to attract and retain a new generation of public health workers.

Public health managers, like other supervisors in the public sector, work within compensation structures that restrict their ability to use financial rewards as a human resource management tool. Public-sector starting salaries are often lower than in comparable private sector positions; not surprisingly, this often impedes recruitment of the best-qualified candidates. Moreover, scheduled public-sector pay increases may be limited or frozen due to financial problems in the entities upon which public health agencies depend for funding. The personnel structures in merit systems may reward time in grade more than quality of performance, a practice that limits the utility of financial incentives for motivating performance and retention. Systems structured to prevent political favoritism or undue personal influence on public personnel actions seriously limit the ability of public health managers to provide significant financial rewards for superior performance. Traditional performance evaluation tends to lose its salience when high ratings are not matched with significant wage increases. The satisfaction that comes with an important job well done has its limits when staff can readily compare their working conditions and salaries with similarly trained employees in other settings.

Historically, aspects of public health employment beyond salary that have fostered **employee retention** have included more generous fringe benefits, strong retirement systems, flexible work hours, and opportunities for professional development. However, rising health insurance costs and new governmental accounting standards for public retirement systems are producing pressures that will probably diminish the extent to which public health managers can rely on distinctions in benefit and retirement packages as **employee recruitment** and retention tools.[14] On the other hand, the shift of the United States economy to service production and the concurrent decline of highly compensated industrial positions, coupled with a trend to market indexing for public-sector salaries, have narrowed the gap between public health agency salaries and comparable salaries in other settings.

Fringe benefits such as health insurance, pensions, paid leave, and employee support services are diminishing in the private sector as corporate managers strive to maximize revenue by cutting employee-related costs. Cost pressures are certainly apparent in public-sector agencies as well, but they have not yet led to dramatic cuts in the availability of fringe benefits. When one spouse is self-employed or a full-time caregiver, access to family health coverage can be a critical element in the decision of the other spouse to forego a higher-wage position that lacks health benefits. Likewise, a single parent may choose a position with a lower salary and higher benefit level to meet family needs. Health insurance is almost unattainable for individuals with expensive care needs, so families with such members also tend to select jobs with generous benefits.

Another attraction of public-sector employment is a high level of access to professional development opportunities. Although some continuing professional education is necessary to retain discipline-specific licensure or credentials, public health agency staff may also look for educational opportunities that support career advancement. Training exercises in emergency preparedness and response have proliferated in recent years, funded by federal support for initiatives to combat bioterrorism and pandemic influenza. A sample of the myriad other training options available at little or no cost is accessible through the TRAIN system maintained by the Public Health Foundation at http://www.train.org.

Working conditions also affect employees' decisions to remain in positions despite higher-wage options. This phenomenon is particularly noteworthy among nurses, who can earn twice as much in some hospitals than in public health agencies, yet choose public health employment because they are not required to work nights or weekends or to take varying shifts on call. Many nurses are also attracted to an atmosphere where prevention is the focus, and there is respect for the ability of professional nurses to promote that central goal. An atmosphere of collegiality and mutual respect is another factor that can partially compensate for a discrepancy in wage rates.

Yet another element in employee retention lies in fostering a sense of shared mission to improve the health and well-being of the community. Celebrating achievements and honoring staff contributions can improve staff cohesion and morale, but managers must be careful to take such steps in a consistent and evenhanded manner. Involving staff representatives in the identification of outstanding projects and individuals helps to avoid the appearance of favoritism.

This is but a sampling of tactics that can be mobilized to promote employee retention. Periodic analysis of hiring and retention patterns is commonly performed by human resource specialists or departments and can assist managers in identifying specific areas that need closer attention.

CONTROLLING

The controlling process of management addresses monitoring and adjusting activities to achieve organizational goals. The process creates standards, monitors activities, compares results with expectations, and takes corrective actions or adjustments to realign activities with organizational goals. Public health professionals are familiar with epidemiologic surveillance as the core function that monitors conditions in the community to identify situations where a public health response or corrective action is needed. The controlling process of management is somewhat analogous but with an internal focus on program activities and performance rather than an external focus on communicable diseases and other health conditions.

Regular, effective, two-way communication between a manager and direct reports is a critical building block of this core management function. Although there is no immutable rule on the subject, most successful managers use a full range of communications options. Commonly used options for communicating with direct reports include one-on-one meetings, group meetings, written reports, phone conversations, and e-mail. There are certainly successful managers who make only one of these options work well for them, but our experience favors a mix of methods. One key to success in this regard is to make some of the communication part of a routine—a regular feature on the calendar, and therefore harder to miss or skip.

It cannot be over-emphasized that communication must flow in both directions. If employees fear retaliation for bringing issues to the attention of management, critical opportunities to avert major problems may be lost. The manager who operates in a cocoon of good news is an all too familiar figure in contemporary public life, and the catastrophic potential consequences should make managers wary of unusually calm, trouble-free periods.

Those submitting reports should be given feedback, even if it is brief. Managers should dedicate a part of every meeting with subordinates to listening and work to do so effectively. The manager who does not listen well is unlikely to carry out the control function well.

Managers are also encouraged to develop means to keep themselves apprised of the general tone and morale of the organization. This should be part of conversations with subordinate managers and supervisors, but experienced managers typically feel the need to cross-validate their impressions.

There are a variety of ways to accomplish this. In 1982, Peters and Waterman popularized an approach they called Management by Walking Around (MBWA).[15] MBWA involves a number of management strategies that go beyond ensuring effective communication, but a key element of MBWA is simply having managers move out of the management suite to circulate among the workforce on a regular basis. Some managers have found periodic lunch sessions with line staff to be an effective way to gauge general employee morale and issues. Most modern general management texts provide information about other approaches to facilitate such communication. The key is for each manager to find a way that works for him or her.

Public health employees as a group are dedicated and conscientious people, but these qualities do not diminish the responsibility of public health management to understand and make clear the performance expectations for public health programs and for public health employees. The complexity of a public health organization means that managers need the help of others to establish appropriate expectations. Categorical grant programs typically come with clearly stated deliverables, and it is the job of project officers to ensure that personnel costs for a grant activity do not exceed their agency's parameters. For clinical activities, especially in the maternal and child health area, some states have developed formal assessment processes that allow local agencies to monitor their activities in a standardized fashion, with the potential for comparison to other departments.

New managers are likely to find that they have inherited a set of standards, whether from their predecessors in office or from the administrative context in which they function. These standards may be explicit, but in some part, they are likely to be unwritten. For example, a certain number of person-hours may be associated with specific functions and serve as the basis for resource allocation. Activity monitoring, in this example, would be an accounting of hours spent on each function, and evaluation would assess the extent to which actual distribution of effort conforms to organizational standards. Where deviations were noted, their causes would be determined and addressed. The control process is subject to its own standards, assessing the adequacy of control mechanisms in terms of their timeliness, economy, comprehensiveness, specificity, objectivity, appropriate allocation of responsibility, and ease of understanding.

Benchmarking is a popular approach to the control function in health care organizations that identifies a desirable performance level in a similar entity and develops strategies to achieve similar outcomes. For example, a state public health agency may develop target rates of immunization, prenatal care, newborn screening, or safety belt use based on rates reported by the highest-performing jurisdictions. Agency managers then identify specific strategies that appear to contribute to the achievement of these target rates and assess their potential implementation within their own environment.

Tools that support the control function include various kinds of charts, such as flowcharts, Gantt charts, spreadsheets, run charts, histograms (common in Total Quality Management), and statistical quality control charts. One popular approach to quality management is the **Plan-Do-Study-Act (PDSA)** quality improvement cycle.[16] It is particularly well-suited to public health agencies because it supports small-scale experimentation and the development of an evidence base in advance of broader action. As noted in Figure 15.2, PDSA is a cycle in which each element provides the manager with an opportunity to learn and adjust before taking the next step. A fully implemented PDSA process for quality improvement can be compared to an expanding spiral because of its potential to affect broader areas of activity in each iteration.

The need for accountability at the public health agency level poses important challenges.[17] Specific sets of performance assessment standards have been used to evaluate the quality of agency performance as well as the adequacy of public health system functions in a given jurisdiction[18,19,20] (see Chapter 16). Currently, there is a movement toward accreditation of public health agencies, and several states have already embarked on accreditation initiatives.[21] However, it remains to be seen if accreditation of public health agencies will actually serve as a quality improvement mechanism. The accreditation movement appears to be driven by national and, in some cases, state organizations. In states where local financing of public health services remains a major part of the funding mix, it is not at all clear that local communities and their elected officials care whether their public health agency is accredited, as long as it delivers the services that they value. Accreditation involves some not-insignificant cost to the agency seeking accreditation. Because the agencies most in need of improvement are often in that position due to lack of funding, accreditation requirements may divert the very

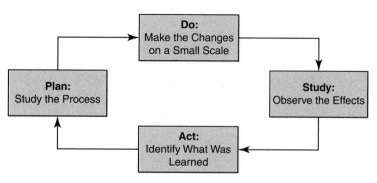

Figure 15.2. The Shewhardt PDSA Quality Improvement Cycle
SOURCE: Delmar Cengage Learning.

resources needed for improvement. Some have suggested that state or federal funding should be withheld from agencies that fail to achieve accreditation after a certain date. But in the absence of resources to help those agencies, funding cuts are unlikely to improve the performance of the agency. It remains to be seen if state health departments or accredited health agencies will be willing or able to take on the responsibility for areas served by unaccredited health agencies. If all that accreditation accomplishes is to give formal recognition to the status quo, it is not likely to be a useful tool for improving public health services.

Although agency performance in relation to benchmarks or standards is a growing focus of public health management, the broader context of population health improvement requires managers to relate to external as well as internal relationships and functions. Optimal performance on the part of a public health agency depends on the quality of community support and systemwide resources at least as much as on excellence in management. As Aday puts it, "public health can most effectively achieve its objectives by mobilizing other stakeholders in the community."[22]

SUMMARY

This chapter is designed as an overview of management concepts and presentation of examples relevant to public health practice. Management techniques vary in the context of each public health organization's goals and environment. Application of the specific concepts associated with the management functions of planning, organizing, and controlling will improve the management of public health organizations. Effective application of management methods creates an opportunity to improve the efficiency and effectiveness of public health organizations.

REVIEW QUESTIONS

1. Describe three types of constraints on public health agency management.
2. Describe steps in the strategic planning process.
3. Why don't public health agencies adopt innovative management structures as often as other health sector organizations?
4. Describe the funding sources reported by local public health agencies in the 2005 NACCHO survey.
5. Describe the modified accrual basis of accounting generally found in government agencies.
6. Discuss factors that can make management of resource prioritization and modification of the service/product mix different for a public health agency than for a private business. Suggest management approaches to address these different challenges.

REFERENCES

1. Gebbie K, Rosenstock L, Hernandez LM, eds. *Who Will Keep the Public Healthy? Educating Public Health Professionals for the 21st Century.* Board on Health Promotion and Disease Prevention, Institute of Medicine. Washington, D.C.: The National Academies Press; 2003.
2. Griffith JR. *The Well Managed Healthcare Organization,* 6th ed. Chicago, IL: Health Administration Press; 2006.
3. Longest BB Jr, Rakich JS, Darr K. *Managing Health Services Organizations and Systems.* Baltimore, MD: Health Professions Press; 2000.
4. Novick LF, Mays G P. *Public Health Administration: Principles for Population-Based Management.* Gaithersburg, MD: Aspen Publishers; 2001.
5. Fleming ST, Scutchfield FD, Tucker TC. *Managerial Epidemiology.* Chicago, IL: Health Administration Press; 2000.
6. Bryson JM. *Strategic Planning of Public and Nonprofit Organizations*, 3rd ed. San Francisco: Jossey-Bass; 2004:32–34.

7. Costich JF, Scutchfield FD. Public Health Preparedness and Response Capacity Inventory validity assessment. *J Pub Health Manag Pract.* 2004; 10(3):225–233.

8. Weick KE, Sutcliffe KM, *Managing the Unexpected.* Ann Arbor: Univ. of Michigan; 2001.

9. Mays GP, McHugh M C, Shim K, et al. Institutional and economic determinants of public health system performance. *Am J Public Health.* 2006;96(3):523–531.

10. Moulton AD, Halverson PK, Honorè PA, Berkowitz B. Public health finance: A conceptual framework. *J Public Health Manage Pract.* 2004;10(5);377–382.

11. National Association of County and City Health Officers. *2005 National Profile of Local Health Departments.* Washington, D.C.: NACCHO; 2006.

12. Governmental Accounting Standards Board White Paper. Why Governmental Accounting and Financial Reporting Is—and Should Be—Different. March 14, 2006. Available at: http://72.3.167 .244/white_paper_full.pdf. Accessed December 29, 2006.

13. Bureau of Health Professions, Health Resources and Services Administration. Public Health Workforce Study. Available at: http://bhpr.hrsa.gov/ healthworkforce/reports/publichealth/default .htm. Accessed January 4, 2007.

14. Government Accounting Standards Board. Other Post-Employment Benefits: A Plain Language Summary of Statements 43 and 45. Available at:

15. Peters TJ, Waterman RH. *In Search of Excellence: Lessons from America's Best-Run Companies.* New York: Harper and Row, 1982.

16. Kelly DL. *Applying Quality Management in Healthcare: A Process for Improvement.* Chicago, IL: Health Administration Press; 2003.

17. Scutchfield FD, Knight EA, Kelly AV, Bhandari MW, Vasilescu LP. Local public health agency capacity and its relationship to public health system performance. *J Public Health Manage Pract.* 2004;10(3),204–215.

18. Corso LC, Wiesner PJ, Halverson PK, Brown CK. Using the essential services as a foundation for performance measurement and assessment of local public health systems. *J Public Health Manage Pract.* 2000;6(5),1–18.

19. Mauer BJ, Mason M, Brown B. Application of quality measurement and performance standards to public health systems: Washington State's approach. *J Public Health Manage Pract.* 2004;10(3),330–337.

20. Mays GP, Halverson PK, Scutchfield FD. Making public health improvement real: The vital role of systems research. *J Public Health Manage Pract.* 2004;10(3),183–185.

21. See, for example, the Michigan Local Public Health Accreditation Program. Available at: http://accreditation.localhealth.net.

22. Aday LA, ed. *Reinventing Public Health.* San Francisco: Jossey-Bass; 2005.

http://www.gasb.org/project_pages/opeb_ summary.pdf. Accessed December 28, 2006.

CHAPTER 16

Performance Measurement and Management in Public Health

Paul K. Halverson, MHSA, DrPH

LEARNING OBJECTIVES

Upon completion of this chapter, the reader will be able to:

1. Assess the internal and external motivations for public health agencies to engage in performance measurement and related quality improvement and accountability activities.
2. Describe the historical development of methods for measuring the performance of public health agencies and systems.
3. Identify key conceptual and methodological issues in applying performance measures to public health agencies and systems.
4. Examine the core skills and capacities needed by public health agencies to engage effectively in performance measurement and improvement initiatives.

KEY TERMS

10 Essential Public Health Services
Accreditation Program
Bias
Confounding
Core Public Health Functions
Inter-Rater Reliability
Measurement Error
Measurement Noise
Measurement Sensitivity
Measurement Specificity
Outcome Indicators
Performance Benchmark
Performance Management
Performance Measurement
Performance Standard
Process Indicators
Public Health System
Reliability
Risk Adjustment
Structural Indicators
Validity

Public health agencies engage in a broad array of activities to protect and improve health at the population level. Unfortunately, studies from the past two decades have found evidence of substantial gaps and wide variation in the ability of state and local agencies to perform essential public health activities. Concerns about such gaps have grown rapidly in response to emerging and resurgent infectious diseases such as SARS and avian influenza, the public health risks presented by both man-made and natural disasters, and the advance of obesity and related chronic diseases. Closing these gaps requires concerted efforts to measure the services produced and results achieved by public health agencies and to develop targeted approaches for improving services and outcomes. The process of developing such measures for a program, organization, or delivery system and comparing them against established goals and expectations has become known as **performance measurement.** Similarly, the practice of using such measures on an ongoing basis to improve an organization's operations and outcomes has become known as **performance management.**

This chapter examines historical and contemporary trends in applying performance measurement concepts and methods to public health agencies and public health delivery systems in the United States. The concept of performance measurement has achieved widespread use in the field of public health only relatively recently, but it has a longer history in other industries. Contemporary methods of performance measurement and management derive from industrial quality improvement concepts that became popular in United States manufacturing industries during the 1980s[1] and later in health care industries and government during the 1990s.[2–5] More recently, public health agencies at local, state, and national levels have begun to use these methods together with basic principles of epidemiological investigation to monitor and improve their operations.[6–9] A review of the practice of performance measurement and management within public health agencies demonstrates that these approaches can serve as useful vehicles for improving the organization, financing, and delivery of public health services.

RATIONALE: WHY MEASURE PUBLIC HEALTH PERFORMANCE?

Performance measurement methods are used in public health settings for a variety of purposes that encompass both intrinsic and extrinsic motivations for public health practice. A public health agency may engage in performance measurement independently to track progress toward internal organizational goals and identify opportunities for improvement. The results of these internally-driven measurement activities may not ever be shared with stakeholders outside the organization. Alternatively, organizations may engage in performance measurement as part of coordinated, multi-institutional initiatives implemented at community, state, regional, or national levels. These activities focus comparing performance across an array of organizations or delivery systems, and often are organized by entities that are separate from and external to those being measured. Participation in these externally-driven activities may be purely voluntary or tied to strong incentives such as funding, contract requirements, or statutorily-defined responsibilities. Whether driven internally or externally, performance measurement activities may aid the field of public health in a number of important ways.

Supporting Management Decision-making

Perhaps the most compelling intrinsic motivation for engaging in performance measurement stems from the value of the information produced.[7,9,10] Equipped with reliable information about how well core activities are performed within an organization or multi-organizational system, public health managers can redesign work processes and reallocate resources to address identified performance gaps. In this way, performance measurement activities function as powerful tools for identifying problems and targeting solutions. Such tools are increasingly important to organizations operating in contemporary public health environments in which health risks and core institutional and financial structures are continually in flux. Public health organizations must adapt their operations on an ongoing basis in response to fluctuations in governmental spending for public health programs, realignments in the constellation of organizations that contribute to public health activities, and shifts in population demographics and disease patterns. In this context, managerial decision making can be compromised substantially without reliable and timely information about an agency's performance and outcomes.

Ensuring Accountability

Performance measurement also provides a means of responding productively to external pressure for greater accountability and transparency in how public resources are used within the field of public health. Organizations that provide financial support or other resources to public health agencies can use performance measurement activities to assess how effectively and efficiently resources are used to meet established expectations and objectives. For this reason, a growing number of state health agencies have developed performance assessment programs for the local public health agencies with which they work.[8] Performance measurement processes can also serve as the basis for performance-based contracting policies and performance-based payment systems that are designed to create incentives for public health agencies to improve the effectiveness and efficiency of their operations.[11,12]

By the same token, public health agencies that depend on external sources of funding can use performance measurement activities to demonstrate their abilities and achievements to governmental policy makers, foundations, and other entities that control the allocation of resources in public health. In this way, agencies can strengthen their ability to secure contracts, grants, governmental appropriations, and other vital resources. Performance measurement activities also can serve as the basis for professional **accreditation programs** that provide organizations with a credential signaling their compliance with identified standards of practice. Several state-based accreditation programs for local public health agencies are currently using performance measurement activities in this way, and an initiative is now underway to develop a national accreditation program for both state and local public health agencies that relies heavily on performance measurement and management approaches. If broadly disseminated, the results of accreditation and related performance measurement activities can help to raise public awareness of and knowledge about the practice of public health, ultimately leading to greater community engagement with and support for public health agencies.[2]

Informing Policy

A third reason for using performance measurement activities in public health stems from the ability to support rational policy development and resource allocation decisions. Public health organizations can use performance measurement activities to identify weaknesses and unmet needs in their operations, and then target resources to address these gaps. The resource allocation decisions informed by such measurement activities may involve funding, deployment of personnel and technology, placement of programs and clinics, and dissemination of information and technical assistance. Policy makers may use performance measurement activities to identify new ways of configuring public health delivery systems to ensure maximum coverage and to achieve operational efficiencies. Performance measures may be used to identify ways of consolidating or coordinating public health programs to pool resources and realize economies of scale. Moreover, performance measurement activities can be used to track and evaluate the effects of resource allocation and policy decisions, thereby creating a feedback mechanism to inform subsequent policy and administrative decisions. In these ways, information produced by performance measurement activities potentially allows for a more efficient and equitable allocation of limited public health resources to populations in need.

Building a Research Base for Practice

A final rationale for using performance measurement activities in public health involves the opportunities for practice-based research and scientific discovery. When rigorously implemented, performance measurement activities can provide a foundation for scientific investigations concerning the impact of a wide array of programs and interventions on public health practice.[7,13] Consistent, longitudinal performance measurement activities can allow researchers to detect how public health practice changes in response to both external and internal stimuli, including organizational changes (e.g., agency mergers, closures, or consolidations), shifts in staffing levels and composition, altered funding levels and sources, modified public health laws and regulations, and quality improvement initiatives. Such practice-based, observational studies have become the hallmark of the health outcomes research efforts carried out in medical care settings, and they have therefore fueled the development of clinical practice guidelines and the practice of evidence-based medicine in these settings.[14] The field of public health has lagged behind in comparable initiatives to develop evidence-based practice standards and guidelines, largely because the science base for public health practice has been slower to develop. Performance measurement activities can produce the information needed to fuel additional practice-based research initiatives in public health. A variety of methodological challenges must be overcome in using these observational databases for scientific investigation.[13] Nonetheless, performance measurement activities potentially create exciting opportunities for investigating the effectiveness of public health programs and policies in actual practice settings.

HISTORY OF PUBLIC HEALTH PERFORMANCE MEASUREMENT

Efforts to measure the outputs and outcomes of public health programs have occurred throughout the twentieth century (for a complete review, see the excellent analysis by Turnock and Handler).[15] The American Public Health Association (APHA) created the foundation for modern public health performance measurement through a series of studies targeted at local public health agencies from the 1920s through the 1940s (Figure 16.1).[16–22] The objectives of these efforts were twofold: developing practice standards for local public health agencies to build public health capacity across the nation, and generating comparative information on public health practice to encourage agencies to improve their performance and to mobilize public and political support for public health practice.[9,15] These objectives have remained paramount for virtually all of the public health performance measurement activities that followed these early efforts.[7,23]

The APHA's initiatives relied on voluntary participation by public health agencies, and most were based wholly on quantitative measures of the outputs produced by these agencies, such as the number of immunizations administered or the number of prenatal home visits delivered. In the initial efforts, measures were collected through site visits made to participating agencies by appraisers. Later, when broad participation became the focus, measures were collected using a self-assessment appraisal form completed by agency administrators. A numerical scoring process was devised to create an aggregate rating of each agency's performance, and ratings were made available to agencies, government officials, and the public to support comparisons across agencies. The APHA's performance measurement instrument was eventually expanded to include some measures of public health outcomes, such as statistics on infant mortality and motor vehicle deaths.[19,21] In the expanded

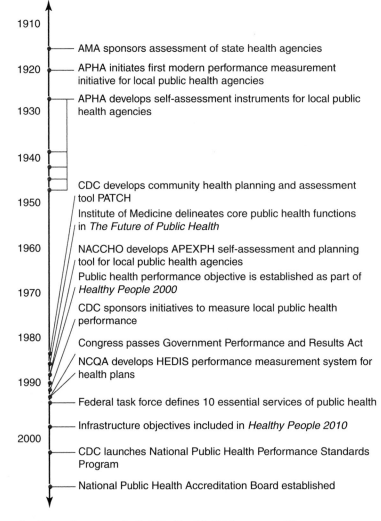

1910

— AMA sponsors assessment of state health agencies

1920 — APHA initiates first modern performance measurement
initiative for local public health agencies

APHA develops self-assessment instruments for local public
1930   health agencies

1940

CDC develops community health planning and assessment
1950   tool PATCH

Institute of Medicine delineates core public health functions
in *The Future of Public Health*

1960   NACCHO develops APEXPH self-assessment and planning
tool for local public health agencies

Public health performance objective is established as part of
1970   *Healthy People 2000*

CDC sponsors initiatives to measure local public health
performance

1980   Congress passes Government Performance and Results Act

NCQA develops HEDIS performance measurement system for
health plans

1990

Federal task force defines 10 essential services of public health

Infrastructure objectives included in *Healthy People 2010*

2000

CDC launches National Public Health Performance Standards
Program

National Public Health Accreditation Board established

Figure 16.1. Historical Developments in Public Health Performance Management

SOURCE: Delmar Cengage Learning.

instrument, performance scores were summarized by size and type of agency to facilitate comparisons among agencies of similar structure. On the whole, public health administrators found these early performance measurement activities to be helpful in managing their programs and organizations.[15] Nonetheless, most of these activities were discontinued in the 1950s as the APHA's interests turned to other issues.[9]

Efforts to measure the performance of state public health agencies have occurred less frequently than those focusing on the local level. The earliest state-level initiative, sponsored by the American Medical Association (AMA) in 1914, relied on a quantitative scoring system that reflected the scope of services provided by state health agencies and the extent of their efforts to develop local public health units.[15,24] Much later, the Association of

State and Territorial Health Officials (ASTHO) and the Public Health Foundation developed a national reporting system that tracked annual trends in state health agency expenditures and services throughout much of the 1970s and 1980s.[9] These efforts supported basic comparisons of state public health infrastructure, but they lacked the detailed and quantitative measures of outputs and outcomes that would be necessary for a more complete analysis of public health capacity and performance.

The early approaches to public health performance measurement were informed by a parallel set of activities developing within the field of medical care. In 1950, Dr. Avidis Donabedian developed a framework for assessing quality of care in medical care settings that focused on three basic domains: (1) measures of structure or capacity, including the physical, human, financial, and technological resources available to deliver care within the setting; (2) measures of process, which reflect the activities undertaken by health professionals to deliver services; and (3) measures of outcome, which reflect the health and well-being of patients treated within the setting. This general framework has become widely used in both medical care and public health assessment initiatives.

A Second Generation of Measurement

The Institute of Medicine's (IOM) 1988 study of the nation's public health system sparked a revival of interest in and support for performance measurement in public health.[25] This renewed interest was fueled not only by the alarming gaps in public health capacity profiled in the report but also by the report's delineation of the concept of "**core public health functions.**"[26] These concepts provided public health researchers and practitioners with a simple and intuitive framework for describing the scope of public health activity, and a framework from which performance measures and performance standards could be derived. IOM's report also raised awareness about elements of organizational capacity that support and inform the delivery of specific public health programs and services, such as surveillance

and assessment, coalition-building, advocacy, public education, policy development, planning and priority setting. As a consequence, the performance measurement activities that developed subsequent to the IOM's report were more reflective of these basic public health activities than previous efforts.[9]

Soon after publication of the 1988 IOM report, the United States Public Health Service established Objective 8.14 as one of its national health objectives for the year 2000, which called for 90 percent of the United States population to be served by a local health department that effectively carries out the core functions of public health.[27] In response to this objective, the United States Centers for Disease Control and Prevention (CDC) sponsored an array of research and development efforts during the 1990s designed to identify the specific practice elements that comprise core public health functions and to develop ways of measuring the extent to which these elements are performed by local public health agencies.

A variety of self-assessment tools and planning protocols were developed during this period to assist public health agencies in improving their performance, many of which used measures of public health processes, outputs, and outcomes to evaluate performance.

This period was also eventful in that there were a number of tools developed to assist communities with community health assessment and health improvement planning. These covered structural features, process and outcomes. One of the firsts was the Planned Approach to Community Health (PATCH), primarily designed by the CDC to assist state health departments in helping communities deal with chronic disease prevention.[28]

The use of the Health People series as a planning and assessment tool was also an important development. The APHA used the *Healthy People 2000* document[29] to establish *Health Communities 2000: Model Standards*. This used the specific objectives and focus areas of Healthy People to allow communities to set their own set of planning targets.

The third major assessment and planning system was developed by the National Association of City and County Health Officials (NACCHO), with support from the CDC, in the early 1990s. This was the *Assessment Protocol for Excellence in Public Health (APEX/PH)*. APEX had three parts that were contained in a workbook.[30] The first part allowed the local health department to ascertain its own capacity to undertake a community health assessment and improvement project. The second part was a community health assessment project, with a set of exercises designed to identify community health needs based on objective information, such as vital statistics, and the community's assessment of their problems. The third part focused on developing solutions to the problems outlined in part two of the program.

All of these tools were actively used during the 90s, however, they fell into more disuse as a new tool became the more commonly used. This new tool was Mobilizing for Action through Planning and Partnerships (MAPP).[31,32] All of these tools are described in more detail in Chapter 12.

The public health assessment and planning tools developed during this period were designed to stimulate improvements in performance within individual public health organizations. Building on these efforts, the CDC sponsored a series of research initiatives during the 1990s to measure and compare performance of core public health functions across the nation's local public health systems to track progress toward Objective 8.14 of *Healthy People 2000*. These initiatives defined **public health systems** broadly to include the full

constellation of organizations that contribute to the performance of essential public health services for a defined community or population. Several of these initiatives were designed around a set of 10 public health practices, each of which was derived from one of the IOM's 3 public health functions by a workgroup convened by the CDC.[33] All of these initiatives relied on measures of public health outputs or processes, such as whether the local population is surveyed routinely for behavioral risk factors, or whether adverse health events are investigated on a timely basis.

One group of studies focused specifically on activities performed by local governmental public health agencies.[34–38] A second group of studies used measures that reflected the activities performed not only by local public health agencies but also those performed by the range of other organizations that potentially contribute to public health activities at the local level.[39–41] Ultimately, indicators from the two groups of studies were combined into a merged set of performance measures and used in several national surveys of local public health performance.[42] Interestingly, all of the national performance measurement studies undertaken during the early and mid-1990s produced similar results indicating that, on average, about half of the activities regarded as important elements of public health practice were performed at the local level (Table 16.1).[15] A more recent study

Table 16.1. Estimates of Local Public Health Performance Produced by Recent Studies

Study	Year	Population/Sample size	Estimate
NACCHO	1990	All U.S. agencies	50%
NACCHO	1992–1993	All U.S. agencies	46%
Miller et al.	1992	Nonrandom selection of local jurisdictions	57%
Turnock et al.	1993	All U.S. agencies	50%
Richards et al.	1993	All local jurisdictions in 6 states	56%
Halverson et al.	1992–1993	Nonrandom selection of local jurisdictions	51%
Rohrer et al.	1995	All Iowa county agencies	61%
Turnock et al.	1994	All U.S. agencies	56%
Mays et al.	1998	All U.S. jurisdictions with at least 100,000 residents	64%
Mays et al.	2006	All U.S. jurisdictions with at least 100,000 residents	70%

SOURCE: Turnock BJ, Handler AS. From measuring to improving public health practice. *Annu Rev Public Health.* 1997;18:261–282.

suggested that performance levels increased moderately between 1998 and 2006, at least among large public health jurisdictions serving 100,000 or more residents.

Individual states also became active in implementing performance measurement activities for their affiliated local public health agencies during the 1990s. In some cases, these activities were developed in response to the demands of state legislatures and other policy makers for greater accountability in the use of public funds. In other cases, these efforts were undertaken as strategies to enhance the capacity of state and local public health delivery systems after weaknesses were exposed by the 1988 IOM report. A 1998 survey of the nation's state health agencies revealed that 22 states currently had a local public health performance measurement process in place, and another 13 states were in the process of developing such a process.[8] More recent studies suggest that that a large majority of state health agencies are now using some form of performance measurement activity regularly with their local public health agencies. However, states vary widely in their approaches to performance measurement and in their strategies for using results in policy and administrative decision making.

Public and Private Sector Stimuli

The movement toward performance measurement in public health was fueled during the 1990s by federal efforts to address concerns about governmental inefficiency and accountability by developing new systems to monitor the activities and results of federal programs. In 1993, Congress passed the Government Performance and Results Act, which required federal agencies to develop systems for measuring the performance of all federally funded programs. In response to this legislation, the United States Department of Health and Human Services (HHS) proposed the creation of Performance Partnership Grants that would require all organizations receiving federal health funds to collect and report performance measures as a means of demonstrating progress toward established

goals. One of the most visible performance measurement processes developed under this policy was the system developed and implemented for state programs funded under the Maternal and Child Health Services Block Grant,[43] which continues to operate successfully today. The National Research Council identified an extensive set of performance measures and data sources that could be used for a wide array of programs in public health, mental health, and substance abuse.[44]

Public health performance measurement activities were also stimulated and informed during the 1990s by a variety of private-sector initiatives to measure and improve the performance of health care providers, building on the earlier work of Donabedian. One of the most visible initiatives has been the Health Plan Employer Data and Information Set (HEDIS), a voluntary performance measurement system developed for health plans in 1991 by a coalition of large health care purchasers that eventually formed the National Committee for Quality Assurance (NCQA). Designed to inform purchasing decisions, the NCQA collects and compares annual measures of health plan performance in areas such as health care effectiveness, accessibility, utilization, cost, and patient satisfaction. The HEDIS system includes detailed standards for data collection, measurement, and auditing that participating plans were required to meet.[45] The HEDIS system has been administered by the NCQA since 1992 and is used as part of the NCQA's accreditation program for health plans.

Another major performance measurement initiative was launched by the Joint Commission on Accreditation of Healthcare Organizations (JCAHO) in 1996 to enhance its accreditation process for hospitals and other health care facilities. Known initially as Project ORYX, the JCAHO's initiative allows participating organizations some flexibility in the types of measures that are used to track their performance. In response to the proliferation of performance measurement activities in health care, several initiatives formed to develop consensus around core sets of measures and to facilitate the dissemination and use of these measures by health care providers, consumers, and purchasers. As the most prominent example, the

National Forum for Health Care Quality Measurement and Reporting was launched in 1999 to develop a coordinated national strategy for performance measurement among health care institutions in the public and private sectors.[46]

IOM provided a major boost to performance measurement activities in medical care with the publication of two landmark studies documenting large gaps and disparities in the quality and safety of health care that most American residents receive: the 1999 report *Crossing the Quality Chasm* and the 2001 report To *Err is Human*. These reports established a framework for measuring performance in health care based on the six constructs of safety, effectiveness, timeliness, efficiency, equity, and patient-centeredness. The IOM reports also ushered in an era of widespread experimentation with programs that collect and publicly report quality-of-care measures for hospitals, physicians, nursing homes, and other health care providers—with both private insurers and public programs such as Medicare and Medicaid sponsoring such activities. More recently, public and private-sector efforts have begun to incorporate performance measures into payment methodologies via "pay-for-performance" programs designed to create financial incentives for quality improvement. Most of these contemporary applications of performance measurement in health care focus on measuring provider adherence to evidence-based clinical practices and guidelines that are strongly linked to improved patient outcomes. As such, these applications focus heavily on the first three of the IOM performance domains: safety, effectiveness, and timeliness of care.

Developing Performance Standards in Public Health

Performance measurement activities have continued to evolve in the public health field as well. Most recently, the CDC and a collection of national public health organizations launched the National Public Health Performance Standards Program in 2002, which includes a set of performance standards for local and state public health systems along with measures and surveillance instruments

that track progress relative to these standards.[7] These standards—which represent expert opinions of activities and practices that high-performing public health systems should follow—were developed through consensus group processes involving a broad cross-section of public health practitioners and researchers. The program is based on the voluntary participation of public health organizations, includes separate but related sets of performance standards and measurement instruments for local public health systems, state public health systems, and public health governing boards. Performance standards and measures are specified at the level of the public health system—which comprises the full range of public and private organizations that contribute to public health—rather than at the level of the individual public health agency. This means that performance standards can be achieved through the actions of the official public health agency and through the actions of other public and private organizations within the system. Each performance standard is linked to one of the **10 Essential Public Health Services** identified by a workgroup of major public health stakeholders in 1994.[47] Participating public health agencies convene a group of major public health stakeholders within their jurisdiction to complete the performance self-assessment instrument and submit their results to the national program for scoring and comparative reporting. As of 2007, more than 10 states and 600 local public health agencies had participated in the program.

Based in part on these performance standards, a series of national health objectives related to public health infrastructure have been included in the *Healthy People 2010* planning document developed by the United States Dept. of HHS.[48] A total of 17 infrastructure objectives were developed, including those related to public health data and information systems, the public health workforce, public health organizations, public health resources, and prevention research. Progress toward these objectives is monitored through a variety of national data sources including data collected through the CDC's National Public Health Performance Standards Program (Table 16.2).

Table 16.2. Public Health Infrastructure Objectives Included in *Healthy People 2010*

Goal: Ensure that federal, tribal, state, and local health agencies have the infrastructure to provide essential public health services effectively.

Objective
Data and Information Systems

23-1   Increase the proportion of tribal, state, and local public health agencies that provide Internet and e-mail access for at least 75 percent of their employees and that teach employees to use the Internet and other electronic information systems to apply data and information to public health practice.

23-2   Increase the proportion of federal, tribal, state, and local health agencies that have made information available to the public in the past year on the Leading Health Indicators, Health Status Indicators, and Priority Data Needs.

23-3   Increase the proportion of all major national, state, and local health data systems that use geocoding to promote nation-wide use of geographic information systems (GIS) at all levels.

23-4   Increase the proportion of population-based *Healthy People 2010* objectives for which national data are available for all population groups identified for the objective.

23-5   Increase the proportion of Leading Health Indicators, Health Status Indicators, and Priority Data Needs for which data—especially for select populations—are available at the tribal, state, and local levels.

23-6   Increase the proportion of *Healthy People 2010* objectives that are tracked regularly at the national level.

23-7   Increase the proportion of *Healthy People 2010* objectives for which national data are released within 1 year of the end of data collection.

Workforce

23-8   Increase the proportion of federal, tribal, state, and local agencies that incorporate specific competencies in the essential public health services into personnel systems.

23-9   Increase the proportion of schools for public health workers that integrate into their curricula specific content to develop competency in the essential public health services.

23-10 Increase the proportion of federal, tribal, state, and local public health agencies that provide continuing education to develop competency in essential public health services for their employees.

Public Health Organizations

23-11 Increase the proportion of state and local public health agencies that meet national performance standards for essential public health services.

23-12 Increase the proportion of tribes, states, and the District of Columbia that have a health improvement plan and increase the proportion of local jurisdictions that have a health improvement plan linked with their state plan.

23-13 Increase the proportion of tribal, state, and local health agencies that provide or assure comprehensive laboratory services to support essential public health services.

23-14 Increase the proportion of tribal, state, and local public health agencies that provide or assure comprehensive epidemiology services to support essential public health services.

23-15 Increase the proportion of federal, tribal, state, and local jurisdictions that review and evaluate the extent to which their statutes, ordinances, and bylaws assure the delivery of essential public health services.

23-16 Increase the proportion of federal, tribal, state, and local public health agencies that gather accurate data on public health expenditures, categorized by essential public health service.

23-17 Increase the proportion of federal, tribal, state, and local public health agencies that conduct or collaborate on population-based prevention research.

SOURCE: U.S. Department of Health and Human Services. *Healthy People 2010: Conference Edition.* Washington, DC: U.S. Dept of Health and Human Services; 2000.

Objective 23-11 directly addresses the ability of the program to engage the nation's public health organizations performance measurement and improvement initiatives, by calling for an increase in "the proportion of state and local public health agencies that meet national performance standards for essential public health services."[48]

From Measuring to Managing Public Health Performance

Performance measures and standards provide important tools for improving public health practice, but by themselves, these tools will not assure changes in practice. Successful performance improvement is likely to hinge on how these tools are used in the day-to-day management of public health agencies and their partner organizations. Recognizing this fact, a national collaborative of public health practitioners and evaluators formed in 1999 to identify successful models for using these tools to improve organizational performance. The Performance Management Collaborative formed as part of the larger *Turning Point Initiative*, an effort sponsored by the Robert Wood Johnson Foundation to strengthen public health system capacity. The collaborative defined performance management as follows:

> Performance management is the practice of actively using performance data to improve

the public's health. This practice involves strategic use of performance measures and standards to establish performance targets and goals, to prioritize and allocate resources, to inform managers about needed adjustments or changes in policy or program directions to meet goals, to frame reports on the success in meeting performance goals, and to improve the quality of public health practice.[49]

The collaborative identified four critical components of a successful performance management system (Figure 16.2):

1. Creating performance standards for public health organizations and systems, including targets and goals and relevant indicators to improve public health practice

2. Developing indicators and collecting measures of the extent to which performance standards are met

3. Documenting and reporting progress over time in meeting performance standards and targets, and sharing this information with relevant stakeholders and the public through feedback mechanisms

4. Implementing processes to improve public health policies, programs, and infrastructure based on performance standards, measurements, and reports

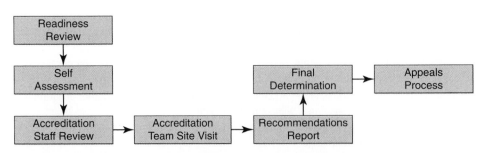

Figure 16.2. Conformity Assessment Process for an Accreditation Program
SOURCE: Exploring Accreditation Steering Committee.

Through the collaborative, the participating states worked actively to implement these components in their respective public health systems and document both facilitators and barriers to implementation. Based on this work, the collaborative identified an inventory of strategies and resources that have proven useful to implementation, including partnership development, communication strategies, information systems development, and managerial processes.[49]

The Move to Accreditation

Several state health agencies have taken their performance measurement activities to the next level by developing formal accreditation programs for local public health agencies that require agencies to document compliance with standards involving key organizational capacities and processes to achieve status as an accredited institution. These existing programs have embedded performance measurement as a key component of the accreditation process, although the specific measures and methods used vary widely across states (refer to Figure 16.2). Some accreditation programs require organizations to collect and submit a standard set of performance measures to the accrediting body as part of a readiness review or self-assessment component of the accreditation process. Other programs have trained assessment staff collect performance measures from organizations during a site-visit component of the process. Still other programs establish accreditation standards that specify how organizations are expected to carry out performance measurement activities within their organizations, including the types of measures used, the frequency of measurement, and the dissemination and improvement processes implemented. Organizations seeking accreditation are then required to document the extent to which they conform to established standards.

An initiative is now underway to develop a nationwide, voluntary accreditation program for state and local public health agencies. The processes and criteria for this national program have yet to be finalized, but they are likely to include a significant role for performance measurement and reporting activities. As these accreditation programs continue to develop, they are likely to generate even greater demand for valid and reliable performance measurement processes that apply to public health organizations. Moreover, these programs are likely to become powerful motivating forces for public health agencies to engage in performance measurement activities as essential steps in preparing for, obtaining, and maintaining their accreditation status.

CONCEPTUAL AND METHODOLOGICAL ISSUES IN PERFORMANCE MEASUREMENT

A variety of measurement issues have come to light during the nation's 80-year experiment with performance measurement activities in public health. These issues include both conceptual problems and methodological challenges that must be considered implicitly or explicitly when designing, managing, or participating in a performance measurement process. Key among these issues are the following:

- The units of measurement (whose performance is measured, and who is accountable for this performance)
- The scope of activity (what domains of performance should be examined)
- The indicators of performance (what activities and practices constitute a high-performing agency or system)
- Performance measures and data (how to obtain reliable and valid information on performance)
- Methods for comparing and evaluating performance (how to differentiate high and low performers)[13,50]

Each of these issues is explored in detail in the following sections.

Unit of Analysis

Public health activities are carried out through an array of important actors and instruments, all of which can be examined through the lens of performance measurement. It is possible to measure and evaluate performance at the level of the individual, the team, the program or division, the organization, and various multi-institutional settings. The appropriate unit of analysis is contingent on the objectives of the performance measurement activity. If the primary goal is to improve performance within a specific program or organization, then measurement should focus on the intraorganizational elements that determine this performance.

A variety of management tools and processes now exist for assessing the function and performance of individuals and teams within an organization, as well as for creating feedback mechanisms and incentive systems to improve performance.[51] The application of such tools is context-specific—highly contingent on the structure and size of the institution, the scope and scale of its production processes, and the composition of its workforce. Alternatively, if the overarching goal of the performance measurement activity is to improve performance on a large (e.g., state or national) scale, it is often desirable to focus measurement activities at the organizational and multiorganizational levels. The rationale for this choice is that performance measurement at these higher levels motivates organizations to undertake interorganizational improvement efforts in ways that are appropriate to their specific institutional contexts.[4,52]

Public health activities are performed by a variety of organizations operating in different institutional, governmental, and geographic settings. Most of the large-scale public health performance measurement activities carried out to date have focused on the activities performed by governmental public health agencies at the local and state levels. In most United States settings, these agencies assume primary responsibility for managing the programs and resources that are dedicated to improving population health. Many important public health activities, however, are carried out by other public and private organizations—either alone or in partnership with governmental public health agencies.[8,41] Performance measures that do not account for these outside contributions may provide an incomplete or biased representation of public health capacity in some settings. Consequently, recent initiatives have focused on measuring performance at the level of the public health system, which is defined as the collection of public and private institutions that contribute to public health for a given population or geographic area.[7,39,41] The appropriate choice between agency-level and systems-level measures ultimately depends on the overall purpose of the performance measurement activity. Agency-level measures may be appropriate for activities that are concerned exclusively with the structure and operation of governmental public health agencies, independent of other actors within the public health system.

To measure performance at the system level, it is first necessary to identify the common population that this system serves. For purposes of epidemiological investigation, populations can be defined in myriad ways, such as by geographic area of residence, sociodemographic characteristics, health status, or characteristics associated with disease risk. For purposes of public health performance measurement, however, the population of interest is typically defined by the geopolitical jurisdiction to which governmental public health agencies are accountable, most often a county, city, or multicounty district.[39] Although these agencies do not directly perform all of the public health activities that occur within their jurisdictions, they are ultimately accountable for these activities (or lack of activities) and their effects on population health. Consequently, public health performance measurement activities typically focus on the jurisdictions served by local and state public health agencies.

Choosing the unit of analysis for a performance measurement process has important implications for the downstream activities of developing specific measures of performance and collecting data for these measures. Measuring the activities undertaken by governmental public health agencies is often straightforward compared to the task of measuring activities undertaken by a loose collection of public and private institutions that comprise a public health system. No single entity within the system is likely to have full and unbiased knowledge about the public health activities performed by all contributing institutions. At the same time, it may not be feasible to collect information from all of the institutions that potentially contribute to public health activities for a given population. For these reasons, each unit of analysis may entail unique sources of bias and measurement error. The choice of unit of analysis must be made with regard to not only the purposes of the performance measurement activity but also to the inherent trade-offs among feasibility, cost, bias, and precision.[13] These issues are revisited in the discussion on measuring indicators of performance.

Scope of Activity

Public health performance is inherently a multidimensional construct because public health organizations and systems do not produce a single product or service.[13] An essential early step in the performance measurement process is to identify the scope of activities that should be performed by the organizations or systems under study. These activities represent general domains of performance for which specific measures and indicators will be developed. These domains should clearly reflect the overall mission, goals, and objectives of the public health programs, organizations, or systems to be covered by the performance measurement system.[4] If the performance measurement process is designed to enhance accountability and outcomes for a specific public health program or funding stream, as is the case for the United States Maternal and Child Health Services Block Grant, these goals and objectives may be relatively narrow and well defined in scope. If, however, the measurement process is designed to improve accountability and outcomes among public health organizations and systems more generally, as is the case for the CDC's National Public Health Performance

Standards Program and many state-level measurement activities, then a broader range of goals and objectives may be required.

In most cases, performance domains are defined to reflect an ideal or expected scope of performance rather than the actual scope of performance, so that measurement initiatives can be used to track progress toward expectations and goals.[51] It is also desirable for performance measurement systems to use a relatively limited number of performance domains, so that the information produced by these systems can be readily understood by public health practitioners, and so that this information creates clear and unambiguous incentives for performance improvement.[4] Nevertheless, performance measurement systems should cover the full scope of activities needed to achieve the overall mission and goals of public health programs, organizations, and systems under study.

The appropriate domains of performance in the field of public health are those activities that are regarded as core elements of practice because of their utility in protecting and improving population health. Perceptions about these core elements may vary over time and across different practice settings; however, several large-scale efforts have been undertaken in recent years to define the ideal scope of activity for public health practice. These efforts have proven very useful in identifying the domains of performance for many current performance measurement activities in public health.

Perhaps the best-known conceptual model of public health practice is the one developed in the IOM's 1988 report on public health.[25] This model consists of three core functions of public health—assessment, policy development, and assurance—to be carried out by public health organizations at every level of practice. The primary limitation of this model for performance measurement activities is its lack of specificity. Each of the core functions potentially encompasses a broad scope of activities and services. To address this limitation, the CDC convened a panel of experts in 1992 to identify a set of specific public health activities that were viewed as components of the core functions defined by the IOM. The result of this effort was a set of 10 public health practices, each of which was linked with one of the core functions.[33] These practices were used as the domains of performance in several large-scale public health performance measurement initiatives conducted at the local level during the 1990s.[37–41]

A more recent model of public health practice was developed by a workgroup convened by the United States Dept. of HHS as part of the national health care reform debates in 1994. This panel of experts identified 10 essential public health services that were considered core components of practice (see Chapter 1).[47] The elements of this model were conceptually similar to the CDC's 10 public health practices and the IOM's core functions, although these elements did not correspond exactly with components of the earlier models. The essential services framework has been used to track public health expenditures in states and localities, and to monitor state expenditures under the federal Maternal and Child Health Services Block Grant.[53] More recently, this framework was used to define domains of performance for the CDC's National Public Health Performance Standards Program described earlier in this chapter.

Another effort to define the scope of public health practice was initiated by the World Health Organization (WHO) in 1997, drawing on the knowledge and experiences of an international collection of public health experts.[54] Using a Delphi process with 145 public health administrators, educators, researchers, and practitioners, the WHO study identified and prioritized a list of 37 essential public health functions that fell within 9 general categories:

- Prevention, surveillance, and control of communicable and noncommunicable diseases
- Monitoring the health situation (health status, determinants, risks, and interventions)
- Health promotion
- Occupational health
- Protecting the environment
- Public health legislation and regulations
- Public health management

- Specific public health services (school health, emergency services, and laboratory services)
- Personal health care for vulnerable and high-risk populations

The conceptual models developed by IOM, CDC, DHHS, and WHO are all quite consistent with each other, but it is unlikely that any one of them represents the final word for defining the complex role of public health in modern society.[26] What matters most for the purposes of performance measurement is not the specific framework used to develop a measurement strategy, but rather the ability to define the overarching mission, objectives, and activities of public health in clear and measurable terms. Various conceptual models can be helpful in accomplishing this task.

Performance Indicators

Another important issue for performance measurement activities involves selection of the specific indicators that are used to measure performance in each domain of activity. Performance indicators can generally be classified into one of three basic types based on Donabedian's framework for assessing quality and performance: indicators of structure or capacity, indicators of processes or outputs, and indicators of outcomes.[55] First, **structural indicators** of public health performance reflect the physical, human, financial, and technological resources used to perform public health activities. Examples of structural indicators in the field of public health practice include the amount and type of human resources available for public health activities; the amount and sources of funding available; the number and types of organizations involved in the public health system; the data, information, and communication systems available to the public health system; and the statutory authority and legal powers granted to governmental public health agencies.

Second, **process indicators** reflect the specific activities performed and outputs produced by the public health system. Examples in public health may include the range of clinical and population-based services provided by public health organizations (e.g., immunizations, screening services, health education programs); the processes used for community health needs assessment and priority setting; and the activities performed for disease surveillance and epidemiological investigation (e.g., frequency, coverage, data collection methods, and scope of diseases included). Ideally, process indicators should reflect activities that, if performed according to expectations, produce desired outcomes such as improvements in health status and reductions in disease and injury risk. In the field of medical care, process indicators often reflect the extent to which evidence-based clinical guidelines and protocols are followed by health care providers, such as the proportion of patients hospitalized for acute myocardial infarction who received aspirin within 24 hours of admission.[56] In the field of public health, the evidence-based guidelines and recommendations such as those contained in the CDC's *Guide to Community Preventive Services* may provide a frame of reference for developing process indicators for performance measurement activities.[57]

Finally, **outcome indicators** capture the effects of public health activities on population(s) of interest. Examples include mortality rates attributable to conditions that can be prevented or controlled through public health measures; incidence rates for preventable diseases and health conditions; and prevalence of behavioral risk factors such as smoking, unsafe sexual activity, physical inactivity, and dependence on alcohol and other drugs that can lead to poor health status. Outcome indicators can also be specified in terms of economic effects (e.g., the costs associated with treating preventable diseases), quality-of-life measures, and measures of public satisfaction or dissatisfaction with public health activities and services.

Effective performance indicators in public health share a number of important attributes. First, indicators should be closely linked to a performance domain or program objective of interest, such as one of the 3 public health core functions identified by the IOM, or one of the 10 Essential Public Health Services identified by the United States

Department of HHS.[4] Indicators having a weak or ambiguous association with performance domains and program objectives may provide very little insight about how well an organization or system carries out its public health responsibilities. In many cases, public health program and policy objectives are defined in terms of population health status goals such as those established in *Healthy People 2010* (e.g., improvements in infant mortality, reductions in the incidence of infectious diseases). For this reason, outcome indicators of performance often have the strongest empirical association with program and policy objectives. Unfortunately, the scientific evidence concerning the association between structural or process indicators of performance and population health status is often quite limited. In these cases, good performance indicators should at least be consistent with expert opinions about the activities and elements that constitute effective public health practice. The indicators and domains used for performance measurement purposes should therefore evolve as standards of public health practice change over time and as new evidence about public health impact becomes available.[13]

Good indicators should also reflect a process or condition that is substantially within the control or influence of the public health organizations under study. This trait helps ensure that indicators are sensitive to changes in public health performance over time and across different organizations or systems (**measurement sensitivity**). This trait also helps ensure that indicators can be used to identify public health performance and distinguish such performance from other phenomena that may independently influence population health (**measurement specificity**). For these reasons, structure and process indicators are used more frequently than outcome indicators in public health performance measurement activities. Population-based health outcome indicators (e.g., statistics on mortality and disease incidence) are influenced by many factors outside the immediate control of the public health system, such as population demographics and mobility patterns, and socioeconomic conditions. Consequently, in some cases, these measures may not be sufficiently sensitive or specific to public health interventions to merit using them for performance measurement purposes. In other cases, it may be possible to adjust these measures using statistical methods to make them suitable indicators of public health performance. Some outcome indicators may also pose problems for performance measurement applications because of the long time lag that may be required for public health activities to exert a measurable impact on the indicator. Mortality statistics, for example, often present this problem. In these cases, process indicators or intermediate outcome measures may be preferred to outcome measures.

Finally, good performance indicators can detect meaningful variation across organizations or jurisdictions and across time. Indicators that are likely to show little variation in the population of interest may not be helpful in distinguishing high-performing and low-performing organizations or systems. Nonetheless, for some applications, it may be useful to include indicators of rare but important events that provide strong evidence of high or low performance. Such sentinel events may include outbreaks of infectious diseases or other public health emergencies that are amenable to prevention and containment by the public health system.

Public health performance indicators can be developed at various levels of detail to measure progress toward program goals and objectives, to achieve the desired attributes of measurement sensitivity and specificity, and to address the constraints of feasibility and cost in data collection. In some cases, indicators are defined around specific health risks and populations at risk, such as the proportion of children age two and younger who are up-to-date on immunizations for vaccine-preventable diseases. Such detailed indicators are often used to track progress toward specific program or policy objectives, such as those specified in the *Healthy People 2010* set of national health objectives.[27] The National Research Council identified a series of such population-specific and disease-specific indicators suitable for use in public health performance monitoring activities (Table 16.3).[4]

In other cases, it may be sufficient to use indicators that capture only general categories of activity, such as whether or not the local public health system surveys the population for behavioral risk factors at least every three years. These types of indicators were used in several performance measurement systems developed during the 1990s to measure progress toward the more generic *Healthy People 2000* objective of increasing the proportion of the population served by a local health department that effectively carries out core public health functions (Table 16.4).[37–42] Generic indicators may be easier to derive from broad program and policy objectives, but they may also be more difficult to measure reliably due to heterogeneity in how such indicators are interpreted by respondents.

Methods for Measuring Performance

The utility of any performance measurement system hinges on its ability to obtain valid and reliable measures of performance indicators. Valid measures capture the information that is expected and intended for the purposes of evaluation and comparison.[58] Reliable measures reflect performance consistently across organizations and over time, thereby enabling meaningful comparisons. Some level of measurement error is unavoidable in most practical applications, but systematic problems with measurement reliability can undermine the utility of the measures that are produced. A number of alternative measurement strategies are possible for collecting useful information about public health performance. Each of these strategies requires a different amount of time and resources to implement, and each entails a different mix of strengths and weaknesses with respect to measurement validity and reliability.[50] Issues of feasibility, validity, and reliability must be balanced carefully when selecting and using public health performance measures.

Self-Assessment Instruments

Most of the performance measurement initiatives that have occurred to date in public health have relied on measures that are self-assessed and self-reported by public health organizations. That is,

Table 16.3. Health Performance Indicators Identified by the National Research Council

Tobacco
- Percentage of (a) persons age 18–24 and (b) persons age 25 and older currently smoking tobacco
- Percentage of persons age 14–17 (grades 9–12) currently smoking tobacco
- Percentage of women who gave birth in the past year and reported smoking tobacco during pregnancy
- Percentage of employed adults whose workplace has an official policy that bans smoking

Nutrition
- Percentage of persons age 18 and older who eat five or more servings of fruit and vegetables per day
- Percentage of persons age 14–17 (grades 9–12) who eat five or more servings of fruit and vegetables per day
- Percentage of persons age 18 and older who are 20 percent or more above optimal body mass index

Exercise
- Percentage of persons age 18 and older who do not engage in physical activity or exercise
- Percentage of persons age 14–17 (grades 9–12) who do not engage in physical activity or exercise

Preventive Screenings and Tests
- Percentage of persons age 18 and older who had their blood pressure checked within the past 2 years
- Percentage of women age 45 and older and men age 35 and older who had their cholesterol checked within the past 5 years
- Percentage of women age 50 and older who received a mammogram within the past 2 years
- Percentage of adults age 50 and older who had a fecal occult blood test within the past 12 months or a flexible sigmoidoscopy within the past 5 years
- Percentage of women age 18 and older who received a Pap smear within the past 3 years
- Percentage of persons with diabetes who had HbA1C checked within the past 12 months
- Percentage of persons with diabetes who had a health professional examine their feet at least once within the past 12 months
- Percentage of persons with diabetes who received a dilated eye exam within the past 12 months

Infectious Diseases
- Incidence rates of selected STDs
- Incidence rates of HIV infection
- Prevalence rates of selected STDs
- Prevalence rates of HIV infection
- Consumer satisfaction with STD, HIV, and tuberculosis treatment programs
- Rates of sexual activity among adolescents age 14–17
- Rates of sexual activity with multiple sex partners among people age 18 and older
- Rates of condom use during last episode of sexual intercourse among sexually active adolescents age 14–17
- Rates of condom use during last episode of sexual intercourse among sexually active adolescents age 18 and older with multiple sex partners
- Rates of condom use during last episode of sexual intercourse among men having sex with men
- Rates of injection drug use among adolescents and adults
- Completion rates of treatment for STDs, HIV infection, and tuberculosis

Immunization
- Reported incidence rate of representative vaccine-preventable diseases
- Age-appropriate vaccination rates for target age groups (children age 2 years; children entering school at approximately 5 years of age; and adults age 65 years and older) for each major vaccine group

SOURCE: Perrin EB, Koshel JJ. *Assessment of Performance Measures for Public Health, Substance Abuse, and Mental Health.* Washington, DC: National Academy Press; 1997.

Table 16.4. Twenty Indicators of Local Public Health Performance

Assessment

1. In your jurisdiction, is there a community needs assessment process that systematically describes the prevailing health status in the community?
2. In the past three years in your jurisdiction, has the local public health agency surveyed the population for behavioral risk factors?
3. In your jurisdiction, are timely investigations of adverse health events conducted on an ongoing basis, including communicable disease outbreaks and environmental health hazards?
4. Are the necessary laboratory services available to the local public health agency to support investigations of adverse health events and meet routine diagnostic and surveillance needs?
5. In your jurisdiction, has an analysis been completed of the determinants of and contributing factors to priority health needs, the adequacy of existing health resources, and the population groups most effected?
6. In the past three years in your jurisdiction, has the local public health agency conducted an analysis of age-specific participation in preventive and screening services?

Policy Development

7. In your jurisdiction, is there a network of support and communication relationships that includes health-related organizations, the media, and the general public?
8. In the past year in your jurisdiction, has there been a formal attempt by the local public health agency to inform elected officials about the potential public health impact of decisions under their consideration?
9. In your local public health agency, has there been a prioritization of the community health needs that have been identified from a community needs assessment?
10. In the past three years in your jurisdiction, has the local public health agency implemented community health initiatives consistent with established priorities?
11. In your jurisdiction, has a community health action plan been developed with community participation to address priority community health needs?
12. In the past three years in your jurisdiction, has the local public health agency developed plans to allocate resources in a manner consistent with community health action plans?

Assurance

13. In your jurisdiction, have resources been deployed as necessary to address priority health needs identified in a community health needs assessment?
14. In the past three years in your jurisdiction, has the local public health agency conducted an organizational self-assessment?
15. In your jurisdiction, are age-specific priority health needs effectively addressed through the provision of or linkage to appropriate services?
16. In your jurisdiction, have there been regular evaluations of the effects of public health services on community health status?
17. In the past three years in your jurisdiction, has the local public health agency used professionally recognized process and outcome measures to monitor programs and to redirect resources as appropriate?
18. In your jurisdiction, is the public regularly provided with information about current health status, health care needs, positive health behaviors, and health care policy issues?
19. In the past year in your jurisdiction, has the local public health agency provided reported to the media on a regular basis?
20. In the past three years in your jurisdiction, has there been an instance in which the local public health agency has failed to implement a mandated program or service?

SOURCE: Turnock, BJ, *Public Health: What It Is And How It Works*, 1997; Jones and Bartlett Publishers, Sudbury, MA. www.jbpub.com. Reprinted with permission.

key respondents within public health organizations are asked to report the extent to which their organization performs core public health activities. A compelling advantage of these types of measures is their ability to be collected relatively quickly and cost effectively, thereby providing timely data with limited respondent burden. Several self-reported performance assessment instruments have been developed for use with the administrators of public health organizations, including those developed by Turnock and colleagues to measure the performance of local public health agencies,[37,38,59] those developed by Miller and colleagues to measure performance within local public health systems,[39,40,42] and those developed for both state and local public health systems and used in the CDC's National Public Health Performance Standards Program.

Performance measures constructed from self-assessed and self-reported data raise important issues of measurement validity and reliability. The **validity** of a measure concerns its ability to produce an accurate reflection of the intended aspect of performance, whereas the **reliability** of a measure concerns its ability to produce a consistent reflection of performance each time it is used. The validity and reliability of self-reported measures depend on whether the appropriate people in the appropriate organizations are consistently recruited to report performance data. To report performance data accurately and consistently, respondents must have sufficient knowledge, expertise, and access rights to the necessary information. Respondent selection is therefore a critically important element of performance measurement. Unreliable performance measures can result from a variety of data collection situations:

- Systematic differences in respondent knowledge and information across organizations or over time (e.g., due to staff turnover within the organizations under study)
- Systematic differences in how respondents interpret performance measures across organizations or over time (e.g., due to incomplete or ambiguous case definitions for measures)

- Systematic differences in the content and quality of information systems used by organizations in reporting performance measures

Efforts to ensure the comparability of respondents and information systems across organizations and over time can help reduce these potential threats. First, clear and specific case definitions should be provided for each measure to reduce differences in how measures are interpreted. Second, performance measurement systems may require respondents to meet detailed reporting standards regarding what information should be used to respond to each measure and how this information should be collected, maintained, and documented by the responding organization. These standards can be periodically verified by audit, as is done in the HEDIS system that monitors health plan performance. Finally, where possible, performance measures should be based on objective, observable criteria rather than on criteria that are subject to the perceptions of the respondents. In the absence of objective information, however, perception-based measures may still offer some insight about practice-patterns and performance among public health organizations and systems.

Performance measures designed to assess the public health contributions of multiple organizations serving a common population are subject to additional validity and reliability issues. One measurement approach is to rely on the governmental public health agency as the key informant about public health contributions made by other organizations.[39–41,60] It is important to recognize that the reliability of such measures is contingent on the agency's access to information about the activities of other organizations. In most cases, the governmental agency may be the best single source for this information. Nevertheless, where information gaps or differences in perception exist, systematic reporting biases may arise. Another strategy for obtaining these measures is to survey directly the range of other organizations that contribute to public health performance, requiring these organizations to report information about their own activities. This strategy is likely to be considerably more

time-intensive and resource-intensive than strategies that target the public health agency only. Additionally, this strategy may encounter problems of
measurement reliability due to systematic differences across organizations in how performance
measures are interpreted.

Reliability tests can be used to detect inconsistencies in performance measure reporting.[61] **Inter-
rater reliability** tests use reports of performance
from multiple independent raters. If these reports
are highly correlated, then measurement reliability
is confirmed. Reliability can also be confirmed
through internal consistency tests. These tests are
carried out by collecting multiple measures of the
same performance dimension from each organization or jurisdiction under study. A high correlation
among the multiple measures suggests sufficient
reliability. Reliability can also be evaluated by collecting repeated observations of the same measure
over time and testing for longitudinal consistency.
Finally, external audits and direct-observation site
visits can be used to confirm the reliability of self-
reported performance measures. These types of reliability tests may be particularly important for performance measures designed to assess the public
health contributions of multiple organizations serving a common population.

To guard against potential reliability problems,
care must be taken in how performance measurement data are used. Self-reported performance measures are particularly vulnerable to problems of
gaming, wherein respondents may inflate their
reported measures to create the impression of high
performance or significant performance improvement over time. The incentives for systematic
reporting bias may be particularly powerful if performance data are publicly disseminated or used
for purposes other than to support internal quality
improvement and practice-based research. For
example, if performance measures are used to allocate resources or enforce contracts, then respondents face clear incentives to inflate their reported
performance levels. Consequently, the implicit
incentives for reporting bias should be considered
carefully when developing and using performance
measures in public health.

Other Measurement Approaches

Public health performance measures can be constructed using a number of other data sources. Secondary data from state vital and health statistics
systems, disease registries, immunization registries,
and notifiable disease reporting systems can be
used to construct a variety of disease-specific and
population-specific process and outcome measures
that may function as valuable components of performance measurement systems.[4] Other potential
data sources include the administrative data systems maintained by federal and state agencies for
specific public health programs (e.g., Medicaid,
WIC), and the hospital discharge data systems
maintained by many state health data organizations. These data elements often do not entail the
same measurement reliability problems that are
commonly encountered in self-reported measures.
Across-state variation in data system structure and
content, however, may introduce new reliability
challenges for performance measurement activities
that span multiple states.[62,63] Additionally, the ability to identify high-performing and low-performing
systems may be complicated when using measures
constructed from secondary data because these
measures may be influenced by many factors outside the control of the public health systems being
studied.

State-level measures relevant to public health
performance can also be constructed from the large
national health surveys conducted periodically by
federal agencies. Among the most widely used surveys for public health applications are the National
Health and Nutrition Examination Survey and the
National Health Interview Survey conducted by
the National Center for Health Statistics, as well as
the Medical Expenditure Panel Survey conducted
by the Agency for Healthcare Research and Quality
(AHRQ). State-level measures of behavioral risk
factors can be obtained from the CDC's Behavioral
Risk Factor Surveillance System. These data sources
are frequently used by initiatives that rank and
compare U.S. states based on measures of health
status and health system performance, such as the

America's Health Rankings report produced annually by the United Health Foundation. Although useful for national- and state-level measurement activities, these national data sources use sampling methods that usually prevent them from being able to produce measures of performance at substate and local levels.[64] For some state and local performance measurement initiatives, it may also be desirable and feasible to establish new primary data collection systems, such as population-based surveys of public health risks and outcomes, or to modify existing surveillance systems to address the need for reliable performance measures. As with any public health surveillance activity, the expected utility of the information obtained from such systems must be weighed against the expected cost of acquiring the information.

Each of the available methods for public health performance measurement offers a different mix of advantages and limitations, whether based on self-reported assessment instruments, population-based surveys, or secondary data sources. The best measurement strategy for a specific application depends upon the types of performance to be measured, the availability of secondary data sources, and the resources available to support data collection and measurement. Where possible, it is often advantageous to use a combination of self-reported measures and measures constructed from objective and verifiable secondary data sources. By avoiding reliance on any single type of measurement strategy, users are better able to detect and address common problems with measurement validity and reliability.

Performance Comparison and Evaluation

The ability to compare performance between organizations and over time is the central objective of most performance measurement activities. Such comparisons allow organizations to chart progress toward established goals and objectives, to benchmark themselves against similar organizations, and to monitor the effects of administrative and policy changes in public health. After valid and reliable measures of public health performance have been developed and collected, a remaining methodological issue concerns how measures are evaluated and compared cross-sectionally as well as longitudinally.[65] A number of methodological issues may complicate the task of evaluating and comparing performance measures, including the following:

- **Measurement error** and **measurement noise:** Some differences in performance measures may result from random variation or from errors in how the data were generated. An important methodological challenge therefore lies in distinguishing this measurement noise from true differences in performance across organizations and systems and over time.

- **Confounding** and **bias:** Observed differences in performance measures across organizations may result from true differences in public health practice, or from underlying, systematic differences in factors outside the control of public health organizations—such as sociodemographic characteristics, economic conditions, and underlying health risks of the populations served by these organizations. Failure to account for systematic differences in these underlying characteristics can lead to incorrect inferences about differences in performance between organizations. Correcting for these potential sources of confounding and bias becomes an additional methodological challenge in comparing performance measures.

Several basic approaches can be used alone or in combination for evaluating and comparing performance measures: using **performance standards** as a basis for comparison; using **performance benchmarks** based on a reference organization or system; and using statistical **risk-adjustment** methods to make cross-sectional and longitudinal comparisons. Each of these approaches is examined in the following sections.

Performance Standards

One common strategy for evaluating performance involves the use of established performance standards. Using this strategy, performance measures are simply compared with *a priori* standards to determine the extent to which these standards are met. Standards can be established using either a dichotomous "pass/fail" metric or a graduated continuum of performance levels that range from low to high. Dichotomous standards are often criticized for creating a ceiling effect such that organizations are not encouraged to pursue additional improvements in performance after achieving the specified threshold.[51] For this reason, graduated performance standards are sometimes preferred as a means for motivating continual improvement. Regardless of the type of standard used, simple bivariate statistical tests can be used to determine whether specific groups of observations exceed a performance standard after accounting for measurement noise. The power of these tests to detect differences in performance depends upon the number of observations included in the analysis and the degree of variation in the performance measure of interest.

Ideally, performance standards are established based on empirical studies that indicate the performance levels needed to achieve desired outcomes, such as the vaccination coverage rates that are required to bring infectious disease risks within certain acceptable ranges, or the purification standards for public water sources that are required to bring waterborne disease risks within acceptable ranges. In the absence of strong scientific evidence, performance standards are often based on professional judgments and norms about expected levels of performance. Standards can be developed, therefore, by convening panels of experienced public health professionals and identifying consensus opinions about appropriate public health practices and expected public health outcomes. A variety of structured group process methods can be used to identify such consensus opinions, with the most widely used methods being the Nominal Group Technique and the Delphi Method—both of which rely on an iterative, anonymous process of generating opinions, rating opinions, and reflecting on the ratings given by other panel members.[66] A variety of electronic technologies are now available to facilitate consensus development processes, ranging from anonymous computerized polling devices to Internet-based discussion forums.[67]

The CDC's *National Public Health Performance Standards Program*, described earlier in this chapter, uses a multiphased process for standards development that relies on consensus conferences and expert panels to define and refine the standards for local and state public health systems.[7] During the initial development phase, the CDC convened a broad range of public health stakeholders to reach consensus about performance standards, including representatives from the National Association of County and City Health Officials, the Association of State and Territorial Health Officials, the National Association of Local Boards of Health, and the American Public Health Association. These consensus panels identified a set of performance standards for each of the 10 essential public health services, with separate standards for local systems, state systems, and governing boards. An ordered continuum of performance levels was identified for each performance standard (for an example standard, see Table 16.5).

The CDC tested the performance standards in both state and local public health settings to confirm their usability, face validity, and relevance to practice. Additionally, the CDC sponsored statistical analyses of the performance data to examine patterns of variation in performance across states and communities. These analyses confirmed the ability of the standards to differentiate between high-performing and low-performing public health systems in multiple domains of activity.[68] Moreover, these analyses demonstrated that performance levels vary with important structural characteristics of the public health system, such as its population size and financial resources (Figure 16.3).[69] The CDC reconvenes its expert panels periodically to review and update performance standards to reflect changes in public health knowledge, technology, and practice.

Benchmarking

Another approach for evaluating performance measures involves comparisons among groups of

Table 16.5. Example Performance Standard Used in the National Public Health Performance Standards Program

Essential Service 1: Monitor Health Status to Identify Community Health Problems

Model Standard 1.1: Population-Based Community Health Profile

To accomplish this standard, the Local Public Health System (LPHS):
- Conducts regular community health assessments to monitor progress toward health-related objectives.
- Compiles and periodically updates a community health profile using community health assessment data.
- Promotes community-wide use of the community health profile or assessment data and assures that this information can be easily accessed by the community.

Indicators

1.1.1   Has the LPHS conducted a community health assessment?

1.1.1.1 Is the community health assessment updated at least every 3 years?

1.1.1.2 Are data from the assessment compared to data from other representative areas or populations?

1.1.1.3 Are data used to track trends over time?

1.1.1.4 Does the LPHS use data from community health assessments to monitor progress toward health-related objectives? In considering 1.1.1.4, do those objectives include:
- Locally established health priorities?
- State-established health priorities?
- *Healthy People 2010* objectives?
- Measures from the Health Plan Employer Data and Information Set (HEDIS)?
- Other health-related objectives?

1.1.2   Does the LPHS compile data from the community health assessment(s) into a community health profile (CHP)? In considering 1.1.1.2, are health status data compared with data from:
- Peer (demographically similar) communities?
- The region?
- The state?
- The nation?

Do CHP data elements include:

1.1.2.1 Community demographic characteristics?

1.1.2.2 Community socioeconomic characteristics?

1.1.2.3 Health resource availability data?

1.1.2.4 Quality-of-life data for the community?

1.1.2.5 Behavioral risk factors for the community?

1.1.2.6 Community environmental health indicators?

1.1.2.7 Social and mental health data?

1.1.2.8 Maternal and child health data?

1.1.2.9 Death, illness, or injury data?

1.1.2.10 Communicable disease data?

1.1.2.11 Sentinel events data for the community?

SOURCE: Centers for Disease Control and Prevention. *National Public Health Performance Standards Program: Local Public Health System Performance Assessment Instrument, Version 2.* Atlanta, GA: Centers for Disease Control and Prevention; 2008.

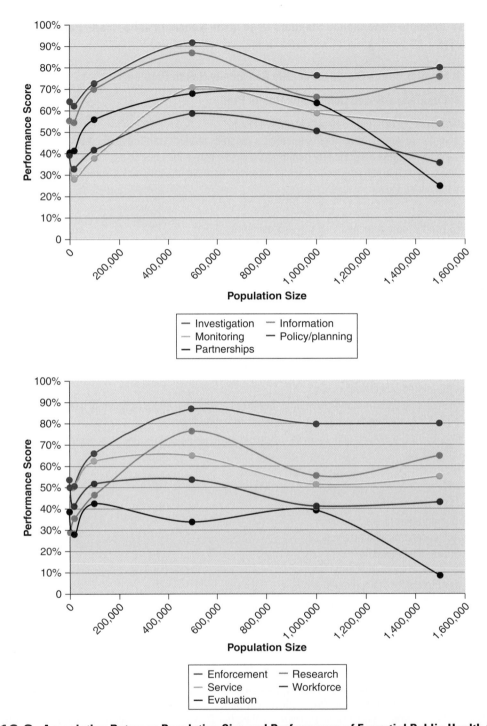

Figure 16.3. Association Between Population Size and Performance of Essential Public Health Services

SOURCE: *American Journal of Public Health,* 2006, 96(3), Institutional and economic determinants of public health system performance, Mays, 523–531.

organizations or systems that are closely related in structure and operation. These benchmarking comparisons are frequently used as part of continuous quality improvement initiatives because they create a "moving target" for organizations to work toward, rather than an absolute standard.[5] Under this approach, organizations are stratified into comparison groups of similar organizations based on observable structural and operational characteristics such as the size and demographic composition of the jurisdiction, and the scope of services offered. Statistical clustering procedures may be used to group organizations based on similarities across multiple characteristics. Performance measures for individual organizations are then compared with norms from the peer group of similar organizations. Bivariate statistical tests can be used to determine whether an individual organization is significantly above or below the average performance level of its peer group. By making comparisons only among similar organizations and systems, this approach reduces the risk of confounding and measurement bias due to unobserved differences across organizations and systems. Consequently, the benchmarking approach offers a potentially powerful strategy for motivating improvements in public

health performance based on empirical observation and comparison.

Researchers at the University of South Florida have developed a community health tracking system for Florida counties that uses this benchmarking strategy for making comparisons among county-level measures of community health resources, processes, and outcomes.[70] This system integrates secondary data from a variety of sources to create measures that can inform local public health decision making. A similar method was used in a recent study to profile measures of public health performance and community health outcomes on a national scale across local public health jurisdictions.[71] For this study, investigators collected measures from all United States local public health departments serving populations of at least 100,000 residents (response rate 71%) at two points in time (1998 and 2006) using a self-reported assessment instrument. After analyzing measures for validity and reliability, a customized report was developed that compared each jurisdiction's measures with United States averages and "peer group" averages (for an example, see Figure 16.4). Peer groups were defined using a statistical clustering algorithm based on jurisdictional

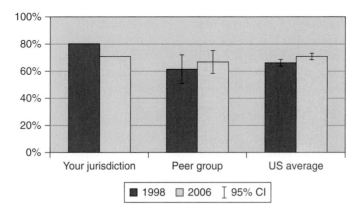

Figure 16.4. **Proportion of Public Health Activities Available in the Jurisdiction**

SOURCE: Mays GP, Scutchfield FD. Summary Report: National Longitudinal Survey of Local Public Health Systems. Little Rock: University of Arkansas for Medical Sciences; 2006.

population size, ethnic composition, and the scope of services offered by the local health department. Reports were sent back to each responding jurisdiction, and follow-up telephone interviews were conducted with a subset of respondents to assess the perceived utility of this benchmarking method. Follow-up interviews indicated that local public health administrators found the comparative results to be useful in developing improvement goals and strategies for their organizations.

If performance measures are collected longitudinally, then another form of benchmarking can be carried out using multiple observations from the same organizations or systems. Simple trend analysis can be used to examine the direction and magnitude of change in performance measures over time, thereby benchmarking an organization or system against itself. Additionally, measures of the magnitude and rate of performance improvement can be computed for each organization and then benchmarked with measures from similar organizations using the methods described previously. For these improvement comparisons, organizations may be grouped based on their baseline performance measures and based on other characteristics. Similar benchmarking methods can be used when multiple cross-sectional measures of performance are collected within the same organizations or systems. In these cases, performance is compared across different domains of activity rather than across different time periods. It is also possible to use longitudinal and cross-sectional benchmarking methods simultaneously, as was done in a recent case study analysis of eight local public health jurisdictions using the performance measurement instrument developed by Miller and colleagues.[72] For this study, performance measures were compared across 10 domains of public health practice as defined in Dyal[33] and across two time periods (1993 and 1996; see Figure 16.5).

Risk Adjustment

Another set of strategies for evaluating and comparing performance measures involves the use of statistical methods to control for potential sources of confounding and measurement bias. In one approach, performance measures are adjusted for factors that influence performance but are fully beyond the control of the public health organizations under study. These factors may include sociodemographic and health status characteristics of the populations served by public health organizations, as well as market and policy characteristics that are determined outside the public health organizations' spheres of influence. These types of controlled comparisons or risk-adjustment methods are especially useful for studies that evaluate the effects of policies and programs that are externally imposed on public health systems.[73] As in most types of observational research, the need to control for a large number of characteristics dictates the use of multivariate statistical methods rather than simple stratified comparisons. These methods can be used to compute adjusted performance scores that then can be compared among organizations or over time using benchmarking techniques. Adjusted performance scores can also be compared with a priori performance standards.

A second method for risk adjustment must be used when analysts want to examine performance variation due to factors that are within the control of the organizations or systems under study. For example, a researcher may want to examine how performance varies with the number of full-time equivalent (FTE) staff available in each organization under study. In these cases, standard statistical modeling techniques often produce estimates that are biased because they do not account for the fact that both public health outputs/outcomes (e.g., vaccination coverage rates) and public health inputs/structures (e.g., staffing levels) are simultaneously determined by the organization under study. In this example, public health agency staffing decisions may be based in part on local economic conditions that also influence health insurance coverage and the demand for health services such as vaccinations. Failure to control for this simultaneous relationship may lead to incorrect inferences regarding the effect of staffing on vaccination coverage. Advanced statistical methods such as structural equation modeling and instrumental-variables

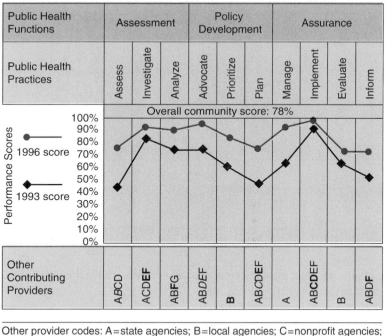

Other provider codes: A=state agencies; B=local agencies; C=nonprofit agencies;
D=hospitals; E=community health centers; F=universities; G=other.
Italics=Contributed in 1993 only
Bold=Contributed in 1996 only

Figure 16.5. **Public Health Performance Profile for a Sample Jurisdiction**

SOURCE: Adapted from Miller CA, Moore KS, Richards TB, and Monk JD. 1994. A proposed method for assessing the performance of local public health functions and practices. *American Journal of Public Health* 84(11): 1743–1749.

analysis can be used to test and control for possible sources of bias due to simultaneous relationships.[74] Specification tests can be applied to help researchers decide whether problems of simultaneity exist in their data and what can be done to address these problems.

This approach was used in one recent study to compare performance measures for local public health agencies that did and did not participate in partnerships with managed care plans.[59] Because such partnerships are at least partly under the control of the public health agencies, a simple comparison of measures between participating and nonparticipating agencies may lead to incorrect

inferences about the effects of partnerships on performance. The main performance measure used for this study was the proportion of 20 public health activities that were performed in the jurisdiction served by each agency, and the study population included all local public health agencies in the United States serving a population of at least 100,000 residents (N = 397, response rate = 71%). Using instrumental-variables estimation, researchers were able to adjust performance measures for the effects of other confounding variables, including the effects of public health agency decisions to form partnerships with managed care plans. Results indicated that performance measures

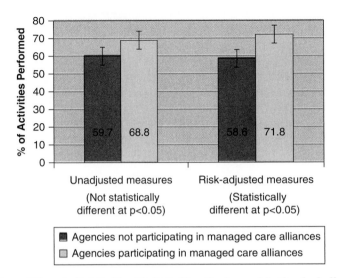

Figure 16.6. **Proportion of Twenty Public Health Activities Performed in the Jurisdictions of U.S. Local Public Health Agencies Serving at Least 100,000 Residents, 1998**

SOURCE: Data from Mays Halverson, and Stevens 2000.

were higher among agencies that formed partnerships with managed care plans and that this difference was statistically significant only when risk-adjusted measures were used (Figure 16.6). These risk-adjustment methods have been developed in the fields of econometrics and health services research, but they are nonetheless readily applicable to performance measurement applications in public health.

A third method of multivariate risk adjustment may be used for applications that collect multiple measures of performance for each organization or system. Rather than analyzing each measure separately, multivariate statistical models can be used to examine the relationships among multiple performance dimensions while simultaneously adjusting for confounding variables that are beyond the control of the public health system. By analyzing multiple performance measures simultaneously, additional statistical power is gained (due to the larger effective sample size) for use in untangling measurement noise from measurement signals.[75] Additionally, by examining the relationships among multiple measures of performance, analysts can

identify and compare patterns of performance across organizations and systems, rather than comparing single performance measures. This type of practice pattern analysis (which is similar in methodology to factor analysis and principal components analysis) can also be useful in identifying common, underlying dimensions of performance that cause multiple measures of performance to covary. For example, one recent study examined 20 different performance measures collected from all United States local public health agencies that serve populations of at least 100,000 residents. Multivariate factor analysis methods were used to identify groups of measures that were strongly correlated after controlling for a variety of confounding variables.[76] This study identified three dominant practice patterns from the measures: one that emphasized ensuring the delivery of health services to populations in need; one that emphasized assessing and prioritizing community health needs; and one that emphasized planning for public health interventions and resource allocation decisions (Table 16.6). Based on these results,

Table 16.6. Practice Pattern Analysis Based on 20 Public Health Performance Measures: Results from a Factor Analysis of Risk-Adjusted Measures

		Factor Loadings (Correlations)		
1.	Community health needs assessment	0.21	0.57**	0.28
2.	Behavioral risk factor survey	0.18	0.50**	0.21
3.	Adverse health events investigation	0.25	0.16	0.03
4.	Laboratory services	0.19	0.10	20.03
5.	Analysis of health determinants	0.23	0.69**	0.11
6.	Analysis of preventive services	0.14	0.41**	0.04
7.	Support and communication networks	0.39	0.16	0.11
8.	Information for elected officials	0.41**	0.13	0.29
9.	Prioritization of health needs	0.25	0.55**	0.38
10.	Implementation of initiatives	0.51**	0.21	0.24
11.	Community action plans	0.12	0.23	0.74**
12.	Plans for resource allocation	0.10	0.13	0.78**
13.	Resources for priority needs	0.43**	0.36	0.35
14.	Self-assessment	0.32	0.06	0.27
15.	Provision/linkage of services	0.37	0.21	0.03
16.	Evaluation of services	0.43**	0.28	0.22
17.	Process/outcome measures	0.41**	0.20	0.13
18.	Public information	0.61**	0.21	0.11
19.	Media information	0.52**	0.01	0.10
20.	Performance of mandated programs	0.13	0.12	0.00
Practice Pattern Grouping:		Assurance-intensive	Assessment-intensive	Planning-intensive

**Statistically significant at p,0.05

SOURCE: Mays GP, et al. *Assessing Organizational Performance in the Nation's Largest Public Health Jurisdictions.* American Public Health Association 126th Annual Meeting. Washington, DC: American Public Health Association; 1999.

additional studies can examine the relative effects of these three practice patterns on specific public health outcomes of interest.

All of the methods available for evaluating and comparing performance measures require good information about the structural and operational characteristics of public health organizations and systems. This information is needed to group organizations and systems for the purposes of benchmarking and to construct statistical controls for confounding sources of variation in risk adjustment models. The information required for such tasks may include data on the geographic extent of public health jurisdictions; the sociodemographic and health status characteristics of populations residing within these jurisdictions; the workforce characteristics of the professionals that staff public health organizations; information on public health funding sources and expenditures; information on the administrative and legal authority of public health organizations, including any governance structures; and information on the array of official and nonofficial organizations that potentially contribute to public health activities. One excellent source of such information is the *National Profile of Local Health Departments* collected periodically by the NACCHO.[31] Similarly, basic sociodemographic and health resources information can be obtained from the *Area Resource File* maintained by the United States Health Resources and Services Administration.[77] Other data elements necessary for these analytic activities may need to be obtained from administrative data systems maintained by individual federal and state agencies. These existing data sources provide a useful starting point for implementing performance measurement activities; however, it is clear that more detailed, comprehensive, and longitudinal data about the nation's public health infrastructure will be needed to support advanced applications in public health performance measurement and evidence-based decision making.

THE FUTURE OF PUBLIC HEALTH PERFORMANCE MEASUREMENT

The movement toward performance measurement activities in public health has been under way for most of the twentieth century. This movement accelerated dramatically during the past decade as public health decision makers faced new pressures to improve the effectiveness, efficiency, and accountability of their organizations. The pressures for performance measurement appear likely to grow in intensity as new and emerging threats to population health continue to develop and as new accountability structures such as accreditation and performance-based payment become more common in the field of public health. Contemporary performance measurement applications have been limited, however, by the types of information that are readily available and easily collected concerning public health structures, processes, and outcomes. New investments in public health information and surveillance systems—which are being made at local, state, and national levels—are steadily overcoming these limitations and expanding the opportunities

for performance measurement. Key among these new developments is the CDC's National Public Health Performance Standards Program, which promises to provide a rich longitudinal data source for public health organizations to use in monitoring their own performance over time, comparing performance with peer institutions, and identifying performance gaps in need of improvement.

These developments uniformly indicate that modern public health organizations require the ability to produce reliable and timely measures of performance for their organizations and jurisdictions and to use these measures appropriately for administrative and policy decision making. To operate successfully in this environment, public health organizations are likely to need a variety of new skills and strategies:

- **Information systems:** Public health organizations require the ability to collect and report verifiable, timely data on the resources consumed, outputs produced, and outcomes achieved in major programs and service areas. The additional costs of such systems may be substantial in some cases, but the benefits of more informed administrative and policy decision making will justify the investment—particularly if these systems are integrated with the organization's other information management and surveillance systems.

- **Interorganizational relationships:** Public health organizations require the ability to measure and monitor the performance of the public health *system* in which it participates, which necessarily entails sharing data and information with the other public and private institutions that contribute to this system. Consequently, the ability to develop and manage effective interorganizational relationships for the purposes of performance measurement becomes essential. Public health administrators must be able to mobilize shared interests in and support for performance measurement among all major stakeholders within the system. Correspondingly, administrators must play key roles in helping these stakeholders understand and use performance measures to achieve their own institutional objectives.

- **Analytical expertise:** To take full advantage of the information generated by performance measurement activities, public health organizations require the analytical expertise necessary to make valid comparisons of performance measures and derive implications for organizational strategy and public health policy. Ideally, this expertise should extend to the technical details of the benchmarking and risk-adjustment methods described earlier in this chapter. Of course, all public health organizations need not maintain this level of analytical expertise in-house, as long as effective mechanisms are in place to obtain this expertise from external sources such as academic institutions and state and federal agencies.

- **Improvement processes:** Public health organizations require the skills necessary to use information generated by performance measurement activities to improve public health operations and outcomes. Successful processes are likely to follow the basic principles of continuous quality improvement, which emphasize active participation by the broad array of stakeholders that influence specific process or outcome under study.[5] Most often, these improvement processes involve iterative cycles of identifying a problem, developing a potential solution, testing and evaluating the solution, and modifying the solution to achieve further improvements in performance. For public health organizations, performance gaps may derive from the work of multiple organizations, which adds additional complexity to the improvement process.[12,78,79]

- **Dissemination, outreach, and marketing strategies:** Finally, public health organizations require the ability to disseminate information on performance measurement activities to internal and external stakeholders that can use this information to improve health-related decision making. These stakeholders may include policy makers involved in resource-allocation decisions in public health; hospitals, community organiza-tions, and other institutions that currently or potentially engage in partnerships with public health organizations; and members of the public that have a general interest in population health and the use of public resources. One important challenge lies in making this information under-standable and usable by such diverse audiences through targeted dissemination and outreach strategies.[80]

Performance measurement applications in public health will continue to evolve in form and function as new data, analytical methods, and information technologies become available. Developing and using these applications will remain key priorities for public health organizations for the foreseeable future, particularly as the field moves toward accreditation, evidence-based practice, and pay-for-performance approaches. More important, however, performance measurement will remain a priority because of the growing imperatives to improve the nation's defenses against existing and emerging public health threats. Public health organizations form the core of the nation's response to problems as varied as new and resurgent infectious diseases, the advance of chronic diseases, persistent disparities in population health, and the looming threat of both natural and man-made disasters. It becomes possible to improve this response only with an accurate and detailed understanding of the work produced and outcomes achieved by the nation's public health organizations. Performance measurement provides the mechanism to achieve this understanding and to prepare for the public health challenges of the future.

REVIEW QUESTIONS

1. Describe three ways in which performance measurement activities can be used internally by public health agencies to improve the management of their organizations.
2. Describe two ways that performance measurement activities can be an asset to an organization that provides financial support to public health agencies.

3. Based on Donabedian's framework for assessing quality and performance in medical care, performance measures can be classified into one of the three basic types. Name the three basic types, and note the strengths and limitations of each type of measure when used for public health improvement activities.

4. Compare the approaches for measuring public health performance at an organizational level versus a system level. Under what circumstances would each approach be useful?

5. Identify three possible sources for establishing benchmarks for evaluating public health performance.

6. Identify three sources of measurement error and measurement bias commonly encountered in public health performance measurement activities.

7. Under what circumstances would a public health administrator want to use risk-adjustment methods as part of a performance measurement and evaluation process? Under what circumstances might it be appropriate to forego risk adjustment?

8. Name three new skills and strategies needed by the public health organizations to engage successfully in performance measurement activities.

REFERENCES

1. Walton M, Deming WE. *Deming Management Method*. New York: Perigee; 1988.

2. Lynch TD, Day SE. Public sector performance measurement. *Public Adm Q*. 1996;19(4): 404–419.

3. Tankersley WB. Performance measurement. *J Public Adm Res Theory*. 1997;7(1):163–171.

4. Perrin E, Durch J, Skillman SM. *Health Performance Measurement in the Public Sector: Principles and Policies for Implementing an Information Network*. Washington, DC: National Academy Press; 1999.

5. McLaughlin CP, Kaluzny AD. *Continuous Quality Improvement in Health Care: Theory, Implementa-* *tion, and Applications*. Gaithersburg, MD: Aspen Publishers; 1999.

6. Scutchfield FD, Zuniga de Nuncio ML, Bush RA, Fainstein SH, LaRocco MA, Anvar N. The presence of total quality management and continuous quality improvement processes in California public health clinics. *J Public Health Manage Pract*. 1997;3(3):57–60.

7. Halverson PK; Nicola RM; Baker EL. Performance measurement and accreditation of public health organizations: a call to action. *J Public Health Manage Pract*. 1998;4(4):5–7.

8. Mays GP, Halverson PK, Miller CA. Assessing the performance of local public health systems: A survey of state health agency efforts. *J Public Health Manage Pract*. 1998;4(4):63–78.

9. Turnock BJ. Performance measurement and improvement in public health. In: Novick L, Mays GP, eds. *Public Health Administration: Principles for Population-based Management*. Gaithersburg, MD: Aspen Publishers; 2000:431–456.

10. Kearney RC, Berman EM. *Public Sector Performance: Management, Motivation and Measurement*. Columbia: Institute of Public Affairs, University of South Carolina; 2000.

11. Byrnes P. Performance measurement and financial incentives for community behavioral health services provision. *Int J Public Adm*. 1997;20(8): 1555–1579.

12. Mays GP, Hatzell T, Kaluzny AD, Halverson PK. Continuous quality improvement in public health organizations. In: McLaughlin CP, Kaluzny AD, eds. *Continuous Quality Improvement in Health Care: Theory, Implementation, and Evaluation*. Gaithersburg, MD: Aspen Publishers. 1999: 360–403.

13. Roper WL, Mays GP. Performance measurement in public health: Conceptual and methodological issues in building the science base. *J Public Health Manage Pract*. 2000;(5):66–77.

14. Clancy CM, Eisenberg JM. Outcomes research: measuring the end results of health care. *Science*. 1998;282(5387):245–246.

15. Turnock BJ, Handler AS. From measuring to improving public health practice. *Annu Rev Public Health*. 1997;18:261–282.

16. American Public Health Association, Committee on Municipal Health Department Practice. First report, part 1. *Am J Public Health*. 1922;12(2): 7–15.

17. American Public Health Association, Committee on Municipal Health Department Practice. First report, part 2. *Am J Public Health.* 1922;12(2): 138–347.

18. American Public Health Association, Committee on Administrative Practice. Appraisal form for city health work. *Am J Public Health.* 1926; 16(1 suppl):1–65.

19. Walker WW. The new appraisal form for local health work. *Am J Public Health.* 1939;29(5): 490–500.

20. Krantz FW. The present status of full-time local health organizations. *Public Health Rep.* 1942; 57:194–196.

21. Halverson WL. A twenty-five year review of the work of the committee on administrative practice. *Am J Public Health.* 1945;35(12): 1253–1259.

22. American Public Health Association, Committee on Administrative Practice. *Evaluation Schedule for Use in the Study and Appraisal of Community Health Programs.* New York: American Public Health Association; 1947.

23. Halverson PK. Performance measurement and performance standards: Old wine in new bottles. *J Public Health Manage Pract.* 2000;6(5):vi–x.

24. Vaughan HF. Local health services in the United States: The story of CAP. *Am J Public Health.* 1972;62:95–108.

25. Institute of Medicine, National Academy of Sciences. *The Future of Public Health.* Washington, DC: National Academy Press; 1988.

26. Miller CA, Halverson PK, Mays GP. Flexibility in measurement of public health performance. *J Public Health Manage Pract.* 1997;3(5):1–2.

27. U.S. Department of Health and Human Services. *Healthy People 2010: Conference Edition.* Washington, DC: U.S. Government Printing Office; 2000.

28. http://www.usmbha.org/Images/Projects/ PromoVision/PATCH.pdf.

29. American Public Health Association. *The Guide to Implementing Model Standards. Eleven Steps Toward a Healthy Community.* Washington, DC: American Public Health Association; 1993.

30. National Association of County and City Health Officials. *Assessment Protocol for Excellence in Public Health (APEXPH).* Washington, DC: National Association of County and City Health Officials; 1991.

31. National Association of County and City Health Officials. *Assessment Planning Excellence through Community Partners for Health* (APEXCPH). Washington, DC: National Association of County and City Health Officials; 1999.

32. National Association of County and City Health Officials. *Mobilizing for Action through Planning and Partnerships (MAPP).* Washington, DC: National Association of County and City Health Officials; 2000.

33. Dyal WW. Ten organizational practices of public health: A historical perspective. 1995; 11(6 suppl):6–8.

34. National Association of County and City Health Officials. 1989–90 *National Profile of Local Health Departments.* Washington, DC: National Association of County and City Health Officials; 1992.

35. National Association of County and City Health Officials. 1992–93 *National Profile of Local Health Departments.* Washington, DC: National Association of County and City Health Officials; 1995.

36. National Association of County and City Health Officials. 1996–97 *National Profile of Local Health Departments.* Washington, DC: National Association of County and City Health Officials; 1997.

37. Turnock BJ, Handler A, Dyal WW, et al. Implementing and assessing organizational practices in local health departments. *Public Health Rep.* 1994;109(4):478–484.

38. Turnock BJ, Handler AS, Hall W, Potsic S, Nalluri R, Vaughn EH. Local health department effectiveness in addressing the core functions of public health. *Public Health Rep.* 1994;109:653–658.

39. Miller CA, Moore KS, Richards TB, McKaig CA. A proposed method for assessing public health functions and practices. *Am J Public Health.* 1994;84(1):1743–1749.

40. Richards TB, Rogers JJ, Christenson GM, Miller CA, Taylor MS, Cooper AD. Evaluating local public health performance at a community level on a statewide basis. *J Public Health Manage Pract.* 1995;1(4):70–83.

41. Halverson PK, Miller CA, Kaluzny AD, et al. Performing public health functions: The perceived contribution of public health and other community agencies. *J Health Hum Serv Adm.* 1996;18(3):288–303.

42. Turnock BJ, Handler AS, Miller CA. Core function-related local public health practice effectiveness. *J Public Health Manage Pract.* 1998;4(5):26–32.

43. Maternal and Child Health Bureau, Health Resources and Services Administration (U.S.). *Guidance and Forms for the Title V Application/Annual Report.* Rockville, MD: Health Resources and Services Administration; 1997.

44. Perrin EB, Koshel JJ. *Assessment of Performance Measures for Public Health, Substance Abuse, and Mental Health.* Washington, DC: National Academy Press; 1997.

45. National Committee for Quality Assurance. *HEDIS 3.0.* Washington, DC: National Committee for Quality Assurance; 1997.

46. Miller T, Leatherman S. The National Quality Forum: A "me-too" or a breakthrough in quality measurement and reporting? *Health Aff.* 1999; 18(6):233–237.

47. Baker EL, Melton RJ, Stange PV, et al. Health reform and the health of the public. Forging community health partnerships. *JAMA.* 1994;272(16): 1276–1282.

48. U.S. Department of Health and Human Services. *Healthy People 2010: Conference Edition.* Washington, DC: U.S. Dept of Health and Human Services; 2000.

49. Public Health Foundation. *From Silos to Systems: Using Performance Management to Improve Public Health.* Seattle, WA: Turning Point National Program Office at the University of Washington; 2002.

50. Eddy DM. Performance measurement: problems and solutions. *Health Aff.* 1998;17(4):7–25.

51. Brannick MT, Salas E. *Team Performance Assessment and Measurement:* Theory, Methods, and Applications. New York: Lawrence Erlbaum; 1997.

52. Kazandjian VA, Lied TR. *Healthcare Performance Measurement: Systems Designs and Evaluation.* Chicago, IL: American Society for Quality; 1999.

53. Barry MA, Centra L, Pratt E, Brown CK, Giordano L. *Where Do the Dollars Go? Measuring Local Public Health Expenditures.* Washington, DC: Public Health Foundation; 1998.

54. Bettcher DW, Sapirie S, Goon EHT. Essential public health functions: results of the international Delphi study. *World Health Stat Q.* 1998; 51(1):44–54.

55. Donabedian A. *The Definition of Quality and Approaches to Its Assessment.* Ann Arbor, MI: Health Administration Press; 1980.

56. Centers for Medicare and Medicaid Services (CMS) and Joint Commission on Accreditation of Healthcare Organizations (JCAHO). *Specifications Manual for the National Hospital Quality Measures, Version 1.04.* Baltimore, MD: CMS; 2005.

57. Taskforce on Community Preventive Services. *The Guide to Community Preventive Services.* New York: Oxford University Press; 2005. Available at: http://www.thecommunityguide.org.

58. Shadish WR, Cook TD, Leviton LC. *Foundations of Program Evaluation: Theories of Practice.* Newbury Park, CA: Sage Publications; 1991.

59. Handler AS, Turnock BJ, Hall W, et al. A strategy for measuring local public health practice. *Am J Prev Med.* 1995;11(supp 2):29–35.

60. Mays GP, Halverson PK, Stevens R. The contributions of managed care plans to public health practice: Evidence from the nation's largest local health departments. *Public Health Rep.* In press.

61. Silva F. *Psychometric Foundations and Behavioral Assessment.* Newbury Park, CA: Sage Publications; 1993.

62. Mendelson DN, Salinsky EM. Health information systems and the role of state government. *Health Aff.* 1997;16(3):106–119.

63. Starr P. Smart technology, stunted policy: Developing health information networks. *Health Aff.* 1997;16(3):91–105.

64. Lee CV. Public health data acquisition. In: Novick L, Mays GP, eds. *Public Health Administration: Principles for Population-based Management.* Gaithersburg, MD: Aspen Publishers; 2000:171–201.

65. Gerzoff RB. Comparisons: The basis for measuring public health performance. *J Public Health Manage Pract.* 1997;3(5):11–21.

66. Patton, MQ. *Qualitative Research and Evaluation Methods.* 3rd ed. Newbury Park, CA.: Sage Publications; 2001.

67. Mays GP, Halverson PK. Conceptual and methodological issues in public health performance measurement: Results from a computer-assisted expert panel process. *J Public Health Manage Pract.* 2000;6(5):59–65.

68. Mays GP, McHugh MC, Shim K, et al. Identifying dimensions of performance in local public health systems: Results from the National Public Health Performance Standards Program. *J Public Health Manag Pract.* 2004;10(3):193–203.

69. Mays GP, McHugh MC, Shim K, et al. Institutional and economic determinants of public health system performance. *Am J Public Health*. 2006;96(3):523–31.

70. Studnicki J, Steverson B, Myers B, Hevner AR, Berndt DJ. A community health report card: comprehensive assessment for tracking community health (CATCH). *Best Practices & Benchmarking in Healthcare*. 1997;2(5):196–207.

71. Mays GP, Halverson PK, Baker EL, Stevens R, Vann JJ. Availability and perceived effectiveness of public health activities in the nation's most populous communities. *Am J Public Health*. 2004; 94(6):1019–26.

72. Mays GP, Miller CA, Halverson PK. *Local Public Health Practice: Trends and Models*. Washington, DC: American Public Health Association; 2000.

73. Iezzoni LI. *Risk Adjustment for Measuring Health Care Outcomes*. Chicago, IL: Health Administration Press; 1997.

74. Newhouse JP, McClellan M. Econometrics in outcomes research: The use of instrumental variables. *Annu Rev Public Health*. 1998;19:17–34.

75. Koopman SJ, Shephard N, Doornik JA. Statistical algorithms for models in state space using SPack 2.2. *The Econometrics J*. 1999;2(1): 107–161.

76. Mays GP, Miller CA, Halverson PK, et al. *Assessing Organizational Performance in the Nation's Largest Public Health Jurisdictions*. American Public Health Association 126th Annual Meeting. Washington, DC: American Public Health Association; 1999.

77. U.S. Health Resources and Services Administration. *Area Resource File 1998*. Fairfax, VA: Quality Resource Systems; 1999.

78. Institute of Medicine, National Academy of Sciences. *Improving Health in the Community: A Role for Performance Monitoring*. Washington, DC: National Academy Press; 1997.

79. Stoto MA. Evaluation of public health interventions. In: Novick L, Mays GP, eds. *Public Health Administration: Principles for Population-based Management*. Gaithersburg, MD: Aspen Publishers; 2000:324–358.

80. Doner L, Siegel M. Public health marketing. In: Novick L, Mays GP, eds. *Public Health Administration: Principles for Population-based Management*. Gaithersburg, MD: Aspen Publishers; 2000: 474–510.

CHAPTER 17

Public Health Workforce

Patricia M. Sweeney, JD, MPH, RN, Kristine M. Gebbie, DrPH, RN, and Hugh Tilson, MD, DrPH

LEARNING OBJECTIVES:

Upon completion of this chapter, the reader will be able to:

1. Identify the roles and professions that comprise the public health workforce.
2. Describe where the public health workforce is employed.
3. Articulate the workforce competencies needed to fulfill the essential public health services.
4. Describe the efforts underway to ensure public health workforce competency and their impact.
5. Identify areas of needed public health systems research.

KEY TERMS

Competencies
Continuing Education
Epidemiology
Health Educator
Multi-Disciplinary Teams
Profession
Sanitarians
Voluntary Health Organizations
Workforce

Effective public health practice is dependent upon the presence of a **workforce** (the population employed in a specified occupation) that is well-prepared and well-matched to the specific community being served. The infrastructure of public health, that upon which all services and programs are built, has three components: accurate, timely data and information; effective systems and relationships; and a competent workforce. It may be true, however, to say that of these three apparent equals, workforce is the most important. This is because people are required for the system to gather and interpret the data to develop meaningful descriptions of health and illness and to organize to deliver strategies for disease prevention and health promotion. Systems and relationships can only be built and maintained by individuals; thus a competent workforce is essential. If the connections made are to serve the health of the public, those making them must understand what public health is, and how it might be achieved.

This chapter provides an overview of the public health workforce from the perspectives of the professions and skills represented in that workforce, the places they are employed, current issues regarding basic and lifelong learning needs, emerging standards for public health practice and areas of needed research. If you are already very familiar with the range of public health practitioners and public health practice may want to concentrate on the latter parts of the chapter; if you are new to the field, the earlier portions are helpful as they introduce the complexities of the field.

WHO PRACTICES PUBLIC HEALTH?

Although often called a **profession** (an occupation that requires specialized education or training that is often available only in a college or university and is usually assessed by a sequence of examinations), public health is unusual because it is not a singular profession in the manner of dentistry or radiation

technology. It is closer to a field of practice as might be described by someone saying "I work in education," or "I work in computers." That is, members of the public health workforce often are defined by their commitment to the goal of disease prevention and health improvement for populations and communities, irrespective of who supplies the paycheck. They do not focus on any one specific body of knowledge such as a specialized approach to diagnosis or treatment of individual problems.

The description of public health provided in a 1988 Institute of Medicine (IOM) report[1] has become well established: "assuring the conditions within which people can be healthy." This description has since been augmented by *Public Health in America*,[2] which identifies the specific responsibilities of public health as being to prevent epidemics and spread of disease, protect against environmental hazards, prevent injuries, promote and encourage healthy behaviors, respond to disasters and assist in recovery, and assure the quality and accessibility of health services. Anyone whose major activities contribute to the fulfillment of these responsibilities of public health through one or more of the essential public health services (see Table 17.1) can be considered a part of the public health workforce.[3] In addition to those discussed further here, there are many who coincidentally contribute to assuring one or more of these services in the course of their work, through activities such as enforcing traffic safety laws and thus reducing injuries, or documenting the epidemiology of injury while delivering acute care in emergency rooms. Table 17.2 illustrates the range of workers encompassed in this scope.

WORKERS AND PROFESSIONALS

This chapter concentrates on the workforce at the professional level, that is, those with at least a baccalaureate degree. This highly educated group requires special attention because of their particular

Table 17.1. Essential Public Health Services

- ✓ Monitor health status to identify community health problems.
- ✓ Diagnose and investigate health problems and health hazards in the community.
- ✓ Inform, educate, and empower people about health issues.
- ✓ Mobilize community partnerships to identify and solve health problems.
- ✓ Develop policies and plans that support individual and community health efforts.
- ✓ Enforce laws and regulations that protect health and ensure safety.
- ✓ Link people to needed personal health services, and assure the provision of health care when otherwise unavailable.
- ✓ Assure a competent public health and personal health care workforce.
- ✓ Evaluate effectiveness, accessibility, and quality of personal- and population-based health services.
- ✓ Research for new insights and innovative solutions to health problems.

Table 17.2. Range of Positions Engaged in Public Health Practice

Health Administrator

Administrative/Business Professional
Attorney/Hearing Officer
Biostatistician
Clinical, Counseling, and School Psychologist
Environmental Engineer
Environmental Scientist and Specialist
Epidemiologist
Health Economist
Health Planner/Researcher/Analyst
Infection Control/Disease Investigator
Licensure/Inspection/Regulatory Specialist
Marriage and Family Therapist
Medical and Public Health Social Worker
Mental Health/Substance Abuse Social Worker
Mental Health Counselor
Occupation Safety and Health Specialist
PH Dental Worker
PH Educator
PH Laboratory Professional
PH Nurse
PH Nutritionist
PH Optometrist
PH Pharmacist
PH Physical Therapist
PH Physician
PH Program Specialist
PH Student
PH Veterinarian/Animal Control Specialist
Psychiatric Nurse
Psychiatrist

Psychologist
Public Relations/Media Specialist
Substance Abuse and Behavioral Disorders Counselor
Other Public Health Professional

Technicians
Computer specialist
Environmental Engineering Technician
Environmental Science and Protection Technician
Health Information Systems/Data Analyst
Occupational Health and Safety Technician
PH Laboratory Specialist
Other Public Health Technician

Protective Service Workers
Investigations Specialist
Other Protective Service Worker

Paraprofessionals
Community Outreach/Field Worker
Other Paraprofessional

Support Workers
Administrative Business Staff
Administrative Support Staff
Skilled Craft Workers
Food Services/Housekeeping
Patient Services
Other Service/Maintenance

Volunteers
Volunteer Health Administrator
Volunteer PH Educator
Volunteer Other Paraprofessional

contribution to public health practice, and the complexities of assuring a steady influx of new professionals to replace those retiring or leaving and those needed to work on newly identified public health challenges. Technical and support workers in public health should not be overlooked, however, by anyone wanting to achieve success in public health practice. These individuals are critical to achieving program goals. They are often the backbone of outreach and community development efforts in maternal and child health or chronic disease prevention and can make or break relationships with the served community. The way in which telephones are answered, arriving citizens greeted, or document requests processed, shape the community's understanding of and appreciation for public health. In addition, many of these individuals, through the process of life-long learning, may themselves form the future workforce (often called the "pipeline") for the professional level. Consequently, all members of the public health workforce must be offered basic public health orientation and public health emergency response training, and be incorporated into all thinking about resources for public health improvement.

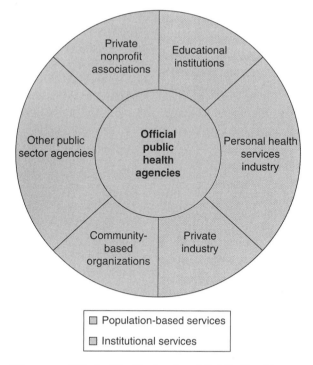

Figure 17.1. The Professional Public Health Workforce: Major Work Settings

SOURCE: Kennedy, et al., Public Health workforce information: A state-level study. JPHMP, 5(3):12 © 1999, Aspen Publishers, Inc.

NUMBERS AND NAMES

Because public health is the vocation of professionals in many work settings, enumeration and assessment of the workforce is a complex endeavor. In the face of such complexities, a landmark report was conducted in 2000 that enumerated the public health workforce. The findings indicated that in 2000, the public health workforce of the United States consisted of at least 448,254 paid individuals augmented by nearly 3 million volunteers.[4] The majority of the employed public health workforce work in local and state health departments, state environmental agencies, and federal departments of health and human services, environmental protection, agriculture, labor, veterans affairs, and the military. The number of volunteers reported comes primarily from the larger community-based voluntary health organizations such as the March of Dimes and the American Cancer Society. Unfortunately, however, the 2000 enumeration acknowledged a serious undercounting of the workforce, particularly in environmental health and in community partner organizations. Figure 17.1 illustrates the complexity of identifying the exact number of public health workers. Although the range of agencies and organizations providing public health services and the use of volunteers have inhibited any regular inventory of public health workers, the major obstacle to an accurate and current count and description of the public health workforce is the failure to assign responsibility (and provide funding) for periodic enumeration to any agency or organization.

Furthermore, public health professionals usually work in **multidisciplinary teams** (work groups composed of or combining several usually separate fields of expertise), to which each brings specific knowledge and a professional or technical world view but within which they share many skills. On a day-to-day basis, it may not be possible to identify the exact professional background in which an individual public health professional was originally trained or to even specify the exact way in which these underlying professional or disciplinary skills contribute to public health practice. That is, the process of doing an outbreak investigation, health facility inspection, or public education program for cancer prevention will be the same regardless of whether the person carrying out the task is a sanitarian, nurse, physician, health educator, nutritionist, or other professional. The strength of public health lies in the fact that when individuals from these various fields gather to explore and interpret results of studies or relationships of findings to communities, each brings a distinct world view that complements the others and enriches the analysis. Despite the complexities of the field and the difficulties arriving at exact numbers, the data indicate that there are just a few professional groups providing the vast majority of public health services. Generally, these groups receive the most attention from those working to improve practice.[5]

Public Health Nurses

Persons with a professional training in nursing comprise the largest group of professionals in the field of public health. The title "public health nurse" at one time was bestowed only on those nurses who had completed a baccalaureate degree program that included public health nursing courses. Some states (e.g., Wisconsin) limit the use of the title to nurses who have verified their level of preparation to the nursing licensing board. The long-standing educational standard for nurses moving into senior roles within public health has been a master's degree in public health or nursing with a concentration in public health. Although these requirements remain the preference, the limited supply and uneven geographic distribution of nurses with public health preparation has meant that many agencies and programs employ nurses with diploma or associate degree preparation for many public health nursing jobs. As public health has developed a larger repertoire of individual health programs in response to access problems and lack of insurance, the clinical skills of these nurses have been well-used. However, as states develop improved health care financing mechanisms and move more personal health and medical care into private practice settings, the clinical skills of this under-credentialed group become less important, and the lack of broader public health knowledge makes transition to other public health responsibilities difficult.

Public Health Physicians

Public health physicians have been described as an endangered species.[6] A part of this problem is the definition: most physicians practicing in public health do not have specialty training in preventive medicine, which is the only medical specialty area recognized by the American Board of Medical Specialties (ABMS) focused on population-based practice. Further, any physician who completes a required reportable disease notification to the local health department, immunizes a child or an adult, reinforces a public health message, or speaks up at the local civic club about the need for proper funding of environmental protection is acting as part of the public health workforce. Some medical specialties are found in explicitly public health practices: obstetrics/gynecology and pediatrics (because of attention to maternal and child health) and internal medicine/infectious diseases (because of the epidemic control responsibilities). More recently, physicians have moved from the field of emergency medicine to public health due to an interest in injury prevention and emergency preparedness and response.

Also, although fewer in number than public health nurses, public health physicians are largely concentrated in management. Many of the physicians working in public health settings have been employed in top leadership positions not because the jurisdiction understood what a physician brought to public health practice, but because state law or local ordinance required it, or because there is a perception that medical training carries with it knowledge of leadership and management and, of course, public health. Because services provided by public health agencies often may include prescribing and administering medications, as in tuberculosis, sexually transmitted disease, or mental health programs, physicians may be seen as essential to these program areas for their prescribing authority. However, this need may be vanishing as advanced practice nurses have been granted prescribing authority and as "mainstreaming" and outsourcing initiatives have resulted in many official public health agencies substantially reducing their provision of personal health services. Physicians originally employed for a specific clinical program within public health may lack the broad understanding of public health's values and skills and may encounter difficulty when making a transition to other public health practice areas. Paradoxically, physicians properly trained in the board-certified specialty of preventive medicine and oriented to intervention at the population level may find themselves under-appreciated by those who employ and pay for their services because of their lack of interest in direct patient care.

At the request of Congress, the IOM recently completed an analysis of the number of physicians needed for careers in public health and the training needed to supply them. The IOM concluded that the currently estimated number of 10,000 should be doubled and that agencies should create the positions needed to add this medical expertise to the public health workforce in official agencies.[7]

Epidemiologists

Epidemiologists study how disease is acquired and transmitted and thus provide the core science for disease prevention, detection, and control. Of the 10 essential public health services, 4 rely directly upon epidemiologic functions, yet fewer than 1 percent of the professional public health workforce are epidemiologists.[5] Furthermore, only about half of the individuals currently working in positions with epidemiologic responsibilities hold a degree in the field. Most have received training on the job or have taken a single course in epidemiology for training.[8] Since 2001, however, federal and state resources have been channeled toward enhancing state health department epidemiologic capacity. A study conducted by the Council of State and Territorial Epidemiologists (CSTE) reported that in 2004, there were 2580 epidemiologists working in state and territorial health departments: a dramatic increase from the 1366 reported in an earlier assessment. This increase in epidemiologic capacity, however, occurred only in the area of bioterrorism preparedness. Epidemiologic capacity in areas such as infectious disease, environmental health, injury, and occupational health have either remained insufficient or have been further compromised since 2001/2002.[8] And the contributions of epidemiologists to the understanding and evidence-based approaches to addressing the chronic diseases have been slow to gain appreciation.[9]

Environmental Health

Environmental health professionals are the most difficult to describe because there is no single entry point for this group. In addition, the separation of many environmentally related functions into agencies with broad natural resource protection responsibilities, has challenged enumeration and development of the environmental health workforce, and has added to the difficulties of a coordinated approach to protecting the public's health.

Sanitarians (persons knowledgeable about sanitary sciences and technically trained to detect environmental risks to health due to such causes as deficiencies in sanitation, ventilation, etc.) are the largest of the environmental health occupations. However, the title *sanitarian* (or Certified Environmental Health Specialist now coming into use) may represent licensure under a state law, certification through the professional association, or simply a convenient job title. Sanitarians are usually prepared at the baccalaureate level in a science (i.e., biology or chemistry) and receive on-the-job training in public health concepts and applications. Many are employed to enforce public health ordinances such as restaurant codes or drinking water standards. And, like nurses and physicians who lack formal public health education, they perform well in many specific program areas but encounter difficulties when asked to change focus or develop new programs due to limited knowledge of the broader theoretical underpinnings of public health practice. A particular challenge for many has been the move from the "command and control" approach of regulation enforcement to collaborative work with licensees to accomplish public health goals.[10] Within the environmental area, engineers bring knowledge of specific components of infrastructure and systems to bear on public health interests such as protection of water supplies, disposal of wastes, and development of safe environments. In addition, nuclear physics supplies professionals for radiation safety.

Health Educators

As with environmental health sanitarians, the title **health educator** (professionals who design, conduct, and evaluate activities to promote wellness and teach individuals and communities about behaviors that encourage healthy lifestyles to prevent disease and injury) may represent completion of a specific course of study or professional certification program, or simply hiring into a position carrying that label. The title Certified Health Education Specialist is bestowed by the major professional association of health educators (National Commission for Health Education Credentialing) as a way of identifying those individuals who have demonstrated understanding of the role and work associated with this field. In actual practice, nurses, nutritionists, social workers, or teachers who have gravitated to health education and information distribution as meaningful work are also called health educators. Some of these have also sought certification as health educators. Historically, the use of health educators has been within specific programmatic areas working with individuals or groups, such as in the Women, Infants, and Children's Nutrition Program (WIC) or well-child clinics. Increasingly, health educators are focused on crafting community-wide efforts to inform and shape public views of critical health issues and stimulate healthy behavior. Recently, the National Commission for Health Education Credentialing has revised the CHES certification exam to incorporate **competencies** (skills, knowledge, and abilities necessary for the practice of public health) that reflect revised areas of health education responsibility. In addition, The Commission is also currently exploring the development of a higher level of certification for those with additional education and experience in health education.[10]

Administrators

Administrators are essential to the organization and success of public health programs. Those assuming administrative roles within public health range from persons who have professional training or degrees in a medical or health discipline who have sought additional training in management and leadership (e.g., master's degrees in business, health administration, or public administration), to persons with a career commitment to management but no formal health preparation, or individuals who rise to leadership positions by virtue of seniority, on-the-job training, and experience. Generally, the highest position in a governmental health agency is filled by appointment by the jurisdiction's chief elected official, who may or may not have restrictions imposed by law (i.e., must appoint a physician, or someone knowledgeable about public health) and may or may not understand the overall roles and responsibilities of the public health agency or its chief professional. Often, the role is understood only in the narrow sense of administrator for an agency rather than as the chief official responsible for helping the jurisdiction fulfill its public health responsibilities through a collaborative public health system.

Agency and program leaders must constantly assess the interests of the body politic as a counterpoint or adjunct to applying the best available public health knowledge. Although many decry the choices of leaders made today,[12] some of the newer appointees have extensive understanding of the political nature of public health work and have facilitated the application of public health principles in difficult situations. For example, the state with the first *Healthy People 2010* plan developed using sound community participation was led by a health director not formally trained in public health administration.

WHERE DO PUBLIC HEALTH WORKERS FIND EMPLOYMENT?

Public health workers can be found in a wide variety of job settings in both the public and private sectors. Some of these settings may not be traditionally characterized as places where public health services are delivered, but services carried out there make important contributions to the public's health nonetheless.

Governmental Employment

At a minimum, public health workers are found in the nation's "official health agencies," the 50 state public health agencies, nearly 3000 local health departments, and the federal Department of Health and Human Services (HHS). This markedly understates the range of employment opportunities, however. Within all three levels of government, public health workers are also found in programs that are concerned with energy, environmental protection, food safety, health insurance (including Medicaid), mental health, occupational health and safety, substance abuse, rural health, traffic safety, welfare, and zoning. Many of these programs, originally developed as part of a department or board of health, have since been relocated or combined as policy makers shift preferences for relating programs and people. For example, pesticide control programs now housed in agriculture were once part of health departments, and the function of assuring access to care for the poor encompassed by Medicaid may have been a part of the jurisdiction

of a board of health. The IOM report[1] described an ideal state health agency that encompasses all of these programs. However, no such agency exists, nor is one likely to arise. Consequently, public health professionals must work collaboratively across program and agency lines and among public and private and voluntary partners.

Nongovernmental Employment

Public health workers can be found in a range of settings beyond governmental public health agencies. For example, school districts and individual schools (public, private, and parochial) employ many public health nurses to assure the health of school-aged children. They may also have nutrition and environmental health professionals working at a district-wide level to assure the healthfulness and safety of school meal programs. Independent water, sewer, or waste management districts also employ public health professionals to assure that standards for public health protection are met.

Hospitals and Health Care Organizations

Many hospitals and health care organizations (including staff-model and other health maintenance organizations) employ public health professionals. Many of the administrators of personal health care services have earned graduate degrees in administration from programs housed in schools of public health, and may have developed a population focus on their work. Among the most common public health workers in these settings are health educators, outreach workers, and epidemiologists. A large institutional system may have its own sanitarians, environmental engineers, and occupational health staff as well. Further, many localities expect that the clinical portion of public health services, such as immunizations or home-based education and outreach, will be housed with other care services rather than in the public health agency and often are incorporated seamlessly into daily practices such as a pediatrician's ongoing care. Conversely, it should be remembered, however, that just providing a health-related service or activity outside the walls of a hospital does not make it a public health activity. The test for whether something should be considered part of public health is the presence of a focus on a population group and on a preventive strategy or a preventable outcome.[13]

Occupational Health

For workforce and other strategic considerations, occupational health is a subspecialty of public health practice that may take workers into almost any other field or endeavor as a part of the organization's infrastructure. These public health professionals include physicians (some board certified in occupational medicine by the American Board of Preventive Medicine), nurses, epidemiologists, and industrial hygienists, and are involved primarily with protection of workers from hazardous working conditions. Some also develop workplace-based health promotion programs or even broader health programs for workers and their families. Workers concerned about their health and safety may also employ public health expertise through unions or professional associations. For example, occupational health advocates on the staff of the American Nurses Association were leading activists in supporting legislation protecting health care workers from occupational exposure to blood-borne pathogens.

Voluntary Organizations

Voluntary health organizations (an industry comprised of organizations that engage in fund raising for health-related research, health education, and patient services) provide another opportunity for public health employment. The American Red Cross is a special case of a voluntary agency, given the public health and care-giving role it plays during emergency response in coordination with local, state, and national officials. It also provides extensive public health education in many localities, for example, through sponsorship of

HIV/AIDS prevention training. Other voluntary organizations with a strong public health presence include the American Lung Association, the American Cancer Society, the American Heart Association, the American Diabetes Association, and Mothers Against Drunk Driving. Although each of these employs public health personnel, they also use extensive networks of volunteers, some of whom are also full-time public health workers in other agencies. For their volunteers who are not public health workers, the training given for volunteer tasks results in expanding the public health knowledge within communities. To illustrate, few communities would be as strict in control of indoor tobacco smoke today were it not for the work of thousands of public health volunteers working through voluntary associations.

HOW DO PUBLIC HEALTH WORKERS KNOW WHAT THEY NEED TO KNOW?

What public health workers need to know is increasingly described in the language of competencies, rather than defined by a listing of relevant degrees. Core competencies for public health practice necessary for the delivery of essential public health services have been defined by the Council on Linkages between Academia and Public Health Practice (see Appendix C), and core areas of knowledge and skill needed by currently employed public health workers were identified through a series of meetings resulting in what has been called the Charleston Charter of needed knowledge (see Table 17.3).

Basic Professional Training

As might be expected from the discussions of who public health workers are and where they work, there is no simple answer to explain how public health professionals gain the knowledge they need

Table 17.3. The Charleston Charter: What Currently Employed Public Health Professionals Need to Know

The nine core curriculum areas for currently employed public health workers are:

1. Public health values and acculturation
2. Epidemiology/quality assurance/economics
3. Informatics
4. Communication
5. Cultural competency
6. Team building/organizational effectiveness
7. Strategic thinking and planning/visioning
8. Advocacy/politics/policy development
9. External coalition building/mobilization

SOURCE: Gebbie KM, Hwang I. Preparing Currently Employed Public Health Professionals. New York: Columbia University School of Nursing; 1998.

for practice. Standards for basic professional training of physicians and baccalaureate nurses include population-based disease/injury prevention and community health knowledge. The accrediting bodies for medical schools and nursing schools have established this expectation, and courses have been offered for many years. However, in medical schools, preventive medicine may no longer be taught by a separate department,[14] and the prevention curriculum is often taught by someone whose primary focus is on individual clinical preventive services rather than the population focus of public health. Although this knowledge is extremely important, it means that essential competencies such as interdisciplinary partnership activities with communities, and the application of **epidemiology** to problem analysis at the community level may be minimized. This means that only the physician going directly into a preventive medicine residency and accompanying master's of public health degree program has a high likelihood of having full public health training prior to employment. Further it means that the assumption that the community-based medical practitioner is well-prepared to assume the role of public health advocate and

partner is also not secure. The IOM committee on physicians in public health careers identified three levels of physician education about public health: basic education for every physician, with all specialty boards urged to identify the public health aspects of that specialty and include it in examinations and continuing education; specific education about public health for physicians engaged in some aspect of public health part of the time due to location or type of practice (e.g., pediatricians and immunizations), and a full range of competency-based training for those working full-time in public health.

For the nursing student, the problem is slightly different, although it has the same ultimate limitation on readiness to practice in or with public health. As some public health agencies have assumed a larger role in providing direct personal health services (usually in response to the growing number of uninsured), the clinical experiences offered students during a public health nursing course may be limited to those associated with homecare services. The competencies required differ little from those required to give the same care in a hospital or other facility, thus there is no opportunity to develop community assessment or partnership skills. Further, the associate degree in nursing curriculum does not include public health theory or practice. In many parts of the country, nurses with associate degrees comprise the largest part of the workforce and are hired by public health agencies because they are the only nurses available to fill vacancies.

Public Health Training

The master of public health degree (MPH) is often described as the basic requirement for professional public health practice. However, only a relatively small proportion of public health workers have this degree prior to beginning employment. Some others go on to earn an MPH after initial exposure to a public health program area, having been employed either as an entry-level generalist or because of some specialized advanced skill needed by a specific program.

The MPH degree may be earned at a school of public health or in one of the growing number of public health programs housed in other schools and departments. The Council on Education for Public Health (CEPH) is the independent agency recognized by the United States Department of Education to accredit schools of public health. Accredited schools and programs awarding the MPH degree must provide course content in biostatistics, epidemiology, environmental health sciences, health services administration, and the social and behavioral sciences.

In addition, CEPH accreditation standards revised in 2002 require each student to participate in a planned, supervised, and evaluated practice experience. The practice experience is intended to provide students with the opportunity to apply the knowledge and skills being acquired through their courses of study. However there is variability among the population-based focus of these experiences. Many programs focus on narrow applications such as administration or biostatistics without addressing how such applications actually apply in communities.

To improve the quality and accountability of public health education and ensure that students earning an MPH degree are acquiring the skills needed to meet contemporary public health challenges, in 2004, the Association of Schools of Public Health (ASPH) developed a set of MPH core competencies that address not only the five core disciplines (Biostatistics, Environmental Health Sciences, Epidemiology, Health Policy Management, and Social and Behavioral Sciences) but also include competencies across seven interdisciplinary, cross-cutting domains (Communication and Informatics, Diversity and Culture, Leadership, Professionalism, Program Planning, Public Health Biology, and Systems Thinking), similar to the eight areas of new knowledge for public health practice presented by the IOM in 2003 (see Appendix C).

The student who adds the MPH skills to an existing health profession should be well prepared to move from an individual focus to a population one, keeping overall population goals in mind even when working with individuals. The person who comes to the MPH with a general science or liberal arts preparation will know a great deal about

public health principles but may still require significant coaching to become an effective public health professional. There is a growing awareness of the special need for this group to receive supplemental curriculum in the biomedical basis for health.

Schools of public health also offer doctor of public health degrees (DrPH) for those interested in continuing to advance the practice field with an additional level of knowledge and research skills. Many schools also offer research degree (PhD) programs in some or all of the public health specialty areas, with the graduates of these programs usually going on to research careers in academic or other settings.

Graduate degrees relevant to public health practice can also be obtained from other schools and departments. Many schools of nursing and medicine offer master's degree programs in public health and community health (a distinction that is often invisible to the observer and may mean little in actual practice). Graduate degrees in environmental areas may be earned in schools of engineering or planning. A narrow focus of the MPH as "the" public health degree stereotypes education for practice and narrows the range of backgrounds from which well-prepared public health practitioners may be recruited.

Furthermore, in recent years, there have been many efforts to increase the level of partnership between schools of public health and public health practice areas, such as establishing practice coordinators in all schools of public health.[15] This is encouraged to assure that the curriculum is relevant to practice and that students have learning experiences relevant to future employment. For those already employed in the field, attainment of advanced education is facilitated. It also helps to fulfill the broader community service mission of training initiatives. The CDC-supported academic health departments and HRSA-supported Public Health Training Centers are examples of efforts to extend and enrich this partnership.

Continuing Education

Given all that has been identified in the preceding, and coupled with the ever-changing nature of the challenges of the field, it should be no surprise that the field of public health is committed to development of a system of *life-long learning* that can assure the newly employed person access to needed core knowledge about public health and facilitate rapid updates of practitioners when the science base for practice advances. Some **continuing education** (specific learning activities generally characterized by the issuance of a certificate or Continuing Education Units [CEU] to document attendance or completion of a course of instruction) comes from academic centers. In addition, many of the professional associations to which public health workers belong offer continuing education. This is done at regular meetings and special educational conferences and through selected sections in professional journals. The American Medical Association, American Nurses Association, American College of Preventive Medicine, National Environmental Association, Public Health Law Association, and American Public Health Association all make efforts to assure that members can remain current in important areas of public health practice.

Through a collaborative effort involving the federal Centers for Disease Control and Prevention and the Health Resources and Services Administration; the Associations of Schools of Public Health, State and Territorial Health Officials, County and City Health Officials, Teachers of Preventive Medicine, and others, a strategic plan for the development of the public health workforce was designed and is being implemented.[15] Figure 17.2 illustrates the cycle of discovery and action needed to assure a fully competent public health workforce.

The responsibility for becoming and remaining competent to perform job functions is one that should be shared by both the individual and the employing agency. That is, anyone who aspires to be recognized by society as a professional should understand that society expects, in return, that the professional is up to date on the full range of information required to deliver the promised level of services. In a complementary way, those employing public health professionals (actually, any employer) should recognize that it is of mutual benefit to make the process of lifelong learning possible without excessive time away from the job and at

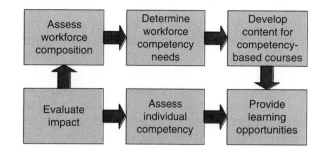

Figure 17.2. Strategic Elements for Public Health Workforce Development

SOURCE: Reprinted from U.S. Department of Health and Human Services, Centers for Disease Control and Prevention. Strategic Plan for Public Health Workforce Development. Atlanta, GA: CDC, Public Health Practice Program Office, 1999.

reasonable cost. In pursuit of this joint goal, the workforce collaboration described in the previous paragraph has moved to make the competencies required for public health practice clear and to encourage the development of a range of both in-person and distance-based learning opportunities. A national network of funded centers for public health workforce development is working in partnership with practice agencies to assure that this comprehensive approach to workforce preparation becomes a reality.[16] As a next step, this developmental opportunity, which has been primarily built around official health agencies, could be extended to all engaged in public health practice, wherever that might be.

Public Health Certification

Following more than two decades of debate regarding the value of credentialing the field of public health, leaders representing public health practice, academia, and professional associations approved the development of an independent National Board of Public Health Examiners (NBPHE) for the purpose of developing and administering a certification exam leading to the credential of Certified in Public Health (CPH). The goals for credentialing include ensuring that graduates from CEPH-accredited schools and programs of public health have mastered the knowledge and skills needed for contemporary public health practice, and to improve the consistency of public health workers nationwide. The NBPHE administered the first CPH exam in the fall of 2008. The Association of Schools of Public Health has created a study guide for those preparing for the examination. The exact nature of recertification and continuing education that may be required in the future is not yet clear.[17]

MAINTAINING PUBLIC HEALTH STANDARDS

Historically, standards for public health practice have taken the form of performance expectations that are tied to federal funding. Some states have had standards for local agencies, but enforcement of these standards has been variable. Because there is no equivalent of the Joint Commission on the Accreditation of Health Care Organizations (JCAHO) for public health, there has been no solid basis for standardization of practice. Acknowledging this, in 2003, the CDC, in partnership with a number of national public health organizations, created a National Public Health Performance Standards Program. Based upon the 10 essential public health services, this voluntary program provides standards that describe optimal public health practice performance rather than minimum expectations and provides a series of instruments that state and local public health agencies and governance boards may use to assess and their performance.[18] Use of these performance standards has grown, with data sets of performance reports now available for scholarly research. Further, an accompanying movement to identify and implement systems and indicators, building on the performance standards to document agency performance and certify those agencies performing

adequately, has demonstrated the utility of agency accreditation.[19]

Workforce Competency

In 2001, the Council on Linkages between Academia and Public Health Practice developed a set of *Core Competencies for Public Health Professionals* that detail the range of skills, knowledge, and attitudes necessary for the broad practice of public health. These competencies encompass skills in analysis and assessment, policy development and program planning, communication and cultural competency, community dimensions of practice, financial planning and management, as well as the basic public health sciences (see Appendix C).

Core competencies have also been established for a limited number of disciplines in public health. There are specific standards of practice for public health nurses, which are the product of collaboration among the ANA (Community Health Nurse Section), Association of State and Territorial Directors of Nursing, Association of Community Health Nursing Educators, and the National League for Nursing. Competencies for the practice of applied public health epidemiology have been drafted by the CSTE and the CDC.[20] Using each of these resources, it is possible to assess the competency of individuals in public health practice in general and nurses and epidemiologists in particular.

Meeting performance and outcome standards, however, can only happen when workers with the requisite competencies are employed. Likewise, because public health practice is based on an ever-enlarging science base, staff members cannot continue to function effectively throughout a career without access to new information and new skills. Therefore, agencies must have mechanisms in place to determine whether staff possess the competencies required for their positions and must have processes in place to facilitate the acquisition of new knowledge and skills.

Recognizing this need for continuing staff development, *Healthy People 2010* set a public health agency infrastructure objective for each agency to incorporate "competencies" into their respective personnel systems.[21] However, data collected during a 2005 national study, which analyzed the extent to which state public health departments have incorporated competencies into their personnel recruiting systems, clearly demonstrated that, although candidates for public health nursing and epidemiology positions are routinely assessed to ascertain their knowledge and skills of the basic public health sciences, assessment of a candidate's cultural competence, or understanding of the community context of practice, virtually never occurs.[22] This makes the roles of managers and leaders in public health extremely critical. Those placed in positions to make employment decisions or to direct the work of others must be knowledgeable about the required public health competencies associated with the program area and skills of employees they hire or direct and must apply that knowledge to their personnel decisions. Furthermore, when applying this knowledge to the process of matching specific workers to specific tasks within the public health mission, attention should be paid to supporting the interdisciplinary collaboration that has always been a strength of public health. Although care must be paid to avoid asking any professional to practice outside his or her legal scope of practice, it is also important to make full use of all of the knowledge and skill each worker brings to the effort, without regard to historic prejudices about who best does what. As an example, in one southern health department, a public health nurse established an exciting role as a troubleshooter and problem solver for environmental health enforcement problems.

There should be ongoing communication between anyone in a supervisory position and his or her staff to identify needed new competencies or emerging science relevant to the practice field. The staff members need to identify ways to gain these new skills, and the supervisor should work to assure that the required learning takes place in a timely way. For small agencies, collaboration with state or national groups serves to reduce the cost for development of training programs. In addition,

distance-based learning approaches show much promise for making the achievement of life-long learning a reality.

Maintaining a Sufficient Workforce

Currently, the average public health worker is 47 years old.[23] It is predicted that over the next decade, approximately half of all state and federal public health workers will either retire or move on to other opportunities. The number of students expected to graduate with public health training will not be sufficient to replace those leaving the field. In addition, the APHA issue brief titled "The Public Health Workforce Shortage: Left Unchecked, Will We Be Protected?" reports an overall decline in the number of public health workers from 220 per 100,000 Americans in 1908, to 158 per 100,00 in 2000, with particularly severe shortages in epidemiology, nursing, laboratory science, and environmental health. Although this presents a very real workforce crisis, it may also translate into opportunity for students and professionals in other fields with interest in population health.[24]

THE UNANSWERED QUESTIONS

This chapter has been written with the assumption that for a community to become healthier, essential public health services must be available, and for essential public health services to be delivered effectively, public health workers must be competent. Further, the competence must be in the areas identified as core public health practice and any of the specific public health practice areas relevant to the population and delivering agency. There is a further assumption that the preferred health outcomes will be achieved more quickly, and more effectively, as staff move from beginning levels of competence to mastery. Although these may be logical assumptions, the public health workforce research base is sufficiently thin that there will be no footnotes to research findings in this section.

The public health community is actively pursuing support for the necessary research on infrastructure and its relationship to public health outcomes. Workforce—along with organization and informatics—is an essential element of infrastructure, and in some ways the most important third. Given the range of public health professions, the variety of practice settings in which they are found, and the immense range of knowledge and skills they bring to bear on solving public health challenges, it is essential that this research be initiated quickly. The human capital of public health is a precious resource that must be developed strategically, deployed thoughtfully, and nurtured responsibly. Knowing more about the connections between who we are and what we can do is critical if we are to deliver on the promises of public health security and a healthy America.

REVIEW QUESTIONS

1. What educational preparation is the basis for public health practice?
2. In what settings do you find the public health workforce?
3. List five key competencies for a public health nurse, physician, administrator, educator, and sanitarian.
4. What are the factors complicating an accurate and consistent enumeration of the public health workforce?
6. What are/should be the linkages between the "essential services" and the competencies of public health workers?
7. Why has it been so difficult for the public health field to generate workforce to population staffing standards?
8. Why are workers employed outside official public health agencies considered part of the public health workforce?
9. The public health workforce includes many individuals in technical and support roles. Identify two categories of such workers and their contribution to public health.

REFERENCES

1. Institute of Medicine, Committee for the Study of the Future of Public Health. *The Future of Public Health*. Washington, DC: National Academy Press; 1988.
2. Public Health Functions Steering Committee. *Public Health in America*. Washington, DC: US Department of Health and Human Services; 1994.
3. Public Health Functions Steering Committee. *The public Health Workforce: An Agenda for the 21st Century*. Washington, DC: US Department of Health and Human Services, Public Health Service; 1997.
4. Health Resources and Services Administration (HRSA), Bureau of Health Professions, National Center for Health Workforce Information and Analysis. *The Public Health Workforce, Enumeration 2000*. Washington, DC: HRSA; 2000.
5. Gebbie, K. *The Public Health Workforce Enumeration 2000*. New York: Center for Health Policy, Columbia University School of Nursing; 2000.
6. Tilson H, Gebbie K. Public health physicians: An endangered species. *American Journal of Preventive Medicine.* 2001; 21(3):223–240.
7. Committee on Training Physicians for Public Health Careers. *Training Physicians for Public Health Careers*. Washington, DC: National Academies Press; 2007.
8. Council of State and Territorial Epidemiologists (CSTE). *National Assessment of Epidemiologic Capacity: Findings and Recommendations*. Available at: http://www.cste.org/Assessment/ECA/pdffiles/ECAfinal05.pdf. Accessed April 2, 2008.
9. Siegel PZ, Huston S, Powell KE, et al. Assessment of chronic disease epidemiology workforce in state health departments—United States, 2003. *Prev Chronic Dis* [serial online]. July, 2007.
10. The National Center for Health Education Credentialing Competencies Update Project (CUP). Available at: http://www.nchec.org/forms/Revised_Areas_of_Responsibility.pdf. Accessed February 16, 2007.
11. Bloom A, Gebbie K. *Preparing currently employed public health environmental professionals for changes in the health systems*. New York: Columbia University School of Nursing, Center for Health Policy and Health Services Research; 1998.

12. Gerzoff R, Richards T. The education of local health department top executives. *Journal of Public Health Management.* 1997; 3(4): 50–56.

13. Gebbie K. Community-based health care: An introduction. In: Brennan P, Schneider S, Tornquist E, eds. *Information Networks for Community Health.* New York: Springer-Verlag; 1997: 3–14.

14. Dismuke S, Sherman L. Identifying population health faculty in US medical schools. *American Journal of Preventive Medicine.* 2001;20(2): 113–117.

15. Centers for Disease Control and Prevention. *Report from the Task Force on Public Health Workforce Development: CDC/ATSDR Strategic Plan for Public Health Workforce Development: Executive Summary and Recommendations.* Washington, DC: US Department of Health and Human Services, Center for Disease Control; 1999.

16. Gordon AK, Chung K, Handler A, Turnock BJ, Schieve LA, Ippoliti P. Final report on public health practice linkages between schools of public health and state health agencies: 1992–1996. *Journal of Public Health Management Practice.* 1999;5(3):25–34.

17. Gebbie K., Goldstein BD, Gregorio D., et al. The National Board of Public Health Examiners: Credentialing public health graduates. *Public Health Reports.* 2007;4:435–440.

18. Department of Health and Human Services Centers for Disease Control and Prevention National Public Health Performance Standards Program. Available at: http://www.cdc.gov/od/ocphp/nphpsp/index.htm. Accessed February 16, 2007.

19. NACCHO National Accreditation website. Available at: http://www.naccho.org/topics/infrastructure/accreditation/national.cfm. Accessed October 31, 2008.

20. Centers for Disease Control and Prevention and the Council of State and Territorial Epidemiologists. Applied Epidemiology Competencies. Available at: http://www.cste.org/dnn/ProgramsandActivities/WorkforceDevelopment/Competencies/tabid/174/Default.aspx. Accessed October 31, 2008.

21. Centers for Disease Control and Prevention. *Healthy People 2010.* Chapter 23 Objective 8. Public Health Infrastructure. Available at: http://www.healthypeople.gov/Document/HTML/Volume2/23PHI.htm#_Toc491137862 Accessed February 16, 2007.

22. Sweeney, PM Workforce recruitment, retention and promotion in the civil service system. Paper presented at the Academy Health annual meeting, Seattle, WA. June 24–28, 2006.

23. American Public Health Association. Strengthening the public health workforce: ensuring a well trained and prepared workforce to respond to future threats. Available at: http://www.apha.org/NR/rdonlyres/0E0166BC-2D70-4352-9FC1-98DF8520861E/0/PublicHealthWorkforceFactSheet.pdf. Accessed January 22, 2008.

24. American Public Health Association. The public health workforce shortage: left unchecked, will we be protected? Available at: http://www.apha.org/NR/rdonlyres/597828BF-9924-4B94-8821-135F665E9D45/0/PublicHealthWorkforceIssueBrief.pdf. Accessed October 31, 2008.

CHAPTER 18

Leadership in Public Health Practice

Cynthia D. Lamberth, MPH, CPH and Louis Rowitz, MA, PhD

LEARNING OBJECTIVES

Upon completion of this chapter, the reader will be able to:

1. Describe historical and current initiatives to provide leadership development to the public health system.
2. Identify and contrast the four salient leadership models for public health.
3. Identify the four competency areas of public health leadership development.
4. Describe collaborative leadership and the methods to achieve effective collaboration.
5. Differentiate between traditional and systems thinking.
6. Identify the five disciplines of a learning organization and how to apply this in the public health practice setting.
7. Identify the four challenges of public health leadership.
8. Identify a set of organizational standards and monitoring mechanisms to manage performance.
9. Describe the approaches and tactics used to advocate for political and or policy changes.

KEY TERMS

Archetype
Balancing Loops
Causal Loop Diagram (CLD)
Coaching
Collaboration
Crisis Leadership
Ecological Leadership
Leadership
Leadership Development
Leverage Points
Mentoring
Meta-Leadership
Mission
Public-Private Alliances
Reinforcing Loops
Servant Leadership
Social Justice
Syndemic Perspective
Systems Leadership
Systems Model of Leadership
Systems Thinking
The Law of the Few (agent)
The Power of Context (environment)
The Stickiness Factor (host)

INTRODUCTION

Being a leader in the business world is clearly different from being a leader in the world of public health. It is not that the tools or the skills needed to function in these areas are widely divergent, but rather that public health leaders need to adapt leadership knowledge, skills, talents, and competencies for them to work in the public sector. Public-sector work requires problem solving and decision making that directly impacts the public good.

In public health, there is a commitment to **social justice,** which is the distribution of advantages and disadvantages within society. This sometimes puts public health professionals at odds with policy makers and the general public. As a result, public health leaders often are forced to attempt to justify actions through a social justice perspective, which includes the philosophy of equal health for all regardless of ability to pay, in an environment that does not value this perspective. Public health leaders use science, research, and practice experiences to make evidence-based decisions.

Public health professionals work within the context of the core functions of assessment, policy development, and assurance. Public health leaders cannot effectively carry out public health activities without an accurate assessment of the health status of their communities. To perform such an assessment, these leaders need to work with their community partners collaboratively within the context of a population-based public health systems model. For example, this community-oriented team might undertake a MAPP (Mobilization for Action through Planning and Partnership).[1] These leaders can use information obtained during the assessment process to develop policies and procedures to enhance the health of the public. Finally, public health through its leaders and partners is responsible for assuring the health of all people through collaborative partnerships, **public-private alliances,** and **meta-leadership** approaches (working across organizations). To assure these things, it is critical that ethical decision making occurs as covered in Chapter 7 of this book. The complexity of all public health problems require a systems approach to problem-solving that extends into numerous organizations, stakeholder groups, and communities. This chapter explores the critical knowledge, skills, competencies, and practices necessary to carry out public health's work through sound and effective public health leadership.

DEFINITION OF LEADERSHIP

Leadership is creativity in action. It is the ability to see the present in terms of the future while maintaining respect for the past. Leadership is based on respect for history and the knowledge that true growth builds on existing strengths.[2]

The **systems model of leadership** (Figure 18.1) defines effective leadership as a synthesis of wisdom, creativity, and intelligence. Public health leaders need creativity to generate ideas, analytic intelligence to evaluate those ideas, practical intelligence to implement the ideas and persuade others of their worth, and wisdom to balance the interests of all stakeholders and to ensure that the actions of the leaders contribute to the common good.[3] As can be seen in the diagram, wisdom is translated into strategic evidence-based programs and policies.

- **creativity** to generate ideas,

- analytic **intelligence** to evaluate those ideas, and

- practical **intelligence** to implement the ideas and persuade others of their worth, and

- **wisdom** to balance the interests of all stakeholders and to ensure that the actions of the leaders seek the common good.

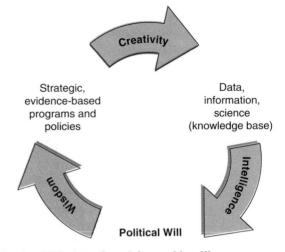

Figure 18.1. The System Model of Leadership: A Synthesis of Wisdom, Creativity, and Intelligence

SOURCE: This model is a blend of ideas from: Sternberg RJ. "A Systems Model of Leadership." *American Psychologist.* 2007;62:34–42.

Richmond–Kotelchuck. *Oxford Textbook of Public Health. Oxford, England: Oxford University Press; 1991.*

This strategic approach allows for creative problem solving that incorporates all types of information into an action perspective. Creativity and intelligence must be joined together to influence policy makers by creating more public value for the activities of public health. Creativity helps generate ideas, analytic intelligence is used to evaluate those ideas, practical intelligence is needed to implement the ideas and to persuade others of their value and worth, and finally wisdom is needed to balance the interests of the internal and external stakeholders to ensure that the actions of the leaders are oriented toward improving the health and welfare of people living in dynamic and growing communities.

PUBLIC HEALTH'S LONG HISTORY OF LEADERSHIP

John Snow, the father of epidemiology, removed the handle from the broad street pump and, with this single act of leadership, proved that contaminated water

indeed spread cholera. This perfectly illustrates the kind of decisive action often required of public health leaders. To this day, Epidemiological Intelligence Service officers at the Centers for Disease Control and Prevention (CDC) will ask the question "Where is the pump handle on this one?" Like Snow, they are looking for the one action or series of actions that can save lives and reduce health inequities.

Recent Calls for Greater Leadership for the Public's Health

Reports and studies on the status of public health personnel in the United States identify some important trends, including increasing demands for a competent workforce and for appropriately educated leadership.[4] Some think enhancing the leadership capacity of the public is one way to ensure the development of and retention of a highly effective public health workforce.[5] The Institute of Medicine (IOM) report, *The Future of Public Health,* called for workforce capacity development to accommodate demands of emerging public health problems and an evolving public health system.[6] The report argued that public health will serve society effectively only if a more efficient, scientifically sound system of practitioner and leadership development is established.

Leadership development is a key factor in organizational effectiveness and infrastructure development. This fact has long been assumed in the private sector. In the *Leadership Matters* Study in 2003, the Haas Foundation was struck by how deeply and systematically the private sector invests in its leaders and by the chronic absence of the same deliberate investment in the nonprofit sector.[7] Barbara Blumenthal states that capacity-building interventions often fail if strong leadership is not in place.[8] This suggests that investing in leadership development may be a necessary precursor to any attempts to build up public health capacity. Over the past decade, public health has recognized that without talented and passionate leaders heading our organizations, we cannot make progress toward our goal of confronting some of the most challenging public health issues facing our society. The IOM report *Who Will Keep the Public Healthy*[9] recommends that schools of public health increase the number of graduates who can assume system-level leadership positions and that they recruit senior-level practitioners and mid-career professionals prepared for leadership positions.

Warren Bennis, a leadership scholar for more than six decades, underscores the importance of leadership today when he predicts that the four most important threats facing the world today are (1) a nuclear or biological catastrophe, whether deliberate or accidental; (2) a worldwide epidemic; (3) tribalism and its cruel offspring, assimilation; and finally, (4) the leadership of our human institutions.[10] Bennis goes on to state that without exemplary leadership, solving the first three problems will be impossible. In the new era of terror prevention and preparedness, public health leadership is at the forefront in preparing and preventing these threats on our society.

Although leaders in public health and in business use many of the same skills and tools, they use their skills and tools in different ways. Business leaders concentrate externally on innovation and profit, whereas public health leaders focus on health status issues in a population. Both types of leaders are concerned with the customer of their programs and services, but public health leaders see the customer within the framework of social justice and population health status.

There are four challenges that a public sector or public health leader must address.[11] First, the public-sector leader works within the framework of laws, rules, and regulations that governmental entities define. These laws, rules, and regulations put restrictions on the public agency executive, and as a result can affect **mission, vision,** performance, and progress in addressing public health issues. Second, the performance of the agency is extremely visible to the outside world through legislative oversight and media scrutiny. Third, the internal and external stakeholders that are affected by the work of public agencies are more numerous than in the business world. Each stakeholder has issues that are unique. This translates into multiple and diverse demands on the work of these public health agencies. There may also be differences in the influence of different stakeholders. Finally, the realities of bureaucracy often impede or delay the ability of leaders to carry out the public's work in an efficient, effective, and timely manner.

The successful ability of public health leaders to handle these challenges creates a framework for their day-to-day work. The public health leader subscribes to the core functions and essential public health services model. This model posits a systems perspective for public health built around the functions of assessment, policy development, and assurance. Public health leadership involves not only managing a public health agency but also viewing public health in a community context. This means that the local or state public health agency is part of a family of local or state resources that address the health needs of the public. In addition, this family of agency resources, also known as the public health system, widens to include public, not-for-profit, and private agencies/stakeholders.

Public health leaders need to be concerned with the organization of the public health system within the context of the communities they serve, while simultaneously maintaining a strong foundation in the principles of public health practice that are discussed throughout this book. This dual understanding is critical for the understanding of all types of traditional and crisis public health issues. Public health leaders[12] need to become proficient in core transformational skills, political competencies, transorganizational or meta-leadership skills, and team-building and collaboration skills.

DEVELOPING EFFECTIVE PUBLIC HEALTH LEADERS: CURRENT APPROACHES

Fortunately, more resources are being dedicated to improve workforce and leadership capacity. The CDC also helps foster a national agenda for public health leadership development, including providing support for public health leadership institutes and the National Public Leadership Development Network (NLN). In 2008, this expanding consortium consisted of 35 state, regional, national, and international institutes providing an integrated system for leadership development.

The National Public Health Leadership Development Network

In 1991, CDC began to support development of public health leaders with the National Public Health Leadership Institute. This created the foundation for what is today a national system of state, regional, and national public health leadership institutes. These one- to two-year programs provide practitioners with access to a unique professional development opportunity to enhance leadership competence in performing essential public health services.

In 1994, CDC also provided support to establish the National Public Health Leadership Develop-

ment Network (NLN). The purpose of the NLN is to improve capacity of and access to leadership development programs through expanding collaboration among academic and practice institute directors, alumni, and representatives of federal, professional, and private organizations. Until 2007, the NLN, through sustained partnerships among schools of public health and state public health departments, was composed of 18 state, 9 regional (multistate), 4 national, and 3 international institutes. In mid 2007, the funding for institutes provided by CDC was changed to support 15 regional institutes and national institutes. This was accomplished by creating partnerships among the single state institutes and adding states to existing regions. The national level institutes include, in order of their establishment, The National Public Health Leadership Institute (PHLI), the CDC Leadership Institute, the National Health Education Leadership Institute, and the National Environmental Public Health Leadership Institute. PHLI provides leadership development for senior public health management and is instrumental in support for the Public Health Leadership Society, an alumni organization serving alumni from all leadership institutes.

Annual NLN conferences and business meetings are held to accomplish strategic objectives. Recent accomplishments include the following:

- Development of a core curriculum that is being used in the National Environmental Public Health Leadership Institute.
- Development of a *Conceptual Model for Leadership Development*[13]
- Development of the *Public Health Leadership Competency Framework*[12]
- Development of an *Evaluation Logic Model*
- Assessment of alumni network and development needs
- Dissemination of best practices, methods, and instruments
- Provision of technical assistance for developing new institutes
- Advocacy for strategic workforce development
- Advocacy for support and resource development

- Formal linkages with national organizations to accomplish objectives

- Creation of the Conceptual Model, the Competency Framework, and models for program evaluation that are fundamental to forming an integrated approach to leadership development[14]

Development of the Leadership Competency Framework

Continuing and professional education has traditionally focused on the practice needs of individuals in their specialized practice area or technical expertise. This form of education has generally led to professional credentials or certification in a field of practice.[15] Concern for the preparation and certification of leadership competence has led to increased demands for education and practice standards for leadership development.[16] Identification of competence requirements is of particular concern because practitioners within public health are prepared in a wide array of professional programs or disciplines.

In 1995, NLN academic and practice members identified the lack of and need to develop a competency framework specific to professional preparation of public health leaders and for those who aspire to or hold public health leadership positions. The objective was set to develop a competency framework for NLN institutes to use as a basis for design of core curriculum modules based on expected performance levels.[17,18] Several existing competency frameworks were identified to begin the process and to confirm the need to develop a specific framework for public health leadership.[19] The framework, consisting of 79 competencies, was developed over a 3-year period. The final set of 79 recommended competencies are divided into the following 4 competency areas:

- **Core Transformational Leadership Competencies:** Personal mastery, including **systems thinking,** which is comprised of analytical and critical thinking processes, visioning of potential futures, strategic and tactical assessment, emotional intelligence, communication and change

dynamics, and ethical decision making and decisive action.

- **Legal and Political Competencies:** Competence to facilitate, negotiate, and collaborate in an increasingly competitive and contentious political environment with complex multilevel crises and emergency events.

- **Trans-Organizational Competencies:** The complexity of major public health problems and crisis or emergency events extend beyond the scope of any single stakeholder group, community sector, profession or discipline, organization, or government unit, thus leaders must have the ability and skills to be effective beyond organizational or system boundaries.

- **Team Leadership and Dynamics:** Facilitation of learning teams or coalitions/networks to develop the capacity and capability to create integrated systems to accomplish mutual objectives.

The NLN serves as an efficient and effective means for producing core competencies and curriculum content from a common framework, determining levels of professional development and prerequisite criteria, and developing measurement and evaluation protocols. Measuring the effectiveness of leadership programs is accomplished through process, impact, and outcome evaluation. Competencies are used to design standards that operationalize teaching objectives and create impact and outcome evaluation models, methods, and instruments. The NLN and several regional and state institutes have conducted various levels of evaluation which show the impact of these leadership efforts on the participants and the public health system.[20,21] In 2005, the NLN created an evaluation logic model for use in design of leadership programs.[22,23] Ultimately, the objective is to measure program impact and outcome to assure competence and performance improvement measured by organizational performance standards.[24]

Efforts to certify and credential the public health workforce are moving forward. There is general agreement that any system designed to accomplish this should be based on fundamental core and universal competency frameworks.[25] There is also an agreement that these competency frameworks should include a set of leadership competencies required as core skills for the public health workforce. If various levels of public health workforce credentials are created, then there should be a distinct category for a high-level leadership credential.

Interest in accreditation of local and state health departments has resulted in development of several voluntary and nonvoluntary models for local and state public health agencies. These models include an emphasis on performance standards and required education and training for specific levels of agency practitioners. Some of these models include a recommended education and training level be implemented for those in leadership positions. These efforts will help solidify the need and impact of leadership development programs in public health.

Leadership Challenges in a Twenty-First-Century Context

The health challenges projected for the coming years are expected to test both the capability and supply of senior leaders in public health. The public health infrastructure and the health status of the population depend upon a viable workforce and skillful leaders.

At a time when the demands of public health leadership are increasing, leaders are in short supply because of demographic changes in the workforce. The baby-boom generation is retiring in record numbers. This is creating a situation where a group of young and relatively inexperienced workers will be asked to take leadership roles early in their careers. These young leaders are typically more technologically savvy than their predecessors, which creates an opportunity to apply some of the latest scientific and technological advances to significantly change the public health system. This group of emerging leaders will be asked to synthesize evidence-based programs and research to meet the needs of the public. These new leaders will also need to embrace and recognize increasing diversity, and design programs and products that are sensitive to cultural differences.

In addition to all these challenges, leaders must also act, think, and make decisions from a global perspective. This is particularly important when considered in light of the looming possibility of pandemic disease and related threats that can transcend traditional geographic boundaries. However, globalization also represents opportunity as well as challenge. The advent of Internet 2.0 tools such a wiki's, blogs, and other mass collaboration sites that are being honed for use in the public health practice and research fields presents the ability to engage in worldwide peer collaboration.

How Effective Leaders Must Respond

Public health leaders are best served by using a systems approach to leadership. The systems leadership model introduced earlier in this chapter (refer to Figure 18.1) gives a basis for change.[26,3] To achieve change, a leader must identify or create strategic, evidence-based programs and policies. These programs and policies should be based on data, information, and science (knowledge base). The leader then must use savvy and skills to mobilize political will for systems change. The four leadership models described in the following sections provide approaches to achieve systems change.

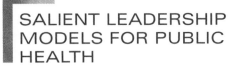

SALIENT LEADERSHIP MODELS FOR PUBLIC HEALTH

Many theories exist related to leadership, which are reviewed extensively in many business leadership books. We will concentrate here on four theories that seem the most relevant to leaders in the public health sector: *transformational leadership, servant leadership, systems leadership,* and *ecological leadership.*

Transformational Leadership

All leadership is about change. Burns[27] has pointed out that leadership is about reciprocity. Leaders are often called on to effect change through creating compromise between partners who may have different values and motivations, and bringing these partners together to collaborate to help reach their goals. The realities of the environment or communities in which these leaders come together also influence these goals. Burns defines two critical kinds of leadership—transactional and transformational. The transactional leader engages others in the reciprocal activity of exchanging one thing for another. Most leadership relationships are related to exchanges of one kind or another. Transformational leaders offer a purpose that transcends short-term goals and focuses on higher order intrinsic needs. This results in followers identifying with the needs of the leader. **Transformational leadership** examines and searches for the needs and motives of others.

In recognizing that public health leaders need to transform the system in which they work and change the understanding and commitment to the work of public health with their internal and external partners, the National Public Health Leadership Development Network sought to define the characteristics and competencies of a transformational leader. The three major activities of the public health transformational leader are; (1) engaging in the development of mission, (2) visioning, and (3) monitoring and facilitating the process of change.

Servant Leadership

The social justice philosophy inherent in public health brings with it a commitment to serve the public to promote health and prevent disease. Greenleaf[28] defines the **servant leader** as an individual who is committed to serving the public. The residents of a community, or professionals in community-based programs, need to actively accept the leadership of the individual who defines leadership in terms of the servant role. Spears, who has served as the Director of the Greenleaf Center for Servant

Leadership in Indianapolis defines 10 characteristics (skills) of a servant leader:[29]

1. Listening
2. Empathy
3. Healing
4. Awareness
5. Persuasion
6. Conceptualization
7. Foresight
8. Stewardship
9. Commitment to the growth (and health) of people
10. Building community

All of these skills are also necessary for the public health leader. Many leadership writers incorporate many of the servant leadership ideas in their own conceptual approaches to leadership.

Systems Leadership: The Five Learning Disciplines

Leaders learn in different ways. Senge[30] has developed a framework that allows us to at least partially understand this process. He pointed out that all traditional organizations need to redefine themselves as learning organizations. **Systems leadership** requires organizational leaders to orient their learning at five different levels. The five learning disciplines are personal mastery, mental models, shared vision, team learning, and systems thinking. At the personal mastery level, leaders will enhance learning for themselves as well as for others within the organization. At the mental model level, leaders will strive to understand the cultural context of the work of public health to see how cultural values and norms shape actions, problem-solving processes, and decision making. With a shared vision perspective, leaders will get a buy-in from partners and other stakeholders to the public health vision for the future. With team learning, leaders see that the combination of perspectives in a team provide a synergistic learning process where outcomes are more than inputs. The fifth level relates to systems thinking and how change gets created in those systems. Not only is change explored but also more effective and efficient ways to implement change processes within a system.

When looking at public health organizations as learning organizations, it helps to think of the collaborative leadership processes that are employed as processes that create "communities of practice." As people develop relationships, a sharing community is formed that is founded on the healthy exchange of ideas.[31] Learning occurs rapidly in communities when that learning helps people improve their own lives.[32] This is also viewed as building communities from the inside out, as members identify the assets within a group, and community residents and their partners build on these assets.[33] These ideas all have important implications that can help shape the development of learning communities in public health.

The public health leader needs to be a systems thinker, and see the whole community as the framework for change. The leader looks for **leverage points**, where the smallest efforts can make the biggest differences, as the system becomes more and more complex. The complexity of problems can interfere with effective decision making.[30] The leader may live in a complex world but must solve problems in as simple a fashion as possible or the decision's key stakeholders may not understand.

Traditional and Systems Thinking

Traditional thinking tends to be more linear, where "A" leads to "B," which leads to "C," in a causal chain.[34] When leaders put events into a pattern, they are moving toward a higher level of thinking. When patterns are combined, systems thinking, or looking at the connections between the patterns occurs.

Basic Language of Systems Thinking

The five major characteristics of a system are[35] listed here:

1. Every system has a purpose (mission), and every system is tied or related to other systems.

2. All parts of a system must be present or the system will not work properly. However, parts can be replaced or adapted to a new level of functioning.

3. The arrangement of the parts is critical if the system is to work.

4. Systems change because they constantly receive information that guides the system's operation (feedback).

5. Systems can remain stable only if they make adjustments based on feedback.

A number of tools have been developed to demonstrate how systems work. The steps of a systems thinking analysis are captured in Figure 18.2. Learning and leverage increases as the leader or team progresses down the pyramid. The analysis starts with the story of the events surrounding the issue. The leader then looks for patterns by identifying the key variables and graphing the trends that help clarify the focusing question. Then the leader examines the structure looking for loops and archetypes. Systems thinkers view their world in terms of two critical types of loops: reinforcing and balancing loops. If leaders develop a program intervention to address a problem, they would expect the intervention to have some impact. This is an example of a **reinforcing loop** (Figure 18.3). In this example, the pressure to restrict public smoking is increasing. As smoking ordinances are passed and enforced, the number of smoking facilities declines, which further decreases the tolerance for public smoking. The example of a balancing loop shows teen pregnancy rates experiencing a reduction but then seeming to level off after a period of time. The leader tries to determine why this new decline is happening. This is an example of a **balancing loop** (Figure 18.4). A grouping of two or more loops can create an **archetype,** which is a pattern seen over and over in many environments.

There is power in the use of the systems archetypes because they provide information and clarification for why things appear to be going right or not so right.[31.] There are eight key archetypes that

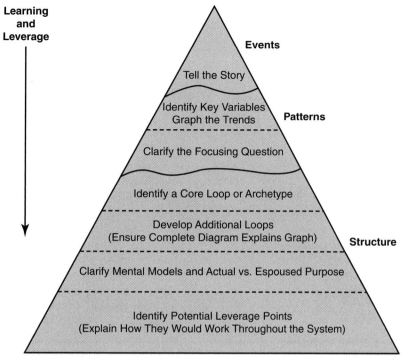

This process is iterative at all levels.

Figure 18.2. The Steps of a Systems Thinking Analysis

SOURCE: With permission of Michael Goodman and David Peter Stroh, www.appliedsystemsthinking.com, © 2007.

■ Reinforcing process loops:
  – virtuous cycles that generate growth or vicious treadmills that create disaster
  – this is an example of a virtuous cycle

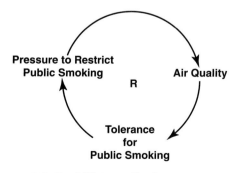

Figure 18.3. A Virtuous Cycle

SOURCE: With permission of Michael Goodman and Peter David Stroh, www.appliedsystemsthinking.com, © 2007.

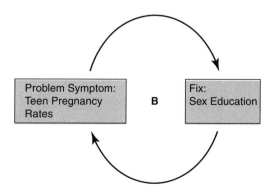

Figure 18.4. Balancing Process Loops

SOURCE: With permission of Michael Goodman and Peter David Stroh, www.appliedsystemsthinking.com, © 2007.

systems analysts use to help understand how the systems work:

1. Drifting Goals
2. Escalation
3. Fixes that Fail
4. Growth and Underinvestment
5. Limits to Success
6. Shifting the Burden

7. Success to be Successful
8. Tragedy of the Commons

An example of how Scholars in the National Environmental Public Health Leadership Institute have used the archetype models to create a causal loop diagram portraying the issues surrounding methamphetamine labs is shown in Figure 18.5. This example shows both balancing and reinforcing loops creating a "fixes that fail" archetype.

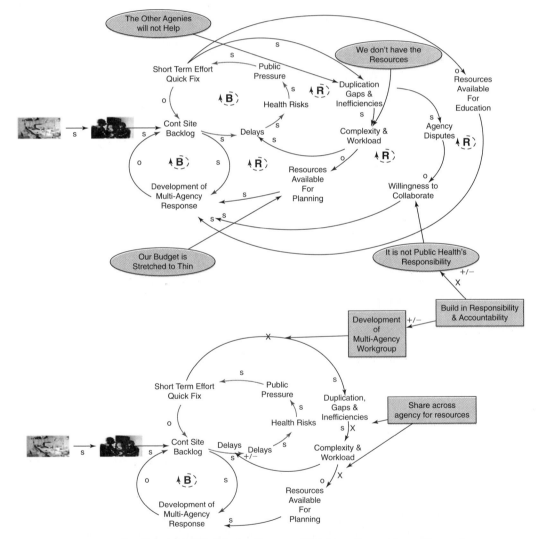

Figure 18.5. Dealing with Meth Labs: Systems Thinking Causal Loop Example

SOURCE: Permission from Connie S. Mendel, BS, RS and David E. Jones, MPH, RS.

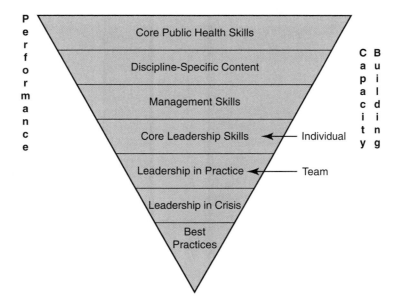

Figure 18.6. Leadership Pyramid

SOURCE: Rowitz L. *Public Health Leadership: Putting Principles into Practice.* Sudbury, MA: Jones and Bartlett; 2001.

Ecological Leadership

Leadership is generally viewed as a life-long learning process.[31,2] Leadership needs to be seen in the context in which the work of leadership takes place. Ecological leaders are professionals who are committed to the development of their leadership skills and competencies throughout their professional careers. These leaders are strongly committed to the appropriate application of these skills to their communities' changing health priorities. Public health leaders recognize that they need training at different times in their careers to address new perspectives and challenges that may arise. The context in which public health takes place is a critical determination of the skills and tools that will be needed. One way to view this is in the leadership pyramid (Figure 18.6).[36] The model shows the leader beginning with core public health skills and discipline-specific knowledge. This is built upon with management and core leadership skills. Practicing these skills as an individual or in a team results in the leader being prepared for crisis and the ability to apply best practices or evidence-based approaches to their work as a leader.

Leaders work at many different levels. They use different skill sets as the landscape of public health changes. Ecological public health leaders search for the training necessary to enhance their knowledge in a changing environment; they will need to synthesize their new skills in a seamless manner to the requirements of the jurisdictions in which they work.

LEADERSHIP ACROSS THE 10 ESSENTIAL PUBLIC HEALTH SERVICES

Since the release of the classic 1988 IOM monograph[37] on the future of public health, the public health community has struggled to apply the public health core functions model (assessment, policy

Essential Public Health Service	Leadership Activities
1. Monitor health status to identify community problems.	Use data for decision making.
2. Diagnose and investigate health problems and health hazards in the community.	Use data for decision making.
3. Inform and educate people about health issues and empower them to deal with the issues.	Engage in mentoring and training, social marketing, and health communication activities; empower others.
4. Mobilize community partnerships to identify and solve health problems.	Build partnerships; share power; create workable action plans
5. Develop policies and plans that support individual and community health efforts.	Clarify values; develop mission; create a vision; develop goals and objectives.
6. Enforce laws and regulations that protect health and ensure safety.	Protect laws and regulations; monitor adherence to laws.
7. Link people to needed personal health services and ensure the provision of health care when otherwise unavailable.	Stress innovation; delegate programmatic responsibility to others; oversee programs.
8. Ensure a competent public health and personal health care work force.	Build a learning organization; encourage training; mentor associates.
9. Evaluate effectiveness, accessibility, and quality of personal and population-based health services.	Support program evaluation; evaluate data collected; monitor performance.
10. Research for new insights and innovative solutions to health problems.	Utilize research findings to guide program development.

Figure 18.7. Essential Public Health Services Leadership Activities

SOURCE: Rowitz L. *Public Health Leadership: Putting Principles into Practice.* Sudbury, MA: Jones and Bartlett; 2001.

development, and assurance) and its pragmatic off-shoot, the 10 essential public health services, to the communities in which they practice (Figure 18.7). The core functions and essential services models are the framework for public health agency work. This presents the public health leader with a series of challenges. Leaders need to develop tools and techniques to put the core functions and essential public health services into practice, to use management and leadership tools to carry out organizational applications of the models and community applications of the model through the use of the MAPP technique and national public health performance standards, and to increase commitment to the models and educate internal and external stakeholders to the models and their use. Each of the 10 essential services also has specific leadership capacities associated with them. Examples of the leadership practices associated with each of the 10 essential services are contained in Figure 18.7.[2]

COMPETENT LEADERSHIP IN ACTION

In addition to the 10 essential public health services, another important perspective can be seen in the Council on Linkages between Academia and Public Health Practice framework,[38] which identified the core competencies of leaders at various levels in a public health organization. This presents eight specific competencies that the Council on Linkages argues are related to leadership and systems thinking skills, and the levels of competency the council feels are necessary for front-line staff, senior-level staff, and supervisory and management staff (Figure 18.8). In addition to specifying a competency requirement for carrying out the essential public health services, the framework recognizes

Specific Competencies	Front Line Staff	Senior Level Staff	Supervisory and Management Staff
Creates a culture of ethical standards within organizations and communities	Knowledgeable to proficient	Proficient	Proficient
Helps create key values and shared vision and uses these principles to guide action	Aware to knowledgeable	Knowledgeable to proficient	Proficient
Identifies internal and external issues that may impact delivery of essential public health services (i.e. strategic planning)	Aware	Knowledgeable to proficient	Proficient
Facilitates collaboration with internal and external groups to ensure participation of key stakeholders	Aware	Knowledgeable to proficient	Proficient
Promotes team and organizational learning	Knowledgeable	Knowledgeable to proficient	Proficient
Contributes to development, implementation, and monitoring of organizational performance standards	Aware to knowledgeable	Knowledgeable to proficient	Proficient
Uses the legal and political system to effect change	Aware	Knowledgeable	Proficient
Applies the theory of organizational structures to professional practice	Aware	Knowledgeable	Proficient

Figure 18.8. **Domain 8: Leadership and Systems Thinking Skills**

SOURCE: Public Health Foundation, Council on Linkages between Academia and Public Health Practice. *Competencies Project*. Available at http://www.trainingfinder.org/comptencies.

the importance of skills related to team-building, collaboration, and organizational learning. The public health leadership wheel (Figure 18.9) demonstrates one way to view the work of public health leaders from a systems perspective.[2] The wheel uses a combination of a planning and an action framework to view public health work. The first spoke of the wheel is team building. When public health faces a challenge from mild to severe and assesses the issue, this triggers a process of bringing together a committee, team, or coalition to address the challenge, study it, create a plan for dealing with it, put the plan into action, and evaluate the result. The next spoke in the wheel is **values clarification**. The team or other group type should first clarify its values and issues. The creation of a mission, a charge, or a determination of the purpose of the team comes next. This mission should be then incorporated into a team vision, to

help determine where the team process will go. Feedback is critical in all parts of the process since corrections or modifications will need to be made along the way.

After the mission and vision are made and written down, goals (long-term) and objectives (short- to mid-term) need to be made. Each goal and objective should reflect the mission and vision. These goals and objectives need to be translated into action steps, which then are incorporated into an implementation plan. Some scenario planning is possible at this stage to explore outcome possibilities. In addition, it is important to estimate the cost of the activities to address each goal and objective. Real costs must be determined for the action and implementation steps in the wheel. Implementation is done primarily in the assurance function of public health. Then, the whole process is evaluated. As the wheel illustrates, all the steps in planning and

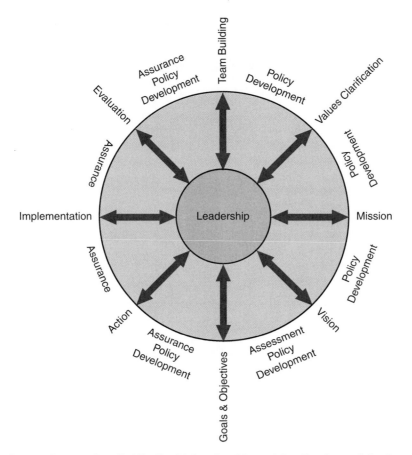

Figure 18.9. A System Approach to Public Health Leadership and Applications of the Core Functions

SOURCE: Rowitz L. *Public Health Leadership: Putting principles into Practice*. Sudbury, MA: Jones and Bartlett; 2001.

action also fulfill the public health requirements of carrying out the core public health functions.

Next we will review several of the most important competencies for public health leaders. These competencies include systems change, collaboration and teambuilding, creative thinking, policy and politics, ethics, performance management, developing others, and crisis leadership. Improved leadership performance strengthens the performance of the public health agency and the public health system as a whole.

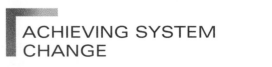

ACHIEVING SYSTEM CHANGE

The important contribution that systems thinking can play in public health leadership cannot be overstated. Keeping this in mind, public health leadership competencies are developed within the context of a community and are not limited to the competencies necessary to run an organization. Leadership is often about how ideas develop and how change and innovation happen. In his book, *The Tipping Point*, Gladwell describes how ideas and innovations spread.[39] The **tipping point** is where "the unexpected becomes expected," where radical change becomes more of a possibility. What was unexpected or rare now becomes reality. Gladwell applies his tipping point model to epidemiology to illustrate the relationship between how epidemics spread and the agent, host, and environment. Gladwell describes three factors that contribute to an epidemic:

1. **The Law of the Few (agent):** The presence of certain types of people called Connectors, Mavens, and Salesmen.

2. **The Stickiness Factor (host):** The "contagiousness" of the message and the ability of the message to gain adherents.

3. **The Power of Context (environment):** Influences how quickly the innovation will spread.

Figure 18.10 shows the relationship of Gladwell's three factors and epidemiology. Often, a few people lead the way to change.

The tipping point model suggests that there might be ways our conscious efforts to create change intentionally tips something. Perhaps public health leaders may be able to tip the scales to avert a potential health crisis and instead promote a healthy condition.

An example of individuals intentionally working to create breakthrough systems change is Ashoka, which is an international effort that supports social entrepreneurs in an effort to increase the reach and scope of their intervention efforts. In the book, *How to Change the World: Social Entrepreneurs and the Power of New Ideas,*[40] David Bornstein describes these innovators and their attempts to change the social canvas. Ashoka Fellows inspire others to adopt and disseminate their innovations, which demonstrate to all citizens that they too have the potential to be powerful change makers and make a positive difference in their communities.

The present landscape of public health and health crises presents a model of complexity.

The Law of the Few (The Agent)
- People who are crucial if an idea is going to be tipped:
  - **Mavens**—"the data banks who are fans of the idea and who understand and appreciate its significance."
  - **Connectors**—"the social glue" who spread the idea throughout their wide circle of acquaintances.
  - **Salesmen**—"the senders" who can persuade from the outside. They influence the "carriers" who receive the message and act on it.

The Stickiness Factor (The Host)
- A determination of the messages that catch on with some of the public and not others.
- Stickiness is the packaging that makes an idea memorable and irresistible.

The Power of Context (The Environment)
- The factors in a community that affect the impact of a problem.
- Epidemics are sensitive to the conditions and circumstances of the times and places in which they occur.
- There are two factors to consider in the power of context, the environmental aspects and our social networks.

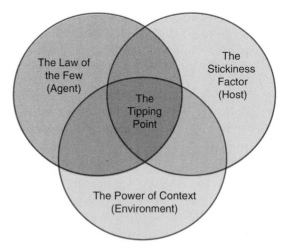

Figure 18.10. The Tipping Point and Epidemiology

SOURCE: Galdwell M. *The Tipping Point.* Boston, MA: Little, Brown; 2000.

Wheatley has stated that there needs to be chaos or disorganization before change occurs.[41] When we view systems, it is necessary to view a system within boundaries that appear to be ordered and somewhat predictable. In fact, many systems thinkers simply seek to examine a system within the context of what it is now. Complexity thinking suggests instead that leaders should look toward the future and envision what systems can be.

Wheatley points out that leadership is about building relationships. It is important to move away from a traditional view of the organization as a machine to a view of structure as something that grows out of the relationship and interaction between partners. Structure limits relationships between people because they put limits on people. Structure should be constantly evolving. Today's structure may be obsolete tomorrow, and things that are unimaginable in the present may guide future evolution of structure. Culture, values and belief systems, ethics, and even vision are all a part of today's chaos that brings new order in the future. This suggests that public health leaders need to be flexible and resilient, particularly since change is constant in the public health system. The syndemic view of health is another important model that can be used as a framework for public health systems change. The syndemic model presents a holistic view of public health and suggests that many public health problems are linked and may aggravate one another. Leaders need to see that many problems that they address cannot be confined to simple one-dimensional public health solutions. Problems that are multi-causal may be more effectively solved through a wider, community-based approach that is better suited to addressing many related conditions. The **syndemic perspective** also suggests that many community partners may need to work together to solve a problem because it may affect many of these partners in complex, interactive ways.

GETTING RESULTS THROUGH COLLABORATION AND TEAMBUILDING

Collaboration and collaboration skills are critical as more of the work of public health occurs outside the walls of public health agencies. According to Winer and Ray, collaboration is a mutually beneficial, well-defined relationship between two or more organizations or individuals that is created to achieve results that would not have occurred if these organizations or individuals had not worked together.[42] Collaboration requires a high level of intensity. Himmelman has pointed out that the ways that people work together go through a series of stages from less intensity to more intensity (Figure 18.11).[43] When people first come together,

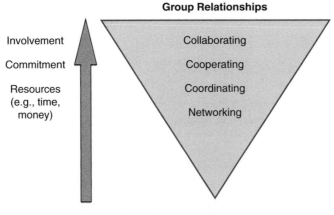

Figure 18.11. Group Relationships

in the networking phase, it is usually to exchange information and to discover what is state of the art at a particular point in time. This involves information exchange that generally benefits all the parties in the relationship. The goal of this informal networking activity is to address a common concern that each of the parties have. As the relationships increase in intensity, they enter a coordinating phase, in which information exchange and the alteration of activities to address the common purpose occurs. Coordinating activities tends to move the relationship of the parties into a more formal relationship. As intensity increases, parties enter a cooperation stage in which the various activities of the partners intensify with some modification of activities occurring, as well as the sharing of resources. These phases lead to the collaboration stage, where all the activities of the earlier stages increase, resources get shared, activities are modified, and the enhancement of the capacity of others occurs. In this collaboration stage, Himmelman points out that the collaborators also share risk, resources, responsibilities, and rewards.

Most discussions of collaboration involve a concern for the structure of the interactions. Just because people work together does not mean that collaboration is occurring. Coalitions tend to operate primarily at the networking level, although attempts at coordination may occur. Alliances and partnerships tend to be more intense and work at the coordination and collaboration levels, although networking and coordination may occur at the earlier stages of work before trust develops.

An important question involves whether public health leaders and other health professionals can learn the skills of collaboration. In 2002, the Turning Point Leadership Development National Excellence Collaborative[44] began the work of developing a curriculum to train public health leaders in collaboration. Several key themes emerged from the work of the collaborative:

- Collaboration and its leadership aspects can best be seen at a local level where there seems to be greater accountability.
- Collaboration is vital to the work of public health, which is a population-based activity.

- Individuals define collaboration differently. Federal, state, and foundation funding sources may also define it differently from local leaders who practice collaboration on a daily basis.
- Because different leadership styles are required for different situations, collaboration may not be the best approach in every circumstance.
- If collaborations are beneficial, it becomes critical to nurture them over time by supporting the various members when they need it.
- Collaboration can be unpredictable in that different members may have different agenda that take precedence to the collaborative activity, or unexpected happenings may occur.
- It is important to deal with team members who are skeptical of collaboration.
- Collaboration skill development needs to be included as a key competency for leadership development programs.

A number of public health leadership institutes and public health emerging leaders programs in the United States have used the six module collaborative leadership curriculum in whole or in part.

Systems thinkers talk about the benefits of creating learning organizations. All experiences provide a learning opportunity. Leaders ideally become proficient at learning. It is possible for the groups in which we work, whether a team, coalition, alliance, or partnership, to serve as a learning organization for team members. Often, as people work together and learn together, they produce better work. Senge, as previously pointed out, presented the five learning disciplines to demonstrate that we learn differently at each of the five levels.[30] It is in our group activities, from networking to collaboration, that learning occurs. If the views of Himmelman, Senge, and others are correct, learning should occur most readily in a collaborative environment.[45] Globalization provides us with the opportunity to collaborate with those in other countries and to create learning communities that cross borders. Working across organizations or countries requires that leaders become meta-leaders.

Using a three-legged stool, Senge[30] sees the learning disciplines for teams as representing aspiration (personal mastery and shared vision), complexity (systems thinking), and reflective conversation (mental models and dialogue). Creating an environment for learning enhances the work of public health and the public health leader. This will be explored in more depth in the next four sections.

The Creative Thinking Process and Envisioning the Future

The ability to think at a systems level also requires that leaders learn to harness their creative energy and use their creativity to build their organizations, find the role of their agencies in the wider context of the public health system, and work with external stakeholders and partners to build and strengthen the public health system. Many leaders solve problems and make decisions by taking the easy way out in their leadership and management approaches. Fritz calls this taking the path of least resistance.[46]

According to Fritz, it is important to create a new model for creatively dealing with challenges. He uses the process of germinating creative ideas and vision for a change, assimilating ideas and increasing momentum, and then eventual completion of the tasks at hand. Thus, creativity is more about process than it is about outcome. There is a creative tension between the path of least resistance and alternate creative processes of change. The leader has a vision of the desired result and an awareness of current reality. This creates tension that wants resolution. Figure 18.12 shows the creative tension that exists between our current reality and that to which we aspire.

DeBono[47] looks for ways to address challenges and creatively generate ideas by developing a process that is different from the way we normally solve problems. We often make our solutions more complex than they need to be. DeBono's process, called the six thinking hats, provides a creative approach that may be used to deal with challenges within our agencies or communities by helping to organize our thinking processes. A group of individuals address the challenge by going through the six thinking hats process.[48] An organizational leader or a professional facilitator leads the group and addresses the challenge, first by defining the

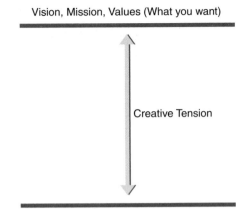

Figure 18.12. Creative Tension
SOURCE: With permission of Michael Goodman and David Peter Stroh, http://www.appliedsystemsthinking.com, © 2007.

issue and the ordering of the hats. Participants only discuss what the hat defines as the tasks at hand. The white hat discussion only relates to the presentation of factual information, the red hat explores the emotions behind the challenge, the black hat reviews the negative side of the possible solutions, the yellow hat reviews the positive aspects of the ideas generated, the green hat is about generating creative ideas and solutions, and the blue hat is the organizing hat. On the surface, the hat exercise appears artificial, but it can reduce the process of generating ideas and solutions significantly.

The responsibility of leadership does not end at the generation of an idea or a solution. It is important to ensure that the ideas are being properly implemented and effectively address the problems that they were meant to solve. Firestein warns leaders who are generating ideas that they need to go beyond generating ideas and be sure to evaluate ideas that have been generated and incorporate them into action plans and implementation strategies.[49]

For the team going through these creativity exercises and approaches, a concern for alignment of the team members around the process is critical.[30] When the team aligns its activities, the energy of the team increases as the team comes to agreement on mission, vision, goals and objectives, and action.

One way to do promote alignment is to spend time on values clarification, as presented in the leadership wheel. Ideally, a value consensus representing an alignment, between personal vision and the shared values that will guide the team into action, will emerge. Senge pointed out that the process involved in team learning is an alignment process with agreement components that increase the ability of the team to get the results that its members will want to support.

The role of the leader is not only to guide and promote the creative process but also to commit and support the outcomes. A systems perspective will also lead to community-based applications and help the agency better related to both its internal and external stakeholders. Leaders are not only the designers of the creative process; they are also the standard bearers for the system that is strengthened through the work of the leader and his or her partners.

To share a vision, it is first important to share and clarify the values of the organization and the community that the individual serves. Both our workplace and our service community are partially made up of the values and beliefs that the members of an agency or community have in common. These values and beliefs guide our individual and collective behavior and help to define the system in which we work. It is important to distinguish between the values that are universal across countries, that is, those values that are significant in our country and the values that impact our profession and our agency's work. It is important to clarify the relationships among personal values, community values, organizational values, and professional values.[2] Leaders need to work with their staffs to merge these different value sets into a meta-value statement for the public health agency. This meta-value statement helps to integrate the internal values of the agency with the value orientation of which the public health agency is a part. Time spent on this meta-value statement is worthwhile because it has the potential to significantly simplify the creation of both a mission for the agency and its vision for the future.

A properly constructed mission ideally is about today, that is, the purpose of an organization and the reason it exists. A properly constructed vision is about tomorrow and creating that road to tomorrow. There are three precursors necessary to the development of a vision.[50] The first precursor is the mission or the reason why the organization exists. The second precursor relates to the strategies that are used to carry out the agency's work. The third precursor relates to the values behind the work of the agency. Using these precursors as core to developing a vision to guide the growth of the agency and the agency's activities, Lipton develops a vision framework.[51] The other elements of the framework include the development of an executive staff, the development of techniques to manage the people processes of the agency, and the creation of what Lipton calls the "growth-enabling culture." It is not enough to put a vision down on paper. It is critical to create a work environment that will make the vision a reality. One of the critical tasks for the executive leadership team is to manage the culture of the agency. The leadership wheel discussed earlier is one way to make the vision a reality in that the wheel ties strategy to action and to results.

POLITICS, POLICY DEVELOPMENT, AND ADVOCACY

Politics play an important role in public health and influence many of the decisions that public health leaders make. Public health is often perceived as only related to the poor or disadvantaged. The philosophy of social justice inherent in public health is seen as "socialistic" and "liberal." Many leaders and citizens question the wisdom and appropriateness of using taxpayer money to help the disadvantaged—"those people". Public health is also equated with "big government"—the local or state public health agency—rather than being equated directly with public health issues. Public health leaders need to understand how the political system works and how to pursue the agendas of public health within our system of government. Politics define many of our official relationships in our community and in our nation at large.[52] Bellah has said that politics involves the translation of the moral consensus of the community into practice.[53] This perspective has profound implications for public health because moral and philosophical arguments are often at the root of decisions public health leaders make. DeLaney points out that a major task for leaders is to work to improve their positions within the system and increase the public value of the issues and positions that they pursue. It is important that the public health leader collaborate with internal and external stakeholders to build social capita, particularly when the infrastructure of public health is put at risk at the national level due to cutbacks in money for social programs.[6] Building social capital is especially important in public health emergencies when these relationships will guide us through the reaction and recovery phase of the crisis.

The 1988 IOM report[54] stated that public health leaders need to develop positive relationships with elected officials and inform these officials of important public health issues. Leaders also need to develop expertise in techniques, such as consensus building, that encourage citizen participation in public health issues. Public health leaders need to partner with health professionals from other sectors to create needed changes in program and develop policies that address public health challenges. Community-wide partnerships need to be constructed, and citizens need to be engaged in efforts to meet public health challenges. The public must be educated about the rationale and desired effects of new policies when they are implemented. This will require that public health leaders to work with grassroots leaders in efforts to address public health issues.

Public health advocacy is an important activity for public health leaders. Although it is true that many local ordinances and state statutes prevent governmental employees from directly contacting elected officials to influence decision making, it is possible to influence public health through our leadership roles in public health professional organizations. For example, the American Public Health Association (APHA) has developed a series of advocacy tips for public health leaders.[55] Leaders can also work with their community constituents and empower them to undertake this advocacy role. Public health leaders need to address the following techniques to empower others to be our advocates:[2]

- Building trust and credibility with community constituents
- Empowering others to be advocates for public health
- Doing background research on health issues
- Drafting policy statements in the language of potential legislative bills and municipal ordinances
- Working with elected or appointed officials on the appropriate legislation

Creating a Culture of Ethical Standards

Many of the health fields have a strong history of ethical deliberation, and have developed a code of ethics. Public health professionals, on the other hand, have come rather late to the creation of a code of ethics. The Public Health leadership Society, an organization composed of the graduates of the national Public Health Leadership Institute, undertook the development of a set of ethical principles for public health. This code is covered in Chapter 7 of this book. The code strongly reflects a belief that people are interdependent, and this interdependence is the critical element in the growth of communities.

A potential limitation to the code, especially when viewed from the perspective of public health as an interactive system, is that the code was intended only for one part of that system, the governmental public health and related agencies in the United States. Nevertheless, the code is an important first step that may help in the development of a more comprehensive code over the next several years. To best address the evolving nature of public health, the code needs to be a living document that can be updated as needed.

PERFORMANCE MEASUREMENT

An important part of the development of leaders and public health professionals in general is performance measurement. A critical link needs to be established between the performance of the individual and the performance of the organization. An important part of **coaching** and **mentoring** as well as general supervisory techniques is encouraging the employee to be part of the process. Many techniques are available to evaluate organizational performance. Harbour[56] says that performance measurement techniques tell an organization where they are in carrying out their goals, the need to set improvement goals on the basis of present performance, methods for determining the gap between goals and present performance, techniques for monitoring progress, how to identify problem areas, and how to use planning to improve performance.

It is important to encourage others and to not criticize them constantly for doing a bad job. Leaders need to encourage others in at least the six following ways:[57]

- Coaching
- Challenging others
- Listening
- Empathizing
- Giving recognition for good ideas and good work
- Rewarding

National Public Health Performance Standards (NPHPS)

Many common performance measurement tools are intended solely to measure the performance of an organization. In the field of public health, performance measurement is directed at the community, rather than primarily at the work of the public health agency. In this vein, The National Public

Health Performance Standards (NPHPS)[58] were developed to assess the status of the public health system. This calls for a community collaborative approach that includes key community stakeholders, as well as the local public health agency. An assessment is undertaken to evaluate the performance of that community in carrying out the core functions and essential services of public health. In spite of the community focus of the NPHPS, public health leaders tend to have oversight over the whole process and are often the driving force in making sure the process is carried out in an organized fashion. The NPHPS also assumes that public health needs to have a customer and community focus that incorporates a continuous quality management model into the standards protocol.

NPHPS includes three instruments. All the instruments use high benchmarks for success rather than baseline standards. One instrument assesses the performance of the state public health system. The second instrument looks at the functioning of the Local Public Health System (LPHS). The third instrument is used to assess governance issues that local boards of health or other governing bodies tend to use. The public health leader can use the results of the various instruments to plan and put into action activities and programs that will allow the state or local community to address essential public health services deficiencies and work to raise performance scores over time. Public health leaders should ensure that performance measurement is carried out on a regular basis.

DEVELOPING OTHERS

One of the important roles for a leader is the mentoring and coaching of others. Mentoring and coaching are important processes in succession planning. However, not all leaders are secure enough or expert enough to carry these tasks off well. And yet, mentoring and coaching includes some of the most important activities of the successful leader. It is the place where our legacy becomes more evident. Coaching is about how to do our jobs better, whereas mentoring is about our careers over the long run. Coaching and mentoring are both interactive. In coaching, the coach and the employee who is being coached want to do two things:[59] they want to solve some performance issue, and they want to develop the abilities of the employee to do the job better. Executive coaching is a high-level set of tasks related to coaching an executive or a leader. The executive coach is usually someone from outside the organization, is well trained for the coaching responsibilities, and may be certified to do executive coaching.

There are four stages in the coaching process. In the *Harvard Business Essentials* book series on coaching and mentoring,[59] these four stages are discussed in detail. In Stage 1 of planning, the coach is observing how the client or supervisee is behaving on the job. One technique used in the training of leaders is shadowing or following employees or leaders as they carry out their work during an average day. Some coaches also use this shadowing model. In Stage 2 of discussion, the coach discusses observations with the client. This needs to be a structured experience. The coach should use an outline to move the discussion along and leave a written summary with the client. In the Stage 3 active coaching of the client, a plan of action is set up that the client or employee will follow. Shadowing and observation may also occur in this stage. In Stage 4, follow-up sessions are done to measure progress. Coaching and executive coaching are very popular in the business world and are now being used more in the public sector as well. An interesting variation of the coaching model can be found in some training programs where the participants in the training bring a problem or personal situation to the training, and the facilitator uses these problems and a peer coaching(other participants in the training help solve the problem) model is employed.

Mentoring is very common in training as well as in situations where individuals are using the experience to develop their personal and team-based skills. The Harvard model defines mentoring as a process in which the goal is to enhance individual development in a career as well as in psychosocial functions. The psychosocial part of the process includes the use of various tools such as Myers-Briggs to help individuals get a better understanding of their personal strengths and weaknesses. Mentoring is about teaching, supporting, encouraging, counseling, and acting as a friend to the individual.[2] A number of state and regional leadership institutes around the country use the mentoring model.

CRISIS LEADERSHIP

Most of our leadership thinking is based on carrying out public health programs in times of normalcy rather than times of crisis. The events of September 11, 2001 have shifted the orientation of many public health agencies to emergency response. A preparedness paradigm was applied to all public health agencies with an understanding that all public health is about being prepared to address any emergencies that may occur in the future. Public health leaders will need to find ways to apply public health approaches rooted in the core functions and essential services model to our preparedness and practice activities. We have not been very successful at doing this thus far.

The shift to preparedness requires that public health leaders become competent in a new set of skills necessary to work in a preparedness environment in addition to the skills needed to function in times of normalcy.[60] Some of these **crisis leadership** skills include the following:

- Advanced systems thinking techniques
- Problem-solving skills
- The ability to work in an environment of complexity
- Communications and emotional intelligence skills
- Knowledge of international, national, state, and local laws
- Risk and crisis communication techniques

- Tipping point awareness and tools
- Forensic epidemiology knowledge and practices
- New methods for collaboration in a crisis environment, and community-building skills
- Emergency management and recovery in a national incident command management system
- Change strategies, and knowledge of new emerging infectious diseases
- Approaches to handling community-based techniques for chronic diseases in an aging American population

THE FUTURE NEEDS OF LEADERSHIP DEVELOPMENT

By 2010, we expect this to be the reality surrounding public health leadership development:

- Intense competition for individuals capable of leading health organizations
- An environment of extreme cognitive complexity, requiring extraordinary strategic thinking skills and the ability to make high-quality decisions quickly in the face of societal pressure and uncertainty
- An emphasis in many organizations on leadership skills—as opposed to technical skills and professional knowledge
- Highly refined communication and talent development skills as critical elements of "leadership"
- An increased priority on executive teambuilding, that is, staffing and mobilizing a team of talented partners—based on the belief that only *teams* of leaders will be capable of creating and implementing strategies that will improve the health status of the population

For this reason, the ability of leaders to convene collaborative teams that can achieve breakthrough systems change to meet these demands is critical for the future.

Faced with impending retirements, normal attrition rates, and a decline in the number of young professionals choosing traditional public health as a career, public health systems across the country are facing a leadership continuity crisis. National estimates have put the number of local health department top executives within five years of retirement at nearly 50 percent. The median age of these top executives is 52, with 88 percent falling between the ages of 40 and 69.[61] Staff with high levels of technical expertise within their respective fields but little or no management and leadership experience are replacing these retiring executives.

Future Challenges for the Field

The aging of public health workforce and the aging of the population in general will place stress on the current system and will require the next generation of leaders to build organizations to meet the health challenges of the population. This will require the use of science, research, and practice experiences to make evidence-based decisions. As we move to the accreditation of local health departments, state health departments, and governance bodies, a clear focus on continuous quality improvement will be imperative. This quality improvement applies to the practitioner as well.

Opportunities and Obligations for Every Practitioner

Leaders in public health have an opportunity to make a difference in the lives of the communities they serve. To be an effective leader, it is important to become a reflective leader and focus on personal mastery. This is accomplished by creating a personal quality improvement plan or personal development planning. This is usually accomplished by participating in assessments and feedback such as a 360-degree feedback instrument that allows your boss, peers, and colleagues to evaluate your abilities as a leader or manager. The leader can then use this information to set goals to build on their strengths and to remediate the weaknesses or areas for improvement. Leaders in public health should always have a self-improvement plan and goals they are striving to obtain to be the optimal resource for their organization and the community. The opportunity to make a huge impact on communities is there; leaders just needs to hone their skills to achieve success.

Leaders are also under a professional obligation to share knowledge and experiences with their colleagues at state and national meetings, to help new health administrators adjust to governmental work through executive coaching and mentoring, and to support training for the public health workforce. The specific activities that occur at this level of leadership include the promotion of the public health profession, the encouragement of staff and direct reports to become involved in state and national public health associations and activities, and to run for office in these organizations. The 16 leadership principles to guide leaders in public health are listed in Figure 18.13.

---

1. Strengthen the infrastructure of public health by utilizing the core functions and essential public health services framework;
2. Improve the health of each person in the community;
3. Build coalitions for public health;
4. Work with leaders from culturally diverse backgrounds;
5. Collaborate with boards for rational planning;
6. Learn leadership through mentoring and coaching;
7. Commit to lifelong learning;
8. Promote health protection for all;
9. Think globally and act locally;
10. Manage as well as lead;
11. Walk the talk;
12. Understand the importance of community;
13. Be proactive and not reactive;
14. See leadership everywhere;
15. Know that leaders are born and made; and
16. Live our values.

Figure 18.13. Leadership Principles to Guide the Public Health Professional

SOURCE: Rowitz L. *Public Health Leadership: Putting Principles into Practice.* Sudbury, MA: Jones and Bartlett; 2001.

REVIEW QUESTIONS

1. Using the systems approach to leadership, how would a leader make changes in the community?
2. Define collaboration, the four stages of interaction, and the commitment of the stakeholders at each stage.
3. What are four theories of leadership that are most relevant to public health?
4. List the four competency areas include in the national leadership competency framework. List at least three specific competencies under each area.
5. Explain how transactional and transformational leadership theory applies to public health.
6. List a least three skills needed in building communities through collaboration.
7. List the 10 essential public health services, and provide leadership practice examples associated with each of the 10 essential services.
8. List the 10 characteristics (skills) of a servant leader.
9. Name the five learning disciplines in a learning organization, and describe how the leader might implement these in public health.
10. Identify the four challenges of public health leadership.
11. What are the National Public Health Performance Standards, and how are they used?
12. Describe the approaches and tactics used to engage community advocates for political and or policy changes.

REFERENCES

1. Mobilizing for Action through Partnerships and Planning. Available at: http://www.naccho.org/topics/infrastructure/MAPP.cfm. Accessed May 15, 2007.
2. Rowitz L. *Public Health Leadership: Putting Principles into Practice.* Sudbury, MA: Jones and Bartlett; 2001.
3. Sternberg RJ. A systems model of leadership. *American Psychologist.* 2007;62:34–42.

4. United States Health Resources and Services Administration. Bureau of Health Professions. *Public Health Workforce Study*. Washington, DC; 2005.

5. Council of State Governments. *Trends alert: Public health worker shortages*. Lexington, KY; 2004.

6. Institute of Medicine. *The Future of Public Health*. Washington, DC: National Academy Press; 1988.

7. Haas Foundation. *Leadership Matters Study*. 2003.

8. Blumenthal, B. Investing in Capacity Building: A Guide to High-Impact Approaches. *Foundation Center;* November, 2003

9. Institute of Medicine. *Who Will Keep the Public Healthy? Educating Public Health Professionals for the 21st Century*. Washington, DC: National Academy Press; 2003.

10. Bennis W. The challenges of leadership in the modern world. *American Psychologist*. 2007;62:5.

11. Daly PH, Watkins M. *The First 90 Days in Government*. Boston, MA: Harvard University Press; 2006.

12. Wright K, Rowitz L, Merkle A, et.al. Competency development in public health. *American Journal of Public Health*. 2000;90(8):1202–1207.

13. Wright K, et al. A conceptual model for public health leadership development. *Journal of Public Health Management and Practice*. 2001;4: 60–66.

14. National Public Health Leadership Development Network website. Available at: http://www .heartlandcenters.slu.edu:16080/nln/. Accessed May 15, 2005.

15. Hunt, ES. Higher education and employment: The changing relationship. Recent developments in continuing professional education. Country study: United States Organization for Economic Cooperation and Development. Report no. OCDE/GD (92) 21. Paris, France; 1992.

16. Senge PM. The leader's new work: Building learning organizations. *Sloan Manage Review*. (1990):7–23.

17. Lovelace BE. A model for evaluating competency-based instruction. Unpublished paper, School of Merchandising and Hospitality Management, University of North Texas. Houston, TX; 1993.

18. Klemp, GO. Identifying, measuring and integrating competence. In: Pottinger P.S., Goldsmith J, eds. *New Directions for Experimental Learning Defining and Measuring Competence*. San Francisco, CA: Jossey-Bass; 1979.

19. Public Health Faculty/Agency Forum, Public Health Competencies, School of Public Health, University of North Carolina, Doctorate in Public Health Leadership Competencies, Johns Hopkins University School of Hygiene and Public Health, Community Based Public Health Competencies, Association of Schools of Public Health Maternal and Child Health Council Maternal, and Child Health Competencies, and Public Health Core Functions and Essential Services.

20. Umble KU, et al. The National Public Health Leadership Institute: Evaluation of a team-based approach to developing collaborative public health leaders. *American Journal of Public Health*. 2005;95(4):641–644.

21. Saleh, SS, Williams D, Balougan M. Evaluating the effectiveness of public health leadership training: The NEPHLI experience. *American Journal of Public Health*. 2005; 94(7):1245–1249.

22. Mains DA, Williams D. An evaluation framework to assess the impact of public health leadership training. Working Paper, August, 2004.

23. National Public Health Leadership Development Network website. Available at: http://www .heartlandcenters.slu.edu:16080/nln/. Accessed May 15, 2008.

24. Strebler MT, Bevan S. *Competence-Based Management Training*. Parkstone, UK: BEBC Distribution. Report no. 302. 1996.

25. Turnock BJ, Handler A. Is public health ready for reform? The case for accrediting local health departments. *Public Health Management Practice*. 1996;2(3):41–45.

26. Richmond JB, Kotelchuck M. *Oxford Textbook of Public Health*. Oxford, England: Oxford University Press; 1991.

27. MacGregor JB. *Leadership*. New York: Harper and Row; 1977.

28. Greenleaf RK. *Servant Leadership*. New York: Paulist Press; 1997.

29. Spears LC. *Insights on Leadership*. Hoboken, NJ: John Wiley and Sons; 1997.

30. Senge PM. *The Fifth Discipline*. New York: Currency Doubleday; 2006.

31. Wheatley M, Kellner-Rogers M. *A Simpler Way*. San Francisco: Berret-Koehler; 1996.

32. Freire P. *Pedagogy of the Oppressed*. New York: Continuum International Publishing Group; 2000.

33. Kretzman, JP, McKnight, JL. *Building Communities from the Inside Out: A Path Toward Finding*

and Mobilizing a Community's Assets. Evanston,
IL: Center for Policy Research; 1993.

34. Kim DH. Introduction to Systems Thinking.
Waltham, MA: Pegasus Communications; 1999.

35. Systems Thinker. What is Systems Thinking?
Waltham, MA; Pegasus Communications; 2002.

36. Lichtveld M, Rowitz L, Cioffi J. The leadership
pyramid. Leadership in Public Health.
2004;6(4):3–8.

37. Institute of Medicine. The Future of Public Health.
Washington, DC: National Academy of Science;
1988.

38. Public Health Foundation, Council on Linkages
between Academia and Public Health Practice.
Competencies Project. Available at: http://phf.org/
link/corecompetenciesdraft.htm.

39. Galdwell M. The Tipping Point. Boston, MA:
Little, Brown; 2000.

40. Bornstien D. How to Change the World: Social
Entrepreneurs and the Power of New Ideas. New
York: Oxford University Press; 2003.

41. Wheatley MJ. Leadership and the New Science.
San Francisco: Berrett-Koehler; 1999.

42. Winer M, Ray K. Collaboration Handbook. St.
Paul, MN: Amherst H. Wilder foundation;
1997.

43. Himmelman A. Collaboration for a Change. Min-
neapolis, MN: Himmelman Consulting; 2002.

44. Turning Point. Collaborative Leadership: Collaborative Leadership Learning Modules. Seattle, WA:
Author; 2004.

45. Friedman TL. The World Is Flat. New York: Farrar,
Straus, and Giroux; 2006.

46. Fritz R. The Path of Least Resistance. New York:
Fawcett Columbine; 1989.

47. DeBono, Edward. Simplicity. New York: Penguin
Books; 1998.

48. DeBono E. Six Thinking Hats. Boston, MA: Back
Bay Books (Little, Brown); 1999.

49. Firestien RL. Leading on Creative Edge. Colorado
Spring, CO: Pinon Press; 1996.

50. Lipton M. Guiding Growth. Boston, MA: Harvard
Business School Press; 2003.

51. Lipton Mark. Guided Growth. Boston, MA:
Harvard Business School Press; 2003.

52. DeLaney A. Politics for Dummies. Foster City, CA:
IDG Books; 1995.

53. Bellah RN. The quest for the self. In: Rubinow P,
Sullivan WM, eds. Interpretive Social Science.
Berkley, CA: University of California Press; 1997.

54. Advocacy Tips for Public Health Leaders. Available at: http://www.apha.org.

55. Rowitz L. Public Health for the 21st Century: The
Prepared Leader. Sudbury, MA; 2006.

56. Harbour JL. The Basics of Performance Measurement. Portland, OR: Productivity Press; 1997.

57. Ramundo M, Shelly S. The Complete Idiot's Guide
to Motivating People. Indianapolis, IN: Alpha
Books; 2000.

58. Centers for Disease Control and Prevention.
National Public Health Performance Standards.
Atlanta, GA; 2003.

59. Harvard Business Essentials. Coaching and Mentoring. Boston, MA: Harvard Business School
Publishing; 2004.

60. Rowitz L. Public Health for the 21st Century: The
Prepared Leader. Sudbury, MA; 2006.

61. National Association of City and County Health
Officers (NACCHO). National Profile of Local
Health Departments. Washington, DC; 2005.

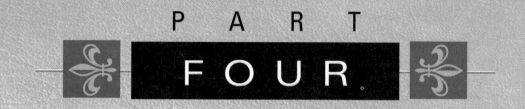

PART FOUR.

The Provision of Public Health Services

CHAPTER 19

Chronic Disease Control

Janet Collins, PhD, Linnea Evans, MPH, and David V. McQueen, ScD*

The findings and conclusions in this chapter are those of the authors and do not necessarily represent the views of the Centers for Disease Control and Prevention.

LEARNING OBJECTIVES

Upon completion of this chapter, the reader will be able to:

1. Identify key data sources for describing the health status of communities, including the distribution and changes in risk factors associated with chronic disease.

2. Summarize major determinants of health and illness, particularly the social, environmental, and behavioral factors known to be associated with chronic disease.

3. Describe the basic concepts and effective models for prevention and control of chronic disease, highlighting program and policy examples from risk factor-, disease-, setting-, and population-based approaches.

4. Articulate some of the critical issues that continue to challenge public health professionals working to address chronic diseases.

KEY TERMS

Applied Research
Behavioral Surveillance
Chronic Diseases
Community
Efficacy
Effectiveness
Health Promotion
Mortality Surveillance
Program Evaluation
Program Intervention
Surveillance
Translation

*The authors would like to thank Carma Ayala, Stephen Banspach, Barbara Bowman, Terry Brady, Cheryll Cardinez, Ralph Coates, Gerald Cook, Deborah Galuska, Bob German, Jennifer Hootman, Rick Hull, Etta Jenkins, Darwin Labarthe, Youlian Liao, Amanda Navarro, David Nelson, and Sam Posner of the National Center for Chronic Disease Prevention and Health Promotion for their reviews and editorial assistance.

In this new century, heart disease, cancer, and other chronic diseases will continue to place a huge burden on global health. By 1990, chronic diseases had already surpassed infectious diseases as the leading cause of death in all areas of the world except sub-Saharan Africa and the Middle East. By 2020, chronic diseases are expected to account for 7 of every 10 deaths in the world, as they already do in the United States. These projections suggest that chronic diseases—and the death, illness, and disability they cause—will soon dominate health care costs and change the role of public health worldwide.[1,2]

In this chapter, the emphasis is on chronic disease in the United States, the special role for behavioral risk factor surveillance, and what is known about effective public health approaches to chronic disease prevention and control. Emerging topics such as border health, global health, and mental health that are closely linked with chronic disease are also discussed.

BURDEN OF CHRONIC DISEASE

Chronic diseases are illnesses that are prolonged, do not resolve spontaneously, and are rarely completely cured. Chronic disease trends in the United States have mirrored the pattern of most advanced industrialized countries. With regard to the two major chronic diseases, rates of cardiovascular disease deaths have declined steadily since the 1960s, and cancer survival rates have improved slightly in recent decades.[3-5] Despite these improvements, more than 1.7 million people die of a chronic disease each year.[6,7] Cardiovascular disease accounts for the largest percentage of deaths (36.3%).[4] Cancer, the second leading cause of death, accounts for about one-fourth of all deaths, and many cancers still have low survival rates. For example, only about 15 percent of people with lung cancer survive for more than five years.[5]

The majority of people who die of chronic diseases are older (60+), but chronic diseases also take a heavy toll on adults who are in the prime of life. Many of the years of potential life lost before age 75 can be attributed to chronic disease (Table 19.1).[8,9] Moreover, chronic diseases, notably cardiovascular diseases are an important cause of premature deaths among African Americans and Hispanics. These conditions account for much of the higher premature death rates observed in African Americans.[6]

Chronic disease morbidity and mortality is often related to health risk behaviors, many that begin before adulthood. Nearly 40 percent of United States deaths have been attributed to smoking, physical inactivity, poor diet, and alcohol use—all risk factors for chronic diseases and all modifiable (Table 19.2).[10,11] Tobacco use has been described as the largest single factor resulting in early deaths in most of the developed world.[12-14] In the United States, it is estimated that more than 430,000 people die each year because of tobacco use. Smokers who die from tobacco-related illness lose an average of 12 years of expected life. It is estimated that an unhealthy diet and lack of physical activity account for at least 300,000 deaths each year in this country. It is clear that one primary mission for public health is to reduce the prevalence of these risk factors.[6]

Deaths alone do not give a complete picture of the chronic disease burden. Millions of people in the United States endure years of pain, disability, and lower quality of life because of chronic diseases such as arthritis and diabetes. Chronic disabling conditions cause major limitations in activity for more than 1 in every 10 Americans. This impact is expected to increase dramatically as baby boomers age. By 2020, an estimated 60 million Americans—or 1 in every 5 persons—will be affected by arthritis, and nearly 12 million of these people will have activity limitations.[6]

Chronic diseases belong at the top of public health concerns because heart disease, cancer, diabetes, arthritis, and mental health are the primary determinants of length and quality of life. Not surprisingly, these conditions also define the vast

Table 19.1. Years of Potential Life Lost Before Age 75 for Selected Causes of Death, United States, Selected Years 1990 and 2003*

	1990	2003*
Diseases of the heart	1,617.7	1,214.1
Cerebrovascular diseases	259.6	207.0
Malignant neoplasms (cancers)	2,003.8	1,628.0
Chronic lower respiratory diseases	187.4	187.8
Influenza and pneumonia	141.5	91.6
Chronic liver disease and cirrhosis	196.9	162.6
Diabetes mellitus	155.9	189.1
Human immunodeficiency virus (HIV) disease	383.8	151.5
Unintentional injuries	1,162.1	1,085.8
Suicide	393.1	344.3
Homicide	417.4	275.4
All chronic disease causes	***4421.3***	***3588.6***
All causes	**9,085.5**	**7,562.0**

*Crude number of years lost before age 75 per 100,000 people under 75 years of age. Italic type denotes chronic diseases.

SOURCE: Centers for Disease Control and Prevention, National Center for Health Statistics. *Health, United States 2006 with Chartbook on Trends in the Health of Americans.* Hyattsville, MD: 2006; 183.

Table 19.2. Actual Causes of Death in the United States in 1990 and 2000

Actual Cause	No. (%) in 1990*	No. (%) in 2000
Tobacco	400 000 (19)	435 000 (18.1)
Poor diet and physical inactivity	300 000 (14)	365 000 (15.2)
Alcohol consumption	100 000 (5)	85 000 (3.5)
Microbial agents	90 000 (4)	75 000 (3.1)
Toxic agents	60 000 (3)	55 000 (2.3)
Motor vehicle	25 000 (1)	43 000 (1.8)
Firearms	35 000 (2)	29 000 (1.2)
Sexual behavior	30 000 (1)	20 000 (0.8)
Illicit drug use	20 000 (<1)	17 000 (0.7)
Total	**1 060 000 (50)**	**1 111 500 (46.3)**

*Data are from McGinnis and Foege. The percentages are for all deaths.

SOURCE: Mokdad AH, Marks JS, Stroup D, Gerberding J. Actual causes of death in the United States. [Published erratum in: *JAMA.* 2005;293:293–294]. *JAMA.* 2004;291:1238–1245.

majority of the $2 trillion spent on health care each year in the United States.[15] Figures from 2001 estimate the care given to people with chronic conditions accounted for over 80 percent of health care spending in this country.[16] Further, these health care costs are increasing at unprecedented rates. Any chance at slowing or containing increasing health care costs will require investment in public health measures to maintain good health, especially among populations at greatest risk, rather than waiting to cope with disease after they are established.

Despite the vast impact of chronic diseases on length and quality of life, there is not always a clear, scientific role for public health action. For any given chronic condition, several factors must be considered before embarking on a response, including whether a science base exists for a population-based approach to prevention or control. It is important that public health's scarce resources be applied to conditions for which interventions have been shown to have proven **efficacy** (an interventions ability to work under ideal circumstances) on a population basis, such as tobacco use prevention and cessation, colorectal cancer screening, physical activity promotion, and high blood pressure control, to name a few. Conditions that are relatively rare, without preventive methods or predictive screenings, and for which highly individualized clinical care provides the greatest hope are not ideal candidates for public health investment.

In a context where health challenges far outpace the resources available to address them, public health investments must be closely aligned to the available science. Strong evidence of **effectiveness** (results obtained under real world circumstances), including cost-effectiveness, should direct our actions and priorities. Likewise, investment in the research endeavor is essential to new and improved public health interventions. Thus, high priority must be given to both scientific discovery as well as putting that science into practice. Investment in science is fruitless in terms of health benefit unless it results in widespread improvements to public health practice. Unfortunately, the history of scientific application suggests that findings such as those

from the Diabetes Prevention Program[17] showing the dramatic impact of a lifestyle intervention on the onset of diabetes may take 20 years or more to be fully implemented. Speeding up the process of **translation,** that is, putting proven public health interventions into practice, is an area in need of scientific study itself.

The magnitude of chronic disease has been well recognized by those working in public health. However, there has not been a proportional investment in this field. Although not logical in a statistical sense, people often tend to be much more fearful of unpredictable, unexpected, and poorly understood risk than they are of more common risks. We seem to adapt or become immune to familiar high levels of disease by developing a certain complacency or faulty sense of inevitability to heart disease, diabetes, and cancer. On the other hand, less familiar risks such as severe acute respiratory syndrome (SARS), bird flu, or anthrax, take precedence in both the "fear factor" and the relative societal investment. There is a lack of a "sense of urgency" with regard to chronic diseases. Creating a sense of "urgency" and "importance" is a challenge to those working in the field of chronic disease prevention.

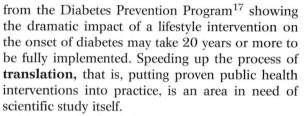

KEY PUBLIC HEALTH STRATEGIES

Many of the same public health strategies essential to efforts in infectious disease, injury, and environmental health apply equally well to work in chronic disease prevention and control, including surveillance, program interventions, applied research, program evaluation, policy, and supportive physical and social environments.

Public Health Surveillance

In public health terminology, **surveillance** refers to the systematic and routine collection of data to help identify and monitor health risks over time. Public health surveillance has a critical role in chronic disease control because it allows us to monitor changes and trends in disease rates, behavior, and social factors over time and in different populations.[18,19] Surveillance provides the information to plan more effective public health interventions and better target program efforts. In addition, surveillance efforts can be used to examine the effects of policies and programs on public health outcomes.

Mortality Surveillance

Mortality surveillance is the systematic and ongoing collection of data on the causes of death for individuals. Mortality surveillance is perhaps the most basic type of surveillance and has been practiced for hundreds of years.[20] Mortality data are one type of vital statistics. In most of the world, including the United States, mortality surveillance is routine. Classification of cause of death is standardized worldwide through an internationally agreed-upon system.[21] Mortality surveillance works best when measures are taken to ensure that the cause-of-death data are highly accurate. This is especially important for chronic disease deaths, which often have multiple causes, thus making classification more difficult.

Surveillance of Behaviors, Physiological Risk Factors, and Disease Outcomes

Behavioral surveillance plays a unique and important role in the field of chronic disease through its relevance to prevention and early intervention. Through behavioral risk factor surveillance, we can examine the relationship between risk behaviors at the population level and disease patterns in the population, and ensure appropriate and useful data to help us plan and evaluate health promotion and risk reduction programs.

When surveys are conducted using standardized methods over many years, such as in the Centers for Disease Control and Prevention (CDC)-supported Behavioral Risk Factor Surveillance System (BRFSS), they are considered a basic surveillance system. The BRFSS is a state-based, random-digit-dialed telephone-based surveillance system tracking noninstitutionalized United States civilians aged 18 years and older; it collects state-level information on adults' health status, use of preventive services, and risk behaviors associated with many of the leading causes of illness and death.

Another basic surveillance system is the Youth Risk Behavior Surveillance System (YRBSS), which collects extensive data from students in grades 9–12 on many of the risk factors that can lead to chronic diseases. The CDC-supported YRBSS includes a national survey as well as surveys conducted by state and local education and health agencies. Two other national survey systems of critical importance to chronic disease planning are the National Health Interview Survey (NHIS) and the National Health and Nutrition Examination Survey (NHANES) (see Table 19.3).

Public health agencies that conduct behavioral surveillance must deal with complexities that can affect the quality and usefulness of the data, and how the data are translated into public health action. In the following sections, we explore some of these issues.

The Importance of Ownership and Partnership in Data Collection for Chronic Diseases

Increasingly, the term *local* is used to refer to smaller geopolitical areas. Whereas some people argue that national data might not reflect state interests, others contend that state data, particularly from large states, might not reflect the perceived and real differences within a state. Perhaps the most notable examples come from states with wide disparities between highly populated urban and low-density rural areas. In planning and assessing public health programs, states want data considered meaningful at a local planning level. Although the BRFSS was designed to produce state-level estimates on health risk behaviors and preventive health practices, CDC is now able to analyze BRFSS data for 175 metropolitan and

Table 19.3. Four Major Survey-Based Chronic Disease Surveillance Approaches

Date Established	BRFSS* 1982	NHIS† 1957	NHANES§ 1960	YRBSS¶ 1991
Outcome	Risk factor data for individual states	Data on health status and risk factors in the U.S.	Risk factor and disease data in the U.S.; focus on diet	Risk factor data on children in schools
Scope	Nationwide, state by state; adults >17 years of age	National sample; primarily adults >17 years of age (some info collected on children residing in household via interviewee)	National sample; individuals up to 74 years of age	National, state, territorial, and local samples; primarily students in grades 9–12
Method	Random-digit-dial household, computer-assisted telephone interview	Household survey	Household interview plus medical exam and lab work	Written survey, self-administered in school
Strengths	Timely, state- and local-level data; monthly data points	Depth of question areas; supplemental surveys	Very comprehensive; objective biochemical and physiological measures	In-depth look at behaviors of students. Additional strength is timely, state- and local-level data
Weaknesses	Lack of depth; telephone-dependent; self-reported data	Self-reported data; data not local	Notably complicated analytical challenges; not timely; only national and regional data	Limited to students in school; self-reported data
Comments	Highly flexible system that allows states to add questions on numerous health topics	The standard for health status data in the U.S.	Extensive information on chronic diseases	Extensive information on risk factors that lead to chronic diseases in later life

*Behavioral Risk Factor Surveillance System.

†National Health Interview Survey.

§National Health and Nutrition Examination Survey.

¶Youth Risk Behavior Surveillance System.

micropolitan statistical areas (MMSAs), which are smaller geographic areas with 500 or more survey respondents. This analysis has shown substantial differences among MMSAs. For example, in 2006, the prevalence of no health insurance ranged from 6.2 percent in the Nassau-Suffolk, NY metropolitan division to 39.1 percent in the El Paso, TX metropolitan statistical area. As another example, the YRBSS provides data for 23 large urban school districts.

Quality of Surveillance Data

Questions of quality go well beyond the standard concerns with validity and reliability.[22] The concerns incorporate concepts of "total survey errors," which take into account errors arising from coverage, nonresponse, sampling, interviewer bias, respondent bias, instrument limitations, mode, and other sources of bias. Two hotly debated issues in behavioral risk factor surveillance are questionnaire content and method of data collection.

Questionnaire content cannot be separated from the theme of ownership. Previously, questionnaire content may have been chiefly determined by academics and government agencies, but now questionnaire development belongs to many different constituencies. Questions in surveillance systems are the product of competing interest groups with many different agendas. The present concern is often not what question to ask, but what the question is going to be used for and who will use it. Thus, good surveillance systems are by necessity responsive to arising needs and flexible enough to adapt quickly to questions dictated by policy needs and shifts in the topics of relevance to public health.

Data collection methodology also has benefited greatly from more than two decades of experience with different data collection approaches. The once accepted "gold standard" of face-to-face interviewing has been replaced with a careful understanding, largely in terms of survey errors and survey costs, of the relative strengths and weaknesses of mail, cell or telephone, paper and pencil, face-to-face and Internet-based strategies.[23]

Program Interventions

The public health response to the large and complicated challenges of chronic disease prevention and control is a relatively recent development. As just one example, the CDC established a center for chronic disease only in 1988, and it was not until 2006 that a Division for Heart Disease and Stroke Prevention was established even though heart disease had been the nation's leading cause of death for decades.

Program interventions designed to prevent and control chronic disease include information, counseling, skill building, medical, and community services delivered through a wide array of settings and the media. The quality of a program can be assessed by considering the reach (the number of persons benefiting from the intervention), cost, effectiveness, including disparity elimination, and sustainability. Programs designed to prevent and control chronic disease are quite varied and include everything from school- and community-based tobacco use prevention programs to training in disease self-management.

Applied Research

As a relatively new field, applied research is a critical part of the public health response to chronic disease prevention and control. **Applied research** examines the efficacy of interventions in an effort to identify ever more powerful and less costly ways to prevent and control disease. Applied research such as the Diabetes Prevention Program sometimes opens entirely new fields of public health work, in this case, the prevention of diabetes rather than just its control.

Program Evaluation

Program evaluation should go hand-in-hand with program delivery to determine whether a given program is actually achieving the intended outcomes. Program evaluation works best when it is included as part of initial program planning and when it provides useful data in a continuous improvement cycle. For example, program innovations such as lay community health workers or promotoras are well worth evaluating because they may give rise to program models with credible evidence of effectiveness that are both affordable and sustainable over time. Too often, programs or policies are instituted without being previously tested (applied research) or evaluated and are nonetheless thought to be effective because the clientele seems to like them. Public health resources are too few and too precious to be used on interventions with no objective evidence of effectiveness.

Policy Interventions

Changes to the policy environment are sometimes the most powerful and cost-effective interventions available because, once established and implemented, they impact large populations over long periods of time. Work on smoking prevention serves as one of the most well-known models of policy intervention, including smoking ordinances, tax increases, enforcement of sales to minors, cessation benefit coverage, and advertising restrictions. Although policy change is often challenging, in part due to local control, there is hardly an area of public health that cannot be influenced in a positive way through formal or informal policy interventions. Policy interventions that are being pursued in the chronic disease area include food labeling for nutrient content, health care benefit coverage, school physical education requirements, worksite health promotion, and transportation and building regulations, to name a few.

Supportive Physical and Social Environments

Changes to the physical environment such as the availability of sidewalks, walking trails, or a safe place to play can make a large difference in the health-related behaviors of a neighborhood or community. Influences to the physical environment can range from a micro level such as the food choices available within a neighborhood to a macro level such as fluoridation of an entire city's water supply. Pricing is a huge consideration within the physical environment. As just one example, healthy food choices such as fruits, vegetables, whole grain products, and low-fat meats and fish tend to be more expensive than high fat, high sugar, calorie-dense foods.

Social support such as a walking group or a tobacco cessation counselor can be the difference between success and failure in initiating and maintaining behavior change. Programs that take the physical and social environment into consideration or better yet that work to ensure that the environment reinforces healthy behaviors are more likely to produce lasting results.

APPLICATION OF CHRONIC DISEASE CONTROL STRATEGIES

Early chronic disease prevention programs within state health departments were generally limited and had difficulty being sustained during tight budget times. As recently as the late 1980s, fewer than half of the states had programs in diabetes control. To some extent, these limitations in funding and infrastructure continue today, with just half of the states funded by the federal government for cardiovascular disease, nutrition, physical activity, and obesity prevention. Furthermore, local health departments, with the exception of some of the largest urban areas, have little infrastructure to tackle chronic disease control.

Some progress has been made in the past 20 years, however. State health departments, which once relied almost exclusively on federal dollars to support their chronic disease control efforts, are garnering more funding from state legislatures and executive branches. States are increasingly aware that chronic diseases—as the leading causes of death and disability—are also the leading source of health care costs. These costs, particularly those related to long-term care, are often born by the states. The financial burden on states will only increase with the aging of the population. Also driving the expansion of chronic disease control efforts are scientific advances and a growing base of interventions that have been proven effective in preventing or substantially delaying illness.

The enormous number of people with well-established risk factors for chronic diseases means that physician-based interventions alone are likely to not reach many of those in need of services. In recent years, public health approaches have emphasized links with community organizations and coalition building as fundamental strategies to leverage resources and, more importantly, to engage a broad set of community settings in chronic disease prevention activities.

For example, the Prevention Research Center at Morehouse School of Medicine[24] has worked hard to solicit community input and support for its projects, which focus on risk reduction and early detection of diseases in African American and other minority populations in Atlanta. Neighborhood groups, schools, youth clubs, health agencies, and organizations serve as links to the target populations. The center has a Coalition Board that is active in setting research priorities and reviewing research projects. The board has defined community values and worked collaboratively to ensure the center's projects are based on these values. Another example is the Cambodian Community Health REACH 2010 project,[25] which is targeting cardiovascular disease and diabetes among Cambodian refugees in Lowell, Massachusetts. The project established a Cambodian Elders' Council to give a voice to older refugees, who often are homebound, isolated, and have limited English skills.

In the sections that follow, we describe interventions that target risk factors and those that target specific chronic diseases. Also discussed are program settings and populations that are the focus of chronic disease control programs.

Programs Targeting Risk Factors

One approach to analyzing risk factors is to determine how modifiable they are. Sex, age, and race are unchangeable. Factors such as education, income, and levels of social support are somewhat modifiable either at an individual or societal level. Diet, physical activity, smoking, and substance abuse are highly modifiable. Chronic disease control programs have targeted a variety of risk factors. The sections that follow focus on important risk factors for chronic disease prevention, including

tobacco use, alcohol use, nutrition, physical activity, and obesity.

Tobacco Use

State health department activities to prevent and control tobacco use have increased markedly in recent years. This growth has resulted from a variety of factors:

- Rising public intolerance of environmental smoke as a health hazard
- State legislation to restrict indoor smoking
- Increased excise taxes on cigarettes
- Funding and support from the National Cancer Institute, the American Cancer Society, the CDC's Office on Smoking and Health, and nongovernmental sources
- Master Settlement Agreement funds from the tobacco industry
- Activism by tobacco consumer groups

In addition, public health activities to prevent and control tobacco use include mass media campaigns, community efforts such as school-based interventions, and tobacco use cessation services.[26] California had much success during the early years after passing Proposition 99, which raised the excise tax on a pack of cigarettes by 25 cents in 1989 and originally designated some of the revenues for tobacco control activities. In the first 5 years after the excise tax was raised, monthly cigarette consumption per person declined 52 percent, from 9.7 packs in 1989 to 6.5 packs in 1993.

The decline was significantly greater in California than in the rest of the United States. No significant declines in cigarette consumption occurred between 1994 and 1996, possibly because of reduced funding for the state's tobacco control program, increased funding for tobacco advertising and promotion, tobacco industry pricing, and political activities.[27,28] Since 1996, however, per capita cigarette consumption has continued to decline, dropping 11.5 percent between 1998 and 1999.[29] Because of the reductions in tobacco consumption observed in California, rates of new lung cancer cases and deaths from coronary heart disease have both declined significantly faster among California residents in recent years than in the rest of the country.[28,30]

Alcohol Use

Excessive alcohol use, either in the form of heavy drinking (drinking more than 2 drinks per day on average for men or more than 1 drink per day on average for women) or binge drinking (drinking more than 4 drinks during a single occasion for men or more than 3 drinks during a single occasion for women) can lead to increased risk of health problems such as liver disease, cardiovascular problems, various cancers, unintentional injuries, and even death.[31] Based on analyses on 2001 data, excessive alcohol use accounts for approximately 75,000 deaths in the United States each year and approximately 30 years of life lost, on average, per alcohol attributable death.[32] Public health has traditionally attempted to prevent and control excessive alcohol use by focusing on the individual. Alcohol use, however, is strongly associated with social, economic, and environmental factors. To curtail excessive alcohol use and its effects, public health will need to take a multifaceted approach, addressing this behavior through educational, behavioral, environmental, and policy approaches. Use of media, school, and community education programs have been used to increase public awareness; screening tools and brief intervention models have been introduced in general, prenatal care, and emergency care settings; and state programs have implemented legal and legislative strategies to reduce the availability of alcohol, especially in the case of minors.

For youth, alcohol presents unique problems, including social and legal problems, disruption of mental and physical development, as well as an increased risk of experiencing motor vehicle injuries, physical or sexual assault, homicide, and suicide.[33,34,35] Recent findings from several national surveys indicate people aged 12 to 20 years drink almost 20 percent of all alcohol consumed in the United States,[36] and over 90 percent of this alcohol is consumed in the form of binge drinking.[37] These findings indicate that targeted measures also need to focus on preventing alcohol use by underage drinkers.

Nutrition

Only in recent years have state nutrition programs expanded beyond their traditional maternal, infant, and childhood nutrition activities, focused primarily on undernutrition. Increasingly, overnutrition is being recognized as the major contemporary nutritional issue in the United States. Most Americans, including children, need to reduce their intake of calories, fat (especially saturated fats and transfats), salt, and sugar, and to increase their intake of grains, fiber-containing foods, fruits, and vegetables. Improved diets help prevent many chronic diseases, including coronary heart disease, hypertension and stroke, type 2 diabetes, and several types of cancer.[38]

As one example, in an effort to promote the health benefits of a diet rich in fruits and vegetables, the National Fruit and Vegetable Program (formerly known as the 5 A Day Program) launched "Fruits & Veggies—More Matters," a public health initiative to reflect the new dietary guideline recommending 2 to 6½ cups of fruits and vegetables a day.[38] The National Program is a public/private partnership (http://www.fruitsandveggiesmorematters .org/) and exemplifies the way government, nongovernmental organizations, and industry can work together to promote healthy eating habits and improve the public's health.

Concerns over the dietary intake of youth and obesity led to the Institute of Medicine (IOM) initiating a study to review and make recommendations on appropriate nutritional standards for the availability, sale, content, and consumption of foods in schools. Notable recommendations from the report, *Nutrition Standards for Foods in Schools: Leading the Way toward Healthier Youth*,[39] advise that federally reimbursable school nutrition programs should be the main source of nutrition at school, opportunities for competitive foods should be limited, and if competitive foods are made available, they should be consistent with the 2005 Dietary Guidelines for Americans. Although this report and the growing concerns over the dietary intake and obesity of youth have prompted schools to review and implement school nutrition policy initiatives, the uptake of these recommendations continues to vary greatly across schools.

Physical Activity

In 1996, the United States Surgeon General reported that a majority of United States adults either were not active enough to achieve health benefits or were sedentary, engaging in no leisure-time physical activity.[40] This trend has not changed substantially. In 2005, more than half of United States adults did not engage in physical activity at a level recommended as beneficial to health, according to BRFSS data. Moreover, 24 percent of United States adults were not active at all in their leisure time.[41] An increasing body of evidence shows that being sedentary is unhealthy and that even moderate amounts of moderate-intensity physical activity improve health outcomes.

Increased physical activity is associated with better outcomes for such diverse conditions as coronary heart disease, diabetes, hypertension, colorectal cancer and other cancers, depression, and osteoporosis.[40] In 2001, the Task Force on Community Preventive Services reviewed literature on physical activity interventions conducted in community settings, producing recommendations for communities, policy makers, and public health providers on effective informational, social and behavioral, and environmental policy approaches to increasing physical activity.[42] Some examples of public health interventions that have been tried and reviewed for evidence of effectiveness include environmental approaches that encourage increased activity as a part of daily life, such as attractive and accessible stairwells and sidewalks, safe neighborhoods, and affordable neighborhood facilities for leisure-time exercise. Mass media campaigns, health provider incentives, school and worksite programs, and activities to increase strength and mobility among older Americans are also compo-

nents of public health interventions to promote physical activity.

Obesity

Evidence has shown a startling increase in the prevalence of obesity in the United States population (Figure 19.1).[43,44] Since the late 1980s, this country has seen a 50 percent increase in the proportion of adults who are obese (body mass index of 30 or more).[45] This increase has been greatest among minority populations and younger adults. The obesity epidemic has spread even faster among children, with a doubling of their rate of overweight between the early 1980s and the early 1990s.[46] This increase is the result of social and environmental changes that foster inactivity and overnutrition.

Trends such as the removal of physical education from schools, increasing portion sizes, and the tendency to eat meals away from home are making it hard for people to maintain normal weight. With the increase in weight, we have seen a parallel increase in the prevalence of diabetes among adults, especially young adults.[47] The twin epidemics of obesity and diabetes represent a critical challenge facing public health, in part because of their scale, affecting so many persons, and also because of their serious disease implications.

To combat obesity, the United States Surgeon General released *A Call to Action to Prevent and Decrease Overweight and Obesity*, detailing the need for a multifaceted public health response highlighting communication initiatives, interventions, and activities, as well as research and evaluation efforts to be employed in conjunction with families and communities, schools, worksites, health care settings, and the media.[48] As highlighted in *The Call to Action*, the critical role of promoting good nutrition and regular physical activity needs to be coupled with initiatives that create supportive environments to encourage and sustain these behaviors. As part of this model, public health practitioners will need to be more advocacy-oriented than in the past, and greater support is needed from other sectors of our society, such as agriculture, transportation, and education, to reverse this epidemic.

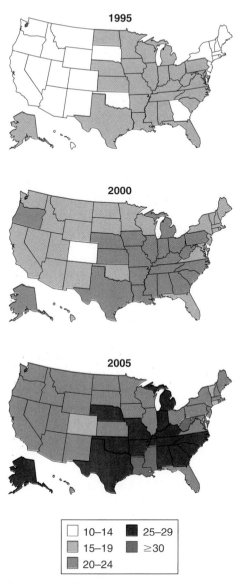

Figure 19.1. Percentage of Adults Who Are Obese (Approximately 30 Pounds Overweight or Body Mass Index of 30 or More)

SOURCE: Centers for Disease Control and Prevention, Behavioral Risk Factor Surveillance System, 1995, 2000, 2005.

PRINTED: Centers for Disease Control and Prevention. State Specific Prevalence of Obesity Among Adults— United States, 2005. *MMWR*. 2006; 55(36); 985–988.

Programs Targeting Diseases

Another approach to chronic disease control is to focus on those priority conditions that are among the leading causes of death and disability. In the following sections, we describe interventions that target the leading causes of death and disability in the United States: heart disease and stroke, cancer, diabetes, and arthritis.

Heart Disease and Stroke

Through a process convened by CDC and the United States Department of Health and Human Services (HHS), key partners, public health experts, and heart disease and stroke prevention specialists came together to develop one of the most detailed and comprehensive public health action plans, *A Public Health Action Plan to Prevent Heart Disease and Stroke*.[49] The National Forum for Heart Disease and Stroke Prevention is helping to implement the action plan and to improve cardiovascular health policies and practices at national, state, and community levels. What is especially compelling about this plan is the breadth of actions that are identified as necessary to both the development of risk factors in the first place as well as to reduce preventable complications from ongoing disease processes. In some ways, the action plan reflects much of what must be done for the entire field of chronic disease-related public health.

Early disease processes such as high blood pressure and high cholesterol are in large measure controllable through lifestyle factors, medication, or both. Yet, such control has been achieved for a small percentage of persons. Although high blood pressure medication is actually available for pennies a day, it is typically much more costly to patients; and 70 percent of those with high blood pressure do not have it controlled.[50] This appalling statistic is largely due to failure to treat and poor compliance and follow-up with medication regimens. Control of high blood pressure (an average reduction of just 12–13 mm Hg in systolic blood pressure over 4 years of follow-up) is estimated to reduce the number of heart attacks by 21 percent and the number of strokes by 37 percent annually.[51] Public health approaches to patient education and clinical care system changes must be applied and perfected to achieve these critical health outcomes.

Cancer

Each year, cancer claims the lives of more than half a million people in the United States.[52] Through the promotion and adoption of healthy practices, such as human papillomavirus vaccination, avoiding tobacco use, increasing physical activity, improving nutrition, achieving and maintaining normal weight, and avoiding sun exposure and tanning beds, many cancers can be prevented. Additionally, increasing access and minimizing the cost of screening and treatment services allows for early detection of various cancers, including breast, cervical, and colorectal cancers, when they are most treatable.[53–56] Screening services for cervical and colorectal cancers can actually detect precancerous conditions and present opportunities to prevent these cancers from ever developing.[55,56]

Through the National Comprehensive Cancer Control Program (NCCCP), with support from the CDC, states, territories and tribes have established programs that encompass the full range of cancer prevention and control activities, from risk reduction through early detection and better treatment to improved cancer survivorship.[57–65] Public health functions include surveillance, research, program and policy initiatives, research, and clinical services, all adapted to their local demographics and infrastructure. Comprehensive cancer control coalitions that include state and local health departments, voluntary associations, academic research centers, community groups, advocacy groups, businesses, and health care providers develop and implement local cancer control plans and work together to strategically coordinate and integrate cancer prevention and control activities.[57–65] CDC also works nationally to educate health care providers and the public regarding colorectal cancer screening practices, and the availability and benefits of available procedures.[66] CDC also supports programs and studies aimed toward determining barriers to colorectal cancer screening and

how best to implement colorectal cancer screening at the community level.

The United States Congress enacted the Breast and Cervical Cancer Mortality Prevention Act of 1990, which established the National Breast and Cervical Cancer Early Detection Program (NBCCEDP).[67,68,69] This program provides uninsured and underinsured women access to breast and cervical cancer screening and appropriate diagnostic follow-up. The program also awards states, tribes, and territories resources to conduct public and provider education about screening for these cancers and to conduct outreach activities to identify women who have never or have rarely been screened. Much of this outreach activity involves working with community-based organizations to get the information out to their constituencies regarding the importance of screening and the availability of financial support. Since program inception in 1991, 7.5 million breast and cervical cancer screening and diagnostic exams have been provided to more than 3.1 million low-income women. Nearly 33,000 breast cancers, nearly 107,000 precursor cervical lesions, and more than 2,000 cervical cancers have been diagnosed. The program now has 68 grantees and operates in all 50 states, the District of Columbia, 5 territories, and 12 American Indian/Alaska Native tribes and tribal organizations. The grantees have always been required to provide cancer treatment referrals to women diagnosed in the program, regardless of ability to pay. In late 2000, Congress enacted the Breast and Cervical Cancer Prevention and Treatment Act (BCCPTA), which allowed for optional Medicaid coverage for breast and cervical cancer treatment for women screened or diagnosed through the NBCCEDP. At this time, this optional Medicaid coverage has been implemented throughout the United States.[69]

Another new area of growth in public health is the establishment of population-wide cancer registries in all states. The National Program of Cancer Registries supports 45 states, the District of Columbia, and 3 United States territories, allowing them to register all cancers by type, stage, and basic demographic information.[70] This data system, covering 96 percent of the United States population, serves as the base for assessing the quality of statewide prevention and control programs. Before, with only mortality data, it was not possible to track trends in incidence or stage of cancer, so the impact of state-level cancer control efforts that would be manifest by declines in breast and cervical cancer diagnosed in the late stages could not be assessed. The increasing use of data systems such as the National Program of Cancer Registries is critical to the evaluation and improvement of state-driven public health control efforts. The *United States Cancer Statistics: Incidence and Mortality* report is updated annually and contains the official federal cancer statistics on cancer incidence from registries having high quality data and cancer mortality statistics for the 50 states and the District of Columbia (http://www.cdc.gov/uscs).

Diabetes

The number of persons with diagnosed diabetes increased substantially during the 1990s, and recent BRFSS interviews indicate that 14.7 million Americans have diabetes.[71] This increase has been greatest among younger adults and minority populations. Fortunately, advancements in science have proven that interventions such as controlling A1C, foot care, and retinal screening can prevent or delay some of the common sequelae of diabetes. Recent studies also have shown that moderate weight loss and physical activity can delay or postpone the development of diabetes for up to 60 percent of persons at highest risk.[17,72,73] The challenge for public health remains one of extending these health promotion practices to all persons in need.

For persons known to have diabetes, public health efforts have influenced systems of care to ensure appropriate services are provided that are known to prevent complications. In some states, public health agencies have convened managed care organizations to agree on standards of care to be provided to all persons with diabetes. The use of a convening/consensus development process has allowed all care organizations to upgrade services on an equivalent basis, not putting any one

organization at a competitive disadvantage. Other states have established reminder systems and tracking programs, some of which have shown promising results, reducing hospitalizations and amputations by more than a third. Others have shown substantial improvement in measures of glucose control, retinal screening rates, and the use of influenza and pneumococcal vaccine among persons with diabetes.

Although significant strides are being made in the care of persons with diabetes, the funnel of persons being diagnosed with the disease is ever widening. Current estimates place the risk at 1 out of every 3 babies born in 2002 receiving a diagnosis of diabetes during their lifetime. That risk grows to 1 out of every 2 for Latino and Hispanic babies. Unfortunately, the nation's obesity epidemic is accelerating the development of diabetes. For public health to succeed in preserving and maintaining the health of Americans, we must not only ensure adequate care of persons with diabetes but also simultaneously slow the pace of new diagnoses. In 2001, results from the Finnish Diabetes Prevention Study and the United States Diabetes Prevention Program gave us renewed hope. Specifically, these studies demonstrated that persons at very high risk could be prevented from advancing to a diagnosis of diabetes and in some cases could achieve a return to normal status of their glucose tolerance. Interestingly, the use of metformin reduced the incidence of diabetes by 31 percent, whereas the lifestyle intervention reduced the incidence by 58 percent.[17] Public health leaders are beginning to explore how to put these important findings into practice now that the clinical trial results are complete. This is one example of the challenges in rapidly applying research findings to practice, especially with limited resources and growing needs.

Arthritis

Arthritis is a relatively new area of emphasis in state public health control programs. It has many characteristics that make it a good choice for intervention. Arthritis is very common, with estimates of more than 46 million Americans having one of the various forms. Arthritis affects people of all ages, and it is the leading cause of physical disability among adults.[74] Research has shown that self-management interventions such as education and exercise can improve pain, function, and mental health among adults with arthritis.

Some people perceive that arthritis is an inevitable consequence of aging and ignore or minimize their arthritis until it interferes with valued life activities. Such misperceptions tremendously understate the importance of arthritis and represent missed opportunities to maintain function and quality of life. State programs are now working to improve the quality of life of people with arthritis by expanding the reach of evidence-based self-management education and exercise programs for persons with arthritis. These state programs are also focusing their efforts on racial and ethnic minorities disproportionately affected by arthritis limitations and severe pain.

Program Settings

The settings where chronic disease control activities take place are diverse. For example, an interventions setting could be a geopolitical area such as a neighborhood or a city. It might be the local school or hospital. It might be a workplace or an area where people spend their leisure time, such as a recreation location or a restaurant. Setting might not refer to a place at all but rather the relationships that people share—for example, people who belong to a social club or who are part of an Internet group. In this chapter, six types of settings are discussed: families, schools, workplaces, communities, health care, and media.

Families

The home is where many health behaviors are established. Family members influence, motivate, and reinforce each other's behaviors and decisions about nutrition, physical activity, health screenings, oral health, and use of tobacco, alcohol, and other substances.[75–78] A family's health can be greatly affected by an intervention, even an activity that targets just one family member. However, health promotion programs can have even greater effectiveness when multiple family members are involved and when links are strengthened between families and other settings such as schools, workplaces, and health care systems.[79]

Schools

School health interventions have the potential for substantial impact for many reasons, including the fact that schools are where children spend much of their time. Schools are ideal sites for environmental interventions such as no-smoking policies, healthy school lunch programs, and quality physical education classes.[80]

Teachers can serve as role models to encourage children to adopt healthy habits, and they can incorporate health messages in their curricula. Numerous curricula for school health education are available, and some schools have integrated health into physical education, science, and math curricula. United States school health programs are placing growing emphasis on preventing tobacco use, violence, and suicide, as well as on identification and school-based management of chronic health conditions among students, according to findings from the School Health Policies and Programs Study 2006. In addition, fewer schools are offering whole milk to students, and the availability of low-fat a la carte foods has increased since 2000.[81]

The IOM and CDC recommend planned, sequential strategies that promote the physical development of children in grades K–12 as well as their emotional, social, and educational development.[82,83] CDC's approach to coordinated school health education includes eight components: (1) health education; (2) physical education curricula; (3) health services that focus on prevention and early intervention; (4) nutrition services; (5) health promotion for school staff; (6) counseling, psychological, and social services for students; (7) a healthy school environment; and (8) activities that encourage parents and community members to support healthy behaviors among students and that link school and community health programs.

Implementing a coordinated school health program faces many hurdles such as overworked teachers, lack of school resources, lack of teacher training in health issues, and competing academic priorities that impede the intervention's success.[80] In some cases, we are actually moving in the wrong direction. For example, the data are clear that fewer and fewer students are participating in daily physical education. In 2005, 67 percent of high school students did not attend physical education classes daily.[84] One of the reasons for the loss of physical education in schools is thought to be the narrowing of the school's focus and curriculum to address intense pressures to raise standardized test scores.[85]

Workplaces

The workplace provides many opportunities for promoting health and preventing disease. Workplace health promotion programs have the potential to influence social norms, establish health policies, promote healthy behaviors, improve employees' knowledge and skills, help them get necessary health screenings and follow-up care, and reduce their on-the-job exposure to injuries and substances that can cause disease.[86] From the employer's point of view, workplace health promotion programs offer the promise of lower health-, life-, and disability insurance costs; reduced workers' compensation costs; reduced absenteeism; increased productivity; improved morale; and less turnover.

For these reasons, most United States employers now provide some type of health-promotion activities.[87] The scope of these activities varies widely by employer. For example, small businesses might provide self-help materials on reducing stress or lowering cholesterol levels, whereas large corporations might have a full-time health promotion staff, on-site facilities, and classes promoting fitness, weight management, nutrition, blood pressure control, smoking cessation, and counseling about drug and alcohol abuse. Most employee health programs aim to change the behaviors of individual employees, but some employers have made policy and environmental changes—for example, by passing and enforcing no-smoking policies and providing healthy food choices in vending machines and in cafeterias. Community outreach is also a part of some workplace health-promotion programs, which offer their expertise and services to employees' families and members of the community.

Unfortunately, few workplace interventions have undergone rigorous, long-term evaluation to determine their effects on employee health or costs. Moreover, measuring the effects of workplace programs is difficult. As Polanyi and colleagues point out, most health indicators used to measure employee health—such as absenteeism, sick leave, and use of benefits—also reflect factors outside the job.[88] The best studied and most cost-effective interventions are those providing work-based monitoring and treatment for high blood pressure. Workplace smoking-cessation programs also appear to be cost-effective.

Communities

There are many definitions for **community.** Some health programs define community as a place, such as a neighborhood with specific geographic boundaries. Other programs define the community as a group of people who share a common bond—for example, a religious congregation or a sports league. However communities are defined, they are a social determinant of health and play an important role in the delivery of health-promotion programs.

Communities linked by geography or social network give health providers access to specific populations, particularly racial and ethnic groups who are at increased risk for chronic disease. Well-designed community interventions involve community members to establish their own health priorities and agendas. Further, health messages are more likely to be effective when they are delivered by someone who is a trusted member of the community, who is socially and culturally similar to community members, and who speaks the same language. Communities also provide the needed social support for healthy behavioral changes.

Health promotion as defined by the World Health Organization (WHO) is the process of enabling people to increase control over, and to improve, their health. The field of health promotion boasts a wide array of successful chronic disease control efforts delivered through community mobilization and empowerment. Importantly, substantial evidence is beginning to accumulate demonstrating the ability of community-based interventions to reduce or even eliminate disparities.[89]

Health Care Settings

Assuring safety and quality of care in health care settings is an important public health priority. Health care settings and health care practitioners play key roles in the detection of risk factors and treatable disease, promotion of healthy lifestyles, and delivery of primary and secondary preventive services. Too often, preventive health care fails to meet established guidelines for care or is delivered to some but not all populations at risk. Quality health care can best be achieved by a strong collaboration between public health and clinical medicine. Public health can assist health care settings in meeting evidence-based guidelines for disease identification and management as well as providing education to ensure that patients are trained in disease self-management and are knowledgeable about the importance of adhering to medication and lifestyle changes. Health care coverage, including strategies to meet the health care needs of uninsured/underinsured populations, remains a daunting public health challenge within this domain.

Media and Technology

Fortune 500 companies spend millions of dollars on media advertising for a reason. Media drives consumer spending, and evidence exists that it can motivate healthy behaviors using the same techniques. As just one example, the CDC-VERB campaign successfully increased physical activity among tweens nationwide through paid TV ads, an interactive Internet site, and guerilla-style marketing.[90] Unfortunately, public health rarely has the resources necessary to purchase paid media. Nevertheless, the innovative use of public service announcements, donated media time, and other inexpensive marketing strategies are still possible. The future of public health will undoubtedly include the involvement of skilled marketers and innovative communication methods, including the

Internet, cell phones, and other high-tech methods to promote health. Attention to cultural differences in media-usage and ensuring that populations at greatest risk are effectively targeted through the media will be key challenges.

Populations

Targeted interventions uniquely designed to meet the needs of populations at greatest risk are the appropriate focus of much of public health.

Racial and Ethnic Groups

Unfortunately, racial and ethnic groups such as African Americans, Native Americans, Alaskan Natives, Asian Americans, Hispanics, and Pacific Islanders often experience higher incidence of chronic diseases, poorer health outcomes, or both. Because chronic illnesses place such a large burden on the population, these conditions contribute greatly to the overall disparity in health between racial and ethnic minority groups and whites. As racial and ethnic minority groups are expected to make up an increasingly larger proportion of the United States population in coming years, the number of people affected by health disparities will likely increase. The *Healthy People 2010* objectives to eliminate racial and ethnic disparities in health reinforce the importance of increased efforts to prevent and control chronic disease in racial and ethnic minority groups.[91] Culturally appropriate, effective, community-driven programs designed specifically to eliminate racial and ethnic disparities, such as those delivered through the congressionally funded Racial and Ethnic Approaches to Community Health (REACH), offer great promise in this area.

Young People

The opportunities for successful intervention are great during youth because many of the behaviors that increase a person's risk for chronic disease are established in late childhood or adolescence. For example, about 80 percent of regular adult smokers began regular tobacco use by age 18,[92] although these statistics are changing as tobacco companies begin to shift their marketing focus to legal age users, especially college-aged youth. Moreover, poor eating habits and low levels of physical activity among children and teenagers are contributing to increasing and earlier rates of obesity and diabetes. Unfortunately, not only do the unhealthy behaviors (such as high fat diets and sedentary lifestyles) get established early but also the related disease processes begin even earlier than we might have imagined. A community-based study found that 61 percent of overweight young people had at least one risk factor for heart disease, such as high cholesterol or high insulin.[93]

Seniors

The aging of the population has led to increasing interest in programs that encourage older adults to engage in healthful behaviors, especially physical activity. Quality of life, independence, and overall functioning are substantially improved when older people become physically active and quit smoking, even late in life. Research is demonstrating that it is never too late to receive some benefit from prevention and that health care savings are possible through reduced hospitalization and prevention of unnecessary complications. Public health planning is also extending to "brain health" or methods of maintaining cognitive health, which is a vital interest of older adults. Helping seniors to stay active and engaged in social, physical, and intellectual pursuits can contribute markedly to quality of life.[94]

CRITICAL TOPICS

The successes of the past century in infectious disease control are balanced by the growing challenges facing public health worldwide. Many of these challenges have direct implications for chronic disease prevention and control, including war and terrorism; migration and urbanization; environmental degradation; inequality in underlying social, economic, and political conditions; and

the role of genomics in personalized medicine and public health.

It is impossible to deal with these challenges in this chapter; however, we briefly touch upon three critical areas for chronic disease in the twenty-first century. First, we address immigration and border health, where the movement of populations play a key role in defining the epidemiological landscape for chronic disease. Second, we cover global connections and how the behaviors that increase people's risk for chronic diseases in the United States—for example, tobacco use and physical inactivity—are spreading to other parts of the world. Finally, we discuss mental health, which needs to be integrated into our understanding of chronic diseases and health promotion.

Immigration and Border Health

Immigration and migration across national boundaries are significant phenomena around the world.[95] One often thinks of such migration as an outcome of war or tragedy and associates it with movement of populations under duress. Although that is certainly true, the impact of immigration in the United States is largely and historically of a different type. It is the result of significant numbers of foreign nationals migrating to the United States to seek work and economic benefits from one of the wealthiest countries in the world. The magnitude of this migration has been most pronounced in the growth of the Hispanic population in the United States during the last decade of the twentieth century. Although this population growth has occurred in many large United States cities, the public health impact has been most notable along the border between the United States and Mexico.[96–100]

The United States–Mexico border region is defined as an area 62 miles (100 kilometers) north and south of the border, as established by the United States–Mexico Border Health Commission. *Healthy Border 2010* is a binational initiative that draws on the United States *Healthy People 2010* program and the National Health Indicators (*Indicadores de Resultados*) Program, which tracks health measures at the national, state, and local levels in Mexico.[96,101] These two programs share 20 objectives, which establish the priority areas for action on health issues in the border region. Several of these shared objectives address chronic diseases, including reducing breast cancer, cervical cancer, and diabetes deaths and diabetes-related hospitalizations. In some cases, health along the border is worse than for the nation as a whole. For example, the cancer death rate in the border region of Mexico is higher than the rate for the rest of Mexico. People in this region are also hard hit by diabetes-related deaths. Age-adjusted mortality rates were 13.7 per 100,000 for United States border residents in 1998 but a striking 74.6 for Mexican border residents in the years 1995–1997. Movement back and forth across the border for employment and health care sets up a fascinating set of public health challenges and opportunities for public health action.

Global Connections

Global interest in the burden of chronic diseases and their risk factors has grown dramatically over the past several years. Several recent WHO reports have noted that chronic diseases are now the leading causes of death and disability-adjusted life years worldwide, and their prevalence is growing rapidly.[1] Although chronic diseases make up a greater proportion of illnesses and deaths in developed countries, the aggregate greatest numbers of chronic disease deaths and illnesses are occurring in the developing world.

We have long known that infectious diseases easily cross borders, given extensive world travel, shipment of goods, and migration of peoples and animals. Thus, solutions have had to be global, and nations have had to cooperate extensively and share responsibility to curtail the spread of infectious diseases. Through mass communications such as television and the Internet, and marketing by multinational companies, patterns of behavior that predict disease (like the use of tobacco) are rapidly communicated across thousands of miles and to millions of people. Knowledge, attitudes, behaviors, and policies spread across borders with greater ease than ever before. Chronic disease problems are global, and solutions will need to be as well.

Mental Health

In the United States, mental health has often been viewed as outside the realm of public health. Although it is readily apparent that many mental health problems such as depression are often long term and chronic, they rarely fall under the rubric of disease. We are beginning to recognize the interrelationship of mental health and chronic disease, and organizations such as the IOM are beginning to apply a public health and population prevention perspective to mental health.[101,103]

Neurological, psychological, and developmental disorders raise some familiar concerns for public health practitioners. Like cancer, HIV/AIDS, and epilepsy, mental illnesses, ranging from depression to schizophrenia, have long suffered from stigma. Thus, the general nature in which these disorders are treated and viewed has itself become a concern for public health activists.

One common aspect of mental health disorders and chronic diseases is the strong emphasis on behavior. Many of the same strategies for prevention that involve supportive physical and social environments may apply to the promotion of mental health. Equally appropriate is the core scientific approach of chronic disease epidemiology. Many mental health problems share a position of comorbidity and causation with chronic illnesses. For example, alcohol abuse can lead to any number of chronic diseases but also to neurological and psychological disorders as well as violence and injury. Thus, the strategies for defining mental health problems as well as the interventions must be integrated with well-established chronic disease and health promotion efforts at the individual, community, and population levels.

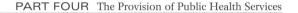

▌SUMMARY

The rising prominence of chronic diseases, now the leading causes of death, can be thought of as one of the great success stories of public health during the twentieth century. Concern with chronic disease reflects our tremendous success in controlling infectious agents with sanitation, safe water, immunizations, and antibiotics. It also reflects improvements in nutrition, living conditions, and income and education, as well as the fact that life expectancy has increased so remarkably that people live long enough to develop and die from chronic illnesses. The growth of chronic illnesses can also be thought of as one of public health's greatest failures, especially of the late twentieth century. The principal known causes of premature death from chronic diseases are tobacco use, poor diet, physical inactivity, overweight, and alcohol use. During the 1970s and 1980s, we made substantial progress in diminishing the toll of tobacco use. Then in the 1990s, rates of tobacco use among children started to climb. Increased calorie consumption and rates of overweight and obesity continue to increase unabated.

On the hopeful side is that a generation of investment in research has led to greater understanding of the causes of these diseases and how to intervene. However, the translation of science into widespread application has been neglected. For example, the recommendation that women should receive mammograms was first announced in the late 1970s, and yet we are only now beginning to see more than 70 percent of women receiving regular screening. Similar stories exist for diabetes, heart disease, stroke, and other chronic illnesses. Delivering what we know to those who need it most will be one of the fundamental challenges for public health in the twenty-first century.

Responding to this challenge will require at least three important actions. First, we must shorten the time it takes to get research widely applied, especially to those in greatest need. Research unapplied serves no real purpose. Second, we must recognize that chronic illnesses will require broad-based societal, environmental, and policy interventions. Individual-level interventions alone have proven to be too slow and costly to address the millions of people at risk. Positive behavioral change must be supported and fostered by supportive environments and policies that help individuals more easily choose and sustain healthful behaviors. Last, and arguably the greatest challenge to public health in the twenty-first century, will be to eliminate health disparities between racial and ethnic groups, and between rich and poor. Although we have made great strides in promoting health, we have made little progress in eliminating disparities, and in some cases those disparities have widened.

Central to our success will be fostering existing partnerships and establishing new partnerships with many sectors of United States society that we have not traditionally worked with. We also will need to be more oriented to advocacy in support of health promotion resources at the local, state, and national levels than ever before.

REVIEW QUESTIONS

1. Describe the major surveys and surveillance systems relevant to chronic disease prevention and control, including their advantages and limitations.

2. Describe a behavior, social or physical condition, or health trend you have noticed in recent years among friends, your community, or society at large that you believe may contribute to chronic disease morbidity and mortality. Using this example, describe potential data sources you might consult to support or refute your observation and discuss if there is a role for public health action. Provide a rationale for your response and the factors you considered when making the decision for or against public health action.

3. If you determined there was a role for public health in the example you provided for question #2, discuss how you might address the issue, illustrating the use of a risk factor-, disease-, setting-, or population-based approach. Provide a rationale on why you chose that particular approach and whom you will need to involve to effectively plan, implement, and evaluate your efforts.

REFERENCES

1. World Health Organization, World Bank. *The Global Burden of Disease*. Cambridge, MA: Harvard University Press; 1996.

2. World Bank. *World Development Report 1993*. New York: Oxford University Press; 1993.

3. Centers for Disease Control and Prevention. *The Burden of Chronic Diseases and their Risk Factors: National and State Perspectives*. Atlanta: US Department of Health and Human Services; 2004.

4. American Heart Association. Heart Disease and Stroke—Statistic Update 2007. *Circulation*. 2007;115(5);e69–171. Available at: http://circ .ahajournals.org/cgi/content/full/115/5/e69. Accessed October 20, 2008.

5. American Cancer Society. *Cancer Facts and Figures—2006*. Atlanta, GA: American Cancer Society; 2006.

6. Centers for Disease Control and Prevention. *Unrealized Prevention Opportunities: Reducing the Health and Economic Burden of Chronic Disease*. Atlanta, GA: Centers for Disease Control and Prevention; 2000.

7. Centers for Disease Control and Prevention. *Chronic Diseases and Their Risk Factors: The Nation's Leading Causes of Death*. Atlanta, GA: Centers for Disease Control and Prevention; 1999.

8. Centers for Disease Control and Prevention, National Center for Health Statistics. *Health, United States 2006 with Chartbook on Trends in the Health of Americans*. Hyattsville, MD: 2006; 183.

9. Centers for Disease Control and Prevention. *Final FY 2003 Performance Plan Revised*. Atlanta, GA: Centers for Disease Control and Prevention; 2002. Available at: http://www.cdc.gov/od/perfplan/ 2002/2002perf.pdf. Accessed October 20, 2008.

10. McGinnis JM, Foege WH. Actual causes of death in the United States. *JAMA*. 1993;270:2207–2212.

11. Mokdad AH, Marks JS, Stroup D, Gerberding J. Actual causes of death in the United States, 2000. [Published erratum in: JAMA. 2005;293: 293–294]. *JAMA* 2004;291:1238–1245.

12. Hahn RA, Teutsch SM, Rothenberg RB, Marks JS. Excess deaths from nine chronic diseases in the United States, 1986. *JAMA*. 1990;264: 2654–2659.

13. US Department of Health and Human Services. *Reducing Tobacco Use: A Report of the Surgeon General*. Atlanta, GA: US Dept of Health and Human Services, Centers for Disease Control and Prevention, National Center for Chronic Disease Prevention and Health Promotion; 2000.

14. Thun MJ, Apicella LF, Henley SJ. Smoking vs. other risk factors as the cause of smoking-attributable deaths. *JAMA*. 2000;284:706–712.

15. Catlin A, Cowan C, Heffler S, Washington B, and the National Health Expenditure Accounts Team. National health spending in 2005: The slowdown continues. *Health Affairs*. 2006;26;1:142–153.

16. Partnership for Solutions, Johns Hopkins University. *Chronic Conditions: Making the Case for Ongoing Care. Update September 2004*. Johns Hopkins University; 2004.

17. Knowler WC, Barrett-Connor E, Fowler SE, et al. *Reduction in the Incidence of Type 2 Diabetes with Lifestyle Intervention or Metformin. N Eng J Med*. 2002;346:393–403.

18. Teutsch SM, Churchill RE. *Principles and Practice of Public Health Surveillance*. New York: Oxford University Press; 2000.

19. Centers for Disease Control and Prevention. Updated guidelines for evaluating public health surveillance systems: Recommendations from the Guidelines Working Group. *MMWR*. 2001; 50(RR-13):1–35.

20. General bill of mortality for the year 1665. In: David FN. *Games, Gods, and Gambling*. London: Griffin; 1962: 101.

21. Centers for Disease Control and Prevention. *International Classification of Diseases, Tenth Revision, Clinical Modification (ICD-10-CM)*. Hyattsville, MD: US Dept of Health and Human Services, Centers for Disease Control and Prevention, National Center for Health Statistics; 2001. Available at: http://www.cdc.gov/nchs/about/ otheract/icd9/abticd10.htm. Accessed October 4, 2001.

22. Jessen RJ. *Statistical Survey Techniques*. New York: John Wiley & Sons; 1978.

23. Lyberg L, Kasprzyk D. Data collection methods and measurement error: An overview. In: Biemer PP, Groves RM, Lyberg LE, Mathiowetz NA, Sudman S, eds. *Measurement Errors in Surveys. Wiley Series in Probability and Mathematical Statistics*. New York: John Wiley & Sons; 1991:237–258.

24. Centers for Disease Control and Prevention. *Prevention Research Centers: Investing in the Nation's Health*. Atlanta, GA: Centers for Disease Control and Prevention; 2001.

25. Centers for Disease Control and Prevention. *Racial and Ethnic Approaches to Community Health (REACH 2010): Addressing Disparities in*

Health. Atlanta, GA: Centers for Disease Control and Prevention; 2001.

26. Centers for Disease Control and Prevention. *Best Practices for Comprehensive Tobacco Control Programs*. Atlanta, GA: US Dept of Health and Human Services, Centers for Disease Control and Prevention; 1999.

27. Pierce JP, Gilpin EA, Emery SL, White MM, Rosbrook B, Berry CC. Has the California Tobacco Control Program reduced smoking? *JAMA*. 1998; 280:893–899.

28. Centers for Disease Control and Prevention. Declines in lung cancer rates—California, 1988–1997. *MMWR*. 2000;49(47);1066–1069.

29. California Department of Health Services. *California Tobacco Control Update*. Sacramento, CA: California Depart of Health Services; 2000.

30. Fichtenberg CM, Glantz SA. Association of the California Tobacco Control Program with declines in cigarette consumption and mortality from heart disease. *New Engl J Med*. 2000;343(24): 1772–1777.

31. Rehm J, Gmel G, Sepos CT, Trevisan M. *Alcohol-related morbidity and mortality. Alcohol research and Health* 2003; 27(1)39–51 or Ashley MJ, Olin JS, le Riche WH, Kornaczewski A, Schmidt W, Rankin JG. Morbidity in alcoholics. Evidence for accelerated development of physical disease in women. *Arch Intern Med*. 1977;137(7):883–887.

32. Stahre MA, Brewer RD, Naimi TS, et al. Alcohol-attributable deaths and years of potential life lost—United States, 2001. *MMWR*. 2004;53(37): 866–870.

33. Mohler-Kuo M, Dowdall GW, Koss M, Wechsler H. Correlates of rape while intoxicated in a national sample of college women. *Journal of Studies on Alcohol*. 2004;65(1):37–45.

34. Abbey A. Alcohol-related sexual assault: A common problem among college students. *Journal of Studies on Alcohol*. 2002;Sup(14):118–128.

35. Institute of Medicine. *Reducing Underage Drinking: A Collective Responsibility*. Washington, DC: National Academies Press; 2004.

36. Foster SE, Vaughan RD, Foster WH, Califano JA Jr. Alcohol consumption and expenditure for underage drinking and adult excessive drinking. *JAMA*. 2003;289(8):989–95.

37. Office of Juvenile Justice and Delinquency Prevention. *Drinking in America: Myths, Realities, and Prevention Policy*. Pacific Institute for Research

and Evaluation in support of the OJJDP Enforcing the Underage Drinking Laws Program: US Department of Justice; November 2001.

38. US Department of Health and Human Services and US Department of Agriculture. *Dietary Guidelines for Americans, 2005*. 6th ed. Washington, DC: US Government Printing Office; January 2005.

39. Institute of Medicine. *Nutrition Standards for Foods in Schools: Leading the Way Toward Healthier Youth. Committee on Nutrition Standards for Foods in Schools*. Washington, DC: The National Academies Press; 2007.

40. US Department of Health and Human Services. *Physical Activity and Health: A Report of the Surgeon General*. Atlanta, GA: US Dept of Health and Human Services, Centers for Disease Control and Prevention, National Center for Chronic Disease Prevention and Health Promotion; 1996.

41. Centers for Disease Control and Prevention. *At a Glance. Physical Activity and Good Nutrition: Essential Elements to Prevent Chronic Diseases and Obesity*. 2007. Available at: http://www.cdc.gov/nccdphp/publications/aag/dnpa.htm.

42. Task Force on Community Preventive Services. Recommendations to increase physical activity in communities. *Am J Prev Med*. 2002;22(4s): 67–72.

43. Centers for Disease Control and Prevention. State Specific Prevalence of Obesity among Adults—United States, 2005. *MMWR*. 2006;55(36): 985–988.

44. Mokdad AH, Serdula MK, Dietz WH, Bowman BA, Marks JS, Koplan JP. The spread of the obesity epidemic in the United States, 1991–1998. *JAMA*. 1999;282:1519–1522.

45. Flegal KM, Carroll MD, Kuczmarski RJ, Johnson CL. Overweight and obesity in the United States: Prevalence and trends, 1960–1994. *Int J Obesity*. 1998;22:39–47.

46. Troiano RP, Flegal KM. Overweight children and adolescents: description, epidemiology, and demographics. *Pediatrics*. 1998;101(3):497–504.

47. Mokdad AH, Bowman BA, Ford ES, Vinicor F, Marks JS, Koplan JP. The continuing epidemics of obesity and diabetes in the United States. *JAMA*. 2001;286(10):1195–1200.

48. US Department of Health and Human Services. *The Surgeon General's Call to Action to Prevent and Decrease Overweight and Obesity*. Rockville,

MD: US Department of Health and Human Services, Public Health Service, Office of the Surgeon General; 2001.

49. US Department of Health and Human Services. *A Public Health Action Plan to Prevent Heart Disease and Stroke: Executive Summary and Overview*. Atlanta, GA: US Department of Health and Human Services, Centers for Disease Control and Prevention; 2003.

50. Centers for Disease Control and Prevention. National Health and Nutrition Examination Survey 1999–2002.

51. He J, Whelton PK. Elevated systolic blood pressure and risk of cardiovascular and renal disease: Overview of evidence from observational epidemiologic studies and randomized controlled trials. *American Heart Journal*. September, 1999; 138(3 Pt 2):211–219.

52. US Cancer Statistics Working Group. *United States Cancer Statistics: 2003 Incidence and Mortality*. Atlanta, GA: US Department of Health and Human Services, Centers for Disease Control and Prevention and the National Cancer Institute; 2006.

53. Institute of Medicine. Curry, SJ, Byers T, Hewitt M (eds). *Fulfilling the Potential of Cancer Prevention and Early Detection*. Washington, DC: Institute of Medicine, National Academies Press; 2003.

54. US Preventive Service Task Force. *Screening for breast cancer: Recommendations and rationale*. AHRQ. August 2002. Available at: http://www .preventiveservices.ahrq.gov. Accessed August 20, 2007.

55. US Preventive Service Task Force. Screening for cervical cancer: Recommendations and rationale. *AHRQ*. January 2003. Available at: http://www .preventiveservices.ahrq.gov. Accessed August 20, 2007.

56. US Preventive Service Task Force. Screening for colorectal cancer: Recommendations and rationale. *AHRQ*. July 2002. Available at: http://www .preventiveservices.ahrq.gov. Accessed August 20, 2007.

57. Coates R, Given L, Lee N, Colditz G. A collaborative, comprehensive approach to fulfilling the promise of cancer prevention and control. *Cancer Causes and Control*. 2005;16(1):1.

58. Given L, Black B, Lowry G, Huang P, Kerner J. Collaborating to conquer cancer: A comprehen-

sive approach to cancer control. *Cancer Causes and Control*. 2005;16(1):3–14.

59. Black B, Cowens-Alvarado R, Gershman S, Weir H. Using data to motivate action: The need for high quality, an effective presentation, and an action context for decision making. *Cancer Causes and Control*. 2005;16(1):15–25.

60. Kerner J, Guirguis-Blake J, Hennessy K, et al. Translating research into improved outcomes in comprehensive cancer control. *Cancer Causes and Control*. 2005;16(1):27–40.

61. Hayes N, Weinberg A, Brawley O, Baquet C, Kaur JS, Palafox NA. Cancer-related disparities: Weathering the perfect store through comprehensive cancer control approaches. *Cancer Causes and Control*. 2005;16(1):41–50.

62. Pollack L, Greer G, Rowland J, et al. Cancer survivorship: A new challenge in comprehensive cancer control. *Cancer Causes and Control*. 2005; 16(1):51–59.

63. Selig W, Jenkins KL, Reynolds S, Benson D, Daven M. Examining advocacy and comprehensive cancer control. *Cancer Causes and Control*. 2005;16(1):61–68.

64. Rochester P, Chapel T, Black B, Bucher J, Housemann R. The evaluation of comprehensive cancer control efforts: Useful techniques and unique requirements. *Cancer Causes and Control*. 2005; 16(1):69–78.

65. True S, Kean T, Nolan P, Haviland S, Hohman K. In conclusion: the promise of comprehensive cancer control. *Cancer Causes and Control*. 2005;16(1):79–88.

66. Centers for Disease Control and Prevention. Centers for Disease Control and Prevention website. Available at: http://www.cdc.gov/cancer/ colorectal. Accessed August 20, 2007.

67. Henson RM, Wyatt SW, Lee NC. The National Breast and Cervical Cancer Early Detection Program: A comprehensive public health response to two major health issues for women. *J Public Health Manage Pract*. 1996;2(2):36–47.

68. Holt H. Progress report: The National Strategic Plan for the Early Detection and Control of Breast and Cervical Cancers. *J Womens Health*. 1998; 7(4):411–413.

69. 106th Congress. *Breast and Cervical Cancer Prevention and Treatment Act of 2000*. Pub L No. 106–354, 114 Stat 1381. H.R. 4386 (S. 662). Approved October 24, 2000.

70. Hutton M, Simpson LD, Miller DS, Weir HK, McDavid K, Hall HI. Progress toward nationwide cancer surveillance: An evaluation of the National Program of Cancer Registries, 1994–1999. *J Registry Manage.* 2001;28(3):113–120.

71. Cowie CC, Rust KF, Byrd-Holt D, et al. Prevalence of diabetes and impaired fasting glucose in adults—United States, 1999–2000. *MMWR.* 2003;52(35):833–837.

72. Tuomilehto J, Lindstrom J, Eriksson JG, et al. Prevention of Type 2 diabetes mellitus by changes in lifestyle among subjects with impaired glucose tolerance. *N Engl J Med.* 2001;344(18):1343–1350.

73. US Department of Health and Human Services. Diet and exercise dramatically delay Type 2 diabetes; diabetes medication Metformin also effective. *HHS News.* August 8, 2001.

74. Centers for Disease Control and Prevention. Prevalence of disabilities and associated health conditions among adults—United States, 1999. *MMWR.* 2001;50:120–125.

75. Bonaguro EW, Bonaguro JA. Tobacco use among adolescents: Directions for research. *Am J Health Promotion.* 1989;4(1):37–41.

76. Nader PR, Sellers DE, Johnson CC, et al. The effect of adult participation in a school-based family intervention to improve children's diet and physical activity: The Child and Adolescent Trial for Cardiovascular Health. *Prev Med.* 1996;25: 455–464.

77. Epstein LH, Wing RR, Koeske R, Valoski A. Long-term effects of family-based treatment of childhood obesity. *J Consult Clin Psychol.* 1987;55: 91–95.

78. Kirschenbaum DS, Harris ES, Tomarken AJ. Effects of parental involvement in behavioral weight loss therapy for preadolescents. *Behav Ther.* 1984;15:485–500.

79. Soubhi H, Potvin L. Homes and families as health promotion settings. In: Poland BD, Green LW, Rootman I, eds. *Settings for Health Promotion.* Thousand Oaks, CA: Sage Publications; 2000.

80. Parcel GS, Kelder SH, Basen-Engquist K. The school as a setting for health promotion. In: Poland BD, Green LW, Rootman I, eds. *Settings for Health Promotion.* Thousand Oaks, CA: Sage Publications; 2000.

81. Kann L, Brener ND, Wechsler H. Overview and summary: School Health Policies and Programs Study 2006. *J School Health.* 2007;77:385–397.

82. Institute of Medicine. *Schools and Health: Our Nation's Investment.* Washington, DC: National Academy Press; 1997.

83. Allensworth DD, Kolbe LJ. The comprehensive school health program: Exploring an expanded concept. *J School Health.* 1987;57(10):409–412.

84. Eaton DK, Kann L, Kinchen S, et al. Youth Risk Behavior Surveillance—United States, 2005. *MMWR.* 2005;55:1–108.

85. President's Council on Physical Fitness and Sports. Washington, DC. *Research Digest.* September 2006;7(3).

86. Davis JR, Schwartz R, Wheeler F, Lancaster RB. Intervention methods for chronic disease control. In: Brownson RC, Remington PL, Davis JR. *Chronic Disease Epidemiology and Control.* 2nd ed. Washington, DC: American Public Health Association; 1998.

87. Biener L, DePue JD, Emmons KM, Linnan L, Abrams DB. Recruitment of work sites to a health promotion research trial: Implications for generalizability. *J Occup Med.* 1994;36:631–636.

88. Polanyi MFD, Frank JW, Shannon HS, Sullivan TJ, Lavis JN. Promoting the determinants of good health in the workplace. In: Poland BD, Green LW, Rootman I, eds. *Settings for Health Promotion.* Thousand Oaks, CA: Sage Publications; 2000.

89. Centers for Disease Control and Prevention. Special Focus Issue—Community Wellness. *Preventing Chronic Disease: Public Health Research, Practice and Policy.* 2007;4(3).

90. Huhman HE, Potter LD, Duke JC, Judkins DR, Heitzler CD, Wong FL. Evaluation of a national physical activity intervention for children: The VERB™ Campaign 2002–2004. *Am J Prev Med.* 2007;32(1):38–43.

91. US Department of Health and Human Services. *Healthy People 2010.* 2nd ed. Washington, DC: US Government Printing Office; November 2000.

92. US Department of Health and Human Services. *Preventing Tobacco Use Among Young People: A Report of the Surgeon General.* Atlanta, GA: US Dept of Health and Human Services, Centers for Disease Control and Prevention, National Center for Chronic Disease Prevention and Health Promotion; 1994.

93. Freedman DS, Serdula MK, Srinivasan SR, Berenson GS. Relation of circumferences and skinfold thicknesses to lipid and insulin concentrations in

children and adolescents: The Bogalusa Heart Study. *American Journal of Clinical Nutrition.* 2006;69:308–317.

94. Centers for Disease Control and Prevention and the Alzheimer's Association. *The Healthy Brain Initiative: A National Public Health Roadmap to Maintaining Cognitive Health.* Chicago, IL: Alzheimer's Association; 2007. Available at: http:www.cdc.gov/nccdphp/publications/aag/aging.htm.

95. United Nations Population Division. *World Population Prospects: The 1998 Revision.* New York: United Nations; 1999.

96. Office of International and Refugee Health. *Health on the US–Mexico Border: Past, Present and Future. A Preparatory Report to the Future United States–Mexico Border Health Commission.* Rockville, MD: US Dept of Health and Human Services; 1999.

97. Bruhn JG, Brandon JE, eds. *Border Health: Challenges for the United States and Mexico.* New York: Garland; 1997.

98. Pan American Health Organization. *Mortality Profiles of the Sister Communities on the United States–Mexico Border.* Washington, DC: Pan American Health Organization; 2000.

99. Power JG, Byrd T. *US-Mexico Border Health: Issues for Regional and Migrant Populations.* Thousand Oaks, CA: Sage Publications; 1998.

100. Mitchell BD, Haffner SM, Hazuda HP, et al. Diabetes and coronary heart disease risk in Mexican Americans. *Ann Epidemiol.* 1992;2: 101–106.

101. US Department of Health and Human Services. *Healthy People 2010.* 2nd ed. Washington, DC: US Government Printing Office; November 2000.

102. Mraazek PJ, Haggerty RJ, eds. *Reducing Risks for Mental Disorders: Frontiers for Preventive Intervention Research.* Washington, DC: Institute of Medicine, National Academy Press; 1994.

103. US Department of Health and Human Services. *Mental Health: A Report of the Surgeon General.* Rockville, MD: US Dept of Health and Human Services, Substance Abuse and Mental Health Services Administration, Center for Mental Health Services, National Institutes of Health, National Institute of Mental Health; 1999.

CHAPTER 20

Reducing Tobacco Use

Michael P. Eriksen, ScD* and Lawrence W. Green, DrPH[†]

LEARNING OBJECTIVES

Upon completion of this chapter, the reader will be able to:

1. Describe the major eras of tobacco consumption in the twentieth century.
2. Identify the major causes of death associated with tobacco.
3. Name the major strategies and policies that account for the decline in smoking during the last third of the twentieth century.
4. Describe the major factors delaying the further decline in smoking.
5. List some leading indicators for progress toward the year 2010 in the United States Healthy People objectives in tobacco control.

KEY TERMS

American Legacy Foundation

Behavioral Risk Factor Surveillance System (BRFSS)

Denormalization

Global Youth Tobacco Survey (GYTS)

Master Settlement Agreement (MSA)

Monitoring the Future (MTF) Study

National Health and Nutrition Examination Surveys (NHANES)

National Health Interview Survey (NHIS)

National Survey on Drug Use and Health (NSDUH)

Nicotine Addiction

Second-Hand Smoke

Smoke-Free Areas

Social Norms

Span of Impact

Surgeon General's Report

Task Force on Community Preventive Services

Youth Risk Behavior Survey (YRBS)

Youth Tobacco Survey (YTS)

*Professor and Director, Institute of Public Health, Georgia State University, Atlanta, Georgia.
[†]Adjunct Professor, Department of Epidemiology and Biostatistics, and Helen Diller Family Comprehensive Cancer Center, University of California at San Francisco.

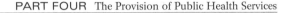

INTRODUCTION

Efforts to reduce tobacco use over the past 50 years have been a study of contrasts. In the 1950s and early 1960s, smoking reached its mid-century zenith. Nearly half of adult men smoked, women's rates of smoking continued to increase, and smoking in public places was the norm. Cigarette advertisements were ubiquitous, including on the most popular television programs. There was virtually no investment in tobacco control, and there was little in the way of regulatory or legislative protection. Research evidence, however, was mounting. By the beginning of the twenty-first century, smoking rates and per capita tobacco consumption had been cut in half. Smoking was socially unacceptable and seen as a habit increasingly limited to lower socioeconomic groups. **Smoke-free areas** had become the norm, with most public places, larger private workplaces, and modes of transportation being completely smoke-free. Combined federal and state resources for tobacco control totaled nearly $1 billion, and there was an intricate web of laws and regulations, primarily at the state and local level, protecting children from becoming exposed to or addicted to tobacco.

The job, however, is far from complete. About one-fifth of adults in the United States continue to smoke,[1] with great variation based on regional, racial, and socioeconomic characteristics. The progress, however, has been undeniable. CDC has declared this progress 1 of the 10 greatest public health achievements of the twentieth century.[2,3]

Both to accelerate achievements in tobacco control further and to export their lessons to other urgent public health challenges, it is important to understand how and why this transformation in the last third of the twentieth century took place. This chapter reviews the current status of tobacco control in the United States with particular emphasis on (1) the continuing harm caused by tobacco use, (2) the current levels and patterns of use, (3) the factors that contributed to the changing tobacco control environment, (4) effective interventions in reducing tobacco use, and (5) future challenges and directions.

THE CONTINUING HARM CAUSED BY TOBACCO USE

The harm caused by cigarette smoking is without precedent. CDC estimates that since the time of the first **Surgeon General's Report** in 1964, 16 million Americans have died as a result of smoking.[4] If current trends continue, another 25 million Americans alive today will be killed by cigarette smoking, including 5 million children.[5] Thus, while progress in the United States and some other countries has been great, the continuing burden caused by tobacco is unacceptable.

Smoking is the leading preventable cause of death in the United States, resulting in more than 440,000 deaths a year and responsible for causing serious illness for 8.6 million people.[6] An estimated one out of two lifetime smokers' lives will be shortened as a result of smoking.[7] On average, a death caused by smoking reduces a person's life expectancy by about 12 years.[8] Although there is a decades-long lag time from the beginning of tobacco use to the manifestation of clinical illness, the harm caused by smoking is not limited to the elderly. Cigarette smoking is a major killer of the middle-aged (45 to 64) and 80 percent of coronary heart disease deaths and a large proportion of the illness, absence from work, and disability in this age group is caused by smoking.[9]

In a perverse way, one can marvel at how many diseases are caused by smoking and how it affects nearly every organ system. Diseases of the pulmonary and cardiovascular systems predominate, with heart disease, lung cancer, and respiratory diseases being most common. Each year, smoking attributes to 249,900 cancer deaths, 898,000 cardiovascular deaths, 188,700 respiratory disease deaths, and 10,060 perinatal deaths.[10]

Lung cancer provides an interesting illustration of the public health impact of cigarette smoking. Cigarette smoking causes at least 30 percent of all cancer deaths and nearly 90 percent of lung cancer deaths.[11] Cigarette smoking and lung cancer are inextricably linked, and their relationship is ironically juxtaposed in Figure 20.1.

At the beginning of the twentieth century, lung cancer was rare. An early medical textbook from 1912 noted:

> On one point, however, there is nearly complete consensus of opinion, and that is that primary malignant neoplasms of the lungs are among the rarest forms of the disease. This latter opinion of the extreme rarity of primary tumours has persisted for centuries.[12]

As cigarette smoking became more popular, the incidence of lung cancer increased dramatically, and its prevalence tracked throughout the century with a consistent lag on the prevalence of smoking. For example, in 1930, the lung cancer death rate for men was 4.9 per 100,000; in 1990, the rate had increased to 75.6 per 100,000.[13] In 1964, on the basis of approximately 7000 articles relating to smoking and disease, the Advisory Committee to the United States Surgeon General concluded that cigarette smoking is "causally related" to lung cancer in men, and a probable cause of lung cancer in women.[14] The committee stated, "Cigarette smoking is a health hazard of sufficient importance in the United States to warrant appropriate remedial action." Today, smokers die more frequently from lung cancer, 123,000 deaths a year, than any other disease caused by smoking. Lung cancer went from being one of the "rarest forms" of cancer to now being the leading cause of cancer deaths for both men and women. Lung cancer surpassed breast cancer as the leading cause of cancer death

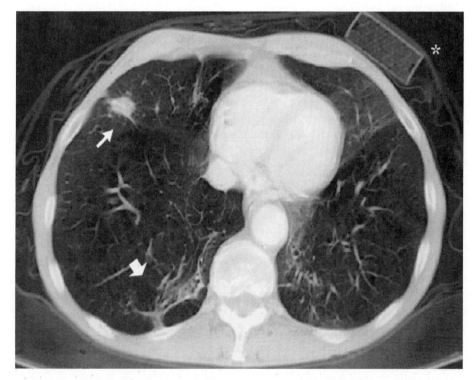

Figure 20.1. Chest Radiograph Showing Causes and Outcomes of Smoking

among United States women in 1987.[15] The American Cancer Society estimates that, in 2006, more than 30,000 more United States women died from lung cancer than from breast cancer.[16] Globally, lung cancer is also the most common cause of cancer death and kills about 1 million people around the world each year.[17]

THE CURRENT LEVELS AND PATTERNS OF USE

The United States is fortunate to have multiple systems to measure and track tobacco use among both adults and children. For adults, the **National Health Interview Survey** (NHIS) is the oldest and most continuous system for monitoring tobacco use, and other critical health behaviors and conditions.[18] The NHIS provides annual national estimates of tobacco use by age, gender, region, and socioeconomic status, as well as providing the opportunity to investigate the relationship between tobacco use and other health behaviors. The **Behavioral Risk Factor Surveillance System** (BRFSS) has provided state-specific data on behavioral risk factors, including tobacco use for the past 20 years, and is now operational in every state. Although it only provides a median national value, the BRFSS provides state-specific and state-owned data, which are valuable for local public health programming and policy setting. The BRFSS data have shown consistently large differences in smoking and smokeless tobacco rates by state, nearly three times as high in tobacco-growing states such as Kentucky, compared to Western states such as Utah or California. The **National Survey on Drug Use and Health** (NSDUH)[19] has recently been expanded, both in sample size and in depth of tobacco questions, as well as having improved computer methodology to obtain valid measures of illicit and private information during interviews in the home. The NSDUH provides valuable information on the incidence of initiation of smoking, the

number of new smokers in a given year, and, most recently, cigarette brand preference among adolescents.

Although tobacco surveillance systems for adults are strong, the systems in place to monitor tobacco use among young people are even more robust. The NSDUH, mentioned previously, obtained more than 68,000 surveys nationally in 2005, 22,500 of whom were 12 to 17 years old. Thus, the NSDUH provides a large and valuable data source for better understanding tobacco use, particularly the initiation of use, and the combination of the use of tobacco with a variety of illicit drugs and alcohol. Because the methodology has been changed many times during the past 10 years, however, it is an inadequate source of data for historical trend analysis. Fortunately, there are multiple sources for trend analysis, particularly from data collected in schools. Most notably, valuable trend data on tobacco use rates among various age groups are provided by the **Monitoring the Future (MTF) Study,** which was conducted by the University of Michigan with support from the National Institute of Drug Abuse (NIDA). These data are complemented by the **Youth Risk Behavior Survey** (YRBS) conducted by the states, like the BRFSS, with the technical assistance and coordination of the CDC.

The MTF survey has been in operation since 1976, tracking the use of tobacco and other substances among high school seniors. In the early 1990s, MTF added eighth and tenth grade samples to its surveys. The YRBS has been operating since 1990, providing national estimates and state-specific estimates in alternating years. Both of these surveys are school-based, providing valid and reliable estimates for those children in school. Because school dropouts are known to have higher smoking rates than children in school, the MTF and YRBS estimates should be considered as conservative estimates of overall smoking rates among young people.

In addition to these federal and state surveys, and as a result of increasing demand for in-depth data on the tobacco control behaviors, attitudes, and perceptions of young people, the CDC and the states developed a new school-based surveillance system called the **Youth Tobacco Survey (YTS)**.[20] The YTS, in contrast to the NSDUH, MTF, and YRBS (which are all multirisk factor surveillance systems) covers just tobacco use. The YTS was developed in response to requests from those state health departments that received early settlements from tobacco industry litigation. The YTS began in Florida, Texas, and Mississippi in 1998, providing valuable data for program planning and evaluation purposes, and is currently being used in 45 states.[21]

The need for in-depth tobacco data was recognized by the **American Legacy Foundation,** which sponsored a national version of the YTS called the National Youth Tobacco Survey (NYTS),[22] and repeated this survey, most recently in 2006. Finally, because of the broad interest in preventing tobacco use among young people, in cooperation with the WHO, the YTS was modified for global use. As of this writing, more than 160 nations have been involved with the **Global Youth Tobacco Survey (GYTS).**[23] Thus, as an outgrowth of the original YTS conducted in a few states in 1998, a true global system of in-depth and comparable tobacco surveillance has evolved, with city and regional, state, national, and international data available for comparison and analysis.

PATTERNS OF USE AMONG ADULTS

Although early tobacco use was primarily ceremonial by Native Americans, with more widespread use of tobacco for pipes, hand-rolled cigarettes, cigars, and chewing, tobacco use today is a highly addicting and habituated behavior. The introduction of blended tobacco that allowed for inhalation, the invention of the safety match, the introduction of mass production of cigarettes, coupled with sophisticated distribution systems (especially to soldiers during WW II) and creative marketing efforts led to the rapid adoption of cigarette smoking during the first half of the twentieth century, peaking in the mid 1960s. A major accomplishment of the past few decades was the reduction in cigarette smoking from a per capita consumption of 4345 cigarettes in 1963,[24] to 1716 in 2005, a reduction of more than 60 percent [25] since the first Surgeon General's Report in 1964.[26]

In addition to the reduction in per capita consumption, which reflects how much smokers are smoking, the United States has also experienced a reduction in adult smoking prevalence, measuring the proportion of people smoking, which dropped from about 43 percent in 1965 to 25.5 percent in 1990.[27] Prevalence then remained fairly flat until 1998,[28] but then subsequently declined to 23.5 percent in 1999, and continued to decline to an estimated 20.8 percent for the first half of 2006.[29] These changes in adult smoking prevalence can be seen in Figure 20.2. Also the percentage of adults who never smoked increased from 44 percent in the mid-1960s to 58 percent in 2005.[30] The net effect produced tens of millions fewer American smokers than would have been expected if earlier rates of smoking continued. All United States population groups, however, have not experienced this progress equally.

Smoking rates vary by demographic characteristics, such as race and ethnicity, level of education, age, poverty status, and region of the country of residence. Despite the very different histories of male and female smoking rates, relatively small differences persist today in smoking prevalence based on gender. In 2005, smoking prevalence of men was at 22.1 percent, which was slightly higher than the smoking prevalence of women at 19.2 percent. That same year[31] found a more than three-fold difference in the likelihood of smoking by race and ethnicity, with the highest smoking rates found among American Indian and Alaska Native populations (32.0 percent), and the lowest among Asians (13.3%).[32] A similar smoking difference with a clear gradient was seen in levels of education. Those with a General Education Development (GED) diploma were more than five times more likely to smoke than those with a graduate degree (43.2% vs. 7.1%, respectively).

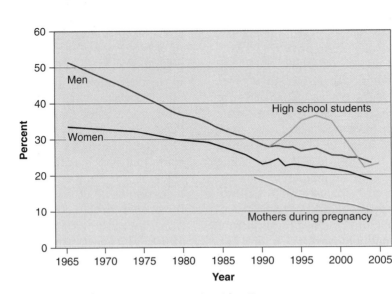

Figure 20.2. Changes Over Time in Adult and Teen Smoking Rates

SOURCE: Centers for Disease Control and Prevention, National Center for Health Statistics, *Health, United States, 2006,* Figure 10. Data from the National Health Interview Survey, Youth Risk Behavior Survey, National Vital Statistics System.

PATTERNS OF USE AMONG YOUNG PEOPLE

The 1994 Surgeon General's Report, *Preventing Tobacco Use Among Young People*,[33] focused intense interest on smoking among youth and young adults. This report emphasized the fact that smoking onset, and **nicotine addiction,** almost always began in the teen years, and provided an early warning of an increase in the use of tobacco products among young adults. In fact, after more than a decade of relatively stable youth smoking rates in the 1980s,[34] cigarette smoking began increasing among high school students in the early 1990s, and peaked in 1996–1997.[35] Their rates have been declining since. According to the MTF Project,[36] the prevalence of daily smoking by twelfth graders peaked at a high of 28.8 percent in 1976, as shown

earlier in Figure 20.2; dropped to 22.2 percent in 1996; and continued to drop to 12.2 percent in 2006. The prevalence rate among this group has significantly dropped but is still showing that approximately 1 out of 9 high school seniors smokes cigarettes every day. The prevalence of current smoking (defined as smoking within the past 30 days) among twelfth graders is also showing a similar pattern, peaking in 1997 at 36.5 percent, and lowering to 21.7 percent in 2006.

Youth smoking rates appear to differ greatly by race and ethnicity, and differently than do the rates for adults. In the late 1970s, there was virtually no difference between smoking rates among youth based on race. In 2002, smoking rates of middle school students continued to be similar among races: white (10.4%), African American (9.4%), and Hispanic (9.1%). Smoking rates in 2002 of high school students, however, do indicate the emergence of disparities: white (25.5%), Hispanic (20.5%), and African American (14.3%).[37]

Data from government surveys clearly demonstrate that more than three-quarters of adult smokers smoke their first cigarette before the age of 18.[38] About 90 percent of adult smokers first tried a cigarette before the age of 19. In the 1994 Report of the Surgeon General, the mean age at which people smoke their first cigarette was calculated to be 14.5. Although some estimates of mean age of first use vary, in every case, the estimated mean age of first use is well below 18 years.

Surveys also clearly show that many smokers become daily smokers before the age of 18. Among adult smokers who have ever smoked daily, about half (53%) began smoking daily before age 18, 71 percent began at ages 18 or younger, and 77 percent began before age 20. According to the latest data from the NSDUH,[39] there were 1.9 million new smokers age 12 years and older in 2002. In 2005, new smokers increased to 2.3 million, of which 63.4 percent were under age 18. Thus, although many measures of smoking rates suggest a reduction in smoking rates among young people, the number of new smokers seems to have increased.

THE FACTORS THAT CONTRIBUTED TO THE CHANGING TOBACCO CONTROL ENVIRONMENT

Recent progress made in tobacco control, besides being noted as one of the 10 greatest public health achievements of the twentieth century,[40] is felt by most Americans. Fewer people are smoking, we seemed to have turned the corner with youth smoking, and most palpably, exposure to **second-hand smoke** has decreased dramatically. Despite these advances, the questions need to be asked—given the magnitude of harm caused by tobacco, the epidemiologic certainty that tobacco is the agent of harm, the fact that illnesses caused by tobacco are completely preventable, and the availability of cost-effective interventions—why has it taken so long for progress to be achieved, and what might limit further progress?

To answer these questions, it is necessary to determine not only the factors that have contributed to our progress but also those that have impeded progress, in what otherwise might have been a fairly simple resolution to a very serious public health problem. It is perhaps even better to look at the second question first, that is, why is continuing progress so difficult. To those in the tobacco control movement, the answer is obvious—the tobacco industry. That the tobacco industry works in its economic self-interest to get as many people to smoke as many cigarettes as possible is a simple matter of economics. What has been most revealing, from a review of industry documents released through litigation, is the revelation of the lengths to which the tobacco industry went to mislead the public, subverting public health, for the purposes of maximizing profits. Thus, it is reassuring and validating for the first major conclusion of the 2000 Surgeon General's Report to read as follows:

> Efforts to prevent the onset or continuance of tobacco use face the pervasive, countervailing influence of tobacco promotion by the tobacco industry, a promotion that takes place despite overwhelming evidence of adverse health effects from tobacco use (page 6).[41]

Besides the industry's behavior, the addictive nature of the product is the other factor that has and continues to impede public health progress in tobacco control. The other question is, despite these impediments, how have we been able to make the remarkable progress that we have? This is more difficult to answer, but has major implications for future progress and perhaps for other public health problems.

Progress in tobacco control has not been the result of any single event or policy, nor has it resulted from a specific public health plan. Rather, progress has been the result of a complex blend of the scientific discovery of the harm caused by smoking, broad dissemination of these findings, very large reductions in smoking rates among opinion leaders (physicians, attorneys, teachers, etc.), and aggressive advocacy by nonsmokers for smoke-free environments. All of these resulted in changes in the social acceptability and public perception of tobacco use. In the 1990s, these changes partially led to and were also built upon by litigation against the tobacco industry for the harm caused by tobacco use, particularly by States' Attorneys General. This litigation resulted in the disclosure of previously secret industry documents, which led, in turn, to an increased distrust of the tobacco industry and further erosion of the acceptability of tobacco use. Some states, notably Florida and California, leveraged this distrust of cynical industry promotions in anti-tobacco campaigns directed variously at adults and youth.

This blending of the scientific documentation of harm, media coverage, public advocacy, changing **social norms,** litigation, and associated disclosure of industry documents has contributed to the major decline of United States tobacco consumption. Fuelling especially the public advocacy and changing social norms was a growing "nonsmokers' rights" movement populated increasingly by former smokers joining never-smokers in the campaigns for smoke-free environments. Although many of these trends are likely to continue, future progress in reducing tobacco use will depend on continued advocacy, as well as the vigorous implementation and monitoring of comprehensive and effective tobacco control programs, including cessation of smoking.

EFFECTIVE INTERVENTIONS IN REDUCING TOBACCO USE

Substantial public health efforts to reduce the prevalence of tobacco use began shortly after the cancer risk was described in 1964. With the subsequent decline in smoking, there have been huge public health improvements. For example, the incidence of smoking-related cancers has declined, with the exception of lung cancer among women (whose smoking rates declined later than men's).[42] Age-adjusted death rates per 100,000 persons for heart disease have decreased from 586.8 in 1950 to 232.3 in 2003.[43] Although the cardiovascular reductions are less singularly attributable to smoking than some of the cancer reductions, it is estimated that between 1964 and 1992, approximately 1.6 million deaths overall caused by smoking were prevented.[44]

Among the many interventions that have been found to be effective in reducing tobacco use and exposure to second-hand smoke are increasing the price of tobacco products, sustained media campaigns, decreasing the out-of-pocket costs for treating nicotine addiction, and restricting indoor smoking. The combination of these has synergistic effects, and the combinations of several into comprehensive programs of tobacco control have yielded the most significant statewide progress in systematic evaluations. Others have been shown to increase the use of tobacco products (e.g., tobacco advertising campaigns targeted to young people, decreases in the price of tobacco products), and yet others have little evidence simply because they have yet to be tried or evaluated (e.g., plain packaging, limits on tar and nicotine levels).

To continue, if not accelerate, this reduction in tobacco use and to concentrate action where it can be most productive, it is essential to know what works, and under what conditions. With this as an objective (and ultimately the title of the 2000 Surgeon General's Report), a multiyear effort was undertaken to identify effective interventions that have been shown to reduce tobacco use and to organize these interventions conceptually to form an intervention typology. The result of this process was *Reducing Tobacco Use: A Report of the Surgeon General*,[45] released in 2000 at the 11th World Conference on Tobacco or Health in Chicago.

The 2000 Surgeon General's Report organized tobacco control interventions into five distinct categories—educational, clinical, regulatory, economic, and social or comprehensive—and reviewed the evidence in support of each category of intervention. Subsequent analysis of these types of intervention conducted in an effort to generalize the tobacco control experience to other public health problems resulted in a modification of the 2000 Surgeon General's Report categories into a new organizing framework for public health interventions,[46] including the following intervention categories:

- The information environment
- The economic environment
- The legal and regulatory environment
- The prevention and treatment environment
- The physical and social environment

The Information Environment

The tobacco industry consistently states that the purpose of spending billions of dollars to market their products is simply to have existing adult smokers smoke "their" brand of cigarettes, and that marketing is not intended to encourage either children or adults to start smoking. Despite this statement, the money spent by the tobacco industry to market and promote tobacco products contributes to new and continued usage by enhancing the appeal, access, and affordability of tobacco products. This issue of whether the tobacco companies purposefully market to children and whether cigarette marketing influences adolescent smoking behavior was a major component of the United States Department of Justice litigation against the tobacco companies. In response to the industry's assertion that marketing was just intended to achieve brand switching or brand loyalty among adult smokers, the government countered that cigarette marketing was aimed at children and was a substantial factor contributing to young people beginning to and continuing to smoke.[47]

In 2003, the United States cigarette companies reported spending $15.15 billion on marketing and promoting cigarettes, the most ever spent, and a 21.5 percent increase from expenditures in the preceding year, which is a much greater increase than the combined inflation and cost of promotions and advertising print space during that

period. The cigarette manufacturers spent $72.9 million on advertisements intended to reduce youth smoking while spending $10.81 billion on price discounts paid to retailers and $1.33 billion on consumer discounts and coupons. Surprisingly, the number of cigarettes consumed in 2003 totaled 19.8 billion, a 5.1 percent decrease from 2002.[48] Restrictions on tobacco advertising form, content, and magnitude are essential for further reductions in tobacco use.

The Economic Environment

Economic interventions include efforts to modify taxation and tariffs and trade policy. The span of impact, as well as the size of impact is very large for both. One of the most effective means of reducing the population prevalence of tobacco use is increasing federal and state excise tax rates. A 10 percent increase in the price of cigarettes can lead to a 4 to 7 percent reduction in the demand for cigarettes. This reduction is the result of people smoking fewer cigarettes or quitting altogether.[49] Studies show that low-income, adolescent, Hispanic, and non-Hispanic black smokers are more likely than others to stop smoking in response to a price increase.[50]

As can be seen in Figure 20.3, the average state excise tax is $1.14 per pack, with 10 states having a tax of $2 or more. The overall highest state tax is in New York ($2.75 per pack), but the overall highest tax in the country is in New York City that has a city tax ($1.50/pack), in addition to the state tax for a total excise tax of $4.25/pack.[51]

The Legal and Regulatory Environment

Laws and regulatory interventions include restrictions on the manufacture and sale of tobacco products, as well as smoking restrictions in public venues and in worksites.[52] The 2000 Surgeon General's Report concluded that regulation of the marketing of tobacco products, particularly products directed at young people, would very likely reduce smoking rates, and that clean air regulations and restrictions of minors' access to tobacco products

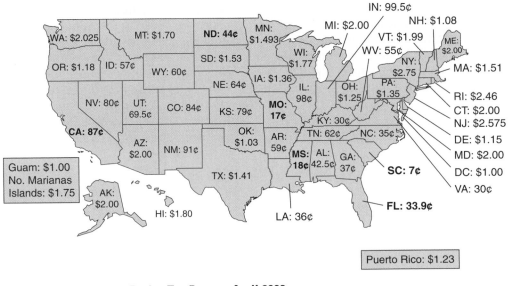

Figure 20.3. **State Cigarette Excise Tax Rates—April 2008**

SOURCE: Delmar Cengage Learning.

contribute to changing social norms against tobacco, and may even reduce tobacco use directly.

Laws have been particularly important in making progress in reducing tobacco use. Laws, most typically at the state and local level, have been particularly effective in providing increased protection from exposure to second-hand smoke. Using data from the **National Health and Nutrition Examination Surveys (NHANES),** Pirkle and colleagues (Figure 20.4) were able to document biologically a 70 percent decrease in serum cotinine levels among nonsmokers over a 14-year period between 1988 and 2002.[53]

Litigation has also been a productive strategy for advancing tobacco control objectives. In many ways, however, reliance on litigation for progress in public health is evidence of the failure of public policy. Requiring individuals and jurisdictions to file litigation to obtain relief and corrective remedies should be the last resort for consumer protection. However, because of the void in appropriate public policy, and the success of the tobacco industry lobby to shape what policy has been passed, the reliance on litigation has resulted in unprecedented

progress in tobacco control, both in providing financial compensation to individuals and states, as well as in providing an unprecedented view of tobacco industry strategy and motives through the release of previously secret documents as a result of the legal discovery process.

Perhaps the best-known tobacco litigation effort was represented by the coordinated litigation of the states' Attorneys General against the tobacco industry for the purposes of recouping state revenue used to pay for diseases caused by tobacco use. After four states settled their claims, in November 1998, the remaining states came to an agreement with the tobacco companies in what has become known as the **Master Settlement Agreement (MSA).**[54] In this agreement, the tobacco companies agreed to pay the states billions of dollars a year and to voluntarily change some of their marketing behavior. In exchange, the states relinquished their claims for reimbursement and agreed not to bring suit in the future. Although both parties indicated their intentions that a substantial portion of the settlement funds be spent on preventing tobacco use among young people, only

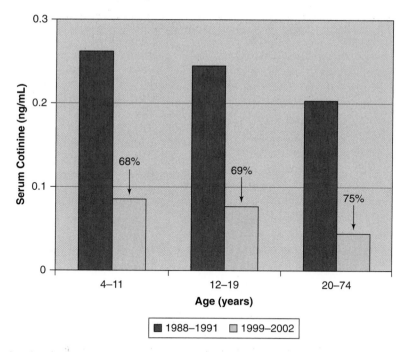

Figure 20.4. **Reduction in Serum Cotinine Levels 1988–1991 and 1999–2002**
SOURCE: Delmar Cengage Learning.

around 5 percent of state MSA payments are used for tobacco control efforts.[55]

Surprisingly, the federal government was not a party to the MSA. In January 1999, however, during his final State of the Union address, President Clinton indicated his intent to file suit against the tobacco companies in a manner similar to that done by the states' Attorneys General. The actual suit was filed in September 1999 and went to trial five years later in September 2004. It was the largest and perhaps costliest litigation in United States government history, with trial testimony concluding in June 2005. In August 2006, in a 1700-page decision, Federal District Court Judge Gladys Kessler found the tobacco companies guilty of RICO violations and defrauding the American public. Judge Kessler ordered the tobacco companies to issue corrective statements and prohibited the use of misleading terms such as "Light" and "Mild"; however, she did not require financial or program-matic remedies because of an earlier Appeals Court ruling. The tobacco companies immediately appealed the overall decision as well as asking the court to allow it to continue to use the terms "Mild" and "Light" around the world. The Federal Appeals court issued a "stay" on all the remedies pending the appeals process, which will likely go to the Supreme Court. However, Judge Kessler rejected the tobacco companies' appeal to use the misleading terms "Mild" and "Light" globally stating in her ruling:

> The Court sees no justification, whether legal or ethical, for concluding that Congress intended to allow a Defendant to continue to tell the rest of the world that "light/low tar" cigarettes are less harmful to health when they are prohibited from making such fraudulent representations to the American public.[56]

In addition to legal and litigation efforts, there is a need to establish meaningful regulation of tobacco products. Tobacco products are escaping meaningful regulation and are expressly exempted from regulation by various federal laws that are otherwise designed to protect consumers, such as the original FDA mandates and the Consumer Product Safety Act.

Analysis of the tobacco product is essential to successful reduction of the harm caused by tobacco use. The cigarette itself has changed dramatically during the past half century and is likely to change even more in the twenty-first century. When cigarettes were first associated with lung cancer in the early 1950s, most United States smokers smoked unfiltered cigarettes. With a growing awareness of the danger of smoking came the first filter, which was designed to reduce the tar inhaled in the smoke. Later, low-tar cigarettes were marketed; however, many smokers compensated by smoking more intensely and by blocking the filter's ventilation holes.[57] Research is needed to determine whether new "highly engineered" products can reduce exposure to toxins and carcinogens, decrease individual risk, or decrease the population harm of tobacco, or whether the mistakes associated with low-tar and nicotine cigarettes will be repeated.[58]

During the late 1990s the FDA attempted to regulate tobacco products as nicotine delivery devices, specifically restricting the marketing and access of tobacco products to young people. As soon as the regulations were issued, the tobacco companies, as well as the advertising industry, sued the FDA, and the case ultimately went to the Supreme Court. In 2000, in a 5 to 4 decision, the Supreme Court decided that, while tobacco products were a deadly product and required regulation, the FDA did not have the authority to regulate tobacco products, and that authority needed to be granted explicitly by Congress. Justice Sandra Day O'Connor, speaking on behalf of the majority, wrote:

> The [FDA] has amply demonstrated that tobacco use, particularly among children and adolescents, poses perhaps the single most significant threat to public health in the United States... [However,] It is plain that Congress has not given the FDA the authority that it seeks to exercise here.[59]

Since that Supreme Court ruling, despite various attempts, Congress has still not granted FDA authority to regulate tobacco products, although bills are currently being considered in both chambers of Congress. It is expected that FDA regulation of tobacco products will receive serious consideration, but the effort is not without continuing controversy.

The Prevention and Treatment Environment

Educational interventions included both school-based curriculum and mass media or other counter-advertising programs. The report concluded that both of these types of interventions have large **spans of impact** and synergistic effects with other interventions, but that the size of their impact when taken alone was either moderate or small. Media campaigns are an effective strategy to change social norms around tobacco use. Sustained media campaigns have been shown to decrease adolescent initiation and increase adult cessation.[60] Of greatest importance, school programs should be conducted in conjunction with community and media-based activities. When this is done, smoking onset can be postponed or prevented in 20 to 40 percent of adolescents. The 2000 Report further noted that current levels of school tobacco prevention practice were not optimal, and more consistent or prolonged implementation was needed, especially in establishing multiyear prevention programs that were coordinated with community and media efforts.

Clinical interventions reviewed included both pharmacologic and behavioral approaches to help smokers quit smoking. They concluded that the span of impact was quite small due to the one-on-one nature of the interventions, and that the size of the impact was moderate to very small for behavioral interventions alone. Having said this, the report concluded that combined pharmacologic and behavioral programs could have success rates of 20 to 25 percent at one-year post-treatment for those smokers who participate in such programs. When pharmacologic interventions such as the nicotine patch are made available over the counter rather than by prescription only, their span of impact or "reach" increases significantly, but the opportunity decreases to couple them with behavioral interventions. The problem, of course, is that although most smokers want to quit smoking, most do not make serious quit attempts involving health professionals. To improve the likelihood that clinical encounters are as successful as possible, in 2000, the Public Health Service published an evidence-based guideline on effective clinical interventions to treat tobacco use and dependence.[61]

The importance of getting existing smokers to quit smoking cannot be overstated. Because many of the health impacts of smoking do not occur until middle age, even if smoking among adolescents could be completely eliminated tomorrow, the impact on morbidity and mortality would take 20–30 years to become evident. For example, the American Cancer Society has set goals for 2015 of a 25 percent reduction in cancer incidence and a 50 percent reduction in cancer mortality rates.[62] The American Cancer Society proposed that 50 percent of that goal could be achieved with a 40–50 percent reduction in smoking prevalence by 2005. Unfortunately, those goals were not achieved by 2005. Multilevel interventions need to be in place to achieve massive changes in behavior among current smokers and in turn reduce smoking prevalence to those levels.

Fortunately there are numerous studies documenting the effectiveness of clinical interventions to enhance quitting, including the Public Health Service guidelines, mentioned previously. It is estimated that if half of the physicians in the United States provided recommended advice to their smoking patients, more than 2 million more smokers would quit each year.[63] These clinical interventions are also highly cost effective.[64] A recent study that prioritized 30 recommended clinical preventive services based upon their impact and the effectiveness and cost-effectiveness of the service

found that treating adult tobacco use ranked second (after childhood immunization).[65] The challenge, however, has been to integrate routine tobacco-use treatment into the health care system, to get practitioners to use them, and to increase access to and payment for effective treatments.

The **Task Force for Community Preventive Services** examined health care system changes that foster effective clinical cessation treatment. This guideline found that reminder systems alone increase the provision of treatment services, and that reminder systems in conjunction with provider training were even more effective. Use of both effective treatments and cessation rates can also be increased by reducing the out-of-pocket costs of treatment and by making cessation counseling more convenient (such as by providing treatment through telephone cessation help lines).[66]

The Physical and Social Environment

One of the most significant factors associated with the progress in reducing tobacco use in the United States has been the dramatic change in social norms. As previously discussed, whereas smoking was once seen as acceptable and even glamorous, it is now seen as socially unacceptable, and nearly as a deviant behavior, practiced generally by those with low levels of education and income, and high levels of co-occurring conditions such as mental illness. Although the **denormalization** of cigarette smoking has contributed to progress in promulgating public policies to increase the price of tobacco products and restrict where smoking can take place, resulting in reductions in smoking and protection of nonsmokers from exposure to secondhand smoke, it must be remembered that most smokers want to quit and consider themselves to be addicted to smoking,[67] and that their addiction is the result of an adolescent decision made in response to a massive marketing campaign. Although increasing social unacceptability of cigarette smoking will likely lead to additional reductions in tobacco use, care should be given to both assist smokers who want to quit and to structure the social environment to prevent nicotine addiction from occurring during the teen years.

Recently, Alamar and Glantz attempted to quantify the magnitude of the impact of the increasing social unacceptability of cigarette smoking on cigarette consumption and estimated that increases in social unacceptability had an effect on cigarette consumption similar to that seen associated with tax increases. Specifically, they estimate that if national public attitudes toward smoking change to resemble those in California, there would be a 15 percent drop in cigarette consumption, similar to the effect from a $1.17 increase in the excise tax on cigarettes.[68] Such findings have fueled renewed efforts to get the film and television industries to place greater restrictions on the appearance of smokers in public entertainment media.

TARGETS FOR TOBACCO CONTROL: LEADING HEALTH INDICATORS AND *HEALTHY PEOPLE 2010* OBJECTIVES

The best manifestation of a United States formal strategy or plan to reduce tobacco use is its explicit objectives for the year 2010 (21 objectives covering tobacco out of 467 for the full range of disease prevention and health promotion goals). These objectives guide the direction and activities not only of the Federal government but also of states, communities, and voluntary organizations. It also has a series of 10 Leading Health Indicators (LHIs) that guide the federal government in setting priorities and monitoring progress in improving public health. LHIs reflect the major health concerns in the United States at the beginning of the twenty-first century. Within this *Healthy People 2010* framework,[69] 3 of the 21 tobacco control objectives are also considered LHIs. Specifically, two prevalence objectives, to reduce current smoking rates by more than half among adults and teenagers, as well as an objective to reduce exposure to second-hand smoke, are

among the LHIs, reinforcing the importance of tobacco control in the nation's overall public health improvement efforts.

Of the 21 tobacco objectives for the year 2010, 4 pertain to patterns of tobacco use, 4 to cessation and treatment, 5 to exposure to second-hand smoke, and 8 to social and environmental changes. The overriding objective is to reduce tobacco use in half, or to 12 percent for cigarette smoking by adults (Objective 27-1), and 16 percent for past month cigarette smoking for high school students (Objective 27-2), for all population groups, by the year 2010. Both of these are also LHIs. The concept of "for all population groups" was emphasized because of the great variation in tobacco use rates by race, ethnicity, and socioeconomic status (see Table 20.1 for examples of groups with comparatively low smoking rates). By adopting the position that all groups should benefit equally (or achieve equally low rates), the *Healthy People 2010* process would go a long way toward eliminating health disparities in the United States. Other objectives that pertain to the use of tobacco products include reducing the initiation of tobacco use among children (Objective 27-3), and increasing the age of first use from 12 to 14 years for adolescents (Objective 27-4).

In 2005, the United States Department of Health and Human Services (HHS) conducted a midcourse review to access the status of the *Healthy People 2010* national objectives.[70] Compared to their

Table 20.1. Groups with Smoking Rates Below the *Healthy People 2010* Goal of 12%

- Adults 25 years and older with at least a bachelor's degree (10.8%)
- Adults 65 and older (~10%)
- Black women 18–24 (10.0%)
- Asian adults (6.7%)
- Hispanic or Latino adults (12.1%)

SOURCE: United States Department of Health and Human Services. *Healthy People 2010. 2nd ed.* International Medical Publishing, Inc.: McLean, VA; 2002.

corresponding baseline, one objective exceeded its target (exposure to environmental tobacco smoke), nine objectives moved toward their targets, one objective moved away from its target, and one objective had mixed progress.

Although there has not been an explicit or official tobacco control "strategy" for the United States, there is a very comprehensive plan of action, embracing behavioral, social, environmental, and policy outcomes. The challenge becomes to develop feasible plans of action necessary to achieve each of the objectives. The Office on Smoking and Health at CDC has undertaken such planning in consultation with the other federal agencies and nongovernmental partners. Achievement of the 21 ambitious objectives, and simply putting in place what we know works, would enable the nation to reach its overall goal of cutting smoking rates in half, for everybody, to no more than 12 percent by the end of the decade; however, cutbacks in funding for programs and enforcement of policies will undermine some of that achievement.[71] Similar plans have been developed for the CDC role in contributing to global tobacco control.

SUCCESSES FROM THE STATES AND FUNDING FOR TOBACCO CONTROL

If the evidence-based interventions that already exist were widely applied, the *Healthy People 2010* objective of reducing tobacco use in half could be achieved. If smoking rates are reduced in half, millions of lives will be saved, and the expenditure of billions of dollars on treating diseases caused by smoking can be averted. Preliminary evidence from California is already demonstrating that sustained implementation of effective tobacco control interventions not only can reduce smoking rates but also can save lives and dollars.[72,73]

The United States is fortunate to have models of successful tobacco control programs within several states. Thanks to citizen initiative and political leadership, the United States enjoys a number of well-funded, evidence-based tobacco control programs. All of these originally emanated from an earmarked portion of an increase in the cigarette excise tax, followed in some states by a dedicated and purposeful use of tobacco industry settlement funds to reduce tobacco use. California was the first state to launch a concerted effort to raise the cigarette excise tax and to devote a substantial portion of the tax revenue to tobacco control, followed most notably by Massachusetts, Arizona, and Oregon. Among states that used their tobacco settlement dollars for tobacco control and have already demonstrated the effectiveness of their program are Florida and Mississippi. As more states launch comprehensive, evidence-based tobacco control programs, even more examples of success can be expected.

The first models of increasing cigarette or tobacco excise taxes and earmarking a portion for tobacco prevention programs came from Canada. More extensive analyses of data from both California and Massachusetts have indicated that increasing excise taxes on cigarettes is one of the most cost-effective, short-term strategies to reduce tobacco consumption, and the ability to sustain or accelerate lower consumption when the tax increase is combined with an antismoking campaign.[74]

Based on the experience of state programs, as well as the published literature, CDC published *Best Practices for Comprehensive Tobacco Control Programs*[75] to guide states in their tobacco control efforts following the implementation of the MSA between states' Attorneys General and the tobacco industry. *Best Practices* provides the research and scientific evidence, together with practice-based experiences in California and Massachusetts, in support of nine elements that should comprise a comprehensive tobacco control program. Because *Best Practices* focused on providing guidance to states on the scientific evidence on public health programs, it did not include policy recommendations on product regulation, pricing, or other nonprogrammatic activities.

In addition, the Task Force on Community Preventive Services[76] established rules of evidence to review the published literature on a variety of tobacco control strategies, including efforts to reduce exposure to second-hand smoke, to increase tobacco use cessation, and prevent initiation. Additional reviews will be forthcoming on pricing, minors' access to tobacco products and media campaigns.

FUTURE CHALLENGES AND CONCLUSIONS

The 2000 Surgeon General's Report, besides reviewing the evidence-base for tobacco control, also identified a number of future challenges, which in many ways, provides an agenda for the future. These challenges include the following:

- Continuing to build the science base of tobacco control
- Understanding the changing tobacco industry
- Implementing a comprehensive approach to tobacco control
- Identifying and eliminating disparities
- Improving the dissemination of state-of-the-art interventions
- Addressing global tobacco use

For continued progress to be achieved, these issues, and perhaps other emerging challenges, must compose our future agenda, particularly attention to global tobacco use.

Although this chapter has focused on the reduction and continued use of tobacco in the United States, the same opportunities and challenges experienced in the United States exist in every country of the world. Unfortunately, the United States and other developed countries have paid the price in untold millions of lives as a result of the cunning and avarice of the tobacco companies for the past century. In fact, Harvard historian Allan Brandt has recently labeled the United States tobacco experience in the twentieth century as "The Cigarette Century."[77] Fortunately, there is intensive global effort to prevent "the cigarette century" catastrophe from occurring in developing countries as it has played out in the United States and other developed countries. Using its treaty-making authority, in 1996, the World Health Assembly adopted a resolution to initiate the development of a Framework Convention on Tobacco Control (FCTC).[78] Formal diplomatic work began in 1999, and a completed tobacco control treaty was unanimously adopted by the World Health Assembly in May, 2003. Today, 154 out of 192 member states have ratified the FCTC, representing over 80 percent of the world's population. Embarrassingly, while the United States government signed the FCTC in 2004, as of mid-2008, the Executive Branch has failed to send the treaty to the Senate for its consideration and ratification.

In large part stimulated by the unprecedented achievement of enacting the first-ever public health treaty, there has been increasing interest in and attention to global tobacco control. There have been increasing efforts to document the burden and scope of the global tobacco epidemic,[79] as well as to disseminate effective interventions and remedies.[80,81] These efforts are all intended either to shorten the period of time it takes to reduce tobacco use from decades to years, or to prevent the tobacco epidemic from occurring in the first place. In either instance, global efforts need to be focused toward complete and strong implementation of the general obligations contained in the FCTC and any future protocols. This focused determination will require an unprecedented investment in global tobacco control, and it is fortunate that major philanthropists, such as Michael Bloomberg and Bill and Melinda Gates have recently stepped forward and dedicated hundreds of millions of dollars for global tobacco control. As we advance our efforts in global tobacco control, we must remember that "the burden is vast, the interventions are proven and the potential for prevention is incalculable."[82]

In summary, despite the achievements over the past few decades, much remains to be done. In 2005, 71.5 million Americans were reported current tobacco users.[83] Cigarette smoking causes approximately 440,000 United States deaths each year—one of every five—and, if current trends continue, approximately 25 million Americans alive today, including 5 million of today's children, will die as a result of smoking.[84] But current trends do not need to continue, and simply putting in place those actions known to reduce tobacco use can halve tobacco use rates. The 2000 Surgeon General's Report,[85] *Reducing Tobacco Use*, documented the scientific evidence of what works, and concluded that if we implement what we know works, we can reduce smoking rates in half, for all population groups. In fact, in 2000, then-Surgeon General David Satcher said:

> It is clear that the major barrier to more rapid reductions in tobacco use is the effort of the tobacco industry to promote the use of tobacco products. Our lack of greater progress in tobacco control is more the result of failure to implement proven strategies than it is the lack of knowledge about what to do. As a result, each year, more than 1 million young people continue to become regular smokers, and more than 400,000 adults die from tobacco-related diseases. Tobacco use will remain the leading cause of preventable illness and death in this nation and a growing number of other countries until tobacco prevention and control efforts are commensurate with the harm caused by tobacco use.[86]

REVIEW QUESTIONS

1. What factors accounted for the progress achieved in United States tobacco control efforts?
2. What could have been done, and what should be done in the future, to accelerate reductions in tobacco use?
3. What is the greatest future challenge to efforts to reduce tobacco use, and what could be done to reduce these challenges?
4. How would you characterize the current patterns of tobacco use in the United States?
5. What is the optimal mix of program and policy to achieve greater progress in reducing tobacco use?
6. Why is cessation, rather than just prevention of the uptake of smoking by youth, essential to the achievement of national objectives for reduction of prevalence and mortality?

REFERENCES

1. CDC. State-specific prevalence of current cigarette smoking among adults and secondhand smoke rules and policies in homes and workplaces—United States 2005. *MMWR*. October 27, 2006;55(42);1148–1151.
2. CDC. Achievements in public health 1900–1999: Tobacco use—United States, 1900–1999. *MMWR*. 1999;48:986–93.
3. Eriksen MP, Green LW, Husten CG, Pederson LL, Pechacek TF. Thank you for not smoking: The public health response to tobacco-related mortality in the United States. In: Ward JW, Warren C. *Silent Victories: The History and Practice of Public Health in Twentieth Century America*. Oxford University Press; New York. 2007.
4. CDC. *A Report of the Surgeon General: 2004*. Washington, DC: The Department of Health and Human Sciences; 2004.
5. CDC. Projected smoking-related deaths among youth—United States. *MMWR*. 1996;45:971–4.
6. CDC. *At A Glance 2006, Targeting Tobacco Use: The Nation's Leading Cause of Death*. Atlanta, GA: National Center for Chronic Disease Prevention and Health Promotion; 2007.
7. Doll R, Peto R, Wheatlet K, Gary R, Sutherland I. Mortality in relation to smoking: 40 years' observations on male British doctors. *BMJ*. 309(6959): 901–911, 1994.
8. CDC. Smoking—attributable mortality and years of potential life lost—United States, 1984. *MMWR*. 1997;46:444–51.
9. Peto R, Lopez AD, Boreham J, Thun M, Heath C. *Mortality from Smoking in Developed Countries 1950–2000*. Oxford, England: Oxford University Press; 1994.

10. CDC. A Report of the Surgeon General: 2004. Washington, DC: The Department of Health and Human Sciences; 2004.

11. American Cancer Society. *Cancer facts and figures—2007.* Atlanta, GA: American Cancer Society; 2007.

12. Adler I. *Primary Malignant Growths of the Lungs and Bronchi: A Pathological and Clinical Study.* London: Longmans, Green and Co.; 1912.

13. Wingo PA, Ries LA, Giovino GA, et al. Annual report to the nation on the status of cancer, 1973–1996, with a special section on lung cancer and tobacco smoking. *J Natl Cancer Inst.* 1999;91:675–90.

14. US Public Health Service. *Smoking and Health.* Report of the Advisory Committee to the Surgeon General of the Public Health Service. US Department of Health, Education and Welfare, Public Health Service, CDC. PHS publication no. 1103; 1964.

15. CDC. Mortality trends for selected smoking-related cancers and breast cancer–United States, 1950–1990. *MMWR.* 1993;42;863–6.

16. American Cancer Society. Cancer Statistics 2006. Available at: http://www.cancer.org/docroot/ PRO/content/PRO_1_1_Cancer_Statistics_ 2006_Presentation.asp. Accessed February 2007.

17. Gazdar AF. DNA repair and survival in lung cancer: The two faces of Janus. *New England Journal of Medicine.* February 22, 2007;356(8):771–773.

18. Green LW, Wilson R, Bauer K. Data required to measure progress on the objectives for the nation in disease prevention and health promotion. *American Journal of Public Health.* 1983;73: 18–24.

19. Substance Abuse and Mental Health Services Administration. Results from the 2005 National Survey on Drug Use and Health: National Findings. Rockville, MD: Office of Applied Studies, NSDUH Series H-30, DHHS Publication No. SMA 06-4194; 2006.

20. CDC. Youth tobacco surveillance—United States, 1998–1999. *MMWR.* 2000;49;No.SS-10.

21. CDC. Youth tobacco surveillance—United States, 2001–2002. *MMWR.* 2006;55;No.SS-3.

22. American Legacy Foundation. Legacy first look report 1: Cigarette smoking among youth: Results from the 1999 National Youth Tobacco Survey, June 2000. Available at: http://www.americanlegacy .org/864.aspx. Accessed October 16, 2008.

23. Warren CW, Riley LA, Asma S, Eriksen MP, Green LW, Yach D. Tobacco use by youth: A surveillance report from the Global Youth Tobacco Survey Project. Bulletin of the World Health Organization. 2000;78:868–876.

24. US Department of Agriculture. *Agriculture Outlook/January–February 2001.* Washington, DC: Economic Research Service/USDA; 2001.

25. US Department of Agriculture. *Tobacco Report.* Washington, DC: Economic Research Service/ USDA; September 2006.

26. US Public Health Service. *Smoking and Health. Report of the Advisory Committee to the Surgeon General of the Public Health Service.* Washington, DC: US Department of Health, Education and Welfare, Public Health Service, CDC. PHS publication no. 1103; 1964.

27. Giovino GA, Schooley MW, Zhu BP, et al. Surveillance for selected tobacco-use behaviors—United States, 1900–1994. In: CDC surveillance summaries. *MMWR.* November 18, 1994;43(No.ss-3): 1–43.

28. CDC. Cigarette smoking among adults—United States, 1998. *MMWR.* 2000;49:881–4.

29. CDC. National Center for Health Statistics. Early release of selected data from the January–June 2006 National Health Interview Survey. Available at: http://www.cdc.gov/nchs/data/nhis/ earlyrelease/200612_08.pdf.

30. CDC. Summary Health Statistics for US Adults: National Health Interview Survey, 2005. Washington, DC: National Center for Health Statistics; December 2006; Series 10;No. 232.

31. CDC. State-Specific Prevalence of Current Cigarette Smoking Among Adults and Secondhand Smoke Rules and Policies in Homes and Workplaces—United States, 2005. *MMWR.* 2006;55: 42;1148–1151.

32. CDC. Tobacco Use Among Adults—United States 2005. *MMWR.* 2006;55:42;1145–1148.

33. US Department of Health and Human Services. *Preventing Tobacco Use Among Young People: Report of the Surgeon General.* Atlanta, GA: US Department of Health and Human Services, Centers for Disease Control and Prevention, National Center for Chronic Disease Prevention and Health Promotion, Office on Smoking and Health; 1994.

34. Johnston LD, O'Malley PM, Bachman JG. *National survey results on drug use from the*

Monitoring the Future study, 1975–1998. Vol 1: Secondary school students. Rockville, MD: National Institutes of Health, National Institute of Drug Abuse; 1999 (NIH publication no. 99–4660).

35. CDC. Trends in cigarette smoking among high school students—United States, 1991–1999. *MMWR.* 2000;49:755–8.

36. University of Michigan. Decline in daily smoking by younger teens has ended. [press release]. Ann Arbor: University of Michigan News and Information Services; December 21, 2006.

37. CDC. Tobacco use among middle and high school students—United States, 2002. *MMWR.* 2003;52:45.

38. US Department of Health and Human Services. *Preventing Tobacco Use Among Young People: Report of the Surgeon General.* Atlanta, GA: US Department of Health and Human Services, Centers for Disease Control and Prevention, National Center for Chronic Disease Prevention and Health Promotion, Office on Smoking and Health; 1994.

39. Substance Abuse and Mental Health Services Administration. Results from the 2005 National Survey on Drug Use and Health: National Findings. Rockville, MD: Office of Applied Studies, NSDUH Series H-30, DHHS Publication No. SMA 06-4194; 2006.

40. CDC. Achievements in Public Health 1900–1999: Tobacco Use—United States, 1900–1999. *MMWR.* 1999;48:986–93.

41. US Department of Health and Human Services. *Reducing Tobacco Use. A Report of the Surgeon General.* Atlanta, GA: US Department of Health and Human Services, Centers for Disease Control and Prevention, National Center for Chronic Disease Prevention and Health Promotion, Office on Smoking and Health; 2000.

42. Wingo PA, Ries LA, Giovino GA, et al. Annual report to the nation on the status of cancer, 1973–1996, with a special section on lung cancer and tobacco smoking. *J Natl Cancer Inst.* 1999; 91:675–90.

43. CDC. Health, United States 2006, With Chartbook on Trends in the Health of Americans, Hyattsville, MD: National Center for Health Statistics; 2006.

44. CDC. Decline in deaths from heart disease and stroke—United States, 1900–1999. *MMWR.* 1999;48:649–56.

45. US Department of Health and Human Services. *Reducing Tobacco Use. A Report of the Surgeon General.* Atlanta, GA: US Department of Health and Human Services, Centers for Disease Control and Prevention, National Center for Chronic Disease Prevention and Health Promotion, Office on Smoking and Health; 2000.

46. Eriksen MP. Lessons learned from public health efforts and their relevance to preventing childhood obesity. In: Koplan J, Liverman C, eds. *Preventing Childhood Obesity.* Institute of Medicine, National Academies of Sciences Press: Washington DC; 2004.

47. Eriksen MP. US Department of Justice. Written Direct Examination, January 27, 2005. Available at: http://www.usdoj.gov/civil/cases/tobacco2/Eriksen%20Written%20Direct%20011705.pdf.

48. Federal Trade Commission. *Cigarette Report for 2003.* Washington, DC; 2005.

49. Chaloupka FJ, Warner KE. The economics of smoking. In: Newhouse J, Culyer A, eds. *The Handbook of Health Economics.* Amsterdam, The Netherlands: Elsevier Science; 1999.

50. Chaloupka FJ, Warner KE. The economics of smoking. In: Newhouse J, Culyer A, eds. *The Handbook of Health Economics.* Amsterdam, The Netherlands: Elsevier Science; 1999.

51. Campaign for Tobacco Free Kids. Available at: http://www.tobaccofreekids.org/research/factsheets/pdf/0222.pdf.

52. Daynard RA, Gottlieb MA, Sweda EL, Friedman LC, Erikesn MP. Prevention and control of diseases associated with tobacco use through law and policy. In: Goodman RA, ed. *Law in Public Health Practice.* Oxford University Press: New York; 2007.

53. Pirkle JL, Bernert JT, Caudill SP, Sosnoff CS, Pechacek TF. Trends in the exposure of nonsmokers in the US population to secondhand smoke: 1988–2002. *Environmental Health Perspectives.* 2006;114:853–858.

54. National Association of Attorneys General. Master Settlement Agreement. Available at: http://www.naag.org/backpages/naag/tobacco/msa/msa-pdf/. Accessed October 16, 2008.

55. US Government Accountability Office. Tobacco Settlement: States' Allocations of Fiscal Year 2005 and Expected Fiscal Year 2006 Payments. *GAO.* 06-502. Washington, DC; April 2006. Available at: http://www.gao.gov/new.items/d06502.pdf.

56. US District Court for the District of Columbia. Memorandum Opinion Civil Action Number 99-2496 (GK), March 16, 2007. Available at: https://ecf.dcd.uscourts.gov/cgi-bin/show_public_doc?1999cv2496-5800.

57. Fielding JF, Husten CG, Eriksen MP. Tobacco: Health effects and control. In: Wallace RB, Doebbeling BN, Last JM, eds. *Public Health and Preventive Medicine*. 14th ed. Stamford, CT: Appleton & Lange; 1998.

58. Warner KE, Slade J, Sweanor DT. The emerging market for long-term nicotine maintenance. *JAMA*. 1997;278:1087–92.

59. Fda V. Brown & Williamson Tobacco Corp. (98-1152) 529 US 120 (2000) 153 F.3d 155, affirmed. Available at: http://supct.law.cornell.edu/supct/pdf/98-1152P.ZO.

60. CDC. Strategies for reducing exposure to environmental tobacco smoke, increasing tobacco use cessation, and reducing initiation in communities and health-care systems. A report on recommendations of the Task Force on Community Preventive Services. *MMWR*. 2000;(No. RR-12):1–11.

61. Fiore MC, Bailey WC, Cohen SJ, et al. *Treating tobacco use and dependence. Clinical practice guideline*. Washington, DC: US Department of Health and Human Services, Public Health Service; 2000.

62. Byers R, Mouchawa J, Marks J, et al. The American Cancer Society challenge goals: How far can cancer rates decline in the US by the year 2015? *Cancer*. 1999;86:715–27.

63. US Department of Health and Human Services. *How to help your patients stop smoking: A National Cancer Institute manual for physicians*. Rockville, MD: USDHHS, National Institutes of Health, National Cancer Institute; 1993. NIH publication no. 93-3064.

64. US Department of Health and Human Services. *How to help your patients stop smoking: A National Cancer Institute manual for physicians*. Rockville, MD: USDHHS, National Institutes of Health, National Cancer Institute; 1993. NIH publication no. 93-3064.

65. Coffield AB, Maciosek MV, McGinnis M, et. al. Priorities among recommended clinical preventive services. *Am J Prev Med*. 2001;21(1):1–9.

66. CDC. Strategies for reducing exposure to environmental tobacco smoke, increasing tobacco use cessation, and reducing initiation in communities and health-care systems. A report on recommendations of the Task Force on Community Preventive Services. *MMWR*. 2000;No. RR-12:1–11.

67. Jones JM. Smoking habits stable; most would like to quit. The Gallup Poll; July 18, 2006.

68. Alamar B, Glantz SA. Effect of increased social unacceptability of cigarette smoking on reduction in cigarette consumption. *American Journal of Public Health*. 2006;96(8):1359–1363.

69. US Department of Health and Human Services. *Healthy People 2010: Understanding and Improving Health*. 2nd ed. Washington, DC: US Government Printing Office; November 2000.

70. US Department of Health and Human Services. *Healthy People 2010: Midcourse Review*. March 2007. Available at: http://www.healthypeople.gov/data/midcourse/pdf/ExecutiveSummary.pdf.

71. Green LW, Eriksen MP, Bailey L, Husten C. Achieving the implausible in the next decade: Tobacco control objectives. *Am J Public Health*. 2000;90:337–9.

72. CDC. Declines in lung cancer rates—California, 1988–1997. *MMWR*. 2000;49:1066–9.

73. Fichtenberg CM, Glantz SA. Association of the California tobacco control program with declines in cigarette consumption and mortality from heart disease. *New Engl J of Med*. 2000;343:1772–7.

74. CDC. Cigarette smoking before and after an excise tax increase and an antismoking campaign. *MMWR*. 1996;45:966–70.

75. CDC. Best practices for comprehensive tobacco control programs—August 1999. Atlanta, GA: US Department of Health and Human Services; 1999; and 2nd ed., October 2007.

76. Zaza S, Briss PA, Harris KW. *The Guide to Community Preventive Services: What Works to Promote Health?* Oxford University Press: New York; 2005 Available at: http://www.thecommunityguide.org/tobacco/default.htm.

77. Brandt A. *The Cigarette Century: The Rise, Fall, and Deadly Persistence of the Product That Defined America*. Basic Books; 2007.

78. World Health Organization. WHO Framework Convention on Tobacco Control. Available at: http://www.who.int/tobacco/framework/WHO_FCTC_english.pdf.

79. Mackey J, Eriksen M, Shafey O. The Tobacco Atlas, 2nd ed. American Cancer Society. Myriad Editions Limited: Hong Kong; 2006.

80. West R. Tobacco control: Present and future. *British Medical Bulletin*. 2006:1–14;DOI: 10.1093/bmb/ldl012.

81. Davis RM, Wakefield M, Amos A, Gupta PC. The hitchhiker's guide to tobacco control: A global assessment of harms, remedies and controversies. *Annual Review of Public Health*. 2007;28: 171–194.

82. Eriksen MP. The potential for prevention. *Health Education Research*. 2006;21(3):303–4.

83. Substance Abuse and Mental Health Services Administration. Results from the 2005 National Survey on Drug Use and Health: National Findings. Rockville, MD: Office of Applied Studies, NSDUH Series H-30, DHHS Publication No. SMA 06-4194.

84. CDC. Projected smoking-related deaths among youth—United States. 1996;45:971–4.

85. US Department of Health and Human Services. Reducing Tobacco Use. A Report of the Surgeon General. Atlanta, GA: US Department of Health and Human Services, Centers for Disease Control and Prevention, National Center for Chronic Disease Prevention and Health Promotion, Office on Smoking and Health; 2000.

86. US Department of Health and Human Services. Reducing Tobacco Use. A Report of the Surgeon General. At-A-Glance, Atlanta, GA: US Department of Health and Human Services, Centers for Disease Control and Prevention, National Center for Chronic Disease Prevention and Health Promotion, Office on Smoking and Health; 2000.

CHAPTER 21

Drug and Alcohol Issues in Public Health

C.G. Leukefeld, DSW, M. Staton-Tindall, PhD, MSW,
Carrie B. Oser, PhD, William W. Stoops, PhD, and J. Mosher, JD

LEARNING OBJECTIVES

Upon completion of this chapter, the reader will be able to:

1. Describe differences in the national prevalence of current use of various drugs.

2. Differentiate between prevalence of drug and alcohol use in the nation and high school students.

3. Examine how emerging drug trends will impact national drug use prevalence, as well as rates of abuse and dependence.

4. Compare traumatic injury and mortality rates associated with either alcohol or other drugs.

5. Identify unique characteristics of female substance users.

6. Present recommendations and implications for public health policy and treatment.

7. Integrate information on criminal justice populations with information on national prevalence of drug use.

8. Assess the overall effects of alcohol and drug use (including prevalence, mortality, and health problems) on public health initiatives.

9. Identify ways practitioners define and "think about" drug and alcohol abuse.

KEY TERMS

Alcohol

Abuse

Criminal Justice

Dependence

Drug

Intervention

Prevention

Treatment

Most public health practitioners and researchers agree that drug and alcohol abuse are chronic and relapsing disorders.[1] This reality is supported by both brain and behavioral research.[2] This chapter focuses on drug and alcohol issues for public health students and practitioners. We included a lot of incidence/prevalence data and policy information because public health officials need to better understand the high levels of drug and alcohol use in the general population as well as in **criminal justice** settings as the same individuals come into contact with public health service providers. Avoidance of drug and alcohol use and related problems may be common in public health settings. We look to future changes in public health policy and practice as substance use, including nicotine, prescription drugs, and current fad drugs such as prescription pain killers, oxycodone preparations, and "home cooked meth," decreases in the United States. Policy is an arena where public health practitioners can impact drug and alcohol use/abuse and addictions with changes in prevention and treatment. A public health approach to drug and alcohol abuse interventions incorporates the interaction of the agent (drug), the host (the individual), and the environment (the community as the place that brings the individual and the drug together, including biological, psychological, social/cultural, and spiritual factors). A community intervention focused on only the agent, the host, or the environment separately may be useful, however, the more useful and successful interventions systematically target all three simultaneously.

INTRODUCTION

Drug and **alcohol** use, abuse, and **dependence** are prominent in the United States. Effective substance use prevention and treatment can reduce problems associated with use, which includes harmful consequences such as relapse, criminal justice involvement, economic instability, and mental health disorders. Drug and alcohol use is the ingestion of a substance that can be distinguished across two dimensions: legal status and purpose of use.[3] The combination of these two dimensions produces four types of use: (1) legal use, (2) illegal use, (3) legal recreational use, and (4) illegal recreational use. *Legal use* includes over-the-counter or prescription drugs (e.g., taking OxyContin with a prescription), whereas, *legal recreational drug use* is the use of government-sanctioned psychoactive substances to achieve a specific mental or psychic state (e.g., drinking alcohol to get intoxicated). *Illegal use* refers to taking drugs without a prescription for some socially sanctioned purpose (e.g., using an amphetamine to work all night). *Illegal recreational use* includes taking drugs without a prescription to achieve a specific mental or psychic state (e.g., taking heroin to get high). Public health practitioners focus on the latter three combinations; however, illegal recreational use currently receives the most attention.

There are a variety of definitions of substance **abuse.** Each definition includes the use of psychoactive substance for a nontherapeutic effect. Medical definitions include the two most commonly used diagnostic tools, the American Psychiatric Association's (APA) Diagnostic and Statistical Manual of Mental Disorders IV and the World Health Organization's (WHO) International Statistical Classification of Diseases and Related Health Problems (ICD). The medical or disease model defines *addiction* as a chronic relapsing medical disorder in which a user/abuser does not have control over his or her drug or alcohol use.

DRUG AND ALCOHOL THEORY

There are gaps in the public health literature on theoretical factors impacting substance abuse. The majority of public health theories are not specific to understanding drug and alcohol use, but focus on explaining health behaviors as a broader category. The traditional public health theoretical foundation of explaining the determinants of health behaviors, such as substance use and abuse, could be improved with a multidisciplinary approach. Although public health practice is biomedically grounded, drug and alcohol use interventions can be enriched with the integration of a variety of psychological[4–6] and sociological theories[7–12] to broaden the traditionally individual-level perspective by including society, culture, and availability.

Health behaviors, including drug and alcohol use/abuse, are usually studied at the individual level. Research should consider interpersonnel processes and organizational factors.[13] Focusing on individual factors alone can promote victim-blaming[13] and personal failure. An ecological theoretical framework developed by Brofenbrenner[14] can supplement an individual focus. For example, a modified version of the ecological framework posits that health behavioral outcomes are influenced by five components: (1) intrapersonal or individual factors, (2) interpersonal processes, (3) institutional factors, (4) community factors, and (5) public policy.[13] *Intrapersonal factors* include demographics as well as individual characteristics such as knowledge, attitudes, behavior, self-concept, and skills. These intrapersonal factors are grounded in psychological behavioral change models, which include the Health Belief Model,[15] Theory of Reasoned Action,[16] and Social Learning Theory.[4] *Interpersonal processes* are the formal/informal social networks and social support systems that can influence behavioral outcomes, whereas *institutional factors* are used to examine the impact of organizational structural characteristics—organizational climate and operational regulations—on behavioral change.[13] *Community factors* include relationships among organizations, institutions, and informal networks within defined boundaries.[13] Health behaviors, including alcohol and drug use, are regulated with policies, procedures, and laws designed to protect the community.[13] *Public health policy* can serve as an impetus for individual behavioral changes.

One model or way of thinking about drug abuse is a bio/psycho/social/spiritual interaction framework. This model presents theoretical grounding to addiction as the interaction of behavior, environment, spirituality, and biology/brain.[17] This frame-

work includes four possible theoretical pathways to addiction:

1. *Biology or genetic* pathways include heritability and biologically conditioned aspects of addiction that represent one foundation for the disease model. The disease model has been criticized because it is "used" by alcoholics and drug users to deny responsibility for their drinking and drugging behaviors, citing that a disease cannot be "controlled."

2. *Psychological* pathways incorporate individual characteristics that contribute to the motivation to use and abuse drugs, expectancies to use, personality factors, and individual "risk" and "protective" factors. However, it is important to keep in mind that a risk factor for one person may be protective for others.

3. *Social and environmental* pathways include laws, culture, familial norms, customs, peer associations, and consequences that have been associated with social learning.

4. *Spirituality* pathways incorporate spiritual beliefs. Although spirituality is related to substance use recovery, it is not without controversy. Controversy focuses on the relationship of spirituality and the idea that religiosity is a protective factor to prevent drug abuse. Theoretical routes to explain alcohol or drug abuse may differ, but the chemical result is the activation of the mesolimbic dopamine system, which serves as the brain's reward or pleasure center.[18]

Theoretical developments can improve community **prevention,** which includes primary, secondary, or tertiary prevention approaches as unique to public health. Primary prevention is directed to preventing the initial use of drugs. Examples of primary prevention include drug-related education programs or anti-drug advertising. Secondary prevention is focused on early identification of drug use and intervention before the progression to drug or alcohol dependence (e.g., drug testing). Tertiary prevention targets an intervention at an advanced state of drug use, such as a rehabilitative approach that focuses on substance abuse treatment. Although prevention ranks low as a federal policy priority, it is important to decrease and delay the substance abuse in the United States.

A Public Health Paradigm

Drug and alcohol use/abuse can also be understood by examining the interaction of three key components of any public health problem: host, agent, and environment. The *host* is usually the individual suffering with a public health problem, and the *agent* (or vector) is what causes harm to the host. The *environment* includes social, economic, physical, political, and cultural settings in which the host and agent interact.[19] Drugs and alcohol can play differing roles within this public health paradigm. For example, with drug-related illnesses such as cirrhosis of the liver, the agent can be alcohol. However, for alcohol-related trauma, the agent or vector is energy (the impact of an automobile hitting a tree), and alcohol is a significant environmental factor increasing the likelihood that an injury from the energy will occur. A high-risk environment creates opportunities for public health harm. For example, environmental change can provide protection to large numbers of people by preventing the agent and host from interacting. A comprehensive public health strategy focuses on all three factors: providing care to those who suffer disease or injury, reducing the harmfulness and availability of particular agents, and addressing dangerous conditions or environments that put people at risk for harm.

A SHIFT IN ALCOHOL POLICY

Until recently, public health principles had limited impact on understanding alcohol and other drug problems. The field has traditionally focused on host and agent factors to the exclusion of an examination of environmental risk factors. During the late 1800s and early 1900s, alcohol policy was dominated by a focus on the individual immorality of drinkers and the need to restrict and eventually prohibit the availability of "demon" alcohol.[20] Dr. Benjamin Rush's pamphlet, entitled "An Inquiry in to the Effects of Ardent Spirits on the Human Mind and Body," as well as other organizations such as the Anti-Saloon League and the Women's Christian Temperance Union (WCTU) contributed to Congress passing the National Prohibition Act (also known as the Volstead Act).[21] Alcohol use changed with alcohol rates higher during wars—the Civil War and the two World Wars. Alcohol use was low during Prohibition, which was passed by Congress in 1919 as a constitutional amendment to prohibit the production and sale of alcohol. Since the repeal of Prohibition in 1933, alcohol use in the United States has been regulated, whereas heroin and cocaine are illegal.

This moralistic perspective continues today in policies addressing many illegal drugs. Following the repeal in 1933, policy shifted to a medical and predominantly host perspective. The primary focus was on identifying and treating alcoholics. Alcohol problems were considered as a limited portion of the population—persons who were predisposed to alcoholism, the disease. With this perspective, policies to address environmental risk factors and controls on alcohol were irrelevant. In fact, they were potentially harmful because they could lead to increased criminal activities and create a "forbidden fruit" status for alcohol.

In the past 25 years, a public health perspective to alcohol use/abuse brought a dramatic shift in assumptions.[22] In part, the shift was associated with prevalence data that alcohol problems were not experienced by a small, discrete subpopulation of alcoholics, but by many others as well. In fact, alcohol problems were reported by those who clearly did not exhibit drinking patterns associated with alcoholism. In addition, individuals can drastically change their problematic drinking patterns over time or experience a spontaneous remission without treatment.[23,24] In addition, researchers became more sensitive to the health problems associated with alcohol in addition to alcoholism: trauma, alcohol-related birth defects, sexual assaults and other violence, cirrhosis of the liver and other long-term health problems, and workplace and school problems, among others.[23-27] Although alcoholics were more likely to report these problems, the problems were also experienced more broadly across the entire society. The diversity of alcohol problems also led to a realization of their complexity. It became apparent that alcohol interacts with and contributes to a wide array of social and health problems; the problems occur in the context of a complex system; and strategies for addressing them must take into account the interaction of a diverse set of factors that put people at risk.

As a result of these shifts in perspective, there is more concern with alcohol availability, drinking environments, and environmental risk factors. The focus shifted to population-based alcohol policies rather than individual-based strategies. In contrast to Prohibition policies, a current focus is to reduce the problems and harm associated with alcohol use.

DRUG POLICY

The illegal drug policies in force in the United States are dominated by the prohibition perspective that was used for alcohol prior to the repeal of Prohibition. The focus has been on individual deviance and immorality and the need to abolish the illegal drug trade. In fact, early illegal drug policies in the United States were targeted on minorities and aimed to eradicate recreational use, rather than medical addiction. For example, during the 1800s, whites were threatened by Chinese immigrants because of the fear that opium smoking would spread to white communities as well as encourage interracial sex.[28] As a result, the Chinese Exclusion Act of 1882 prohibited the immigration of Chinese laborers for 10 years, and the Smoking Opium Exclusion Act of 1909 decreased the accessibility of opium. Another example of a racially targeted policy is the Marihuana Tax Act, 1937. The Marihuana Tax act essentially banned the possession and sale of marijuana products until 1970, when it was replaced with the passage of the Comprehensive Drug Abuse Prevention and Control Act.[29]

During the late 1800s opiate and cocaine preparations were inexpensive and were widely used in over-the-counter preparations. Legislation was passed to reduce opiate and cocaine availability and consequent use. Beginning in the late 1800s and continuing into the early 1900s, there was increased government regulation to decrease physician-prescribing practices to reduce opiate and cocaine use. As a result, opiate and cocaine use decreased during World Wars I and II and during the Depression. The use of heroin, an opiate derivative, increased dramatically in the late 1950s and 1960s in major United States cities. Although illicit drug use increased and peaked in the general United States population during the 1970s, the abuse of most drugs remained stable during the 1980s. However, there was increased crack/cocaine use in the mid-1980s and increased heroin use in the 1990s, which was also the case for methamphetamine and prescription drugs into 2000 and beyond with raves, club drugs, meth cooking, and the abuse of prescription drug like OxyContin.

Even with a federal drug czar who, as a cabinet-level official, coordinates federal law enforcement and drug prevention/treatment activities, Americans continue to use mind-altering drugs. The drug czar's Office of National Drug Control Policy (ONDCP) is responsible for developing and updating the *National Drug Control Strategy*, (http://www.state .gov/documents/organization/30228.pdf). Like other strategies, the 2004 drug strategy focuses on *supply reduction* (law enforcement) and *demand reduction* (prevention and treatment). The current national priorities are (1) Stopping use before it starts, (2) healing America's drug users, and (3) disrupting the market. Even though the drug war is no longer called a war, the strategy focuses on illicit drugs—not tobacco or alcohol, which also have major health-related consequences. The strategy ignores the idea that motivations to "get high" or to "cope" may be simple but have complex roots that range from having better sex, to getting away from the realities and stresses of everyday life, to studying more efficiently, and to expanding awareness or increasing creativity.

President George W. Bush's National Drug Control Strategy budgeted $12.5 billion for fiscal year

2006 for drug control; however, there was a decrease in five-year budget allocations from $18 billion in 2001 to $12.5 billion in 2006.[30,31] Data demonstrate that the United States has exceeded the goal of reducing past-month, or "current," use of illegal drugs by 10 percent in two years.[32] Because we are incarcerating more drug abusers, these areas are budgeted with approximately 61.7 percent of the funds for law enforcement costs, primarily prison construction, criminal justice costs, drug interdiction programs, and other Department of Justice programs. Only 14.6 percent of the 2006 fiscal year budget was for prevention, and 23.7 percent for treatment. In addition, there has been a decrease in the percentage of federal spending for both treatment and research, whereas the percentage of budget for law enforcement has increased.[31–33]

An environmental approach to preventing illegal drug problems focuses on two overall risk factors: the availability of illegal drugs, and the broader family, community, social, cultural, and political contexts in which illegal drug problems occur. The United States legal-illegal drug policy creates different responses that have little or no relationship to the relative risks to public health that the drugs pose.[34] If a drug is legal, it is generally widely available at relatively low prices because economic interests push for increasing markets and lower prices. In response to these economic pressures, legal drug policies generally focus on individual deviance. If a drug is illegal, criminal justice strategies dominate availability policy, with primary attention given to controlling the distribution network and punishing illegal drug users, who are seen as morally weak.

DRUG POLICY STRATEGIES

United States drug policies have changed in the past several decades, sometimes dramatically, with emphases on law enforcement strategies to lock up drug users and drug prevention and treatment to help drug users. Drug policies have been shaped by planned as well as spur-of-the-moment political, moralistic, and media-inspired responses to three illicit drugs—heroin, marijuana, and cocaine—and to a lesser extent, two legal drugs—alcohol and nicotine. Like heroin, cocaine and crack-cocaine, methamphetamine (meth), and prescription drugs are the most recent drugs to be spotlighted by the media. From one point of view, the United States drug policy has been successful because of only marginal increases and decreases in drug use. However, from another point of view, increased stimulant use, particularly cocaine and crack cocaine use, is overflowing United States prisons and jails with mandatory/minimum fixed sentencing. Drug abuse has been a major national issue for more than 30 years with the rhetoric of a "War on Drugs." Congresses, presidents, and both major political parties fought the war, with increased federal spending as the armament to fight the chronic and relapsing nature of drug addiction.

Different ideas and approaches continue to influence drug policy. *Enforcement/police approaches* focus on arresting and locking up drug pushers and users. *Treatment providers* emphasize helping those affected become drug free. *Public health officials* encourage harm-reduction approaches to make needles available to injectors, such as needle exchange programs to decrease the spread of HIV/AIDS, which has been described by others as encouraging drug abuse by making needles available. *Educators* have historically denied there is a drug problem in their school and have developed drug-free zones around schools to prevent drug use at school. There are also those who support the idea that drugs should be legalized to eliminate profits from drug sales while others say that drug abusers need to "pull themselves up by their bootstraps." Given the limited consensus about drug abuse and the lack of a quick fix or instant cures, our shifting United States drug policies are a reality.

PUBLIC HEALTH INFLUENCE

Drug abuse prevention and interventions continue to be influenced by public health thinking. A major public health milestone was the 1979 Surgeon

General's Report on health promotion and disease prevention, titled *Healthy People*. This report encouraged a second public health revolution that emphasized prevention and extended the first revolution that targeted infectious diseases.[35] Alcohol and drug abuse prevention were identified as challenges for public health with the high prevalence of alcohol and drug abuse among United States youth. The report established five major goals that focused on lifecycle stages: healthy infants, healthy children, healthy adolescents/young adults, healthy adults, and healthy older adults. Early successful smoking prevention efforts[37] were a key factor for drug prevention. Almost immediately, this approach was adapted as Just Say No, which was encouraged by First Lady Nancy Reagan, even though research data were less than complete.

More recently, community-based drug courts expanded to respond to the overlap of drug abuse and crime and to provide treatment for drug abusers. Drug court is a court-managed drug treatment approach designed to provide an alternative to traditional criminal case processing. The interest in drug courts increased and the number grew to over 1200 in 2004.[32] Unlike Just Say No, the benefits of drug courts have been described in the research literature as reduced recidivism, decreased drug use, increased birth rates of drug-free babies, high program retention, and cost-efficient treatment.[38]

SUPPLY REDUCTION

United States supply reduction policies have focused on two major approaches to reduce drug supply: law enforcement to arrest drug dealers, and increasing United States border control. Law enforcement policies include searches and seizing drug dealers' property, as well as mandatory sentencing. Federal efforts target reducing drugs from other countries with border control, which is called *interdiction*. Interdiction includes interrupting the flow of drugs high in the drug-dealing pyramid to decrease sales. The idea is that large-scale arrests of drug dealers increase the street price of illicit drugs, which lowers the demand and use of illicit drugs. Several federal agencies are involved in supply reduction and interdiction, including Alcohol Tobacco and Firearms (ATF), the Drug Enforcement Agency (DEA), United States Customs, the Food and Drug Administration (FDA), Homeland Security, and, to a lesser extent, the Federal Bureau of Investigation (FBI). During the past 30 years, United States national strategies have been implemented to improve supply-reduction policies. Presidents Nixon, Ford, Reagan, Bush, Clinton, and Bush consistently increased the visibility of interdiction and other law enforcement efforts. These supply-reduction policies, while generally politically popular, have not been as effective in reducing overall drug use in the United States. When these policies are compared to risk reduction and harm reduction policies in other western countries with similar drug problems, there is general support for the idea of the overall effects of harm-reduction policies. However, United States lawmakers have favored "get tough" enforcement policies to increase the street prices of illicit drugs; however, the relationship between increased drug costs and drug use is not as clear for illicit drugs.[39]

DEMAND REDUCTION

Decreasing use during a drug abuser's addiction career can include community treatment, coerced treatment, incarceration, pharmacotherapy, and 12-step and other self-help groups. Research has consistently supported the effectiveness of drug abuse treatment. For example, the National Institute of Drug Abuse (NIDA) reported that drug treatment reduces drug use by 40 percent to 60 percent.[40] Effective drug abuse treatment can also reduce the spread of the human immunodeficiency virus (HIV) among injecting drug abusers.

Prevention: A Public Health Tradition

Lifestyle risk reduction emphasizes that alcohol and drug problems are a result of the interaction of biological risk with the quantity and frequency of alcohol or drug use.[41] Prevention includes no use or abstinence, as well as reducing high-risk use. Individual choices about quantity and frequency are a key to preventing alcohol and drug problems. Quantity/frequency choices determine how much a person uses, how often alcohol or drugs are used, and whether a person's threshold for alcohol is reached. Environmental/social and psychological factors establish risk by influencing whether, how much, and how often a person uses alcohol or drugs. This interaction among biology, individual choice, and setting determines the degree of intoxication, risk for problems, and the degree of later physiological damage or risk. Lifestyle risk reduction programs incorporate five conditions for effective drug prevention: (1) It could happen to me—my choices matter; (2) I know what to do to reduce risk; (3) People around me support low-risk choices; (4) I want to make low-risk choices; and (5) I have the skills I need. Biology establishes an individual threshold for intoxication, addiction, and diseases such as liver damage. Prevention strategies can be most effective if they first target personal vulnerability by establishing the belief that high-risk choices are likely to cause alcohol/drug-related personal health or impairment problems.

Treatment

Drug abuse **treatment** can be as effective as other treatments for long-term, relapsing illnesses, if it is well delivered and targeted. Without treatment follow-up or continuing treatment, former users can return to drug use. **Intervention** options can range from drug testing to intensive behavioral/biological treatment. Nevertheless, some believe that substance abuse treatment does not work from personal experiences with friends or family members. However, it becomes clear for these individuals that the proper blend of treatment combined with follow-up supervision, relapse prevention, and self-help groups such as Alcoholics Anonymous were not used, or participation was minimal.

Drug abuse treatment includes detoxification where a patient can get drugs out of his or her system. Detoxification can be either medical detoxification where medication is used for withdrawal, or social detoxification without medication. Detoxification periods are short and have limited success. Patients are usually referred to treatment, including inpatient treatment, therapeutic/residential treatment, or outpatient treatment. Inpatient hospitalization for detoxification usually focuses on multiple drug use, dual diagnosis, or medical complications.

Residential treatment targets social skills, including relapse prevention, individual/group counseling/education, and family therapy. Residential treatment is generally no more than 30 days. Facilities can be private and insurance driven. Therapeutic communities incorporate a community approach that focuses on changing behaviors over a longer period through "graduation." Lengths of stay are structured to focus on behavioral change within planned stages of change. Therapeutic community treatment is now popular in prison settings. Halfway houses are less structured than therapeutic communities but are more structured than outpatient treatment. "Halfway" settings can serve as a transition between institutions, such as prisons, and independent living, to help individuals become integrated into the community. Services include individual/group sessions, aftercare, and resource supports. Outpatient treatment is the most common drug treatment. Outpatient treatment involves individual and group sessions that are usually held weekly. Intensive outpatient treatment includes participating in structured daily "programming" in community treatment, while participants live on their own.

Pharmacotherapy approaches incorporate using prescription drugs to maintain drug abstinence and reduce drug craving. The most commonly used pharmacotherapy is methadone, a synthetic narcotic used primarily for heroin/opiate detoxification and maintenance. Methadone blocks the effects of heroin. Methadone is controlled by federal regulations like other pharmacotherapy drugs. Disulfuram is often the pharmacotherapy used for alcohol treatment. When taken orally, it gives the user a severe reaction to using alcohol, including nausea and irregular heartbeat. Compliance with taking disulfuram is minimal because patients do not want to take something that makes them sick if they use alcohol. Other currently approved pharmocotherapies for opiate and alcohol dependence include naloxone, buprenorphine, and acamprosate. However, there are no currently approved pharmacotherapies for cocaine or methamphetamine addiction, although modafinil and *d*-amphetamine have shown promise.

THE PREVALENCE OF ALCOHOL AND OTHER DRUG PROBLEMS

Alcohol and other drug use are present throughout society among all social and economic classes, ethnic and racial groups, and geographic regions. Rates of use vary by type of drug, with alcohol by far the most commonly used drug among all groups. The use of other drugs varies by group and availability; however, marijuana, prescription pain reliever, and cocaine use represent the highest illicit drug use nationwide.[42]

NATIONAL DRUG USE

According to the 2005 National Survey on Drug Use and Health (NSDUH), the most recent survey for which data are available, nearly 52 percent of the population over 12 years of age uses alcohol at least once a month, compared to 8.1 percent for those who report illicit drug use as shown in Table 21.1. A majority of illicit drug use can be attributed to marijuana, with approximately 6 percent of the population reporting current use (i.e., in the past month). Rates of other illicit drug use are relatively low, however, these rates have been stable over the past few years, indicating that efforts to decrease use of these drugs have not met with great success.

Table 21.1. Household Population: Past Month Alcohol and Selected Illicit Drug Use for 2003, 2004, 2005

	Percent of Population		
	2003	2004	2005
Alcohol use	50.1	50.3	51.8
Heavy alcohol use*	6.8	6.9	6.6
Any illicit drug	8.2	7.9	8.1
Marijuana use	6.2	6.1	6.0
Cocaine use	1.0	0.8	1.0
Heroin use	0.1	0.1	0.1
Methamphetamine use	0.3	0.2	0.2
Pain reliever use	2.0	1.8	1.9
Tranquilizer use	0.8	0.7	0.7

*Five or more drinks on the same occasion, five or more times in the past 30 days.

SOURCE: National Survey on Drug Use and Health, 2003. National Survey on Drug Use and Health, 2004. National Survey on Drug Use and Health, 2005. Substance Abuse and Mental Health Services Administration, US Department of Health and Human Services. Available at: http://www.samhsa.gov.[42–46]

PREVALENCE IN YOUNG PEOPLE

Drug use among high school seniors has been measured for more than 30 years with the Monitoring the Future (MTF) Survey. This survey examines trends in drug use and provides a picture of emerging illicit drug use among American youth. Alcohol is the commonly used drug, although the percentage of high school seniors reporting current alcohol use is lower than nationwide levels. Data from the MTF Survey indicate that larger percentages of high school seniors report current (i.e., past month) illicit drug use than the population in general. For example, use of marijuana, cocaine, prescription narcotics, and tranquilizers is much higher in this group than nationwide averages. These data indicate that drug use is indeed a problem for the youth of America and will likely remain so, given the relatively stable rates of use over the past few years (see Table 21.2).

Ethnic and Racial Group Variations

Table 21.3 shows rates of drug use by ethnic and racial group. Whites are more likely to use alcohol than blacks, Hispanics, American Indians, or Asians. However, illicit drug use may be more prevalent in blacks and American Indians. Interestingly, illicit drug use appears to be less common in Hispanics and Asians. The reasons for these differences are unknown but could be due to socioeconomic status, access to alcohol or drugs, or cultural norms.

Despite these differences across ethnicities and races, minorities, in general, may experience greater problems related to substance use disorders. For example, one recent study found that although Asians have lower levels of alcohol disorders overall, Asians with alcohol disorders are significantly more likely to be diagnosed with co-morbid personality disorders.[50] Another study indicates that minorities suffer more greatly than whites at any given level of alcohol consumption.[51] In addition, treatment disparities for alcoholism are quite

Table 21.2. High School Seniors: Past Month Alcohol and Selected Illicit Drug Use for 2003, 2004, 2005

	Percent of Seniors		
	2003	2004	2005
Alcohol use	47.5	48.0	47.0
Been drunk	30.9	32.5	30.2
Any illicit drug use	24.1	23.4	23.1
Marijuana use	21.2	19.9	19.8
Cocaine use	2.1	2.3	2.3
Heroin use	0.4	0.5	0.5
Methamphetamine use	1.7	1.4	0.9
Narcotic use	4.1	4.3	3.9
Tranquilizer use	2.8	3.1	2.9

SOURCE: Monitoring the Future Reports 2003, 2004, 2005. US Department of Health and Human Services. Available at: http://www.monitoringthefuture.org.[47–49]

Table 21.3. Percentage of Respondents Reporting Past Month Alcohol and Selected Illicit Drug Use by Selected Race/Ethnicity: 2005

	Percent of Population				
	White	**Black**	**Hispanic**	**American Indian**	**Asian**
Alcohol use	56.5	40.8	42.6	42.4	38.1
Any illicit drug	8.1	9.7	7.6	12.8	3.1
Marijuana use	6.1	7.6	5.1	9.8	1.6
Cocaine use	1.0	1.1	0.8	0.5	0.1

SOURCE: National Survey on Drug Use and Health, 2005. Office of Applied Studies, Substance Abuse and Mental Health Services Administration, US Department of Health and Human Services. Available at: http://www.samhsa.gov.[42]

prevalent between those available for minorities as compared to whites.[51]

These disparities are not solely related to alcohol use, however. One study surveyed health care use in inner city drug users (verified via a positive heroin or cocaine screen) and found that blacks report more Emergency Department (ED) visits than whites, and that blacks have more ED episodes than Hispanics.[52] In addition, blacks were more likely to be diagnosed with cardiovascular disease, alcohol use disorders, and sexually transmitted diseases, whereas Hispanics were more likely to be diagnosed with HIV, dental problems, or drug overdose.[52] Other research has elucidated perceived or real barriers to health care or drug abuse treatment in minority groups.[53,54]

EXCLUDED POPULATIONS

The NSDUH and Monitoring the Future surveys are the primary sources for data on alcohol and other drug use in the United States, as the preceding discussion suggests. Unfortunately, these data sources are incomplete because they do not reflect the entire population. The NSDUH does not include individuals who reside in hotels, hospitals, and prisons/jails, or who are homeless. The school-based surveys do not include young people who have dropped out of school before graduation or

who are absent the day of the survey. Various fragmentary studies suggest that alcohol and other drug use within these populations is significantly higher than in the general population.[19]

Public Health Consequences of Alcohol and Other Drug Use

Differences in the rates of alcohol and other drug use are reflected in data reporting public health and societal problems, with alcohol problems far more prevalent than illicit drug problems. The nature and definition of the problems also differ, reflecting in part the social responses that emerge from their legal or illegal status. These differences make accurate comparisons between problems associated with alcohol and problems associated with other drugs difficult. In general, illicit drug use itself is defined as a problem, while alcohol use is usually defined as problematic only when it leads to specific behavioral or physical harm.

TRAUMATIC INJURY AND MORTALITY

Alcohol was the cause of approximately 85,000 deaths in the year 2000 and 76,000 deaths in 2001.[55,56] Alcohol-related traffic fatalities and liver disease comprise the largest groups of deaths, totaling approximately 14,000 and 12,000 deaths in 2001, respectively.[56] Alcohol is also implicated in other forms of traumatic deaths, including homicide, suicide, burns, poisoning, drowning, and falls as well as other forms of alcohol-related disease, such as esophageal and otolaryngeal cancers.[56]

In addition, alcohol is a major contributor to traumatic injury. Alcohol-related motor vehicle injuries are by far the largest category of these, causing approximately 17,000 deaths and 260,000 serious injuries in 2002,[57] and costing $51 billion dollars (estimated for 2000).[58] Alarmingly, although the number of alcohol-related deaths overall decreased from 2000 to 2001, the number of alcohol impaired driving incidents increased from 1999 to 2002.[59] In general, the higher the blood alcohol content of the person causing the injury, the more serious the injury. The CDC estimates the years of potential life lost attributable to alcohol to be approximately 2.3 million for 2001.[26]

Data on illicit drug-related deaths are not nearly as reliable or precise as those available for alcohol. The Drug Abuse Warning Network (DAWN) estimates that in 2003, drug-related deaths ranged from 53 per 1,000,000 people to 206 per 1,000,000 in a sampling of areas across the United States.[45] Decedents in this study were most likely to be male and between the ages of 35 and 54.[45] The most common drugs associated with death were cocaine, opiates, antidepressants, and benzodiazepines.[45]

DAWN also provides data regarding illicit drug episodes reported in ED visits.[46] Approximately 940,953 emergency room episodes involving illicit drugs were reported in 2004. Among these drugs, cocaine was mentioned 383,350 times, marijuana was mentioned 215,665 times, heroin was mentioned 162,137 times, and other stimulants (including amphetamine and methamphetamine) were mentioned 102,843 times. The overall number of illicit drug-related episodes represents an increase from drug-related ED visits from 2000, which was approximately 545,000 (see Table 21.4). DAWN does not provide a means to compare these data with data on alcohol-related ER episodes but does report 461,809 mentions of the use of both

Table 21.4. **Percentage of Drug-Related Emergency Department Visits by Alcohol and Selected Drugs: 2000, 2004**

Category	2000	2004
Any drug related	1.0	2.0
Alcohol combined with other drugs	0.2	0.4
Cocaine	0.2	0.3
Marijuana	0.1	0.2
Heroin	0.1	0.2
Pain relievers	0.2	0.1

SOURCE: Drug Abuse Warning Network Estimates of Drug Related Emergency Department Visits, 2004. Office of Applied Studies, Substance Abuse and Mental Health Services Administration, US Department of Health and Human Services, 2006. Available at: http://www.samhsa.gov.[46]

illicit drugs and alcohol. Based on estimates of alcohol-related traumatic events, it is probable that alcohol accounts for several times the numbers reported for illicit drugs.

ILLICIT DRUG AND ALCOHOL DEPENDENCE AND ABUSE

The 2005 NSDUH found that nearly 22.2 million individuals were dependent on or abusing illicit drugs or alcohol in the United States. In 2005, 15.4 million Americans were dependent on or abusing alcohol but not illicit drugs, whereas 3.6 million people were dependent on or abusing illicit drugs but not alcohol.[42] Approximately 3.3 million individuals were classified as dependent on or abusing both illicit drugs and alcohol.[42] In terms of illicit drug dependence or abuse, individuals were most likely to meet this classification for marijuana (4.1 million), cocaine (1.5 million), or prescription pain relievers (1.5 million).[42] Younger individuals (i.e., ages 18–25) were more likely to be dependent on or abuse illicit drugs or alcohol relative to other age groups. Specifically, 21.8 percent of this group was classified into these categories, whereas 8 percent of individuals aged 12–17 and 7.1 percent of individuals aged 26 or over fell into these groups. In addition, males (12%) were more likely to be dependent on or abuse illicit drugs or alcohol relative to females (6.4%).

RELATED PUBLIC HEALTH PROBLEMS

Alcohol and other drug use is associated with a wide array of other public health problems. Alcohol use prevalence among pregnant women has been estimated at about 10.1 percent.[60] Alcohol use during pregnancy is associated with a constellation of birth defects called Fetal Alcohol Syndrome (FAS). FAS results in long-term physical, psychological, and intellectual developmental problems and delays.[61] The use of other drugs can also result in developmental delay or birth complications. For example, in one study, infants exposed *in utero* to methamphetamine were 3.5 times more likely to be small for their gestational age relative to those that were not.[62] In addition, children of mothers that use drugs during pregnancy may be more likely to use drugs themselves than those with mothers that did not use drugs.[63]

ALCOHOL, OTHER DRUGS, AND THE CRIMINAL JUSTICE SYSTEM

Alcohol and other drug use has an enormous impact on the criminal justice system. In 1999, an estimated 5.4 million violent crimes and 8 million property crimes involving alcohol or illicit drug use occurred.[64] These crimes cost an estimated $71.5 billion in tangible costs.[64] From 1994 to 2003, the number of arrests related to drug abuse violations increased by 24.2 percent.[65] The large majority of these arrestees are adults, however, approximately 12 percent of the arrestees in 2003 were juveniles.[65] Arrests for drug abuse violations in this group are largely related to marijuana, but cocaine, opium, narcotics, and nonnarcotics are also prevalent in this group.

Use of alcohol and other drugs also contributes to crimes other than drug abuse violations. For example, alcohol and illicit drug use has often been tied to sexual assault. One study found that pre-offense drinking by an offender predicted victim injury.[66] Other research indicates that drug use contributes to criminality, which includes methamphetamine users who were more likely to self-report criminal behavior and have higher numbers of criminal offenses than nonusers.[67] In addition, drug urine screens taken from arrestees indicate that drug use may be increasing in criminal justice populations. For example, the 2000 Arrestee Drug Abuse Monitoring (ADAM) report indicated that a median of 64.2 percent of arrestees had drug-positive urine screens.[68] The number for the 2003 ADAM report was 67 percent.[69] Although this does not appear to be a large increase, the overall rate of current drug use in arrestees, as verified by urine drug screens is much higher than that of the general population.

The most recent ADAM report[69] indicates that drug use in arrestees may vary by gender. Table 21.5 presents median percentage of drug positive urines in adult male and female arrestees for 2003. As noted earlier, drug use in both of these groups is more prevalent than in the general population.

Table 21.5. Median Percentage of Drug Positive Urines Adult Male and Female Arrestees by Selected Drug: 2003

Drug	Males	Females
Marijuana	44.1	31.6
Cocaine	30.1	35.3
Opiates	5.8	6.6
Methamphetamine	4.7	8.8
Multiple drugs	23.4	23.8

SOURCE: Zhang, 2004.[69]

Interestingly, males were more likely to have urine screens positive for marijuana, whereas females were more likely to have urine screens positive for cocaine, opiates, and methamphetamine. These data suggest that female arrestees may have more illicit drug use problems than males.

ECONOMIC COSTS OF ALCOHOL AND ILLICIT DRUG PROBLEMS

As the data in this section suggest, alcohol and other drug problems create staggering costs for society. The impact is enormous for individuals, families, communities, and institutions within communities, as well as for society as a whole. Costs for alcohol use in 1998 were estimated to be more than $186 billion.[70] The large majority of these costs were due to lost productivity; however, health and criminal justice costs also contributed significantly. This estimate represented a 25 percent increase over costs for 1992.

The estimated economic costs in 2002 for illicit drug abuse were more than $180 billion.[71] As in 1998, the large majority of these costs were due to lost productivity, however, health costs made up nearly 9 percent of the economic costs of drug abuse. These costs are spread across a number of drugs; for example, costs related to prescription opioid analgesic use in 2001 were estimated to be $8.6 billion, with about 33 percent of costs being health related and 50 percent of costs being work related.[72] Alarmingly, overall cost of drug abuse has increased since 1992, when costs were estimated to be more than $107 billion.

EMERGING DRUGS

Illicit drug use changes over time in cycles as fad drugs. Each year, the Department of Justice, National Drug Intelligence Center (NDIC) publishes a National Drug Threat Assessment, which predicts the drug use cycles for the coming year. The most recent Drug Threat Assessment was published in October 2006 for 2007 and indicates that the leading drug threats to the United States are cocaine, heroin, marijuana, methamphetamine, and MDMA (ecstasy). According to this report, the majority of these drugs are being smuggled into the United States rather than being produced here. In particular, there is evidence to suggest that local "cooking" of methamphetamine is decreasing and that it is increasingly being smuggled into the United States from Mexico. Another threat identified in this assessment is the diversion and abuse of prescription drugs, particularly opiate pain medications, sedatives/tranquilizers, and stimulants. The sources of these drugs range from pharmacy robberies to Internet pharmacies. Although this assessment reports data at a national level, it also provides information regarding drug threats in specific areas of the country. For example, the greatest drug threat in the Pacific, Southwestern, and Central Western United States is methamphetamine. For other areas of the United States, cocaine, heroin, and marijuana appear to be greater drug threats at this time, although methamphetamine is still a concern. Given the emergence of different drug threats across the country, and mounting evidence that drug use may vary by environmental setting (i.e., urban versus rural),[73,74] it appears that illicit drug use prevention and intervention strategies will need to be adapted for the needs of specific areas and communities

WOMEN, DRUG AND ALCOHOL USE, AND INCARCERATION

Much of what is known about the public health consequences of drug and alcohol use and abuse is based on clinical and research conducted with males. With the release of a landmark report by the Public Health Service Task Force on Women's Health Issues in 1985, it became apparent that there were a number of unique health, mental health, and substance use issues faced by women.[75] This report indicated the following:

- Social and environmental conditions can be risk factors for women's health.

- Certain health conditions are more prevalent among women (such as reproductive health problems).

- There are differences in health problems and risk factors across the lifespan from adolescence to elderly.

- Women are more susceptible to the risks associated with alcohol and drug use.

- Women have increased mental health issues compared to men.[75]

Due to the findings from this report, along with growing anecdotal evidence on the health, mental health, and substance abuse problems among women, a research agenda emerged for the first time with a mandate by the National Institutes of Health (NIH) in October 1986 to include women in federally funded research trials.[76] The priority placed on including women sparked the growth of a developing body of literature in the past two decades focused on differentiating the effects of alcohol and other substances for women and men.

Women and Social roles

Research has increased in the past several years on gender differences and substance use. One factor that may contribute to gender differences in substance use and subsequent consequences is the importance of social roles. These roles were typically to rear children, take care of homes, and in general, to maintain and enhance relationships. This thinking is supported in the substance abuse literature because women with substance abuse problems are less likely to be employed and stay at home[77] than men who are more competitive and assertive, and less relational.[78] In addition, drug and alcohol related consequences for women are more likely to affect family life and social networks.[79,80] Along the same lines, women are generally expected to adhere

more closely to pro-social, nonsubstance using norms, suggesting that women who use drugs and alcohol may be viewed with a higher level of scrutiny when compared to men. The resulting guilt and stigma, associated with using drugs or alcohol, can lead to a denial of a substance abuse problem and less treatment seeking.

Women's Biological Differences

Evidence has emerged about the clear biological differences related to substance use between men and women. For example, women have a higher concentration of body fat, which leads to a higher concentration of alcohol in body tissue when a woman consumes an equal amount of alcohol as a man.[75] Women are also more susceptible than men to the adverse effects of alcohol due to a decreased level of the metabolizing enzyme, gastric alcohol dehydrogenase.[81] The physical health consequences of alcohol and drug use, which include HIV, hepatitis, severe headaches, dental problems, hypertension, emphysema, and asthma, are also often more severe for women than for men.[82,83] When women enter drug treatment, they report more co-occurring mental health issues, including high levels of psychological distress, increased incidence of trauma and abuse, and a propensity for diagnosable disorders, such as post-traumatic stress disorder (PTSD).[84]

Relational Differences

An additional factor that may differentially contribute to drug and alcohol use among men and women is social relationships. Having a history of problem relationships and social support systems has been consistently reported among substance using women. In fact, women's episodes of use, abstinence, and relapse are related to their significant opposite-sex relationships[85] as drug and alcohol use may be a coping mechanisms to deal with abusive family situations.[86] In addition, women receiving substance abuse treatment are more likely than men to have a spouse or family member with a substance abuse problem.[77,87] Relationships, particularly for women, with others who use drugs or alcohol may influence the severity of substance use. Many male partners of female substance abusers often have extensive histories of substance abuse.[88]

Drug and Alcohol Use and Incarceration

Much of the literature on female prisoners has focused on incarcerated women who are drug and alcohol abusers. Drug/alcohol use and abuse have been consistently reported as major contributing factors in the increasing population of female prisoners.[85] In fact, a large number of female inmates, reported as high as 98 percent, have a history of substance abuse, and nearly half of incarcerated women indicate that they were under the influence of alcohol or drugs at the time of their offense.[89–91] There are unique public health and treatment issues to be considered among incarcerated female substance users.

Sexually Transmitted Diseases

Sexually transmitted diseases (STDs), which include chlamydia, human papillomavirus, herpes simplex, cystic and mymatic conditions, dysmenorrhea, and chronic pelvic inflammation,[83] are more common among female prisoners than the general population.[92] In addition, a higher percentage of incarcerated women, compared to men, are diagnosed as HIV positive (3.5% vs. 2.2%)[93] with the rate of HIV infection about six times higher among male and female prisoners than in the general United States population.[94] HIV risk behaviors have been consistently reported by females, which include sharing drug injection equipment, having unprotected sex with drug-injecting partners, having sex with multiple partners, exchanging sex for money and drugs, reporting a history of a diagnosed STD, using condoms inconsistently with multiple sex partners, and using alcohol and other noninjection drugs.[91,95] HIV and related risk behaviors are serious health concerns for female drug abusers.

Mental Health

Female substance abusers experience a variety of mental health issues, which often co-occur with substance abuse.[96–99] For example, about two-thirds (64%) of incarcerated women reported lifetime psychiatric disorders that include drug abuse or dependence, alcohol abuse or dependence, personality disorders, major depressive episodes, and dysthymia.[100] Depression and anxiety are the most common mental health issues, and in some cases, the symptoms are severe. A high percentage of women present characteristics associated with suicide risk (defined as a history of psychiatric treatment, previous suicide attempts, alcohol or drug abuse, social and economic disadvantages, or a history of physical or sexual abuse).[101]

Victimization and Violence

Many drug-abusing women have detailed histories of physical, mental, and sexual abuse.[102–104] For example, over half (57%) of incarcerated women reported experiencing at least one lifetime incidence of physical or sexual assault.[93] Among the general population of female prisoners, it has been estimated that 33 percent of female inmates reported abuse by an intimate partner, but other studies have found that 72 percent of incarcerated women reported being beaten by a boyfriend or a spouse, whereas 44 percent had been abused by one or both parents.[102] The association between experiences of victimization and violence, particularly as a child, significantly impacts adult experiences of health and mental health problems.[105]

Children, Parenting, and Incarceration

Estimates indicate that a high percentage of women in jails (70%), state prisons (65%), and federal prisons (59%) have young children.[93] In 1997, more than two-thirds of incarcerated women had a child under age 18 and about 5 percent were pregnant at the time of incarceration.[93] Being a prisoner separates mothers from their children and this loss increases a woman's sense of inadequacy, despondency, and fear of permanently losing her children.[106] Additionally, most of these mothers feel intense guilt and shame, and experience fear of being rejected by their children,[106] particularly if they have a history of substance use that created family tension and strain. Dealing with involuntary separation from their children has increased consequences for drug-abusing women because mothers can face a variety of reunification issues. This stress can increase a woman's risk for relapse.

Women and Treatment

Female substance abusers can experience a complexity of treatment issues that can be compounded by involvement in the criminal justice system. Women have specific needs that require gender-specific services that are designed with knowledge and expertise to address special issues, including mental health, victimization and violence history, relationship issues, and physical health. These specialized services should be developed with a continuum of care that is tailored to addiction severity and treatment need. One approach is to more effectively target at-risk women as they enter publicly funded health care centers. For example, targeted assessments and outreach to at-risk women as they enter health departments and emergency rooms could enhance services for female drug users. Increased community linkages with substance abuse treatment should be a priority. An additional focus of substance abuse programs for women should be HIV prevention. Intervention programs should target decreasing risk-taking behaviors, including sex exchange, sex with multiple partners, inconsistent condom use, and unprotected oral sex.[91]

CONTROVERSIES

In many ways, drug and alcohol use, substance abuse, and addictions are value laden with moralistic undertones and controversies that shape current approaches. These controversies include the following.

Drugs and Crime

The relationship between drugs and crime remains controversial in spite of a documented relationship. For example, a survey of inmates in state and federal correctional institutions indicates that 83 percent of state prisoners reported drug use.[107] In fact, two-thirds of United States prisoners are drug abusers, whereas over 60 percent of persons who come into contact with jails and lock-ups reported using a drug other than alcohol at the time of arrest.[108] Controversy focuses on how law enforcement officials and community treatment providers conceptualize drug abuse treatment and law enforcement control as opposites with treatment on one side, and criminal justice control on the other side. Many community treatment providers suggest that criminal justice authority is disruptive to the therapeutic relationship for those who are court ordered to treatment. However, drug offenders, under criminal justice authority, usually remain in treatment as long as others.

There are other ways of thinking about treatment and control because interventions can incorporate both treatment and control. For example, a therapeutic community/residential treatment facility is very high in treatment and control with criminal justice—judicial—referrals, whereas outpatient drug treatment is low in both treatment exposure and control unless a participant is court ordered. Nevertheless, treatment and control are usually discussed as opposites, which depend upon ideology, perceived public interest, and political needs. Part of the controversy is the idea that drug abusers have limited internal motivation and need to be externally motivated to enter drug treatment in order to change. Behavior change is expected to include reduced arrests, reduced crime, and no drug use. It is important to keep in mind that, from both a criminal justice point of view and the treatment point of view, no drug use is expected. Consequently, substance offenders who have limited internal motivation to change their behaviors can be externally motivated in treatment, using authority from the criminal justice system. This authority includes probation, parole, diversion, and drug courts.

Pharmacotherapy Treatment

Using physician-prescribed drugs to treat drug and alcohol abuse has been controversial in the United States. Examples of prescribed drugs include methadone, which blocks the effects of heroin and opiates; naltrexone, which blocks the effects of alcohol and cocaine; and disulfuram, an antagonist that makes alcohol abusers sick when they use alcohol. Controversy centers on the idea, which is supported by self-help groups such as Alcoholics Anonymous (AA) and Narcotics Anonymous (NA) as well as law enforcement officials and judges, that drug abusers should not use any drugs. Although clinical and randomized studies report on the utility of pharmacotherapies, their use in the United States is more limited than in other countries.

Drug Testing

Drug testing can be part of getting a job. Periodic and random drug testing can also be used to monitor employee drug use. Drug testing remains controversial because protecting individual rights should be balanced to safeguard society. Proponents of drug testing say that individuals should not be on drugs while on duty or on the job. This includes pilots, police officers, military personnel, and production workers. Nonsupporters of drug testing advocate individual rights and stress that what a person does when not working should not be "controlled" by an employer. Courts support the use of urine testing, blood testing, breath testing, saliva testing, hair testing, and legal sanctions for those who use at work.

Harm Reduction and HIV/AIDS and Drug Injecting

Perhaps a forgotten part of HIV/AIDS is transmitting the HIV virus with contaminated drug injection equipment or sharing needles, syringes, water, cotton, and cookers. About one-third of HIV cases in the United States continue to be related to injecting drug users. In fact, the reason a number of women become HIV infected in the United States involves their sex partners who are injecting drug users. However, United States HIV prevention initiatives have been limited by federal policy to the distribution of bleach to drug injectors to clean needles, although selected jurisdictions support needle and syringe exchange programs. Clearly, harm-reduction approaches to control the spread of HIV among injecting drug users is limited in the United States. Harm-reduction approaches have roots in Britain and in the Netherlands. More common harm-reduction approaches in the United States include designated drivers, cigarette warning labels, smoke free areas, and seat belts.

Decriminalizing Marijuana

There is almost universal agreement that marijuana should not be used by children and adolescents as they develop physically and emotionally. Marijuana use is illegal except in states that allow use for medical purposes, such as nausea reduction related to cancer treatment. There are lobby groups that support the use of marijuana, including the National Organization for the Reform of Marijuana Laws (NORMAL) and media outlets such as *High Times* magazine. The controversy surrounding marijuana legalization, with enforcement policy grounded in the Marihuana Tax Act of 1937, is targeting small growers and users rather than distributors. With current minimum-mandatory sentencing, marijuana users are helping to crowd prisons and jails. An argument for legalization is that it would save taxpayers money and resources. On the other side of the issue, which is perceived to be the opinion of most Americans, legalizing marijuana would give the wrong message to adolescents and others—that it is okay to use a mind-altering drug. Opponents of legalization point out that marijuana is a "gateway" drug to the use of other illegal drugs, which are called "hard drugs"—cocaine and heroin. There is also controversy about growing hemp, the fiber from the marijuana plant for use in making cloth for blue jeans and rope. In spite of the country's drug czar and others who condemn the medical use of marijuana, as well as the United States Supreme Court's decision, medical marijuana is currently legal with a physician's prescription in Alaska, California, Colorado, Maine, Minnesota, Mississippi, Nebraska, Nevada, New York, North Carolina, Ohio, and Oregon (http://www.norml.org/index.cfm).

The Media and Drug Use

The media continues to have a powerful and sometimes controversial role in shaping perceptions about drugs and drug use. This is underscored by the level of advertising and product promotion for alcohol and prescription drugs. Controversy surrounds the degree to which advertising should be controlled.

IMPLICATIONS

Drug and alcohol public health implications are clear. Simply stated, more public health attention and involvement is necessary in drug and alcohol abuse policy development and practice. This involvement must not only focus on drug and alcohol behaviors but also incorporate drug and alcohol use generally as a behavior that is associated with a constellation of problem behaviors or other high-risk behaviors such as accidents, sexually transmitted infections, maternal and child health, and violence associated with criminality. These high-risk behaviors deserve community-based attention by local public health departments to target the "whole person" rather than disassociated community interventions for each problem behavior, which can needlessly label drug and alcohol users as deviants. This focus includes tailored community-wide policy developments such as enhancing disease prevention and community health promotion activities. However, these kinds of holistic public health approaches are generally limited and

fractured by funding or statutory and traditional agency responsibilities.

This chasm for public health is deepened by United States prevention and treatment policies that largely focus on "no use" rather than an acceptance of varied interventions and approaches such as harm reduction. In other words, the overall United States policy focuses on law enforcement or *supply* reduction more than *demand* reduction activities, including prevention and treatment. This focus is evident in our National Drug Control Strategy, which identifies fewer resources for "stopping drug use before it starts" and "healing America's drug users" with over half (61.7%) of the 2006 fiscal year budget allocated to law enforcement and related activities.

Although drug/alcohol incidence and prevalence data suggest an overall stabilization and decrease for some illicit drugs, other illicit drug use is increasing. These increases include "fad drugs" such as "home cooked meth" and prescription pain medications. Disrupting the illicit drug market is very important. However, there is also a need for additional resources to support community public health drug/alcohol prevention and treatment. For example, with our current judicial sentencing practices, our prisons and jails are filled with drug and alcohol users. However, there are limited treatment and health promotion interventions in our jails and prisons. Community public health practitioners can target incarcerated drug-abusing women and their high-risk children. This should be in addition to increasing preventative services for both female and male drug users who are incarcerated in local jails and lock-ups, and who are at high risk for a variety of Sexually Transmitted Infections (STIs) such as HIV.

Increasing our public health knowledge base will be enhanced with academic and practitioner thinking to develop multidisciplinary and comprehensive theories that explain addiction and can be used to better examine drug/alcohol use, abuse, dependency, and addiction. This enhanced and broadened theoretical foundation will facilitate targeting and tailoring public health interventions on the whole person, including biological, psychological, and social factors. One possibility to consider, for example, is additional public health education and training for law enforcement officials as well as cross-training on the public health and law enforcement consequences of alcohol and drug addiction.

Drug and alcohol policies as well as practice can be controversial, within and across communities. Controversies include real and perceived differences between harm-reduction public health approaches, including providing clean needles and syringes for drug injectors, and criminal justice strategies to lock up drug abusers. However, many drug abusers are now diverted from prisons and jails by being court-ordered to community-based drug abuse treatment as part of a Drug Court, for example. An additional controversy is the use of prescribed medications—pharmacotherapies—to treat drug abusers. Methadone maintenance treatment is an example. Although mandatory drug testing in the workplace is generally accepted, it remains controversial for some—but not as controversial as decriminalizing marijuana. Clearly, a challenge for public health policy makers and practitioners is not only how to provide holistic services to drug and alcohol users/abusers but also how to work with law enforcement officials and substance abuse treatment provides so patients and services are not stigmatized.

REVIEW QUESTIONS

1. What are some ways drug and alcohol abuse affect minorities differently they affect non-minorities?
2. Describe populations that are included or excluded from national surveys on drug and alcohol use. Why is it important to understand the impact of excluding certain individuals from these surveys?
3. What are some ways that drug and alcohol abuse impact the national economy? How can these costs be reduced?
4. How do public health professionals approach drug abuse?
5. Name at least two theories that are used to explain drug and alcohol abuse.

6. Give the two approaches to United States drug abuse policy used in the past decades. What kinds of intervention strategies are most commonly used?
7. Are there similarities or differences in education/prevention and treatment interventions?
8. Name three theoretical perspectives that help to explain the unique differences in substance use and public health consequences of substance use among women.
9. Name at least three gender-specific treatment needs that incarcerated female substance users commonly experience.
10. Describe at least one barrier to the development of public health focused "holistic approaches" to treatment.
11. Describe the strengths and weaknesses of traditional public health theoretical approaches used to explain substance abuse.
12. Identify the components of an ecological framework and provide examples of each component to apply how this framework impacts substance abuse treatment outcomes. From a public health perspective, explain which component has the most influence and which component has the least influence on substance abuse treatment outcomes.
13. Summarize the differences between the United States policies on alcohol versus illegal drugs.

REFERENCES

1. Institute of Medicine. *Pathways of Addiction: Opportunities in Drug Abuse Research.* Washington, DC: National Academy Press; 1996.
2. Leshner AE. Addiction as a brain disease, and it matters. *Science.* 1997;278(3):45–47.
3. Goode E. *Drugs in American Society. 6th ed.* New York: McGraw Hill; 2005.
4. Bandura A. *Social Foundations of Thought and Action: A Social Cognitive Theory.* Englewood Cliffs, NJ: Prentice-Hall; 1986.
5. Jessor R, Jessor S. *Problem Behavior and Psychosocial Development: A Longitudinal Study of Youth.* New York: Academic Press; 1997.

6. Kaplan H. Self-Attitudes and Deviant Behavior. Pacific Palisades, CA: Goodyear; 1975.

7. Akers R, Kron M, Lanza-Kaduce L, Radosevich M. Social learning and deviant behavior: A specific test of a general theory. *American Sociological Review*. 1979;44:6363–655.

8. Becker H. *Outsiders: Studies in the Sociology of Deviance*. New York: Free Press; 1963.

9. Hirschi T. *Causes of Delinquency*. Berkeley: University of California Press; 1969.

10. Gottfredson M, Hirschi T. *A General Theory of Crime*. Stanford, CA: Stanford University Press; 1990.

11. Lindesmith A. A sociological theory of drug addiction. *American Journal of Sociology*. 1938; 43:593–613.

12. Merton K. *Social Theory and Social Structure*. New York: Free Press; 1968.

13. McLeroy KR, Bibeau D, Steckler A, Glanz K. An ecological perspective on health promotion programs. *Health Education Quarterly*. 1988;15(4): 351–377.

14. Brofenbrenner U. *The Ecology of Human Development*. Cambridge, MA: Harvard University Press; 1979.

15. Janz NK, Becker MH. The health belief model: A decade later. *Health Education Quarterly*. 1984;11(1):81–92.

16. Ajzen I, Fishbein M. *Understanding Attitudes and Predicting Social Behavior*. Englewood Cliffs, NJ: Prentice Hall; 1980.

17. Leukefeld CG, Leukefeld S. Primary Socialization Theory and A Bio/Psycho/Social/Spititual Model for Substance Abuse. *Substance Use and Abuse*. 1999;34(7):983–991.

18. Doweiko, H. *Concepts of chemical dependency*. 5th ed. Pacific Grove, CA: Wadsworth; 2002.

19. Mosher J, Yanagisako K. Public health, not social warfare: A public health approach to illegal drug policy. *J. Public Health Pol.* 1991;12:278–323.

20. Levine HG. The alcohol problem in America: From temperance to alcoholism. *Br J Addict*. 1984;79:109–119.

21. White W. *Slaying the dragon: The history of addiction treatment and recovery in America*. Bloomington, IL: Chestnut Health Systems; 1998.

22. Center for Substance Abuse Prevention. *Environmental Prevention Strategies: Putting Theory into Practice. Training and Resource Guide*. Rockville, MD: Center for Substance Abuse Prevention,

Substance Abuse and Mental Health Services Administration; 2000.

23. Cahalan D. *Problem Drinkers: A National Survey*. San Francisco, CA: Jossey-Bass; 1970.

24. Walters G. Spontaneous remission from alcohol, tobacco, and other drug abuse: Seeking quantitative answers. *American Journal of Drug & Alcohol Abuse*. 2000;26(3):443–460.

25. Humphreys K, Tucker J. Toward more responsive and effective intervention systems for alcohol-related problems. *Addiction*. 2002;97(2): 126–132.

26. Moore M, Gerstein D, eds. *Alcohol and Public Policy: Beyond the Shadow of Prohibition*. Washington, DC: National Academy Press; 1981.

27. Weschler H, Davenport A, Dowdall G, Moeykens B, Castillo S. Health and behavioral consequences of binge drinking in college. A national survey of students at 140 campuses. *JAMA*. 1994;272(21): 1672–1677.

28. Courtwright D. *Dark Paradise: Opiate Addiction in America Before 1940*. Cambridge, MA: Harvard University Press; 1982.

29. Musto D. *The American Disease: Origins of Narcotic Control*. New York: Oxford University Press; 1999.

30. National Drug Control Strategy. *FY 2003 Budget Summary*. Washington, DC: Office of National Drug Control Policy; 2002.

31. National Drug Control Strategy. *FY 2007 Budget Summary*. Washington, DC: Office of National Drug Control Policy; 2006.

32. National Drug Control Strategy. *FY 2005 Budget Summary*. Washington, DC: Office of National Drug Control Policy; 2004.

33. National Drug Control Strategy. *FY 2006 Budget Summary*. Washington, DC: Office of National Drug Control Policy; 2005.

34. Mosher J. Drug availability in a public health perspective. In: Resnik H, ed. *Youth and Drugs: Society's Mixed Messages*. OSAP Prevention Monograph 6. Rockville, MD: Office of Substance Abuse Prevention; 1990:129–168.

35. Healthy People: *The Surgeon General's report on health promotion and disease prevention*. Washington, DC: US Government Printing Office; 1979.

36. Evans RI, Rozelle RM, Mittelmark MB, Hansen WB, Bane AL, Havis J. Deterring the onset of smoking in children: Knowledge of immediate physiological peer pressure, media pressure, and

parent modeling. *Journal of Applied Social Psychology.* 1978:8;126–135.

37. Evans RI, Rozelle RM, Maxwell SE, Raines BE, Dill CA, Guthrie TJ. Social modeling films to deter smoking in adolescents: results of a three-year field investigation. *Journal of Applied Psychology.* 1981:66;399–414.

38. Belenko S. Research on Drug Courts: A Critical Review. *National Court Institute Review.* 1998:1:1;1–30.

39. Musto DF. *The American Disease.* 2nd ed. New York: Oxford University Press; 1987.

40. National Institute on Drug Abuse. *Principles of Drug Addiction Treatment: A Research-Based Guide.* NIH Publication No. 06-5316; 1999.

41. Daugherty R, Leukefeld C. *Reducing the Risks for Substance Abuse: a Life Span Approach.* New York and London: Plenum Press; 1998.

42. Substance and Mental Health Services Administration. US Department of Health and Human Services. *National Survey on Drug Use and Health*; 2005. Available at: http://www.samhsa.gov.

43. Substance and Mental Health Services Administration. US Department of Health and Human Services. *National Survey on Drug Use and Health*; 2003. Available at http://www.samhsa.gov.

44. Substance and Mental Health Services Administration. US Department of Health and Human Services. *National Survey on Drug Use and Health*; 2004. Available at http://www.samhsa.gov.

45. Substance Abuse and Mental Health Services Administration. *Drug Abuse Warning Network, 2003: Area Profiles of Drug-Related Mortality.* Rockville, MD; 2005.

46. Substance Abuse and Mental Health Services Administration. *Drug Abuse Warning Network, 2004: National Estimates of Drug-Related Emergency Department Visits.* Rockville, MD; 2006.

47. US Department of Health and Human Services. *Monitoring the Future Report*; 2003. Available at: http://www.monitoringthefuture.org.

48. US Department of Health and Human Services. *Monitoring the Future Report, 2004.* Available at: http://www.monitoringthefuture.org.

49. US Department of Health and Human Services. *Monitoring the Future Report, 2005.* Available at: http://www.monitoringthefuture.org.

50. Mosher J. Alcohol and poverty: Analyzing the link between alcohol-related problems and social policy. In: Samuels S, Smith M, eds. *Improving the Health of the Poor: Strategies for Prevention.* Menlo Park, CA: Henry J. Kaiser Family Foundation; 1992: 97–121.

51. Huang B, Grant BF, Dawson DA, et al. Race-ethnicity and the prevalence and co-occurrence of Diagnostic and Statistical Manual of Mental Disorders, Fourth Edition, alcohol and drug use disorders and Axis I and II disorders: United States 2001–2002. *Compr Psychiatry.* 2006:47; 252–257.

52. Schmidt L, Greenfield T, Mulia N. Unequal treatment: Racial and ethnic disparities in alcoholism treatment services. *Alcohol Res Health.* 2006:29; 49–54.

53. Bernstein J, Bernstein E, Shepard DS, et al. Racial and ethnic differences in health and health care: Lessons from an inner-city patient population actively using heroin and cocaine. *J Ethn Subst Abuse.* 2006:5;35–50.

54. Jemmott LS, Brown EJ. Reducing HIV sexual risk among African American women who use drugs: Hearing their voices. *J Assoc Nurses AIDS Care.* 2003:14;19–26.

55. MacMaster SA. Experiences with and perceptions of barriers to substance abuse and HIV services among African American women who use crack cocaine. *J Ethn Subst Abuse.* 2005:4;53–75.

56. Mokdad AH, Marks JS, Stroup DF, Gerberding JL. Actual causes of death in the United States, 2000. *JAMA.* 2004:291;1238–1245.

57. Centers for Disease Control. Alcohol-attributable deaths and years of potential life lost—United States, 2001. *Morbidity and Mortality Weekly.* 2004:53;866–870.

58. National Highway Traffic Safety Administration. *Traffic Safety Facts, 2002.* US Department of Transportation; 2003.

59. National Highway Traffic Safety Administration. Alcohol: *Traffic Safety Facts 1999.* US Department of Transportation; 2000.

60. Quinlan KP, Brewer RD, Siegel P, et al. Alcohol-impaired driving among US Adults, 1993–2002. *Am J Prev Med.* 2005:28;346–350.

61. Centers for Disease Control. Alcohol consumption among women who are pregnant or might become pregnant—United States, 2002. *Morbidity and Mortality Weekly.* 2004:53;1178–1181.

62. Merrick J, Merrick E, Morad E, Kandel I. Fetal alcohol syndrome and its long-term effects. *Minverva Pediatr*. 2006:58;211–218.

63. Smith LM, LaGasse LL, Derauf C, et al. The infant development, environment, and lifestyle study: Effects of prenatal methamphetamine exposure, polydrug exposure, and poverty on intrauterine growth. *Pediatrics*. 2006:118;1149–1156.

64. Alati R, Najman JM, Kinner SA, et al. Early predictors of adult drinking: A birth cohort study. *Am J Epidemiol*. 2005:162;1098–1107.

65. Miller TR, Levy DT, Cohen MA, Cox KL. Costs of alcohol and drug-involved crime. *Prev Sci*. 2006. Epub ahead of print.

66. US Department of Justice. *Arrest of Juveniles for Drug Abuse Violations from 1994 to 2003*. 2004. Available at: http://www.fbi.gov/ucr/cius_04/special_reports/arrest_juveniles.html.

67. Ullman SE, Brecklin LR. Alcohol and adult sexual assault in a national sample of women. *J Subst Abuse*. 2000:11;405–420.

68. Stoops WW, Tindall MS, Mateyoke-Scrivner A, Leukefeld C. Methamphetamine use in nonurban and urban drug court clients. *Int J Offender Ther Comp Criminol*. 2005:49;260–276.

69. National Institute of Justice. *Drug and Alcohol Use and Related Matters Among Arrestees 2000*. 2003. Available at: http://www.ojp.usdoj.gov/nij/topics/drugs/adam.htm.

70. Zhang Z. *Drug and Alcohol Use and Related Matters Among Arrestees 2003*. National Institute of Justice; 2004.

71. Harwood H. *Updating Estimates of the Economic Costs of Alcohol Abuse in the United States: Estimates, Update Methods, and Data*. Report prepared by The Lewin Group for the National Institute on Alcohol Abuse and Alcoholism; 2000. Based on estimates, analyses, and data reported in Harwood H, Fountain D, Livermore G. *The Economic Costs of Alcohol and Drug Abuse in the United States 1992*. Report prepared for the National Institute on Drug Abuse and the National Institute on Alcohol Abuse and Alcoholism, National Institutes of Health, Department of Health and Human Services. NIH Publication No. 98-4327. Rockville, MD: National Institutes of Health; 1998.

72. Office of National Drug Control Policy. *The Economic Costs of Drug Abuse in the United States, 1992–2002*. Washington, DC: Executive Office of the President; 2004.

73. Birnbaum HG, White AG, Reynolds JL, et al. Estimated costs of prescription opioid analgesic abuse in the United States in 2001: A societal perspective. *Clin J Pain*. 2006:22;667–676.

74. Havens JR, Walker R, Leukefeld CG. Prevalence of opioid analgesic injection among rural nonmedical opioid analgesic users. *Drug Alcohol Depend*. 2006. Epub ahead of print.

75. Knudsen HK, Johnson JA, Roman PM, Oser CB. Rural and urban similarities and differences in private substance abuse treatment centers. *J Psychoactive Drugs*. 2003:35;511–518.

76. Public Health Service. Report of the public health service task force on women's health issues. *Public Health Reports*. January–February 1985:100; 73–107.

77. NIH. National *Institutes of Health Guide for Grants and Contracts*. US Department of Health and Human Services. October 24, 1986:15(22).

78. Westermeyer J, Boedicker AE. Course, severity, and treatment of substance abuse among women versus men. *American Journal of Drug and Alcohol Abuse*. 2000:26(4);523–539.

79. Eagly AH. *Sex differences in social behavior: A social-role interpretation*. Mahwah, NJ: Lawrence Erlaum Associates. Mahwah, NJ; 1987.

80. Lex BW. Gender differences and substance abuse. *Advances in Substance Abuse*. 1991:4;225–296.

81. Naegle M. Substance abuse among women: Prevalence, patterns, and treatment issues. *Issues in Mental Health Nursing*. 1988:9(2);127–137.

82. Lieber CS. *Women and alcohol: Gender differences in metabolism and susceptibility*. Women and Substance Abuse. New York: Ablex Publishing; 1993.

83. Ingram-Fogel C. Health problems and needs of incarcerated women. *Journal of Prison & Jail Health*. 1991:10(1);43–57.

84. Ross PH, Lawrence JE. Health care for women offenders. *Corrections Today*. 1998:60(7); 122–127.

85. Hall S. Drug abuse treatment. In: Blechman EA, Brownell KD, eds. *Behavioral medicine & women: A comprehensive handbook*. York, PA: Guilford Press; 1998: 420–424.

86. Henderson DJ. Drug abuse and incarcerated women. *Journal of Substance Abuse Treatment*. 1998:15(6);579–587.

87. Greene S, Haney C, Hurtado A. Cycles of pain: Risk factors in the lives of incarcerated mothers and their children. *The Prison Journal*. 2000: 80(1);3–23.

88. Pelissier BM, Camp SD, Gaes GG, Saylor WG, Rhodes W. Gender differences in outcomes from prison-based residential treatment. *Journal of Substance Abuse Treatment.* 2003:24;149–160.

89. Laudet A, Magura S, Furst RT, Kumar N, Whitney S. Male partners of substance-abusing women in treatment: An exploratory study. *American Journal of Drug and Alcohol Abuse.* 1999:25(4);607–628.

90. BJS. *Bureau of Justice Statistics. Prison Statistics, Summary Findings December 31, 2002.* 2002. Available at: http://www.ojp.usdoj.gov/bjs/prisons.htm. Accessed September 11, 2003.

91. Brewer VE, Marquart JW, Mullings JL, Crouch BN. AIDS-related risk behaviors among female prisoners with histories of mental impairment. *Prison Journal.* 1998:78(2);101–118.

92. Cotton-Oldenburg NU, Jordan K, Martin SL, Kupper L. Women inmates' risky sex and drug behaviors: are they related? *American Journal of Drug and Alcohol Abuse.* 1999:25(1);129–149.

93. Hammett TM, Harmon P. Sexually transmitted diseases and hepatitis: Burden of disease among inmates. In *1996–1997 Update: HIV/AIDS, STDs, and TB in correctional facilities.* National Institute of Justice, NCJ 157642. Washington, DC: US Department of Justice; 1999.

94. Greenfield L, Snell, T. Bureau of Justice Statistics. *Women Offenders.* Washington, DC: Bureau of Justice Statistics; 2000.

95. Maruschak LM. HIV in prisons and jails, 1996. In *1996–1997 Update: HIV/AIDS, STDs, and TB in correctional facilities.* National Institute of Justice, NCJ 157642. Washington, DC: US Department of Justice; 1999.

96. Hankins CA, Gendron S, Handley MA, Richard C, Lai Tung MT, O'Shaughnessy M. HIV infection among women in prison: an assessment of risk factors using a nonnominal methodology. *American Journal of Public Health.* 1994:84(10); 1637–1640.

97. Sacks JY. Women with co-occurring substance use and mental disorders (COD) in the criminal justice system: A research review. *Behavioral Sciences & the Law.* 2004:22(4);449–466.

98. Staton M, Leukefeld C, Webster JM. Substance use, health, mental health: Problems and service utilization among incarcerated women. *International Journal of Offender Therapy and Comparative Criminology.* 2003:47(2);224–239.

99. Teplin LA, Abram KM, McClelland GM. Mental disorders of women in jail: Who receives services? *American Journal of Public Health.* 1997:87(4); 604–609.

100. Young DS. Health status and service use among incarcerated women. *Family Community Health.* 1998:21(3);16–31.

101. Jordan BK, Schlenger WE, Fairbank JA, Caddell JM. Prevalence of psychiatric disorders among incarcerated women. *Archives of General Psychiatry* 1996:53;513–519.

102. Liebling A. Suicide amongst women prisoners. *The Howard Journal.* 1994:33(1);1–9.

103. Bond L, Semaan S. At risk for HIV infection: Incarcerated women in a county jail in Philadelphia. *Women & Health.* 1996:24(4);27–45.

104. Sheridan MJ. Comparison of the life experiences and personal functioning of men and women in prison. *Families in Society: The Journal of Contemporary Human Services.* 1996:77;423–434.

105. Staton M, Leukefeld C, Logan TK. Health service utilization and victimization among incarcerated female substance users. *Substance Use & Misuse.* 2001:36(6&7);701–716.

106. Messina N, Grella C. Childhood trauma and women's health outcomes in a California prison population. *American Journal of Public Health.* 2006:96(10);1842–1848.

107. Coll CG, Surrey JL, Buccio-Notaro P, Molla B. Incarcerated mothers: Crimes and punishment. In: Coll CG, Surrey JL, Weingarten K, eds. *Mothering Against the odds: Diverse voices of contemporary mothers.* New York: The Guilford Press; 1998: 255–274.

108. Bureau of Justice Statistics. *Substance Abuse and Treatment of State and Federal Prisoners, 1997; 2002.* Available at: http://www.ojp.usdoj.gov/bjs/pub/press/satsfp97.pr. Accessed January 30, 2007.

109. Office of National Drug Control Policy. *The National Drug Control Strategy: 1996 Budget Summary.* Washington, DC: US Government Printing Office; 1996.

CHAPTER 22

Infectious Disease Control

Alan R. Hinman, MD, MPH

CHAPTER OBJECTIVES

Upon completion of this chapter, the reader will be able to:

1. Describe the methods of transmission of infectious diseases.
2. List the steps in outbreak investigation.
3. Recognize the impact and nature of immunization programs in the United States.
4. Describe the impact and methods for control of sexually transmitted diseases in the United States.
5. Describe the impact and methods for control of tuberculosis in the United States.
6. Describe the nature and impact of food-borne and waterborne diseases in the United States.
7. Explain the nature and potential impact of emerging/reemerging diseases and antibiotic diseases in the United States.
8. Describe the potential impact of bioterrorism in the United States.

KEY TERMS

Airborne Transmission
Direct Transmission
Epidemic
Food-Borne Illness
Immunization
Indirect Transmission
Model of Transmission
Outbreak Investigation
Sexually Transmitted Diseases (STDs)
Tuberculosis
Surveillance
Vaccines
Vaccine Efficacy
Vector-Borne Transmission
Vehicle-Borne Transmission
Waterborne Illness

Historically, infectious diseases have been the major killers of humans. It is only within the last century that they have been replaced by chronic diseases and injuries as primary killers in the United States. Worldwide, however, infectious diseases still account for approximately 20 percent of all deaths.[1] The major advances in infectious disease control to date have been through protection of food and water and through immunizations. This chapter begins with general considerations of infectious disease transmission, surveillance, and investigation, and then considers specific topics of immunization, sexually transmitted diseases (STDs, including human immunodeficiency virus [HIV] infection), tuberculosis (TB), food-borne and water-borne diseases, emerging/reemerging diseases, and antibiotic resistance.

GENERAL CONSIDERATIONS

This section introduces general principles of infectious disease transmission. It also discusses how surveillance and outbreak investigation help control the spread of infectious diseases.

Transmission

The four means by which infectious diseases are transmitted are direct transmission, indirect transmission, vehicle-borne or vector-borne transmission, and airborne transmission. **Direct transmission** may occur as a result of "touching, biting, kissing, or sexual intercourse, or through direct projections (droplet spread) of droplet spray onto the conjunctiva or onto the mucous membranes of the eye, nose, or mouth during sneezing, coughing, spitting, singing or talking (usually limited to a distance of about 1 meter or less)."[2] Sexually transmitted diseases and measles are conditions spread by direct transmission. **Indirect transmission** may be vehicle-borne or vector-borne. **Vehicle-borne transmission** may occur as a result of "contaminated inanimate materials or objects (fomites) such as toys, handkerchiefs, cooking or eating utensils, water, food, milk, or blood. The agent may or may not have multiplied or developed in or on the vehicle before being transmitted."[2] **Vector-borne transmission** may be mechanical or biological. Mechanical vector-borne transmission includes "simple mechanical carriage by a crawling or flying insect through soiling of its feet or proboscis, or by passage of organisms through its gastrointestinal tract. This does not require multiplication or development of the organism."[2] With biological vector-borne transmission, "propagation (multiplication), cyclic development, or a combination of these is required before the arthropod can transit the infective form of the agent to humans."[2] **Airborne transmission** involves the "dissemination of microbial aerosols to a suitable portal of entry, usually the respiratory tract. Microbial aerosols are suspensions of particles in the air consisting partially or wholly of microorganisms. They may remain suspended in the air for long periods of time, some retaining and others losing infectivity or virulence."[2] For example, patients in a hospital several rooms away from a patient with varicella have become infected,[3] and measles has been transmitted to a patient visiting a physician's office approximately one hour after the source case had left the office.[4]

Surveillance

Surveillance is key to understanding the epidemiology of infectious diseases. Surveillance is "the process of systematic collection, orderly consolidation, analysis, and evaluation of pertinent data with prompt dissemination of the results to those who need to know, particularly those who are in a position to take action."[2] A simpler definition of surveillance is "information for action."[5] Surveillance information is used to develop and modify interventions and monitor their success. In addition, surveillance may identify clusters of cases or outbreaks that warrant further investigation.

Outbreak Investigation

Outbreak investigation involves seven major steps, many of which may be carried out simultaneously:

1. Confirm whether there truly is an epidemic. The definition of an **epidemic** is "the occurrence, in a defined community or region, of cases of an illness (or an outbreak) with a frequency clearly in excess of normal expectancy."[2] Obviously, it is necessary to know not only how many cases there are but also how many are expected. A single case of paralysis due to wild poliovirus occurring in the United States, for example, would be considered a potential epidemic because there have been no such cases reported since 1979.[6] Two cases associated in time and place would be sufficient evidence of transmission to be considered an epidemic.

2. Identify the illness involved, often by establishing a clinical case definition if a definitive diagnosis has not been established.

3. Enumerate all cases and characterize them according to time, place, and person. Characterization as to time typically involves construction of an epidemic curve depicting the number of cases by time of onset (by hour, day, week, or month, as appropriate). A common vehicle outbreak with a point contamination of the vehicle typically has an epidemic curve with a single sharp peak centered on the median incubation period following exposure (typically a few hours to a few days). Person-to-person direct transmission is generally accompanied by an epidemic curve in which there is a gradual buildup of cases, often with a typical incubation period between "generations" of cases, and a gradual decline as susceptibles are exhausted, in the absence of measures to interrupt transmission. Characterization by place often involves constructing a map showing residence (or worksite) of individual cases to identify any geographic localization. Characterization by person involves the obvious—age and gender—but may also entail race/ethnicity, occupation, behavioral characteristic, or other variables.

4. Confirm the diagnosis in the laboratory or by other means.

5. Formulate a hypothesis about the cause of the epidemic and the means of transmission, and test that hypothesis through further investigation or interview of cases, culture of suspected vehicle, or other means.

6. Take control measures to end the epidemic.

7. Prepare and disseminate a report about the epidemic, either through formal publication in the literature or through an administratively circulated report. This last step, which is the one most often ignored, is essential to learn from the current situation and prevent recurrences.

IMMUNIZATION

Immunization is one of the most important interventions for the control and prevention of infectious diseases. Globally, immunization has resulted in the eradication of smallpox and the near-eradication of poliomyelitis as well as preventing millions of deaths due to other diseases. This section addresses vaccines impact, safety, and effectiveness; immunization coverage; immunization schedules; and the immunization infrastructure in the United States.

Vaccines

Vaccines are suspensions of live (usually attenuated) or killed microorganisms (bacteria or viruses) or fractions thereof administered to induce immunity and prevent infectious disease or its sequelae. Live, attenuated vaccines consist of living organisms that have been adapted in the laboratory to reduce their ability to cause disease while still stimulating an immune response. They are believed to induce an immunologic response more similar to that resulting from natural infection than do inactivated vaccines. Inactivated or killed vaccines may consist of:

- Inactivated whole organisms (e.g., cholera, whole cell pertussis)
- Soluble capsular material alone (e.g., pneumococcal polysaccharide)
- Soluble capsular material covalently linked to carrier proteins (e.g., *Haemophilus influenzae* type b [Hib] conjugate)
- Purified extracts of some component or components of the organism (e.g., hepatitis B, acellular pertussis)

Toxoids are modified bacterial toxins (e.g., diphtheria, tetanus) that have been rendered nontoxic but retain the ability to stimulate the formation of antitoxin. They are often included in the general category of vaccines.[7]

Impact of Vaccines

Introduction and widespread use of childhood vaccines have had a dramatic effect on the reported incidence of infectious diseases in the United States. The United States is currently enjoying historic low levels of disease incidence and historic high levels of vaccine coverage. Table 22.1 shows the typical number of cases reported of childhood vaccine-preventable diseases in the years preceding introduction of vaccines and the number of cases of those diseases reported in 2006.[8] There has been a reduction in excess of 95 percent in virtually every one of the conditions. Some of the reductions are quite recent—the Hib conjugate vaccine was introduced in the United States for use in infants in 1990, but its widespread use led to virtual elimination of HiB disease in this country within a period of less than 10 years.[9] Transmission of measles and rubella has been interrupted in the United States, and these are no longer endemic diseases; all cases arise as a result of importation from another country.[10,11]

Table 22.1. Typical Pre-Vaccine and Current Morbidity from Vaccine-Preventable Diseases, United States

Disease	Typical	2006	Percentage Decline
Diphtheria	175,885	0	−100
Hib (<5)	20,000	29	−99.86
Measles	503,282	55	−99.99
Mumps	152,209	6,584	−95.67
Pertussis	147,271	15,632	−89.38
Polio (paralytic)	16,310	−0	−100
Rubella	47,745	11	−99.98
CRS	823	1	−99.88
Tetanus	1,314	41	−96.88

Immunization Coverage

Table 22.2 shows the 2006 nationwide levels of vaccine coverage in 19- to 35-month-old children.[12] The levels are not uniform throughout the country. For example, in 2005, state-specific levels of measles vaccination ranged from 82.7 percent (OR) to 97.0 percent (MA). In the past, there has been

Table 22.2. Vaccination Coverage Levels Among Children Aged 19–35 Months, United States, 2006

Vaccine/Dose	Coverage (%)
DTP ≥ 3	95.8
DTP ≥ 4	85.2
Polio ≥ 3	92.0
Hib ≥ 3	93.4
MMR ≥ 1	92.4
Hepatitis B ≥ 3	93.4
Varicella	89.3
Combined series	
4 DTP/3 Polio/I MMR	83.2
4 DTP/3 Polio/1 MMR/3 Hib	82.3
4 DTP/3 Polio/1 MMR/3 Hib/3 Hep B	80.6
4 DTP/3 Polio/1 MMR/3 Hib/3 Hep B/1 varicella	77.0

significant racial variation in coverage rates, with blacks having lower rates than whites. In 2005, for the first time, this disparity had been eliminated. Unfortunately, it again appeared in 2006.

Immunization rates in adults are not as high as those in children. For example, in 2005, only 63.3 percent of adults 65 years of age or older had received influenza vaccine in the preceding year, and 63.7 percent had ever received pneumococcal vaccine.[13] Both vaccines have been recommended for all persons 65 or older (and for younger persons with certain conditions) for decades.

Immunization Schedules

Recommendations for immunization of children in the United States are developed principally by the Public Health Service's Advisory Committee on Immunization Practices (ACIP)[7] and the American Academy of Pediatrics' (AAP) Committee on Infectious Diseases (Red Book Committee).[14] Along with the American Academy of Family Physicians (AAFP), these committees develop harmonized immunization schedules for children and adolescents (Figures 22.1 and 22.2). Immunization of all children and adolescents in the United States is currently recommended against 16 diseases: diphtheria (D), hepatitis A, hepatitis B, Hib, human papilloma virus, influenza, measles, meningococcal disease, mumps, pertussis (P), pneumococcal disease, poliomyelitis, rotavirus, rubella, tetanus (T), and varicella.[7,15]

Figure 22.3 shows 2008 immunization recommendations for adults, who may have special needs for vaccines because of increased risk of illness or death resulting from age, occupation, behavior, or chronic illness.[15] ACIP recommendations for children, adolescents, and adults are revised annually and are posted at http://www.cdc.gov/vaccines/

Vaccine ▼ Age ►	Birth	1 month	2 months	4 months	6 months	12 months	15 months	18 months	19–23 months	2–3 years	4–6 years
Hepatitis B[1]	HepB	HepB	see footnote1		HepB						
Rotavirus[2]			Rota	Rota	Rota						
Diphtheria, Tetanus, Pertussis[3]			DTaP	DTaP	DTaP	see footnote3	DTaP				DTaP
Haemophilus influenzae type b[4]			Hib	Hib	Hib[4]	Hib					
Pneumococcal[5]			PCV	PCV	PCV	PCV				PPV	
Inactivated Poliovirus			IPV	IPV		IPV					IPV
Influenza[6]						Influenza (Yearly)					
Measles, Mumps, Rubella7						MMR					MMR
Varicella[8]						Varicella					Varicella
Hepatitis A[9]						HepA (2 doses)				HepA Series	
Meningococcal[10]											MCV4

■ Range of recommended ages   ■ Certain high-risk groups

This schedule indicates the recommended ages for routine administration of currently licensed childhood vaccines, as of December 1, 2007, for children aged 0 through 6 years. Additional information is available at www.cdc.gov/vaccines/recs/schedules. Any dose not administered at the recommended age should be administered at any subsequent visit, when indicated and feasible. Additional vaccines may be licensed and recommended during the year. Licensed combination vaccines may be used whenever any components of the combination are indicated and other components of the vaccine are not contraindicated and if approved by the Food and Drug Administration for that dose of the series. Providers should consult the respective Advisory Committee on Immunization Practices statement for detailed recommendations, including for high-risk conditions: http://www.cdc.gov/vaccines/pubs/ACIP-list.htm. Clinically significant adverse events that follow immunization should be reported to the Vaccine Adverse Event Reporting System (VAERS). Guidance about how to obtain and complete a VAERS form is available at www.vaers.hhs.gov or by telephone, 800-822-7967.

Figure 22.1. Recommended Immunization Schedule for Persons Aged 0–6 Years, 2008
SOURCE: Delmar Cengage Learning.

Vaccine▼ Age▶	7–10 years	11–12 years	13–18 years
Diphtheria, Tetanus, Pertussis[1]	see footnote 1	Tdap	Tdap
Human Papillomavirus[2]	see footnote 2	HPV (3 doses)	HPV Series
Meningococcal[3]	MCV4	MCV4	MCV4
Pneumococcal[4]	PPV		
Influenza[5]	Influenza (Yearly)		
Hepatitis A[6]	HepA Series		
Hepatitis B[7]	HepB Series		
Inactivated Poliovirus[8]	IPV Series		
Measles, Mumps, Rubella[9]	MMR Series		
Varicella[10]	Varicella Series		

■ Range of recommended ages   ☐ Catch-up immunization   ▦ Certain high-risk groups

This schedule indicates the recommended ages for routine administration of currently licensed childhood vaccines, as of December 1, 2007, for children aged 7–18 years. Additional information is available at www.cdc.gov/vaccines/recs/schedules. Any dose not administered at the recommended age should be administered at any subsequent visit, when indicated and feasible. Additional vaccines may be licensed and recommended during the year. Licensed combination vaccines may be used whenever any components of the combination are indicated and other components of the vaccine are not contraindicated and if approved by the Food and Drug Administration for that dose of the series. Providers should consult the respective Advisory Committee on Immunization Practices statement for detailed recommendations, including for high-risk conditions: http://www.cdc.gov/vaccines/pubs/ACIP-list.htm. Clinically significant adverse events that follow immunization should be reported to the Vaccine Adverse Event Reporting System (VAERS). Guidance about how to obtain and complete a VAERS form is available at www.vaers.hhs.gov or by telephone, 800-822-7967.

Figure 22.2. Recommended Immunization Schedule for Persons Aged 7–18 Years, 2008

SOURCE: Delmar Cengage Learning.

recs/acip/default.htm. Recommendations have also been developed for health care workers.[16]

Immunization Infrastructure

Most children in the United States currently receive their immunizations in the private sector, from pediatricians or family physicians. A significant minority receive immunizations in the public sector, typically from local health departments. There is considerable variation around the country.[17]

Since 1962, the federal government has supported childhood immunization programs through a grant program administered by the Centers for Disease Control and Prevention (CDC). The grants support purchase of vaccine for free administration at local health departments and also support immunization delivery, surveillance, and communication/ education.

At 2007 prices, the cost for vaccines alone (irrespective of physician fees) is approximately $1700 in the private sector (CDC, unpublished data). Most employer-based insurance plans now cover childhood immunizations. Children who are uninsured, covered by Medicaid, or are Alaska natives/ American Indians can receive vaccines free of charge through the Vaccines for Children program enacted in 1993.[18] Underinsured children (those whose parents have insurance that does not cover immunizations) may also receive the vaccines free at Federally Qualified Health Centers (most Community Health Centers).

Immunization efforts in the United States have been significantly aided by the enactment and enforcement of laws in each state that require immunization before first entry into school. Since 1980, all states have had such laws in place. As a result, at least 95 percent of children entering school are fully immunized.[19]

Although immunization levels are currently at record high levels and vaccine-preventable disease incidence is at record low levels, there is continuing

Vaccine ▼　　Age Group ▶	19–49 years	50–64 years	≥65 years
Tetanus, diphtheria, pertussis (Td/Tdap)[1,*]	1 dose Td booster every 10 yrs Substitute 1 dose of Tdap for Td		
Human papillomavirus (HPV)[2,*]			
Measles, Mumps, Rubella (MMR)[3,*]	1 or 2 doses	1 dose	
Varicella[4,*]	2 doses (0, 4–8 wks)		
Influenza[5,*]	1 dose annually		
Pneumococcal (polysaccharide)[6,7]	1–2 doses		1 dose
Hepatitis A[8,*]	2 doses (0, 6–12 mos or 0, 6–18 mos)		
Hepatitis B[9,*]	3 doses (0, 1–2, 4–6 mos)		
Meningococcal[10,*]	1 or more doses		
Zoster[11]		1 dose	

*Covered by the Vaccine Injury Compensation Program.

■ For all persons in this category who meet the age requirements and who lack evidence of immunity (e.g., lack documentation of vaccination or have no evidence of prior infection)

■ Recommended if some other risk factor is present (e.g., on the basis of medical, occupational, lifestyle, or other indications)

Figure 22.3. **Recommended Adult Immunization Schedule, 2007–2008**

SOURCE: Delmar Cengage Learning.

cause for concern about immunizations in the United States:

- There are approximately 4 million births each year (11,000 per day), and each of these children requires immunization.

- The population is quite mobile. Approximately 16 percent of Americans change address in any given year, and at least 25 percent of children receive immunizations from more than one provider. This mobility creates problems in record-keeping.

- The immunization schedule is increasingly complex as new vaccines or additional doses are recommended.

- Both parents and providers overestimate the immunization levels of their children/patients. Most parents feel their children are fully immu-

nized and so do physicians. However, several studies have demonstrated that pediatricians typically overestimate coverage in their patients by 20 percent or more.

- Few physicians use reminder or recall systems to notify their patients of immunizations due (reminder) or overdue (recall).[20]

All of these factors support the need for automated mechanisms to keep track of children's immunization status and notify parents and providers about needed immunizations. The National Vaccine Advisory Committee (NVAC) has called for a nationwide network of population-based immunization registries, and the *Healthy People 2010* objectives call for 95 percent of children 0–6 to be enrolled in population-based immunization registries by 2010.[21]

The Institute of Medicine (IOM) report *Calling the Shots* discussed the appropriate role of the federal government in supporting immunization programs.[22] It called for an increase in both federal and state support for immunization programs and greater stability in that funding as well as an increased level of support for global immunization programs.

Vaccine Safety and Efficacy

Modern vaccines are safe and effective; however, they are neither perfectly safe nor perfectly effective. Some individuals who receive a vaccine will not be protected against disease, and some will suffer adverse consequences. Adverse events may range from minor inconveniences such as discomfort at the injection site or fever to serious conditions such as paralysis associated with oral poliovirus vaccine (OPV). The goal is to achieve maximum safety and maximum efficacy.

The fact that vaccines are not perfectly effective means that some vaccinated individuals will develop disease on exposure. A common situation in the United States in recent years has been that approximately half of the people who develop a disease (e.g., measles) give a history of vaccination. This leads many persons to question the efficacy of the vaccine.

A simple formula exists to determine **vaccine efficacy** (VE)

$$VE = (ARU - ARV)/ARU \times 100$$

where ARU is the attack rate of disease in unvaccinated individuals, and ARV is the attack rate in vaccinated individuals.[23] A nomogram has been constructed, as shown in Figure 22.4, to demonstrate the relationship between the proportion of

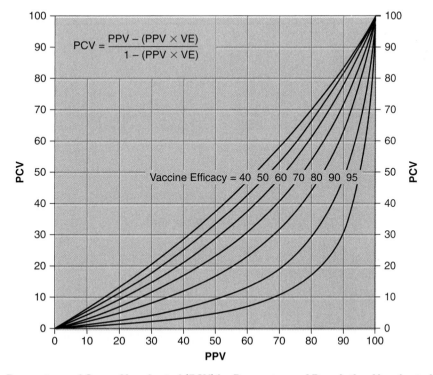

$$PCV = \frac{PPV - (PPV \times VE)}{1 - (PPV \times VE)}$$

Vaccine Efficacy = 40 50 60 70 80 90 95

Figure 22.4. Percentage of Cases Vaccinated (PCV) by Percentage of Population Vaccinated (PPV), for 7 Values of Vaccine Efficacy (VE)

SOURCE: Delmar Cengage Learning.

cases with a history of vaccination (PCV) and the proportion of the population vaccinated (PPV) at varying levels of vaccine efficacy (VE). Simply put, if 90 percent of the population has been vaccinated, and half the cases give a history of vaccination, this is consistent with high efficacy for the vaccine (approximately 90%).

Decisions about use of vaccines are based on the relative balance of risks and benefits. This balance may change over time. For example, recipients of oral polio vaccine (OPV) and their close contacts have a risk of developing paralysis associated with the vaccine of 1 in approximately every 2.4 million doses of vaccine distributed. This risk is quite small and was certainly outweighed by the much larger risk of paralysis due to wild polioviruses at the time they were circulating in the United States. However, because wild polioviruses no longer circulate in the United States, and the risk of importation of wild viruses has been greatly reduced by the global effort to eradicate polio, the balance has shifted.

There has not been a case of paralysis in the United States due to indigenously acquired wild poliovirus since 1979, and the entire Western Hemisphere has been free of wild poliovirus circulation since 1991.[24] The ACIP recommended, in 1997, that children receive a sequential schedule with two doses of inactivated polio vaccine (IPV, which carries no risk of paralysis) followed by two doses of OPV. In 2000, the recommendation was made to switch to an all-IPV regimen.[25] Vaccine-associated paralysis has essentially disappeared in the United States.

It is often difficult to ascertain whether an adverse event that occurs after immunization was caused by the vaccine or was merely temporally related and caused by some totally independent (and often unknown or unidentified) factor. This is particularly a problem during infancy, when a number of conditions may occur spontaneously. In a given instance it may be impossible to determine whether the vaccine was responsible.[26] Particularly when dealing with rare events, it may be necessary to carry out large-scale case-control studies or review comprehensive records of large numbers of infants to ascertain whether those who received a vaccine had a higher incidence of the event than those who did not. The CDC operates a large linked database involving several large health maintenance organizations. This Vaccine Safety Datalink project includes more than 6 million persons (approximately 2% of the United States population) and has proved to be an invaluable resource in attempting to determine causality.[27]

One result of the extraordinary success of immunization efforts has been the fact that today's young parents (and young physicians) have never seen many of the diseases against which they are being urged to have their children vaccinated. Consequently, they may not be as motivated as were parents and physicians in the past. In the absence of disease, the infrequent known (or alleged) adverse events associated with vaccines assume greater prominence. This imbalance has led some parents (and even some physicians) to question whether use of some (or all) vaccines is still warranted. The rise of the Internet has made it easier for opinions about vaccines to be disseminated, whether based in science or not. This increases the obligation on public health authorities to explain fully the risks and benefits of vaccines.[28] The occasional occurrence of previously unrecognized adverse events actually caused by the vaccine (as with intestinal intussusception and rotavirus vaccine) adds to the complexity of the explanation.[29]

SEXUALLY TRANSMITTED DISEASES (STDS)

All **sexually transmitted diseases** (STDs), including human immunodeficiency virus (HIV) infection, are historically, biologically, behaviorally, economically, and programmatically related.[30] Intimate sexual contact is the common (but not exclusive) mode of transmission of the causative organisms. Several dozen bacterial, viral, parasitic, and fungal infections are now recognized as being commonly (or predominantly) transmitted by sexual contact. In general, they share the characteristic that women suffer disproportionately from their effects. This is a result of a variety of factors, including the fact that women are generally less able to prevent exposure to STDs than men because of the relative lack of safe, effective, female-controlled preventive measures. Women also are frequently unable to negotiate the conditions under which sexual intercourse occurs. In addition, complications of STDs in women are likely to be more severe: pelvic inflammatory disease (PID), infertility, ectopic pregnancy (the leading cause of maternal mortality in the United States), and cancer.[31]

Efforts to control STDs have been guided by both the magnitude of the problem and the availability of diagnostic and therapeutic measures. The United States began the twentieth century focusing on one dominant STD—syphilis—which could be diagnosed with newly developed serologic techniques and treated with a suppressive (but not, at the time, curative) therapy. Subsequent improvements in the ability to detect and treat syphilis led to a striking decline in its incidence. In 1999, CDC, in collaboration with other partners, launched a National Plan to Eliminate Syphilis from the United States.[32] Elimination was defined as the absence of sustained transmission (i.e., no transmission more than 90 days after the report of an imported index case). National targets for 2005 included reducing primary and secondary (P & S) syphilis incidence to fewer than 1000 cases (0.4 cases per 100,000 population) and increasing the number of syphilis-free counties to 90 percent. In 1999, there were 6675 cases of P & S syphilis reported (2.5 cases per 100,000), and 79.4 percent of counties reported no cases of P & S syphilis. The South had the highest rates in the country. The incidence rate in blacks (15.2 per 100,000) was 30 times the reported rate in whites (0.5).[33] Unfortunately, however, after reaching a low point in 2000 (5979 cases), cases of primary and secondary syphilis began to rise and reached 9756 in 2006. The South continued to have the highest rates in the country, but the gap in incidence rates between blacks and whites narrowed, with blacks having 5.9 times the reported rate in whites. Reported rates in males were 5.7 times the reported rates in females, reflecting the predominance of cases in men who have sex with men.[34] Figure 22.5 shows the trends in incidence of primary and secondary syphilis in the United States, 1987–2006.

In 2006, CDC reframed the Syphilis Elimination Effort and set the following interim elimination targets for 2010: reduce rates of primary and

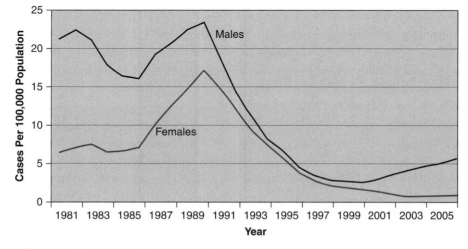

Figure 22.5. Reported Primary and Secondary Syphilis Rates; United States, 1988–2006, by Gender
SOURCE: Delmar Cengage Learning.

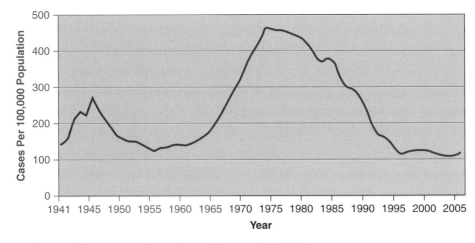

Figure 22.6. Reported Gonorrhea Rates; United States, 1941–2006

SOURCE: Delmar Cengage Learning.

secondary syphilis to fewer than 2.2 per 100,000 population (from 2.8 in 2004), reduce congenital syphilis to fewer than 3.9 per 100,000 live births (from 8.8 in 2004), and reduce the black:white racial disparity ratio to less than 3.0 (from 5.9 in 2006).[35]

Growing awareness of the serious individual and social implications of gonorrhea, accompanied by improvements in diagnostic techniques, led the United States to embark on a major program to control gonorrhea in the 1970s. Reported gonorrhea incidence reached an all-time high in 1975 and progressively declined, although incidence has been relatively stable since 1997. In 2006, 358,366 cases were reported (120.9 cases per 100,000 population).[34] Figure 22.6 shows trends in reported incidence of gonorrhea in the United States from 1941–2006.

In the early 1980s, the spectrum of STDs expanded with recognition of the acute syndromes (and long-term consequences) caused by a number of other conditions, including *Chlamydia trachomatis*, *Trichomonas vaginalis*, herpes simplex virus, and human papillomavirus. These were all overshadowed by the discovery of a new STD, acquired immunodeficiency syndrome (AIDS), in 1981.[36]

The United States began the twenty-first century focusing on a new dominant STD, HIV/AIDS, for which there was an effective serologic diagnostic technique and suppressive but not curative therapy. It is hoped that advances in development of preventive and therapeutic measures will enable major progress to be made against this STD in the current century as occurred with syphilis in the twentieth century.[37]

Following the first report of AIDS cases in June 1981, there was a rapid increase in the number of cases and deaths reported during the 1980s followed by substantial declines in new cases and deaths in the late 1990s.[38] The decline in new cases represents the effect of HIV prevention efforts and increases in societal awareness of, and response to, the AIDS epidemic. The decline in numbers of deaths reflects both the decline in incidence as well as the impact of antiretroviral therapies. As of December 31, 2006, 1,014,797 persons had been reported with AIDS in the United States, at least 55 percent of whom had died[39] (Figure 22.7).

Approximately one-half of the cases in the United States have occurred in men who have sex with other men, and one-quarter have been associated with injection drug use. This is to be contrasted with the situation in the developing world, where the vast majority of cases are associated with heterosexual contact. Nearly all transmission of HIV through transfusion of blood or blood

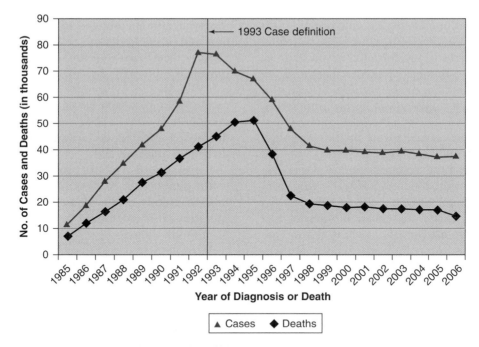

Figure 22.7. Estimated AIDS Cases and Deaths Among Adults and Adolescents with AIDS; United States, 1985–2006

SOURCE: http://www.cdc.gov/hiv/topics/surveillance/resources/slides/epidemiology/slides/EPI-AIDS.pdf.

products occurred before screening of the blood supply for HIV antibody was initiated in 1985.

Model of STD Transmission

Anderson and May have developed a simple and very useful **model of transmission** of STDs based on earlier work by themselves and by Yorke and Hethcote.[40] It is based on the assumption that a disease can sustain itself only when the reproduction rate is greater than one, that is, when each infected person on average transmits the disease to at least one other person. If the reproduction rate is less than one, transmission of the disease cannot be sustained and it will die out. The formula for the reproduction rate is

$$R = B \times c \times D$$

where **R** is the reproduction rate (the number of new infections produced, on average, by an

infected individual); **B** is a measure of transmissibility (the average probability that an infected individual will infect a susceptible partner given exposure); **c** represents the average number of different partners the infected individual has per unit time; and **D** represents the duration of infectiousness of the disease. These three determinants of the reproductive rate are influenced by the interplay of biological and behavioral variables for each STD.

The values for each parameter may vary depending on the STD and the type of sexual contact; estimates have been made for several of them. For example, for gonorrhea, the overall estimate for **B** is 50 percent (50–90 percent for male-to-female transmission and 20–50 percent for female-to-male transmission). For syphilis, **B** is estimated at 20–30 percent and for HIV at 1–10 percent.[41] Additionally, HIV transmissibility is apparently higher for penile-anal intercourse than for penile-vaginal intercourse.

Because not all members of a given population have the same number of sex partners, a refinement can be made in the formula for variable **c,** using the median number of sex partners and the variance in the number of sex partners instead of a simple average. It appears that a core population of highly sexually active persons (with many different partners) plays a major role in the continued transmission of STDs.

The duration of the infectious period, **D,** is also quite different for the different STDs, ranging from a few days for gonorrhea (in men), to a lifetime for HIV infection. There are other biological and behavioral factors affecting **D,** such as health care seeking behavior, and compliance with treatment, among others.

Elements of STD Control Programs

Control strategies may aim to modify any of the factors in the equation of transmissibility. In general, control programs include public information and education, professional education and training, screening, prompt diagnosis and therapy, counseling, partner notification, and surveillance. No approach by itself is likely to prevent the spread of STDs, but each contributes to the overall effort. CDC publishes *Sexually Transmitted Diseases Treatment Guidelines.* The most recent revision was in 2006.[42]

The aim of public information and education, counseling, and partner notification is to reduce factors **B, c,** and **D** by encouraging changes in sexual and health care related behaviors. Given the differential importance to overall STD transmission of those who have few and those who have many sex partners, targeted behavior change among core group members may have much greater impact on transmission than would behavior changes in non-core group members.

Through partner notification, the sex (and needle-sharing) partners of persons with STDs are contacted, notified of their risk of exposure (without disclosing the identity of the original patient), educated about risky practices and prevention methods, and encouraged to come in for examination and possible treatment. This activity can affect all three factors in the equation: persons can reduce transmissibility (**B**), for example, by eliminating receptive anal intercourse or insisting on the use of condoms in all sexual activity; they can reduce the number of their sexual partners (**c**); or they can be diagnosed and treated early in the progression of their own infection (**D**).

Surveillance is essential to assess the magnitude of the problem, identify groups at particular risk, monitor trends, and evaluate the impact of control programs. It is (or should be) a major determinant of program direction.

With particular regard to HIV, it must be recognized that the HIV epidemic is not a monolithic event. Rather, it is a number of epidemics with varying primary means of transmission and different rates of spread in different areas and in different segments of society.[43] These may call for different approaches. Freedom from discrimination and guaranteed confidentiality are essential. Current HIV prevention efforts focus on preventing initiation of the behaviors and conditions that put individuals at risk of acquiring or spreading the virus (e.g., delaying onset of sexual activity, not starting to use drugs) and modifying behaviors to reduce the likelihood of transmission if exposure occurs (e.g., condom use, assurance of clean needles and syringes). Other specific approaches include screening donated blood, treating HIV-infected pregnant women to prevent mother-to-child transmission, treating other STDs, treating tuberculosis, providing contraceptive services, and using highly active antiretroviral drugs in HIV-infected individuals to maintain their health and to reduce the levels of circulating virus (thereby reducing the likelihood of transmission). Another important component is the education of health care workers in the use of universal precautions to reduce the risk of nosocomial transmission. In 2003, CDC announced a new initiative Advancing HIV Prevention (AHP)[44] with four new strategies:

- Make HIV testing a routine part of medical care.[45]

- Implement new models for diagnosing HIV infections outside medical settings.

- Prevent new infections by working with persons diagnosed with HIV and their partners.

- Further decrease perinatal HIV transmission.

Tuberculosis (TB)

Tuberculosis (TB) is caused by *Mycobacterium tuberculosis,* a bacterium primarily transmitted through inhalation of airborne bacilli or droplet nuclei. Initial infection is usually not noticed but is accompanied by an immune response manifested by development of a positive reaction to purified protein derivative (PPD) applied intradermally.

Only 5–10 percent of immunocompetent persons infected with TB ultimately go on to develop TB disease at any time in their lives. However, for those with impaired immune systems, the risk of developing active TB is much higher (on the order of 7–10% per year for those with HIV infection).[46] Clinical manifestations of TB commonly involve fever, weight loss, and cough, reflecting pulmonary infection. Persons with pulmonary TB may develop cavitary lesions visible on a chest x-ray and may excrete large numbers of organisms when they cough or sneeze.

For those excreting large numbers of bacilli (who are presumably most infectious), it may be possible to visualize characteristic acid-fast bacilli (AFB) on direct smear of the sputum. For others, however, diagnosis of TB is made difficult by the fact that the causative organisms are slow growing. Even with newer techniques, it may take more than one week for a culture to become positive and then another week or more to determine antibiotic susceptibility. Using older techniques, this period could extend to two or three months. During this time, the patient may remain infectious if not started on appropriate therapy.

TB Prevention and Control

The approach to TB prevention and control in the United States has two major components. One is the identification and treatment of persons with TB disease. This both cures their infection and prevents transmission to others. The other is the identification and treatment of those with TB infection to prevent their subsequent development of TB disease.

Management of TB disease (or latent infection) is made difficult by the fact that treatment (either for infection or disease) involves six months or more of medication. Consequently, patient adherence to therapy is a major problem, and inconsistent adherence to therapy may result in the emergence of organisms resistant to the drugs being administered. Fortunately, directly observed therapy (DOT), in which a health worker personally gives each dose of medication to the patient and observes that it is taken, has been shown to be a highly effective way of ensuring completion of therapy.[47]

TB in the United States

At the beginning of the twentieth century, TB was the leading cause of death in the United States. Reported mortality from TB declined steadily during the first half of the century, in the absence of specific therapy, as a result of improvements in nutrition and housing, and the isolation of infected individuals in sanatoriums. TB first became reportable on a nationwide basis in 1952, and from that time until 1985, there was a steady decline in reported incidence, averaging 4–5 percent per year (Figure 22.8). The overall decline from 1953 to 1985 was 74 percent. In 1985, there were 22,201 cases reported (9.3 cases per 100,000 population). The decline was so impressive that it was believed that TB could be eliminated from the United States, and, in 1989, CDC and the Advisory Council for the Elimination of Tuberculosis (ACET) issued "A Strategic Plan for the Elimination of Tuberculosis in the United States."[48]

The plan established a national goal of TB elimination by 2010, defined as a case rate of less than 1 per 1,000,000 population. The plan described three components: (1) more effective use of existing prevention and control methods; (2) development and evaluation of new prevention, diagnostic, and treatment technologies; and (3) rapid transfer of

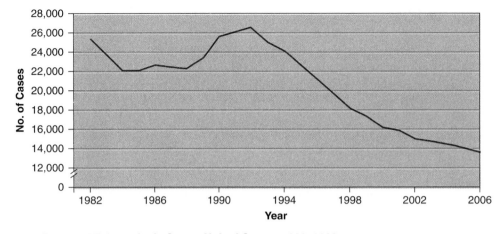

Figure 22.8. Reported Tuberculosis Cases; United States, 1982–2006
SOURCE: Delmar Cengage Learning.

newly developed technologies into clinical and public health practice.

The plan was widely endorsed and increased resources were made available to TB control programs, although not in the amounts necessary to fully implement the elimination program. In the late 1980s, the incidence of TB began to rise, reaching a peak in 1992, when 26,673 cases were reported. There was a 20 percent increase in reported numbers of cases between 1985 and 1992. Assuming that the reported incidence should have continued to decline at the rate it did from 1980 to 1985, it is estimated that more than 63,000 excess cases of TB occurred during the period 1986–1992.

The increase during the period 1986–1992 was ascribed to at least four factors: (1) deterioration of the public health infrastructure; (2) immigration of persons from countries with high prevalence of TB; (3) the HIV epidemic; and (4) outbreaks of TB (particularly multidrug-resistant TB [MDR-TB]) in congregative settings such as hospitals, correctional facilities, and shelters for the homeless, among others.[49]

In response to the outbreaks of MDR-TB, a national task force was formed and developed the *National Action Plan to Combat Multidrug-Resistant Tuberculosis,* first released in April 1992.[50] Commitment of significant federal, state, and local resources to combat TB and implement the MDR-TB plan resulted in a rapid turn-around in incidence, and the number of reported TB cases in the United States has decreased steadily since 1992, reaching a record low of 13,779 in 2006, representing a 45 percent decline since 1993.[8] The reduction is attributed to more effective implementation of "standard" TB control strategies.[51] However, TB in immigrants remains an important issue, as does TB and HIV. In 2006, 56 percent of all cases occurred in persons born in another country; a high proportion occurred within five years of arrival, indicating they probably arrived in this country infected with TB. In addition, CDC estimates that 9 percent of all cases and nearly 16 percent of cases of TB in persons aged 25–44 years occur in HIV-infected individuals.[52]

Given the resurgence of TB in the late 1980s and the return to control in the 1990s, the ACET revisited the prospects for TB elimination and reaffirmed its call for the elimination of TB in the United States.[53] The IOM examined issues relating to TB control in the United States and issued a report *Ending Neglect,*[54] which endorsed the prospects for eliminating TB in the United States if sustained commitment to resources could be provided and if the United States increased its involvement in global TB control (to reduce the threat of imported TB).

WATERBORNE AND FOOD-BORNE DISEASES

A variety of parasitic, bacterial, and viral diseases can be transmitted through food and water. Disease results either from infection or from intoxication. Some diseases, such as giardiasis and typhoid fever, result from ingestion of small numbers of microorganisms that subsequently multiply and cause disease, either local or invasive. Others, such as cholera and diarrhea caused by enterotoxigenic *Escherichia coli,* result from ingestion of living bacteria that multiply and elaborate toxins, which act on intestinal mucosa to cause diarrhea. Some conditions such as botulism or Clostridium *perfringens* food poisoning result from ingestion of toxins formed by organisms multiplying in the food before it is eaten. Finally, some fish and shellfish may contain toxins that cause neuromuscular symptoms. Food and water can also carry natural or synthetic toxins (e.g., metals, plant toxins, and insecticides).

These illnesses may vary greatly in symptoms. Some are characterized by mild nausea, vomiting, and diarrhea (e.g., most *Salmonella* infections). Others may be associated with life-threatening profuse diarrhea (cholera), hemorrhagic diarrhea with hemolytic-uremic syndrome (E. coli 0157:H7), sepsis (typhoid), infectious hepatitis (hepatitis A), miscarriage (*Listeria monocytogenes*), or cranial nerve and respiratory paralysis (botulism).

Waterborne Diseases

Waterborne illness is now relatively uncommon in the United States as a result of the protection of water supplies, prevention of cross-connections between water and sewage systems, and chlorination. If municipal water supplies become contaminated, large numbers of persons may become ill. During a 1965 outbreak of waterborne salmonellosis in Riverside, California, an estimated 16,000 persons became ill.[55] More than 400,000 persons became ill with waterborne cryptosporidiosis in Milwaukee in 1993.[56]

During 2003–2004, CDC received reports on 36 outbreaks (from 19 states) associated with drinking water or water not intended for drinking, causing more than 2000 persons to become ill. The causative agent was identified for 25 (83.3%) of the outbreaks—17 involved pathogens (13 bacterial, 1 parasitic, 1 viral, and 2 mixed), and eight involved chemical/toxin poisonings. Additionally, there were 62 outbreaks (from 28 states) attributed to recreational water exposure, also affecting more than 2000 persons. Thirty of these were outbreaks of gastroenteritis that resulted from infectious agents, chemicals, or toxins; 13 were outbreaks of dermatitis; 7 were outbreaks of acute respiratory illness; 4 represented single cases of amebic meningoencephalitis, meningitis, leptospirosis, and otitis externa; and 8 represented mixed illnesses.[57]

Food-Borne Diseases

Prevention of **food-borne illness** involves preventing initial contamination; cooking foods properly to destroy organisms that are present; preventing cross-contamination or recontamination (as can occur when cooked foods are sliced with a knife or on a cutting board contaminated by raw food or are placed back in containers from which they came before cooking); preventing incubation of microorganisms by keeping cold foods cold and hot foods hot; and ensuring other appropriate food-handling practices.

Food-borne illness remains common and has been estimated to cause 6.5 million cases of human illness and 9000 deaths annually in the United States.[58] However, only a small proportion of the outbreaks estimated to occur are actually reported. During 1998–2002, a total of 6647 outbreaks of food-borne disease were reported to the CDC, causing 128,370 persons to become ill.[59] The etiology was known for only 33 percent of the reported outbreaks; these accounted for 54 percent of reported illnesses. Of the outbreaks with known etiology, 55 percent were caused by bacterial pathogens, 31 percent by viral pathogens (primarily norovirus),

10 percent by chemical agents, and 1 percent by parasites.

During the period 1998–2002, fully half of the outbreaks were associated with restaurants or delicatessens. Several different types of outbreaks were reported, including multistate outbreaks caused by ground beef contaminated with *E. coli* 0157:H7; and fresh produce contaminated with *Salmonella*, *E. coli* 0157:H7, *Cyclospora cayetanensis*, or hepatitis A. Multidrug-resistant strains of *Salmonella* caused outbreaks linked to unpasteurized milk and ground beef. A large multistate outbreak of listeriosis caused by contaminated deli meat led to one of the largest food recalls in the United States.[60] The factors most commonly reported as contributing to the outbreaks included improper (bare-handed) handling of food, improper holding temperatures of foods, and inadequate cooking of food.

Table 22.3. Examples of New Disease/Organism Recognition

Year	Condition
1973	Rotavirus
1975	Parvovirus
1976	*Cryptosporidium parvum*
1977	Ebola virus
1977	*Legionella pneumophila*
1977	Hantaan virus
1980	HTLV-1
1981	Toxin-producing S. aureus
1982	*E. coli* 0157:H7
1982	*Borrelia burgdorferi*
1983	HIV
1983	*Helicobacter pylori*
1988	HHV-6
1989	Hepatitis C
1992	Bartonella henselae
1993	Sin nombre virus
1995	HHV-8

EMERGING/REEMERGING DISEASES AND ANTIBIOTIC RESISTANCE

Although we are making progress against many infectious diseases, we continue to recognize new diseases or discover infectious causes for already known conditions. Table 22.3 shows the year of recognition of selected new diseases or etiologic agents over the past 30 years. In 1973, rotaviruses were recognized as major causes of childhood diarrhea. Ebola virus was first recognized in the late 1970s, as were *Legionella pneumophila* (causative agent of Legionnaire's disease and Pontiac fever) and toxin-producing *Staphylococcus aureus* (causative agent of toxic shock syndrome). *E. coli* 0157:H7 (cause of hemorrhagic colitis and hemolytic-uremic syndrome) was first recognized in 1982, and HIV was first identified in 1983. It has only been in the past 25 years that we have learned that *Helicobacter pylori* is the primary cause of duodenal ulcer disease.[61]

Diseases known to occur in one part of the world may be introduced to other parts of the world with devastating consequences, as occurred during the European colonization of the Americas, when significant proportions of the indigenous population were killed by smallpox and measles. Modern transportation means that virtually any infectious disease is only an airplane ride away. Other diseases, for example, West Nile virus, may be introduced from other countries by means which are yet unknown.[62]

In addition to the recognition of new diseases, diseases once under control have an ability to reemerge. This happened in the United States with TB in the late 1980s as a result of lack of continued application of effective control measures. Changing ecological circumstances can also favor increases in new or old infectious diseases. Some of these factors include population growth, crowding, migration, urbanization, changes in behavior, changes in ecology, and modern travel and trade.

Development of resistance to antibiotics has led to the reemergence of some previously controlled conditions. Major factors leading to resistance are the indiscriminate, inappropriate, inadequate, incomplete, and inconsistent use of antibiotics. Each of these factors can result in selection of strains of microorganisms that are resistant to the drugs being used. *Streptococcus pneumoniae*, the causative agent of pneumococcal pneumonia and pneumococcal meningitis, was initially exquisitely sensitive to penicillin. However, a study of United States medical centers in 1997–1998 found that 29.5 percent of strains were at least partially resistant to penicillin, and 12.1 percent were fully resistant.[63]

Prevention of the emergence of additional strains of antimicrobial-resistant microorganisms will require concerted action to ensure that antibiotics are used appropriately.

BIOTERRORISM

Biological agents have long been used in warfare, and their use has presumably come to an end as a result of international accords. As concerns about biological warfare have decreased, concerns about **bioterrorism** have come to the fore. The prospect exists that individuals or groups could use biological agents as political weapons, and there have been isolated incidents in which this has been documented.[64] CDC convened a workgroup that developed a strategic plan for preparedness and response to biological and chemical terrorism.[65] The plan outlines a series of steps to prepare public health agencies for biological attacks, focusing on surveillance, education, and communication. Development of new diagnostic tests and stockpiling appropriate vaccines and drugs were also recommended. The agents/diseases thought most likely to be used as bioterrorism weapons included smallpox, anthrax, plague, botulism, tularemia, and viral hemorrhagic fevers (e.g., Ebola, Lassa). The purposeful spread of anthrax through the mail on the East Coast of the United States in the Fall of 2001 verified the necessity for improving capacities at all levels to identify and respond to biologic agents dispersed as weapons of terror.[66] (See especially Chapter 23, but also Chapters 3, 11, 13, 29, and 31.)

SUMMARY

Voltaire's phrase "the best is the enemy of the good"[67] applies to HIV prevention and to other infectious disease prevention and control measures. In some situations, the insistence on only the "best" solution to a given health problem may interfere with the incremental, partially effective steps that are collectively necessary in mounting effective (but not perfect) prevention programs. In fact, if the imperfect approach is more acceptable to the target population than the perfect one, it may ultimately have a greater effect on the occurrence of disease.

The HIV epidemic and other major infectious disease health problems do not happen in the same way or at the same rate in all groups. Nor are they uniformly susceptible to any single intervention. Controlling the HIV epidemic and solving other problems will require different, mutually reinforcing techniques to reach the myriad groups in this pluralistic society. Until more effective (or even "perfect") approaches are available, partially effective approaches should be more fully implemented. The world is not a perfect place, and the quest for solutions must reflect that fact.[68]

Infectious diseases remain significant causes of morbidity and mortality in the United States and are even greater problems in developing countries. The current favorable situation in the United States is a reflection of the active prevention and control measures that have been applied. However, it must be remembered that infectious diseases are merely being kept at bay. Unless they are eradicated, relaxation of control efforts can and will lead to a resurgence of disease. In addition, new infectious diseases are being recognized that pose new threats to health and necessitate maintenance of surveillance and response capability.[69]

REVIEW QUESTIONS

1. What are the four means by which infectious diseases are transmitted?
2. What are the seven major steps of outbreak investigation?
3. How are immunization recommendations developed in the United States?
4. How do you assess vaccine efficacy?
5. What are the elements of STD control programs in the United States?
6. What are the components of TB prevention and control in the United States?
7. What are the primary approaches to prevention of food-borne illness?

REFERENCES

1. World Health Organization. Health systems: Improving performance. *World Health Report 2000*. Geneva, Switzerland: WHO; 2000.
2. Heymann DL, ed. *Control of Communicable Diseases Manual*. 18th ed. Washington, DC: American Public Health Association; 2005.
3. Gustafson TL, Lavely GB, Brawner ER Jr, et al. An outbreak of airborne nosocomial varicella. *Pediatrics*. 1982;70:550–556.
4. Bloch A, Orenstein WA, Ewing WM, et al. Measles outbreak in a pediatric practice: Airborne transmission in an office setting. *Pediatrics*. 1985; 75:676–683.
5. Orenstein WA, Bernier RH. Surveillance: Information for action. *Pediatr Clin North Am*. 1990;37: 709–734.
6. Strebel PM, Sutter RW, Cochi SL, et al. Epidemiology of poliomyelitis in the United States one decade after the last reported case of indigenous wild virus-associated disease. *Clin Infect Dis*. 1992;14:568–579.
7. Centers for Disease Control and Prevention. General recommendations on immunization: Recommendations of the Advisory Committee on Immunization Practices (ACIP) and the American Academy of Family Physicians (AAFP). *MMWR*. 2006;55(RR1):1–48.
8. Centers for Disease Control and Prevention. Final 2006 reports of notifiable diseases *MMWR*. 2007;56:851–863.
9. Centers for Disease Control and Prevention. Progress toward eliminating *Haemophilus influenzae* type b disease among infants and children— United States, 1987–1997. *MMWR*. 1998;47: 993–998.
10. Katz SL, Hinman AR. Summary and conclusions: Measles elimination meeting, 16–17 March 2000. *JID* 2004;189(Suppl 1):S43–S47.
11. Centers for Disease Control and Prevention. Achievements in public health: Elimination of rubella and congenital rubella syndrome—United States, 1969–2004. *MMWR*. 2005;54:279–282.
12. Centers for Disease Control and Prevention. National, state, and urban vaccination coverage levels among children aged 19–35 months— United States, 2006. *MMWR*. 2007;56: 880–885.
13. Centers for Disease Control and Prevention. Influenza and pneumococcal vaccine coverage among persons aged >65 years—United States, 2004–2005. *MMWR*. 2006;55:1065–1068.
14. American Academy of Pediatrics. *Report of the Committee on Infectious Diseases*. 27th ed. Elk Grove Village, IL: American Academy of Pediatrics; 2006.
15. Centers for Disease Control and Prevention. Immunization schedules. Available at: http:// www.cdc.gov/vaccines/recs/schedules/default .htm. Accessed February 7, 2008.
16. Centers for Disease Control and Prevention. Immunization of health-care workers: Recommendations of the Advisory Committee on Immunization Practices (ACIP) and the Hospital Infection Control Practices Advisory Committee (HICPAC). *MMWR*. 1997;46(RR18):1–42.
17. Orenstein WA, Rodewald LE, Hinman AR, Schuchat A. Immunization in the United States. In: Plotkin SA, Orenstein WA, Offit P, eds. *Vaccines*. 5th ed. (Chapter 67). Philadelphia, PA: Saunders Elsevier; 2008.
18. Centers for Disease Control and Prevention. Vaccines for Children program. Available at: http://www.cdc.gov/programs/immun10.htm. Accessed November 6, 2006.
19. Centers for Disease Control and Prevention. Vaccination coverage among children in Kindergarten—United States, 2006–2007 school year. *MMWR*. 200;56:819–821.
20. National Vaccine Advisory Committee. Development of community and state-based immunization registries, January 12, 1999. Available at:

http://www.cdc.gov/vaccines/programs/iis/pubs/nvac.htm. Accessed January 9, 2008.

21. US Department of Health and Human Services. *Healthy People 2010*, Objective 14–26. Washington, DC; US Dept of Health and Human Services; 2000.

22. Institute of Medicine. *Calling the Shots: Immunization Finance Policies and Practices*. Washington, DC; National Academy Press; 2000.

23. Orenstein WA, Bernier RH, Dondero TJ, et al. Field evaluation of vaccine efficacy. *Bull WHO*. 1985;63:1055–1068.

24. Robbins FC, de Quadros CA. Certification of the eradication of indigenous transmission of wild poliovirus in the Americas. *J Infect Dis*. 1997; 175(suppl 1):S281–S285.

25. Centers for Disease Control and Prevention. Poliomyelitis prevention in the United States: Updated recommendations of the Advisory Committee on Immunization Practices (ACIP). *MMWR*. 2000;49(RR05):1–22.

26. Centers for Disease Control and Prevention. Update: Vaccine side effects, adverse reactions, contraindications, and precautions. Recommendations of the Advisory Committee on Immunization Practices (ACIP). *MMWR*. 1996;45(RR12): 1–35.

27. Chen RT, DeStefano F, Davis RL, et al. The Vaccine Safety Datalink: Immunization research in health maintenance organizations in the USA. *Bull WHO*. 2000;78:186–194.

28. Hinman AR. Children, vaccines, and risks. *J Children's Health*. 2003;1:309–321.

29. Centers for Disease Control and Prevention. Intussusception among recipients of rotavirus vaccine—United States, 1998–1999. *MMWR*. 1999;48:577–581.

30. Cates W Jr, Hinman AR. Sexually transmitted diseases in the 1990s. *N Engl J Med*. 1991;325: 1368–1370.

31. Hinman AR, Wasserheit HN, Kamb MI. Potential impact of STD prevention programmes. In: Rashad H, Gray R, Boerna T, eds. *Evaluation of the Impact of Health Interventions*. Liège, Belgium: International Union for the Scientific Study of Population; 1995.

32. Centers for Disease Control and Prevention. *The National Plan to Eliminate Syphilis from the United States*. Atlanta, GA: US Dept of Health and Human Services, CDC, National Center for HIV, STD, and TB Prevention; 1999: 1–84.

33. Centers for Disease Control and Prevention. Primary and secondary syphilis—United States, 1999. *MMWR*. 2001;50:113–117.

34. Centers for Disease Control and Prevention, STD Surveillance 2006. Available at: http://www.cdc.gov/std/stats/toc2006.htm. Accessed October 21, 2008.

35. Centers for Disease Control and Prevention. Syphilis elimination effort (SEE). Available at: http://www.cdc.gov/stopsyphilis/SEEexec2006.htm. Accessed November 10, 2006.

36. Centers for Disease Control and Prevention. Pneumocystis pneumonia—Los Angeles. *MMWR*. 1981;30:250–252.

37. Sepkowitz KA. AIDS—the first 20 years. *N Engl J Med*. 2001;344:1764–1772.

38. Centers for Disease Control and Prevention. HIV and AIDS—United States, 1981–2000. *MMWR*. 2001;20:430–434.

39. Centers for Disease Control and Prevention. HIV/AIDS basic statistics. Available at: http://www.cdc.gov/hiv/topics/surveillance/basic.htm. Accessed October 21, 2008.

40. Anderson RM. The transmission dynamics of sexually transmitted diseases: The behavioral component. In: Wasserheit JN, Aral SO, Holmes KK, Hitchcock PJ, eds. *Research Issues in Human Behavior and Sexually Transmitted Diseases in the AIDS Era*. Washington, DC: American Society of Microbiology; 1992:61–80.

41. Brunham RC, Ronal AR. Epidemiology of sexually transmitted diseases in developing countries. In: Wasserheit JN, Aral SO, Holmes KK, Hitchcock PJ, eds. *Research Issues in Human Behavior and Sexually Transmitted Diseases in the AIDS Era*. Washington, DC: American Society of Microbiology; 1991:38–60.

42. Centers for Disease Control and Development. Sexually Transmitted Diseases Treatment Guidelines, 2006. *MMWR*. 2006;55(RR-11):1–94.

43. Hinman AR. Strategies to prevent HIV infection in the United States. *Am J Public Health*. 1991;81:1557–1559.

44. Centers for Disease Control and Prevention. Advancing HIV prevention: New strategies for a changing epidemic. Available at: http://www.cdc.gov/hiv/topics/prev_prog/AHP/resources/factsheets/progress_2005.htm. Accessed November 13, 2006.

45. Centers for Disease Control and Prevention. Revised recommendations for HIV testing of

adults, adolescents, and pregnant women in health-care settings. Available at: http://www.cdc .gov/mmwr/preview/mmwrhtml/rr5514a1.htm. Accessed November 13, 2006.

46. Selwyn PA, Hartel D, Lewis VA, et al. A prospective study of the risk of tuberculosis among intravenous drug users with human immunodeficiency virus infection. *N Engl J Med.* 1989;320:545–550.

47. American Thoracic Society. Intermittent chemotherapy for adults with tuberculosis. *Am Rev Respir Dis.* 1974;110:374–375.

48. Centers for Disease Control and Prevention. A strategic plan for the elimination of tuberculosis in the United States. *MMWR.* 1989;38(S-3):1–25.

49. Cantwell MF, Snider DE, Cauthen GM, Onorato IM. Epidemiology of tuberculosis in the United States, 1985 through 1992. *JAMA.* 1994;272: 535–539.

50. Centers for Disease Control and Prevention. National action plan to combat multidrug-resistant tuberculosis. *MMWR.* 1992;41(RR-11):1–48.

51. McKenna MT, McCray E, Jones JL, et al. The fall after the rise: Tuberculosis in the United States, 1992 through 1994. *Am J Public Health.* 1998; 88:1059–1063.

52. Centers for Disease Control and Prevention. The deadly intersection between TB and HIV. Available at: http://www.cdc.gov/hiv/resources/ factsheets/hivtb.htm. Accessed February 4, 2008.

53. Advisory Council for the Elimination of Tuberculosis (ACET). Tuberculosis elimination revisited: Obstacles, opportunities, and a renewed commitment. *MMWR.* 1999;48(RR09):1–13.

54. Institute of Medicine. *Ending Neglect: The Elimination of Tuberculosis in the United States.* Washington, DC; National Academy Press; 2000.

55. Collaborative Report: A waterborne epidemic of salmonellosis in Riverside, California, 1965. *Am J Epidemiol.* 1971;93:33.

56. MacKenzie W, Hoxie N, Proctor M, et al. A massive outbreak in Milwaukee of Cryptosporidium infection transmitted through the public water supply. *N Engl J Med.* 1994;331:161–167.

57. Centers for Disease Control and Prevention. Surveillance for waterborne-disease and outbreaks associated with recreational water—United States, 2003–2004 and Surveillance for waterborne disease and outbreaks associated with drinking water and water not intended for drinking—United States, 2003–2004. *MMWR.* 2006;55(SS-12): 1–65.

58. Bennett JV, Holmberg SD, Rogers MF, Solomon SL. Infectious and parasitic diseases. In: Amler RW, Dull HB, eds. Closing the gap: The burden of unnecessary illness. *Am J Prev Med.* 1987; 3(suppl):102–114.

59. Centers for Disease Control and Prevention. Surveillance for foodborne-diseases outbreaks— Untied States, 1998–2002. *MMWR.* 2006; 55(SS-10):1–38.

60. Centers for Disease Control and Prevention. Outbreak of listeriosis—Northeastern United States, 2002. *MMWR.* 2002;51:950–951.

61. Committee on International Science, Engineering, and Technology. Infectious Disease—A global health threat. Washington, DC: US Government Printing Office; 1995.

62. Nash D, Mostashari F, Fine A, et al. The outbreak of West Nile virus infection in the New York City area in 1999. *N Engl J Med.* 2001;344:1807–1814.

63. Doem GV, Brueggemann AB, Huynh H, et al. Antimicrobial resistance with Streptococcus pneumoniae in the United States, 1997–1998. *Emerg Infect Dis.* 1999;5:757–765.

64. Torok TJ, Tauxe RV, Wise RP, et al. Large community outbreak of salmonellosis caused by intentional contamination of restaurant salad bars. *JAMA.* 1997;278:389–395.

65. Centers for Disease Control and Prevention. Biological and chemical terrorism: Strategic plan for preparedness and response. Recommendations of the CDC Strategic Planning Workgroup. *MMWR.* 2000;49(RR-4):1–5.

66. Centers for Disease Control and Prevention. Update: Investigation of anthrax associated with intentional exposure and interim public health guidelines, October, 2001. *MMWR.* 2001;50: 889–893.

67. Kaplan J, ed. *Bartlett's Familiar Quotations.* 16th ed. Boston: Little Brown & Co; 1992: 306.

68. Cates W Jr, Hinman AR. AIDS and absolutism: The demand for perfection in prevention. *N Engl J Med.* 1992;327:492–494.

69. Lederberg J, Shope RE, Oaks SC Jr, eds. *Emerging Infections: Microbial Threats to Health in the United States.* Washington, DC: National Academy Press; 1992.

CHAPTER 23

Public Health Preparedness

Linda Young Landesman, DrPH, MSW, Isaac B. Weisfuse, MD, MPH, and Susan Waltman, JD, MSW

LEARNING OBJECTIVES

Upon completion of this chapter, the reader will be able to:

1. Describe types of disasters.
2. Describe the types of public health problems caused by disasters.
3. Understand the key components of health system preparedness.
4. Describe the role of local departments of health in preparing and responding to emergencies.
5. Understand the assets that the federal government is able to provide in response to an emergency.

KEY TERMS

All-Hazards Plans
Biodetection
Command Center
Community Mitigation
Covert
Disasters
Emergency Management Assistance Compact (EMAC)

Emergency Management
Emergency Management Authority (EMA)
Emergency Support Functions (ESF)
ESF 8
Emergency System for the Advance Registration of Health Professions Volunteers (ESAR-VHP)
First Responder
Hazard Vulnerability Analysis (HVA)
Hospital Incident Command System (HICS)
Incident Command System (ICS)
Incident Commander
Incident Action Plan (IAP)
Job Action Sheets
The Joint Commission
Laboratory Response Network (LRN)
Mitigation
Mutual Aid
Medical Reserve Corps (MRC)
National Incident Management System (NIMS)
National Response Framework (NRF)
National Disaster Medical System
Disaster Medical Assistance Teams
Disaster Mortuary Operational Response Teams (DMORT)

Disaster Portable Morgue Unit Team

National Nurse Response Team

National Pharmacy Response Teams

Veterinary Medical Assistance Teams

Overt

Pandemic Influenza

Point of Distribution Sites (PODs)

Preparedness

Presidential Disaster Declaration

Recovery

Redundancies

Response

Seasonal Influenza

Sectors

Sentinel

Span of Control

Stafford Act

Strategic National Stockpile (SNS)

Syndromic Surveillance

Vulnerable Populations

Warning or Forecasting

WHAT IS A DISASTER?

Disasters have been defined as natural or man-made hazards that result in ecologic disruptions, or emergencies, of such severity and magnitude that they result in deaths, injuries, illness, or property damage that cannot be effectively managed by the application of routine procedures or resources and that result in a call for outside assistance. Historically, preparedness and response activities have been organized around the events before the disaster (pre-impact), while it is occurring (impact), and during recovery (post-impact). Injury, illness, or death can be reduced or prevented by the actions taken by public health professionals, emergency management officials, and the population at risk during all three periods.

The basic phases of disaster management include mitigation or prevention, warning and preparedness, response, and recovery. **Mitigation** includes actions to reduce the harmful effects of a disaster, such as those that may prevent further loss of life, disease, disability, or injury. **Warning,** or **forecasting,** refers to monitoring events for indicators that signify when and where a disaster might occur and what its magnitude might be. In **preparedness,** officials or the public plan a response

to potential disasters and, in so doing, lay the framework for recovery.

Across the globe, mankind is experiencing an increase in both natural and technological disasters, as evidenced by both events in recent years[1,2] and statistical trends.[3] A disaster that requires external international assistance occurs, on average, once a day, somewhere in the world. In 2005 alone, approximately 1.5 million people were affected worldwide and $100 billion was lost in property damage as a consequence of these disasters.[4] One of the deadliest disasters in modern history occurred on December 26, 2004, when the Sumatra-Andaman earthquake struck the Indian Ocean. This earthquake, the fourth largest since 1900, with a magnitude of 9.15, generated a tsunami that destroyed coastal areas in 14 countries in South Asia and as far away as East Africa, killing more than 225,000 people.[5] The tsunami, like the other major disasters, resulted in the need for public health intervention with diverse populations for prolonged periods.

Natural Disasters

In the past century, 8.1 million people were affected by more than 600 natural disasters, or naturally occurring events, that struck the United States.[6] Large portions of the population in the United States, located in every region of the country, are at risk today from just three types of natural disasters: earthquakes, floods, and hurricanes. While most people think of California as the most earthquake-prone state, 39 states containing more than 70 million residents are seismically active. More than 6,000 developed communities, with populations of 2,500 or more persons, are located in flood plains.[7] Further, it is estimated that by 2010, more than 127 million people, more than one-third of the population, will live in coastal areas of the United States, including the Great Lakes region.[8] The significance of this concentration is evident when the risk posed just by hurricanes is examined. The National Oceanic and Atmospheric Administration has noted an increasing trend in hurricane activity since 1995, consistent with a multi-decadal climate pattern that is predicted to last for many more years. The 2005 Atlantic hurricane season was the most active season on record, with 28 storms, including 15 hurricanes. More than half of the seven "major" hurricanes that season (Dennis, Katrina, Rita, and

---

EXHIBIT 23-1 Hurricane Disaster: Floyd

On September 16, 1999, Hurricane Floyd struck the North Carolina coastline with high winds and 20 inches of rainfall. More than 2 million people were affected by widespread flooding along the area's five rivers. The flooding, exacerbated by a previous and then a subsequent hurricane, most severely affected rural inland counties, destroying agriculture and livestock farms, and drowning millions of chickens and hundreds of thousands of pigs. Floodwaters swept through sewage plants, contaminating the water supply. Ten states were declared disaster areas, more than 7,000 homes destroyed, and more than two million people were evacuated.

Public Health Implications: Hurricane Floyd and its associated flash flooding caused more than 50 deaths and many injuries. Most deaths resulted from drowning when occupants were trapped in submerged vehicles. Other causes included motor vehicle accidents, heart attacks, burns and trauma suffered during escape attempts, hypothermia, electrocution, and falls. Injuries were caused by clean-up and debris. Illnesses during the recovery stage included asthma and diarrhea, which were associated with the mold and mildew damage to homes and with outbreaks in shelters. This natural disaster is also believed to have caused a significant increase in suicides, dog bites, febrile illnesses, basic medical needs, dermatitis,

arthropod bites, diarrhea, violence, and hypothermia. Following the storm, there was a high demand for first responders and increased need for public health surveillance.

Public Health Interventions: Communities around the state responded by initiating evacuations, opening shelters, and issuing public service announcements about the dangers of driving on flooded roads. Public health response teams conducted daily surveillance, in hospitals, shelters, and the community, to track communicable diseases, injuries, and environmental issues, such as ground, water, and air pollution. The North Carolina Department of Health (NCDOH) coordinated its efforts with numerous governmental agencies (e.g., health and environment, emergency management, cooperative extension, and building inspectors). NCDOH also issued guidelines to prevent outbreaks, manage chemical hazards, control for mosquitoes and other vectors, bury animal carcasses, and deal with mental health issues. Key activities were assurance of safe housing, drinking water, and sanitation. Home inspections were conducted to test flooded wells and general water supplies. Local departments of health (DOH) provided instruction on disinfecting wells and issued guidelines for the reopening of restaurants and other food service institutions.

EXHIBIT 23-2 Cold Weather Disaster: New England Ice Storm

In January 1998, an ice storm struck the Northeastern United States. In Maine, 3 days of rain and below-freezing ground temperatures resulted in heavy accumulations of ice on trees and electric power lines. An estimated 600,000 persons lost electrical power, and 50,000 households still were without power 9 days after the storm. All 16 Maine counties were declared federal disaster areas.

Public Health Implications: The hospital emergency departments (EDs) in the heaviest hit area treated nearly 50 percent more patients in the post-storm period compared to the same time period the previous year. The increase in visits to the ED was attributed in part to "provider shifting," because many physicians' offices were closed due to loss of power. The lack of utilities in the middle of winter produced dangerous situations for those whose homes were heated with electricity as people turned to alternative power sources, for example, gas-powered generators. As a result, many people required emergency medical

treatment for CO poisoning. In addition, incidences of cold exposure, burns, lower respiratory tract infection, and cardiac conditions increased.

Public Health Interventions: The initial community response focused on the mobilization of town and county road crews, utility workers, EMS personnel, the National Guard, and volunteer organizations to clear roads, restore utilities, and relocate people (on a volunteer basis) to heated shelters, particularly those most vulnerable, such as the elderly, the disabled, and families with young children. In addition, the Centers for Disease Control and Prevention (CDC) and the Maine Bureau of Health (MBOH) conducted a needs assessment and morbidity surveillance in the area EDs. On learning that only a fraction (8 percent) of households with power outages reported having a working CO detector, and given the increase in CO poisonings, MBOH initiated public service announcements about the hazards of CO coupled with community outreach and CO monitoring in cooperation with the local fire departments.

Wilma) struck the United States, with catastrophic consequences.[9] Hurricane Katrina claimed approximately 1200 lives and caused damages estimated at $75 billion just in the New Orleans area.[10] More than two years later, the region has barely recovered.

Manmade or Technological Disasters

Like natural disasters, manmade or technological disasters, events caused by human action or technological breakdown, have also increased worldwide with devastating impacts on the public's health.[11] In the past century, the United States alone experienced more than 300 technological accidents that killed 14,558 people and injured 24,481.[6] The aging and crumbling infrastructure of U.S. cities

increases our vulnerability for disruptions of daily life that can range from water main breaks, which release asbestos, to bridge collapses. Technological or industrial accidents, such as the 1984 chemical accident in Bhopal or the 1979 partial nuclear accident at Three Mile Island, could easily have been as devastating as the nuclear plant meltdown at Chernobyl in 1986. The 1992 civil unrest in Los Angeles caused 53 deaths, more than 2000 injuries, and the destruction or closure of 15 county health centers, 45 pharmacies, and 38 medical and dental offices. There were also significant impacts to the quality of water, to hazardous materials and solid waste, and to protecting sources of food. Because widespread burning, as occurred during the civil unrest, can release hazardous materials into the air, almost 3000 sites were surveyed for the release of hazardous waste.[12]

EXHIBIT 23-3 Technological Disaster: Oklahoma City Bombing

On April 19, 1995, at 9:02 a.m., a bomb destroyed the Alfred P. Murrah Federal Building in downtown Oklahoma City, Oklahoma. This domestic terrorist act killed 168 people, including 19 children and 1 rescue worker; injured more than 800 people; and damaged or destroyed more than 300 surrounding buildings. A third of the city's residents knew someone who had been killed or injured in the blast.

Public Health Implications: Residents who lived near the site were displaced. Services were disrupted. The injured sought care en masse at local hospitals. Rescue workers were exposed to toxic smoke and other hazards, causing injuries

and illness. The community, rescue workers, and survivors, especially the children who had survived, experienced long-term mental health disorders.

Public Health Intervention: The medical response to the catastrophe was swift. Medical personnel from local hospitals ran to the scene. External teams were on site within hours setting up search-and-rescue and medical operations. Victims were quickly assessed, triaged, and treated or transported for appropriate care. Public health professionals conducted surveillance for injuries and illness and monitored the rescue workers for exposure-related illness and injuries.

Despite previous high-profile disasters in the United States, the most shocking manmade disaster occurred in 2001, when the World Trade Center in New York City and the Pentagon were attacked, resulting in the collapse of the World Trade Center's twin towers. More than 2600 people died at the World Trade Center, 125 died at the Pentagon, and 256 died on the four planes involved in this coordinated, multipronged attack.[13]

The actual and potential effects of manmade disasters will continue to escalate, generating an increased need for public health intervention as the world's population grows, population density increases, and technology becomes more sophisticated. The need for public health information has spurred the development of readily available guidance.[14,15]

Bioterrorism and Pandemic Influenza as an Emerging Infectious Disease

In recent years, health care professionals around the world have recognized the potential peril from bioterrorism and other emerging threats, such as Severe Acute Respiratory Syndrome (SARS) and

pandemic influenza. Should a massive infectious disease outbreak occur, public health professionals and the health sector would have difficulty containing and responding to the masses of people who would become sick or die.[16] Terrorist activity both within the United States and globally is increasing, and a number of experts suggest that the likelihood of a chemical or biological warfare (CBW) attack is also increasing.[17] In response to growing concerns for public safety in the face of these impending disasters, federal funding has been allocated to help the country prepare, including funding dedicated to bolstering the role of public health, discussed later in this chapter.

Bioterrorism Agents

To help prioritize preparedness efforts, the Centers for Disease Control and Prevention (CDC) developed a list of critical agents and grouped them into three categories. Category A agents are those with high impact and require the greatest preparedness. Category B has a lesser requirement for preparedness. Category C can be handled within current public health capacity. Of these diseases, only five Category A agents (anthrax, smallpox, plague, botulism, and tularemia) are considered serious threats. The

EXHIBIT 23-4 Emerging Infection Disaster: Severe Acute Respiratory Syndrome

Severe acute respiratory syndrome (SARS) is an emerging respiratory disease that resulted in thousands of diagnosed cases and worldwide mortality shortly after the turn of the twenty-first century. While SARS first presented as atypical pneumonia in China in 2002, the Chinese government did not report the new disease to the World Health Organization (WHO) until secondary cases had spread. Within a few months, cases were reported in other countries in Asia and in Canada. The disease rapidly spread around the globe, and its case fatality rate ranged from 9 to 17 percent.

Public Health Implications: SARS spreads quickly by close person-to-person contact, such as having cared for or lived with someone with SARS or having direct contact with respiratory secretions or body fluids of a SARS patient. The virus is thought to be transmitted by respiratory droplets when an infected person coughs or sneezes. The virus can also spread when a person touches a surface or object contaminated with infectious droplets and then touches his or her mouth, nose, or eye(s). SARS cannot be treated with antibiotics.

Patients are supported with antipyretics, oxygen, and ventilatory support as needed. Management includes strict isolation of suspected cases, preferably in negative-pressure rooms, with full barrier precautions for anyone coming in contact with these patients.

Public Health Interventions: By coordinating with governments, health care officials, workers, and scientists from around the globe, WHO spearheaded a model public health response to the SARS outbreak. The emphasis was international cooperation and rapid response to an emerging infectious disease. In the search for the responsible etiologic agent, a novel human coronavirus, SARS Hco-V, was discovered through genetic sequencing of case isolates. The outbreak was controlled by the development of a diagnostic case definition, detailed case reporting and contact tracing, and implementation of strict infection control protocols and international quarantine procedures. Governments around the world imposed restrictions on travel to and from the infected area, including total prohibition, and varying types of quarantines.

diseases can be categorized in three ways. The first is those diseases (anthrax, plague, and tularemia) that can be spread by an aerosolized release of bacteria producing pulmonary disease. The second category includes illness that is transmitted person-to-person, such as smallpox. The last category includes diseases caused by contaminated food, water, or other ingested material, such as botulinum toxin.

Overt and Covert Release

If the release of a biological agent is announced by those releasing it, the release is called **overt**. It is possible to assess overt threats and initiate a timely response to them, preventing most disease out-

breaks. The **covert,** or unannounced, release of a biologic agent, however, would present as illness in the community, and the initial release combined with contagious agents (people), would create the potential for large-scale spread of disease before detection. Covert dissemination of a biologic agent is most likely to be a terrorist act, providing little opportunity for early recognition and treatment before the onset of disease. Planners assume that exposed individuals will leave the scene of the release and not show signs of illness for hours, days, or weeks.

The first response to bioterrorism is at the local level, with detection dependent on public health surveillance and the integration of the health sector. Subsequent public health and health sector management is coordinated at local, state, and federal levels in predefined plans. For some diseases, early recognition and diagnosis of the disease is essential for preventing devastating outcomes, such as anthrax, for which treatment is usually effective only before the onset of severe symptoms. A release in an airport or among a highly mobile population could disseminate a highly infectious pathogen, such as smallpox, throughout most of the world before the epidemic would be recognized. To bring such an epidemic under control, a major multifocal international response would need to be activated.

Pandemic Influenza

Seasonal influenza, a common but frequently serious disease known as "flu," annually results in more than 200,000 hospitalizations, 36,000 to 40,000 deaths, and $1 billion to $3 billion in direct costs for medical care in the United States.[18] Influenza spreads rapidly and can be transmitted by those who are infected but asymptomatic, resulting in simultaneous escalating outbreaks in multiple communities. Influenza infections are responsible for secondary complications such as pneumonia, dehydration, and exacerbations of chronic respiratory and cardiac problems. Most individuals have some immunity to the circulating viruses either from previous infections or from vaccination, often moderating the spread or impact of the seasonal influenza virus.

Pandemic influenza, flu that spreads quickly around the world, occurs, on average, every three to four decades. Pandemics occur when a novel strain of the flu emerges. These unique viral strains are capable of causing significant morbidity and mortality because people have no immunity against them. Using projection models, public health authorities predict that the next influenza pandemic has the potential to infect 30 percent of the population of the United States, resulting in between 209,000 and 1.9 millions deaths.[19] Scientists and epidemiologists are currently concerned about a potential pandemic caused by the H5N1 virus, commonly referred to as the *avian flu.* To date, H5N1 avian influenza has primarily affected birds and has not been broadly transmitted among humans. However, the human mortality rate in those struck by avian flu is more than 50 percent, and sustained transmission from person-to-person would require a massive global response.

Three pandemics occurred in the last century— in 1918, 1957, and 1968. In past pandemics, influenza viruses spread worldwide within months. It took 2 months for the 1918 influenza to spread from American soldiers stationed in Europe to the citizens of their host countries. The 1957 Asian Flu spread to the United States within 4 to 5 months after detection in China. The spread of the 1968 pandemic was even quicker—it was detected in the United States only 2 to 3 months after being discovered in Hong Kong. In future pandemics, modern travel patterns will result in even faster spread. Importantly, the 2002–2003 pandemic outbreak of SARS demonstrated that countries worldwide must be ready to immediately implement their response plan once pandemic viruses have begun to spread.

While the spread of seasonal flu is contained by vaccination each year, the production and distribution of seasonal flu vaccine has not always guaranteed a timely or sufficient supply across the United States. Public health officials are concerned about the production and distribution of a vaccine for a novel influenza virus. Using current technology, the manufacture of a vaccine effective for a virus capable of causing a pandemic would take 6 to 8 months. Because seasonal flu vaccine is currently developed in advance, it may not match the virus strains that eventually circulate. In a pandemic, it is not certain whether manufacturers could produce enough vaccine even if an exact match were found. Further, the distribution system for influenza vaccines has been decentralized, making it difficult for public health officials to control the planning for or provide advanced direction about redistribution should a vaccine shortage occur. In an effort to alleviate some of these concerns, the federal government has earmarked more than $1 billion to develop cell-based vaccine and manufacturing capacity in the United States.[20]

THE PUBLIC HEALTH IMPLICATIONS OF DISASTERS

Disasters create public health challenges that require special preparation beyond the routine practice of disease prevention or health care delivery. Some tasks require the provision of emergency health care, such as triage and distribution of casualties, or having to function within a damaged or disabled health care infrastructure. Other tasks, such as warning and evacuating residents and reaching out to those with disabilities or other special needs, involve coordination with both private sector organizations and with multiple jurisdictions at all levels of government. To be effective managers and to respond effectively, public health professionals must work proficiently with emergency management and must be competent in the specialized set of skills needed for disaster related problems. For example, while temporary deficiencies in resources may occur in any disaster, in the United States, the problem with resources during disasters frequently is one of how assets are used or distributed, rather than one of deficiencies.[21] As a result, among other tasks, public health professionals could coordinate volunteers and manage the storage and distribution of relief materials. The **Strategic National Stockpile (SNS),** a federal source of medicine and medical supplies, has been used to supplement local provisions during public health emergencies.

Communities can experience public health consequences following all types of disasters. While not all disasters result in the same types of problems, commonalities exist in the interventions required in response to the most devastating events. Disasters cause a wide range of morbidity and mortality. As an example, storms, such as hurricanes and tornados, can result in broken bones; crush injuries, and other trauma; dehydration from being trapped without access to drinkable water; injury from cleanup activities; and death.

Floods can result in contamination from mold or mildew, drowning, diarrheal, skin, and waterborne diseases due to exposure to contaminated water or hazardous waste, and vector-borne diseases. In addition, there may be food shortages secondary to flooding. During heat waves people suffer cramps, dizziness, heatstroke, loss of consciousness, myocardial infarction (heart attack), stroke, and even death. Technological or manmade disasters can result in skin and respiratory exposure to hazardous agents, and in burns, injury and death.

Commonalities also exist in the types of services needed during a response. Many natural disasters disrupt the health care system, creating a greater need for the emergency provision of medical care for chronic health conditions, pregnancy and preterm deliveries, and even prescriptions, walking aides, and eyeglasses. Following the 1993 floods in the Midwest, victims increased their use of primary health care and experienced long-term impediments to their access to health care.[22] Local DOH in Missouri experienced interorganizational impediments to an effective response, such as burdensome coordination and difficulties in collecting and using assessment information.[23] Mass casualty events can result from earthquakes and explosions. Short-term humanitarian needs often occur as a result of all these events, including those for water, medicines, sanitation, shelter, food, logistics, and epidemiological surveillance. Long-term development and recovery needs also exist and vary depending on the extensiveness of the damage.

After a disaster has occurred, public health officials and emergency managers will determine the nature of relief efforts after reviewing a complex set of data. Response activities may vary depending on the demographic characteristics of the affected area; the assessment of casualties, including deaths, injuries, and selected illnesses; and the needs of the displaced population. During the 1995 heat wave in Chicago, high mortality demonstrated the need for standardized methodologies so that geographic comparisons could be made across the country.[24]

THE MENTAL HEALTH IMPACTS OF DISASTERS

Public health agencies and public health professionals are heavily involved in addressing the social and psychological impacts of disaster, and attention to these issues represents a core part of the public health profession's response to disaster.[25] All events have the potential for mental health sequelae, especially for widespread mental health risks for children and the elderly. Research shows that mental health problems can result from exposure to both natural and technological disasters.

The social and psychological impacts of a disaster can greatly exceed the number of physical injuries as these effects are less visible and have historically affected the functioning of individuals and communities for years postimpact. In general, the transient reactions that people experience after a disaster represent a normal response to a highly abnormal situation. Disasters are highly stressful, disruptive experiences which expose people to situations that are well outside the bounds of everyday experience.[26] While most individuals exposed to a disaster experience transient stress reactions,[76] a portion of the population may suffer more serious, persistent effects. The more persistent psychological problems include acute stress disorder (ASD), posttraumatic stress disorder (PTSD), depression, substance abuse, anxiety, and somatization. Other kinds of problems, including domestic violence, physical illness, and problems in daily functioning, have also been documented.[28] The extent to which disasters cause serious, long-lasting mental health impacts varies by the nature of the disaster and by the community.

Planning for mental health programs and services should be an integral part of the public health response to a disaster. Implementation should include informational and educational support about normal reactions, ways to handle reactions, and early treatment where indicated,[27] in addition to the many types of services required at family assistance centers and in long-term treatment.[15] Disasters can also profoundly affect the social health of communities. The Buffalo Creek dam failure in 1972 demonstrated that post-disaster efforts must include interventions to restore support networks and the health of the community as a whole. Following the flooding that dislocated 4000 people, an ill-conceived relocation effort effectively destroyed the social support system that held together the formerly tight-knit community.

Natural Disasters, Manmade Disasters, and Mental Health

Natural and manmade disasters, although differing in origin, have equally profound impacts on the mental health of victims and responders. While both types of events have in common the immediate threat of and the potential for ongoing disruption, there is a huge discrepancy between humans' perceived and actual control over these two kinds of disaster. People tend to see natural disasters simply as part of nature, over which we have no control. In contrast, manmade disasters are, in principle, preventable. Because we expect to be able to control technology, manmade disasters often produce higher levels of anger and distrust than natural disasters, because victims can direct blame and responsibility to those associated with causing the events.[28] Technological acts are also very scary because we may not know when the consequences caused by the event are over, making it difficult for those affected to move on.

THE PUBLIC HEALTH ASPECTS OF ENVIRONMENTAL SERVICES DURING DISASTERS

Following natural disasters, the infrastructure to prevent disease or provide safe water and food may be intact but not working, or it may be destroyed.

This is often the result of the destruction or inoperability of barriers, such as sewage plants and water-treatment operations, that protect populations from exposure to environmental hazards. The inventory of potential environmental exposures following a disaster is far-reaching, ranging from issues such as sanitation to hazardous materials. Public health professionals' task is to protect or to restart the protective barriers that exist, or to promote changes in behavior through educational messages that will compensate for the disrupted barriers. Examples of these messages include orders to boil water before using it, warnings about foods that may have spoiled during electrical outages, or announcements regarding where potable water will be provided. For displaced populations, all basic services usually need to be restarted from scratch.

Sanitation and Personal Hygiene

Disasters can disrupt or destroy sewage treatment plants. One of the first activities in disaster response should be re-establishing a sanitation system, if the system has been destroyed or interrupted. The use of latrines or other excreta-containment facilities has been shown to prevent diarrheal illness more than any other environmental measure following an emergency. While specific instructions for the re-establishment of sanitation systems are beyond the scope of this chapter, the appropriate type of facility varies among settings and cultures.

Hand washing, particularly after defecating and before preparing food, has been shown to protect against fecal–oral illnesses (including diarrhea). Therefore, soap should be provided in whatever latrine facilities are put in place, and public education should emphasize the importance of personal hygiene. Education alone, however, is not sufficient to change behavior, so any efforts to promote hand washing should be accompanied by a simple monitoring component to ensure that increased hand washing is actually occurring.[29]

Water: Quantity and Quality

After a disaster, ensuring the availability of safe drinking water is critical to preventing disease outbreaks. Once it has been determined that water service to an area has been affected by the disaster, public health professionals should arrange for the water to be lab tested, arrange for emergency distribution of bottled water, and educate the public about the necessary steps to take to ensure that water is safe.

The United Nations High Commissioner for Refugees (UNHCR) recommends that people need at least 4–5 gallons of water (15–20 liters) of water per person per day to maintain human health. During a crisis, available water and water consumption by each person should be estimated at least weekly. In areas with piped water, surveys can quickly determine which areas are lacking in water service. Where water service is expected to be inoperable, water often can be transported to the area by vehicle.

Lab testing can determine water quality, usually through detection of fecal coliforms, a bacterial measure that indicates whether water is safe to drink. Although these bacteria are not pathogenic, their presence is an early indication of fecal contamination and the likely presence of other pathogens. While the UNHCR considers water with less than 10 fecal coliforms per 100 mL to be reasonably safe, the current USEPA drinking water standard is either "positive" or "negative" for total coliform. Other indicator bacteria include *E. coli*, fecal streptococci, and total coliforms. Although water sources may provide water of variable quality, in many, even most, settings, proper handling and storage of water are critical. Studies have shown that water quality deteriorates over time after water is initially collected and that water contamination occurs where household buckets are dipped into water for distribution. The best way to ensure clean water is to add a chlorine residual to the water. This means that in unsanitary settings, or during times of outbreaks, it may be appropriate to chlorinate safe-source water.

Food and Shelter

Like ensuring the availability of safe water, providing food and shelter is also an essential component of disaster preparedness and response.

When electrical service is lost, refrigerated food is vulnerable to becoming spoiled. At such times, public health advisories and intervention are critical in protecting a population against foodborne disease. Advisories can be issued about food safety, spoilage, and how to properly handle food to avoid illness. Proper food handling includes correct storage, adequate cooking, and sufficient washing of hands and all utensils.

After a disaster, people who have lost or been evacuated from their homes must be sheltered. Evacuation or establishing shelters will be coordinated with local agencies, such as the American Red Cross (ARC). For people who cannot or do not evacuate, however, and remain in their homes, several things can be done to reduce their hardship. People in very cold climates, for example, can be given high-energy foods, blankets and sleeping bags, and plastic sheeting to cover windows and unused doorways. If possible, several people or households can share a common heated place. Also, where fuel is burned as a source of heat, public health officials should disseminate educational messages to warn people about the signs of carbon monoxide poisoning and to provide information on checking for gas leaks. In warmer climates, opaque plastic sheeting can be distributed to keep people dry during rainstorms and provide shade from the sun.

Vector Control

The disruption of the environment in a disaster often results in the growth of vector populations, increasing the risk of disease. Public health officials should assess a region after a disaster has struck it to determine whether potential environmental hazards exist, such as the growth of mosquito habitats or rodent- and fly-breeding sites. In the United States, mosquito spraying and monitoring can be major components of a post-hurricane public

health program. Mosquito monitoring is widespread in the United States and can be a useful tool following storms and floods for assessing the risks of mosquito-borne illnesses. Reducing mosquito-breeding sites, spraying, and providing area residents with netting and repellant are effective illness-prevention measures. Rat control may also be required, particularly where food is stored. Most food warehouses attempt to control rats with poisons, traps, or cats. Because garbage collection may be interrupted after a disaster, garbage should be stored in plastic bags and in containers that have tight-fitting lids, where possible.

Assessments for Other Environmental Hazards

The potential environmental problems posed by a disaster vary and include compromised air quality and accidental releases of toxic agents and radiation. In order to prepare effectively for all environmental risks, communities should undertake a *hazard vulnerability analysis* (HVA). An HVA analyzes and accounts for the probability and severity of various events that might occur in a locality as the result of a disaster, including potential impact on humans, property, and business. An HVA also projects the response needed and assesses internally and externally available resources. These community assessments enable residents to know in advance of hazards that could affect the health and safety of the community.

HOW DISASTER RESPONSE IS ORGANIZED

In the United States, the response to disasters is organized through multiple jurisdictions, agencies, and authorities that function at local, state, and federal levels. The term *emergency management* is used to refer to response activities. Emergency management groups organize their activities by **sectors,** such as fire, police, and emergency medical services

(EMS). Public health and health care organizations are part of the **health sector.**

After a disaster, a multi-organizational public health response is required because disasters typically generate needs beyond the mission of any one health care organization. The **response** phase of a disaster necessitates relief followed by recovery, including reconstruction of the community. Emergency relief activities include saving lives, providing first aid, restoring emergency communications and transportation systems, and providing immediate care and basic needs to survivors, such as food and clothing or medical and emotional care. **Recovery** includes actions for returning the community to normal, such as repairing infrastructure, damaged buildings, and critical facilities.

All states and many localities have an **emergency management authority (EMA),** sometimes called an office of emergency preparedness (OEP). It is the responsibility of the EMA, under the authority of each state's governor's office, to coordinate the use of all state assets during an emergency or disaster. These assets may be expansive and include the state's DOH, housing and social services agencies, and public safety agencies. While the organization of each state's EMA is unique, commonalities exist among EMAs. For example, each EMA coordinates statewide integration with federal agencies and local governments, and manages and coordinates information needed for response operations. Also, state and local agencies follow the procedures established in their disaster plans. The local and state EMAs establish a **command center** whose function is to coordinate the response of representatives from each of the numerous pertinent agencies. Called the **emergency operations center (EOC),** this command center is located away from the disaster site and oversees the emergency response. The DOH participates in the command center activities as a full partner.

The overriding jurisdictional principle in disaster response is that emergencies are local, and localities having primary responsibility for managing the response unless and until they request assistance or become overwhelmed. When the resources of a local jurisdiction are insufficient to respond to a disaster, the coordinating agency can seek help, called **mutual aid,** from surrounding jurisdictions or can escalate a request to the state or federal level, or both. States in many regions of the country are forming multistate, regional mutual aid compacts or consortia. These consortia can provide relatively rapid response throughout the area due to geographic proximity. Similar to these consortia, but larger, the **Emergency Management Assistance Compact (EMAC)** is a mutual aid agreement among all states in the United States. On request by the affected state(s), EMAC can rapidly facilitate the interstate provision of personnel and supplies to the affected areas. Using EMAC, professional liability and reimbursement are worked out in advance.

When response to events requires additional resources, federal aid is available through a **presidential disaster declaration,** which is enacted 40–70 times a year. This federal assistance for managing major disasters and emergencies is authorized through the **Stafford Act,** passed by Congress in 1988.[31] Under the Stafford Act, the president may approve allocation of federal resources, medicine, food and other consumables, manpower and services, and financial assistance. Requests for federal assets are initiated at the local level of government and forwarded to the state. The governor of a state makes the formal request for federal assistance, activating the declaration and initiating the flow of federal aid. While most presidential declarations are made immediately after a disaster strikes, a state's governor may submit a request before the disaster has occurred in situations where the consequences are imminent and warrant predeployment of assets to limit catastrophic impacts. Where indicated, the president has the authority to expedite the conveyance of federal resources by declaring a disaster prior to a state's request.

The Emergency Medical Services (EMS) System

For most disasters that occur suddenly, the initial medical response is provided by a local or regional

EMS system. In most parts of the United States, EMS is provided by semiautonomous local agencies with regional or state oversight. The EMS includes the pre-hospital system (e.g., public access, dispatch, EMTs/medics, and ambulance services) and the in-hospital system (e.g., emergency departments and inpatient care). EMS provides medical care known as **basic and advanced life support.** Basic life support includes noninvasive first aid and stabilization for a broad variety of emergency conditions, and semiautomatic defibrillation for cardiac arrest victims. Advanced life support, provided by paramedics, includes sophisticated medical diagnosis followed by on-site, protocol-driven medical treatment prior to and during transport to hospitals.

Incident Command Systems

In responding to a disaster, the effective coordination and management of the numerous activities and agencies are crucial. Drabek et al. found that the coordination of organizations, multiple activities, and local and external resources was among the most difficult and crucial challenges in managing a disaster response.[32] The **incident command system (ICS)** is the standard management structure used in disaster response across the United States.

ICS was developed by the California fire service after a difficult season indicated the need for better organization and management, and it facilitates multiple agencies working in coordination. While initially used by **first responders,** such as fire and police, and emergency management agencies, the ICS is now the system used by all health care organizations and agencies, including DOH, to organize their response.[33]

The goal of the ICS is to support an efficient and timely response by integrating communication and planning among many agencies, thereby eliminating duplicate efforts. Principles of the ICS include use of a common terminology, a modular organizational approach that may contract and expand depending on the needed response, management by objective, and accountability of personnel and resources. The ICS is flexible enough to be used in any type of incident. Key to the success of the ICS is its organization of tasks and functions into manageable components, known as *span of control.*

In the ICS, one individual from a facility or from an agency is in charge of the emergency response and decision-making process. This individual is referred to as the **incident commander.** The person who assumes this responsibility may vary depending on the response skills needed and the time and type of incident. Regardless of the type of incident, someone will assume the role of the incident commander.

Under an ICS framework, a number of additional standardized roles and positions are assigned depending on the incident. This standardization of roles within ICS facilitates effective communication among the different sectors involved in the response. A typical ICS structure includes operations, logistics, planning, and finance sections reporting to an incident commander. Individuals are designated for each function and each function has a predetermined list of duties and responsibilities. The tasks associated with each function are described in **Job Action Sheets.**

An **incident action plan (IAP),** or objectives and strategies for responding to the events, is usually established by the incident commander and planning section. An IAP for each operational period (e.g., 12 or 24 hours) helps focus the use of available resources for the highest priorities as the response activities change.

THE PREPAREDNESS OF THE FEDERAL GOVERNMENT

The federal government sets standards for public health emergency preparedness through the legislative process, allocation of funds, and oversight by the Department of Health and Human Services (DHHS) and Department of Homeland Security (DHS). In December 2006, the Pandemic and All-Hazards Preparedness Act (The Act) was passed,[34] consolidating responsibilities for public health emergency preparedness within the DHHS, under an Assistant Secretary for Preparedness and Response (Secretary). The Act mandates that benchmarks to measure preparedness be developed with funds potentially withheld from jurisdictions that do not meet these benchmarks. For the first time, starting in 2009, jurisdictions will need to report their monetary contribution to emergency preparedness. The Act tasks the Secretary to create near real-time, electronic situational awareness to provide information of emerging public health threats. Finally, it establishes a Biomedical Advanced Research and Development Authority to facilitate development of medical countermeasures including new drugs and vaccines.

There have been extensive federal preparations for emergency response. The DHS provides the framework for policy and operational directions during an emergency through its **National Response Framework (NRF)**.[35] The NRF delineates the roles of federal response agencies to "incidents of national significance," utilizing an ICS-based system called **National Incident Management System (NIMS)** for incident management. During the response, a federal coordination center called the Joint Field Office works with local and state authorities as an on-site federal presence.

The NIMS standards, promulgated by the DHS, provide guidance for coordinating all levels of governmental response across the country. Although NIMS is geared toward governmental agencies, it

---

EXHIBIT 23-5 Earthquake Disaster: Izmit, Turkey

During the early morning of August 17, 1999, an earthquake registering 7.4 on the Richter scale hit northwestern Turkey. The temblor struck a densely populated and industrialized region with inferior building construction, resulting in an estimated $6.5 billion in infrastructure damage, 17,000 deaths, and injuries to 44,000 people. The earthquake resulted in the simultaneous release of multiple hazardous materials (i.e., anhydrous ammonia, acrylonitrile, naphtha, and liquid petroleum) into air, soil, and water. Further, the earthquake generated a tsunami that caused serious coastal flooding.

Public Health Implications: In addition to the massive damage to the country's infrastructure, and the loss of more than 200,000 residential buildings and 30,500 businesses, the earthquake displaced approximately 600,000 individuals. More than 120 tent cities were erected to provide emergency temporary housing. To limit morbidity and further mortality, it was critical that disaster relief officials ensured proper sanitation, provided safe water and food, established medical care, limited overcrowding, and isolated individuals with communicable illnesses. The quake damaged the public health infrastructure,

so medical care was provided primarily through relief agencies and aid workers.

Public Health Interventions: The Turkish government and military responded by providing search-and-rescue teams and establishing emergency medical field stations and temporary tent cities to shelter displaced persons. Many international, national, and nongovernmental organizations assisted. The Turkish government requested that the U.S. Centers of Disease Control and Prevention (CDC) determine the immediate needs of the affected population. The CDC then conducted a needs assessment and morbidity surveillance that assessed food, water, housing, heating, and health care needs, as well as prevalent medical conditions. While the CDC found that the overall condition of the tent cities was good and the number of illnesses and injuries was low, its assessment identified potential improvements in the availability and distribution of medications for chronic conditions, the availability of social services (including mental health assistance), and the reporting of morbidity and mortality data to regional health offices.

also provides guidance for coordination with hospital based systems. Compliance with NIMS standards is now a requirement for receipt of any federal funding for emergency preparedness.

Emergency Support Functions (ESF) within the NRF provide detailed guidance for the actual response and delineate the roles and responsibilities of participating federal agencies. **ESF 8**—the Public Health and Medical Services Annex—covers public health emergencies and is overseen by the DHHS, which must assess the need for assistance on a number of issues such as surveillance, deployment of supplemental medical care personnel, worker health and safety, and patient care. Support comes from many other agencies, including DHS; the Departments of Defense, Energy, and Veterans Affairs; the Environmental Protection Agency; and the American Red Cross.

Voluntary Agencies

A vast array of voluntary agencies participate in disaster response with functions that contribute significantly to public health outcomes. Under the coordination of the Federal Emergency Management Agency, the American Red Cross (ARC) provides mass care, which includes providing shelter, food, emergency first aid, and family reunification, as well as distributing emergency relief supplies to disaster victims. ARC responds first through its local chapters, then through state and regional chapters, which may call on national-level ARC resources if necessary. Public health works closely with the ARC in the temporary shelters.

Numerous other voluntary agencies are involved in disaster response. Many of these are church affiliated, such as the Salvation Army, the Mennonite

---

EXHIBIT 23-6 Tornado Disaster: Alabama, 1994

A series of storms swiftly moved through five southern states on Sunday, March 27, 1994. One tornado, measuring F4 on the Fujita scale, raced through several Alabama counties, destroying three churches during their Sunday morning services. Thunderstorm warnings had been issued by the National Weather Service approximately 30 minutes before the event. However, because of the storm's speed, warnings were not issued to the public by local television and radio stations until mere minutes before the tornado touched ground. While the warnings urged citizens to seek shelter immediately, less than a third of those who heard the warnings were protected. More than 400 people were injured and 47 died, including 20 who were attending church.

Public Health Implications: In less than an hour, 144 people were seeking emergency medical care in a local hospital, and 57 of these required hospitalization. A survey of the effectiveness of the tornado warning system found significantly more

people learned of the tornado warning from a siren than from television or radio.

Public Health Intervention: Passing motorists helped transport the injured from the churches to nearby hospitals for treatment. While the local health care infrastructure remained intact, outside assistance was required from regional facilities in order to respond to the sudden, overwhelming demand on resources in local emergency departments. A makeshift morgue was erected at a National Guard armory. The town civic center was transformed into a shelter for the victims' families. Unfortunately, the response to the disaster was not well coordinated and rescue efforts were hampered by the lack of power and phone service. As a result, in 1996 a regional trauma system was implemented in the Birmingham, Alabama, Regional Emergency Medical Services System. This system covers a six-county area, which includes some of the counties hardest hit by the 1994 tornado.

Central Committee, and Catholic Relief Services. Some are dedicated solely to disaster-related functions, but most have more routine public service and emergency functions that are activated according to the needs of a specific disaster.*

A FRAMEWORK FOR HEALTH SECTOR PREPAREDNESS

Health care system preparedness depends heavily on the existence of a strong framework for regional collaboration and coordination among health care providers, medical and public health agencies, and emergency management authorities. It is important that individual providers and institutions, such as hospitals and outpatient clinics, are well trained in identifying, containing, and treating medical conditions that result from disasters. However, health care providers cannot prepare or respond effectively in isolation. It is essential that they work closely with local, state, and federal agencies and other organizations. The term *provider* is used here to refer to both individuals and health care institutions in the health sector.

Within the preparedness framework, many domains are the same for both health care facilities and DOH. Their specific tasks, however, are different. Hospitals have to be ready to provide medical care to many more people than normal. Sometimes that care is complicated by the type of emergency and the exposures that patients have had. DOH have to be ready to provide guidance, investigate population-wide issues and provide preventive care. In all instances, they should work in partnership to provide an effective and prompt response to the emergencies that they face.

The following sections describe how hospitals and DOH approach the same types of issues in ways that are consistent with their mission. The framework presented reflects the New York City region's approach to preparing for and responding to emergencies.**

Regional Collaboration

A primary step in disaster preparedness is for providers to actively participate in a **local coordinating committee or council.** These councils are designed to regularly bring together regional providers, public health agencies, and emergency management authorities for planning purposes. Such a forum allows providers to prepare more effectively for disaster response by understanding the broader emergency management system, how other agencies organize their roles and responsibilities, and how they as providers can obtain needed information and resources during an emergency.

Often, local emergency management agencies meet among themselves, but fail to include health care providers and other private entities. Providers should insist on being included in such planning efforts. If no such committee or planning process exists, providers should proactively create such a framework and strongly encourage the participation of all health care organizations that might be involved in a response. In addition, providers should be represented in their region's emergency operations center (EOC). As part of the jurisdiction's formal response structure, providers can stay abreast of developments during an emergency, seek assistance when necessary, and better coordinate their response efforts and resources. Representation through professional associations or local provider groups has been shown to be effective.

Risk and Preparedness

Like the community in which they live, health care providers should also undertake a hazard vulnerability analysis (HVA), which was discussed previously. Through the use of this tool, providers carry out analyses about the possibility of natural events, such as hurricanes; technological events, such as electrical failures; human-related events, such as mass casualty incidents; and events involving hazardous materials.

Once the probability and the severity of the various hazards are understood, providers can address preparedness needs. Providers should perform seven types of activities in preparing for and responding to any emergency. In general, these categories include the following:

1. Developing the basic emergency management plan
2. Ensuring communications to mobilize staff
3. Monitoring and evaluating external sources of information
4. Addressing staff availability and supporting their needs
5. Ensuring effective internal and external communication during the emergency
6. Ensuring the availability of equipment, supplies, and services
7. Ensuring security.[†] For example, providers should seek supplemental manpower to deliver care and necessary support, such as medical equipment vendors and pharmaceutical suppliers.

Emergency Management Programs: Emphasis on All-Hazards Planning

Anticipating and planning for the most probable types of events in a particular locality is the next step in disaster preparedness. A strong, well-thought-out emergency plan that provides a road map for providers' response is critical to effective relief action. Comprehensive emergency plans are often referred to as **all-hazards** plans because they provide a framework for preparing for and responding to the broadest range of events, disasters, and emergencies. It is important that providers have a plan that is both extensive and flexible so that it provides guidance for an efficient and effective response to many types of emergencies. An "all-hazards plan can guide the response for unanticipated events or events that unfold in an unanticipated way.

At a minimum, the disaster plan should address areas identified as priorities in the hazard vulnerability analysis. Building on this general plan, providers can add components that address event-specific issues, such as actions by the emergency and infection control departments, the workforce, and security. Components of the all-hazards plan include:

- Activation of the response plan,
- Internal and external communications,
- Designation of the incident commander for different types of disasters,
- Identification of external resources and how they should be obtained, and
- Security mechanisms to implement.

Incident Command Systems

The primary goal of preparedness and response is to effectively manage and respond to an emergency. In order to accomplish this goal both within and across multiple health care organizations, the organizations must have a common approach. Incident command systems (ICS) provide this structure in hospitals, just as they do for other emergency response agencies. ICS fit neatly into an all-hazards approach to planning because they allow different entities to respond similarly and to speak a common language, regardless of the type of event or disaster.

Health care providers have historically modeled their approach to ICS after the Hospital Emergency Incident Command System, or HEICS, which was developed by the San Mateo [California] County Emergency Medical Services Agency. That system evolved into the current version, called the **hospital incident command system,** or **HICS.**

Regulatory and Accreditation Requirements for Health Care Institutions

While provider emergency management plans reflect the operational imperatives of their institution, these plans are also based on the requirements of regulatory agencies and accrediting bodies. For example, most states provide direction regarding health care facilities' emergency plans, drills, and general emergency response procedures.[36] Similarly, federal regulations that set forth the conditions for hospitals to participate in the federal Medicare and Medicaid payment programs require that hospitals have certain emergency systems and procedures.[37]

The Joint Commission, a nonprofit, nationwide organization that accredits many kinds of health care providers, has specific preparedness requirements. In its standards for "Management of the Environment of Care," the Joint Commission requires hospitals to have an emergency management plan that comprehensively describes its approach to emergencies in the hospital or in the community. In the "Elements of Performance" related to this standard, the Joint Commission outlines a number of components that should be included in such emergency management plans as well as in the planning process. Some of these components are the functioning of the hospital's command structure, conducting a hazard vulnerability analysis, conducting drills, and undertaking community-wide planning.[38]

Developing Mechanisms for Effective Communication

Effective communication during an emergency facilitates the providers' understanding of the scope of an emergency, the steps necessary to respond to it, the care of patients, and protection of staff and community. To effectively communicate, health care systems need both equipment (e.g., radios, cellular phones, etc.) and advance planning that identifies with whom to communicate with, how to communicate, and for what purposes. This section discusses the mechanisms and systems necessary to ensure effective communication among providers before and during emergencies.

Building Redundant Systems

Providers should develop a number of methods for communicating both internally and externally. Different types of emergencies affect or undermine communication systems differently, causing communication systems to fail. Further, all personnel need to be kept informed of events as they are unfolding, their specific role and tasks in the situation, and how to communicate with all response partners.

To fully understand the limitations and vulnerabilities of their communication systems, providers should specifically assess the systems' sensitivity to power outages and to being overwhelmed during times of heavy call volume. A disruption in electricity will affect landline phone switches, computers, and other aspects of communications, causing cell-phone lines to become overwhelmed. Knowing that your facility is vulnerable to such disruption necessitates a specific plan to ensure that communication systems will be protected by backup power (e.g., emergency generators) and to create built-in system **redundancies.** Redundant systems assemble multiple methods of communication, so that should one or more systems fail, at least one will work. Many providers have organized redundant communication devices (e.g., telephones, cellular phones, pagers, satellite phones, wireless Internet, and radio-operated devices, such as Blackberries) to ensure their ability to send and receive information during emergencies.

Radios. Providers commonly purchase radios that enable simultaneous conversations about the status of an emergency and information-sharing about needs and resources. Local EMA often have 800 megahertz (or other frequency) radios that enable them to talk among themselves. The radios can be programmed with channels that allow simultaneous conversations without interfering with each other. Some communities have a dedicated health channel on which providers can talk among themselves and with emergency responders in order to stay abreast of events and better respond to and manage the emergency.

Providers also can use ham, or amateur, radio, if other communication options fail. This can be accomplished by identifying who on their staff might be a ham radio operator and ensuring that they are coordinating with the local Amateur Radio Emergency Services system.

Telephone numbers
Mobile phone numbers
Email addresses
Fax numbers
Pager numbers
Satellite phone numbers
Direct connect phone/radio numbers
Radio capabilities
Who maintains the radios
Ham radio information
Information about each provider's or agency's emergency
   operations center

Figure 23.1. Information collected for emergency directory

Communications Directories

In addition to redundant or multiple means of communicating, providers should compile directories that identify every method of reaching key personnel, other providers, essential vendors, and the agencies on which the provider might depend during an emergency. This broad-based information should be compiled so that key contacts can be reached during business and nonbusiness hours. The information that should be collected is listed in Figure 23.1.

To ensure that the most current contact information is always available, such information should be regularly updated and distributed to everyone on the list.

Mechanisms for Rapidly Transmitting Information

In addition to contact information, providers should establish mechanisms for rapidly transmitting information to everyone who needs it. Examples include call-down systems for reaching staff, telephone trees, blast emails, text messaging, global messaging, paging systems, intranet messages, or call-in numbers with recorded messages that instruct staff on when to report to work and what actions to take.

Monitoring Information

Providers must ensure that alert systems are in place to monitor or receive information critical to managing the response. These systems often are maintained by local, state, and federal jurisdictions to provide information about emergencies and the changing community health and public health needs needs. Health care systems should assign someone to regularly monitor these systems. Providers who subscribe to or participate in alert systems must ensure that the relevant authority has their current contact information in its communication directory so that key personnel can be reached during both business and nonbusiness hours.

Systems for Collecting/Sharing Information Needed to Manage an Emergency. The health care institutions located closest to the site of an emergency are typically overwhelmed with patients seeking care. As a result, they may need assistance from other providers in areas such as increased staffing, supplies, and bed capacity. Further, larger disasters can simultaneously affect many providers in the same region. To provide support to overwhelmed hospitals and to organize the effective allocation of needed resources, a system should be developed by area providers for the prompt collection and dissemination of information regarding an emergency. This will enable health and emergency management agencies to identify and meet particular needs by locating other providers who can supplement available services and resources.

For example, the New York Department of Health worked with the Greater New York Hospital Association's Emergency Preparedness Coordinating Council to develop a system, called the Health Emergency Response Data System (HERDS), to determine statewide health care system capacity. While initially designed to collect data that had been requested during the New York City region's response to the World Trade Center attacks in 2001, HERDS has since been expanded to accommodate many needs and uses.

The initial goals in designing HERDS were (1) to identify in advance and to agree on specific data elements that would be required during an emergency in order to minimize confusion about data requests, and (2) to create an efficient and prompt mechanism for the collection of these data. In general, the data that can be collected by HERDS fall into three broad categories: (1) bed, staffing, supply, and equipment needs and availability; (2) event-related visits, including emergency department visits, admissions, mortalities, and unidentified patients; and (3) patient locator information that can be used to identify and locate individuals who seek care from or are taken to hospitals. Specific data requests can be tailored to each emergency so that providers will be asked only for information pertinent to each situation. In addition, the system allows for the development of unanticipated data requests.

HERDS includes mechanisms for alerting facilities and for delivering emails to ensure that providers know when the system is activated so that they can log on to obtain and input information. It also collects weekly data on bed occupancy, to undertake surveys on available facility assets, and to collect other information as needed, for example, vaccine supplies and infection control procedures. This approach enables New York to collect the real-time information required to oversee the health care system and helps providers become familiar with the system through regular use.

Training and Education

Regular training and education are essential to ensuring that hospital personnel and other health care responders are familiar with the basics of identifying, containing, and treating public health threats and other emergencies. While extensive training is provided to clinicians who will be responsible for patient care during an emergency and to those who will hold leadership positions during an emergency, all hospital personnel should have sound working knowledge of the hospital's emergency management plan, Incident Command System, evacuation procedures, security protocols, and system for accessing information during an emergency. Many facilities provide all employees with basic information but make more extensive information, tailored to specific situations, available during an emergency. This allows employees to access what they need, when they need it.

The more-extensive clinician training often covers the particular types of patient health care needs that clinicians might encounter during an emergency, such as trauma, burns, and injuries caused by explosions. In addition, given increased concerns about terrorism, extensive training is often provided about nuclear, radiological, biological, and chemical injuries. Extensive training materials are available on government websites and do not, in all cases, need to be locally developed. For example, the CDC offers toolkits and materials describing key elements of public health emergencies that hospital personnel might encounter.

Columbia University's Center for Public Health Preparedness, Mailman School of Public Health, and Center for Health Policy in its School of Nursing, in collaboration with the Greater New York Hospital Association, developed a set of core competencies for the hospital workforce to guide the development of emergency preparedness and response training for both hospital workers and leaders. These competencies help ensure that staff know what is expected of them and address concerns that the workforce might have about reporting to or staying at work during emergency situations.[39]

Drills and Exercises

Drills and exercises are an integral part of effective emergency management in that they test the effectiveness of emergency management plans and identify where additional planning may be required. They are also an important aspect of collaborative planning because they can help participants better understand each other's roles and responsibilities during emergencies. Effective emergency management plans should include the four phases of emergency management (mitigation, preparedness, response, and recovery), so drills and exercises ideally should test as many of these phases as possible, though not necessarily all at the same time. Facilities accredited by the Joint Commission are required to conduct drills regularly to test emergency management plans. In addition, many state regulations require hospitals to conduct drills.

The following section borrows from the Greater New York Hospital Association's brochure *Effective Emergency Management Drills and Exercises* and defines some of the terms used with respect to drills and exercises.

Drill

A *drill* is defined as a supervised activity with a limited focus to test a procedure that is one component of an organization's overall emergency management plan. For example, an organization might conduct a drill for its radio operators on the use of a radio system.

Tabletop Exercises

A *tabletop exercise* uses written and oral scenarios to evaluate the effectiveness of an organization's emergency management plan and procedures and to highlight issues of coordination and assignment of responsibilities. Tabletop exercises do not physically simulate specific events, utilize equipment, or deploy resources. During a tabletop exercise, a facilitator usually coordinates discussion.

Functional Exercises

A *functional exercise* simulates a disaster in the most realistic manner possible without moving real people or equipment to a real site. A functional exercise utilizes a carefully designed and scripted scenario, with timed messages and communications between players and simulators. The emergency operations center—the facility or area from which disaster response is coordinated—is usually activated during a functional exercise and actual communications equipment may be used.

Full-scale Exercises

A *full-scale exercise* is often the culmination of previous drills and exercises. It tests the mobilization of all (or as many as possible of) the response components, takes place in real time, employs real equipment, and tests several emergency functions. In the hospital context, a full-scale exercise often involves pre-hospital as well as hospital responses, and usually involves actors simulating patients and

the activation of the emergency operations center (EOC). It may also include other health care facilities in order to test mutual aid agreements. *Controllers,* who maintain order and ensure that the exercise proceeds according to plan, are also usually used. Full-scale exercises are generally intended to evaluate the operations capability of emergency management systems in a community and to evaluate interagency coordination.[40]

AN OVERVIEW OF HEALTH DEPARTMENT RESPONSIBILITIES

The events of September 11, 2001, and the subsequent anthrax attack focused nationwide attention on the public health aspects of emergencies. Compared to hospitals and pre-hospital care organizations, where emergency preparedness and care is routine, public health agencies had not successfully integrated emergency management into their responsibilities before then. Therefore, many departments of health, both local and state, had to rapidly expand and improve their emergency preparedness staffing and activities, initially without either the resources or best practice models to guide them.

Fortunately, the federal government realized that supporting public health was essential to this process, and passed the Public Health Security and Bioterrorism Preparedness Response Act of 2002, which allocated an immediate $918 million for emergency preparedness to state and local DOH. Since then, allocations have decreased slightly, and grant requirements have evolved; nonetheless, these funds provide a great boost to preparedness in the United States. Notable public health emergency initiatives or responses since 2001 in which DOH have played a role include the August 2003 blackout in the Northeastern United States; Hurricane Katrina in 2005, which impacted the Gulf Coast Region; the smallpox vaccination campaign

EXHIBIT 23-7 Flood Disaster—Iowa

In the spring and summer of 1993, excessive rainfall triggered near-record flooding in nine Midwestern states. In Iowa, 2.7 million people were affected and every county in the state reported flood damage. The entire state was declared a disaster area.

Public Health Implications: In Iowa, health care and public health infrastructures were strongly affected. Numerous primary-care physician offices were closed, including 200 offices in Polk County alone. Flood-related hospitalizations in seven counties included cases of carbon monoxide poisoning, hypothermia, electrocution, wound infections, and exacerbations of chronic illnesses. Eight counties experienced interruptions of the public health services, including vaccination and STD clinics, and WIC (Women, Infants, and Children) programs. More than a third of the population suffered disruptions of safe water and sewage services. Further, more than half the population was exposed to an increase in the number of rats and mosquitoes. In addition, 2 percent of the counties reported an increase in post-flooding hospitalization for substance abuse

and nine counties reported increased admissions to mental health facilities.

Public Health Interventions: More than 54,000 people were evacuated. As the floodwaters receded, the communities opened shelters, served meals, and provided clothing as many residents whose homes were destroyed had evacuated without personal belongings.

The Iowa Department of Public Health (IDPH) conducted a rapid health assessment and ongoing surveillance. Working with the Centers for Disease Control and Prevention (CDC), the IDPH conducted weekly surveillance through submission of weekly data from the medical, mental health, substance abuse facilities and county sanitation departments. In addition, it participated as part of a multidisciplinary team (medical, environmental, social service, government, emergency preparedness, and hospital) to determine the response to the disaster. During recovery, the IDPH conducted public education programs regarding food and water safety, home cleanup, and sanitation and personal safety.

in 2002; and pandemic influenza planning; as well as numerous local emergencies.

THE PREPAREDNESS OF LOCAL AND STATE DEPARTMENTS OF HEALTH

This section provides an overview of the basic activities that all state and many local DOH must engage in to prepare for emergencies, and describes specific response activities carried out by DOH personnel during an emergency. Because local

responders play a critical role in the immediate response, their activities are emphasized.

Organizational Preparedness

The single most important resource for a DOH is an engaged, trained and well-informed workforce. Therefore, the first task in organizational emergency preparedness is to inform, educate, and test all current public health employees on their roles and responsibilities during an emergency. The core competencies for emergency preparedness[41] are useful starting points for matching personnel with their emergency roles. Existing staff may question the need for their participation, or not understand the role of public health during emergencies. All newly hired staff should be oriented to these responsibilities. Minimum requirements for all staff include understanding the role of the agency during an emergency, basic information on incident command, knowledge of their response role, how to use communication equipment, and how to communicate within the organization. Specific response roles for employees should mirror their everyday tasks as much as possible. All employees should create an emergency plan for their families, which will help alleviate their concerns about their families' safety when they are asked to leave their families to respond to a community emergency. These responsibilities may be emphasized as a required part of an employee's annual performance evaluation. For example, participation in agency preparedness activities, such as planning or drills, may be assessed for each employee.

Like hospitals and other emergency response agencies, DOH have adopted an ICS structure for organizing their emergency response activities. ICS may present a cultural challenge to DOH that traditionally rely on a slower, consensus-building approach, rather than on the hierarchical, streamlined decision making that is a hallmark of ICS systems. These challenges can be overcome by regular training and exercises, however.

Partnerships

Relationship building is another vital part of emergency preparedness. Public health officials should not meet their agency counterparts for the first time during an emergency. Relationships with organizations that are not traditional public health partners should be actively developed. These organizations may include police departments, fire departments, local FBI offices, ambulance or emergency medical services, state or local emergency management offices, local or state environmental organizations, veterinarians, local transportation agencies, and the American Red Cross. The purpose of building relationships with such organizations is to better understand the role each group plays in emergency response; to jointly prepare for emergencies, including participation in tabletops and drills; and

to develop the personal familiarity that will enable the group members to work together effectively during a crisis.

Hospitals are key partners to public health professionals. Their preparedness activities are funded through the federal government and currently are being coordinated through state DOH, with the exception of four cities (Los Angeles, Chicago, New York City, and Washington, D.C.) whose preparedness activities are directly funded. Hospital preparedness was detailed above.

Preparedness Activities

Over the past several years, departments of health have been asked to develop response plans for a variety of emergencies, including outbreaks of smallpox and pandemic influenza. A better strategy than this specific approach, however, is for DOH to view plan development from a broader more generic perspective, the all-hazards approach, as health care facilities do. This approach looks at the overall management of any emergency, and might include an ICS, list the specific roles and responsibilities of employees, detail notification protocols, note the legal jurisdiction for emergency actions, and discuss how a health department works with other governmental agencies during an emergency.

Department of Health Exercises

Only after a plan has been written and staff have been educated about it, is it worth spending the time and funds required to conduct exercises to test the plan. Exercises are valuable for testing employee awareness of a plan and for identifying problems by challenging the integrity of the plan. These tests usually are tabletop exercises, in which participants are confronted with a hypothetical emergency that they then need to notionally coordinate a response to, or drills which involve actually demonstrating some part of the activity needed for response. (See the section on Tabletop Exercises for more information.) They may vary in complexity from an exercise involving a single subunit of the health department to one where many agencies and stakeholders participate. Any tabletop exercise or drill should result in an *after-action report* that summarizes the exercise and lists any required remediation steps, the parties responsible for remediation, and a proposed time line for resolution. National standards for exercise design are established by the Department of Homeland Security's exercise and evaluation program.[42]

Notification and Mobilization of Staff

Notification and mobilization of personnel are key initial response activities, so DOH must have mechanisms for notifying staff 24 hours a day, 7 days a week. Depending on the size of the health department, these may range from a simple telephone tree to electronic notification systems that can simultaneously phone hundreds of employees. As mentioned previously, in the discussion of emergency communications in health care facilities, redundant communication mechanisms are important, generally, for events during which telephone land or cell-phone lines may be compromised, such as a blackout or an explosion.

Mobilizing personnel may require the use of health department vehicles, or the resources of local police, fire, or emergency management groups.

The Oversight Role of Departments of Health

State DOH have fiscal and programmatic oversight of the federal cooperative agreements for emergency preparedness within their states, with the exception of the four cities listed above that are directly funded. It is challenging, however, to provide statewide solutions to local emergencies because local DOH across a state may vary in size and ability and may serve very different populations, whether rural, suburban, or urban. Federal funding should directly support the local health department's activities.

State DOH face additional oversight challenges when they must work with tribal authorities located within the state and with regional metropolitan areas that cross state boundaries. It is critical that a process for communication and mutual aid be worked out as part of everyday preparedness. States

located on the Mexican or Canadian borders may also need to work with these countries to coordinate emergency response in cross-border regions.

Surveillance

Surveillance is the backbone of public health. This is especially true during emergencies, where a premium is placed on the earliest possible identification of a threat in order to mitigate its health consequences. Existing surveillance systems have been reviewed to assess whether they can meet the complex challenges posed by disasters. New systems have been created to address the diagnosis and reporting delays inherent in older systems. Much of this work has been done in response to the threat of a bioterrorism event.

Traditional systems that passively collect information from health care providers and laboratories continue to be important parts of emergency preparedness. During the anthrax cases that occurred in 2001, the first case was diagnosed and reported by an astute clinician, as were subsequent cases. Despite this excellent work by individuals, traditional surveillance suffers from a number of deficiencies that create barriers to the rapid diagnosis and reporting needed for quick identification of an outbreak. These deficiencies may include clinicians' lack of understanding of reporting requirements, the lack of a mechanism to report to DOH, and the lack of clinicians' ability to recognize rare infectious diseases or unusual clusters of diseases. DOH should work with community physicians to resolve these problems by sponsoring educational sessions on the roles of physicians in emergency preparedness, distributing educational materials to clinicians to encourage reporting, and creating 24/7 rapid-response teams who can accept and act on suspicious reports in real time.

New surveillance systems, generally called **syndromic surveillance,** have been created in part to address the recognition delays inherent in traditional surveillance. The new systems rely on recognizing patterns of symptoms or behavior (such as buying anti-flu medications or absenteeism among large groups of people) rather than on diagnoses of specific diseases among individuals. This approach is useful because many bioterrorism agents, such as anthrax, cause nonspecific flu-like illnesses early in the course of the infection, before the patient presents with more classical signs and symptoms of a disease. In this way, a signal, such as a large number of patients complaining of flu-like illness, may be identified and investigated as early as possible, thus potentially providing an earlier opportunity for medical intervention. However, it is unlikely that syndromic surveillance systems will detect a bioterrorism incident if only small numbers of people become ill from the attack.

Like traditional surveillance systems, syndromic systems benefit where baseline information is available to establish the normal patterns for a particular population leading to better understanding of seasonal variation. Syndromic surveillance generally relies on information collected electronically for purposes other than surveillance, and needs to be analyzed quickly and routinely. Examples of data sources include ambulance transport chief complaints, reasons for visits to hospital emergency departments, pharmacy purchases of over-the-counter and prescription drugs, employee absenteeism for large employers or school districts, visits to clinics, and phone calls to medical help lines.

During syndromic surveillance, information is collected daily, reviewed, and analyzed to identify patterns or increases in symptoms that could signify the outbreak of an infectious disease, a possible terrorism event, or another event. (For example, increased rates of respiratory and gastrointestinal symptoms trigger suspicion.) Recently, the federal government has funded Biosense, a program whose purpose is to collect such information across the United States and centrally monitor such trends. These automatic reporting systems, however, do not replace the need for providers to be vigilant and to report suspicious symptoms and situations.

A further extension of traditional and syndromic surveillance is **biodetection,** which uses environmental monitoring to identify the release of bioterrorism agents, in hopes of identifying an attack as early as possible. Several biodetection initiatives have been employed. The first, Biowatch, involves the collection of airborne particles onto filters that are collected and tested for agents of bioterrorism. Biowatch detectors have been deployed in many cities across the United States. A second program, the Bioagent Detection System (BDS), has been deployed in mail-sorting facilities across the United States, in an effort to identify any letter containing anthrax as soon as it goes through a sorting machine. BDS enables pathogen testing, using polymerase chain reaction assays, within the system and sets off an alarm when anthrax is detected.[43]

When either of these systems is used, it is crucial that public health authorities understand how to manage a positive laboratory result, i.e., how to engage their mandated partners, explain the result, and act appropriately on the result.

Several more sophisticated biodetection systems are in development, and it is likely that in the future more of these systems will be deployed in diverse locations.

Laboratory Preparedness

In 2001, departments of health were overwhelmed with environmental and clinical specimens for *B. anthracis* screening. This incident focused attention on the fragility of our public health laboratories. Two years earlier, the CDC formed the **Laboratory Response Network (LRN),** which linked hospital, state and local health, CDC, FBI, local law enforcement, and other reference labs. The LRN was formed to enhance the timeliness of lab testing, to establish common protocols for testing, and to foster communication among the various players involved in emergency response. Specific LRN objectives include training **sentinel,** or clinical, labs to rule out, recognize, or refer potential select agents to the Public Health Lab; establishing packaging and requirements for shipping between the LRN labs to ensure the safe transport of specimens; establishing biosafety level 3 facilities within each state for safe testing of dangerous specimens; and enhancing security requirements for dealing with bioterrorism agents.

Laboratories should create plans to enable continued operations in the event of an emergency, which is important to all aspects of public health, but is critical to labs, because of their dependence on appropriate laboratory space, reagents, equipment, and properly trained staff. Laboratories should establish emergency within their jurisdictions, so that they can meet the anticipated surge in the submission of specimens during emergencies. In addition to establishing backup facilities, labs can cross-train staff so that each staffperson can perform a variety of tests. Other preparedness activities may include testing Biowatch specimens and membership in the Food Emergency Response Network (FERN), which coordinates lab testing in response to a terrorist attack involving the contamination of the food supply.

Laboratories are critical to surveillance. However, traditional laboratory reporting has inherent problems that may impede the rapid identification of emergency disease threats. Physicians may not order the correct tests, and definitive diagnostic tests may be available only in public health laboratories through the LRN. In addition, timely reporting to DOH may be delayed. Many DOH have instituted electronic laboratory reporting systems linking commercial and hospital laboratories to DOH to improve the timeliness of reporting. DOH have also worked with these labs to quickly identify and safely ship specimens for definitive testing. Public health laboratories, in turn, work with laboratories at the CDC to perform testing confirming bioterrorism agents.

Communication

Departments of health have a critical role, different from that of health care facilities, in communicating with the public and with other responding agencies during emergencies. Therefore, it is critical that DOH position themselves as trusted sources of information in everyday situations, so that the public will turn to them during public health emergencies. DOH should proactively build and maintain relationships with critical community partners, including the media, other governmental agencies,

nonprofit and community organizations, elected officials, unions, faith-based organizations, disability and other advocacy groups, community health centers, hospitals, health care providers, and businesses and others in the private sector. DOH should also disseminate preparedness information to stakeholders to enable them to educate their constituents, and to solicit their feedback. Communication issues should be a part of tabletop exercises and drills.

DOH should establish mechanisms for communicating with the public in advance of an emergency. The most critical task is maintaining regularly updated contact information for media, community, and government partners that should work closely with DOH during an emergency response. It is also critical that DOH develop a cache of easily adaptable public information tools, including press releases, fact sheets, talking points, and call center scripts. In addition to ensuring the ability to contact mainstream media, nontraditional media partners, such as ethnic media, must be engaged in advance of an emergency—especially because their key audiences may be inherently distrustful of government and advance relationship building helps establish credibility of DOH. Other preparedness activities include developing rapid translational capabilities to provide information to non–English-speaking populations, and to identify and train subject matter experts both within and outside of government.

Risk communications and media relations are critical during emergencies. The tenets of risk communication are sharing information about what is known, acknowledging what is not known, and explaining how the government is working to fill knowledge gaps. Effective risk communication includes delivering what you promise and not over-reassuring people in the face of uncertainty. It is also important for DOH to prepare public messages about how people can protect themselves, their families, and their communities from whatever threats exist or are imminent.

Public health officials should be trained in risk communication and media relations so that they can provide useful information to the public about an unfolding crisis, despite whatever uncertainty exists about the outcome of events. For example, DOH should help their leaders prepare for emergencies by educating them about risk communication; this training should include role-playing practice.

Mechanisms to enhance communication with health care providers are essentialThese may take the form of monthly newsletters, grand round presentations at local hospitals, email alert systems, or timely conference calls with hospitals. Even when there is no emergency, these activities promote traditional surveillance and improved communication and often provide life-saving medical advice.

Medical Countermeasures

Departments of health have been tasked with developing strategies to provide medical countermeasures to health threats—in other words, to rapidly treat or provide prophylaxis to large populations during medical emergencies. Such strategies, for example, might include supplying antibiotic prophylaxis following exposure to anthrax, or smallpox vaccination following a smallpox outbreak. The federal government's Strategic National Stockpile[44] plays a key role in these strategies. The SNS is maintained at secure locations across the United States and has two components: the first is a "push pack" of antibiotics, and other medicines and medical equipment needed for immediate response. The second is *vendor managed inventory*, which provides longer-term support. Push packs can be deployed to any location in the United States within 12 hours after the request from the governor of the affected state. DOH need to formally accept the SNS and then develop their own intrastate distribution plan.

DOH may be involved in other stockpiling and distribution activities. Chempack, for example, is a federal-state initiative to predeploy chemical nerve agent antidotes to hospitals. Most states have recently decided to purchase medications for treatment or prophylaxis for pandemic influenza. Several jurisdictions are also considering bolstering supplies of critical-care-related equipment, such as ventilators, by creating stockpiles.

Points of Distribution Sites

Once material reaches the local cities or counties from the Strategic National Stockpile, it is distributed to the affected population. This occurs at **points of distribution** sites (PODs), places where the well public comes to receive preventive medical interventions. Because hospitals' and clinics' capacity is likely to be overwhelmed during a crisis, PODs are usually located in other facilities. PODs staff quickly assess attendees and provide the appropriate intervention. PODs are not designed to diagnose and treat illness, however. Because of the enormous difficulties in accessing an entire population for prophylaxis, especially in urban areas with large populations, the CDC has created a City Readiness Initiative to provide increased funding for this activity. In addition, alternatives to PODs are being explored. In one such initiative, the United States Postal Service would deliver needed antibiotics through the mail. Other alternatives may include drive-through PODs or working with nursing agencies to provide antibiotic prophylaxis to the homebound.

Volunteers

All medical countermeasures rely on the availability of a sufficient number of well-trained health care personnel. In an attempt to ensure sufficient personnel during emergencies, the **Medical Reserve Corps (MRC)** enrolls health care personnel as volunteers, so that they can supplement local workforces during a variety of crises. MRC volunteers were deployed following Hurricane Katrina, for instance. Training MRC volunteers, however, can be a challenge. The nature of emergencies, of course, is that they are unpredictable. So, the training a volunteer receives may not be appropriate to a specific crisis, or the training may occur so far in advance of an emergency that the volunteer does not remember the training by the time a crisis occurs. Therefore, many jurisdictions have created just-in-time training plans that can be activated when the nature of the emergency and the needed countermeasures are known. A related initiative, the **Emergency System for the Advance Registration of Health**

Professions Volunteers (ESAR-VHP), has established guidelines to allow states to register, credential, and privilege health professional volunteers to provide a supplemental workforce during an emergency.

Mental Health

Responding to mental health issues in populations affected by disaster is a prominent part of emergency response. This is true of any disaster, but is especially true of crises caused by terrorist attacks, because terrorism often targets the mental health of the affected population. Therefore, strategies to address a community's mental health should be integrated into the initial responses and the public communication used to address the situation. Many emergencies require the provision of crisis counseling to victims and the families of the deceased. Therefore, a cadre of trained mental health providers with expertise in grief counseling needs to be created and maintained. The American Red Cross plays a key role in supply and training these providers in many communities.

Members of the public are not the only ones affected by disasters, however. First responders, including public health staff, may be profoundly affected by their work, so attention to their psychological needs should be planned for as well. Public health leadership should be sensitive to the well-being of those from their agencies who respond to disasters, and employee counseling services should be available to these responders during and after an emergency.

Community Preparedness

The ability of government to respond to an emergency is largely dependent on the willingness of communities to prepare in advance and to respond to instructions as events unfold. Unfortunately, recent surveys have found that the public is not prepared, and may not follow instructions during times of crisis,[45] because of lack of trust and lack of knowledge of emergency planning efforts.

Many institutions have published basic emergency preparedness booklets for communities that serve as a useful resource. DOH and emergency management organizations should work together to emphasize to the public the need for individual, family, and community preparedness.

Emergencies may result in the prolonged disruption of access to health care in a community. This disruption, in turn, may increase the burden on emergency medical services. For example, persons who no longer have access to their routine medications may become ill from a chronic medical condition that is usually well-maintained but no longer is. In the aftermath of Hurricane Katrina, problems in obtaining medical care (23.3 percent of those polled), and prescription medicines (9.4 percent)[46] were common, and it became difficult to get medical care for chronic health conditions because so many medical records were lost. DOH and community providers should emphasize to the public and to their patients, respectively, the importance of patients maintaining a list of their prescription medications and several days' worth of reserved pharmaceuticals and medical supplies.

The Hurricane Katrina response also focused attention on evacuation and shelters. Providers' plans for evacuation of facilities, such as hospitals and nursing homes, and of individual persons with disabilities, for example, need to be coordinated with first-responder agencies. Triage protocols to determine whether evacuees require shelters, referral to hospitals, or other special needs facilities should be developed and drilled. Public health professionals should work with local providers to support the medical and psychological needs of residents living in evacuation shelters and other housing arrangements. Arrangement for pet care and veterinary service also need to be considered.

DOH must plan for the quarantine of people who are exposed to communicable diseases, such as SARS or pandemic influenza, but who are not yet ill, and for the isolation of those who have become ill. In regards to quarantine procedures, DOH need to work with the CDC's Division of Quarantine to identify sick passengers who may arrive in their jurisdiction by plane or ship. Similarly, medical monitoring systems should be created to identify persons who have been exposed to and have developed an illness, so that they can be isolated from the rest of the population.

Planning for quarantine and isolation must consider a broad range of circumstances, such as identifying facilities to house those who are not from the community (i.e., those on business or visiting). Other scenarios call for caring for people at home. Procedures for the medical, social, and psychological support of these populations should be created.

The term *community mitigation* refers to measures that might be instituted to decrease the spread of a highly contagious disease, such as pandemic influenza, usually by discouraging unnecessary gatherings, or, in other words, by encouraging what is called *social distancing*. These measures may include cancelling large gatherings such as entertainment events or civic gatherings, or instituting the prolonged closure of schools. This latter measure is difficult to implement, however, because schools supply social support (such as school meals) and because students may re-congregate in other settings (such as malls). To successfully carry out a prolonged school closure, DOH need to plan for this contingency with their community's school districts.

Vulnerable Populations

Meeting the needs of **vulnerable** populations during emergencies cannot occur without prior planning. Vulnerable populations may include the elderly, the homebound, the homeless, immigrants, children, prison populations, persons on renal dialysis, the mentally ill, the chronically ill, and others. These populations may have difficulty in accessing information, resources, or medical care. They may lack the ability to respond to governmental recommendations, such as an order to evacuate, or to report to a POD. Some vulnerable populations, such as children or persons with disabilities, may have medical and emotional needs that are different from those of other vulnerable populations.

DOH should consult with agencies and individuals who routinely provide care to these populations and with social service providers to create special arrangements for these populations. These providers also need to be prepared to deal with emergencies, to help ensure continuity of services during a crisis, and to better understand effective communication mechanisms and strategies with each of these populations.[47]

Mass Fatality Planning

The ability to properly handle and identity a large number of decedents following a disaster is another aspect of emergency preparedness. DOH need to work with hospitals, coroners, medical examiners, police and clergy, and others to help coordinate this facet of response. If a communicable disease outbreak is responsible for a large number of deaths, it may not be safe for people to gather at large funerals, and alternatives may have to be considered.

Legal Issues

State and local DOH must review their jurisdictions' existing legislation to determine whether it is adequate to meet the needs of a large-scale emergency, such as one caused by bioterrorism. Specifically, laws covering surveillance (methods as well as specific diseases), isolation and quarantine, and control of property may require revision. Local and state governments need to understand their emergency powers and need to formulate plans for emergency regulatory relief (such as hospital regulations). Because epidemiologic investigations of incidents of terrorism require that DOH coordinate with local law enforcement, agreements on confidentiality, information sharing, and joint investigatory protocols should be formulated and practiced between these agencies. A Model State Emergency Public Health Powers Act has been created that provides a template for comparison to existing legislation, and may enhance the ability of public health authorities to respond to emergencies.[48]

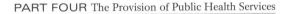

EMERGENCY RESPONSE OF LOCAL AND STATE DEPARTMENTS OF HEALTH

The specific response of local and state departments of health depends on the nature and extent of the event, as well as on the capabilities and resources of the affected area. Therefore, this section focuses on general, rather than specific, response activities.

Organizational Response

When notified of an emergency, DOH must quickly determine whether the event has public health implications. Public health officials may need to travel to the location of an event or to a hospital to better assess the situation and to make initial recommendations. Determining the existence of a public health problem and confirming the diagnosis are of the utmost importance. Depending on the nature of the problem, other immediate responses may include radiologic measurements or other environmental assessments.

Once it is determined than an emergency has a public health component, internal agency notification should commence and a decision should be made about activating the agency's incident command system. If the ICS is activated, an emergency operations center is usually opened either at the local/state emergency management agency or at the DOH. In addition to deciding the scale and type of response, the agency will need to determine which of its routine activities will be continued during the emergency. Also, because it may be necessary for responders to work through the night, support for employees may include provision of food, sleeping arrangements, and transportation. All expenditures, including overtime costs, should be tracked to facilitate subsequent reimbursement. When the acute part of the emergency is mitigated, a decision to de-escalate the response needs to be made, although the recovery phase may be extended. An after-action review should occur as soon as possible after the de-escalation. The after-action review should be followed by the **after-action report,** which should make specific recommendations about how to improve the response process, in order to better prepare the organization for future emergencies.

Surveillance

New surveillance systems may need to be created to enable public health officials to understand the health impact of the emergency. For example, emergency department surveillance may be needed to identify casualties of a bombing or building collapse, or a system may be required to measure survivors' health care needs. For example, following Hurricane Katrina, new surveillance systems were set up to help health care professionals assess the incidence of communicable diseases among evacuation center residents, the mental health needs of returning residents, and the extent of mold problems in homes in New Orleans.[49] In some emergencies, existing systems may be relied on, but additional provider education may be needed to enhance reporting. Follow-up may be necessary to measure the long-term health effects of the emergency; this may be accomplished through the establishment of a registry. A good example is the World Trade Center Registry,[50] the largest environmental health registry in history, which attempts to identify long-term (20-year) medical and psychological outcomes for building evacuees, first responders, and other groups that were closely associated with the 9/11 disaster.

Mental Health

As public health professionals prepare for and engage in emergency response, they should think of ways to reduce any unintended mental health consequences of the emergency among the public. For example, language used in press releases may inadvertently concern or even panic the public. So, mental health experts should review these communications before they are distributed or broadcast. In addition, providing psychological support services to victims, responders, and the general population may decrease the incidence of mental health symptoms. Mental health responders should be mobilized and deployed to sites servicing victims, responders, or the public, such as hospitals or PODs. If this is not immediately possible, as may be the case during a large-scale disaster, efforts should be made to ensure that crisis counseling, assessments, and referrals are provided after the event to help identify and treat mental health symptoms among the population.

Environmental Response

Environmental issues are an aspect of many emergencies. Following a disaster, environmental staff should be mobilized to assess the size of any affected area, help establish or evaluate standards for personal protective equipment for those who enter it, and begin planning for the cleanup and re-occupancy of the area. These are general activities, but other, event-specific responses but may include restaurant and food safety inspections (including food service facilities for responders), radiologic assessment, safe drinking water assessment, environmental sampling activities, and hazardous waste removal. Many of these responses occurred following the World Trade Center disaster. At the time, new monitoring systems had to be created to determine the composition and extent of the huge debris-and-dust plume, to formulate cleanup recommendations and standards for personal protective equipment, to inspect and clean abandoned restaurants, and to enhance mosquito- and rodent-abatement activities.[51]

Communication

When a disaster occurs, public health officials and government leaders need to explain the nature and extent of the emergency as quickly as possible to the public. These announcements may take the form of press conferences or releases, and their frequency may vary. Early in the emergency, however, they may take place every few hours or as important information becomes available. Departments of health should designate spokespersons in advance and make them available to the media. Press coverage should be monitored to quickly identify rumors or misinformation that would need to be immediately corrected. It is important that DOH integrate communication strategies within the **joint information center,** a centralized site typically organized by the jurisdiction's emergency management agency to disseminate the most up-to-date information about the emergency. Other methods of providing information to the public also should be activated, including telephone hotlines and area or door-to-door leafleting. Communication among public health officials, health care providers, and hospitals should begin immediately and include health alerts, conference calls, or providing updated clinical information on websites.

Medical Recommendations

Departments of Health need to quickly determine or evaluate needed prophylaxis or treatment approaches for a disaster. This should be followed by rapid communication with the local health care system. Public health leadership and emergency management agencies must determine whether it is necessary to access the Strategic National Stockpile and communicate that decision to the state's governor's office.

Laboratory Services

If laboratory testing is a prominent part of the DOH emergency response, public health labs need to quickly evaluate the situation, launch their business continuity plan, determine the need for reagents and equipment for specimen testing, and activate their plans for deploying additional personnel. If confirmatory testing is needed by a reference laboratory, such as the CDC, mechanisms to quickly package and transport specimens, including by plane, need to be worked out.

THE FEDERAL GOVERNMENT'S RESPONSE

In addition to the Strategic National Stockpile, the federal government has created the **National Disaster Medical System,**[52] which can deploy critical assets during an emergency and has several components. These include **Disaster Medical Assistance Teams,** which consist of trained and equipped medical personnel who can be quickly mobilized to provide emergency medical care at the site of an emergency. **Disaster Mortuary Operational Response Teams (DMORT)** can recover, identify, and process the deceased victims of a disaster. The **Disaster Portable Morgue Unit Team,** in turn, helps DMORTs by setting up and running mortuary operations. **National Pharmacy Response Teams** assist in large-scale POD operations and in other activities requiring pharmacists. The **National Nurse Response Team** also assists in POD operations and provides nursing care in response to an event involving weapons of mass destruction. Finally, **Veterinary Medical Assistance Teams** provide veterinary services during emergencies.

Although not a federal resource, the Medical Reserve Corps may be deployed to sites of emergencies through the Emergency Management Assistance Compact.[53] MRC members from across the United States were deployed through EMAC to the Gulf States following Hurricane Katrina, for example.

SUMMARY

Public health professionals have markedly increased their emergency management expertise since September 11, 2001. Maintaining and enhancing this expertise will be a challenge, however. Continued federal support, in terms of both leadership and resources, is a critical component of future progress. Likewise, measurable and meaningful benchmarks need to be developed to evaluate future progress. More work needs to be done to meet the needs of society's vulnerable populations. Finally, Schools of Public Health should develop programs to educate their students on emergencies, so that the next generation of public health leadership can further the work of today's leaders.

DISCUSSION QUESTIONS

1. How should public health professionals prepare for emergency response?
2. What are the potential environmental, behavioral, and physical impacts of disasters?
3. What are incident command systems, and how do they work together?
4. What is an all-hazards plan, and why is it useful in disaster response?
5. Which federal assets are utilized in response to an emergency, and when and how are they used?
6. What are the activities carried out by a local department of health in response to an emergency?
7. What do all health department employees need to know about
   a. their response role during an emergency?
   b. mental health counseling techniques?
   c. how to interpret surveillance data?
   d. the principles of risk communication?

REFERENCES

1. Nishenko SP & Bollinger GA. Forecasting damaging earthquakes in the central and eastern United States. *Science.* 1990;249:1,412–16.
2. Gray WM. Strong association between West African rainfall and US landfall of intense hurricanes. *Science.* 1990;249:1,251–56.
3. Universite Catholique de Louvain. EM-DAT: The Office of Foreign Disaster Assistance/CRED International Disaster Database. http://www.em-dat.net/. Accessed 23 Dec 2006.
4. Universite Catholique de Louvain. EM-DAT: The Office of Foreign Disaster Assistance/CRED

International Disaster Database. http://www
.em-dat.net/documents/2005-disasters-in-
numbers. Accessed 23 Dec 2006.

5. http://earthquake.usgs.gov/eqcenter/eqinthenews/
2004/usslav/#summary. Accessed 5 November
2008.

6. http://www.emdat.be/Database/CountryProfile/
countryprofile2.php#summtable Accessed 5
November 2008.

7. L.R. Johnston Associates. *Floodplain Management
in the United States: An Assessment Report. Volume
2 Full Report. Prepared for the Federal Interagency
Floodplain Management Taskforce. FIA-18/June
1992.* Washington, DC: U.S. Federal Emergency
Management Agency, Federal Interagency Floodplain Management Taskforce, 1992.

8. Culliton TJ, et al. *50 Years of Population Change
along the Nation's Coasts, 1960–2010* (Coastal
Trends Series, Report 2). Rockville, MD: National
Oceanic and Atmospheric Administration; 1990.

9. U.S. Department of Commerce. National Oceanic
and Atmospheric Administration. NOAA Predicts
Very Active North Atlantic Hurricane Season.
Available at: http://www.noaanews.noaa.gov/
stories2006/s2634.htm. Accessed 9 June 2006.

10. U.S. Department of Commerce. National Hurricane Center. National Oceanic and Atmospheric
Administration. *Hurricane History.* Available at
http://www.nhc.noaa.gov/HAW2/english/
history.shtml. Accessed 5 November 2008.

11. http://www.em-dat.net/documents/figures/
tech_dis_trends/05/tdnumber0005.gif. Evans CA.
Public health impact of the 1992 Los Angeles
unrest. *Public Health Reports.* 1993;108(3):
265–72.

12. Nation's Commission on Terrorist Attacks upon
the United States. The 9/11 commission report
final report of the nation's commission on terrorist attacks on the United States executive summary.
Available at: http://www.9–11commission.gov/
report/911Report_Exec.htm. Accessed 23
December 2006.

13. Centers for Disease Control and Prevention.
*Public Health Emergency Response Guide for
State, Local, and Tribal Public Health Directors.*
http://www.bt.cdc.gov/planning/responseguide
.asp. Accessed 23 December 2006.

14. Landesman LY. *Public Health Management of Disasters: The Practice Guide.* 2nd ed. Washington,
DC: American Public Health Association, 2005.

15. Trust for America's Health. *Ready or Not? Protecting the Public's Health from Disease, Disasters,
and Bioterrorism, 2006.* Available at: http://
healthyamericans.org/reports/bioterror06/
BioTerrorReport2006.pdf. Accessed 23 December
2006.

16. Hood E. Chemical and biological weapons: new
questions, new answers. *Environmental Health
Perspectives.* 1999;107(12):931–32.

17. Heinrich J. *Infectious Disease Preparedness—
Federal Challenges in Responding to Influenza
Outbreaks.* United States Government Account-
ability Office, September 28, 2004.

18. Department of Health and Human Services. Pandemic flu planning assumptions Available at:
http://www.pandemicflu.gov/plan/pandplan.html.
Accessed 9 June 2006.

19. American Public Health Association. *Developing
a Comprehensive Public Health Approach to
Influenza Vaccination.* Washington, DC:
November 2006.

20. Auf der Heide E. *Community Medical Disaster
Planning and Evaluation Guide.* Dallas, TX: American College of Emergency Physicians; 1996.

21. Axelrod C, et al. Primary health care and the
Midwest flood disaster. *Public Health Rep.* 1994;
109(5):601–05.

22. Gautam K. Organizational problems faced by the
Missouri DOH in providing disaster relief during
the 1993 floods. *J Public Health Manag Prac.*
1998;4(4):79–86.

23. Whitman S, et al. Mortality in Chicago attributed
to the July 1995 heat wave. *Am J Public Health.*
1997;87(9):1,515–18.

24. Gerrity ET & Flynn BW. Mental health consequences of disasters. In: *Public Health Consequences of Disasters,* EK Noji ed. New York:
Oxford University Press; 1997:101–21.

25. Young BH, et al. *Disaster Mental Health Services:
A Guidebook for Clinicians and Administrators.*
Menlo Park, CA: National Center for Post-
Traumatic Stress Disorder; 1998.

26. Ursano RJ, et al. Trauma and disaster. In: Ursano
RJ, et al., eds. *Individual and Community
Responses to Trauma and Disaster: The Structure
of Human Chaos.* Cambridge, UK: Cambridge
University Press; 1994:3–27.

27. Green BL Solomon SD. The mental health impact
of natural and technological disasters. In: Freedy
JR, Hobfoll SE, eds. *Traumatic Stress: From Theory*

to Practice. New York: Plenum Press; 1995: 163–80.

28. Esrey S, et al. Effects of improved water supply and sanitation on ascariasis, diarrhoea, dracunculiasis, hookworm infection, schistosomiasis, and trachoma. *Bull World Health Organ.* 1991;69(5): 609–21.

29. "Mortality among Newly Arrived Mozambican Refugees—Zimbabwe and Malawi. *Morb Mortal Wkly Rep (MMWR).* 1992;42(24):468–77.

30. *Robert T. Stafford Disaster Relief and Emergency Assistance Act.* Public Law 93–288.

31. Drabek TE, et al. *Managing M multiorganizational Emergency Response: Emergency Research and Rescue Networks in Natural Disaster and Remote Area Setting.* Boulder, CO: Natural Hazards Information Center, University of Colorado; 1981.

32. Greater New York Hospital Association. *Emergency Preparedness Resource Guide.* New York: GNYHA; 2005.

33. http://www.govtrack.us/congress/bill.xpd? bill=s109–3678.

34. http://www.dhs.gov/xprepresp/committees/ editorial_0566.shtm.

35. 10 New York State Code, Rules and Regulations Section 405.24(g).

36. 42 Code of Federal Regulations Section 482.41.

37. Joint Commission on Accreditation of Healthcare Organizations. *Comprehensive Accreditation Manual for Hospitals: The Official Handbook* (EC 1.6, EC 2.5, EC 2.9, EC-5, EC-6, EC-12, EC-13, EC-25, EC-26, EC-49, EC-50, HR 1.25 (draft), HR 4.35 (draft), Oakbrook Terrace, IL: 2005.

38. Greater New York Hospital Association. *Emergency Preparedness Resource Guide.* New York: GNYHA; 2005.

39. Greater New York Hospital Association. *Effective Emergency Management Drills and Exercises.* New York: GNYHA.

40. http://www.cumc.columbia.edu/dept/nursing/ chphsr/pdf/btcomps.pdf.

41. https://hseep.dhs.gov.

42. Centers for Disease Control and Prevention. Responding to detection of aerosolized Bacillus anthracis by autonomous detection systems in the workplace. *MMWR.* 2004;53(RR-7):1–11.

43. http://www.bt.cdc.gov/stockpile/.

44. Lasker RD. *Redefining Readiness: Terrorism Planning Through the Eyes of the Public.* New York: The New York Academy of Medicine, 2004.

45. Centers for Disease Control and Prevention. *Assessment of Health-Related Needs After Hurricanes Katrina and Rita—Orleans and Jefferson Parishes, New Orleans Area, Louisiana, October 17–22, 2005. MMWR.* 2006;55(02):38–41.

46. Misrahi JJ, Matthews GS, Hoffman RE. Legal authorities for interventions during public health emergencies. In: Goodman RA, Rothstein MA, Hoffman RE, Lopez W, Matthews GW, eds. *Law in Public Health Practice.* New York: Oxford University Press; 2003.

47. Eisenman DP, Cordasco KM, Asch S, Golden JF, Glik D. Disaster planning and risk communication with vulnerable communities: lessons from Hurricane Katrina. *Am J Public Health.* 97 (Suppl 1):S109–15.

48. Centers for Disease Control and Prevention. Public health response to Hurricanes Katrina and Rita—Louisiana, 2005. *MMWR.* 2006;55(02): 29–30.

49. Centers for Disease Control and Prevention. Surveillance for World Trade Center disaster health effects among survivors of collapsed and damaged buildings. In: *Surveillance Summaries, April 7, 2006. MMWR.* 2006;55(SS-2):1–18.

50. Holtz TH, Leighton J, Balter S, et al. The public health response to the World Trade Center disaster. In: Levy BS, Sidel VW, eds. *Terrorism and Public Health.* New York: Oxford University Press; 2003.

51. http://www.oep-ndms.dhhs.gov/.

52. http://www.emacweb.org/.

CHAPTER 24

Environmental Health in Public Health

Alan M. Jacobs, PhD and DuWayne Porter, MPH, RS

LEARNING OBJECTIVES

Upon completion of this chapter, the reader will be able to:

1. Discuss the human needs, sources, environmental threats, and ways to protect our water supplies.

2. Identify atmospheric stratification, helpful and harmful gases, human oxygen needs, and air pollutants.

3. Evaluate the threats to our food supplies from the growth of pathogens and contamination by chemicals that the body may not be able to safely metabolize and excrete.

4. Recognize and appraise common hazards in the workplace and living areas.

5. Describe how waste has been mismanaged resulting in unacceptable risks to human health.

6. Discuss a chronology of environmental events in the latter half of the twentieth century that led to the establishment of regulatory safeguards.

7. Distinguish between natural and man-made environmental disasters. Evaluate whether it is possible to prevent or mitigate human impacts from such disasters.

8. Identify the role of chemicals and alternate methods to reduce pests and disease from nonhuman populations.

9. Discuss the various environmental issues that are global in scope, such as acid rain, climate change, ozone, chemical spills, and international terrorism.

10. Synthesize the various environmental health issues and evaluate how public health agencies can help to lessen adverse impacts to human health.

KEY TERMS

Acid Rain

Aquifer

Biochemical Oxygen Deficit (BOD)

Bioconcentrate

Bioremediation

Building Related Illness (BRI)

Chloro-Fluorocarbons (CFCs)

Conduction

Convection

Free Radical

Greenhouse Gases

Integrated Pest Management

Maximum Contaminant Level (MCL)

Plume

Point Source

Radon

Sick Building Syndrome (SBS)

Smog

Stratosphere

Wetlands

Zoonosis

INTRODUCTION

Humans try to maintain a healthy and safe environment in spite of fluctuating environmental conditions. We try to protect ourselves against adverse natural conditions: temperature extremes, floods and droughts, disease vectors, radiation, earthquakes, volcanic eruptions, tsunamis, and landslides. We also protect ourselves against adverse conditions resulting from our own actions: pollution, poor sanitation, poor working conditions, havoc from war and terrorism, and problems resulting from our tampering with natural fluctuations.

Civilization has survived to this point in time in a relatively healthy and safe condition through the evolution of an immune system that provides, to some extent, built-in resistance to diseases and sensitivities to allergens. If our ancestors had not had these resistances, they would not have survived to perpetuate the human species. In other words, former humans without these resistances died without their legacy of immunity.

Extra layers of protection have been added where natural immunity has not developed or kept pace with environmental change. Civilization has survived and flourished to this point in time also because of the development of an infrastructure that provides medical, public safety, and waste management services, using scientific, technical, and educational initiatives. It is the role of the public health agencies to monitor and manage this infrastructure for the protection of human populations.

Environmental health, the field dedicated to health and safety concerns in the public interest, is an important part of the mission of public health

agencies. The multidisciplinary, scientific approach that helps agencies monitor and understand environmental health problems is called *environmental health science*. The steps used by agencies to protect society from environmental health problems form the basis of *environmental health practice*.

With each environmental health concern noted in this chapter, we present the *principles* of environmental health science followed by *procedures* that public health agencies practice to protect the public.

CLEAN WATER: PRINCIPLES

Of the entire water budget ($\sim 1.5 \times 10^9$ km^3) of the earth, only 2.5 percent is fresh (not salty or brackish).[1] Our freshwater needs are further limited by its availability. Two percent of the entire water budget are in glaciers, and therefore are unavailable. Finally, the remaining 1/2 percent of available freshwater can become contaminated, rendering it unfit for human use. Consequently, public health agencies must be concerned about water supply and water quality.

Hydrologic Cycle

The hydrologic cycle is a closed system because the amount of water on the Earth is fixed, except for slight additions of ice from impacting comets. Within this system, water is present in oceans, clouds in the atmosphere, rivers, lakes, glaciers, snow fields, water-bearing strata (aquifers) in the ground, artificial ponds, soil moisture, wetlands, humid air, water vapor spewed by volcanoes, living creatures, hydrous minerals and other natural compounds, and manufactured items that combine water in their chemical makeup during processing. Each of these places (compartments) where water is found can change compartments at varying rates, so that ocean water can evaporate to form clouds, resulting in water precipitating to form snow, that compacts into glacial ice, that melts into rivers, is impounded in lakes, seeps underground into aquifers, resurfaces as springs, flows overland to the sea, and recycles—changing from compartment to compartment along different paths or the same path.

Water in the various compartments can naturally be cleansed by filtration (e.g., through **aquifers** and **wetlands**), by evaporation, by dilution (e.g., by rainwater), by adsorption (e.g., by carbon or clay in soils), by dispersion (e.g., in rivers), and by the action of organisms that consume contaminants (**bioremediation**). Water in the various compartments also can become contaminated from hazardous materials and wastes. Human actions can treat contaminated water or protect fresh water from contamination or can cause additional contamination.

Water Needs

Human adults need to consume three liters of water at least every few days.[2] Our body consists of about two-thirds water. We need this water internally for digestion, for circulation of bodily fluids, and for elimination of waste products.

Aside from ingestion, we use water for bathing, cooking, cleaning and sanitation, cooling, food production, power generation, and manufacturing. Volumetrically, our greatest personal use (misuse) of drinking water, ironically, is the flushing of toilets.

We derive almost all of our fresh water supply from surface water impoundments (4%) and groundwater aquifers (96%), depending on the regional geology and climate. The presence of productive aquifers allows nearby communities to rely on pumping from groundwater supplies for their water needs. The presence of fresh-water lakes or streams that can be dammed allows nearby communities to rely on surface water supplies. These sources of water can be put at risk in a number of ways, however. For example, evaporation can deplete surface water supplies, especially in arid regions; over-pumping of fresh-water aquifers near seacoasts can cause saltwater intrusion of the aquifer, and surface impoundments (reservoirs) can become silted in resulting in a loss of volume of the reservoir.

As human populations increase in size, water conservation grows in importance, but actions that waste water are all too common.[2] These actions range from nonessential water usage (e.g., watering lawns and golf courses, and filling swimming pools in arid areas) to losing unused water (e.g., dripping faucets, leaking pipes, malfunctioning or over-flushed toilets, and broken water mains). Allowing water to become contaminated is tantamount to wasting it at the source. Water supplies can be contaminated by its mixing with wastewater from improperly designed or functioning septic systems, from leaking wastewater conduits, or from manufacturing or waste disposal operations. Water pollution can be from **point sources** (identifiable waste stream outlets) or from nonpoint sources (runoff from agricultural fields or pavements).

Water can cause health problems if it contains pathogens (e.g., bacteria, viruses, and parasites). Contaminants that cause adverse health effects are usually invisible to the naked eye and lack scents or tastes. There are a number of common health problems resulting from the use of contaminated water, especially in the so-called "developing world." Chief among them is diarrhea, a common cause of death globally, especially in children, from dehydration. Other health problems from poor-quality water can include bloody stool, constipation, fever, headache, and muscle pains. Examples of diseases that can be transmitted by contaminated water are listed here:

- Bacteria: Typhoid fever, Cholera, Dysentery, Salmonellosis, pathogenic *E. coli*.
- Viruses: Hepatitis A, Poliomyelitis.
- Protozoa: Giardiasis, Cryptosporidiosis.
- Flukes: Schistosomiasis.

Water containing toxic chemicals can also cause health problems. A large number of metals and organic compounds at doses exceeding safe levels can cause defects during pregnancy (teratogens), genetic defects (mutagens), cancers (carcinogens), nerve damage (neurotoxins), and organ failure. Common toxic substances in water that cause health problems include high levels of arsenic, lead, pesticides, industrial solvents, PCBs, nitrates, and disinfectant byproducts.

Regulation

Public water supplies, serving groups of families and whole communities, are monitored and regulated under the scrutiny of the federal and state Environmental Protection Agencies (EPAs). The most frequently monitored contaminants, coliform bacteria, are indicators of contamination of water supplies by sewage.[2] Although most coliform bacteria themselves do not cause disease, sewage contamination may contain other pathogens from people with serious diseases (typhoid fever, polio, etc.). A strain of *E. coli* bacteria (O157:H7) will be discussed with respect to pathogens in foods. Although private water supplies (wells, cisterns, and springs) may be regulated to construction and health standards, in most cases, quality control and ongoing monitoring is the responsibility of the owners. Such private wells are notoriously contaminated, and contamination may be unnoticed. Some suppliers of water conditioning equipment may test the water for some contaminants, but this testing does not always include EPA-approved coliform testing.

Regulations developed in the 1970s to implement the Clean Water Act and later the Safe Drinking Water Act, finally put an end to the "right" to pollute water. In the 1980s, maximum permissible levels of contaminants **(Maximum Contaminant Levels, or MCLs)** were established in water supplies.[3] These levels are not totally health protective but were a big first step in monitoring drinking water. Truly health protective routine testing may be too costly and technically unfeasible, rendering the price of water too high for most communities. In

cases when contamination is suspected, however, the EPA can demand additional testing.

Many sewage systems combine wastewater derived from toilets and residential and commercial drains with stormwater drainage from streets and roadways. All of this wastewater is directed to the municipal sewage treatment plants, POTWs (Publicly Owned Treatment Works). This sounds like a good approach; both sources of wastewater will get treated before being released to the environment. Unfortunately, the conduits transporting all this drainage cannot accommodate all of the sewage, especially the increased storm drainage during intense storm events. What happens to the discharge that cannot be accommodated? The system, called Combined Sewage Overflow (CSO), is designed to release all the sewage in excess of the capacity of the conduits directly to the streams without treatment (see Figure 24.1). This results in raw sewage, including feces and soiled toilet paper, being discharged to surface streams.

Clean Water: Procedures

Public health agencies play a key role in the prevention of contamination in both surface and groundwater. Although these agencies are prepared to respond to emergencies created by contamination, prevention is their goal. Poorly constructed and maintained water wells have been a notorious source for groundwater contamination. Consider the infamous "Broad Street Pump." In London in 1854, Dr. John Snow analyzed fatalities associated with a cholera outbreak. He isolated the source as a common use pump located on Broad Street in Soho, London. The well had been contaminated by a nearby cistern/cesspool. By removing the pump handle and thus ending access to the water supply, the outbreak ceased. Not only did he prove the groundwater was the source of contamination, but he had proven that cholera was a waterborne illness. His findings provide one of the first examples of applied epidemiology, an approach that has become the backbone of public health investigations.

All supplies of water for human usage at the surface (natural lakes, surface impoundments,

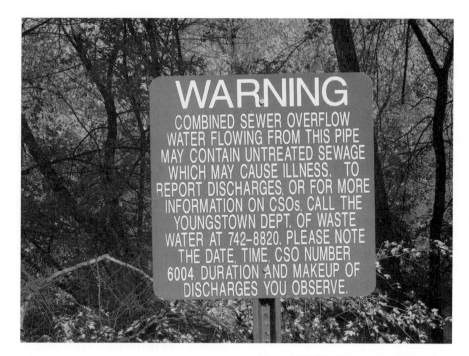

Figure 24.1. **Warning sign near Combined Sewage Overflow (CSO) Outlet Pipes**
SOURCE: Photo by Alan M. Jacobs.

rivers, and wetlands) and even underground water-bearing strata (aquifers) that are shallower than 25 feet can become easily contaminated. Public health agency private water well rules address the construction and sealing of wells to prevent this cross contamination. Many public health agencies require permits to install private water supplies. The permit process allows for evaluation of the site conditions prior to installation, inspection of the private water system after construction, testing for bacterial contamination, and, finally, the maintenance of records of test results. Groundwater wells are traditionally tested for coliform bacteria, which serve as indicator organisms. Coliform bacteria are not naturally occurring in groundwater, and their presence indicates that surface contamination has entered the well. The further presence of *E. coli* indicates wastewater contamination. Inspection by local health agencies ensures that the improper construction or maintenance of water wells is quickly addressed before entire aquifers are contaminated. In many instances of contamination, the problem can be easily solved by disinfecting the water well and the distribution system.

Public health agencies must also be involved with the proper sealing of water wells when they are no longer in use ("abandoned"). Because they are built by drilling a hole through protective layers of earth, water wells provide a direct route for contamination of underground aquifers when they are not properly maintained or are abandoned without being sealed.

Surface water protection is a more difficult endeavor. Surface water is easily contaminated through surface spills, airborne contaminants, watershed runoff, and animal or human waste. Public health agencies often get involved with surface water contamination when complaints or concerns are brought to the agency's attention. Public health agencies will test and monitor these waters and evaluate potential sources for contamination if they are requested to do so, or if a problem is discovered by agency surveillance.

Protecting our water supplies is typically a joint agency cooperative venture that may involve environmental protection agencies, departments of natural resources, local health departments, and public and private utilities. Surface water protection is essential. The United States Geological Survey (USGS) estimates that 79 percent of our water supplies are obtained from surface water, leaving only 21 percent obtained from groundwater wells. Without the surveillance provided by the public health agencies noted previously, assuring that drinking water supplies remain uncontaminated by chemical or biological agents would be impossible. These agencies are required to educate the public about the importance of acting in a manner that minimizes water contamination.

CLEAN AIR: PRINCIPLES

Above the ground surface, we are surrounded by gases that comprise the atmosphere.[1] These gases change in composition, pressure, and temperature from the ground surface upward. Except for people needing supplied oxygen or oxygen supplements, most humans rely on natural gases found near the ground surface. These gases include nitrogen (78%), oxygen (21%), argon (0.9%), carbon dioxide (0.03%), and trace amounts of others. Among those gases, humans can directly use only the oxygen, and must have approximately 20 cubic meters per day of air containing more than 19.5 percent oxygen. Oxygen deprivation of less than that percentage can cause brain damage and death.

The most abundant of gases near the ground surface is nitrogen.[3] Although our body needs nitrogen to live (proteins are compounds that contain nitrogen), we cannot use nitrogen directly from the atmosphere. We obtain nitrogen from foods and must rely on nitrogen-fixing bacteria (found growing on the roots of legumes and in other plants) or on the manufacture of chemical fertilizers for our nitrogen needs. Commercial fertilizers contain compounds of fixed nitrogen (and phosphorus and

potassium). Fixed nitrogen in the form of ammonia, nitrates, and nitrogen oxides, therefore, is an important soil nutrient. It is vital to plants and other biota higher in the food chain, including humans.

Other gases in the atmosphere that affect our lives include air pollutants near ground surface that can irritate our respiratory system, attack our internal organs through the lungs and bloodstream, and cause disease (e.g., emphysema, lung cancer, pneumonia).[4] Carbon monoxide, a byproduct of incomplete combustion (burning with a deficiency of oxygen), can attach to our blood hemoglobin in place of oxygen and starve our bodies of needed oxygen. Rain water can dissolve sulfur and nitrogen oxides in the atmosphere and form acids. When the acid rain water impacts the surface, it can destroy leaves, erode building exteriors, and make metallic contaminants in aqueous environments more able to dissolve. Compared with the metals in solid form, dissolved metals that are ingested are more easily absorbed in the body with an increased risk of toxic effects.

Chronic exposure to lead can cause anemia and neurological dysfunction.[5] Mercury poisoning can interfere with cell function, cause neurological dysfunction, and produce birth defects.[6] In the atmosphere at high altitudes, greenhouse gases can trap heat energy and cause global warming. Also, ozone can accumulate in the **stratosphere** (17–50 km) to absorb ultra-violet radiation from sunlight to reduce potential eye and skin damage.

The atmosphere is also responsible for weather phenomena, which indirectly affects our health and safety. Weather events are caused by atmospheric circulation powered by solar heating of the atmosphere and influenced by ocean circulation, the earth's rotation, and topographic barriers. Severe weather-related events can take the form of hurricanes (or typhoons), monsoons, tornadoes, and floods and drought.

The air in our buildings containing chemicals from fabrics, paints, machinery; and outside contaminated air from intake vents, and cracks in basements or slabs can cause discomforts such as headache, nausea, disorientation, and upset stomach. When a feeling of sickness from being in a building ceases upon exiting the building, and the sick feeling cannot be traced to a cause, we call that situation **Sick Building Syndrome (SBS).**[2] When a cause for the illness can be traced, we call this **Building Related Illness (BRI).** A serious form of BRI results from chronic exposure to **radon.** Radon gas (radioactive) can seep up from rock strata and collect in houses, where it can be inhaled to come in contact with lung tissue, causing cancer in some. Explosive gases such as methane can also seep into houses from abandoned underground coal mines and from landfills.

Clean Air: Procedures

The role of public health in both indoor air quality (IAQ) and outdoor air quality has continued to expand. The responsibilities have increased as the number of ailments associated with poor air quality has grown. Public health's role is to identify and monitor these hazards, and ensure that appropriate preventive and corrective measures are taken to maintain air quality. Examples of air pollution issues that have recently affected human health include radon, urea formaldehyde, airborne asbestos, sick building syndrome, automobile exhaust, ozone depletion, and mold.

Standards adopted under the Clean Air Act and amended in 1990[7] have proven to be cost effective. For those health and ecological benefits that could be quantified and converted to dollar values, EPA's best estimate is that in 2010, the benefits of the Clean Air Act programs will total about $110 billion. This estimate represents the value of avoiding increases in illness and premature death, which would have prevailed without the clean air standards and provisions required by the Amendments. By contrast, the detailed cost analysis conducted for this new study indicates that the costs of achieving these health and ecological benefits are likely to be only about $27 billion, a faction of the benefits.[8]

As early as 1881, cities such as Chicago and Cincinnati enacted clean air laws by federal, state, and local authorities. The development of clean air laws was slow but gradual as the twentieth century progressed. **Smog** issues in Donora, Pennsylvania (and elsewhere) brought air quality issues to the forefront. In Donora, a small industrial town south of Pittsburgh, on the night of October 26, 1948, a cloud of industrial gases and dust covered the town while the residents slept. Twenty residents died, and another 7,000 were hospitalized.[9] The poisonous cloud came from the smokestacks of the local zinc smelter, the major employer in the area. The United States legislature passed the Air Pollution Control Act of 1955, which was the first in a series of air quality laws that are in place today.

Because testing, monitoring, and correcting air pollution requires specific training, specialized agencies are best able to address these tasks. Regulation of the large geographic areas that can be affected by air pollution requires regional air agencies with multijurisdictional authority for best results. Multi jurisdictional authority allows for enforcement in more than one legal district, crossing state, city, or county lines. The agencies may analyze and monitor solid and gaseous air pollutants, respond to citizen complaints, issue air permits, issue air pollution alerts and pollen counts, and monitor air regulation compliance.

Furthermore, monitors must be installed over a wide geographic area to track the sources and direction of movement of **plumes,** which can travel long distances. Routine monitoring of ozone and particulates (less than 2.5 microns) is performed and evaluated regionally to determine which regions should reduce industrial air emissions, institute inspection of auto exhaust systems, alert the public to restrict refueling and grass mowing to certain times of the day, warn the elderly or those with respiratory problems to stay indoors, restrict outdoor activities during smog alerts, and so on.

SAFE FOOD SUPPLY: PRINCIPLES

Paracelsus (1493–1541), the Father of Toxicology, is credited with the notion that everything is a poison at the proper (improper) dose. Our food is no exception. We think we are eating pure nutrients with every bite. Unfortunately, there can be traces of pesticides, feces, food additives, growth hormones, precipitants from air pollution, pathogens, parasites, drug residues, allergens, and nutrients in quantities that carry risk when consumed. Poisons are not only added to foods or crops; plants themselves can produce their own "natural" pesticides to keep from being eaten.

Our own immune system can handle most contaminants using our in-bred resistance. Humans can withstand and counteract natural poisons. Our organs can metabolize harmful chemicals using enzymes into other less toxic chemicals and into chemicals that are easier for the body to excrete.[10]

However, newly manufactured chemicals (in the past 130 years), especially those whose chemical structure is rare in the natural world, may not be metabolized in this beneficial manner. Our bodies are not equipped with enzymes that can handle all chemicals. In fact, odd chemicals may be metabolized into less toxic chemicals, more toxic chemicals, or not metabolized at all. For example, toluene, a component of gasoline, can reach and impair the nervous system. The liver contains enzymes that convert toluene into benzoic acid, which is less toxic and more easily excreted from the body. Benzene, another and major component of gasoline, cannot be converted in this manner, so it cannot be detoxified. It is a known carcinogen. The manufactured chemical bromobenzene can be either metabolized into a chemical (bromobenzene epoxide) that can lead to cell death or to excretion depending on the concentration of bromobenzene.[10] Finally, polycyclic aromatic hydrocarbons (components of soot) are not carcinogenic in themselves.[11] Rather, through a series of biochemical processes in which the body "tries" to convert benzo[a]pyrene (a PAH) into a more water-soluble compound for ease of excretion, it "mistakenly" creates a very stable charged particle that is carcinogenic.

Why can't existing enzymes detoxify some synthetic chemicals? Although the grouping of atoms is similar among many natural and synthetic organic compounds, there are subtle differences.[10] For example, the group of manufactured solvents called chlorinated hydrocarbons (e.g., trichloroethylene [TCE] and perchloroethylene [PCE]), contains carbon-chlorine bonds, which are relatively rare in

nature. These solvents replaced formerly used solvents that were flammable (and toxic). Chlorinated hydrocarbons are not flammable, but they have adverse health effects and can **bioconcentrate** in fatty tissue in the body. Chemically, these compounds are more soluble in the fatty tissue than in water by factors of several hundreds to almost a thousand times more. This means that if you drank water having a PCE concentration of only one-thousandth of 1 percent, and the PCE were completely absorbed by the fatty tissue, the concentration of PCE in your fatty tissue would be almost 1 percent. Furthermore, if we ate fish that swam in water having a PCE concentration of 0.001 percent, the PCE would be bioconcentrated in the fatty tissue as well at 1 percent concentrations. As certain fish are eaten whole (sardines, smelts, etc.), including their livers, the ingestion of fish that swim in contaminated waters can result in absorbing even higher concentrations of contaminants.

In the past 130 years, chemists have created hundreds of thousands of synthetic chemicals, many of which have commercial uses. The toxic inventory maintained under TSCA (Toxic Substance Control Act) lists approximately 60,000 chemicals that were in commercial use by 1976.[12] Too often, these substances are marketed and used without a clear understanding of their ultimate impact on the environment and human health.

Food services and suppliers self regulate by preventing spoilage to protect their inventories. No one will buy foods that look, smell, or taste rotten. Most people can identify spoiled canned foods whose containers are bloated, and detect bad produce or dairy products that show evidence of mold. However, food that looks, smells, and tastes good can still be problematic.

Under certain conditions, food can be unsafe. Microorganisms that can make food unsafe include bacteria, viruses, parasites, and fungi. Microorganisms produce toxins that damage cells. As they grow, the quantity of toxins increases.

FAT TOM is an acronym to help us remember conditions conducive for growth of bacteria: Food (proteins and carbohydrates), Acidity (pH of 4.6–7.5), Temperature (danger zone TDZ = 41°F to 140°F), Time (>4 hrs in TDZ), Oxygen (varies), and Moisture (water activity of 0.85 or higher).

Food-borne illnesses from bacteria include *E. coli*, Salmonellosis, Shigellosis, Listeriosis, Gastroenteritis, and Botulism, among others. Bacteria causing these diseases can be found in a variety of foods, both animal and plant derived. A strain of *E. coli* bacteria (O157:H7), furthermore, has been the cause of serious outbreaks of food poisonings at food establishments. This strain, which produces a powerful toxin, can be found in cattle farms and petting zoos.

Food-borne illnesses causing infection from viruses include Hepatitis A, Norwalk Virus Gastroenteritis, and Rotavirus Gastroenteritis. They do not reproduce in food although they can be found in food (and water) and on food-contact surfaces.

Food-borne illnesses causing infection from parasites include Trichinosis, Giardiasis, and Intestinal Cryptosporidiosis. These parasites are found mostly in animals and fish.

Food-borne illnesses causing infection and intoxication from fungi (molds, yeasts, and mushrooms) cause spoilage and illness (from the toxins produced).

Safe Food Supply: Procedures

Public health agencies have a major role in the protection of our food supplies. This role begins with food processing and ends with consumption. It is difficult to declare that the enforcement of food service (restaurants) and food establishment (groceries) rules decrease the number of food-borne illness because their role is prevention and education.

Each year, more than 75 million people in the United States are struck with food-borne illness with 5,000 deaths.[13] Yet, most food-borne illness remains preventable through safe food handling, which is best guaranteed by training food handlers and educating consumers.

Episodes of food-borne illness can have serious economic as well as health impacts. A recent example occurred in late October of 2003, when emergency room physicians in Beaver County, Pennsylvania, reported an unusually high number

of hepatitis A virus cases. Health department investigators found that those that had become ill had eaten at a Chi Chi's Restaurant at the Beaver Valley Mall. The source was determined to be fresh, uncooked green onions imported from Mexico. Over 650 confirmed cases affecting residents of 6 other states were linked to this outbreak.[14] More than 9,000 persons who had eaten at the restaurant that had potentially been exposed were inoculated with immune globulin to protect against the hepatitis A virus. The nationally known chain of Chi Chi's Restaurants never fully recovered and filed for bankruptcy. The chain is no longer in business. This single food-borne outbreak required the collaboration of federal (United States Food and Drug Administration), state (Pennsylvania Department of Health), and Beaver Medical Center Emergency Room physicians to understand and correct.

The federal food safety laws require local health departments to inspect according to the potential food hazards associated with each food service or food establishment. This Hazard Analysis and Critical Control Point (HACCP) program analyzes hazards and identifies critical control points to once again prevent food-borne illness. Critical control points are those points in the food preparation and service of food at which control can be applied. Control is essential to prevent or eliminate a food safety hazard or to reduce it to an acceptable level. Such inspections involve measuring temperatures of stored foods, potential for drippings to cross-contaminate foods, presence of vermin or mold in food preparation or storage areas, hand-washing protocols of food-establishment staff, and so on.

HEALTHFUL WORKING AND LIVING CONDITIONS: PRINCIPLES

Health issues in the working and living environment include indoor or outdoor air quality, work activities that may be repetitive or require exertion, exposure to chemicals, potential hazards that can cause injury or disease, and freedom from fear (the psychological environment) by employees for their safety through right-to-know and risk communication programs.

A working environment for employees should be free of unhealthy and unsafe conditions. This environment should be monitored or inspected to determine compliance with permissible limits, as discussed later in this chapter. If unhealthy or unsafe conditions are identified, these conditions should be eliminated or controlled.

Control of unhealthy or unsafe conditions includes engineering controls, administrative controls, personal protective equipment (PPE), and employee training. For example, engineering controls can include changes in ventilation, lighting, addition of handrails, and noise absorbing wall or ceiling panels. Administrative controls can include warnings using signs or labels, reduction of time employees spend in hazardous areas, scheduling of training sessions, and health and safety communica-

tions (health and safety plans, spill prevention and control plans, and evacuation plans). Employees should wear personal protective clothing and use PPE and monitoring devices (gloves, hardhats, steel-toed boots, eye and ear protection, and contaminant detectors). Depending on tasks performed, employees should be properly trained, including the satisfactory completion of periodic refresher courses.

Healthful Working and Living Conditions: Procedures

Public health's role in the home and workplace has increased dramatically over the past two decades. We are now familiar with workplace and home ailments such as legionnaire's disease, sick building syndrome, black mold, radon poisoning, urea formaldehyde poisoning, asbestosis, and carbon monoxide poisoning. It was not so long ago that most of these environmental situations were not considered problems (Figure 24.2). Before the discovery of a potential association with mold and the

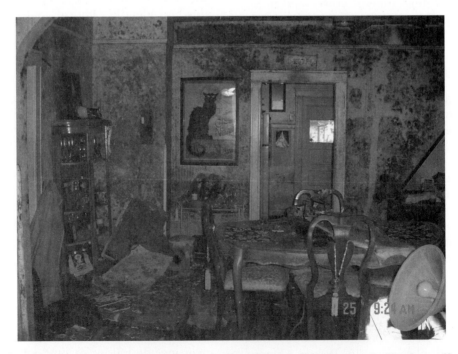

Figure 24.2. Mold growth in a residential home in New Orleans after damage by Hurricane Katrina
SOURCE: Photo by John Rindy.

"bleeding lung syndrome," mold in the home was considered an allergen problem but not a public health threat. Mold can grow on food and on building surfaces as long as there is moisture, a food source, and a temperature conducive for growth. In the aftermath of Hurricane Katrina, damage to residences in New Orleans included the growth of mold in interior building surface (see Figure 24.2). The greatest health threats are from toxins from the mold that could be ingested, that is, those on food. Mold that grows on building surfaces can cause property damage, and mold spores can spread to breathing zones and food.

The Occupational Safety and Health Act of 1970 created both the National Institute for Occupational Safety and Health (NIOSH) and the Occupational Safety and Health Administration (OSHA). OSHA is responsible for enforcing and developing workplace safety and health regulations, and NIOSH was established to help assure safe and healthful working conditions by providing research, information, education, and training in the field of occupational safety and health.

Although most local public health agencies are not involved in industrial and commercial business, they may play a part in residential health and safety issues. Many departments inspect for radon, urea formaldehyde issues, asbestos, and mold. However, it is becoming increasingly more difficult to maintain qualified staff in these areas as requirements for individuals with specific knowledge, skills, and abilities because of the increase in personnel costs and the need for detailed training.

WASTE MANAGEMENT: PRINCIPLES

Waste is generated from manufacturing, commercial, residential, mining, governmental, nongovernmental organizations, and even health facilities. It can take the form of wastewater, discharge to bodies of water, air emissions, stormwater, municipal solid waste, construction and demolition waste, hazardous chemical waste, radioactive waste, and infectious waste. Waste is land filled, incinerated, transported, stored temporarily, processed chemically or physically (to be less mobile, toxic, or have less volume), recycled, reused, injected into deep rock strata, or isolated in repositories (radioactive waste from nuclear power plants and nuclear weapons). Proper management of waste is required under various laws and regulations (discussed later in this chapter). Even today, some waste still is illegally dumped on vacant land, on highway right of ways, in streams, in shallow depressions, in lakes and oceans, and so on.

Waste that is not properly managed can cause adverse health effects from the release of toxic substances into the environment. A risk to public health exists if there is a source of waste that is transported through the environment to receptors, and exposures exceed acceptable risk levels. Unacceptable risk levels may vary among individuals in the population. Those who are elderly, very young, pregnant, sick, or sensitive to allergens can be more susceptible to disease than are other members of the general population.

WASTE MANAGEMENT: PROCEDURES

Waste management is a priority in the environmental health programs of public health agencies. From federal agencies such as the EPA, the Agency for Toxic Substance and Disease Registry, the Small Flows Clearing House, and many state and local public health agencies, the development and implementation of waste management programs has always been an ongoing task. Both liquid and solid waste may contain hazardous chemicals and materials as well as pathogens and disease vectors. The improper disposal of these wastes can threaten public health.

Field operations in waste management may pose a health and safety risk to the workers in the contaminated work areas. Government agencies responsible for occupational health and safety require workers to be protected during waste management operations. They must be trained, wear health and safety clothing (see Figure 24.3), be familiar with decontamination procedures, use health and safety monitoring equipment, operate under approved health and safety plans, undergo medical examinations, be protected under Right-to-Know laws, and be supervised by managers who have undergone health and safety training.

Wastewater related to sewage disposal is a particularly difficult problem. Inadequately treated sewage effluent can contain dangerously high levels of pathogenic bacteria. The management of sewage waste disposal ranges from small residential onsite treatment systems to large municipal treatment facilities. Untreated wastewater with concentrations of dissolved oxygen (**biochemical oxygen deficit [BOD]**) that is released directly into streams and lakes can reduce populations of fish in the vicinity and downstream of the release.

Recycling solid waste has become a major educational program in an effort to decrease the volume of residential and commercial solid waste while ensuring its proper containment and disposal. Recycling and decreasing unnecessary packaging are two approaches that will diminish the volume of future waste requiring disposal.

The improper management of solid waste became news worthy when, in 1978, the story of Love Canal hit the news media. Love Canal was a one-mile stretch of a proposed canal meant to connect the Niagara River with Niagara Falls. The Canal was never completed and was purchased by the City of Niagara Falls in 1920. The City began using the Canal as a landfill for chemical waste disposal. In 1942, the Hooker Chemical and Plastics Corporation acquired the land for its own use. The company is known to have buried tons of toxic waste in the area. The site was closed in 1952. The City of Niagara School Board bought the property with full knowledge of the chemical waste landfill. The City also constructed sewer lines through a portion of the site. In 1978, it was discovered that the residents of the area had a high rate of cancer, and birth defects were prevalent. In the five-year period between 1974 and 1978, a study financed by the Love Canal Home Owners Association indicated a 56 percent birth defect rate (9 of 16 births.[15]) On May 21, 1980, President Jimmy Carter declared a state of emergency at Love Canal, and the EPA agreed to evacuate 700 families temporarily. Eventually, the government relocated more than 800 families and reimbursed them for their homes. Hooker Chemical's parent corporation, Occidental Petroleum, was sued by the EPA and in 1995 agreed to pay $129 million. Solid waste disposal facilities have no longer been overlooked by government regulators.

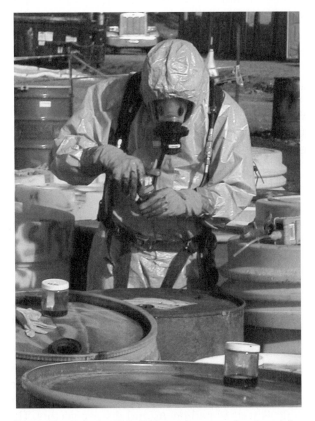

Figure 24.3. This EPA worker, wearing Level A protection gear, samples this barrel to determine its contents

SOURCE: United States Environmental Protection Agency.

ENVIRONMENTAL LAWS AND REGULATIONS: PRINCIPLES

Although awareness of environmental degradation and its effect on human health predates the twentieth century, health-protective environmental laws and regulations did not develop until recently. The 1960s witnessed anti-establishment movements that asked a question: "Are we pursuing wealth at the expense of health?" One important influence in this movement was the publication of *Silent Spring* in 1962 by Rachel Carson.[16] Carson alerted us to the health dangers of chemical pesticides, used to increase food production.

Most laws and regulations addressed the management of wastes that caused pollution of the environment.[17] Other laws pertain to hazardous materials prior to their becoming wastes. Federal laws have been augmented by state and local environmental laws, and the laws (acts or statutes of legislative bodies) have been codified into regulations (by regulatory agencies). Regulatory agencies of the federal government include the Environmental Protection Agency, the Nuclear Regulatory Commission, Departments of the Interior, Agriculture, Defense, Transportation, Labor, and others. The following list forms a brief chronology of the federal laws and newsworthy events that contributed to the environmental movement.

- 1947 FIFRA-insecticide, fungicide, and rodenticide
- 1948 CWA-Clean Water Act
- 1962 Publication of *Silent Spring*.
- 1955 CAA-Clean Air Act
- 1963 CAA, Title 2 (motor vehicles)
- 1965 SWDA (solid waste disposal)
- 1967 AQA (Air Quality Act)
- 1969 Cuyahoga River Fire (June 21)
- 1969 NEPA (National Environmental Policy Act) for federal projects
- 1970 UNITED STATES EPA established

- 1970 CAA Amendments of 1970
- 1970 OSHA (occupational safety and health)
- 1972 CWA
- 1973–74 More CAA Amendments
- 1974 SDWA (drinking water)
- 1974 Ozone "layer" discovered
- 1975 HMTA-hazardous materials transportation regulations (Department of Transportation [DOT])
- 1976 TSCA (toxic substance control)
- 1976 RCRA (resource conservation and recovery)
- 1977 More CAA Amendments
- 1970–80 Solid and Chemical Waste Acts
- 1978 Love Canal area evacuated
- 1979 Three-Mile Island nuclear accident
- 1984 Bhopal India pesticide leak disaster
- 1986 Chernobyl nuclear accident
- 1986 EPCRA (emergency planning and community right-to-know)
- 1987 Montreal Protocol (limiting CFC production)
- 1989 Exxon Valdez Oil Spill
- 1990 Pollution Prevention Act
- 1990 Oil Pollution Act
- 1991 Persian Gulf War oil dump
- 1992 Earth Summit, Rio de Janeiro
- 1994 U.N. Conference on Population, Cairo, Egypt
- 1997 Kyoto, Japan Accord (global warming)

ENVIRONMENTAL LAWS AND REGULATIONS: PROCEDURES

Through identification and clarification of a problem, public health agencies can best determine situations that require legislative redress. After this is done, public health agencies must convince politicians to introduce enabling legislation to establish laws and rules that will allow enforcement of compliance. These laws and rules allow for public health agencies to inspect and insure compliance by homeowners as well as commercial and industrial corporations. These inspections allow for the development of documentation to request compliance and, if necessary, prepare for legal action. It is imperative that public health agencies have these laws and regulations to complete the protection and fair implementation of environmental and public health programs under which they have enforcement jurisdiction.

DISASTER PREPAREDNESS: PRINCIPLES

Cataclysmic events that are "natural" or "man-made" can have negative impacts on public health and the environment. Natural disasters, such as tsunamis, hurricanes, tornadoes, earthquakes, volcanic eruptions, meteorite impacts, landslides, naturally ignited forest or range fires, and avalanches, cannot be easily prevented or their impact easily mitigated. Disasters that are basically natural can be exacerbated by ignoring natural consequences from lack of education, avoiding the necessary costs of safeguards, or fatalism. Living in tornado-prone areas in trailer parks and in other houses without basements can leave the public unable to take shelter in time to safely weather the storm. Too many people build in areas where natural disasters are predictable or build without safeguards. There can be serious consequences from floods on floodplains, from earthquakes in seismically active areas, from floods in coastal areas where hurricanes are common, and so on. Do humans have the right to live wherever they want and expect the public to bale them out whenever natural disasters strike? Public health efforts should encourage the population, through education, to live in the environmentally safest areas.

Disasters that are solely initiated by human action, namely war, carelessness, and terrorism, should be mitigated by public action through education and preparation for such disasters. Preparedness for potential human atrocities (before the disaster occurs) is a growing responsibility of public health.

DISASTER PREPAREDNESS: PROCEDURES

Environmental technology, government regulations, and early warning can mitigate the impact of the construction and maintenance of levees, flood-control dams, and artificial wetlands, sea walls, and barrier islands. For example, flood damage from earthquakes can be reduced by adherence to building codes, construction of "shock-absorbing" foundations (aseismic bearing pads), and zoning laws. Landslides can be prevented by dewatering, terracing, and buttressing unstable slopes. Volcanic eruptions and offset movements of the Earth's crust can be handled by restrictive zoning and evacuations. Violent storms can "be weathered" by directing people to emergency shelters.

On September 11, 2001, the reality of terrorism struck home in the United States and found a nation unprepared. The reality of the event and the inadequate nature of our disaster preparedness became evident. The heroes were there, but many agencies lacked the equipment and training necessary to address disasters of this magnitude. The federal government began pouring in much needed dollars to fortify the capacity of responsible agencies. Public health was not forgotten. Resources were made available for both equipment and training. Public health began a new era in disaster preparedness. The Incident Command System (ICS) was introduced and implemented throughout public health agencies. ICS is an on-site tool to manage all emergency response incidents. It can be used for natural, chemical, biological, and other man-made disasters. This training was never more evident than the hurricane Katrina disaster. In August of 2005, Katrina, a category 5 hurricane, devastated much of the north-central Gulf Coast of the United States. It hit the city of New Orleans especially

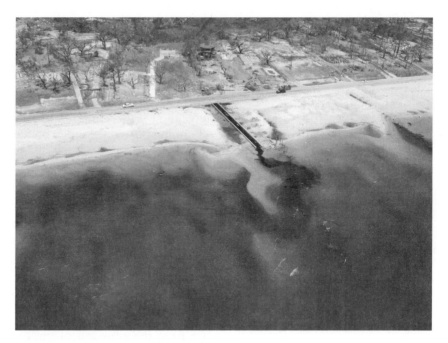

Figure 24.4. Shoreline Pollution, Hurricane Katrina
SOURCE: United States Environmental Protection Agency.

hard, flooding 80 percent of the city. More than 1,800 people were lost and estimates of damage costs exceed \$81 billion.[18] Public health was there. Volunteers streamed in from all over the United States and the public health response was coordinated by the CDC in Atlanta, Georgia. Attempts were made to use the ICS, but lack of individuals trained in its use did not allow for the system to function as desired. Training in ICS is now required of those most likely to implement this management tool in the case of future disasters.

In addition, public health has taken one more step toward disaster preparedness and established Medical Reserve Corps throughout the United States. This Corps will provide pools of volunteer health professionals ready to respond to local emergencies when needed.

Katrina had a profound effect on the environmental health of the area. When flood waters receded, the residual water contained sewage, bacteria, industrial chemicals and pesticides that had been mixed with the flood waters (Figure 24.4). All segments of the environment were impacted:

human, animal, and plant. The residual waters were pumped from the city and environmental health professionals evaluated the conditions for the safe return of the residents. Health education became the most important tool in ensuring the safety of the citizens of New Orleans. This effort will continue for many years.

PEST AND VECTOR CONTROL: PRINCIPLES

Pest control involves elimination of weeds, rodents, insects, and fungi. Such pests can cause disease or allergic reactions. Vectors (carriers of disease) can include mosquitoes, flies, rodents, dogs, cats, raccoons, birds, horses, and other living creatures. Some of these carriers can get the disease, whereas others are only carriers and unaffected themselves. A disease that is transmissible from animals to humans is called a **zoonosis.**[19]

Chemicals are used to control these pests and vectors that spread disease and consume commercial farm plants. Such chemicals can also enter the environment and lead to human exposure. The chemical can be the cause of toxic and allergic reactions if exposure to the public is above acceptable risk levels. Runoff from farm fields can carry excess pesticides that had been applied to the croplands. Runoff can enter water supply reservoirs and aquifers.

DDT, now banned since 1974 in the United States, is a pesticide that was used to combat malaria, spread by mosquitoes. Indiscriminate spraying of DDT, even on people and food supplies, had toxic repercussions exacerbated by the fact that DDT remains in the environment long after its application. Some pesticides that target certain pests, that are applied judiciously, and that decompose quickly cause fewer environmental and health problems.

PEST AND VECTOR CONTROL: PROCEDURES

Public health's role in pest control is one of prevention. How do we eliminate the pathway to the human population? Indiscriminate use of pesticides or untried alternatives often leads to environmental complications. For example, the indiscriminate use of DDT, a very good wide-ranging pesticide, eliminated pests but had effects on wildlife (e.g., thinning of shells of birds' eggs) that dictated the discontinuance of DDT.

Environmental health professionals now use **Integrated Pest Management.** This is a tool that coordinates the use of pest and environmental information along with the best available pest control methods. These methods include biological (natural predators, parasites, and disease organisms), cultivation, genetic, and a minimum of chemical control measures. The use of one or a combination of these controls can provide us with the safest, most economical, and effective control measures. Most environmental health professionals in this area are certified pest control operators in the jurisdiction in which they work.

GLOBAL ISSUES: PRINCIPLES

Global issues include acid rain, global warming/greenhouse gas emission, ozone depletion, ocean dumping of wastes, spills, pandemics, and international terrorism. After these discussions, the role of public health departments will be presented.

Acid Rain

During combustion of sulfur-containing materials (e.g., high sulfur coal), sulfur oxides are discharged into the atmosphere, where, combined with moist air, they produce rain containing sulfuric acid. A similar process occurs with combustion at very high temperatures producing nitrogen oxides and nitric acid. Precipitation of this acid rain can occur far from the emission of the gaseous oxide pollutants, often across state and national borders.

Acid rain falling upon the land surface can damage crops and forests by destruction of plant tissues. The acid rain can also dissolve metallic mineral grains in the stream and lake sediment, causing toxic metals to dissolve. Metals in solution are more available for absorption by aquatic life, land animals, and humans ingesting this water, thus facilitating immediate toxic effects, and easy entry into the food chain.

Global Warming

The emission of **greenhouse gases** (carbon dioxide, methane, water vapor, chlorofluorocarbons, and ozone) increases the tendency of the atmosphere to warm up. Solar (radiant) heat energy can pass down through the greenhouse gases onto the Earth where the rays are absorbed on the Earth's surface and passed on to other objects by contact (**conduction**). Also, the energy can be transmitted about the Earth by air or water currents (**convection**). The greenhouse gases diminish the ability of conductive/convective heat energy to penetrate back up through the atmosphere away from the Earth. This causes a buildup of heat, as in an unventilated greenhouse.

The Earth would be a frozen planet without the benefit of the greenhouse gases. Without the greenhouse gases, the Earth would maintain an average daily temperature of only negative 17°C (1.4°F). With these gases, we maintain an average daily temperature on Earth of +14°C (57.2°F). What's the problem? We are experiencing a gradual warming above this level, which may lead to significant warming of the Earth. This could result in a significant melting of the ice caps (namely, continental glaciers on Antarctica and Greenland). If sufficient melting occurs, sea level will rise, flooding coastal areas up to about 100 meters. Warmer temperatures also could have other effects, both positive and negative as discussed later.

Is the cause of the global warming mainly the result of human discharge of greenhouse gases or natural processes? Discharge of greenhouse gases can come from volcanoes, wetlands, and natural forest fires. Or . . . what is the influence of variations in the intensity of incoming radiation from the sun? How about the changes in reflectivity (albedo) of the Earth's surface? What is the effect of variations in the Earth's orbit?

Geologists have evidence that the Earth has experienced ice ages for the past two million years (way before the Industrial Revolution), where interglacial warming periods were warmer than today (Cypress trees in southern Illinois, from pollen records).[20] Correlation of upward trends of carbon dioxide and Earth temperatures from ice cores in Greenland seem to rise in tandem, but such correlations do not prove cause and effect. In fact, the rise in carbon dioxide could be caused by natural global warming. With global warming, there would be a reduction of land areas subject to frost and an increase in the duration of frost periods. The population of decomposer organisms would increase. The warmer and frost-free climate would allow decomposer organisms to cause an increase in the decay of vegetation and dead organisms. This, in turn, would release more carbon dioxide into the atmosphere.

We tend to dwell on the adverse effects of global warming that may cause an increase in average world temperatures of a few centigrade degrees. Such effects can include coastal flooding and the increase in tropical diseases and insect vectors. However, a shift in the warmer climatic zones poleward may result in smaller areas of permanently or partially frozen ground, larger areas of croplands, grasslands, and wetlands, and longer crop-growing seasons.

Could we stop the global warming by reducing industrial emission? We don't know. Could we start it up again, if we find global cooling would trigger another ice age? Is the natural global warming just a minor warming period in an overall cooling period? Answers to these questions are not at hand. The belief by some scientists that industrial emissions are the prime cause of global warming is not shared by all. Many geologists and other Earth scientists who have studied climate change prior to the Industrial Revolution still argue that global warming has occurred long before human influence. Variations in solar energy input on Earth through cyclic changes in solar output, orbital and axial changes (wobble) of planet Earth, changes in the reflectivity of the Earth's surface (snow covered and non-snow covered), and changes in ocean currents that distribute heat in the ocean basins.

What we do know is that the Earth is currently warming up. We also know that increased air emissions from industry cause poor air quality and resultant adverse health effects. So the answer is to reduce or don't increase air emissions, and monitor the warming trend.

Ozone Depletion

There is good ozone and bad ozone. The bad ozone is present in ground-level smog. Here we need ozone depletion. The good ozone is found in the stratosphere above jet aircraft cruising altitudes. Here the ozone molecule (3 oxygen atoms) is formed by lightning discharge from a normal oxygen molecule (2 oxygen atoms). Stratospheric ozone absorbs some of the ultra-violet radiation, which if unabsorbed causes damage to eyes and causes skin cancer. Depletion of stratospheric ozone in parts of the stratosphere has been caused by the discharge of **chloro-fluorocarbons (CFCs)** into the atmosphere. Here, with the action of a chlorine **free radical,** the ozone molecule (3 oxygen atoms) reverts back to the normal oxygen molecule (2 oxygen atoms), which does not have UV-radiation absorption characteristics. CFCs were manufactured as refrigerants and propellants, and have since been banned or phased out by the Montreal Protocol.[2]

Spills

Crude petroleum, petroleum products, chemicals, and liquid wastes are transported by tanker ships, trucks, railroad cars, and pipelines to refineries, chemical plants, fuel distribution points, and waste treatment, storage, and disposal sites (TSDs). On route, accidents have happened that have resulted in spillage into the environment.

Major spills of crude oil have occurred that have severely damaged the environment. The Exxon *Valdez* ran aground on a rock ledge in Prince William Sound, Alaska, in 1989, and spilled 260,000 bbls. The Torrey *Canyon* spilled 700,000 bbls of oil in 1967 off the coast of Great Britain. The Amoco *Cadiz* spilled 1.1 million bbls of oil off the coast of France in 1978. The largest oil spill, and no accident, occurred at the end of the first Gulf War in 1991, when 6 million barrels of oil were intentionally dumped into the Persian Gulf.

Less dramatic spills occur when trucks or railroad cars leak liquids that run off into streams and lakes. Highways are closed, cleanup crews are dispatched, and in some cases, evacuations occur after each accident. Each inland spill is not global in nature, but the totality of occurrences worldwide has global significance. These spills degrade the environment because spilled contaminants foul water supplies and soils.

Global Concerns

Human boundaries that separate nations, ethnicity and race, linguistic differences, economic and social classes, religious beliefs, educational levels, and politics, are transparent to environmental health impacts. For example, air emissions from power plants in the Midwest United States and the resulting acid rain can drift eastward to Atlantic seaboard states and into southeast Canada. Waste from ocean dumping can be carried by marine currents to far-away shores. Contagious diseases can be passed through the populations worldwide and can cause pandemics (bird flu, SARS, HIV/AIDS, etc.). Foods containing parasites and chemical contaminants can be shipped worldwide to distant receptors. Tsunamis generated from offshore earthquakes can travel thousands of miles and destroy distant coastal communities. Environmental health problems can start in localized areas but can spread globally.

These human boundaries, however, can affect how we view the environment and how we solve or choose to ignore the environmental health problems and potential problems. Therefore, environmental problems of a global nature must be addressed by national governments and international accords. Monitoring of agreed upon solutions to these environmental problems, nevertheless, should be aided by local or regional health agencies.

These human boundaries, furthermore, can separate and alienate groups of individuals, resulting in acts of international terrorism. For example, the spread of anthrax pathogens through the United States mail and release of sarin gas in the Tokyo subways alerted us to the possibility that other terrorists could spread other harmful substances. Human exposure to these substances could be a threat to public health. Fears of poisoning our water supplies, damaging of flood protection dams, discharge of smallpox viruses, and detonation of dirty bombs (radioactive), emphasize global environmental threats to public health. Key factors that make an environmental hazard a potential weapon for terrorists are the virulence of the hazard and the ease of spreading the hazard through the population.

GLOBAL ISSUES: PROCEDURES

Health agencies can be helpful in preparing the public for potential attacks to water supplies, spread of pathogenic organisms, food poisoning, and release of air toxins.

In general, environmental health risks are present when all of the following are present: a source of contamination or disease, an environmental pathway between source and receptor, and human (or zoonotic) receptors. Pubic health agencies can remove the source, block the pathway, or evacuate or immunize the receptors. Removing any one of these can significantly reduce the health risk to the receptors. This strategy is more helpful regarding terrorism and contaminant spills. Acid rain, ozone depletion, and global warming can be mitigated only by removal of sources, namely in regard to air pollutants. Air pollutants, including sulfur and nitrogen oxides, chlorofluorocarbons (CFCs), and greenhouse gasses can be dispersed beyond a regional boundary to cause global effects, and, therefore, can only be controlled through the cooperation of global authorities.

REVIEW QUESTIONS

1. To promote good health and to prevent disease, public health agencies must work toward mitigating the impacts of potential environmental hazards. Discuss five environmental hazards and, in this context, specify how the agencies should deal with these impacts.
2. What is the difference between SBS (Sick Building Syndrome) and BRI (Building Related Illness), and how should the public health agencies respond to complaints?
3. What is the significance of finding coliform bacteria in drinking water?
4. Should food safety be treated as an environmental health issue? Explain.
5. Discuss the positive and negative potential health effects of global warming.

REFERENCES

1. Cunningham WP, Cunningham M, Saigo BW. *Environmental Science: A Global Concern.* 8th ed. Boston, MA: McGraw-Hill; 2005.
2. Nadakavukaren A. *Our Global Environment; A Healthy Perspective.* 5th ed. Prospect Heights, IL: Waveland Press, Inc.; 2000.
3. Moore GS. *Living with the Earth; Concepts in Environmental Health Science.* 2nd ed. Boca Raton, FL: Lewis Publishers; 2002.
4. Friis RH. *Essentials of Environmental Health.* Sudbury, MA: Jones and Bartlett Publishers; 2007.
5. Newman MC. *Fundamentals of Ecotoxicology.* Boca Raton, FL: Lewis; 2002.
6. Philp RB. *Ecosystems and Human Health, Toxicology and Environmental Hazards.* 2nd ed. Boca Raton, FL: Lewis; 2001.
7. United States Environmental Protection Agency. Available at: http://www.epa.gov/air/caa/.
8. United States Environmental Protection Agency. Benefits and Cost of the Clean Air Act. Available at: http://www.epa.gov/air/sect812.
9. Public Broadcast System (PBS). The Donora Smog Disaster. Available at: http://www.pbs.org/now/science/smog.html.
10. Rodricks JV. *Calculated Risks—the Toxicity and Human Health Risks of Chemicals in our Environment.* Cambridge: Cambridge University Press; 1992.
11. Baird C. *Environmental Chemistry.* 2nd ed. New York: WH Freeman; 1999.
12. US Environmental Protection Agency. Available at: http://www.answers.com/topic/toxic-substances-control-act.
13. Centers for Disease Control and Prevention. Available at: http://www.cdc.gov/ncidod/dbmd/diseaseinfo/foodborneinfections_g.htm.
14. USA Today. Available at: http://www.usatoday.com/news/health/2003-11-21-onions-outbreak_x.htm.
15. Fact Pack P001. Center for Health Environment and Justice. P.O. Box 6806, Falls Church, VA.
16. Carson R. *Silent Spring* Boston: Houghton Mifflin; Cambridge, MA: Riverside Press; 1962.
17. Bregman JI, Edell, RD. *Environmental Compliance Handbook* Boca Raton, FL: Lewis Publishers; 2002.
18. Science Daily. Available at: http://www.sciencedaily.com/releases/2005/06/050609234408.htm.
19. Last JM. *A Dictionary of Public Health.* New York: Oxford University Press; 2007.
20. Grueger, E. The development of the vegetation of southern Illinois since late Illinonian time (preliminary report). *Revue Geographie Physique et Geologie Dynamique.* 1970;12:143–148.

CHAPTER 25

Primary Care and Public Health

Michael R. King, MD, MPH, Kevin A. Pearce, MD, MPH, and
Samuel C. Matheny, MD, MPH

LEARNING OBJECTIVES

Upon completion of this chapter, the reader will
be able to:

1. Describe the concept of primary care as it
   relates to health care services and public
   health services.

2. Describe the value of primary care to individual and population health as well as to
   the performance of a health care system.

3. Examine the workforce of primary care,
   including trends in specialty care of
   physicians, contributions of nonphysician
   providers, and the maldistribution issues of
   health care providers.

4. Show the unique contribution of health
   centers in providing primary care services
   to the underserved, especially rural
   populations.

5. Examine the role of governmental and
   policy interventions in providing for
   and supporting primary care to the
   underserved, including policies that
   influence the workforce, training,
   placement, and payment of primary
   care providers.

6. Explain the synergy and tension between
   primary care and public health regarding
   individual and population health.

7. Describe the utility and opportunities of
   population-based data on actual medical
   care with regards to primary care and
   public health.

8. Describe the conceptual model of COPC as
   a way of integrating primary care and public
   health activities.

9. Demonstrate the role of primary care and
   public health in providing preventive
   services.

10. Illustrate the role and potential of primary
    care providers as a public health sentinel.

KEY TERMS

Community Oriented Primary Care (COPC)

Federally Qualified Health Center (FQHCs)

National Health Service Corps (NHSC)

Primary Care

Primary Care Health Professional Shortage
    Areas (HPSAs)

Primary Health Care

Primary Medical Care

Primary Prevention

Public Health Sentinel

Secondary Prevention

Tertiary Prevention

Primary care and public health are inexorably linked, though not congruent. Clean air, potable water, public safety, and national defense are all public health functions distinct from primary care. But what about childhood immunizations, the prevention of heart disease, or the treatment of battered women? Is screening for breast cancer a public health function, a primary care function, or both? Despite areas of overlap, and some areas of conflict, the link between public health and primary care is an important one because of the role primary care providers play in providing essential health care services.

The overarching goals of *Healthy People 2010* are to increase quality and years of healthy life, and eliminate health disparities. Primary care services and providers play a central role in achieving these objectives. It has been well established that primary care provides effective, high quality, accessible care that the population needs to treat their health problems and maintain their health. Primary care practice intersects with nearly every focus area and leading health indicator set forth by *Healthy People 2010*. Monitoring health services delivered through the primary care workforce provides a way to both measure the health of a population and link population needs to available services. The strong linkages between primary care and public health provide natural opportunities for community partnerships, research, and policy development to solve or improve health problems. Understanding the value of primary care, barriers to obtaining primary care, and the associated implications for the medical workforce are all necessary to fully understand the health of local communities, especially in rural or medically underserved communities.

PRIMARY CARE AND ITS IMPACT ON POPULATION HEALTH

Primary care is not a new concept, but its definition and manifestation in the general context of medical care have been sequentially modified over the past 50 years. The Declaration of Alma-Ata stated in 1977 that "primary health care is . . . the first level of contact of individuals, the family, and community with the national health system, bringing health care as close as possible to where people live and work, and constitutes the first element of a continuing health care process." This Declaration, which placed primary care as the central piece of the system of health care, was part of the World Health Assembly Global Strategy of Health Care for All by 2000.[1] More recently, the Institute of Medicine (IOM) defined primary care as "the provision of integrated, accessible health care services by clinicians who are accountable for addressing a large majority of personal health care needs, developing a sustained partnership with patients, and practicing in the context of family and community."[2]

The distinction has been made between primary medical care and primary health care. **Primary medical care** is concerned with the issues of accessibility of medical and preventive services from health care workers; **primary health care** is a social concept concerned with populations and involving a wider variety of individuals than simply health care workers.[3] Vuori states that primary health care can be interpreted in four ways: as a set of activities, as a level of care, as a strategy of organizing health care, or as a philosophy of care.[4]

Primary care is usually, but not always, the portal of entry through which individuals obtain medical services, and most Americans report having a primary care physician.[5,6] Individual health care services routinely delivered through primary care include health promotion, disease prevention, health maintenance, counseling, patient education, and the diagnosis and treatment of both acute and chronic illnesses. Other key responsibilities of primary care providers is the coordination of individuals' health care services, advocacy for the individual as they navigate the health care system, and focus on achieving safe, high quality, cost-effective care. Public health also feels some responsibility to these individual health services but more as they relate to the population's health. It has been said that primary care is an essential service, and when the population needs dictate it, many public health agencies take on providing personal health services or primary care services; often becoming the provider of last resort for underserved and disadvantaged populations.[7]

Within the spectrum of individual health care services, primary care medical services have a powerful impact on public health, especially for younger populations[7] and those people living in poverty.[8] Twenty years of research has provided evidence that proves that a primary care-based health system matters. Individuals, populations, and countries with adequate access to primary care realize a number of health and economic benefits (see Table 25.1). Primary care decreases long-term morbidity and mortality, reduces cost and overuse of health care resources, and reduces health disparities.[15] Specifically, an increase of 1 primary care physician per 10,000 population results in a decrease of 14.4 deaths per 100,000 with an enhanced effect on racial disparities.[9] When analyzing physician types and population health, not all physician providers are equal. Higher concentrations of primary care, in contrast to specialty to

Table 25.1. Evidence Supporting the Benefits of Access to Primary Care Services

Reductions in:
- Overall mortality[9,10]
- Overall premature mortality[10]
- Stroke[11] and heart disease[10]
- Pulmonary disease (asthma, bronchitis, emphysema, and pneumonia)[10]
- Cervical[12] and colon cancer[13]
- Health costs overall and with acute and preventive care[14]
- Emergency Department use[15]
- Hospitalizations[15]
- Reduced health disparities related to race,[9] income inequality,[11,16–18] and rural (nonurban) status[18]

Improved:
- Reporting of good health[8]
- Preventive care[14]
- Detection of breast cancer[19]

care, has proven to lower mortality and achieve more equitable health for populations at the county, state, national, and international levels.[20,21] Whether or not primary care is labeled as such is less important than an emphasis on the principles of primary care in the medical services infrastructure. Having a primary care physician as a usual source of care is associated with better health outcomes than receiving care only from nonprimary care specialists and is a stronger predictor of good health outcomes than insurance status.[8] Among primary care specialties, only Family Medicine was consistently associated with lower mortality when controlling for other factors.[15]

PRIMARY CARE PROVIDERS, PAST AND PRESENT

During the first part of the twentieth century, the majority of medical care was provided by general practitioners to those who could afford it, or by the public wards of larger city hospitals to some who could not. At that time, general practitioners represented 85 percent of all the physicians in practice. By the end of the World War II, specialization within medicine had accelerated and was further stimulated by the emergence of the federal government as the major source of funding for medical education in the postwar years.

As Stevens points out, unlike Great Britain, the United States had never developed a formal structure for primary care. Although a professional relationship had developed early in the twentieth century between generalists and specialists in Great Britain, in the United States, it was common for all physicians to compete against each other, and general practice was becoming a "residual field." This was encouraged by the lack of a governmental national health policy in the United States. The American patient, by the middle of the twentieth century, had grown accustomed to the idea of direct access to specialists, not necessarily by referral from the primary care physician.[24]

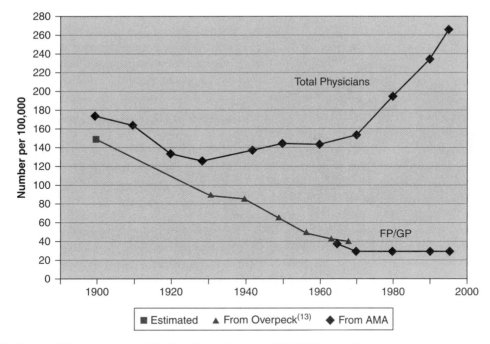

Figure 25.1. Total Physicians and Family Physicians per 100,000 Population

SOURCE: Reprinted with permission from: Council on Graduate Medical Education. *Compendium; Update on the Physician Workforce.* August 2000. Mentioned in Figure: Overpeck MD. Physicians in family practice 1931–67. *Public Health Rep* 1970; 85(6):485–494.

By the 1950s, the status of the general practitioner, and the numbers of medical students entering general practice, had reached an all-time low. Concern about adequate provision of first-line care had reached high levels among the American public and within the health professions. Two reports, *The Graduate Education of Physicians* (Millis, 1966) and *Meeting the Challenge of Family Practice* (Willard, 1966) reached essentially the same conclusion and called for the development of a new discipline to meet the needs of primary care in the United States. In 1969, Family Medicine became the 20th medical specialty, a primary care one that was designed to specifically meet this need. Other specialties such as Internal Medicine and Pediatrics, which train both generalists and subspecialists, also began to focus on primary care by creating special tracts for training primary care physicians within their programs.

As a result of this physician workforce policy shift, the rapid expansion of Family Medicine training over the past four decades has halted the decline in generalist physicians. In 2004, there were over 76,000 family physician in the United States,[25] with approximately 460 Family Medicine residency programs graduating about 3300 new family physicians each year.[26] Despite this progress, there has been little actual gain in primary care physicians due to the overall growth of the total number of physicians over the past 20 years (see Figure 25.1).[27] Three specialties, Family Medicine, general Internal Medicine, and general Pediatrics, constitute the main physician primary care workforce, 36 percent of active physicians (see Figure 25.2).[25] These numbers, however, do not reveal the major problem of maldistribution of physicians that has persisted in the United States health care system for some time. This problem is most evident

Total Active Physicians 620,627

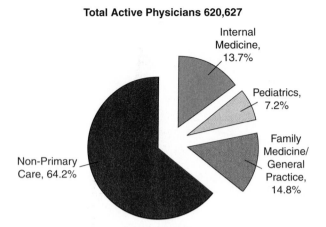

Figure 25.2. Primary Care Versus Nonprimary Care Physicians in 2004

in the rural and inner-city areas of the United States. The maldistribution of physicians, and how it impacts public health, will be discussed in greater detail in the next section of this chapter.

It is important to note that physicians are not the only primary care providers in the United States health care system. Over the past quarter-century, the training of nonphysician clinicians (NPCs) such as nurse practitioners (NPs) and physician assistants (PAs) has rapidly developed and grown partly in response to projected physician shortages. As of 2006, there are around 115,000 NPs and 61,600 PAs in clinical practice with each field respectively training 6000 and 4300 graduates annually.[25,28] Reportedly, about 80 percent of all NPs and 38 percent of all PAs are involved in primary care, but NP data is not precise for true practice.[25,29] Despite the growing number of states allowing independent practice of NPCs, there is an increasing preference in the past 10 years toward subspecialty practice given that in 1996 over 50 percent of PAs practiced in primary care.[28] There is also evidence that NPCs, unlike family physicians, do not necessarily practice or settle in areas of greatest need, but follow the trend of physician placement and practice in the areas where there are already the greatest number of practitioners.[30] Recent reports suggest that NPC training programs have peaked and now appear to be declining year to year in the number of

graduates produced per year. As a result, it is uncertain to know how many NPCs will contribute to the primary care workforce if recent trends toward subspecialization and a declining number of new NPCs yearly persist.[31]

SUPPLY AND DISTRIBUTION OF PRIMARY CARE SERVICES

A medical home or a regular source of primary care is essential to improve the health status of populations, control costs, and improve long-term health outcomes. People with no usual source of primary care do not fare as well. In many developed nations, physician distribution and the proportion of the medical infrastructure devoted to primary care services are both reasonably well balanced. This is not the case in the United States, which ranks 15th among all nations in health care, according to the multidimensional WHO Index, but 1st in the world in annual health care expenditures per capita.[22,23] Two major features of the organization and financing of health care in the United States largely explain this gap between health care expenditures and major health indicator outcomes:

- A high ratio of subspecialty physicians to primary care physicians
- Geographic physician maldistribution resulting in overabundance of health care services in most metropolitan and suburban areas, with physician shortages in rural areas and inner-city areas

There are several ways to identify physician shortages and thus effectively identify access to health services for an area or population. One of the most commonly used method for mapping out physician shortages is the United States government's Health Professional Shortage Areas (HPSA) designation. **Primary care HPSAs** are defined as having fewer than 1 full-time-equivalent (FTE) primary care physician for each 3500 residents. This threshold ratio can be raised under circumstances (e.g., poverty or language) that increase barriers to medical care.[32] Approximately one-fourth of United States counties are wholly designated as primary care HPSAs, with at least one part of another 60 percent of counties so designated.[29,32] Currently about 20 percent of the United States population resides in primary care HPSAs.

Another prominent method of identifying shortages of primary care services is the geographic area based Medically Underserved Areas (MUAs) or the population-specific Medically Underserved Populations (MUPs) within an area that experiences significant barriers to care. MUA/Ps criteria incorporate poverty levels, population over age 65, infant mortality rates, and providers per 1000 population. More than 34 federal programs depend on these 2 methods for program eligibility and funding,[32] some of the most prominent have a large impact on the medically underserved and will be discussed later in the chapter.

The accessibility of health care for rural and underserved areas has been adversely affected by the declining generalist tradition and increased specialization within health care. Approximately 20 percent of the United States population lives in rural areas, but only 9 percent of physicians practice there. Over 75 percent of counties designated as HPSAs or MUAs are in rural areas.[27] It appears clear that nothing influences practice choice site of physicians more than specialty choice, and this is particularly true for rural areas. Primary care physicians distribute themselves geographically according to the population better than subspecialists do even when accounting for the large population referral base that each subspecialist usually needs. Primary care physicians constitute the main bulwark against catastrophic physician shortages in rural and underserved areas in the United States. Even within primary care specialties, preferences exist that affect distribution as well. Pediatricians, general internists, and obstetrician-gynecologists rarely settle in rural or inner-city areas. Among all specialties, only Family Medicine distributes its residency graduates equally and in virtually exact accordance with the United States population in terms of rural, urban, and suburban communities (see Figure 25.3).[27] The gravity of this problem is easily

substantiated when analyzing HPSA data. If all family physicians were withdrawn from the workforce, 58 percent of United States counties would become primary care HPSAs. In contrast, if other primary care specialties, general internists, general pediatricians, and obstetricians-gynecologists combined were withdrawn, only 8 percent of counties would become primary care HPSAs.[26,31] It is not surprising to learn that in rural areas, over 50 percent of the care is provided by family physicians.

It is important to remember that the expertise and practices of subspecialty physicians are important to public health. But health care systems that emphasize subspecialty care at the expense of primary care demonstrate worse health status in their populations compared with systems that emphasize primary care. Although experts in the past have recommend a 1:1 ratio of primary care physicians to all subspecialists combined, only about one-third of United States physicians are primary care physicians, and the ratio is not improving.[32] Most current physician workforce policies suggest future shortages in physicians due to the growing United States population, an aging of the population, the increased use of services, changing physician practice styles, and an aging physician workforce. These workforce polices do not specifically endorse an increase in the number of primary care physicians, and in some cases, there is a push to increase subspecialty workforces given market demands.[25] These recent trends and policies suggest concern regarding the primary care workforce given that there has been a declining interest in all primary care specialties among medical graduates over the past decade.[26]

Despite past and future workforce policies, it is clear that an unbalanced ratio of primary care to subspecialty physicians, coupled with geographic maldistribution of physicians, has led to and perpetuates widespread shortages of primary care medical services in the United States. Changes in medical education that successfully produce more family physicians and other primary care physicians, coupled with improved incentives for new residency graduates to settle in rural and inner-city areas, can be expected to have very positive impacts on public health.

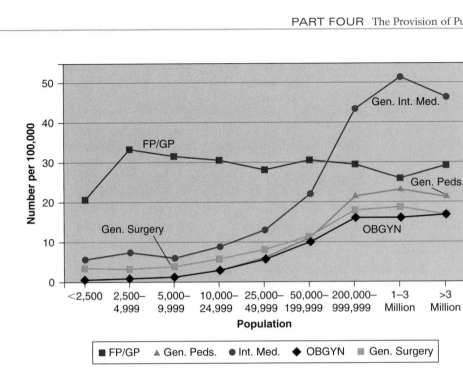

Figure 25.3. Physicians per 100,000 Population by Specialty, by County Size in 1997

SOURCE: Reprinted with permission from: Council on Graduate Medical Education. *Compendium; Update on the Physician Workforce.* August 2000.

PUBLIC PROGRAMS SUPPORTING PRIMARY CARE

Over the past 35 years, a number of programs have been instituted at various levels of government to address several areas of concern with the American health care system. These issues relate to the consistent findings of (1) a maldistribution of physicians in the United States; (2) widespread shortages of primary care physicians throughout the United States; and (3) restricted access to care for people with absent or inadequate health insurance without other resources to pay for health care, even in areas of adequate physician supply. The combination and magnitude of these issues have never been more important given the growing number of uninsured in American. In 2005, 1 in 7 (46.1 million) Americans was uninsured providing

a significant barrier to accessing health care, especially in rural areas.[33]

The *Tenth Report* of the Council of Graduate Medical Education[32] identified five major types of efforts used to address these problems with the United States health care system: (1) interventions to provide access to needy populations, (2) deployment of health professionals to underserved areas, (3) educational interventions to encourage redistribution of new health professions graduates, (4) economic incentives, and (5) research and policy development for primary care services. There are obvious areas of overlap for access, educational, and economic interventions because, in most cases, they cannot be successful without each other.

Intervention to Provide Access to Needy Populations

In the 1960s, Medicaid legislation was passed that provided reimbursement to providers for poor and near poor individuals. Since that time, there have numerous initiatives such as independent funding or enhanced reimbursement rates to provide care for the uninsured and underserved. In many cases, health departments had been providing primary health care services and those that already provided primary care services, along with others, saw the potential for a new funding stream from Medicaid. In response, many health departments assumed roles as "providers of last resort" for their communities in an effort to improve access to care for the uninsured and underserved. As Medicaid moved to managed care in the 1990s, patients receiving primary care at those health departments migrated to private physicians, truncating the Medicaid funding stream into the health departments, and leaving those reliant on that funding in a difficult situation.

The issue of whether or not health departments should be providing primary medical care remains controversial. The IOM report titled *The Future of Public Health* reflects that ambivalence. Many suggest that the health department must fulfill this function, as there is not an alternative system that can or will assume responsibility for primary medical care for the indigent. Others suggest that this function draws resources that are intended to provide population-based services to the care of a relatively few individuals. Despite this controversy, there is no doubt that effective and accessible primary care services are necessary to enhance public health.

One of the most highly recognized attempts at providing access to health care for the millions of low-income or medically underserved Americans was the creation of community health centers in 1965 as part of the "war on poverty."[34] Today, these centers are part of the **Federally Qualified Health Centers (FQHCs)** program funded under Section 330 of the Public Health Service Act (Consolidated Health Center Program). Community Health Centers (CHCs) make up 82 percent of all FQHCs and serve the medically underserved and low-income populations. The Migrant Health Centers, Homeless Health Centers, and Public Housing Health Centers are the other types of FQHCs. These health centers are local, nonprofit, community owned, and located in HRSA-designated MUA/P. These health centers serve as medical homes to more than 15 million people in 2005 by providing afford-

able comprehensive primary and preventive care services with many with onsite dental, pharmaceutical, mental health, and substance abuse services. Service are provided without regard for patients' ability to pay, and fees are based on a proportioned sliding scale that depends on patients' family size and income.[35] Primary care physicians composed 95 percent of the physician staffing for these centers, with more than half being family physicians.[36] These centers have variable relationships with state and local health departments, and they vary widely in their distribution throughout the United States. Over one- third are in rural counties.[32] Overall, FQHCs probably account for around 4 percent of all primary care visits nationally but routinely serve the most vulnerable populations. FQHCs see a disproportionately larger number of ethnic minorities who are either insured by Medicaid or completely uninsured compared with other sources of primary care.[37] The success and impact of FQHCs has been tremendous, further proving that effective primary care services improve health outcomes, control cost, and reduce disparities (see Table 25.2).

Other federal, state, and local programs and initiatives, such as the Rural Health Clinic Program, FQHC "Look Alikes," state-funded health centers, independent community clinics, private not-for-profit clinics, and local health department primary care clinics, all have enhanced primary care services and provide a safety net to underserved populations as well. Many of these programs meet criteria for enhanced reimbursement through Medicaid given the geography and populations they serve. There is evidence that these "community health clinics" perform as well as private physicians or HMOs in the delivery of preventive services to lower income populations.[38] Overall, these programs and FQHCs provide care for a significant proportion of low-income patients along with private physicians (see Figure 25.4).

Deployment of Health Professionals to Underserved Areas

The **National Health Service Corps (NHSC)** is the main health professional deployment program

Table 25.2. Facts on Federally Qualified Health Centers (FQHCs), Their Patients, and Impact[35]

Health Centers:	
Service	15 million people nationally.
Facilities	Over 1000 Community, Migrant, and Homeless Health Centers in over 5000 service delivery sites.
Patients:	
Income level	92% low income ($\leq$200% Federal Poverty Level)
	71% $\leq$ 100% Federal Poverty Level
Insurance	40% uninsured
	36% Medicaid/SCHIP
Race/ethnicity	2/3 racial or ethnic minorities
	36% Hispanic/Latino
	23% African American
Rural status	Approximately 50%
Impact:	
Access	CHC uninsured are more likely to have a usual source of care.
Prevention	Local community uninsured are less likely to have unmet medical needs and visit ERs or be hospitalized.
Cost-effectiveness	30% annual savings on its Medicaid beneficiaries.
	Reduced specialty referral, 11% less hospitalizations, 19% less ER use.
Quality care	Evidence suggest equivalent or improved quality of care compared to other sources of care.
Health disparities	Do not exist, even when controlling sociodemographics.
Chronic care	Meets or exceeds national standards, improved outcomes, lower cost.
Birth outcomes	10% lower infant mortality compared to non-CHC communities.

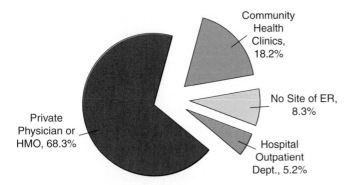

Figure 25.4. Safety-Net Site for Persons Over 50 and Under 200% of Poverty Threshold

instituted by the federal government to help balance geographical access to primary care. Since its inception in 1970, more than 21,000 health professionals (physicians, PAs, and NPs) have participated in this program, and more than 2000 health professionals yearly receive either direct scholarship assistance or loan repayment. In exchange, the providers incur a defined service commitment to initially practice in specific underserved areas (HPSA designation). Nearly half of all these health professionals annually are placed in federally funded CHCs. Family physicians comprised 78 percent of the NHSC primary care physician FTEs in 1999 and nearly 70 percent of nonfederal physicians in whole-county HPSAs.[36] The NHSC has faced criticism given low retention rates after service commitments are over; however, evidence supports that NHSC participants are more likely to locate in underserved communities, in or near their service commitment, compared to non-NHSC providers.[39]

Because of the success of the NHSC, most states have developed their own loan repayment and scholarship programs with varying degrees of success in recruitment and retention. Federal grant funds are available to support these efforts and will match funds for primary care providers to HPSAs through the State Loan Repayment Program. Since its inception in 1987, 38 states have participated in the program.[40]

Another program, called the J-1 Visa Waiver Program, allows graduates of foreign medical schools to obtain a waiver of the J-1 visa home-residence requirement provided they deliver health care services for three years in primary care or mental health HPSAs or MUA/Ps.[41] In some rural areas, this program outperforms scholarship and loan programs that look to attract United States physicians to similar areas.

Educational Interventions

In addition to its support for expansion of medical schools, since the 1970s, the federal government has supported the growth and expansion of programs in primary care medical education, such as Family Medicine, primary care Internal Medicine, and primary care Pediatrics. Funding from Title VII, section 747 of the Public Health Service Act has transformed the landscape of primary care training and practice. Greater emphasis has been placed on primary care medical student education, graduate education, departments of Family Medicine, and related faculty development programs. Title VII programs produce 2 to 5 times more graduates that are minority and disadvantaged students, which are 3 to 10 times more likely to practice in medically underserved communities, thus expanding the diversity of the health care workforce and impacting underserved communities. Studies have consistently shown that these minority and disadvantaged graduates are more likely to establish practices that serve the needs of both the urban and rural underserved. Title VII and similar federal grant funds have also supported the education of nurse practitioners and physicians' assistants to increase the number of these providers in the past decade.[42]

A novel approach to addressing the maldistribution of physicians has been the creation of rural community-based Family Medicine residency programs.

These programs place an average of 76 percent of their graduates into rural areas[43,44] compared to the 21–25 percent nationwide average of traditional programs.[32,45] A related strategy has been the creation of comprehensive selection and training programs with a clear mission to produce rural primary care physicians. Such programs can be conceived as "pipelines" that begin at the high school level, extend through formal medical training, and encompass recruitment, placement, and retention of residency-trained physicians in areas of need.[43] One example is the Physician Shortage Area Program (PSAP) of Jefferson Medical College, which, since 1974, has involved only 7 percent of graduates yearly but now accounts for 21 percent of Pennsylvania's Family Physicians in rural practices.[46]

The Area Health Education Centers (AHECs) are another important program to enhance rural training of health care providers through academic-community partnerships. Forty-five states use match funds to support federally funded AHECS. Yearly, AHECs train 37,000 health professions students in community-based sites and work with approximately 1500 FQHCs, 800 health departments, and 180 NHSC sites. AHECs improve the supply, distribution, diversity, and quality of the health workforce, ultimately increasing access to health care in medically underserved areas. They also provide health career enhancement and recruitment activities to high school students.[47]

Along with federal support, more than 40 States have created special grant programs for primary care and family physician training. State governments support medical education through direct funding to medical schools and indirect support of Graduate Medical Education (GME) though Medicaid payments despite a formal obligation to do so. State Medicaid is second only to Medicare, which has a statutory requirement, as a payer of GME. State budget deficits and constraints have and will continue to adversely affect this funding given that Medicaid accounts for 30 percent or more of the budgets.[42]

Because of the ongoing concern with physician maldistribution and the unmet needs of Medicaid beneficiaries, as many as 10 states require that Medicaid GME payments be linked to state policy goals related to health care workforce, such as training primary care or using community and rural sites for education. Several states' innovative approaches to GME financing to address health workforce needs could serve as new models for national GME financing given the ongoing state financial constraints. Independent state educational commissions to monitor workforce and training needs and distribute direct state GME funding have been established and use matching of federal funds. Other states have set up state-wide community-based Family Medicine residency programs; some work collaboratively with AHECs to achieve success. There are increasing examples of creations of trusts or diversified pooling of multiple payer sources (commercial insurers) to fund GME. There are even longstanding examples of private-sector GME financing that created Family Medicine residencies within their medical groups, such as Group Health of Washington and Kaiser-Permanente in California. All of these show that states and private insurers understand what primary care services and the training of these providers mean to their populations.[42]

Economic Incentives

An important federal incentive for physicians providing care in urban and rural HPSAs was the establishment of Medicare bonus payments in 1989. This measure, along with designations at the state and federal levels that allow a near cost-based reimbursement via the Medicare and Medicaid mechanism, have added to the financial incentive to practice in the HPSAs and MUA/Ps and participate in programs that enhance the care and access to care for underserved populations. These enhanced payments as well as other direct funding of programs or benefits help to form the economic basis of success of federal programs (see Table 25.3).[32] Another more recent provider incentive is the Physician Scarcity Area (PSA) payments that became effective in 2005 as a result of the Medicare Modernization Act. PSA Medicare bonuses are a 5 percent quarterly payment based on what Medicare actually pays the providers for their services, and the designation is different from that used for HPSAs and MUA/Ps.[48]

Research and Policy Development

The Office of Rural Health Policy (ORHP) was established by Congress in 1988 through the Public Health Services Act. ORHP established a network of rural health research centers that research the problems and impact of rural geographic maldistribution. ORHP also supports the development and dissemination of telemedicine for rural areas. Another part of Health and Human Services that is becoming increasingly important in primary care research is the Agency for Healthcare Research and Quality (AHRQ). AHRQ has as part of its mission "to support research designed to improve the

Table 25.3. Federal Programs for Enhancing Care of Underserved Areas[32]

Programs	Benefit	Designation
National Health Service Corps	Provider scholarship and loan repayment	HPSA
Medicare Incentive Program	10% Medicare bonus to physicians	HPSA
Medicare Telehealth	Teleconsultation Medicare reimbursement	HPSA
FQHC/Community Health Centers reimbursement	Federal funding (Section 330, PHS Act), Enhanced Medicare/Medicaid	MUA/P
FQHC Look Alikes	Enhanced Medicare/Medicaid reimbursement	MUA/P
Certified Rural Health Clinics	Enhanced Medicare/Medicaid reimbursement	HPSA or MUA
J-1 Visa Waiver Program	International Medical Graduate recruitment	HPSA or MUA/P

outcomes and quality of health care."[49] Within AHRQ, there is a Center for Primary Care Research that funds research projects specifically related to primary care issues. Both of these entities are helping to shape health workforce policy by analyzing access to care and underserved issues.

SYNERGIES AND TENSIONS BETWEEN PRIMARY CARE AND PUBLIC HEALTH

Using the IOM's definition of primary care,[2] and envisioning primary care as being directed to care of the individual in a broader context, large areas of overlap and synergy between primary care and public health emerge.[50] But areas of tension also exist. In some cases, health care oriented to the individual can easily be combined with health care oriented to populations because of common goals.

In other situations, health care with the goal of the best possible outcome for an individual may actually conflict with other health-related goals for the population.

The following case studies are meant to illustrate these concepts, and serve as springboards for discussion.

Treatment of Individuals and Community Health

The following two case examples show the overlap of primary care and public with regards to maintaining the health of the public as it intersects with a patient's right to medical confidentiality. Other examples of overlap include the reduction of high-risk behavior of all age groups as a primary prevention strategy to control diseases such as STDs. Primary care and public health play a similar role in both the primary prevention of chronic disease as well as the secondary prevention to manage those diseases, thus reducing the disease burden within the population.

CASE #1: TREATMENT AND CONTROL OF CURABLE INFECTIOUS DISEASE

John S. was a 48-year-old street vendor whose primary care physician diagnosed him with pulmonary tuberculosis that had been symptomatic for at least two months. John shared a cramped apartment with his mother, sister, and his sister's four children. He had a girlfriend who lived at a different address. John's doctor started anti-tubercular treatment. He also referred him to the Tuberculosis Control Clinic at the local health department for assistance with identification, surveillance, and, if necessary, treatment of his close contacts. The services directed to his family, girlfriend, and other close contacts were obviously in the interest of public health but did not compromise his own treatment. The requirement that others be told about his tuberculosis

was, for John, outweighed by the fact that this breach of confidentiality directly helped his friends and loved ones. John's physician was able to explain all of this to him, and he was grateful for all of the services.

This example of synergy between individual and public health care goals and services relies on the patient's perception of his disease as not having very negative social consequences and being highly preventable and treatable. Had John been suffering from an infection with greater social implications, such as gonorrhea, tensions would probably have arisen between what was the best course of action for him alone, versus the best actions for the health of the community.

CASE #2: DIAGNOSIS AND TREATMENT OF HIV/AIDS

Tom W. was a 38-year-old bisexual physical therapist whose physician diagnosed him with HIV infection that had not yet progressed to AIDS. Tom discussed confidentiality issues with his physician. He wanted comprehensive HIV treatment and strict confidentiality about his diagnosis. Tom felt that letting anyone else know that he had HIV would disrupt important relationships and compromise his ability to maintain his career. In this case, the physician's obligation to serve as the best advocate possible for his patient's individual health met with the conflict of the physician's other obligation to public health. Specifically, many would argue that the physician had the responsibility to take reasonable actions to see that Tom's sexual contacts were informed of his diagnosis. Although the physician may have seen no need to notify the employer, one of Tom's past sexual partners worked at the same hospital, and Tom was sure that the "word would get out" if that partner were informed. Such disclosure would lead to terrible discomfort for him at work, and he felt that his employer would then find a reason to lay him off. That would cut off Tom's health insurance when he needed it most.

A state law requiring the reporting of new HIV cases to the local public health department might have facilitated identification and notification of at-risk contacts but did little to resolve the moral dilemma faced by Tom's physician.

Individual Versus Collective Use of Medical Resources

Tensions between what is best for the individual and what is best for the population often arise over the fair and equitable distribution of medical resources. In certain situations, such as the treatment and control of infectious disease, resources spent at the individual level directly benefit the broader population at risk of contracting a given disease. Problems of resource allocation draw public attention when payment for individual medical care comes from tax-based public funds (such as Medicaid), but these problems are common whenever people pool their funds for health care. Although they may not label it as such, most Americans have become quite aware of resource allocation problems as the medical insurance industry has heightened its efforts to control costs and maintain profits through managed care.

Numerous examples exist regarding appropriate and necessary use of health care resources. Others to consider are the preferences patients may have for newer medications or the desire of patients with terminal disease to pursue experimental and unproven treatments.

PUBLIC HEALTH AND THE SCIENTIFIC BASIS FOR PRIMARY CARE

Evidence related to disease etiology, prevention, diagnosis, and treatment derives from studies of individuals, small groups, and large populations. Such evidence is sometimes appropriately applied from populations to individuals or vice versa but may also be inappropriately extrapolated, especially when evidence gathered from one subpopulation is applied to another without consideration of pertinent differences. Furthermore, when physicians attempt to apply evidence derived from groups to individual patients, personal biases, fears, expectations, and resources come into play. The translation of research findings into actual

⚜ CASE #3: EXPENSIVE TESTS

Alison P. was a 32-year-old mother of four with headaches and dizziness. After interviewing and examining her, her physician thought that these symptoms were responses to stresses in her life, and that a brain tumor or other intracranial pathology was very unlikely (but not impossible). In fact, Alison was quite frightened that she had a tumor, and her personal physician was unable to reassure her otherwise. He understood that ordering expensive (but safe) tests to completely rule out a tumor would erase the shadow of doubt that he could not otherwise fully remove and that this would help his patient. He was also aware that each time he ordered expensive tests that were medically unnecessary, he contributed to the rapid rise in health care expenditures overall and that this indirectly reduced the health care resources available to the population at large. Alison's physician finally rationalized that he would actually save medical resources by doing an expensive test because without it, his patient would continue to feel ill, and she would keep seeking medical consultations until she got her brain scan.

medical practice requires much more than the flow of information.

Primary medical care is ideally guided by evidence derived from appropriate populations that are generalizable. For most primary care issues, the reliability and validity of the available evidence are proportional to the number of people studied and the variety of settings and situations represented. Public health data sets inclusive of large numbers of people and settings have much to contribute to primary care. This is especially true for disease etiology and certain aspects of health promotion and disease prevention. However, such population-based data sets are few. Furthermore, because the United States does not have an integrated system of health care, population-based data reflecting actual medical care and outcomes in community physicians' practices are altogether lacking.[50,51]

The potential, but untapped, power of standardized data collection on disease screening, diagnosis, treatment, and outcomes during routine primary care is enormous. Imagine physicians being able to query databases fed by hundreds of thousands of patients (and their physicians) as to the power of a given test to diagnose or rule out a disease, the efficacy of a given screening strategy, or the effectiveness and patient-acceptance (balanced against risks) of a treatment. Glimpses of this power can be found in studies conducted by large, closed-panel health maintenance organizations.[51,52] But the promise of large, clinically useful datasets becoming commonplace as managed care organizations took control of the United States health care market in the 1990s has not been realized. This is probably due to the lack of financial incentives for data collection beyond that necessary for licensure, accreditation, and competition.[50]

Practice-based research networks (PBRNs) represent a grassroots approach to studying health and disease in the context of routine health care. For the past 25 years, primary care PBRNs have been operating in the United States, Canada, and Europe.[53] The funding for PBRNs has been miniscule compared with other types of medical "research laboratories," and their impact has been limited. A few PBRNs have steadily produced reports of significant original research directly applicable to primary care physicians and their patients. One of the largest and most successful has been the National Network for Family Medicine and Primary Care Research.[54,55] Primary care PBRNs have garnered support from the federal government through the Agency for Healthcare Research and Quality (AHRQ), the Health Resources and Services Administration (HRSA), and most recently the National Institutes of Health (NIH). It remains to be seen whether these networks of primary care providers will be able to significantly improve public health through their research efforts.

For now, the overall failure to collect data on the processes and outcomes of individual health care constitutes a missed opportunity for both public health and primary care.[50,51] Understanding how individual preferences and limitations interplay with disease risks, detection, treatment, and prevention would greatly enhance the effectiveness of public health initiatives. Such information can be obtained only through the collection of data related to personal health care services.[50]

Lacking the ideal sources of information discussed previously, physicians turn to two other major sources of evidence to guide their decisions for individuals: (1) limited observational data available from surveillance of large groups, and (2) data from controlled clinical trials that usually involve small, selected groups. The following cases illustrate strengths and weaknesses of this approach.

Why the conflicting information? Jean's physician relied on expert advice derived from large observational, public health-oriented studies of postmenopausal women.[56] The data were not based upon a general sample of postmenopausal women visiting their primary care physician (like her). The available studies had problems with confounding (perhaps women who took ERT were more health-conscious than those who did not), as well as questionable applicability to individual patients and settings that differed from those studied. The media, and the friend's physician, were responding to two randomized clinical trials, involving selected women who had to meet multiple special criteria related to heart disease.[57,58] In fact, the evidence about ERT was mixed, the best course for women in Jean's situation was unclear, and reliable high-quality evidence, collected from large groups of women similar to Jean, was not available.

In this case, there was population-based evidence plus clinical evidence from selected patients, and the two sources were congruent. Johnnie and his physician could thus make decisions about managing his high cholesterol with greater confidence than was possible for Jean and her physician regarding ERT.

Bringing Research-Based Evidence to the Point of Medical Care

The slow dissemination and flow of new evidence to practicing physicians impedes the progress toward evidence-based primary care as much as does the lack of pertinent data and research findings. If one

⚜ CASE #4: CONFLICTING INFORMATION AND DATA LIMITATIONS

Jean W. was a 54-year-old librarian who consulted her physician about postmenopausal estrogen replacement therapy (ERT). Although she was not at high risk for it, Jean was especially concerned about the prevention of heart disease. Based on the published advice of multiple experts over the past two decades, Jean's doctor educated her about the various benefits and risks of ERT. He advised her that because heart attacks were the number one killer of women in the United States, and large studies had shown a protective effect from ERT, the benefits of its use outweighed any risks. Jean's trust in her physician was eroded when she heard news reports that ERT did not protect against heart attacks and might even increase the risk in certain women. Jean's friend told her that her physician advised against ERT. Jean stopped taking ERT and quietly switched physicians.

CASE #5: POPULATION-BASED DATA SUPPORTED WITH CLINICAL TRIALS

Johnnie H. was an actuary for an insurance company whose physician informed him that he had very high cholesterol and advised he change his diet plus take medicine to get it under control. Johnnie had heard for years that high cholesterol increased the risk of heart attack. But now that he had the problem, he questioned his physician about the evidence that high cholesterol was truly bad and that lowering cholesterol was good for the heart. The advice Johnnie's physician gave was informed by population-based, public health-oriented observational studies, plus practice-oriented controlled clinical trials.[32] The population-based data showed a strong and consistent causal relationship between high blood cholesterol and heart attack, and the more narrow clinical trials of diets and medicines showed that lowering cholesterol prevented heart attacks by the amount expected from the observational studies.[60]

accepts the premise that good primary care is good for public health, then well-developed systems for enhancing the flow of evidence and information related to medical decision making should have high priority.

At present, multiple technologies and methods are being brought to bear on the problem of improving clinicians' access to information and evidence that they need, when they need it. The general approach to this problem is to create methods for prompt, systematic, and critical reviews of new research, and feed these reviews into electronic medical literature databases that are extensively cross-referenced. Technology must make this information readily available and manageable at the point of medical care. The access of this evidence by clinicians must be very rapid with minimal input steps. Among the many challenges to this goal is prioritization of which types of information and evidence to monitor, filter, critique, rate, store, cross-reference, and disseminate. Major efforts are under way to meet the human and technological challenges inherent to bringing high-quality information to the point of medical care. Notable examples are the Cochrane Project devoted to putting the results of clinical trials into usable evidence-bases,[61] support of medical informatics, evidence-based practice centers and technological assessments by the AHRQ,[62] and the Family Physicians Inquiries Network, funded by the American Academy of Family Physicians.[63]

COMMUNITY-ORIENTED PRIMARY CARE

The model for medical care in most of the Western world for the twentieth century has been that of separate sectors of care rather than an integrated system. Public health programs, hospitals, and ambulatory or primary care services have usually developed without any real coordination among these areas. Further fragmentation of mental health services and substance abuse treatment worsened the division of areas of responsibilities. There have been attempts through the past century to merge these health care sectors into an integrated system, with the premise being that only by doing so could health care providers benefit from the knowledge obtained in one sector being transmitted most effectively to another for the greatest health benefits.

By 1919, early attempts had been made by the Commissioner of Health of New York to accomplish this, but they came to no avail. Similar attempts were followed in Britain in 1920, but not until 1921 was an actual model devised and constructed along these lines by Dr. John Grant in China. The Karks followed in 1940 with the development of their pioneer model in rural Natal, and later in Israel.[64] With the advent of the National Health Service in Great Britain, increasing strides were made to coordinate the preventive and primary care health services throughout the country. Cuba made one of the first major attempts at the merging of public health and primary care with a new initiative in 1974 called Medicine in the Community, which was expanded and altered to emphasize Family Medicine access for all residents in the 1990s. Physicians in Cuba have both personal and public health responsibilities for the communities they serve, with concomitant dramatic improvements in the health status indicators for that country.[22] Training in Community Medicine as a discipline began at the University of Kentucky in the 1960s, and the concept of merging preventive and primary care medicine became a center for the newly developed Community Health Centers, first funded by the United States federal government in the late 1960s.[64]

The best-known conceptual model of this merger of care has been called **Community-Oriented Primary Care (COPC).** As defined by Nutting, COPC is "a variation of the primary care model in which major health problems of a defined population are identified and addressed through modifications in both primary care services and other appropriate community health programs."[65] The COPC process, in its simplest form, consists of the following four stages: (1) identification and definition of the community, (2) identification of community health problems, (3) development of some intervention in the health care program, and (4) evaluation of the effectiveness of the program. This approach is designed to define communities, and through the use of various forms of data, identify areas of special concern to a specific community or practice. The intervention may have various forms, but frequently, it is designed to facilitate the delivery of care or provide a measure of preventive services in an attempt to improve the overall health status of the community. One of the other important features of community-oriented primary care is that representatives of the community itself should be involved with prioritizing the areas of emphasis in this model.

This model has been attempted for a number of years in community health centers, the Indian Health Service, Family Medicine residency programs, and in individual and group practices. Some reported projects have included programs to reduce rural neonatal mortality rates,[66] initiatives to reduce teenage substance abuse,[67] and statewide interventions for prevention of cardiovascular disease.[68]

However, the COPC model has been slow to fulfill expectations in its early days of development. Several reasons for this are evident. It has been difficult, up to the present time, to accurately obtain community-level information on health and to develop the resources to integrate this information into that of a specific practice. COPC programs require time, and in a fee-for-service model, time allocations for community-based approaches have not been readily compensated. Critics have also expressed concern that the evaluations of program effectiveness have been sketchy at best.[69] New innovations with integrated health information systems, such as interfaced electronic health records systems or electronic health networks could provide the population data repository for community-level preventive and disease interventions. Once established, it could also be used for tracking outcomes. This of course would need to be a state or national priority to become realized. State and federal interests in enhancing chronic disease care and reporting quality care measures provide the policy emphasis to one day realize large-scale community health data sets that can be used to drive public health and primary care interventions for populations of people, instead of delivering the majority of health care one patient at a time.

PREVENTIVE SERVICES

Preventive services can be conceptualized as primary, secondary, or tertiary. In general, **primary prevention** refers to steps taken to prevent disease, injury, or illness from ever beginning. **Secondary prevention** is conceived as stopping subclinical or symptomatic disease before it becomes symptomatic or is transmitted to others. **Tertiary prevention** is aimed at ameliorating disease or illness after it has become symptomatic and limiting its negative effects on quality or quantity of life. Tertiary prevention encompasses curative and palliative medical treatments.

Public health classically has played a major role in primary prevention. This domain cannot be delivered solely through individual clinicians. It includes societal infrastructures related to clean water, clean air, crime control, highway safety, and food safety, as examples. But primary prevention also includes counseling to eliminate or mitigate exposure to disease risk. These sorts of services are also within the domain of individual medical care, especially primary care. Examples include counseling on safe sexual practices, counseling and treating for smoking cessation, counseling and education about seat belt use, lactation consultation, and the prevention of drug and alcohol abuse. Immunizations are also an example of primary prevention often pursued through individualized clinical services.

Secondary prevention falls squarely on the shoulders of individual clinical services. For the most part, large-scale public health-based screening programs, such as the use of mobile x-ray units to screen for tuberculosis, have disappeared. Today in the United States, most screening for disease, plus treatment and amelioration of the subclinical disease thereby detected, is accomplished through individual services, mainly through primary care clinicians.[50,70] If these clinicians accept the responsibility for secondary prevention, how can they target appropriate preventive services? For example, in America's technologically developed medical system, how is the physician to determine what battery of tests or prophylactic treatments to recommend to each patient, and at what frequency?

To do his best to promote Janet's health, her physician had to weigh the accuracy of tests (taking into account the probability that Janet has each asymptomatic disease considered), the effectiveness of early detection and treatment of each disease in question, and the risks of each test. Cost-effectiveness had to be considered if he accepted any responsibility for the health of the community, or if Janet had to pay out of her pocket for preventive services. He also had to identify her personal health risks and target his advice to modifiable behaviors related to those risks. Finally, he had to explain his advice to her and answer her questions.

Until the past two decades, there was little scientific evidence to guide physicians in their selection of screening tests or appropriate counseling related to health risks. Since then, there has been a blossoming of research and subsequent evidence to guide the preventive efforts of health care providers. Evidence-based guidance would have been severely hampered without epidemiology and biostatistics, and without the use of large public health databases. Clinical preventive services now have a better scientific basis than most other segments of clinical medicine, thanks to the application of these public health sciences. This is important because the threshold for trying unproven treatments to help a patient in distress is usually much lower than the threshold for pursuing unproven tests, changes

⚜ CASE #6: CLINICAL PREVENTIVE SERVICES

Janet T. was a 48-year-old advertising executive who went to her family physician for a "physical." She had been too busy to see a physician for the past 4 years. She felt well but had finally scheduled a complete checkup to be sure she was healthy.

She wanted "everything tested," and requested a "complete blood profile," a pap smear, mammogram, a brain scan, a colon exam, a chest x-ray, a bone scan, a urine test, shots, and anything else the physician thought was necessary.

in lifestyle, immunizations, or medications for people who feel well.

Several evidence-based guidelines for preventive services have been developed.[71] The most comprehensive of these is the United States Preventive Services Task Force's *Guide to Clinical Preventive Services*.[72] Using these guidelines, physicians can efficiently target appropriate clinical services to patients based on their age, gender, and characteristics that define risks for various common disease states. Clinical preventive services are thus tailored to the individual but with background population in mind. The ability to improve the health of individuals, and by extension, populations, is core to the selection of preventive services. Health risks, risks associated with tests and treatments, potential risk-reduction, allocation of health care resources, and individual patients' beliefs and resources all come into play.

Screening services that might detect a disease early, but for which treatment would not have altered the length or quality of life, should not be pursued. An example is periodic chest radiography in asymptomatic smokers. Screening services with high potential for detection of early disease amenable to eradication must also be acceptably safe, not too uncomfortable, and cost-effective. Thus, even though colonoscopy under sedation is highly effective for detecting and treating precancerous or cancerous colon polyps, its inherent costs, discomforts, and risks have hampered its widespread use in the general population at average risk for colon cancer.

Despite the near perfect marriage of public health and primary care in terms of disease prevention, some areas of tension do exist. Prominent among these is the question of who should provide preventive services for the medically indigent. Similarly, the question commonly occurs of who should provide preventive services that are not reimbursed by third-party payers.[50] Third-party payers are less motivated to provide preventive services that are in the public interest. Enrollees in health plans change their health plans often enough that third-party payers find it difficult to prove that they can profit from covering preventive services, despite the fact that these services are cost-effective when looking at larger populations under a single payer.

PRIMARY CARE PHYSICIANS AS PUBLIC HEALTH SENTINELS

A basic tenet of pubic health is the identification and control of epidemics. For epidemics to be identified in an early stage, **public health sentinels** must be present and alert. In our current system, there are not enough public health officials distributed throughout the country to effectively institute an early-warning or early-detection system for disease. Even if there were sufficient public health personnel, a large proportion of early-onset epidemic illness would present first to primary care physicians. Thus, to effectively halt or mitigate epidemics at an early stage, primary care physicians need to be alerted to their probability and be able to recognize rare patients who may be early victims. Epidemic detection and control will always be an area of great potential synergy between public health and primary care, but there are significant barriers that still prevent the realization of that potential.

Dr. William Pickles beautifully illustrated the power of a general practitioner being a sentinel and amateur epidemiologist and effectively tracing the source of an epidemic in the 1920s.[74] Since Dr. Pickles's time, medical care and society have changed in ways that make such accomplishments difficult. Dr. Pickles was able to be very sensitive to changes around him because of the relative isolation and permanence of his surrounding rural community. He basically knew everybody. In American society today, physicians and the public are so mobile that, in most communities, Dr. Pickles's approach is impractical.

Infrastructures to support primary care physicians as public health sentinels are needed. Our main advantage in the twenty-first century rests on new and efficient methods of communication. Computerized medical records, other computerized practice functions, the Internet, and e-mail have taken the potential efficiency of the sentinel function to a new level. The negative public health effects of societal changes that have loosened the bonds between primary care physicians and their communities can be partially offset by new capabilities for detection and communication during an emerging epidemic. The sentinel function of primary care is poised to be a realistic contribution to public health, if properly stimulated and supported. However, that potential has yet to be tapped in any significant way. Time and resources of public health personnel and primary care physicians remain a major stumbling block, and there are currently insufficient incentives to overcome these barriers. Future incentives should include time-saving alerts and access to medical information delivered electronically to member sentinel physicians.

If these infrastructures were realized, the effects during an epidemic would be profound because of the overall impact on health services. Primary care services during an epidemic are crucial to provide education, screening and triaging of patient concerns and symptoms as well as the acute illness, hospital, and follow-up care that would be needed for affected individuals. Recent concerns with disaster preparedness after Hurricane Katrina, bioterrorism, and potential epidemics or pandemics of influenza show the importance of a responsive public health and primary care workforce in preparation for, and during, these crises.

THE FUTURE OF PRIMARY CARE AND PUBLIC HEALTH

Four major forces are likely to shape the future of primary care as it relates to public health: changes in health care organization and finance, technological innovations, an aging society, and population (and cultural) migrations.

Health Care Organization and Finance

In the early 1990s, rising health care costs helped to usher in the "managed care revolution," and within five years, the majority of American's employer-based insurance was through managed care. Selective provider networks and negotiated payment rates helped to bring cost-containment to health care providers. Access to care, services, and therapies became more controlled and scrutinized. By the end of the decade, consumer backlash had begun, and tight labor markets made less restrictive plans available by employers. As managed care weakened, financially strained hospitals and health care organizations began expanding services to compete in the evolving market for patients. This reemergence of the "medical arms race" has focused on high-margin services and health care costs have continued to rise.

Although managed care continues to dominate as a strategy, it has a diminished ability to control costs and promote quality. Rising health care costs and insurance premiums are an enormous challenge for individuals and for employers trying to provide health insurance benefits. Eighty percent of the medically uninsured people are employed. Since 2001, 70 percent of the decline in employer-based insurance coverage was due to the loss of the employer's sponsorship of coverage in general, the altering of eligibility for health benefits, or the loss of a dependent's coverage.[33] Consumers themselves now have to assume more cost responsibility for their care as the use of consumer-driven health care plans and health savings accounts have increased. Cost-conscious consumers could potentially forgo care that is preventive or routine for managing disease, thus potentially leading to increased health disparities and worsening downstream cost if they are chronically ill.

Rising health care cost (as a percent of gross domestic product) has continued to stress employers, jeopardizing the ability to remain competitive in the market, as well as individuals who or continuing to assume more cost even with health care insurance. These financial impacts as well as the continued increase in the number of uninsured since 2000 has once again brought on policy considerations for universal health care.[33] Health care reforms for universal coverage have begun to be debated and implemented in many states as a potential solution to the uninsured and access to care problems. State government policy initiatives and national debates on health care reform may provide a new direction to be realized in the United States health care system. The rebuilding and redesign of the health care system in New Orleans after Hurricane Katrina has provided many plans from the city, state, and federal governments that prefer a primary care-based model. The goal would be to have a less fragmented, more efficient health infrastructure that relies on primary and preventive care as well as electronic medical records that are accessible for everyone.[73] Success with these new policies and plans could mean a renewed emphasis for primary care and public health in the United States health care system.

Technological Innovations

As technological advances open doors and empower health care professionals, they also usually raise costs. Most people who pay for health care, whether directly or through insurance premiums, are conscious of continuously rising costs that outstrip inflation. They often benefit from new medications, new diagnostic and monitoring tools, or improved surgical techniques. But what proportion of their income, or of the gross national product, should be spent on health care? How will we define cost-effectiveness in the future, and who will decide on resource allocations? As we have seen, positive health indicators or outcomes are not proportional to the amount spent on health care, whereas the degree to which health systems use primary care is positively associated with desirable health outcomes.

What will be the best blend of technological advances and primary care, in terms of public health? Which technologies hold the most promise for primary care and public health? Unable to predict the future, we can still make educated obser-

vations. The human genome project has enormous potential as a tool through which preventive services can be highly tailored to individuals via accurate risk-profiling, with huge increases in their cost-effectiveness. Information technologies are poised to bring all kinds of critical information to the point of an individual's medical care, greatly reducing medical errors and oversights as they guide clinicians to the best tests and therapies for the individual at hand. Properly applied, these technologies will probably enhance the healing powers of physicians and improve public health more than anything seen since the advent of antibiotics. But to wield that much power, technologies must be widely available at a relatively low cost. Very expensive technologies with severely limited scopes of use cannot be expected to have appreciable impacts beyond the few individuals who access them.

An Aging Society

As the population in developed countries ages, there will be an increased use of health care resources for managing chronic disease. How will the health care system deal with this increased use of health care services for diagnosis and management of a growing and aging population needing diagnosis and management of multiple chronic conditions? For what proportion of the population can an economy support multiple subspecialty medical services used chronically? There is no doubt that primary care physicians can expect a growing need for their services in this area, given the access to care issues, maldistribution of physicians, and the need for physicians who are skilled at caring for people with a multitude of chronic conditions, not just a specialty-specific disease. Appropriate, high-quality, cost-effective disease management will be highly important for primary care as will the effective use of public health and community-based resources for chronic disease care.

Population (and Cultural) Migrations

Population and cultural migrations have occurred throughout history, often bringing sweeping waves of change. Large migrations are usually driven by strife, and the arriving immigrants are usually poor. The United States has experienced and absorbed such waves many times in its history, quite often with marked strains on public health systems. What roles will primary care providers play in mitigating the suffering of future waves of impoverished immigrants? How will they reach across barriers of language and culture? Cultural competence training is becoming mainstream in primary care residency programs, with unknown impacts so far. Will (or should) more public funds be appropriated for health care for illegal or undocumented immigrants? If efforts are increased to provide care to medically indigent immigrants, will their care be perceived mainly as a function of specially funded (and vulnerable) centers? Or will it be distributed through the health care system? One thing seems certain: inattention to the health of medically indigent immigrants threatens the public health of all Americans.

In summary, many forces are at work that should compel the integration of primary care and public health. The primary care provider may be the individual of first contact in the identification of public health threats, such as environmental exposures, disasters, or bioterrorism. Implementation of accepted screening measures to prevent illnesses, particularly chronic diseases, may best be accomplished with primary care and should be greatly aided by the advent of vastly improved informational systems. There is also an increased interest in challenging the way in which we organize and deliver health care through the traditional "silos" of physical health, mental health, substance abuse, and public health. On the other hand, health care in the United States, at least, remains fragmented, and millions are uninsured. Significant changes in the economy may have a profound effect on funding for public health and underserved populations. It is difficult to predict the impact of the changing demographics of the American population. Nevertheless, it is important to continue to work for the improvement of the health care of the population. Success may depend on the willingness of the forces of public health and primary care to work together.

REVIEW QUESTIONS

1. What individual health care services are routinely delivered by primary care providers?
2. What health and economic benefits do individuals, populations, and countries realize with adequate access to primary care services?
3. What percentage of total active physicians are primary care, and what three physician specialties make up primary care and deliver primary care services?
4. What four types of health centers comprise the Federally Qualified Health Center (FQHCs) program that is funded through Section 330 of the Public Health Service Act?
5. What are three methods used to designate or map physician shortages in the United States?
6. What physician workforce issues have led to and perpetuate widespread shortages of primary care medical services in the United States?
7. What five major types of interventions have been developed to address the shortages of primary care and lack of access to care for the uninsured?
8. What type of data sets would be most useful to public health and primary care to improve individual health?
9. What types of preventive services (primary, secondary, or tertiary) have the greatest overlap between public health and primary care?
10. What are four major forces that are likely to shape the future of primary care as it relates to public health?

REFERENCES

1. Declaration of Alma-Ata. International Conference on Primary Health Care, Alma-Ata, USSR, September 6–12, 1978.
2. Institute of Medicine. *Primary Care: America's Health in a New Era.* Donaldson MS, Yordy KP, Lohr KN, Vanselow NA, eds. Washington, DC: National Academy Press; 1996.

3. Ashton J. Public health and primary care: Towards a common agenda. *Public Health*. 1990;104:387–398.

4. Vuori H. Primary health care in Europe—Problems and solutions. *Community Med*. 6;221–231.

5. Graham Center for Policy Studies in Family Practice and Primary Care. Utilization patterns and usual source of care. Policy Center One-Pager #2. Available at: http://www.aafp.org/afp/20061001/graham.html. Accessed December 1999.

6. Green LA, Fryer GE Jr, Yawn BP, Lanier D, Dovey SM. The ecology of medical care revisited. *N Engl J Med*. 2001;344:2021–2025.

7. Starfield B. Public health and primary care: A framework for proposed linkages. *Am J Public Health*. 1996;86:1365–1369.

8. Leiyu S, Starfield B. Primary care, income inequality, and self-rated health in the United States: A mixed-level analysis. *Int J Health Serv*. 2000;30:541–555.

9. Shi L, Macinko J, Starfield B, Politzer R, Xu J. Primary care, race, and mortality in US states. *Soc Sci Med*. July 2005;61(1):65–75.

10. Macinko J, Starfield B, Shi L. The contribution of primary care systems to health outcomes within Organization for Economic Cooperation and Development (OECD) countries, 1970–1998. *Health Serv Res*. June 2003;38(3):831–865.

11. Shi L, Macinko J, Starfield B, et al. Primary care, income inequality, and stroke mortality in the United States: A longitudinal analysis, 1985–1995. *Stroke*. 2003;34(8):1958–64.

12. Campbell RJ, Ramirez AM, Perez K, Roetzheim RG. Cervical cancer rates and the supply of primary care physicians in Florida. *Fam Med*. 2003;35:60–4.

13. Roetzheim RG, Gonzalez EC, Ramirez A, Campbell R, van Durme DJ. Primary care physician supply and colorectal cancer. *J Fam Pract*. 2001;50:1027–31.

14. Forrest C, Starfield B. The effect of first-contact care with primary care clinicians on ambulatory health care expenditures. *J Fam Prac*. 1996;43:40–48.

15. Phillips RL, Jr., Starfield B. Why does a US primary care physician workforce crisis matter? *Am Fam Physician*. October 15, 2003;68(8):1494, 1496–1498,1500.

16. Shi L, Macinko J, Starfield B, Wulu J, Regan J, Politzer R. The relationship between primary care, income inequality, and mortality in US States, 1980–1995. *J Am Board Fam Pract*. September–October 2003;16(5):412–422.

17. Shi L, Macinko J, Starfield B, Politzer R, Wulu J, Xu J. Primary care, social inequalities, and all-cause, heart disease, and cancer mortality in US counties, 1990. *Am J Public Health*. April 2005;95(4):674–680.

18. Shi L, Macinko J, Starfield B, Politzer R, Wulu J, Xu J. Primary care, social inequalities and all-cause, heart disease and cancer mortality in US counties: a comparison between urban and non-urban areas. *Public Health*. August 2005;119(8):699–710.

19. Ferrante JM, Gonzales EC, Pal N, Roetzheim RG. Effects of physician supply on early detection of breast cancer. *J Am Board Fam Pract*. 2000;13:408–14.

20. Starfield B, Shi L, Grover A, Macinko J. The effects of specialist supply on populations' health: Assessing the evidence. *Health Aff (Millwood)*. January–June 2005; Suppl Web Exclusives:W5-97-W95-107.

21. Starfield B, Shi L, Macinko J. Contribution of primary care to health systems and health. *Milbank Q*. 2005;83(3):457–502.

22. Starfield B. Is US health really the best in the world? *JAMA*. 2000;284:483–485.

23. World Health Organization. *The World Health Report 2000. Health Systems: Improving Performance*. Available at: http://www.who.int/whr/2000/en.

24. Stevens R. The Americanization of Family Medicine: Contradictions, challenges, and change, 1969–2000. Formal discussion papers from Keystone III. The Role of Family Practice in a Changing Health Environment: A Dialogue. Robert Graham Center, 2001. Chapter 1: 19–41.

25. Green LA, Dodoo MS, Ruddy G, et al. *The physician workforce of the United States: A Family Medicine perspective*. Washington, D.C.: Robert Graham Center; 2004.

26. Pugno PA, McGaha AL, Schmittling GT, Fetter GT, Jr., Kahn NB, Jr. Results of the 2006 National Resident Matching Program: Family Medicine. *Fam Med*. October 2006;38(9):637–646.

27. Council on Graduate Medical Education. Update on the physician workforce. Rockville, MD: US Department of Health and Human Services; August 2000.

28. American Academy of Nurse Practitioners. What is an NP? FAQs about Nurse Practitioners. Available at: http://www.aanp.org/Default.asp. Accessed October 26, 2006.

29. American Academy of Physician Assistants. Data and Statistics. Available at: http://www.aapa.org/research/index.html. Accessed October 26, 2006.

30. Cooper R, Laud P, Dietrich C. Current and projected workforce of nonphysician clinicians. *JAMA*. 1998;280(19):788–794.

31. Fryer GE, Green LA, Dovey SM, Phillips RI Jr. The United States relies on family physicians unlike any other specialty. *Am Fam Physician*. 2001;63:1669.

32. Council on Graduate Medical Education. *Tenth Report. Physician Distribution and Health Care Challenges in Rural and Inner-City Areas*. Washington, DC: US Dept of Health and Human Services; 1998.

33. Kaiser Commission on Medicaid and the Uninsured. *The Uninsured: A Primer*. Washington, DC: Kaiser Family Foundation; October, 2006. Available at: http://www.kff.org/kcmu.

34. HRSA Bureau of Primary Health Care. *About Health Centers*. Available at: http://bphc.hrsa.gov/success/criticalconnections.htm. Accessed November 16, 2006.

35. National Association of Community Health Centers. *America's Health Centers, Fact Sheet #0206*. Washington, DC: National Association of Community Health Centers; August 2006.

36. Physician Workforce: The Special Case of Health Centers and the National Health Service Corps. *American Family Physician*. 2005;72(2):235–235.

37. Forrest C, Whelan E. Primary care safety-net delivery sites in the United States: A comparison of community health centers, hospital outpatient departments, and physicians' offices. *JAMA*. 2000; 284(16):2077–2083.

38. O'Malley AS, Mandelblatt J. Delivery of preventive services for low-income persons over age 50: a comparison of community health clinics to private doctors' offices. *J Community Health*. June 2003;28(3):185–197.

39. Holmes, GM. Does the National Health Service Corps improve physician supply in underserved locations? *Eastern Economic Journal*. 2004;30(4): 563–581.

40. HRSA Bureau of Health Professions. *State Loan Repayment Program*. Available at: http://nhsc .bhpr.hrsa.gov/join_us/slrp.asp. Accessed November 16, 2006.

41. *Tools for Monitoring the Health Care Safety Net*. AHRQ Publication No. 03-0027. Rockville, MD: Agency for Healthcare Research and Quality; September 2003. Available at: http://www.ahrq .gov/data/safetynet/tools.htm.

42. Council on Graduate Medical Education. *State and Managed Care Support for Graduate Medical Education: Innovations and Implications for Federal Policy*. Washington, DC: US Dept of Health and Human Services; July 2004.

43. Geyman JP, Hart LG, Norris TE, Coombs JB, Lishner DM. Educating generalist physicians for rural practice: How are we doing? *J Rural Health*. 2000;16:56–80.

44. Bowman RC. Continuing Family Medicine's unique contribution to rural health care. *Am Fam Physician*. 1996;54:471–480.

45. Rosenthal TC. Outcomes of rural training tracks: A review. *J Rural Health*. 2000;16:213–216.

46. Rabinowitz HK, Diamond JJ, Markham FW, Hazelwood CE. A program to increase the number of family physicians in rural and underserved areas: impact after 22 years. *Jama*. January 20, 1999;281(3):255–260.

47. HRSA Bureau of Health Professions. *Area Health Education Centers*. Available at: http://bhpr.hrsa .gov/ahec/. Accessed November 16, 2006.

48. Centers for Medicare & Medicaid Services. *HPSA/PSA (Physician Bonuses)*. Available at: http://www.cms.hhs.gov/HPSAPSAPhysician-Bonuses. Accessed November 20, 2006.

49. Agency for Healthcare Research and Quality. Mission Statement. Available at: http://www.ahrq .gov/about/budgtix.htm.

50. Welton WE, Kantner TA, Katz SM. Developing tomorrow's integrated community health systems: A leadership challenge for public health and primary care. *The Milbank Q*. 1997;75:261–288.

51. Pollock AM, Rice DP. Monitoring health care in the United States—A challenging task. *Public Health Rep*. 1997;112:108–13.

52. Barlow WE, Davis RL, Glasser JW, et al. The risk of seizures after receipt of whole-cell pertussis or measles, mumps, and rubella vaccine. *N Engl J Med*. 2001;345:656–661.

53. Nutting PA, Beasley JW, Werner JJ. Practice-based research networks answer primary care questions. *JAMA*. 1999;281:686–688.

54. Green LA, Hames CG Sr, Nutting PA. Potential of practice-based research networks: Experiences from ASPN. *J Fam Pract.* 1994;38:400–405.

55. American Academy of Family Physicians. Academy begins national research network. Family Physicians Report, October 1999. Available at: http://www.aafp.org/fpr//991000fr/all.html.

56. Sharp PC, Konen JC. Women's cardiovascular health. *Primary Care.* 1997;24:1–14.

57. Hulley S. Randomized trial of estrogen plus progestin for secondary prevention of coronary heart disease in postmenopausal women. *JAMA.* 1998; 280:605–613.

58. Herrington DM, Reboussin DM, Brosnihan KB, et al. Effects of estrogen replacement on the progression of coronary-artery atherosclerosis. *N Engl J Med.* 2000;343(8):522–529.

59. Gaziano JM, Herbert PR, Hennekens CH. Cholesterol reduction: Weighing the benefits and risks. *Am Coll Physicians.* 1996;124:914–918.

60. Expert Panel on Detection, Evaluation, and Treatment of High Blood Cholesterol in Adults. *The Third Report of the National Cholesterol Education Program (NCEP) Expert Panel on Detection, Evaluation, and Treatment of High Blood Cholesterol in Adults (Adult Treatment Panel III).* Available at: http://www.nhlbi.nih.gov/ guidelines/cholesterol/.

61. Becker L. Helping physicians make evidence-based decisions. *Am Fam Physician.* 2001;63: 2130–2136.

62. Agency for Healthcare Research and Quality. Clinical Information. Available at: http://www .ahrq.gov/clinic/.

63. Dickinson WP, Strange KC, Ebell M, Ewigman BG, Green LA. Involving all family physicians and Family Medicine faculty members in the use and generation of new knowledge. *Fam Med.* 2000; 32:480–490.

64. Kark S. Community-oriented primary health care: A review. *COPaCETIC.* 1998;5(1):1–6.

65. Nutting P. Community-oriented primary care: An integrated model for practice, research, and education. *Am J Prev Med.* 1986;2:140–147.

66. Marquardt D. Improvement in rural neonatal mortality: A case study of medical community intervention. *Fam Med.* 1993;23:269–274.

67. Frame P. Is community-oriented primary care a viable concept in actual practice? An affirmative view. *J Fam Pract.* 1989;28:203–208.

68. Mittelmark M, Luepker R, Grimm R, et al. *The Role of Physicians in a Community-Wide Program for Prevention of Cardiovascular Disease: The Minnesota Heart Disease Program.* Public Health Reports. 1988:103(4):360–365.

69. O'Connor P. Is community-oriented primary care a viable concept in actual practice? An opposing view. *J Fam Pract.* 1989;28(2):206–209.

70. American Academy of Family Physicians. The importance of primary care physicians as the usual source of health care in the achievement of prevention goals. Center for Policy Studies in Family Practice and Primary Care One-Pager. Available at: http://www.graham-center.org/ x159.xml. Accessed February 21, 2000.

71. National Guideline Clearinghouse. Available at: http://www.guidelines.gov/.

72. US Preventive Services Task Force. *Guide to Clinical Preventive Services.* 2nd ed. Baltimore, MD: Williams & Watkins; 1996.

73. National Association of Community Health Centers. *Legacy of a Disaster: Health Centers and Hurricane Katrina, One Year Later.* Washington, DC: National Association of Community Health Centers; 2006.

74. Pickles WN. *Epidemiology in Country Practice.* Bristol, England: John Wright & Sons Ltd; 1949.

75. Lesser C, Ginsburg P, Devers K. The End of an Era: What Became of the "Managed Care Revolution" in 2001? *Health Services Research.* 2003;38(1):337–355.

CHAPTER 26

Maternal and Child Health

Carol Hogue, PhD, MPH

LEARNING OBJECTIVES

Upon completion of this chapter, the reader will be able to:

1. Describe the maternal and child health impact of 8 of the 10 major public health accomplishments of the twentieth century.

2. Relate these accomplishments to the 10 essential public health services.

3. Describe the major federal programs that fund maternal and child health services, with respect to their history and current function.

4. Apply this understanding to twenty-first century maternal and child health problems, such as asthma and childhood obesity.

5. Describe the interplay among advocacy, public opinion, public policies, and public health as applied to family planning services and child health and welfare services in the twentieth century.

6. Apply this understanding toward framing effective public health advocacy, surveillance, and related programs for the twenty-first century.

KEY TERMS

Asepsis

Family Planning

Infant Mortality

Maternal Deaths

Maternal Mortality

Maternal Mortality Review (MMR) Committees

Neonatal Mortality

Neonates

Oral Contraceptives

Preterm Deliveries

Replacement

Sepsis

Stillbirth

Women, Infants, and Children (WIC)

In 1999, the Federal Centers for Disease Control and Prevention published a series of articles under the general heading "Ten Great Public Health Achievements—United States, 1900–1999."[1] These achievements were chosen because they reflect major contributors to death and disability that can be effectively reduced through efforts to prevent them. It is notable that 8 of the 10 achievements directly address maternal and child health issues. These include achievements that were targeted directly at improving maternal and child health (healthier mothers and babies and family planning), as well as those that improved the overall health of women and their children (safer and healthier foods), and those that addressed specific childhood diseases and health risks (control of infectious diseases and vaccination, motor-vehicle safety, fluoridation of drinking water, and recognition of tobacco use as a health hazard). A review of the history, current status, and future needs of the two targeted areas provides a framework for discussing the scope of maternal and child health problems and the programs designed to alleviate them. Toward the latter part of the twentieth century, improvements in maternal and infant survival stalled or were reversed. Further improvement in maternal and child health during the twenty-first century will require attention to effective implementation of the 10 essential public health services particularly for vulnerable populations, with particular attention to an examination of the rationale for public health actions and focused research on the remaining major threats to maternal and child health.

TWO GREAT TWENTIETH-CENTURY PUBLIC HEALTH ACHIEVEMENTS

During the twentieth century, two major public health achievements were important to the United State's health status. The first was a focus on the health of mothers and babies, and the second was family planning.

Healthier Mothers and Babies

Early in the twentieth century, childbirth was extremely dangerous, with more than 800 **maternal deaths** recorded for every 100,000 live births in the United States. A death is defined as maternal if it occurs during pregnancy or delivery or shortly after delivery, as a result of complications of the pregnancy or delivery. **Sepsis** (blood stream infection) related to unsafe delivery practices and illegal abortions (voluntary termination of pregnancy prior to the possibility of survival outside the womb) accounted for 40 percent of the deaths, but most of these could have been prevented then if known principles of **asepsis** (i.e., infection control procedures) at the time of the delivery had been uniformly applied. The death rate for infants was even higher, with as many as 30 percent of babies in some urban areas dying before their first birthday.[2] Many of these deaths were also preventable but required improvements in living conditions, drinking water safety, nutrition, and pasteurized milk supplies.

Recognizing these critically important needs, social reformers concerned about child labor as well as high infant mortality rates formed coalitions with public health workers, pediatricians, and obstetricians to advocate for milk pasteurization (first introduced in Chicago in 1908) and, later, for improved housing, nutrition, sanitation, income, and access to medical care. Their efforts led to the establishment of the federal Children's Bureau in 1912, which focused attention on the link between poverty and maternal and infant health risks and advocated for comprehensive welfare services for pregnant women and their babies, including prenatal, delivery, and postpartum home visits by health care providers. In 1921, this integrated approach was formulated into law in the Maternity and Infancy Act (also known as the Sheppard-Towner Act for its congressional sponsors). The provisions of this act included federal matching funds to establish maternal and child health divisions in state health departments, with missions not only to provide maternity care services, health education, and nutrition counseling but also to deliver household assistance, especially for poor and immigrant inner-city populations. However, the emphases on public funding of health care, involvement in family life, and prevention over cure proved to be controversial, and the Act was defeated in 1929, despite its apparent effectiveness. During the 1930s, as the Great Depression deepened, Congress passed the Social Security Act of 1935, which was modeled after the Maternity and Infancy Act. However, rather than integrating social welfare and health care, it separated the two into income assistance for indigent families (the forerunner of Aid to Families with Dependent Children, which is now Temporary Assistance for Needy Families [TANF]) and maternal and child health services under Title V.

These efforts paid off in immediate reductions in infant deaths; from 1915 to 1929, **infant mortality** (deaths in the first year of life per 1000 live births) declined by almost one-third. It wasn't until the 1930s, however, that public awareness led to effective action and a dramatic drop in maternal deaths. In 1933, the White House Conference on Child Health Protection, Fetal, Newborn, and Maternal Mortality and Morbidity report[3] documented the association between poor obstetric practices and maternal deaths. Although not the first to make this association, this report catalyzed state medical associations to establish maternal mortality review committees to assess the preventability of each maternal death. Over the next two decades, these efforts led to guidelines for obstetrics and delivery services as well as qualifications for physicians delivering in hospitals. At the same time, the proportion of births occurring in hospitals increased from about 50 percent to 90 percent of all deliveries, and **maternal mortality** (maternal deaths per 100,000 live births) dropped from about 700 to about 100 per 100,000—a decline of more than 85 percent between 1930 and 1950. Infant mortality also continued its steep improvement, declining another 50 percent during this period.

During the last half of the twentieth century, improvement in both infant and maternal mortality slowed considerably. Although the century saw a 93 percent drop in infant mortality, more than two-thirds of that occurred prior to 1950. Public concern about infant health reached a nadir during the 1950s and 1960s. The Children's Bureau was weakened in 1946 and eliminated in 1969. Although some argued that infant mortality had reached an irreducible level, the United States ranked below most developed and several developing countries in infant survival, and dramatic differences in infant mortality rates among sociodemographic groups in the United States pointed to vulnerable populations with many preventable infant deaths. Gradually public awareness grew that more could be done, especially for high-risk **neonates** (babies younger than 28 days) whose survival depended on intensive care in state-of-the-art facilities. During the late 1960s and early 1970s, a coalition of public health providers, advocacy groups such as the March of Dimes, and medical care providers effectively lobbied to establish regional perinatal centers to care for high-risk mothers and infants. Largely through technological advances and access to them with regionalized services, **neonatal mortality** (neonatal deaths per 1000 live births) dropped 41 percent from 1970 through 1979. Over the same period, concern grew about the continued high proportion of babies being born weighing less than 2500g (about 5½ pounds), who are at greatly increased risk of morbidity and mortality when compared to larger babies. Maternal and child health advocates argued successfully in 1989 for improved access to prenatal care to prevent low birth deliveries through expanded Medicaid eligibility. However, although more women have been able to enter prenatal care early, the low birth weight rate has not declined, and **preterm deliveries** (<37 weeks' gestation) have actually increased (discussed later in this chapter).

Two other developments contributed substantially to improvement in infant mortality in the 1980s and beyond. One was a medical advance— the introduction of artificial pulmonary surfactant to increase lung maturation among premature infants as a means to prevent respiratory distress syndrome. The other was a public health advance—the recognition that placing infants on their backs to sleep could prevent sudden infant death syndrome (SIDS) in some infants. The "back to sleep" movement to educate the public is credited with a greater than 50 percent drop in SIDS rates during the 1990s.

Only 15 percent of the dramatic drop in maternal mortality during the twentieth century occurred after 1950. The first 85 percent decline was mostly attributable to improved delivery practices, whereas the last 15 percent was largely owing to improved abortion practices during the 1960s and 1970s. No improvement in maternal mortality has occurred since 1982, and many state maternal mortality review committees have been disbanded. However, recent studies have determined that maternal mortality has not reached an irreducible limit. Rather, about half of the 300–400 deaths per year of otherwise healthy women—in the prime of their lives and with families to care for—could be prevented with the uniform application of good obstetrics practices.[4]

Family Planning

Both maternal and child health are affected by fertility levels. The likelihood that babies will be born healthy is greatest when pregnancies are spaced two to four years apart. For women, childbirth risks are minimized if pregnancies occur no sooner than two years after their first menses. The more children a woman has, the greater her likelihood of experiencing major morbidity or mortality from childbirth. Childbirth risks increase with increasing maternal age, particularly for women in their mid-30s or older. Thus, the timing of pregnancies as well as the number of children born affects both maternal and child health. **Oral contraceptives,** which are the most popular form of nonpermanent birth control, also have noncontraceptive health benefits, including reduced rates of pelvic inflammatory disease, endometrial and ovarian cancer, recurrent ovarian cysts, benign breast cysts and fibroadenomas, and menstrual cramp discomfort.[5]

Family planning is the deliberate effort by women and couples to determine the number of conceptions the woman will have and the timing of those conceptions. The need for universal access to family planning services was a major public health issue during the twentieth century in the United States. During the nineteenth century, family size in the United States had already declined 50 percent to an average of 3.5 births per woman in the age range 15 to 44. However, the knowledge about and practice of family planning was largely denied poor and immigrant families, owing to federal and state "Comstock" laws passed during the 1870s, which outlawed the distribution of information about contraception or the provision of contraceptive services. As part of the social reform movement of the early 1900s, Margaret Sanger and colleagues sought to overcome this barrier. Sanger opened the first family planning clinic in Brooklyn, New York, in 1916. She was promptly jailed, and the clinic was shut down. However, her efforts focused public attention on the plight of the poor. Over the next three decades, she successfully challenged the laws and gradually won public acceptance for provision of family planning services to married couples. Some public health departments began offering services in the 1930s, when fertility dropped to nearly **replacement** (the number of children needed to replace the current generation), despite the lack of modern contraceptive methods. Available methods of birth control at that time included the condom, douching, withdrawal, cervical diaphragms (introduced in 1925), and "rhythm" methods with correct knowledge of ovulation and the fertile period (established in 1928). Abortion was widely practiced, although it was largely illegal and often conducted under dangerous conditions. Deaths associated with abortion contributed substantially to maternal mortality until the late 1960s.

With the return of prosperity during World War II, average family size increased in the United States to a peak in 1957 of 3.7 children per woman of reproductive age. Fertility had already begun to decline again before the introduction of modern contraceptives—the first oral contraceptive pill and the first intrauterine device—in 1960. Concern for continued high abortion rates and lack of access to modern contraceptives for poor women led efforts to eliminate the remaining Comstock laws. In 1965, the Supreme Court nullified all remaining state laws prohibiting contraceptive use by married couples. By 1980, all Comstock laws had been declared unconstitutional, clearing the way for contraceptive services to all, irrespective of marital status. To improve contraceptive access to poor and underserved women and men, Congress passed the Family Planning Services and Population Research Act in 1970, which created Title X of the Public Health Service Act with funding targeted at establishing family planning services at an affordable price. One of the bill's sponsors was the future President George H.W. Bush. By 1988, publicly supported family planning clinics had proven to be highly cost-effective in providing contraceptives to women and men who might otherwise not be able to afford them. However, over time these clinics have been called upon to provide more comprehensive reproductive and other primary care with ever-decreasing funds, while federal monies for contraceptive services have been reallocated in part to abstinence-only programs that have been proven to be ineffective in reducing unintended pregnancies.

THE 10 ESSENTIAL PUBLIC HEALTH SERVICES FOR THE HEALTH OF WOMEN, INFANTS, AND CHILDREN

So far we have focused on the two major public health achievements of the twentieth century that contributed the greatest to the remarkable improvements in the health of women and infants. These achievements were social and public health programs that (1) drastically reduced infant and maternal mortality and (2) improved technology and access to safe family planning practices. Of the other eight major public health achievements

highlighted by CDC, the following six had significant impact on reducing morbidity and mortality for children and, to a lesser extent, for mothers as well:

- Safer and healthier foods
- Control of infectious diseases
- Vaccination
- Motor-vehicle safety
- Fluoridation of drinking water
- Recognition of tobacco use as a health hazard

What is common to all these achievements is that success was accomplished through application of the 10 essential public health services. Although it is not possible in the scope of this chapter to document how each success came about or how progress will be maintained, it is possible to illustrate how the 10 essential public health services contribute to this process.

The same essential services are required to achieve success against the twenty-first century challenges to maternal, infant, and child health, particularly chronic diseases including asthma, obesity, HIV/AIDs, mental illness, and stress related to socioeconomic disparities. Asthma is a chronic respiratory disease that causes periodic inflammation and narrowing of small airways. Asthma attacks, which can vary from mild to life-threatening, are triggered by allergens, infections, exercise, weather changes, and irritants such as tobacco smoke. Over the past two decades, asthma prevalence has increased, and is highest among children. In 2005, an estimated 8.9 percent of United States children suffered from asthma.[6] Asthma often requires emergency room visits (e.g., 750,000 among children with asthma in 2004) and interferes with daily activities, such as school attendance; children with asthma missed nearly 13 million school days in 2003. People living in poverty and members of minority groups have an approximately 25 percent higher prevalence of asthma than the rate for non-Hispanic white persons.

Medical care professionals view the management of chronic diseases as "the major challenge for health care professionals who care for infants, children and young adults and for those who will treat them as they age into adulthood. . . ."[7] Public health professionals see a parallel challenge in preventing chronic diseases or postponing their onset. Obesity is an underlying cause of many chronic diseases, such as diabetes, that are now appearing at far younger ages than before. A major prevention effort is underway to reverse the trend toward ever increasing prevalence of obesity in infancy and childhood. Intervention studies designed to increase physical activity and improve nutrition have begun at the individual, family, community, and environmental levels of impact. If the obesity trend is not reversed, it is widely believed that this generation of children will have a lower life expectancy than their parents and grandparents.

Another major child health problem that has only recently begun to receive widespread attention is promoting mental health and caring for those with mental health issues. It is estimated that by the year 2020, childhood neuropsychiatric disorders will become one of the top five causes of morbidity, mortality, and disability among children.[8] Already, mental illness that is severe enough to cause some level of impairment affects about 10 percent of United States children, but only about 20 percent of them receive mental health care services. The National Agenda for Action, which grew out of a series of conferences, calls for engaging all 10 essential public health services toward prevention, screening, diagnosis, and adequate treatment.

Briefly described next are some of the ways that the 10 essential public health services contribute singly and in combination to combat the maternal and child health issues that were "left over" from the nineteenth and twentieth centuries as well as those that emerged in the latter half of the twentieth century and are becoming major public health challenges in the twenty-first century.

Enforcing Laws and Regulations to Protect Health and Safety

Vulnerable infants and young children benefit when evidence-based laws and regulations to protect their health and safety are enforced. Major examples include protection of food and water, protection from vaccine-preventable infectious diseases, protection from motor vehicle injuries and death, and prevention of dental caries through fluoridation of water supplies.

The Pure Food and Drug Act was passed in 1906, in part because of the public awareness raised by Sinclair Lewis' novel, *The Jungle*, which exposed highly unsanitary meat-packing processes in Chicago. Through attention to hand washing, sanitation, refrigeration, pasteurization, and pesticide application practices, illness and deaths attributable to food-borne diseases have been drastically reduced. Over the same time period, increased understanding of basic nutritional needs has virtually eliminated nutritional deficiency diseases such as rickets, scurvy, beri-beri, pellagra, and goiter. Maternal and child health advocates have taken the lead in these efforts, beginning with the 1921–1929 Maternal and Infancy Act, which provided funds for state health departments to employ nutritionists. Nutritional programs, such as the Special Supplemental Food Program for **Women, Infants, and Children (WIC),** have reduced iron-deficiency anemia among vulnerable populations, and most recently neural tube defects associated with folic acid deficiency are decreasing because of food fortification.

The sharp decline in deaths attributable to infectious diseases was driven in part by strategic vaccination campaigns and earmarked programs to increase vaccination coverage, particularly for poor children. Since the Vaccination Assistance Act of 1962, federal funds support the purchase and administration of a full range of childhood vaccines. Most recently, the human papilloma virus (HPV) vaccine has been introduced, which provides protection not only against one of the most common sexually transmitted diseases, but more importantly against 70 percent of cervical cancer causes by HPV infection. One of the deadliest remaining infectious diseases scourges is HIV/AIDs for which no vaccine has yet been proven effective. However, screening and treatment of pregnant women infected with HIV/AIDs has greatly reduced the risk of maternal-to-infant transmission and the number of newly infected infants in the United States.

One of the greatest scourges among children and youth during the twentieth century was deaths caused by motor vehicle accidents. Motor-vehicle-related deaths were the leading cause of death for those aged 1–24 years in 1996.[9] Yet the rate would have been much higher had there not been sustained, comprehensive efforts to increase highway safety. Over the twentieth century, the overall highway death rate declined 90 percent, from 18 per 100 million vehicle miles traveled (VMT) in 1925 to 1.7 per 100 million VMT in 1997.

Supporting Policies and Plans to Achieve Health Goals

As outlined earlier, public policies have had a major impact on reducing maternal, infant, and childhood morbidity and mortality since the beginning of the twentieth century. The continued expenditure of public funds to improve maternal and child health and welfare requires a political demand for community action. In turn, political demand derives from a shared understanding of the problem and the approach to its solution. Over the course of the twentieth and early twenty-first centuries in the United States, there were major shifts in both problem definitions and agreed-upon solutions to those problems. Those shifts drove changes in the amount, scope, and nature of public expenditures for maternal and child health and welfare services.

As described previously, early twentieth century social reformers who represented the Progressive Movement defined the problem as poverty and the solution as a global attack on the causes and consequences of poverty. The Sheppard-Towner Act, which funded maternal and child health divisions in state health departments, reflected this paradigm. Programs administered through maternal and child health agencies included not only prenatal care, nutritional counseling, and health education but also household assistance for poor and immigrant families and family counseling. Then the Progressive Movement lost popular support, while at the same time health care was increasingly becoming professionalized with less emphasis on prevention than on cure. The stage was set for the demise of the Sheppard-Towner Act, reduced public funding for health and welfare programs, and a bifurcation of programs into health and social arenas that still persist.

The Great Depression of the 1930s once again revealed the needs of poor families and needy children, with public recognition of a federal obligation to provide charity for vulnerable groups. As part of the Social Security Act of 1935, Title V institutionalized federal funding for maternal and child health services in poor and underserved areas, as well as targeted services for "crippled" children and children in need of protective services. Another part of the Social Security Act provided for income assistance for poor families, which served as the forerunner for Aid to Families with Dependent Children (AFDC), and later, Temporary Assistance for Needy Families (TANF).[10]

Another major paradigm shift occurred as part of the civil rights movement of the 1960s and 1970s. Public health programs were now viewed as required to achieve equality and eliminate disparities that had been caused by generations of racial injustice. The progressive approach re-emerged in the form of neighborhood health centers with broad mandate to provide primary care, create employment opportunities, improve nutrition, reduce lead exposure, and so on. Maternal and infant care projects were funded to improve health care in targeted communities. Federal funds were distributed to states under mandates for uniform program enactment, which was understood to protect against politically motivated disparities within the states.

At the same time, advocacy groups for specific problems became more influential, giving rise to a checkerboard of programs with narrow goals. These included family planning services previously discussed, as well as WIC, school lunch programs, Title I educational assistance, and PL 94–142, which guaranteed the right to education for handicapped children.

Funding for these programs and for Medicaid (Title XIX), which is the primary government funding mechanism for health care for poor women and children and which was enacted in this era, reflects a popular view that only certain women, infants, and children should receive financial help. Eligibility for assistance is strictly defined and varies from program to program. Unlike Medicare, which covers health care costs for virtually all United States citizens aged 65 and older, these programs vary in their coverage from state to state and from program to program. Program participation is further limited in some states because funds are insufficient to cover all eligible citizens. Despite these limitations, numerous evaluations of WIC and other programs have concluded that most are cost-effective and beneficial.

Another major shift in public support of maternal and child health services occurred as an outgrowth of the Reagan administration's new federalism in the early 1980s. The emphasis was on saving money and improving efficiency, through distributing a smaller amount of federal funds to the states in the form of block grants, with fewer "strings" attached. The Maternal and Child Health (MCH) block grant consolidated federal funds for children with special health care needs and children eligible for Supplement Security Income, maternal and child health, lead-based paint poisoning prevention, sudden infant death syndrome, adolescent pregnancy prevention, genetic disease testing and counseling, and hemophilia diagnostic and treatment centers. The goal of achieving efficiency was achieved by some states, but the impact of reduced funds for programs as well as lack of assurance of equal access to programs within and across states has not yet been determined.[11] As the block grant system has matured, however, the Health Resources and Services Administration (HRSA), which administers the program, has gradually developed and implemented performance measures aimed at assessing these impacts.

In the 1990s, public policies continued to shift away from governmental support for poor families, with the dismantling of the AFDC Program, which was replaced with TANF in 1997. The Personal Responsibility and Work Opportunity Reconciliation Act of 1996 established a five-year lifetime limit for cash assistance for most eligible families and required that assistance recipients participate in welfare-to-work programs. Consistent with the new federalism, states were given more discretion over eligibility and other regulations. The result was a rapid decrease in the number of families receiving assistance. The impact of this significant shift in public policy on the health and welfare of the least economically advantaged groups in this country has yet to be determined.

At the same time, access to medical insurance was increased for poor and near-poor children through Title XXI of the Social Security Act, which established the State Children's Health Insurance Program (SCHIP). In 2005, 41 percent of deliveries were paid for through Medicaid.[12] Nearly 90 percent of children ages 0–18 were covered by health insurance. Of these, 30 percent were enrolled in either Medicaid or SCHIP, and 70 percent were privately insured. However, only two-thirds of children eligible for Medicaid/SCHIP were enrolled. Of the 8.9 million uninsured children, 45 percent were eligible for Medicaid, 24 percent were eligible for Title XXI State Programs, and 30 percent remained ineligible for any subsidized health care insurance plan. There is strong public policy advocacy for universal health care insurance, beginning with full coverage for children, which is likely to dramatically decrease the uninsured population in the near future.

A competing trend, however, is the large and growing population of undocumented residents who do not qualify for publicly funded services. All babies born in the United States are automatically citizens, which creates fissures in health care access between parents and children. How the public resolves immigration policies in this century remains to be seen.

Linking People to Needed Personal Health Services

Personal health services for many pregnant women, infants, and children are provided through public health clinics in many states, with a combination of federal and state funding. Other states pay private providers for MCH personal health services, primarily through Medicaid and SCHIP. The United States Constitution reserves authority for health to the states, which means that each state decides how to organize these services and administer these programs. Some of the key programs are briefly described in the following sections.

Title V

Title V is administered at the federal level by HRSA and provides block grant funds for shaping and linking personal health services. States match the federal funds on a formula basis and must demonstrate that they will use the funds for objectives within the scope of the Public Health Service's *Healthy People 2010* objectives.

WIC

The Supplemental Food Program for Women, Infants, and Children (WIC) is a federal program administered by the United Stares Department of Agriculture and each state. WIC participation has been found to improve pregnancy outcome and to increase the likelihood that infants will receive scheduled vaccinations. Eligible pregnant and breastfeeding women and children up to five years of age receive food vouchers, infant formula, nutrition education, and referrals to other maternal and child health services. Eligibility is determined by income and risk of poor nutrition. This is not an entitlement program, which means that benefits depend on the availability of funds, and, at times, funds run out before the end of the fiscal year in some states.

EPSDT

The Early Periodic Screening, Diagnosis, and Treatment Program (EPSDT) is part of Medicaid. It provides funding for preventive services for children up to age 21 who are enrolled in Medicaid. These services include well-child screening, outreach to inform eligible families of this service, and travel assistance as needed.

Family Planning

The history of family planning was discussed earlier. Currently family planning services are funded through Title X, Medicaid, and Title V as well as state funds. Most federal funds for contraceptives are now distributed to the subset of all women in need of them who also qualify for Medicaid. Some states have expanded Medicaid coverage of family planning services through federally approved waivers to expand eligibility. Based on the experiences of these states, it has recently been estimated that if Medicaid coverage for contraceptive services were to be expanded to all United States women whose incomes were at or below 250 percent of the federal poverty level, there would be 722,600 fewer unintended pregnancies and 291,200 fewer abortions—a 23 percent reduction to the overall number of abortions.[13]

Monitoring Community Health Status Through Surveillance and Surveys

Several surveillance systems are maintained by the states, with federal sponsorship and funding administered by the CDC. These systems include the Behavioral Risk Factor Surveillance System (BRFSS), the Pregnancy Nutrition Surveillance System (PNSS), the Pregnancy Risk Assessment Monitoring System (PRAMS), and the Pediatric Nutrition Surveillance System (PedNSS). BRFSS and PRAMS are ongoing, population-based surveys, whereas PNSS and PedNSS are program-based systems that use routinely collected data from federally funded public health programs.

Behavioral Risk Factor Surveillance System (BRFSS)

Begun in 1984, BRFSS is the world's largest, ongoing telephone health survey system. BRFSS samples adults at random in each state. Participants respond to questions about their general health, as well as specific health issues such as asthma, diabetes, and hypertension. They are also asked about access to preventive health care and various health-related practices such as smoking, alcohol use, weight, nutrition, family planning, and more. Information from BRFSS is used to assess the prevalence of smoking, obesity, sedentary behavior, and other behavioral health risks.

Pregnancy Risk Assessment Monitoring System (PRAMS)

PRAMS samples women identified from birth certificates as recently having given birth. Some high-risk pregnancies, such as low-birth-weight births, are over-sampled. In each state, from 1300 to 3500 women chosen for the sample each year are sent mailed questionnaires; if they do not respond, they may be contacted by telephone. As of 2007, 37 states plus New York City and the Yankton Sioux Tribe in South Dakota were participating in PRAMS. PRAMS provides data not available from other sources about prenatal care, maternal complications during pregnancy delivery and the first few months postpartum, breastfeeding practices, infant health in the early months, and much more. Information from PRAMS has been used to identify women and infants at high risk for health problems (such as domestic violence), to monitor trends in health care (such as access to early prenatal care) and status (such as maternal obesity), and to track progress in achieving national and state public health goals (such as percentage of births that were intended at conception). For example, using PRAMS data for Georgia and other information, Collier[14] estimated that 13 percent of cases of cerebral palsy and 14 percent of cases of mental retardation could be prevented each year if all unwanted pregnancies were prevented. An additional 2.5 percent of cases of cerebral palsy and 0.8 percent of cases of mental retardation could be prevented among pregnancies that are wanted, if no pregnant women smoke. As an example of how both PRAMS and BRFSS have been used to monitor maternal and infant health status, Huber and colleagues[15] estimated the risk of oral contraceptive failure associated with obesity with data from the 1999 BRFSS and the 2000 PRAMS surveys in South Carolina. They found that, compared to normal-weight women, overweight women (body mass index [BMI] of 25–29.9 kg/m^2) and obese women (BMI of $\geq$30) may have an increased risk of oral contraceptive failure resulting in a live birth.

The Pregnancy Nutrition Surveillance System (PNSS) and the Pediatric Nutrition Surveillance System (PedNSS)

Unlike BRFSS and PRAMS, which are ongoing, population-based surveys, PNSS and PedNSS use readily available program data from the major federally funded maternal, infant, and child health programs to monitor health status and assess program impact for the population eligible for such services. PNSS uses data from the Special Supplemental Nutrition Program for Women, Infants, and Children (WIC) and Title V MCH programs. PNSS data include information on approximately 750,000 low-income, pregnant, and postpartum women. PedNSS data cover more than seven million children from birth to their fifth birthday. In some states, data from the Early and Periodic Screening, Diagnosis, and Treatment (EPSDT) Program of Medicaid are combined with WIC and Title V data to provide information on children and adolescents to age 20. With these data, program analysts can track trends in the prevalence of nutritional problems such as anemia, health practices such as breastfeeding, and risk factors such as obesity among the program participants.

Occasional Surveys

In addition to the rich data sources of these ongoing surveillance systems, maternal and child health status may be monitored less frequently but in greater depth through occasional surveys, such as the 2001 National Survey of Children with Special Health Care Needs[16] and the 2002 National Survey of Family Growth (NSFG).[17] Since 1973, the National Center for Health Statistics of the CDC has periodically conducted the NSFG. This is a multipurpose survey of a nationally representative sample of reproductive-aged women (15–44) living in households. In-depth interviews are conducted in person, by interviewer and computer-assisted interviewing techniques. In 2002, the NSFG included a separate sample of 4928 men, as well as a sample of 7643 women. The results of the NSFG are used to track contraceptive use, access to family planning services, information about HIV/AIDs and other sexually transmitted diseases, and highly detailed information about family formation. Of particular interest is the prevalence of unwanted and mistimed pregnancies, which account for half the pregnancies in the United States, unlike other developed countries. Approximately one-half of these unintended pregnancies are terminated by induced abortion. Women with unintended pregnancies are also at increased risk of initiating prenatal care later than desired, and to give birth to children with developmental problems. Unwanted fertility also may lead to family dissolution.[18] Between 1995 and 2002, when the latest two NSFG surveys were conducted, births from unwanted pregnancy actually increased, and fewer fertile women who reported that they did not want to become pregnant were using contraception.[19] Although contraceptive use among sexually active teens had improved, contraceptive use among sexually active adults had deteriorated. These disturbing trends suggest the need for increased attention to contraceptive use among adult women in the United States.

The category of children with special health care needs (CSHCN) has been defined by the Maternal and Child Health Bureau as ". . . those who have or are at increased risk for a chronic physical, developmental, behavioral, or emotional condition and who also require health and related services of a type or amount beyond that required by children generally." Using this definition, the random, national survey of nearly 39,000 families in 2000 and 2001 found that 12.8 percent of children meet this definition. Encouragingly, 95 percent of these children had health insurance at the time of the survey; 82 percent reported receiving all the services they needed. However, 20 percent of these children live in households with financial problems caused by their condition. This is partly due to the fact that nearly 30 percent of parents of these children indicated that they have had to cut back on work or stop working to care for their children. The federal authorities concluded that "these indicators paint a picture of an adequate system of care for CSHCN that meets the needs of the majority of these children. However, room for improvement still exists, especially where systems serve the most vulnerable children, such as those for low-income families and those who receive insurance coverage through public programs."

Investigating and Diagnosing Health Problems and Hazards

Investigating and diagnosing health problems and hazards is similar to monitoring community health status through surveillance and surveys in that it is based on analysis of data. However, surveillance depends on large data sets with uniform data definitions, collected over time, whereas health problem investigation is focused on individual cases, examined with great specificity. **Maternal mortality review (MMR) committees** were highly effective during the middle third of the twentieth century through application of this methodology. Each maternal death was examined for whether it could have been prevented, and if so, how it could have been prevented. Health care providers modified their practices accordingly.

Based on this successful model, HRSA in conjunction with the American College of Obstetricians and Gynecologists and state and local health departments launched a movement in the 1990s known as Fetal and Infant Mortality Review (FIMR). There are key differences between FIMR and MMR committees that reflect an understanding of the complexities involved in reducing infant mortality rates. First, health care providers may not be the most important change agents. The major causes of infant deaths are associated with preterm delivery and birth defects, and current knowledge regarding how to prevent these deaths through health care alone is highly limited. Rather, in FIMR, the underlying assumption is that currently preventable fetal and infant deaths are those in which support systems, such as family planning and prenatal care programs, are inadequate to meet the demand for services or are of insufficient quality.[20] The FIMR process includes a Community Action Team, whose job is to assure that public program and services are responsive to the recommended remediation of the Case Review Team. Evaluation of the FIMR process found that better performance of the essential MCH services was associated with the presence of a FIMR program,[21] suggesting that the FIMR process may improve infant outcomes when fully implemented.

Informing and Educating People Regarding Health Issues

The information age has transformed health education and information systems. With Internet access now nearly universal, it is possible for most citizens to access highly accurate information about specific health problems and issues. The CDC, including the National Center for Health Statistics, NIH, and other governmental-sponsored websites at federal, state, and local levels provide a wealth of data and information about programs. Of particular use for maternal and child health issues is the HRSA-sponsored website http://www.mchlibrary.info. Also, the Maternal and Child Health Bureau produces an annual snapshot of maternal and child health, with data on MCH from all Title V recipients, at https://perfdata.hrsa.gov/mchb/mchreports/snapShot.asp.

Numerous nongovernmental organizations maintain websites with easily accessible, relevant information. Here are just a few of the key ones:

- **http://www.citymatch.org (CityMatCH):** Among other topics, includes detailed information about the National Perinatal Periods of Risk (PPOR) tool.

- **http://www.kff.org (Kaiser Family Foundation):** Serves as a nonpartisan source of data and information about women's and children's health and other issues, including data collected and analyzed by the Foundation, geared to policy makers, the media, the health care community, and the public.

- **http://www.marchofdimes.com/peristats (March of Dimes Perinatal Data Center):** Provides free access to maternal and infant health-related data gleaned and analyzed from 12 government agencies and organizations and presented at the national, state, county and city level, including easy-to-access PowerPoint slides.

- **http://www.guttmacher.org (The Alan Guttmacher Institute):** Focuses on sexual and reproductive health in the United States and worldwide, with easy-to-access fact sheets, PowerPoint presentations, and interactive data bases at the state level.

- **http://www.aecf.org/MajorInitiatives/KIDSCOUNT.aspx (Annie E. Casey Foundation):** Provides access to the annual KIDS COUNT Data Book, with national- and state-level information on the child well-being indicators.

- **http://www.nwlc.org/publication.cfm?section=infocenter (National Women's Law Center):** Makes the counterpart document for women's health indicators, "Making the Grade on Women's Health," available for ordering.

Mobilizing Partnerships to Solve Problems

Coalitions and partnerships are a hallmark of maternal and child health advocacy. The Healthy Mothers/Healthy Babies Coalition has functioned for several decades in all states and serves in many areas as a potent force for public policy review and legislation. One of the most recent coalitions has formed around the need to assure women's health status prior to their pregnancies. Known as Preconception Care,[22] the problem that needs to be solved is defined somewhat differently by different members of the partnership. As a known means to improve pregnancy outcome, this effort is supported by child advocacy groups such as the National March of Dimes. As a means of improving women's health irrespective of whether they become pregnant, this effort is supported by women's health advocacy groups as well. Whether this movement becomes successful will rely, in part, on keeping these somewhat disparate partners together in their advocacy goals.

Ensuring a Skilled, Competent Public Health Workforce

As part of a larger effort to improve the public health workforce, CDC and HRSA have focused efforts on increasing the number and competence of maternal and child health epidemiologists, as well as nurses, health technicians, and primary care providers at all levels. Numerous educational programs have been established, including distance learning programs that address the needs of individuals already in the workforce who have a need to upgrade their skills and competencies.

Maternal and child health educators also emphasize the need of the public health workforce for cultural literacy to address the needs of an increasingly diverse population in need of services. Skills in conducting community-based participatory program development are also stressed to assure that services meet the needs of the specific community being served.

Evaluating Effectiveness, Accessibility, and Quality of Health Services

Examples of program evaluations have been provided previously in other sections of this chapter. These are keys to the appropriate and best use of public resources. Another level of evaluation is to consider the impact of policies on the health issues they were designed to address. An example of this type of evaluation is the impact of increasing Medicaid eligibility for prenatal care and deliveries, which was enacted in 1989 as a means to reduce the stubborn rates of premature delivery and infant mortality. In a comprehensive review of the published studies of this question, Howell[23] determined that the policy did increase the proportion of pregnant women receiving Medicaid-paid prenatal and deliveries services, and that some women entered prenatal care earlier than they would have otherwise done. However, there is very little evidence that this policy change resulted in improved birth outcomes. Improved access to prenatal care may have other benefits that justify the expense, but the solutions to

the ongoing problems of premature delivery and birth defects remain elusive.

Researching and Applying Innovative Solutions

What solutions to the persistent (and increasing) risk of preterm delivery should be explored? This was the topic of a recent Institute of Medicine (IOM) study, *Preterm Birth: Causes, Consequences, and Prevention*.[24] Recommendations for research spanned health care of the pregnant woman and preterm infant, as well as epidemiologic investigations of the complex and interrelated potential causes of preterm birth. This should be a key goal for maternal and child health research in the twenty-first century.

Stillbirth (death in the womb of a fetus of at least 20 weeks gestation), which now accounts for almost one-half of deaths of babies from 20 weeks' gestation through the first year of life, is currently the topic of a large, population-based, case-control study sponsored by the Eunice Kennedy Shriver National Institute of Child Health and Human Development. Data derived from this study will provide information about the scope and causes of stillbirth and may also supply some answers to the cause of preterm delivery.

In addition, a comprehensive study of the impact of environment, stress, genetics, and chronic diseases on human growth and development has long been a high priority of maternal and child health researchers. Fortunately, this ambitious dream is being fulfilled, in the form of the National Children's Study, which will involve recruiting a random sample of more than 100,000 women and following them through conception, pregnancy, and delivery and their offspring up to age 21.[25]

▌SUMMARY

The twentieth century saw an unprecedented improvement in maternal and child health in the United States (and throughout the globe). However, much of this improvement occurred during the first half of the century. Renewed and continued progress will require focus on rigorous application of the 10 essential public health services, particularly evaluation of the impact of ongoing programs to solve current problems, such as the obesity epidemic and asthma, and research into the causes of preterm delivery, birth defects, asthma, and other persistent health issues.

REVIEW QUESTIONS

1. Why are there so few maternal mortality review committees currently in existence?
2. What impact on health would you expect because of the fundamental differences in maternal mortality review committees (MMR) and fetal/infant mortality review (FIMR)?
3. Why is there a difference in eligibility criteria between Medicaid and Medicare? Are these differences likely to remain throughout the twenty-first century? Why or why not?
4. What impact on maternal and child health (positive and/or negative) is likely with the increased public health emphasis on preconception care?
5. How can policy claims be framed to increase political support for improved access to contraceptive services?
6. How can the 10 essential public health services be used to stem the childhood obesity epidemic?

REFERENCES

1. Ten Great Public Health Achievements—United States, 1900–1999. *MMWR*. 1999;48(12): 241–243.
2. Meckel RA. Save the babies: American public health reform and the prevention of infant mortality, 1850–1929. Baltimore, MD: The Johns Hopkins University Press; 1990.
3. Wertz RW, Wertz DC. Lying-in: A history of childbirth in America. New Haven, CT: Yale University Press; 1989.
4. Berg CJ, Harper MA, Atkins SM, et al. Preventability of pregnancy-related deaths: Results of a state-wide review. *Obstetrics & Gynecology*. 2005;106: 1228–1234.
5. Peterson HB, Lee NC. The health effects of oral contraceptives: Misperceptions, controversies, and continuing good news. *Clinical Obstetrics and Gynecology*. 1989;32:339–355.
6. Akinbami L. Asthma prevalence, health care use and mortality: United States, 2003–05. Centers for Disease Control and Prevention, Office of Analysis and Epidemiology; November 2006.
7. DeAngelis CD, Zylke JW. Theme issue on chronic diseases in infants, children, and young adults: Call for papers. *JAMA*. 1006;296:1780.
8. US Department of Health and Human Services. *Report of the Surgeon General's Conference on Children's Mental Health: A National Action Agenda*. Washington, DC; 2001.
9. Division of Unintentional Injury Prevention, National Center for Injury Prevention and Control, CDC. Achievements in public health, 1900–1999. Motor-vehicle safety: A 20th century public health achievement. *MMWR*. 1999;48(18): 369–374.
10. Lesser AJ. The origin and development of maternal and child health programs in the United States. *Am J Public Health*. 1985;75(6): 590–598.
11. Rosenbaum S. The maternal and child health block grant act of 1981: Teaching an old program new tricks. *Clearinghouse Rev*. August/September 1983:400–414.
12. Tang S-f S. Fact sheet: Children's health insurance. American Academy of Pediatrics. April 16, 2007.
13. Frost JJ, Sonfield A, Bold RB. Estimating the impact of expanding Medicaid eligibility for family planning services. Occasional Report No. 28. August 2006.
14. Collier S, Hogue C. Modifiable risk factors for low birth weight and their effect on cerebral palsy and mental retardation. *Maternal and Child Health Journal*. 2007;11:65–71.
15. Huber LRB, Hogue CJ, Stein A, Drews C, Zieman M. Body mass index and risk of oral contraceptive failure: A case-cohort study in South Carolina. *Ann Epidemiol*. 2006;16:637–643.
16. Maternal and Child Health Bureau, Health Services and Research Administration, US Department of Health and Human Services. *The National Survey of Children with Special Health Care Needs Chartbook*. Washington, DC; 2001.

17. For reports of the two most recent surveys, see Abma J, Chandra A, Mosher M, Peterson L, Piccinino L. Fertility, family planning and women's health: New data from the 1995 National Survey of Family Growth. National Center for Health Statistics. *Vital Health Stat.* 23(19):1997; Chandra A, Martinez GM, Mosher WD, Abma JC, Jones J. Fertility, family planning, and reproductive health of US women: Data from the 2002 National Survey of Family Growth. National Center for Health Statistics. *Vital Health Stat.* 23(25):2005.

18. Hogue CJR. Consequences of unintended pregnancy. In: Sarah S. Brown and Leon Eisenberg, eds. *The Best Intentions: Unintended Pregnancy and the Well-Being of Children and Families.* Washington, DC: National Academy Press; 1995: 50–90.

19. Gaydos L, Hogue C, Kramer M. Riskier than we thought: Revised estimates of women at risk for unintended pregnancy. *Public Health Reports.* 2006;121:155–159.

20. Hogue CJR. Whither FIMRs? *Maternal and Child Health Journal.* 2004;8(4):269–271.

21. Strobino D, Baldwin K, Grason H, et al. The relation of FIMR programs and other perinatal systems initiatives with maternal and child health activities in the community. *Maternal and Child Health Journal:* 2004;8(40):239–249.

22. Preconception Care. Available at: http://www.cdc.gov/ncbddd/preconception/. Accessed November 14, 2008.

23. Howell EM. The impact of the Medicaid expansions for pregnant women: A synthesis of the evidence. *Medical Care Research and Review.* 2001;58(1):3–30.

24. Behrman RE, Stith Butler A, eds. *Committee on Understanding Premature Birth and Assuring Healthy Outcomes.* Board on Health Sciences Policy, Institute of Medicine. Washington, DC: The National Academies Press; 2007.

25. National Children's Study. Available at: http://www.nationalchildrensstudy.gov/.

CHAPTER 27

Injury Control

María Seguí-Gómez, MD, ScD and Susan P. Baker, MPH, ScD (Hon.)

LEARNING OBJECTIVES

Upon completion of this chapter, the reader will be able to:

1. Define the term *injury.*
2. Communicate the dimension and magnitude of the problem and its relationship with other public health problems.
3. Justify the application of the public health model to injuries.
4. Describe William Haddon's framework and proposed countermeasures.
5. Describe other conceptual frameworks for injury prevention.
6. Be aware of the axioms guiding injury prevention.
7. Defend the role of individual and institutional public health practitioners to prevent injuries.

KEY TERMS

Accident

Energy

Event

"Iceberg" or "Pyramid"

Injuries

Injury Prevention

Vehicles (or Vectors)

ACKNOWLEDGEMENTS: We thank Dr. Sleet and Dr. Rosenberg for their contribution in the first edition of this book. Partial support for the writing of this chapter was provided by a CDC grant to the Johns Hopkins Center for Injury Research and Policy (R49/CCR302486) and structural funds from the European Center for Injury Prevention at the University of Navarra (MSG).

We normally think of health problems or diseases as those conditions associated with exposure to infectious agents (e.g., HIV, malaria), environmental agents (e.g., tobacco, lead), chronic degenerative processes, or those due to genetic disorders. Yet, the leading cause of years of potential life lost, one of the top five causes of death, and a major source of disability in the United States population and worldwide, has nothing to do with those conditions. These deaths and morbid and disabling conditions relate to exposure to some form of **energy** (kinetic, potential, electrical, or other) in amounts that exceed the individual's tolerance threshold or in amounts released in too short of a time period, therefore resulting in injuries. This is a health problem as old as humankind.

Given the magnitude of this problem, it seems natural, then, that as public health practitioners, we should turn our attention to injuries and their control. Unfortunately, this has not always been the case.

Injuries and their prevention have not traditionally been embraced as a public health issue. One obstacle has been the belief that injuries are the result of **accidents,** which has caused them to be considered by many as unpredictable and therefore unpreventable. In the instances in which they were "investigated," the conclusion was often that they were primarily due to some irresponsible behavior on the part of the injured individual or someone else. As a result, injury control has been retarded by the "accident" folklore, including the notion of reckless, selfish, careless, and intoxicated people as primarily responsible for injuries.[1] Thus, until the last quarter of the twentieth century, the field of injury control was characterized by misunderstanding, lack of progress, and scarcity of relevantly trained scientists.

Fortunately, current public health thinking embraces injury prevention, and all the 10 essential public health services and the Core Competencies for Public Health Professionals are applicable to this major public health problem.[2–3] In this chapter, we will provide a brief overview of the injury problem. The chapter is designed to provide a general orientation, rather than an exhaustive discussion. The goal is to facilitate a clearer understanding of the role of the public health practitioner and public health agencies in the reduction of the burden related to injuries. To achieve that goal, we will present useful definitions and conceptual frameworks, a summary of the magnitude of the problem, and examples of the use of public health tools in its prevention. Emphasis is placed on the preventability of these injuries, and wherever possible, we have provided examples of prevention efforts. It is not our intent to provide a detailed account of the epidemiology of injuries, nor the effectiveness or efficiency (or lack thereof) of all interventions tested to date. Many other references are available to the reader interested in those matters.[4–7]

DEFINITION OF INJURY

We will use the term *injury* to describe any damage to the body due to acute exposure to amounts of thermal, mechanical (kinetic or potential), electrical, or chemical energy that exceed the individual's tolerance for such energy, or to the absence of such essentials as heat or oxygen. We have, therefore, adopted the broad definition first described in *Injury Prevention*[8] and endorsed by the Institute of Medicine (IOM),[9] which includes intentional injuries (e.g., homicide, suicide) as well as unintentional injuries. The chapter does not address psychological damage as a result of, for example, violence or motor vehicle crashes. This chapter also encompasses injuries regardless of where they occur (e.g., outdoors, at home, or at school), the activity that was taking place when the injurious event happened (e.g., occupational, recreational, sports-related), and the object that was involved in the energy transfer (e.g., motor vehicle, gun). Table 27.1 lists energy types, their frequency as the source of fatal injuries in the United States population, the **vehicles (or vectors)** that most frequently transfer the energy, and the most common types of resulting injuries.

Table 27.1. Examples of Energy, Vehicle, Injury Types and Their Proportion of Injury Deaths in the United States, 2004, Fatally Injured Population (N = 167,184)

Etiology of Injury	Vehicle (vector)	Type of Injuries	Percentage of Deaths
Kinetic energy	Motor vehicle, train, other vehicles, guns, knives, machinery	Abrasions, contusions, sprains, strains, dislocations, fractures, concussion, blunt, open wounds (cuts, piercing), crushing	58.2
Chemical energy	Drugs, cleaning products, poisonous animals	Poisonings, chemical burns	16.3
Absence of oxygen	Water, foreign objects	Strangulation, suffocation, drowning	10.7
Potential energy*	Falling person	Same as kinetic	11.8
Thermal energy	Fire, heat	Burns, heat stroke	2.3
Electrical energy	Wires, appliances	Electrocution	<1
Absence of heat		Frostbite	<1
Ionizing radiation	Radioactive materials	Burns	<1

SOURCE: CDC NCHS, Compressed mortality file 1999–2004. CDC WONDER On-line Database, compiled from Compressed Mortality file 1999–2004 Series 20 No. 2J, 2007. Query date: June 11, 2007. Available at: http://wonder.cdc.gov.

*It has been argued, however, that potential energy causes injury only when transformed into kinetic energy.

DIMENSIONS AND MAGNITUDE OF THE PROBLEM

In the United States in 2004, 167,184 people died because of injuries, amounting to a rate of 5.7 per 100.000. Injuries are among the five leading causes of death in our population, right behind cancer, heart, cerebrovascular, and respiratory diseases (Table 27.2). As seen in Table 27.2, unintentional injuries are the fifth leading cause of death for individuals of all ages combined, and the leading cause of death for individuals ages 1 through 44. Intentional injuries (whether suicide or homicide) are the second to fourth leading causes of death for ages 1 to 54. Therefore, injuries become the most important cause of Years of Potential Life Lost (YPLL), almost 80 and 100 percent higher than the YPLLs (before age 65) associated with cancer and cardiovascular diseases, respectively (Figure 27.1).[10]

In addition to deaths, injuries result in some 2 million hospital admissions (95% Confidence Interval 1,594,930–2,354,046), which implies a rate of 672 per 100,000 and 48 million emergency department contacts every year.[11] The relationship between mortality and morbidity (or different degrees of severity) is referred to as the **"iceberg" or "pyramid"** of injury (Figure 27.2), and the actual ratio between each of the levels of that pyramid varies depending on the specific injury or the specific injury mechanism because some injuries are more lethal than others. Table 27.3 further illustrates this point by presenting the crude death and hospitalization rates per 100,000 population by several mechanisms of injury. In the table, drowning/near drowning has a death:hospitalization ratio of 1:0.6, whereas homicide/legal interventions have a ratio of 1:6, and fall-related injuries have a ratio of 1:36.

Injuries are also a leading source of short- and long-term disability. It is estimated that some 7 percent of individuals who are injured sustain some degree of disability, which means some 4 million new cases per year.[12]

Table 27.2. Five Most Common Causes of Death by Age Category, United States 2004. All Races, Both Sexes

Rank	<1	1–4	5–9	10–14	15–24	25–34	35–44	45–54	55–64	65+	Total
1	Congenital Anomalies 5,622	Unint. Injuries 1,641	Unint. Injuries 1,126	Unint. Injuries 1,540	Unint. Injuries 15,449	Unint. Injuries 13,032	Unint. Injuries 16,471	Malignant Neoplasms 49,520	Malignant Neoplasms 96,956	Heart Disease 533,302	Heart Disease 652,486
2	Short Gestation 4,642	Congenital Anomalies 569	Malignant Neoplasms 526	Malignant Neoplasms 493	Homicide 5,085	Suicide 5,074	Malignant Neoplasms 14,723	Heart Disease 37,556	Heart Disease 63,613	Malignant Neoplasms 385,847	Malignant Neoplasms 553,888
3	SIDS 2,246	Malignant Neoplasms 399	Congenital Anomalies 205	Suicide 283	Suicide 4,316	Homicide 4,495	Heart Disease 12,925	Unint. Injuries 16,942	Chronic L. Resp. Disease 11,754	Cerebro-vascular 130,538	Cerebro-vascular 150,074
4	Maternal Complications 1,715	Homicide 377	Homicide 122	Homicide 207	Malignant Neoplasms 1,709	Malignant Neoplasms 3,633	Suicide 6,633	Liver Disease 7,496	Diabetes Mellitus 10,780	Chronic L. Resp. Disease 105,197	Chronic L. Resp. Disease 121,987
5	Unint. Injuries 1,052	Heart Disease 187	Heart Disease 83	Congenital Anomalies 184	Heart Disease 1,038	Heart Disease 3,163	HIV 4,826	Suicide 6,906	Cerebro-vascular 9,966	Alzheimer's Disease 65,313	Unint. Injury 112,012

SOURCE: CDC NCHS. Office of Statistics and Programming. National Vital Statistics Systems. WISQARS™. Available at: http://www.cdc.gov/ncipc/wisqars/. Accessed June 11, 2007.

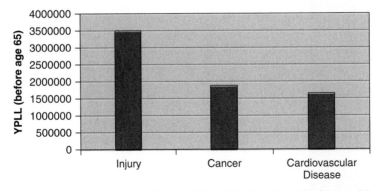

Figure 27.1. Years or Potential Life Lost* by Cause of Death Before Age 65. Adapted from the CDC NCIPC National Center for Health Statistics Vital Statistics System. U.S., all genders, both sexes, 2004.

*Years of Potential Life Lost calculated up to age 65.

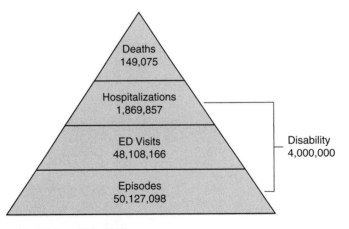

Figure 27.2. The Pyramid of Injury U.S. 2000

SOURCE: Adapted from Finkelstein EA, Corso PA, Miller TR, et al. *The Incidence and Economic Burden of Injuries in the United States*. New York: Oxford University Press; 2006.

When one combines mortality, morbidity, and disability in a metric such as the Disability Adjusted Life Years (DALYs), injuries are responsible for approximately *15 percent* of all DALYs lost in the world. As of 2002, injuries due to motor vehicle crashes, interpersonal violence, or suicide are the 8th, 15th, and 17th leading causes of DALYs lost worldwide, respectively. Worse yet, it is estimated that by the year 2030, their burden will increase to make them causes number 4, 13, and 14 of lost DALYs.[13]

The economic impact of injuries is significant also. It is estimated that the aggregate lifetime costs of all injuries produced in 2000 will amount to $326 billion dollars; $80 billion of which will relate to costs of health care, and the remaining will be associated with lost productivity resulting from premature death and disability.[14]

Last, a summary of the impact of injuries cannot be complete without reference to the largely unmeasured but immense burden that they impose on families and communities. The literature in this field is peppered with evidence of higher divorce rates among parents of injury victims, higher school dropout rates among siblings of victims, and higher alcohol and drug involvement among relatives and others.[15]

Table 27.3. Crude Rates of Deaths and Hospitalizations Due to Injury per 100,000 Population. United States 2004. All Ages, Both Sexes

	Deaths	Hospitalizations	Ratio death:hospitalizations
Motor Vehicle	15.4	121.7	1:7.9
Falls	6.7	242.8	1:36.2
Drowning/near drowning	1.4	0.9	1:0.6
Fires/flames	1.3	6.0	1:4.6
Poisonings	10.3	118.4	1:11.5
Homicide/legal intervention	6.0	35.1	1:5.9
Suicide/self-harm	11.5	97.8	1:8.5
Total	56.9	672.4	1:11.8

SOURCE: Office of Statistics and Programming. National Vital Statistics Systems. WISQARS™. Available at: http://www.cdc.gov/ncipc/wisqars/. Accessed June 11, 2007.

THE ROLE OF PUBLIC HEALTH

As with any other population health problem, we can apply the public health model of a scientific approach to prevention (Figure 27.3).

During the remainder of this chapter, we will follow this model. Under "Epidemiological Framework," we will discuss issues related to the definition of the problem: data collection and surveillance, the identification of causes and risk factors, and the development of interventions. Under "Choice and Evaluation of Countermeasures," we will present issues related to the testing and selection of interventions. Issues that relate to the last step of the public health model will be presented in the "Axioms to Guide Injury Prevention" section and in our discussion of the roles of public health practitioners and public health agencies.

Epidemiological Framework

Injury epidemiology allows for investigation of the interaction among the host (or individual injured), the etiological agent (energy), the vehicle or vector that transmits the energy, and the physical and socio-cultural environment where the interaction occurs. (*Vehicles* are the inanimate objects that transmit the energy [e.g., cars, matches, guns], whereas *vectors* are the plants, animals, or persons that transmit the energy [e.g., biting animals, poisonous snakes, human fists].) The use of epidemiology has helped demonstrate that injuries, like diseases, display long-term trends and demographic, geographic, socioeconomic, and seasonal patterns. However, it was not until 1949 that Dr. John Gordon first acknowledged that injury occurrence and severity, much like any other health condition, could be measured and related to different characteristics of individuals, the sources of injuries, and their environments. It was only in 1961 that Dr. James Gibson separated the role of the vehicles or vectors from that of the energy they transmit, thus enabling the application of the analytical framework of epidemiology to the study of injuries. (Readers interested in a more extensive review of the history of injury control are referred to the work of J. A. Waller.[16])

Data Collection and Surveillance

As identified in the essential public health services[2] and in several of the specific competencies outlined in the first domain (Analytic Assessment Skills) of the Core Competencies for Public Health

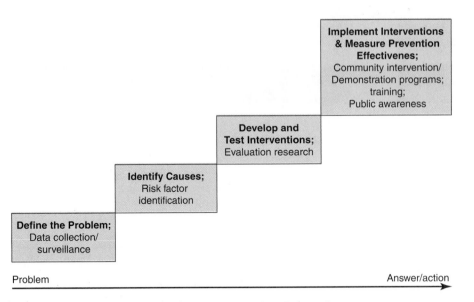

Figure 27.3. **Public Health Model of a Scientific Approach to Prevention**

SOURCE: Adapted from the National Center for Injury Prevention and Control, Centers for Disease Control and Prevention.

Professionals,[3] see Appendix C effective control of injury (or any other disease, for that matter) requires collection of appropriate detailed data (e.g., frequency, location) related to the injury under study and the events or circumstances surrounding that injury. The analysis of such data helps us to understand the epidemiological patterns of these problems, identify risk factors, suggest causal factors, and guide us in the development of preventive interventions. At times, researchers develop unique data collection efforts to better address the issues under investigation. Most commonly, however, existing datasets are used, despite the fact that most of these datasets are administrative in nature and tend to be oriented either toward the injuries (i.e., the medical aspects) or toward the events (i.e., the incidents or "accident" aspects), and rarely include enough detailed information for both. Several United States government and private agencies maintain data systems that collect injury data on a continuous basis as part of their public health practice. Table 27.4 lists some of the most commonly used data systems, as well as their website addresses.

Identification of Causes and Development of Interventions

We have indicated, thus far, that injuries involve an unfavorable interaction between etiologic agents and the individual. Therefore, the essence of injury prevention involves keeping the etiologic agent from reaching the potential host at all (i.e., preventing the interaction) or from reaching it at rates and in amounts that would produce damage (i.e., minimizing the consequences). Under some circumstances, prevention is aimed at modifying the agents; under others, at reducing exposure to the agent or the susceptibility of individuals. Several conceptual models have been developed over the past 30 years to facilitate the understanding of injury-producing events and possible countermeasures. Before we present these models, let us revisit the sequence of injury events.

We live in a particular environment. In this environment, we conduct our lives: we walk, drive, exercise, prepare meals, and do countless other things. On each occasion, we are exposing ourselves to the possibility of undergoing an event that may lead to

Table 27.4. **Selected Surveillance Systems Used in Injury Control**

Data System	Acronym	Federal Agency	Web Address
Census of Fatal Occupational Injuries	CFOI	Bureau of Labor Statistics	http://www.bls.gov
Survey of Occupational Injuries and Illnesses	SOII	Bureau of Labor Statistics	http://www.bls.gov
Survey of Workplace Violence Prevention	—	Bureau of Labor Statistics	http://www.bls.gov
National Crime Victimization Survey	NCVS	Bureau of Justice Statistics	http://www.ojp.usdoj.gov
National Ambulatory Medical Care Survey	AMCS	Centers for Disease Control and Prevention	http://www.cdc.gov/nchswww
National Hospital Ambulatory Medical Care Survey	NHAMCS	Centers for Disease Control and Prevention	http://www.cdc.gov/nchswww
National Hospital Discharge Survey	NHDS	Centers for Disease Control and Prevention	http://www.cdc.gov/nchswww
National Health Interview Survey	NHIS	Centers for Disease Control and Prevention	http://www.cdc.gov/nchswww
National Vital Statistics Systems—Current Mortality Sample	NVSSS	Centers for Disease Control and Prevention	http://www.cdc.gov/nchswww
National Vital Statistics Systems—Final Mortality Data	NVSSF	Centers for Disease Control and Prevention	http://www.cdc.gov/nchswww
Behavioral Risk Factor Surveillance System	BRFSS	Centers for Disease Control and Prevention	http://www.cdc.gov/brfss/
Youth Risk Behavioral Surveillance System	YRBSS	Centers for Disease Control and Prevention	http://www.cdc.gov/nccdphp/dash/yrbs
National Traumatic Occupational Fatality Surveillance System	NTOF	Centers for Disease Control and Prevention	http://www.cdc.gov
National Electronic Injury Surveillance System	NEISS	Consumer Product Safety Commission	http://www.cpsc.gov
Law Enforcement Officers Killed and Assaulted	LEOKA	Federal Bureau of Investigation	http://www.fbi.gov
National Incident Based Reporting System	NIBRS	Federal Bureau of Investigation	http://www.icpsr.umich.edu/NACJD/NIBRS
Uniform Crime Reporting System—Supplemental Homicide Report	UCRSHR	Federal Bureau of Investigation	http://www.fbi.gov

(*continued*)

Table 27.4. (*continued*)

Data System	Acronym	Federal Agency	Web Address
Nationwide Personal Transportation System	NPTS	Federal Highway Administration	http://www.bts.gov/ntda/npts
Healthcare Cost and Utilization Project	HCUP	Agency for Health Care Policy and Research	http://www.ahcpr.gov/data
Healthcare Finance Administration	CMS	US Dept. Health & Human Services	http://www.cms.hhs.gov
Indian Health Service— Ambulatory Care System	IHSACS	Indian Health Service	http://www.ihs.gov
Indian Health Service— Inpatient Care System	IHSICS	Indian Health Service	http://www.ihs.gov
National Data Archive On Child Abuse and Neglect	NDACAN	National Center for Child Abuse and Neglect	http://www.ndacan.cornell.edu
Fatal Accident Reporting System	FARS	National Highway Traffic Safety Administration	http://www-fars.nhtsa.dot.gov
National Accident Sampling System— Crashworthiness Data System	NASS CDS	National Highway Traffic Safety Administration	http://www-nrd.nhtsa.dot.gov/Pubs/NASS94.PDF
National Accident Sampling System—General Estimates System	NASS GES	National Highway Traffic Safety Administration	http://www-nrd.nhtsa.dot.gov
National Occupant Protection Use Survey	NOPUS	National Highway Traffic Safety Administration	http://www-nrd.nhtsa.dot.gov
Monitoring the Future Study	MTFS	National Institute of Drug Abuse	http://monitoringthefuture.org
Drug Abuse Warning Network	DAWN	Substance Abuse and Mental Health Services Administration	http://dawninfo.samhsa.gov/
Census of Agriculture—	BCCOA	Bureau of the Census	http://www.nass.usda.gov/Census_of_Agriculture/index.asp
National Fire Incident Reporting System	NFIRS	Fire Administration	http://www.nfirs.fema.gov
Web Based Injury Statistics Query and Reporting System*	WISQARS	CDC National Center for Injury Prevention and Control	http://www.cdc.gov/ncipc/wisqars/

*It contains multiple of the data sources identified in this table and provides user-friendly access to its data.

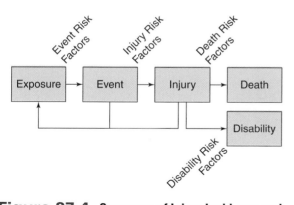

Figure 27.4. Sequence of Injury Incidence and Outcomes

SOURCE: Delmar Cengage Learning.

an injury. This is what could be referred to as the *exposure* component of the chain of events. For example, consider every minute a child spends enjoying a playground. Every so often, a potentially injurious **event** may happen. Following our example, the child falls from the swing; but only a fraction of such falls lead to any *injury*. Some of these injuries, however, may be severe enough to cause death or disability. This chain of events is depicted in Figure 27.4. This sequence of events is very similar to what has been labeled as the Domino Model[17] because of the linear relationship between the different components of this model. **Injury prevention** consists of intervention(s) aimed at blocking the progression of the events. In our example, we could have prevented the event from happening by eliminating the swings from the playground area or by designing them in such a manner that prevents ejection of the child. We could have minimized the impact of the fall by using an energy-absorbing flooring underneath the swing. Finally, we could have minimized the consequences of the injury by providing quick care at a pediatric facility with expertise in head injury.

The Haddon Matrix

Dr. William Haddon, Jr., a pioneer in the field of injury prevention, proposed a framework that integrates the role of the *individual,* the vehicle or

vector carrying the energy, and the *environment* in which the interaction occurs with the sequence of events associated with the injury.[18]

Individuals, vehicles (or vectors), and environments play different roles at different times. The sequence of events over time is divided into three phases: *pre-event* (i.e., preventing the event or incident from occurring), *event* (i.e., preventing injury while the event is happening), and post-event (i.e., minimizing the adverse results after the event has occurred). For example, interventions aimed at eliminating motor vehicle crashes or falls from windows, suicide attempts, or shootings are pre-event interventions. Event-phase interventions are aimed at either preventing the injury or at reducing the resulting injury by minimizing its severity. Examples of interventions at this stage include bicycle helmets, bullet-proof vests, or pills with smaller medication doses so that they are not as toxic if ingested. The variety and effectiveness of countermeasures at this event stage highlight the point that even if the event (e.g., crash) is not prevented, damage to passengers and occupants can be reduced or eliminated. Post-event interventions can be directed to two goals: reducing any further damage or restoring the health of the individual who sustained injuries.

In Table 27.5, we have listed potential interventions to prevent motor vehicle-related injuries using the Haddon Matrix.

Haddon's 10 Basic Strategies

In addition to developing the matrix, Haddon described 10 basic strategies for injury control, presented here with examples relating to injury produced by chemicals (in parentheses):

1. Prevent the initial marshaling of the agent. (Do not produce lead paint.)

2. Reduce the amount of the agent marshaled. (Package medicine in small quantities.)

3. Prevent release of the agent. (Use childproof caps on bottles of medicine.)

4. Modify rate or spatial distribution of release of agent from its source. (Devise containers that release poison at limited rates.)

Table 27.5. Haddon Matrix with Selected Examples of Motor Vehicle Occupant Injury Prevention Interventions

	Host (Child and Adult Occupants)	Vehicle (Car)	Environment Physical (road)	Socioeconomic
PRE-CRASH	Avoid distracting technology and behaviors Driver's drug or alcohol use, and fatigue	Antilock brakes Speed control Daytime running lights	Improve traffic patterns Increase visibility of hazards	Children in rear seats Legislation regarding child restraint Speed limits, licensing laws
CRASH	Use adequate child restraint Use safety belts, airbags	Seating position Built-in child car seats Vehicle speed, size and mass Interior surfaces	Separation from other lanes Energy-absorbing roadside fixtures	
POST-CRASH	Exercise and other health enhancement to reduce comorbidity	Crash detection systems that notify EMS (and indicate type of occupants on board) Designs to facilitate extrication Improve location of fuel tank	Designated lanes for emergency vehicles Reduce distance from EMS	**Trauma** system EMS system prepared to handle children Societal acceptance of residual disabilities

5. Separate, in space or time, the agent from the susceptible person. (Keep children out of orchards while spraying.)

6. Separate the agent from the susceptible person with a material barrier. (Use gas masks.)

7. Modify the contact surface, subsurface, or basic characteristics of the agent. (Reformulate detergents to make them less caustic.)

8. Strengthen the resistance of the person who might otherwise be damaged. (Immunize susceptible people against insect stings.)

9. Counter the continuation and extension of the damage. (Provide and make use of first-aid treatment and poison control centers.)

10. Repair and rehabilitate. (Institute intermediate and long-term therapy.)

Obviously, there are some commonalities between these 10 countermeasures and the matrix described in the previous section. Several of these countermeasures relate to the host (strategies 5, 6 and 8), some to the vehicle or vector (strategies 1 through 4, and 7), and some to the environment (strategies 5, 6, 9, and 10). They could also be classified as pre-event, event, or post-event. Actually, countermeasures 1 through 3 could be described as pre-event interventions, 4 through 8 as event

interventions, and 9 and 10 as post-event interventions, although Haddon himself disagreed with such categorization because each strategy is broadly relevant. For example, countermeasure 1 could also be an event intervention, and countermeasure 5 could also be considered a pre-event intervention.

Human Performance and Environmental Demands Model

Another system-oriented model was described in the ergonomics literature by Blumenthal.[19] His model is centered on the dynamic interaction between the subject and the environment (Figure 27.5). The lower line represents the variable demands of a particular task, for example, driving a car, and includes the limitations and deficiencies in the vehicle and the environment (including other drivers). The upper line represents the performance of the subject of interest. The injurious event occurs when the system demands increase or the subject performance decreases simultaneously to levels at which they overlap. At times, it is the individual's behavior that fails dramatically, such as in the situation of a driver who suffers a myocardial infarction or stroke. At other times, it is the system that becomes overwhelming, as in the case where another vehicle on

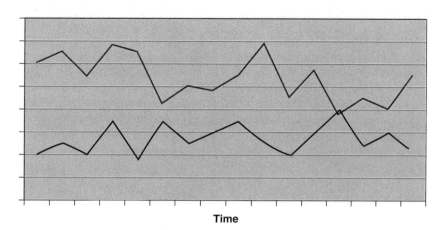

Time

Figure 27.5. Hypothetical Localized System Failure
SOURCE: Adapted from Blumenthal 1968.

the road has a tire blowout. The third, and most common situation, involves neither cataclysmic human failure nor overwhelming demands but rather a simultaneous decrease in performance and increase in task demand. Such would be the situation where an intoxicated driver (who may be able to drive in a straight line) fails to negotiate an unexpected curve, or a teenager who is distracted by a passenger.

Historically, efforts in injury prevention have focused on the individual's performance. It is only recently that attention has been focused on reducing demands of the task.

Regardless of which specific model of injury causation one prefers, data from the data systems described in the previous section (and others) can and should be rigorously examined using public health science methods such as those listed under the sixth domain (Basic Public Health Sciences Skills) of the Core competencies,[3] for example, social sciences, biostatistics, and epidemiology, to better characterize the exact contribution of each possible factor involved in the occurrence of an injury.

Choice and Evaluation of Countermeasures

The role of epidemiology in identifying modifiable risk factors is closely related to the identification of countermeasures. Modifiable risk factors become the basis for intervention design. Note that factors playing an important role in minor injuries are not necessarily the same as factors that are important in severe or fatal injuries. Consequently, the choice of countermeasures may change as the severity of injuries changes. Also, countermeasures should not be determined by the relative importance of causal or contributing factors or by their earliness in the sequence of events. Rather, priority and emphasis should be given to measures that will most effectively and efficiently reduce injury losses. For example, although psychological factors may be important in the initiation of motor vehicle crashes, it does not follow that psychological screening of drivers would be fruitful.

It is also important to discuss the assumption that anything that sounds reasonable will be effective; this has been the rationale for countless programs, from "defensive driving" training to holiday death counts. Safety programs not only may lack effectiveness, but under certain circumstances, they could even increase the number or severity of injuries, as in the case of driver education programs that enable teenagers to drive at an earlier age than they otherwise would.[20]

Numerous safety measures have been adopted without proof of their effectiveness or without being evaluated. The resulting entrenchment of untested measures makes improvement difficult and comparison with alternatives impossible. Millions of dollars can be wasted in unsuccessful safety campaigns, and without adequate preplanned evaluation, no one will ever know whether a campaign was effective and guidance for the future will be lost. The importance of effectiveness evaluation across all public health problems is emphasized both in the Essential Services[2] and as "monitoring program performance" under the seventh domain of the core competencies.[3]

In contrast, many other interventions have been evaluated. Table 27.6 lists selected injury control interventions that have been proven effective. For a review of the issues involved in evaluating more detailed prevention interventions, refer to Dannenberg and Fowler's article in *Injury Prevention*.[21]

Another issue to keep in mind when selecting countermeasures is that, very frequently, a "mixed strategy" should be employed, incorporating countermeasures that address complementary aspects. Here the challenge will be in choosing the right type, intensity, and order of interventions to make the "combined" countermeasures most efficient. For example, whether airbags should be designed to protect even unbelted occupants in a frontal collision or as a supplement to safety belts became the issue of a long and intense dispute among motor vehicle safety specialists in the early 1980s. After it was decided that they should be supplemental restraints, the issue of which crashes were severe enough to warrant airbag deployment in a belted occupant became the new topic of debate.[22]

Table 27.6. Examples of Injury Prevention Strategies of Known Effectiveness

Motor vehicle	Child passenger restraint
	Child passenger restraint laws
	Safety belts
	Safety belt laws
	Sobriety check points
	Laceration protective windshields
	Nighttime curfews for teenage drivers
	Pedestrian-friendly front end of automobiles
	Minimum drinking age laws
	Breakaway utility poles
Firearm	Absence of handguns in homes
Fires/burns	Manufacture of fire-safe cigarettes
	Smoke detectors
	Automatic sprinklers
	Fire-resistant pajamas for children
	Legislation regulating flammability of children's clothing
	Fire exits and fire drills
Recreational	Four-sided barriers around swimming pools
	Bicycle helmet use
	Promoting bicycle helmet use (e.g., laws)
	Breakaway bases for softball
Sports injuries	Mouthguards
	Protective equipment (e.g., knee and elbow pads, wrist pads for inline skating)
Falls	Window guards in high-rise buildings
	Weight-bearing exercise among elderly
	Fall-cushioning materials underneath playground equipment
	Protective hip pads for elderly
	Prevention or treatment of osteoporosis in women
Poisonings	Packaging of children's aspirin in sublethal doses
Farm	Rollover protective structures on farm tractors
Choking and suffocation	Legislation and product design changes (e.g., safe refrigerator disposal, warning labels on thin plastic bags)
Shootings	Having no firearms in the home
All injuries	Minimum drinking age of 21
	Increase in excise tax for alcohol
	911 response systems

Choices must be made, by default if not consciously, on such matters as these or on the question of how many dollars to spend in preventing a given number of lost days or injury hospitalizations or deaths. More complicated still are decisions as to how many hundreds of drivers a state will attempt to take off the road in an effort to prevent one of them from killing himself or herself or someone else. This conscious weighing of alternatives is often lacking in the safety field.

AXIOMS TO GUIDE INJURY PREVENTION

Over the years, enough experience has been gathered to establish several axioms that can help guide efforts in controlling injuries:

Injury Results from Interactions between People and the Environment

The agent of injury will cause little damage if the amount of energy reaching tissues is below human tolerance levels. For example, tap water temperature of less than 120 degrees Fahrenheit is not likely to acutely damage human tissue, although higher temperatures or lengthy immersion may. The importance of this interaction is reflected in approaches that control the environment by reducing hot water temperatures at the tap and that simultaneously target the elderly and parents of small children for education about hot water scald risk.

Injury-Producing Interactions Can Be Modified through Changing Behavior, Products, or Environments

Modifying the weakest or most adaptable link in the chain of causation can reduce injuries. Unsanctioned swimming in a home swimming pool is more easily reduced by placing an isolation fence or barrier between the child and the pool than by supervising the child's behavior all the time. During sanctioned swimming, supervision is the most important strategy. Changing the environment, the laws, the person, or the product can each lead to reductions in injuries.

Environmental Changes Have the Potential to Protect the Greatest Number of People

Changes to the environment that automatically provide protection to every person have the potential to prevent the most injuries. Automatic protection includes, for example, bullet-proof windows in liquor stores, automatic sprinkler systems in buildings, energy-absorbing steering wheel columns in vehicles, fuses in homes, and child-resistant packaging of consumer products.

Effective Injury Prevention Requires a Mixture of Strategies and Methods

The primary strategies—behavior change (whether by education or by legislation) and technology/engineering are widely recognized as potentially effective in preventing injuries. Individual behavior change, product engineering, public education, legal requirements, law enforcement, and changes in the physical and social environment work together to reduce injuries. The challenge in intervention planning is to select the most efficient combination of strategies to produce the desired results. Identifying target populations and deciding on the proper combination of strategies are not exclusive to injury prevention but are part of the fundamental competencies of a public health professional, as outlined in several of their second domain (policy development/program planning) skills.[3]

Public Participation Is Essential for Community Action

Effective public policy requires the support and participation of community members. This is, again, reflected both in the Essential Services[2] and under the fifth domain (Community Dimensions of Practice Skills) of the Core Competencies.[3] Local conditions and resource availability often determine the direction of injury prevention programs. Injury prevention is most successful when there is public participation, support for, and understanding of injury prevention methods. Without public support, laws that are designed to protect the public, such as laws requiring the use of bicycle or motorcycle helmets, or safety belt use, may be ignored or repealed. This was clearly seen in the Massachusetts legislature regarding mandatory safety belt use; the law was repealed by popular vote in 1986, 11 months after the legislation had been enacted, and enacted again in 1994.

Cross-Sector Collaboration Is Necessary

Injury prevention requires coordinated action by many groups. Participation by community leaders, in addition to health officials, is necessary in planning and implementing injury prevention programs. There are a number of ways that other community members can contribute to a program's success, ranging from identifying problems to mobilizing community action and evaluating intervention effectiveness.

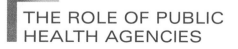

THE ROLE OF THE PUBLIC HEALTH PRACTITIONER

Public health professionals can play a vital role in injury prevention from a variety of positions.

Research

Public health practitioners are particularly well positioned to collect and analyze local data to identify injury patterns, trends, and risk factors. They are also well positioned to introduce scientific methods to injury control by insisting that new countermeasures be evaluated and that, where relevant, they first be subjected to testing in the field.

Service

Public health practitioners can assist community organizations in analyzing data and choosing countermeasures that are known to be effective.

Education

It is essential to educate not only individuals in the community but also, and even more important, the public and private decision makers (e.g., legislators, designers, executives, builders) whose decisions affect the risk of injury for large numbers of individuals. Every day, these decision makers are confronted with issues such as whether to delay implementation of vehicle standards; whether to make an appliance safer or depend upon users always to follow directions; or whether to promote products on the basis of their potential for reducing injury, as opposed to assuming that "you can't sell safety." Public health practitioners can be of great assistance in these processes. It is also particularly important to educate the members of the media.

Influencing Legislation and Regulation

Public health practitioners are particularly well positioned to assist (or initiate) local policy discussions and assist in evaluating the appropriateness or quality of the facts presented by the different parties involved in policy discussions. For a public health practitioner to be successful in all these areas, he or she must also be aware of the barriers to the implementation of injury prevention activities, including funding limitations, organizational difficulties, and turf battles.[7]

THE ROLE OF PUBLIC HEALTH AGENCIES

The growing awareness that injuries can be reduced through the application of public health principles to populations has expanded expectations for national, state, and local public health agencies to increase their activities in injury control.

Information Collection

Effective injury control depends on adequate information systems. National agencies play a major role in the response to injury-related issues, but the quality of their basic data is determined, predominantly, at the local level. Health departments should stimulate uniform reporting and prompt analysis of injury data and make appropriate use of injury data in administration. Numerous issues that are related to injury definition, coding, case inclusion criteria, event definition and coding and its standardization remain unresolved and prevent further advance of the injury field.

National public health agencies must also reinforce these activities by ensuring that information developed from local data eventually gets back to the local level.

Regulation and Legislation

Safety standards have long been applied to many kinds of products and operations. Standards may be descriptive in nature, specifying such things as materials, design, and process, or they may be performance standards, indicating what a product should do (and what it should never do) no matter how it is made. For safety purposes, performance standards are generally preferable, although both types sometimes contribute little except a false sense of security. Most commonly, standards are voluntary and industry-wide. Yet, voluntary standards are often insufficient. When public attention is drawn to an industry's failure to keep its products from being unreasonably hazardous, the government may consider issuing regulatory standards.

In addition to product and environmental standards, laws regulating human behavior are also intended to reduce injuries. As with other regulations, whether they succeed depends upon whether they are enforced, whether the penalties are effective, and whether the basic assumptions underlying the regulations and their enforcement are valid. State-level safety belt laws provide a wonderful example of this point. As of 2007, all states except New Hampshire have some form of safety belt law for motor vehicle occupants. The degree of coverage, details, and enforcement of these laws varies widely from state to state; however, one of the most distinguishing factors of these laws' effectiveness is whether they are primary (i.e., not wearing safety belts is reason enough for arrest and punishment) or secondary (i.e., some other offense is needed for the safety belt regulation to be enforced). Figure 27.6 shows safety belt use as reported from observational surveys by state. States with secondary safety belt laws have significantly lower safety belt use.

Emergency Systems

When primary prevention strategies fail, secondary and tertiary strategies become imperative. Municipal, state, and federal agencies are taking an increasing interest in emergency care and transport. Local and regional planning is required for successful organization of emergency communication systems, transportation, trauma units, poison control centers, and specialized units such as those for burns. Public health agencies have a role in organizing such systems, for example, by categorizing emergency facilities on the basis of what kind of injury cases they are equipped and staffed to treat, so that seriously injured patients can have the optimum chance of receiving adequate care. Lately, this role has expanded into development of triage criteria and establishment of regionalized trauma systems where not only the emergency facilities are categorized, but hospitals are too.

Education

Even though we have said before that priority in injury prevention should be given to measures that require little or no human action or cooperation, education must supplement some forms of injury control.[29] Public health agencies must devise and implement educational efforts directed to the general public that address all three phases of the injury sequence: pre-event, event, and post-event. Another very important function of education is to convince the public as well as private and public organizations that the hazards of their environment can be controlled, reduced, or eliminated. Public support is often needed before a preventive measure can be introduced; for example, people must be persuaded of the benefits of a motorcycle helmet law before they support it. Finally, individuals (e.g., legislators, regulators, administrators) whose decisions can determine the likelihood of injury to thousands of people need to be educated to take advantage of their role in injury prevention.

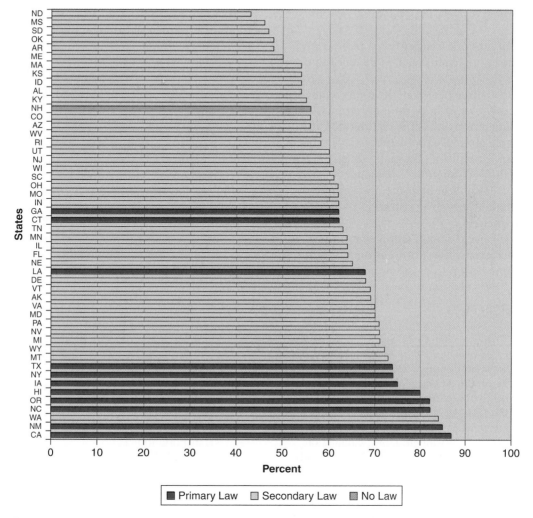

Figure 27.6. State Safety Belt Use Rates by Law Type. United States, 2006

SOURCE: National Highway Traffic Safety Administration. Traffic Safety Facts: Safety Belt Use in 2006—Use Rates in the States and Territories. DOT HS 810690. Washington, DC; 2007.

SUMMARY

Injury is a public health problem that can be controlled with the application of public health tools such as epidemiology, program design and implementation, and evaluation. Major achievements over the past 30 years or so reinforce this point. Further reductions in both unintentional and

intentional injuries and their associated medical, psychological, and economic burden will require continued efforts by the public health community in surveillance and research, in building partnerships with public and private organizations, and in the development of state and local health department injury control programs. Those public health practitioners who understand the issues and scientific concepts involved in injury occurrence can contribute effectively to substantially reducing this huge problem.

REVIEW QUESTIONS

1. If the bumper of a car strikes a pedestrian, fracturing the femur, what is the etiologic agent?
2. Name the three phases of the injury sequence.
3. What is the most important criterion when choosing among possible countermeasures to reduce an injury problem?
4. Give an example of automatic ("passive") protection of automobile passengers.
5. True or False: Seat belts are an example of automatic ("passive") protection of automobile passengers.
6. True or False: Primary enforcement of a seat belt law means that not wearing a seat belt is sufficient reason to arrest someone.

REFERENCES

1. Baker SP. Injury control. In: Sartwell PE, ed. *Preventive Medicine and Public Health*. 10th ed. New York: Appleton Century-Crofts; 1973.
2. Public Health in America. Available at: http://www.health.gov/phfunctions/public.htm.
3. Council on Linkages Between Academia and Public Health Practice. *Core Competencies for Public Health Practice*. Washington, DC: Council on Linkages Between Academia and Public Health Practice; 2001. Available at: http://www.phf.org/link/corecompetencies.htm.
4. Baker SP, O'Neill B, Li G, Ginsberg M. *The Injury Fact Book*. 2nd ed. New York: Oxford University Press; 1992.
5. Laflamme L, Svanstrom L, Schelp L, eds. Safety Promotion Research: *A Public Health Approach to Accident and Injury Prevention*. Stockholm, Sweden: Karolinska Institutet; 1999.
6. Gielen AC, Sleet DA, DiClemente RJ. *Injury and Violence Prevention: Behavioural Science Theories, Methods and Applications*. San Francisco: John Wiley & Sons; 2006.
7. Christoffel T, Scavo Gallagher S. *Injury Prevention and Public Health: Practical Knowledge, Skills and Strategies*. 2nd ed. Gaithersburg, MD: Aspen Publishers; 2006.
8. National Committee for Injury Prevention and Control. Injury prevention: Meeting the challenge. *Am J Prev Med*. 1989;5(3, supp l):297.
9. Bonnie RJ, Fulco CE, Liverman CT, eds. In: IOM report *Reducing the Burden of Injury: Advancing Prevention and Treatment*. Washington, DC: National Academy Press; 1999.
10. CDC NCHS, Office of Statistics and Programming. Vital statistics system for numbers of deaths. WISQARS. Available at: http://www.cdc.gov/ncipc/wisqars/. Accessed June 11, 2007.
11. CDC NCHS, Office of Statistics and Programming. Vital statistics system for numbers of deaths. WISQARS. Available at: http://www.cdc.gov/ncipc/wisqars/. Accessed June 11, 2007.
12. Warner M, Barnes PM, Fingerhut LA. Injury and poisoning episodes and conditions; National Health Interview Survey. *Vital Health Stat*. 2000; 10(202).
13. Mathers CD, Loncar D. Projections of global mortality and burden of disease from 2002 to 2030. *PLOS medicine*. 2006;3;2011–2029.
14. Finkelstein EA, Corso PA, Miller TR, et al. *The Incidence and Economic Burden of Injuries in the United States*. New York: Oxford University Press; 2006.
15. Segui-Gomez M. *Literature Search for Psychological and Psychosocial Consequences of Injury*. NHTSA DOT HS 808 527. National Highway Traffic Safety Administration, US Dept of Transportation; 1996.
16. Waller JA. Public health then and now: Reflections on a half century of injury control. *Am J Public Health*. 1994;84:664–670.
17. Heinrich HW. *Industrial Accident Prevention. A Scientific Approach*. 4th ed. New York: McGraw-Hill; 1980.
18. Haddon W Jr. A logical framework for categorizing highway safety phenomena and activities. *J Trauma*. 1972;12:193–207.
19. Blumenthal M. Dimensions of the traffic safety problem. *Traffic Safety Res Rev*. 1968;12:7.
20. Vernick JS, Li G, Ogaitis S, MacKenzie E, et al. Effectiveness of high school driver education on motor vehicle crashes, violations, and licensure. *Am J Prev Med*. 1999;1S:40–46.
21. Dannenberg AL, Fowler CJ. Evaluation of interventions to prevent injuries: An overview. *Inj Prev*. 1998;4:141–147.
22. Graham JD. *Preventing Automobile Injury: New Findings from Evaluation Research*. Dover, MA: Auburn House Publishing Co; 1988.

CHAPTER 28

Oral Diseases: The Neglected Epidemic

Myron Allukian Jr., DDS, MPH

LEARNING OBJECTIVES

Upon completion of this chapter, the reader will be able to:

1. Explain why oral health is a neglected epidemic and a public health problem in need of a public health solution.

2. Explain why oral health is important, in terms of overall health, social cost, and economic cost.

3. Describe the major oral diseases, their prevalence, and their public health significance.

4. Define the role of health departments and community oral health programs in improving oral health using the 10 essential public health services.

5. Describe the importance of community water fluoridation as the foundation for improving the oral health of communities.

6. Describe the community and individual preventive measures for dental caries and compare the five effective community prevention programs for dental caries.

7. Describe what actions are needed on the local, state, and national level to improve oral health.

8. Describe the types and roles of dental personnel, the importance of less-restrictive state dental practice acts for dental hygienists and assistants, and the need for new mid-level providers such as the Alaska Dental Therapist.

9. List the different resources available to improve oral health.

KEY TERMS

Cleft Lip/Cleft Palate

Community Water Fluoridation

Craniofacial Anomalies

Dental Caries

Dental Fluorosis

Denturists

Endodontics

Fluoride

Gingivitis

Malocclusion

Oral and Pharyngeal Cancer

ACKNOWLEDGEMENTS: The author would like to thank Dr. Stephen B. Corbin, formerly the Chief Dental Officer of the U.S. Public Health Service, and Dr. Alice M. Horowitz, former Senior Scientist at the National Institute of Dental and Craniofacial Research, for their assistance with this chapter in the first edition of this book, and Ms. Natalie Grigorian and Mr. Juho Whang for their assistance with this chapter in the third edition of this book.

Oral health is an essential component of general health and well-being.[1] Yet oral diseases are a neglected epidemic, and millions of Americans suffer unnecessarily from them, even though many oral diseases are preventable.[2] The combination of high prevalence, high morbidity, and relative inattention from the health community and society makes oral diseases a significant public health problem in need of a public health solution.

Public health practitioners have the responsibility and opportunity to include oral health as an integral component of health in the development of policies and programs. When a needs assessment is done of a community or group of individuals, oral health must be included. As C. Everett Koop, MD, the former U.S. Surgeon General, has said, "You're not healthy without good oral health."

This chapter explains why oral health is a neglected epidemic, why oral health is important, and how public health can help promote good oral health. It also describes the epidemiology of oral disease and discusses preventive programs that can improve oral health. It concludes with a discussion of dental personnel in the United States.

BACKGROUND

Beginning in the early 1800s and due to a variety of factors, health sciences, education, and practice viewed the mouth as being disconnected from the rest of the body. After the founding of the first dental school in the world, the Baltimore College of Dental Surgery, in 1840, dentistry became a separate health profession from medicine, with separate schools, organizations, institutions, and programs. As dentistry evolved, many physicians, nurses, and even public health professionals were left without an understanding or appreciation of the impact oral diseases have on individuals and society.

When public health practitioners properly assess the major health needs of a target population, they usually find that the need for better oral health is a significant public health problem from the perspectives of both prevention and treatment. Major oral diseases and conditions include:

- **dental caries** (tooth decay)
- periodontal diseases (gum diseases)
- **malocclusion** (crooked teeth)
- edentulism (complete tooth loss)
- **oral and pharyngeal cancer**
- **craniofacial anomalies**, including **cleft lip/ cleft palate**
- **soft tissue lesions**
- **orofacial injuries**
- **temporomandibular dysfunction (TMD)**

Dental expertise is also of value in promoting and protecting the general health of communities. Examples of health concerns in which dental public health expertise has been invaluable to society are infection control, mercury toxicity, tobacco control, school-based programs, maternal and child health, primary care, AIDS/HIV, hepatitis B, tuberculosis, occupational health, needs assessment, policy development, quality assessment, community organization, and prevention on both the individual and community levels.

THE NEGLECTED EPIDEMIC

Although there has been substantial improvement in oral health on a national level in the last 20–30 years, due to water fluoridation, **topical fluorides,** and an emphasis on prevention, oral diseases are still pandemic in the United States, as the following statistics show:

- Twenty-five percent of 12- to 17-year-old adolescents have had **orthodontic treatment.**[3]

- Sixty percent of adolescents experience gum infections.[4]

- Seventy-seven percent of 16- to 19-year-old adolescents have had tooth decay, with an average of six affected surfaces.[5]

- Ninety-six percent of adults aged 50 to 64 have had tooth decay, with an average of 54 affected surfaces.[5]

- Twenty-seven percent of those aged 65 and older have no teeth at all.[5]

- More than 34,000 Americans are diagnosed with oral and pharyngeal cancer each year and approximately 7,500 die annually.[6]

- One out of 700 Americans are born with cleft lip/cleft palate.[7]

For vulnerable populations, such as children, minorities, the elderly, and those with low incomes, oral diseases are especially problematic.[8] Selected studies have shown that up to 97 percent of the homeless need dental care.[9] More than half of some Head Start children have had early childhood caries.[10] Almost half of abused children have orofacial trauma.[11] Sixteen percent of emergency department visits are for orofacial injuries.[12] Low-income seniors aged 65 to 74 are almost four times as

likely to be edentulous than high-income seniors.[13] African American, low-income, and American Indian and Alaska Native children aged 2–4 years have about two to six times more untreated tooth decay than their peers.[8,14] More than 50 percent of the homebound elderly have not seen a dentist for 10 years.[15] Finally, people without health insurance have four times the rate of unmet dental needs as those with private insurance.[16]

Fortunately, most oral diseases can be prevented. Unfortunately, once they occur, they usually do not resolve themselves without the physical intervention of a dental provider. Two exceptions to this are an incipient carious lesion, which is reversible when exposed to **fluoride,** and mild **gingivitis.**

Untreated dental caries usually progresses to an infection of the nerve and blood supply from the involved tooth, which may result in an abscess, cellulitis (an infection of the soft tissue), and sometimes even death.[17,18] When dental caries is treated, a dentist must physically remove the bacterial infection, reshape the infected area of the tooth, and then restore the tooth with an artificial substance to retain its function. Restored teeth are weaker than intact healthy teeth and subject to fracture and additional caries attack.

IMPORTANCE OF ORAL HEALTH

Oral health is an integral component of total health. The maintenance of good oral health is important for:

- freedom from pain, infection, and suffering
- the ability to eat and chew food for proper digestion and nutrition
- the ability to speak properly
- social mobility
- employability
- self-image and self-esteem
- quality of life and well-being

Studies have shown associations between periodontal disease and premature low-birth-weight babies, and between oral infections and heart disease and stroke.[19–25] Poor oral health may also compromise individuals in school, work, or daily living.[2,26] People with poor oral health may suffer unnecessarily with pain, have difficulty in interpersonal relationships, and have diminished job opportunities. One study estimated that approximately 20 percent of Americans experience orofacial pain in a 6-month period.[27] Good oral health is critical to the ability of the young, elderly, and medically compromised to function and thrive.

The Social Cost of Oral Disease

The social cost of oral diseases to the individual and society are great. For example, in 1989, among school-age children, more than 51 million hours of school were lost due to oral health problems, almost 1.2 hours per school child.[28] Also in 1989, more than 164 million hours were missed from work, an average of 1.48 hours per employed adult.[28] In 1991, school-age children had almost 4.8 million restricted activity days and 2.2 million bed days.[29] In 1994, low-income children had almost 12 times more days of missed school due to dental problems than higher-income children.[30] In 1996, employed persons 18 years and older had more than 9.7 million restricted activity days and more than 4.6 million bed days.[2]

The Economic Cost of Oral Disease

The economic cost of oral diseases is also significant. Dental services consumed about $91.5 billion, or 4.1 percent of all health expenditures, in 2006.[31] Dental expenditures are expected to reach $167.3 billion by the year 2015, or about 4.1 percent of personal expenditures.[31] Most dental expenditures are paid by private sources, such as private insurance, or are out-of-pocket. Only about 51.6 percent of the United States population has some form of dental insurance/benefit plan.[32] Of the enrolled individuals, 43 percent are in indemnity plans, 17.9 percent are in dental health management organizations (HMOs), 31.2 percent are in preferred provider organizations (PPOs), and 7.5 percent are in other types of plans. About 30.7 percent of all dental patients are self-payors and 5.4 percent are on public assistance.[32]

Public programs providing dental insurance are few. Medicaid includes dental services, primarily for children as part of the Early Periodic Screening Diagnosis and Treatment (EPSDT) Program. In 2005, dental Medicaid expenditures were about $4 billion, or 1.38 percent of the $289.3 billion spent for all Medicaid personal health care expenditures.[33] Only 15.7 percent of Medicaid-eligible children actually received treatment in 2004.[34] In addition, many Medicaid programs do not adequately reimburse for effective preventive procedures such as dental sealants. Dentistry is an optional service for adults under Medicaid, and many states provide only limited services to adults. Unfortunately, Medicare, which provides health care to individuals over age 65, does not include dental services at all unless they are related to trauma or oral cancer.

AN OVERVIEW OF ORAL HEALTH PROBLEMS

Major oral health problems include dental caries, periodontal diseases, and oral/pharyngeal cancer. The prevalence and public health significance of these problems are addressed next.

Dental Caries

Dental caries, or tooth decay, is the most prevalent oral disease in the United States. It is a bacterial infection that is influenced by a variety of factors in the host, agent, and environment.

Prevalence

The prevalence of dental caries increases with age, especially during the first two decades of life, as shown in Table 28.1 for decay rates in 1986–1987.

Table 28.1. Prevalence of Tooth Decay and Mean Number of Permanent Tooth Surfaces Affected, United States School Children, 5 to 17 Years of Age, 1986 to 1987[35]

Age	% Prevalence	Mean Number Affected Tooth Surfaces
5	2.7	0.07
6	5.6	0.13
7	15.8	0.40
8	25.0	0.71
9	34.5	1.14
10	44.3	1.69
11	55.0	2.33
12	58.3	2.66
13	66.0	3.76
14	72.3	4.68
15	78.2	5.71
16	80.0	6.68
17	84.4	8.04
all ages (5 to 17)	49.9	3.07

Table 28.2. Prevalence of Tooth Decay and Mean Number of Permanent Tooth Surfaces Affected by Age Group, United States, 1999–2004[5]

Age Group	% Prevalence	Mean Number Affected Tooth Surfaces
6–8	10.16	0.33
9–11	31.36	1.32
12–15	50.67	2.85
16–19	67.49	5.79
20–34	85.58	13.39
35–49	94.30	31.46
50–64	95.62	53.87
65–74	93.25	69.88
75+	92.70	74.08

At age 6, when the 32 permanent teeth usually begin erupting, only about 5.6 percent of school children had tooth decay in their permanent teeth.[35] Not only does the prevalence of the disease increase with age, but the number of affected tooth surfaces also increases. By age 17, 84 percent of adolescents have had tooth decay, with an average of 8 affected tooth surfaces, and by age 40 to 44, almost 99 percent of adults have had tooth decay, with an average of 45 affected tooth surfaces.[35,36] For all children in the United States, 75 percent of the dental caries actually occurs in only about 25 percent of children.[35] More recent data, for the years 1999–2004, with the ages grouped, shows similar trends, although there are fewer permanent teeth affected by tooth decay (see Table 28.2). For 6- to 8-year-olds, prevalence increased from 10.16 percent with 0.33 affected surfaces to 95.62 percent for ages 50–64 with 53.87 affected tooth surfaces.[5]

Types of Caries

There are three general types of tooth decay: coronal, which occurs on the crowns of teeth; **root surface,** which occurs on the roots of teeth; and **recurrent,** which is reoccurring tooth decay. Root surface decay usually occurs in older individuals. A study of New England elders showed that 52 percent of individuals over age 70 years had root caries. For 22 percent of them, the disease was untreated.[37] In a national study of individuals over age 75 years, almost 60 percent had root caries with 3.1 affected tooth surfaces.[38] More recent data shows a decrease in root caries prevalence for this age group to 42 percent.[5] The level of untreated dental caries is much higher among minorities and those with low income and less education. People who have lived in fluoridated communities since birth experience much lower rates of dental caries.

Early Childhood Caries

The 20 primary teeth begin erupting at about 6 to 9 months of age, and by about 2 years of age they have all erupted. *Early childhood caries* (ECC), formerly called *baby bottle tooth decay,* is tooth decay that occurs primarily in the upper anterior primary teeth when a baby is given a bottle, whose contents contain sugar, at bedtime or nap time. Juices or milk alone can cause ECC if they are given over extended periods of time.

About 8.3 percent of children in the United States age 2–5 years still use a baby bottle, and of these, 48.3 percent were reported as having gone to bed with a bottle containing something other than water.[39] The prevalence of ECC has averaged as high as 53 percent for Head Start children who were rural Native Americans or Alaskan Natives, and up to 11 percent for children in urban areas. ECC is higher in preterm, low-birth-weight infants and those that are malnourished. This may be due to poor tooth development of the fetus in utero when the mother is malnourished. Other possible causes include bacteria transferred from the caregiver after birth and improper baby feeding practices. Although dental caries in permanent teeth decreased nationally over the years, the most recent national study shows an increase in caries in primary teeth in children age 2–5 years.[5]

ECC may be painful and expensive. The treatment may cost about $3,000 to $8,000 per child because general anesthesia and, therefore, the use of an operating room are often required. It is much more cost effective to prevent ECC. It can be prevented by educating parents and caregivers about the dangers of giving infants bottles for prolonged periods unless they contain plain water. Bottle-fed infants should not be given bottles with juices, milk, or sweetened fluids when they are going to bed or otherwise using the bottle as a pacifier. Once a child has been fed by bottle, the teeth should be wiped clean. In general, breast-feeding should be encouraged over bottle-feeding, and parents should be taught to wean from the breast to the cup, rather than to the bottle, at around age 1 year. If ECC is prevalent in a given population, widespread prevention requires the development of a comprehensive, multidisciplinary, community-oriented education program.[10]

Periodontal Diseases

There are essentially two types of infections of the soft tissues (gums) surrounding a tooth: gingivitis and periodontitis. Both are quite common.

Gingivitis

Gingivitis is a localized infection or inflammation of the soft tissues surrounding a tooth that results in swelling and bleeding of the gums. It may or may not be self-limiting. Poor oral hygiene is the major contributing factor to gingivitis; therefore, good self-care is important in its prevention. Some forms of gingivitis, such as acute necrotizing ulcerative gingivitis (ANUG), or **trench mouth,** can be extremely painful. ANUG is often associated with stress, lack of sleep, poor nutrition, and poor oral hygiene.

Gingivitis occurs in about 60 percent of adolescents and about 48 percent of adults.[4,8] Among certain high-risk populations, the prevalence is higher. For Native American and Alaskan Natives, as many as 98 percent may have the disease, and it is found in up to 64 percent of Mexican Americans and 50 percent of low-income individuals.[8]

Periodontitis

Periodontitis is an infection or inflammation of the soft tissues and of the supporting alveolar bone around teeth with loss of periodontal attachment. When left untreated, periodontitis usually results in teeth becoming loose, necessitating extensive treatment and possible removal. In persons with AIDS or HIV infection, periodontitis can progress quite rapidly.

The prevalence of periodontitis increases with age. About 22 percent of people aged 35 to 44 have periodontitis, with the prevalence higher in high-risk populations such as minorities and low-income individuals.[8]

Prevention

Successful prevention of periodontal disease is oriented more to the individual than to the community. Prevention measures are similar for gingivitis and periodontitis, but gingivitis responds better to preventive measures. Patient compliance with proper oral hygiene procedures and regular mechanical removal of dental plaque with a toothbrush and floss helps prevent periodontal disease. It also usually responds well to a thorough professional cleaning, prophylaxis, **scaling**, and **root planing** performed by a dentist or dental hygienist.

Educational programs need to be developed as part of comprehensive health education for school children to reinforce the importance of good oral hygiene. Public awareness also needs to be increased so that individual compliance is improved in the use of proper oral hygiene practices and periodic dental visits.

Oral and Pharyngeal Cancer

More than 34,000 new cases of oral and pharyngeal cancer and 7,500 deaths from oral and pharyngeal cancer were estimated for the United States for 2007.[6] It is the seventh most common cancer for men, who are more than two times at risk than women. More Americans die from oral cancer than from cervical cancer. Tobacco and alcohol use are associated with more than 70 percent of oral cancers, and they occur most often in men over the age of 40.[40] The increase in the use of **spit (smokeless) tobacco**, especially among teenagers, may result in more individuals with oral cancer in the future. The 5-year oral and pharyngeal cancer survival rate for Euro-Americans is 61 percent compared with 40 percent for African Americans.[6] This is the second-largest cancer survival rate disparity between these two races.

Early detection and treatment of oral cancer results in higher survival rates. In 1998 only 13 percent of adults over age 40 in a national survey reported that they had ever been examined for oral cancer.[8] One study showed that for the two years prior to being diagnosed with oral cancer, patients had a median of 7.5 to 10.5 health care visits, yet 77 percent of the eventual diagnoses were for late-stage cancer.[41] Most of these visits were with physicians considered to be their regular source of care.

It is apparent that physicians and other health care providers need to be motivated and trained in early recognition of oral cancer. Health education programs for children and adults should emphasize the dangers of spit (smokeless) tobacco, cigarette smoking, and alcohol use. Policies should be implemented to discourage youth from tobacco and alcohol use. For example, in 1994 the National Collegiate Athletic Association (NCAA) banned student athletes and coaches from using smokeless or any other tobacco product during practices and games.[42] Periodic dental visits should also be promoted for early detection and treatment.

THE UTILIZATION OF DENTAL SERVICES

The utilization of dental care varies with age, income, and race,[13] as shown in Table 28.3. It also varies by insurance status.[13] In 1989 approximately 57 percent of the population in the United States over age

Table 28.3. Percent of Persons 2 Years of Age and Older Who Had Dental Visits in the Past Year and Number of Visits per Person per Year, by Age, Race, and Income: United States, 1989[13]

	Persons Who Visited in Past Year	Visits per Person per Year
Characteristics		
Age	**Percent**	**Number**
All ages	57.2	2.1
2–4 years	32.1	0.9
5–17 years	69.0	2.4
18–34 years	57.0	1.8
35–54 years	57.4	2.3
55–64 years	54.0	2.4
65 years and over	43.2	2.0
Race		
African American	44.5	1.2
Euro-American	59.3	2.2
Family income		
Less than $10,000	40.9	1.3
$10,000–$19,999	43.4	1.5
$20,000–$34,999	58.3	2.0
$35,000 and over	73.0	2.8

Table 28.4. Percentage of Children Ages 2–17 Who Had at Least One Dental Care Visit, 2003[44]

Characteristics	Percentage Who Visited at Least Once (Ages 2–17)	Average Number of Visits (Ages 2–17)
Total	50.9%	2.6
Race/Ethnicity		
Hispanic	36.7%	2.1
White single race	59.6%	2.8
Black single race	36.8%	1.8
Other single race/multiple race	45.3%	2.6
Gender		
Male	49.5%	2.5
Female	52.5%	2.7
Income		
Poor/Near poor	35.8%	1.9
Low/Middle income	37.4%	2.3
High income	60.1%	2.8

2 years had seen a dentist in the past year, for an average of 2.1 visits per year. For 5- to 17-year-olds, 69 percent had been to a dentist in the last year, as compared with only 43 percent of persons over age 65. For individuals with a family income of more than $35,000 a year, 73 percent had visited a dentist in the last year compared with 40 percent with family incomes of less than $10,000. Approximately 59 percent of Euro-Americans saw a dentist in the past year, with 2.2 visits on average, as compared with 44 percent of African Americans, with an average of 1.2 visits.[13]

Dental utilization is the lowest for those over age 65 years, but this age group has been increasing its visits to the dentist over the years. For those over age 65 in nursing homes, the unmet needs are even greater, and access to care is limited. The Omnibus Budget Reconciliation Act (OBRA) of 1989 has regulations requiring an oral examination of patients in long-term–care facilities within 14 days of admission and annually thereafter. These regulations became effective in 1992. OBRA's regulations have had a limited impact due to the lack of proper training to perform an oral assessment of nursing home staff or the necessary accountability to ensure compliance with these regulations.[43]

More recent data for children ages 2–17 is given in Table 28.4, which shows that 50.9 percent had been to a dentist in the last year with an average of 2.6 visits. Utilization varies based on race, sex, and income.[44]

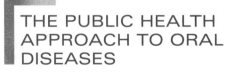

THE PUBLIC HEALTH APPROACH TO ORAL DISEASES

The oral disease epidemic presents a unique challenge to the public health professional, who has the responsibility to prevent as much disease as possible and to improve access to care for those least able to obtain such services. A population-based approach centered on the three core functions—assessment of dental needs, policy development for dental disease prevention and treatment, and assurance of access to needed services—is most likely to make an impact on oral disease.[45]

Every local, state, and federal health agency and department should have a dental public health program with properly trained staff to address this neglected epidemic. The national oral health objectives for the year 2010 as defined in *Healthy People 2010* can be achieved more easily with dental public health expertise and the appropriate resources.[8] Smaller local health departments should also utilize such dental expertise. Schools of public health and dental, medical, and nursing schools should also include dental public health expertise to help educate health profession students about oral health needs and programs from the public health perspective.

Dental Public Health

Expertise in dental public health is essential to respond to the oral disease epidemic in a meaningful and effective way. Dental public health has been defined by the American Board of Dental Public Health as:

> . . . the science and art of preventing and controlling dental diseases and promoting dental health through organized community efforts. It is that form of dental practice which serves the community as a patient rather than the individual. It is concerned with the dental health education of the public, with applied dental research, and with the administration of group dental programs, as well as the prevention and control of dental diseases on a community basis.[46]

Dental public health is the second smallest of the nine dental specialties recognized by the American Dental Association. Public health dentists are trained in program and policy development, management and administration, research methods, health promotion, disease prevention, and delivery of care systems. The competency objectives and competencies for dental public health have been delineated,[47,48] and this expertise is unique in dentistry because of its population-based approach.

Public health dentists have improved the oral health of millions of Americans by their initiatives. There are about 2,032 dentists in the United States who work in public health roles, of which about 1,000 have at least 1 year of advanced education and more than 600 have 2 years.[49] In 2006, 155 dentists were board-certified and active in dental public health.[50]

The American Board of Dental Public Health is the certifying board for this specialty, which requires a dental degree, a master's degree in public health, a 1-year residency, 2 years' experience in dental public health, and then the successful completion of a comprehensive 3-day examination.

Health Departments and Community Oral Health Programs

Based on the ten essential public health services, *A Model Framework for Community Oral Health Programs* (see Table 28.5) was developed by the American Association for Community Dental Programs.[51] The purpose of this framework is to provide guidelines for public health officials to develop oral health programs and services at the community level. It provides a context for local health officials in which to consider their responsibilities as they relate to oral health. It is a resource for local officials who do not have oral health expertise as well as oral health professionals and community boards who are involved in the planning, implantation, and enhancement of community oral health programs. Of the approximately 2,900 local public health agencies in our country, less then 700 (24 percent) have oral health programs.

A Guide to Developing a Community Oral Health Program

A Guide for Developing and Enhancing Community Oral Health Programs[52] is designed to assist local public health agencies and other interested parties to develop, integrate, expand, or enhance community oral health programs. This guide is a supplemental document to *A Model Framework for the Community Oral Health Programs: Based Upon*

Table 28.5. A Model Framework for Community Oral Health Programs: Based on the Ten Essential Public Health Services

1. **Monitor health status to identify community health problems.**
   a. Obtain and share data that provides information on the community's oral health (e.g., prevalence of early child-hood caries and dental caries, untreated caries, and oral cancer rates).
   b. Determine access to oral health care for the uninsured or underinsured, and determine community capacity to meet oral health needs.
   c. Analyze data to identify trends and population oral health risks (e.g., poverty levels, undocumented immigrants, lack of water fluoridation, adverse pregnancy outcomes, and cardiovascular disease).
   d. Review national, regional, and state oral health data for comparison and planning purposes.
   e. Conduct efforts or contribute oral health expertise to community health assessments to develop a comprehensive picture of the public's oral health (e.g., Title V needs assessment).
   f. Integrate oral health data with other health-assessment and data-collection efforts conducted by the public health system (e.g., Youth Risk Behavior Survey).
   g. Develop relationships with oral health professionals and others in the community who have information on diseases and other conditions relevant to public health, and facilitate information exchanges (e.g., among Head Start programs, community heath centers, schools, nursing homes, and hospital emergency units).

2. **Diagnose and investigate identified health problems and health hazards in the community.**
   a. Identify oral health problems and environmental hazards to general health (e.g., improper fluoride levels and amalgam disposal).
   b. Track trends and behaviors that identify emerging oral health problems (e.g., diabetes mellitus, obesity, lack of dental insurance, inadequate Medicaid/State Children's Health Insurance Program [SCHIP] coverage, and insufficient number of oral health professional participating in Medicaid/SCHIP).
   c. Participate in local public health agency (LPHA) planning for emergency preparedness.

   d. Identify and advocate for changes in social and economic conditions that adversely affect the public's oral health.
   e. Maintain access to laboratory expertise and capacity to help monitor and report on community and environmental health status (e.g., water plant operations and private well monitoring).

3. **Inform, educate, and empower people about health issues.**
   a. Share oral health and related information with individuals, community groups, agencies, and the general public to improve understanding of the issues affecting public health (e.g., social, economic, educational, and environmental issues).
   b. Provide information that is appropriate for the cultures and literacy levels of various audiences to help individuals understand the decisions they can make to promote their own oral health and the actions agencies can take to promote oral health.
   c. Conduct health-promotion activities to improve the oral health status of the community (e.g., tobacco-cessation activities and oral-cancer-detection activities).
   d. Mobilize the community to advocate for policies and activities that will improve the public's oral health (e.g., community water fluoridation policies).
   e. Work with the media to convey information of oral health significance (e.g., the relationship between diet and oral health).

4. **Mobilize community partnerships to identify and solve health problems.**
   a. Contribute oral health expertise to a comprehensive planning process that engages the community in identifying, prioritizing, and solving their public health problems and establishing oral-health-related goals.
   b. Support and implement strategies that address identified oral health problems through the development and maintenance of partnerships of public and private organizations, government agencies, businesses, schools, and the media.
   c. Develop partnerships to generate interest in and support for improved community oral health status.

Table 28.5. (*continued*)

d. Identify potential advocates and organizations that represent populations effected by oral health problems and disparities (e.g., Head Start participants, individuals with developmental disabilities, families who are homeless, and senior citizens).

e. Develop advocates (i.e., "champions") to support the development of community oral health programs.

5. Develop policies and plans that support individual and community health efforts.

a. Serve as a primary oral health resource to guide federal, state, and local elected and appointed officials to establish and maintain sound public health and oral health policies, practices, and capacity (e.g., fluoridation, oral services in Medicaid/Medicare, state dental practice acts, MCH block grant, tobacco policy, comprehensive school health programs, and oral health services for high-risk populations).

b. Provide oral health expertise to policy development efforts to improve physical, social, and environmental conditions in the community that adversely affect public health (e.g., school lunch programs/beverage contracts, long-term–care and correctional facilities, and tobacco-free public places).

c. Engage in LPHA strategic planning to develop a vision, mission, and guiding principles for the agency that is responsive to the community's oral health needs.

d. Develop community oral health vision and mission statements and guiding principles that reflect the community's oral health needs.

6. Enforce laws and regulations that protect health and ensure safety.

a. Monitor laws, ordinances, regulations, and policies that impact oral health, and take steps to ensure their enforcement to maintain or improve oral health in the community (e.g., Medicaid/Early and Periodic Screening, Diagnosis and Treatment requirements; Head Start program performance standards; nursing home oral examination requirements; fluoridation laws; and blood-borne pathogen standards).

b. Educate policymakers on gaps in public health law, ordinances, regulations, and policies needed to

protect the public's oral health (e.g., adult Medicaid oral services).

c. Inform and educate individuals and organizations about the purpose, meaning, and benefit of public health laws, ordinances, regulations, and policies that impact oral health.

d. Determine whether modifying, repealing, or developing new laws, regulations, ordinances, or policies is needed to maintain or improve the community's oral health, and take appropriate steps to effect change.

e. Monitor and respond to proposed legislation, regulation, ordinances, and policies that may impact community oral health.

7. Link people to needed personal health services and ensure the provision of health care when otherwise unavailable.

a. Lead or join efforts to increase access to comprehensive culturally competent oral health care that includes health promotion, prevention, and treatment services.

b. Partner with the community to establish systems and programs to meet oral health treatment needs (e.g., for individuals with special health care needs, for families who are homeless).

c. Partner with the community to identify and establish systems and programs that include preventive services (e.g., school-based/linked dental sealant and fluoride programs, mouth guard programs, and early-childhood-caries-prevention programs).

d. Link individuals to appropriate oral health services (e.g., using care coordination mechanisms, and patient navigators).

8. Ensure a competent public health and personal health care workforce.

a. Ensure appropriate presence of community oral health programs in the LPHA and state organizational structure and decision-making processes.

b. Apply appropriate public health competencies to the recruitment, training, and development of the community oral health director and workforce.

(continued)

Table 28.5. (continued)

c. Assess the dental public health competencies of community oral health program staff, and promote these competencies through training, continuing education, and leadership development activities.

d. Provide expertise in developing and implementing public health curricula through partnerships with academia (e.g., public health/dental/medical/allied health students).

e. Provide educational experiences in community oral health for the future oral health workforce.

f. Recruit, train, develop, and retain a diverse and culturally competent oral health workforce.

g. Promote the use of effective oral health practices among all professionals and agencies engaged in public health interventions.

h. Promote the use of effective preventive services among oral health professionals and other health professionals in the community.

i. Provide the community oral health program workforce with access to the training and resources needed to develop and maintain their competencies.

j. Identify and provide strategies for addressing public- and private-sector shortages in the oral health care workforce (e.g., dental health professional shortage area designations, utilization of National Health Service Corps, and loan repayment mechanisms).

k. Identify and address barriers to the utilization of oral health services (e.g., transportation, financial, health literacy, and language).

9. **Assess the effectiveness, accessibility, and quality of personal and population-based health services.**

a. Evaluate the effectiveness of strategies implemented through the comprehensive health-planning process to achieve the identified goals for the community oral health program.

b. Evaluate the effectiveness and quality of all community oral health programs and activities against evidence-based criteria, and use the information to improve performance and outcomes (e.g., community oral health programs and community health centers).

c. Review the effectiveness of oral health interventions provided by other health professionals (e.g., physicians and nurses) and agencies (e.g., Head Start, maternal and child health, and WIC).

10. **Research for new insights and innovative solutions to health problems.**

a. Use current data and research findings to develop evidence-based community oral health programs.

b. Collaborate with researchers to actively involve the community in oral health research.

c. Develop research activities in a collaborative fashion so as to provide mutual benefit to all parties.

d. Provide data and expertise to support research that benefits the community's oral health.

e. Involve the community in developing, conducting, and disseminating research.

f. Ensure confidentiality and safety for community members participating in research.

g. Contribute to the evidence base of community oral health programs and the identification of best practices by sharing results of research and program evaluations.

---

the Ten Essential Public Health Services, discussed previously. The guide describes the six steps necessary to develop community oral health, as follows:

1. Mobilize community support
2. Assess needs and resources
3. Determine priorities and plan the program
4. Implement the program
5. Evaluate the program

6. Participate in policy development and research

National Dental Public Health Associations

The five major national dental public health associations are the:

1. American Association of Public Health Dentistry

2. American Board of Dental Public Health

3. American Public Health Association, Oral Health Section

4. American Association of Community Dental Programs

5. Association of State and Territorial Dental Directors

The American Association of Public Health Dentistry and the Oral Health Section of the American Public Health Association are the two major dental public health membership organizations. The Association of State and Territorial Dental Directors (ASTDD) is made up of state dental directors, and the American Association of Community Dental Programs consists of local dental directors. In addition, the National Network for Oral Health Access (NNOHA), the Community and Preventive Dentistry Section of the American Dental Education Association (ADEA), and the Behavioral Sciences and Health Services Research Group of the American Association of Dental Research (AADR) have strong community orientations. NNOHA membership is primarily made up of community and migrant health center dentists; the ADEA section consists primarily of educators, and the AADR researchers. Some dental hygienists also have training in public health and are an important resource for improving the oral health of the public.

Individuals trained in dental public health have the knowledge and education to respond to the oral disease epidemic. Public health leaders and programs can utilize these national public health associations as well as the U.S. Public Health Service for assistance if they do not have access locally to the expertise of public health-trained dentists or hygienists.

Healthy People 2010

Healthy People 2010 includes oral health as one of 28 priority areas. This area contains 17 objectives and numerous subobjectives.[8] The goal of the oral health objectives is to prevent and control oral and craniofacial diseases, conditions, and injuries, and to improve access to related services. The 17 objectives cover the following:

1. Dental caries experience

2. Untreated dental decay

3. No permanent tooth loss

4. Complete tooth loss

5. Periodontal diseases

6. Early detection of oral and pharyngeal cancers

7. Annual examinations for oral and pharyngeal cancers

8. Dental sealants

9. Community water fluoridation

10. Use of oral health care system

11. Use of oral health care system by residents in long-term-care facilities

12. Dental services for low-income children

13. School-based health centers with oral health component

14. Health centers with oral health service components

15. Referral for cleft lip/cleft palate

16. Oral and craniofacial state-based surveillance system

17. Tribal, state, and local dental programs

Examples of complete objectives for the year 2010 are as follows:

1. Increase the proportion of children who have received dental sealants on their permanent teeth (target, 50 percent; baseline, children age 8, 23 percent; adolescents aged 14, 15 percent).

2. Increase the proportion of the United States population served by community water systems with optimally fluoridated water (target, 75 percent; 1992 baseline, 62 percent).

3. Increase the proportion of long-term-care residents who use the oral health care system each year (target, 25 percent; 1992 baseline, 19 percent).

4. Increase the proportion of low-income children and adolescents who received any preventive dental service during the past year (target, 57 percent; baseline, 20 percent).

5. Increase the proportion of local health departments and community-based health centers, including community, migrant, and homeless health centers, that have an oral health component (target, 75 percent; baseline, 34 percent of local health departments and 60 percent of community health centers had oral health components in 1997).

6. (Developmental) Increase the number of tribal, state (including the District of Columbia), and local health agencies that serve jurisdictions of 250,000 or more persons that have in place an effective public dental health program directed by a dental professional with public health training.

The Surgeon General's Report

The first-ever U.S. Surgeon General's Report on Oral Health was released in the year 2000.[1] This report raised the visibility of the oral health crisis in the United States and delineated the importance of oral health. It also discussed the status of oral health in the United States, the relationship between oral health and general health, how oral disease is prevented, and the needs and opportunities to enhance oral health. The report called the oral health crisis "a silent epidemic" and highlighted the disparities of oral health between the haves and the have-nots. The report also called for action on the national level to prevent oral diseases, improve access to services, and reduce oral health disparities among different population groups.

The major findings of the report are:

1. Oral diseases and disorders in and of themselves affect health and well-being throughout life.

2. Safe and effective measures exist to prevent the most common dental diseases-dental caries and periodontal diseases.

3. Lifestyle behaviors that affect general health such as tobacco use, excessive alcohol use, and poor dietary choices affect oral and craniofacial health as well.

4. There are profound and consequential oral health disparities within the United States population.

5. More information is needed to improve America's oral health and eliminate health disparities.

6. The mouth reflects general health and well-being.

7. Oral diseases and conditions are associated with other health problems.

8. Scientific research is key to further reduction of the burden of diseases and disorders that affect the face, mouth, and teeth.

A framework for action was outlined by the Surgeon General's Report as follows:

1. Change perceptions regarding oral health and disease so that oral health becomes an accepted component of general health.

2. Accelerate the building of the science and evidence base and apply science effectively to improve oral health.

3. Build an effective health infrastructure that meets the oral health needs of all Americans and integrates oral health effectively into overall health.

4. Remove known barriers between people and oral health services.

5. Use public-private partnerships to improve the oral health of those who still suffer disproportionately from oral diseases.

The *Guide to Community Preventive Services*

Chapter 3 of this book discusses the *Guide to Community Preventive Services* and the work of the independent, nonfederal Task Force on Community Preventive Services. The community guide was developed with the support of the U.S. Department of Health and Human Services working with private and public parties. The publication includes an oral health component that delineates effective population-based preventive measures. It will be helpful to local and state health departments and other health personnel who wish to improve the oral health of a community or population group.

PREVENTION

Many oral disease prevention measures prevent the disease before it occurs, which is called primary prevention, as well as control or respond to the disease after it occurs, which is called secondary or tertiary prevention. Because dental caries is the most common oral disease, and because the prevention methods for caries have such a well-documented scientific basis and are cost effective, the focus here is on dental caries prevention.

COMMUNITY AND INDIVIDUAL PREVENTIVE MEASURES

Dental caries can be prevented on the community or individual level, as shown in Table 28.6. Community prevention programs are more effective than individual prevention programs because they are population based.

The most effective, economical, and practical preventive measure for dental caries is community water fluoridation.[53,54] The most significant contribution a public health professional can make to improve the oral health of a community is to help that community become fluoridated if natural fluoride levels are too low to be effective. Individual prevention measures are not as effective as community prevention measures in general because they rely on the individual to carry them out, decreasing the effectiveness of these measures on a population or group basis. However, individual prevention

Table 28.6. Effective Community and Individual Preventive Measures for Dental Caries

Measure	Method of Application	Target	Period of Use
Community Programs			
Community water fluoridation	Systemic	Entire population	Lifetime
School water fluoridation	Systemic	School children	School years
School fluoride tablet program	Systemic	School children	Age 5–16 yrs
School fluoride rinse program	Topical	School children	Age 5–16 yrs
School sealant program (professionally applied)	Topical	School children	Age 6–8, 12–14 yrs
Individual Approach			
Prescribed fluoride tablets or drops	Systemic	Children	Age 6 months–16 yrs
Professionally applied fluoride treatment	Topical	Individual need	High-risk populations
Over-the-counter fluoride rinse	Topical	Individual need	High-risk populations
Fluoride toothpaste	Topical	Entire population	Lifetime
Professionally applied dental sealants	Topical	Children	Age 6–8, 12–14 yrs

SOURCE: This was published in *Jong's Community Dental Health*, fifth ed., Allukian, Jr, M. and Horowitz, A.M., Effective Community Prevention Programs for Oral Diseases, p. 237–276, Copyright Mosby Press, St. Louis (2002).

measures should be continuously recommended and reinforced in all programs to improve individual compliance.

Systemic and Topical Fluorides

Fluoride may be provided **systemically** or **topically,** as shown in Table 28.6. Preventive measures that provide fluoride to the teeth systemically by ingestion, such as water fluoridation or fluoride tablets, strengthen the teeth *while they are developing* and protect the teeth after they have erupted into the oral cavity and throughout life. Continued exposure to fluoridated water and fluorides after tooth eruption are also beneficial.

Children who live in communities that do not have fluoridation should be given a daily dietary fluoride supplement beginning at 6 months of age. In 1989, about 15.1 percent of children under the age of 2 used a fluoride supplement in the United States.[55] There are major differences in dietary fluoride supplement use by race, income, and education, as shown in Table 28.7. About 16.6 percent of Euro-American children use fluoride supplements as compared with 6.5 percent of African American children and 12.9 percent of Hispanic children. Only 6.4 percent of children below the poverty level use fluoride supplements compared with 18.2 percent at or above the poverty level. Some of the geographic variation in fluoride supplement use may be due to water fluoridation status.

Professionally applied fluoride treatments, school and over-the-counter fluoride rinses, and fluoride toothpaste protect the teeth by providing fluoride to the teeth topically after they have erupted into the oral cavity. These fluorides provide an additional benefit to systemic fluoride, especially for high-risk individuals. The direct application of fluoride helps in the **remineralization,** or repair, of tooth enamel that is in the early stages of tooth decay. Professionally applied fluoride treatments need to be done periodically as long as the individual is at high risk for dental caries. Fluoride toothpaste should be used by people of all ages at least twice a day, after breakfast and before going to sleep at night. About 93.7 percent of school-age

Table 28.7. Percent of Children in the United States Under 2 Years of Age by Selected Characteristics Who Use a Dietary Fluoride Supplement, 1989

	%
All children	15.1
Parents' Education:	
Some college	19.8
High school or less	10.8
Race/Ethnicity:	
African American	6.5
Euro-American	16.6
Hispanic	12.9
Non-Hispanic	15.5
Region:	
North	20.6
Midwest	7.9
South	10.4
West	20.6
SES Status:	
At/above poverty level	18.2
Below poverty level	6.4

SOURCE: Wagener DK, Nourjah P, Horowitz A. *Trends in Childhood Use of Dental Care Products Containing Fluoride: U.S. 1983–1989.* Hyattsville, MD: National Center for Health Statistics; 1992. Advance data from Vital and Health Statistics no. 219.

children 5 to 17 years of age in the United States use a fluoride-containing toothpaste.[55]

Due to the widespread use of fluorides in water supplies, dental offices, and over-the-counter dental products, there has been a national decline in tooth decay in the last 20–30 years.

Dental Sealants

Because fluorides prevent dental caries most effectively on the smooth surfaces of the teeth, now almost two-thirds of tooth decay occurs on the chewing surfaces of teeth.[35] Dental sealants, however, effectively prevent tooth decay on these surfaces. Dental sealants are thin plastic coatings that are placed as liquid plastics on the pits and fissures of the chewing surfaces of teeth and then polymerized. Ideally, susceptible tooth surfaces should be sealed soon after the tooth has erupted. This painless and noninvasive procedure does not require anesthesia or the cutting of tooth structure. A good school-based prevention program should use both fluorides and sealants. A recent national study showed an increase in the prevalence of dental sealants on the permanent first molars of 8-year-olds, especially among non-Hispanic black and Mexican American populations. The prevalence increased from nearly 23 percent in 1988–1994 to about 32 percent in 1999–2004. For all adolescents, the prevalence of dental sealants increased from about 18 percent in 1988–1994 to 38 percent in 1999–2004, regardless of demographic subgroups.[5]

Dental Fluorosis

With the increasing use of fluorides there has been an increase in **dental fluorosis**. This is a chronic, fluoride-induced condition in which enamel development is disrupted and the enamel is hypomineralized.[56] It occurs when the teeth are forming, primarily from birth to 6 years of age, due to excessive fluoride intake. A confirmed history of fluoride exposure is needed to validate this diagnosis. In the 1980s, a series of studies showed that the prevalence of fluorosis had increased in both fluoridated and nonfluoridated communities.[56] Fluorosis appears clinically as a bilateral, chalky white appearance of the teeth. In severe forms the teeth may be discolored or pitted. Most of the increase in fluorosis is of a very mild or mild form that would probably be noticed only by a dentist. Fluorosis is not a health problem, but may be considered an individual cosmetic problem in its more severe forms. It is correctable with dental treatment.

Individuals and populations with varying levels of dental fluorosis have less decay than those without fluorosis. Fluorosis may be due to inappropriate prescriptions of dietary fluoride supplements, ingestion of fluoride toothpaste by children younger than 6 years of age, infant formula reconstituted with fluoridated water, and communities fluoridated naturally at higher than the recommended level. In 1978, manufacturers of infant formulas, cereals, and juices voluntarily began processing their baby-food products with water containing minimal amounts of fluoride. In 1979, a revised lower fluoride supplement schedule was adopted for children younger than 2 years of age by the American Academy of Pediatrics following the guidelines of the American Dental Association. In 1994, the recommended fluoride supplement schedule was revised again lowering the dosage for children younger than 6 years of age.[57] To prevent fluorosis, health professionals and their patients need to be educated about the proper use of fluoride-containing products, particularly for children 6 years of age and younger.

Community Water Fluoridation

Community water fluoridation should be the foundation for improving the oral health of every community. Community water fluoridation is defined as the upward adjustment of the fluoride content of a community water supply for optimal oral health. It is the most cost-effective preventive measure for preventing tooth decay.[53] Fluoridation is safe, economical, and practical.[53,54,56,58–60] It has been estimated that for each dollar spent on fluoridation, there is a $25–$80 savings in dental treatment costs.[61,62] Today, fluoridation can be expected to prevent tooth decay in both primary and permanent teeth by up to 40 percent. Before the widespread use of fluorides, fluoridation prevented tooth decay by 50 to 60 percent. It is still a public health bargain, however. Because it has demonstrated benefits for adults, everyone reared in a fluoridated community benefits, regardless of age, income, education, race, gender, or access to dental care.

All water supplies contain some fluoride naturally but generally not enough to prevent dental caries. The recommended fluoride level is 0.7 to 1.2 parts per million (ppm), depending on the mean maximum daily air temperature over a 5-year period.[63] Most water supplies in the United States are fluoridated at about 1.0 ppm. At the recommended level in the water supply, fluoride is odorless, colorless, and tasteless. The mean national weighted cost of fluoridation in 1989 was $0.51 per capita with a range of $0.12 to $5.41, depending on the size of the community and the complexity of its water distribution system.[53] In 2005 dollars, the range was $0.32–$3.37, with an average of $0.72 a person. In 2005 dollars, for communities with more than 10,000 persons, the range was $0.32 to $0.58 per capita, and for communities with less than 10,000 persons, it was $ 1.31 to $3.37.[64] Once a community is fluoridated, fluoride levels in the water supply must be monitored on a regular basis so that the population served receives the maximum health and economic benefits at little or no risk.[63]

A Historical Perspective on Fluoridation

Fluoridation's effectiveness was first demonstrated in the United States, and the history of its discovery is one of the great public health success stories. For generations, millions of Americans lived in communities that were naturally fluoridated, though not necessarily at the recommended level. Communities then sought to duplicate the benefits that had been demonstrated by nature. In 1945, the first communities implemented adjusted fluoridation on a study basis, and in 1950, *adjusted fluoridation* was endorsed by the U.S. Public Health Service and then the American Dental Association as a public health measure. Fluoridation is now recognized as one of the great public health achievements of the twentieth century.[65]

Fluoridation in the United States Today

In 2006, about 184 million people or 69.2 percent of the United States population on public water supplies lived in fluoridated communities,[66] as compared to 162 million Americans or 65 percent in 2000.[66,67] The United States has the largest number of people in the world living in fluoridated communities and about 8 million of the 184 million

are fluoridated naturally at the recommended level.[66]

Variation in Fluoridation Rates by State and City

Table 28.8 shows the percentage of the public water supply population that uses fluoridated water for each state. Water supplies of 43 of the 50 largest cities in the United States are fluoridated. The 7 cities of the largest 50 that are not fluoridated have a total population of about 4.2 million people. These cities are listed in Table 28.9. Los Angeles, the second largest city in the United States, became fluoridated in 1999. The most recent large city to implement fluoridation was San Antonio, Texas, in 2002.[68]

Fluoridation Laws

Eight states have long-standing laws that require fluoridation, although these laws vary from state to state. The eight states and their national rank for percent of the population with a fluoridated public water supply are listed in Table 28.10. Illinois and Minnesota have the most comprehensive legislation requiring fluoridation. In the fall of 1995, the California legislature passed a law requiring fluoridation of all public water systems with at least 10,000 service connections, depending on funding and in 2006 Pennsylvania passed a law requiring communities to fluoridate. Fluoridation laws usually help facilitate public health policy to implement fluoridation, depending on the nature of the law and whether or not it is enforced. On the other hand, a referendum is required by the public in the following five states before fluoridation can be initiated: Delaware, Maine, Nevada, New Hampshire, and Utah. These states rank from 22 to 42 in terms of the percent of population with fluoridated public water.

Mandatory referenda shift the responsibility for public health policy from the legislature or board of health to the voting public. This is an ineffective way to determine public health policy as shown by the low ranks of these states. It is essential that legislators, community leaders, and health policy makers are educated about the benefits of fluoridation.[69]

Table 28.8. Percentage of a State's Population on Public Water Supplies with Community Water Fluoridation and Their National Rank, 2006[66]

Location	Percent	National Rank Fluoridation	Location	Percent	National Rank Fluoridation
United States overall	69.2		Montana	31.3	46
Alabama	82.9	20	Nebraska	69.8	31
Alaska	59.5	35	Nevada	72.0	30
Arizona	56.1	38	New Hampshire	42.6	42
Arkansas	64.4	33	New Jersey	22.6	49
California	27.1	48	New Mexico	77.0	25
Colorado	73.6	26	New York	72.9	29
Connecticut	88.9	17	North Carolina	87.6	18
Delaware	73.6	27	North Dakota	96.2	4
Florida	77.7	24	Ohio	89.3	16
Georgia	95.8	5	Oklahoma	73.5	28
Hawaii	8.4	50	Oregon	27.4	47
Idaho	31.3	45	Pennsylvania	54.0	40
Illinois	98.9	2	Rhode Island	84.6	19
Indiana	95.1	6	South Carolina	94.6	9
Iowa	92.4	12	South Dakota	95.0	7
Kansas	65.1	32	Tennessee	93.7	11
Kentucky	99.8	1	Texas	78.1	23
Louisiana	40.4	43	Utah	54.3	39
Maine	79.6	22	Vermont	58.7	37
Maryland	93.8	10	Virginia	95.0	8
Massachusetts	59.1	36	Washington	62.9	34
Michigan	90.9	14	Washington, DC	100.0*	
Minnesota	98.7	3	West Virginia	91.7	13
Mississippi	50.9	41	Wisconsin	89.7	15
Missouri	79.7	21	Wyoming	36.4	44

*Not a state.

Comparison of Effective Community Prevention Programs

Community prevention programs are difficult to compare due to wide variation in the studies that have been done. Table 28.11 compares five different community programs that have been shown to be effective. Most of the information (except the data on practicality) comes from the Michigan Conference on Cost Effectiveness on Caries Prevention in Dental Public Health.[53]

It is difficult to determine the absolute effectiveness of specific fluoride programs because of the widespread use of fluoridation and fluorides, and the halo or diffusion effect through processed foods and beverages, all of which result in overlapping benefits and a national decline in dental caries in children.[70] For any given community, a thorough analysis of the literature, consultation with a dental public health expert, and review of the community's needs and resources should be done to determine which type of program is best for that community. As shown in Table 28.11, community

Table 28.9. The Seven Cities of the Fifty Largest Cities in the United States That Are Not Fluoridated, 2006

City	Rank in Size	Population (1,000s)
San Diego, CA*	6	1,238
San Jose, CA	11	867
Portland, OR	26	503
Tucson, AZ**	31	466
Fresno, CA*	39	404
Honolulu, HI	41	395
Wichita, KS	50	335
		4,208

*In 2007, the single largest expansion of community water fluoridation in the United States occurred when water systems for 18 million residents of 26 cities became fluoridated in southern California, in the counties of Los Angeles, Orange, Riverside, San Diego, and Ventura (Crozier S. Fluoridated water comes to 18 million southern Californians. *ADA News*, June 16, 2008). This reached only 9 percent of San Diego residents, however. In June 2008, the San Diego City Council voted to fluoridate San Diego, the largest nonfluoridated city in the United States. This should be implemented by 2010 (Crozier S. Water milestone: San Diego authorizes fluoridation. *ADA News*, June 16, 2008).

**Voted for fluoridation in 1992.

Table 28.10. States With Long-Standing Mandatory Fluoridation Laws

State	National Rank	State	National Rank
Connecticut	17	Minnesota	3
Georgia	5	Nebraska	31
Illinois	2	Ohio	16
Michigan	14	South Dakota	7

fluoridation is the most effective and economical of the five effective community prevention programs for dental caries.[53] It is also the most practical.

For communities without a public water supply, a school water supply fluoridation program or a school dietary fluoride supplement program would probably be the fluoride preventive measure of choice, depending on the dental health of school children and the community's resources. School-based dental disease prevention programs and clinics are effective because they work with population groups who have not yet had the disease, are readily accessible, and can be reached on a group basis with proven prevention programs. School prevention programs also reinforce the importance of good, regular oral hygiene.

School Fluoridation

School fluoridation is the adjustment of the fluoride content of a school's water supply to prevent dental caries. The school water supply is fluoridated at 4.5 times the level recommended for community fluoridation because children are in school only for a limited amount of time during the year. Studies have shown that school fluoridation prevents tooth decay by 20–30 percent over 12 years for children aged 5 to 17.[53] This figure may now be high, as there have been no recent studies since the national decline in dental caries due to the impact of more widely available fluorides. In 1992, 117,430 children in 330 schools and 12 states in the United States were receiving the benefits of school fluoridation.[a]

School Dietary Fluoride Supplements

School dietary fluoride supplement programs, such as fluoride tablet programs, are done on a daily basis during the school year only for children who live in nonfluoridated communities. School dietary fluoride supplements are effective because children are assured of receiving fluoride on a regular basis. These programs should begin at the earliest age possible and continue until the age of 12 to 14 years. The programs are easy to implement and require

[a]*Fluoridation Census, 1992*. Atlanta, GA: Centers for Disease Control and Prevention, U.S. Public Health Service; 1993.

Table 28.11. Comparison of Five Effective Community Prevention Programs for Dental Caries*

Program	Effectiveness (percent)	Adult Benefits	Cost per Year	Practicality
Community fluoridation	20–40	demonstrated	$0.72 per capita[a]	excellent; most practical; no individual effort necessary
School fluoridation	20–30[b]	expected but not demonstrated	$1.19–13.83 per child	good, if there is no central community water supply; no individual effort necessary
School dietary fluoride daily supplement program	30	expected but not demonstrated	$1.13–7.56 per child	fair; continued school regimen required for 8–10 years
School fluoride mouth rinse program	25–28[b]	not expected	$0.73–2.49[c] per child	fair; continued daily or weekly school regimen required
School sealant program	51–67[d]	expected but not demonstrated	$18.30–39.72 per child	good; primarily done for children age 6–8 and 12–14 years

*This table is a simplified comparison of these prevention programs. A thorough analysis of the literature should be done to understand the relative merits of these programs.

[a]In 1999 dollars, see text for range.

[b]This range may now be high; no recent studies.

[c]Includes using volunteer personnel.

[d]First molar chewing surfaces only over a 5-year period.

SOURCE: American Assn Public Health Dentistry.

little classroom time, although achieving compliance in the middle school years can be a challenge.

School Fluoride Mouth Rinses

Topical fluoride programs such as **school fluoride rinse programs** can be done in nonfluoridated communities, those recently fluoridated, or those with children at high risk for dental caries. The effectiveness of school fluoride rinse programs is no longer clear in communities where the amount of new tooth decay is already low due to the widespread use of fluorides in general.

School rinse programs are usually carried out weekly for ease of administration. Nondental personnel may supervise both fluoride tablet and rinse programs. They are easy to carry out and require little classroom time, approximately 3–5 minutes per procedure. Approximately 1 in 10 school children, 5 to 17 years of age, participate in a school-based fluoride mouth rinse program.[55]

School Sealant Programs

School sealant programs are recommended in both fluoridated communities and nonfluoridated communities for children age 6 to 8 and 12 to 14 years. School sealant programs are important because they target the 6- and 12-year molars, which are highly susceptible to decay. The 6-year molars are the most important teeth for maintaining the dental arch.

These programs are more cost-effective when sealants are placed by dental hygienists or dental assistants rather than dentists. In 1991, 48 states allowed dental hygienists to place sealants, and 15 states allowed dental assistants to place sealants, under various degrees of supervision by a dentist. About 43 percent of state dental practice acts did not require a dentist to be physically present at all when sealants were placed by auxiliaries in public programs, and 29 states reported having a community-based sealant program. In addition, Medicaid reimbursement for sealants was provided in 42 states.[71] In 2001, all states allowed dental hygienists to place sealants and in 2004, 26 states allowed dental assistants to do so.[72,73]

Sealants are generally applied to a tooth surface only once, but sometimes they need to be replaced, so they should be checked periodically. Five-year studies show a 51 to 67 percent reduction in tooth decay of the chewing surfaces of first molars to which sealants have been applied.[53] Targeted, school-based dental sealant programs have been shown to reduce racial and economic disparities in caries prevalence among schoolchildren.[74] School sealant programs should be done in conjunction with fluoride prevention programs to obtain the maximum protection for children.

Oral Health Education

Oral health education should be incorporated into school curricula beginning in kindergarten to reinforce in children the importance of individual and community dental preventive measures and the need for periodic dental visits. Parents, teachers, health professionals, community leaders, and the public in general also need to be informed about dental disease prevention and the significance of oral health.

Physicians, nurses, and other health providers, in addition to dental health providers, play an important role in educating the public about oral health. The United States Clinical Preventive Services Task Force included counseling to prevent dental disease and screening for oral cancer in its recommendations to physicians.[75] All patients should be encouraged to visit a dental care provider on a regular basis. In addition, primary care clinicians should counsel patients regarding daily tooth brushing and dental flossing, the appropriate use of fluoride for caries prevention, the importance of avoiding sugary foods, and risk factors for developing early childhood tooth decay. For children living in communities with inadequate water fluoridation, dietary fluoride supplements should be prescribed. While examining the mouth, clinicians should be alert for obvious signs of oral disease.

Screening for Oral and Pharyngeal Cancer

Routine screening of asymptomatic persons for oral cancer by primary care clinicians is not recommended by the U.S. Preventive Services Task Force, but it may be prudent for clinicians to carefully examine for cancerous lesions of the oral cavity in patients who are over age 40 or who use tobacco or excessive amounts of alcohol, as well as those with suspicious symptoms or lesions detected through self-examination. Also, all patients should be counseled to receive regular dental examinations, discontinue the use of all forms of tobacco, and limit consumption of alcohol. In addition, persons with increased exposure to sunlight should be advised to take protective measures to protect their lips and skin from the harmful effects of ultraviolet rays.[75]

From the community-wide perspective, strategies for action to prevent oral and pharyngeal cancer have been recommended by the National Strategic Planning Conference for the Prevention and Control of Oral and Pharyngeal Cancer in five major areas:[76,77]

- Advocacy, collaboration, and coalition building
- Public health policy
- Public education
- Professional education and practice
- Data collection, education, and research

Other Prevention Programs

It is beyond the scope of this chapter to discuss the full range of prevention programs related to oral health. Briefly, however, other examples of successful programs range from mouth-guard programs for high school athletes in contact sports[78] to programs to educate dentists about children suffering from abuse or neglect[79] or how dental care providers may help the users of cigarettes and spit (smokeless) tobacco quit.[80] Clearly, a range of oral health programs exists to improve oral health, and these can be utilized in any community depending on its needs and resources.[81–86]

ORAL HEALTH—AN ESSENTIAL COMPONENT OF HEALTH AND PRIMARY CARE

Oral health is an essential component of total health and primary care.[87] Dental and oral diseases may well be the most prevalent and preventable conditions affecting Americans.[2,8,86,88] When any health or primary care program is being developed or considered for implementation, an oral health component should be included. As oral diseases affect most of the population, community-based prevention should always be a very high priority.[2,8,86] Unfortunately, the United States does not have national disease prevention or treatment programs, or national health insurance. Regardless of whether an evolving health care system emphasizes oral health services, public health professionals have the responsibility and opportunity to make meaningful contributions to the public's health by including oral health in health programs.

VULNERABLE POPULATIONS

Vulnerable populations, such as low-income groups, minorities, migrants, persons with HIV, and the institutionalized, homeless, homebound, elderly, and medically compromised, have the greatest dental needs and poorest access to dental services. Health programs targeted to vulnerable and high-risk populations must have an oral health component. Although some dental programs are provided by local, state, and federal agencies for vulnerable populations, they are usually inadequate.

Low-income groups and minorities suffer a disproportionate share of untreated oral diseases.[2,8,89] Community-based prevention, health care reform, and primary care dentistry can help address inequities and access issues for vulnerable populations.[90]

CALL TO ACTION

In response to the *Surgeon General's Report on Oral Health*[1], A Call to Action[2] includes the following six recommendations:

1. Oral health must become a much higher priority at the local, state, and national levels, so that oral health disparities can be improved and resolved.

2. The federal government must be a role model and set the example that oral health is an integral and important component of all health programs.

3. Promotion and use of effective individual and population-based prevention services and programs must become a much higher priority at the local, state, and national levels, especially for children and high-risk populations.

4. The oral health component of Medicaid and the Child Health Insurance Program must be upgraded and improved.

5. All communities with a central water supply must have fluoridation.

6. The oral health workforce needs to be modified and augmented.

Action Initiatives

Examples of action initiatives as part of A Call to Action have also been suggested by the author. They include:[2]

a. Funding and development of an effective dental public health infrastructure at the local, state, and national levels to provide guidance in responding to these needs.

b. The oral health needs of the underserved must be more effectively met by community and migrant health centers; the National Health Service Corps; Head Start; maternal and child health agencies; Healthy Start; the

Special Supplemental Nutrition Program for Women, Infants, and Children; area health education centers; school-based health centers; and other such programs.

c. Tobacco settlement funds must also be used to develop and institutionalize effective prevention programs because of the relationship between tobacco use and oral diseases. These services and programs can include school, community, or institutional prevention initiatives that provide fluorides, dental sealants, early childhood caries prevention, and oral and pharyngeal cancer examinations.

d. The accountability of state officials involved in dental Medicaid and the Child Health Insurance Program must be increased.

e. An effective statewide distribution of safety-net providers must be available in every state.

f. The U.S. Department of Health and Human Services must play a much stronger leadership role, working with local and state agencies and organizations to promote and support community water fluoridation.

g. More dentists, including those of minority backgrounds, should be trained in dental public health.

h. State practice acts must also be less restrictive and more responsive to the needs of the public in such areas as national reciprocity for licensees and delegation of duties for dental hygienists and assistants.

DENTAL PERSONNEL

The total number of dental personnel is adequate to meet the current demand for oral health services but not the need. There is also a maldistribution of dental personnel in certain parts of the United States, with many inner-city and rural areas left underserved. Access to dental care for vulnerable populations and Medicaid recipients is a serious problem in the United States. In 2007, there were 3,559 dental health professional shortage areas for a population of 46.2 million people needing 9,054 dentists to achieve a 1:3,000 dentist-to-population ratio.[91]

If health care reform in our country were to include reimbursement for oral health needs, the demand for service would increase and stress the capacity of the existing dental care delivery system. The best response to the growing need in those circumstances would be to increase the use of dental auxiliaries and incorporate oral health services into existing programs for vulnerable populations. The public health professional, as a leader and policy maker, can play a key role in helping to meet oral health needs by not only drawing on the four categories of dental personnel for assistance (dentists, dental hygienists, dental assistants, and dental laboratory technicians), but also supporting the expansion of duties for all dental personnel and supporting new dental personnel, such as the Alaska Dental Therapist.

Dentists

Dentists have a minimum of 2 years of college before going to dental school, and most have a college degree. In 2007, there were 56 dental schools in the United States, all had a 4-year curriculum, except for one school, University of the Pacific, which had 3-year program.[92] For the 2005–2006 academic year, there were 10,731 applicants and from those, 4,558 were enrolled.[92] In the year 2004, there were an estimated 175,705 professionally active dentists, of which 162,181 (92.3 percent) were in private practice.[93] Due to the closure of seven dental schools since 1985, a decrease in the applicant pool, and the increasing cost of a dental education, the number of dental school graduates dropped from 5,550 in 1980 to about 4,075 in 2000.[94,95] The ratio of active dentists to population is expected to drop to 52.7 per 100,000 by 2020 from 58.3 in 2000.[95] Most dentists in the United States are general practitioners who work in private practice, and they had an average net income of about $185,940 in 2004.[96] About

21 percent of dentists are active specialists. Only about 14.1 percent of professionally active dentists are women and 14 percent are people of color, of which 7 percent are Asian/Pacific Islander, 3.4 percent African American, 3.3 percent Hispanic and 0.1 percent Native American.[95] The nine dental specialties are dental public health, **endodontics,** oral and maxillofacial surgery, oral pathology, orthodontics, pediatric dentistry, periodontics, **prosthodontics,** and radiology.

Dental Hygienists

Dental hygienists primarily provide preventive services to patients, usually including screening, prophylaxis (cleaning), scaling, root planing, taking radiographs, health education, and topical fluoride and dental sealant application. Most hygienists have 2 years of education and training after high school. In 1998, there were 237 dental hygiene schools in the United States with a total of 6,087 first-year students, and in 2006, there were 286 schools.[95,97] Once hygienists are licensed by the state, they are known as registered dental hygienists (RDHs). Some hygienists have 4 or more years of education. Hygienists who work in public health policy or administration usually have a master's or doctoral degree in public health or health sciences.

In 1990, there were about 98,000 hygienists with active licenses in the United States of which about 81,000 were in active practice.[94] In 2005, there were about 161,140 RDHs.[97] Dental hygienists are one of the fastest growing health occupations in the United States. Dental hygienists are an excellent resource for public health initiatives for promoting and implementing prevention programs, health education, screening and referral, school-based programs, community outreach, and improved access to the underserved. In 2004, the American Dental Hygienists Association initiated the Advanced Dental Hygiene Practitioner concept to help respond to the oral health needs of our country. Some state dental practice acts unnecessarily restrict what hygienists may do, resulting in access problems, lower efficiency, and higher costs for providing oral health services.

Table 28.12. Scope of Practice Allowed by States for Dental Hygienists, 2006

SCOPE OF PRACTICE	Number of States
General supervision*	43[102]
Local anesthesia	40[102]
Nitrous oxide	25[102]
Direct access	20[102]
Independent practice**	19[103]
Directly bill Medicaid	12[104]

*In all allowed settings.
**Independent Practice includes various forms of unsupervised practice or less restrictive supervision.

A recent national study showed that the utilization of oral health services and oral health of the population increases where professional practice environments for dental hygienists are more favorable.[98] It has also been known for years that expanded function auxiliaries benefit the public and dentists.[99] Table 28.12 indicates the scope of practice allowed for dental hygienists by the number of states. In 2007, Wisconsin and Pennsylvania allowed dental hygienists to have less supervision and the South Carolina Supreme Court ruled that the state dental board was committing restraint of trade by limiting the scope of practice of dental hygienists.[100,101]

Alaska Dental Therapists

The Alaska Dental Therapist program began in remote rural Alaska in 2005, with four practicing therapists. This program was developed by the Alaska Native Tribal Health Consortium, a native-owned, nonprofit agency, with funding from the U.S. Department of Health and Human Services, private foundations, and private organizations.[105] The therapists provide oral health education, preventive services (fluorides, sealants, and cleaning), drilling, fillings, and simple extractions. These therapists received their training in the 2-year New Zealand Dental Therapist Training Program followed by a 400-hour preceptorship under the direct supervision of the dentists. These therapists are Native Alaskans and they work in isolated rural communities that lack roads, electricity, public water supplies, and dentists. This innovative program has been a very helpful resource for these remote communities. The American Public Health Association (APHA), the American Association of Public Health Dentistry, the American Association of Community Dental Programs, and the National Rural Health Association passed resolutions supporting the ANTCH program. (See the APHA Resolution in Exhibit 28.1.)

EXHIBIT 28-1 Support for the Alaska Dental Health Aide Therapist and Other Innovative Programs for Underserved Populations, APHA Policy, 2006

The American Public Health Association (APHA) views access to preventive and therapeutic oral health services as vitally important for all Americans; and APHA desires to foster effective broad-based policies and programs to help alleviate oral diseases.

Oral health is an integral part of overall health and well-being. According to the 2000 U.S. Surgeon General's report, *Oral Health in America*, the burden of oral problems is extensive and may be particularly severe in vulnerable populations. There are profound and consequential oral health disparities within the U.S. population; and reducing disparities requires wide-ranging approaches that target populations at highest risk for specific oral diseases and involves improving access to existing care.

Many populations, such as the 85,000 Alaska Natives living in 200 remote and isolated villages spread out over about 400,000 square miles, have overwhelming unmet oral health needs that have been longstanding and require prompt action to prevent further unnecessary pain and suffering. In most of these villages, the only health care provider available on a routine basis is the community health aide who provides services out of a small clinic, many of which lack even running water or a piped sewer. In many instances, Alaska Native patients must travel by bush-plane, boat, or snow machine in order to obtain dental services. Alternatively, children, or adults with toothaches, can only access care during itinerant visits from dentists working in the tribal programs, but these visits are very limited and can be sporadic.

Children and adolescents of Alaska Natives have dental caries rates that are 2.5–5.0 times the rate of children in the U.S. general population; 60 percent of Alaska Native children under age five years suffer from severe early childhood caries; dentists serving in rural Alaska remark that it is not uncommon for Alaska Native adults to be completely edentulous by the age of 20 years.

There is an inadequate supply of dentists to provide regular and continuous oral health care for the Alaska Natives in the remote and isolated villages. There is a 25 percent annual vacancy rate and a 30 percent average annual turnover rate for dentists in Alaska's tribal programs. There are more than 20 vacancies for dentists in the Alaska tribal programs.

Recognizing the plight of the Alaska Native population, applications for Dental Clinical Preventive and Support Centers by the Indian Health Service, USPHS [U.S. Public Health Service] were sent out in FY 2000. Emphasis for awarding funding was placed upon collaborative efforts between tribal programs and IHS-managed programs that were designed to meet the perceived needs of the areas. The Alaska Dental Health Aide Program proposal received a favorable review for technical and scientific merit, by a panel of nonfederal experts and tribal health staff, and was one of the successful grants funded that year. The Alaska Native Tribal Health Consortium, in compliance with federal law,[13] developed the Dental Health Aide Therapist (DHAT) program as part of that comprehensive initiative to respond to these overwhelming dental needs in an established and effective way, which ensures program continuity and year-round services in isolated, under-served communities. The DHAT program is an expansion of the successful Community Health Aide Program, initiated about 37 years ago, that provides overall primary health care to Alaska Natives using community health aides. DHATs are trained and educated in a certified program with professional supervision to perform primary prevention services, including health education as well as routine fillings and extractions which organized dentistry has referred to as "irreversible procedures." Evaluation of the program is an integral component and a recent independent evaluation has shown that the DHATs are providing competent and safe dental care to Alaska Natives. It is stressed in the evaluation document that dental health aides must meet the same standard of care, for those procedures that they perform, as dentists or any other provider in our system. There are not two standards of care.

DHATs have been used successfully in 42 other countries, including New Zealand, for over 84 years. In Saskatchewan, Canada, where DHATs have been employed for over 30 years, there have been no incidents of malpractice or any complaints reported to the Regional Disciplinary Board, and one study demonstrated that "the quality of restorations placed by dental therapists was equal to, but more often better than . . . those . . . by dentists."

In spite of the evidence supporting the effectiveness and safety of dental therapists, the American Dental Association (ADA) and Alaska Dental Society (ADS) are opposed to non-dentists performing "irreversible" procedures and have taken extraordinary action to block the Alaska DHAT program, such as full-page advertisements in the Alaska newspapers attacking the program and lobbying and testifying in Congress. Reasons given by the ADA for their opposition to DHATs include lack of supervision by dentists, that DHATs are acting illegally, that DHATs deliver second-class care, that DHATs are inadequately trained and educated, that only dentists should perform irreversible procedures and that volunteer dentists can fill the need. In January 2006, the ADA filed a lawsuit in Alaska State Court seeking a court order against the Alaska Native Tribal Health Consortium and the individual dental therapists under which their practice would be barred since it is not licensed by the State, even though the Alaska State Attorney General had already ruled that dental therapists may perform these procedures under Federal law. The ADA has proposed alternative mechanisms for improving access to care for this population that are not viewed as providing a more suitable alternative by the Alaska Native Tribal Health Consortium. The ADA has recognized the unavailability of dentists in remote villages of Alaska as far back as 1987. Attempts to encourage private practicing dentists to provide dental care in these settings has not proved to be successful.

The First evaluation of the DHAT program provides evidence that the concerns raised by the ADA have not materialized. The training of the DHATs appears to be sufficient to safely and effectively provide the services for which they have been trained. DHATs are under the general supervision of a dentist who is responsible for writing the standing orders and being the point of contact for the therapist. The supervising dentist also conducts periodic reviews of the therapist that include both chart review and patient examination.

The Alaska Federation of Natives, the Alaska Public Health Association,[37] the American Association of Public Health Dentistry, the National Rural Health Association,[39] the American Association of Community Dental Programs, Alaska Primary Care Association and the APHA Governing Council[41] have passed resolutions or support Dental Health Aides and Therapists; and the APHA Governing Council has supported the use of innovative programs to expand access to oral health care through expanded duties/functions/roles for dental hygienists and assistants at least four times since 1966. This resolution does not supplant these four resolutions, but builds upon them.

(continued)

EXHIBIT 23-4 (continued)

There is a need for other innovative programs to expand access to oral health care that can reduce disparities.[46] The Association of State and Territorial Dental Directors has developed a Best Practices Approach for State and Community Oral Health Programs that includes, ". . . expanding the traditional delivery system, developing community-based collaborative innovative and integrated delivery systems, increasing the health care workforce, and assuring sustainability through adequate and long-term funding." In addition, ". . . Dental auxiliary duties, responsibilities, and services may need to be expanded [and] the provision of selected dental services by nontraditional providers, such as physicians and nurses, should be explored . . ."; and ". . . changes in federal and state statutes and policies need to be implemented to enable and sustain the elimination of barriers for universal access to oral health care."

Examples of such innovations can be seen in various states, in addition to the Alaska Dental Health Aide program. In Colorado, legislation has been enacted to permit direct billing to Medicaid by dental hygienists, and in Minnesota, legislation was passed for expanded functions dental auxiliaries. Iowa's Department of Public Health and Department of Human Services implemented the EPSDT Exception to Policy, allowing regional Title V child health contractors to be reimbursed by Medicaid for oral screenings and fluoride varnish application provided by dental hygienists to Medicaid children in areas with a demonstrated lack of access to dental providers. In Connecticut, OPEN WIDE is an oral health training program for non-dental health and human service providers including physicians, nurses, nutritionists, childcare and community health workers. The program training enables non-dental providers to recognize and understand oral diseases and engage in anticipatory guidance and prevention intervention. In North Carolina, Into the Mouths of Babes, a statewide program in which pediatricians, family physicians, and providers in community health clinics are reimbursed by

Medicaid to provide preventive dental services for children (risk assessment, screening, referral, fluoride varnish application) and caregivers (counseling). In 35 states, dental hygienists can administer local anesthesia and in 21 states can administer nitrous oxide.

Other models have been developed for improving access to oral health care for under-served populations, such as FirstHealth of the Carolinas, Community DentCare Network in Harlem, and the New Mexico Health Commons model, offering basic oral health services in connection with community-based primary care services to ensure comprehensive health care for the most vulnerable and underserved populations, where few dentists participate in publicly assisted programs. Where there is a shortage of dental providers, communities are looking to medical providers to provide screening and preventive care.

Given the evidence of the safe and effective oral health care delivered by Dental Health Aide Therapists and the need for such services for populations in remote and under-served areas and the support for having those oral health services, therefore, the American Public Health Association:

1. Actively supports the Dental Health Aide Therapist (DHAT) Program and other innovative programs and practices to help prevent and alleviate the great unmet oral health needs of Alaska Natives;
2. Encourages the Governor of Alaska and other administrative and legislative leaders in Alaska to recognize and support the Dental Health Aide Therapist Program as a legitimate, practical and responsible program to help meet the needs of Alaska Natives;
3. Urges key members of the Congress, the administration, federal and Alaska health agencies, and Alaska dental, public health and Native Tribal organizations and other groups to support the Dental Health Aide Therapist program.

4. For other underserved populations in other parts of the United States, resolves to strongly support DHAT and other innovative and effective programs, aimed at improving access to preventive and therapeutic oral health services for other underserved populations in the United States;

5. Supports efforts to inform, as needed, national and state health, public health and dental organizations and agencies and legislative and judicial bodies, and the general public, of APHA's support of such programs;

6. Urges the Congress, the administration, and federal agencies to improve oral health policies, programs, and funding so that fluoridation, health education, preventive and therapeutic dental services are provided for all underserved individuals and communities who lack these services in the United States.

References: Not included, but available on the APHA website, http://www.apha.org.

Unfortunately, organized dentistry, including the Alaska Dental Society and the American Dental Association, have vigorously opposed this program by buying full-page print media ads, lobbying Congress, lobbying state decision makers, and, finally, filing a lawsuit in 2006 against the Alaska Native Tribal Health Consortium (ANTHC) and the individual Alaska Native therapists, even though the Alaska Attorney General stated that the program is legal. In 2007, the Alaska Superior Court ruled in favor of ANTHC, and as part of the 13 terms of the settlement agreement, the ADA agreed to pay the ANTCH foundation $537,500 to support its efforts to promote preventative oral health in remote Alaska.[106] It is unfortunate that the ADA and ADS opposed a program that responds to an overwhelming, unmet dental need for a very-high-risk population in very remote areas. Creative and responsive programs such as the Alaska Dental Therapist Program are needed to respond to the great unmet dental needs of underserved populations.

Dental Assistants

A formally trained dental assistant usually has 1 year of training after high school. Many dentists have trained their assistants on the job, but this is not recommended given the technological advances and challenges in dentistry, including the need for following the Centers for Disease Control and Prevention's guidelines for infection control. Dental assistants usually assist the dentist or hygienist when treatment is provided to the patient. Their duties include but are not limited to history taking, selecting and sterilizing instruments, mixing dental materials, and taking and developing radiographs.

Studies have shown that the productivity of dentists can be improved dramatically by the proper use of dental assistants. When dental assistants are allowed to perform expanded duties, the productivity of dentists increases even more.[96,108] Many state practice acts unnecessarily restrict what dental assistants are allowed to do, thus constraining dental productivity. In 2005, there were about 270,720 active dental assistants in the United States, for a ratio of 1.54 active assistants per active dentist.[97] In 2003, there were 255 accredited dental assisting schools with 4,990 graduates.[109]

Dental Laboratory Technicians

On receiving a prescription from a dentist, dental laboratory technicians construct **prostheses** for the dentist to provide to the patient. These include but are not limited to dentures, crowns, bridges, and space maintainers. Lab technicians usually do not have direct contact with patients. In a few states, such as Oregon, dental laboratory technicians, known as **denturists,** are allowed to make dentures directly for the public. Lab technicians may have a 1- to 2-year training period after high school, but many are trained on the job. In 1990, there were about 70,000 laboratory technicians in the United States,[94] in 1996 there were about

53,000 technicians and in 2003, there were 24 accredited schools for laboratory technicians with 322 graduates.[109,110]

SUMMARY

Oral diseases are a neglected epidemic in our country. The public health professional has the responsibility and opportunity to respond to this epidemic. Oral health is an essential component of total health for both the individual and the community. The challenges to the public health professional for the future have been clearly delineated.[1,2,8,111] The *Healthy People 2010* national health objectives include 17 objectives that address oral health, and oral health must be included in the 3 public health core functions of assessment, policy development, and assurance, and in the 10 essential public health services.

Most oral diseases can be readily assessed and prevented. Cost-effective individual and community preventive measures are available and must be used. Community water fluoridation must be the foundation for better oral health for all communities. Every local, state, and federal health department and agency must have dental public health expertise to respond effectively to this epidemic. Every health initiative or program must include an oral health component, from targeted programs for infants, pregnant women, persons with HIV, or the homeless, to health centers, managed care, and local, state, and national programs, including health care reform. The oral health needs of the American people must be addressed by the public health professional for healthier communities and a healthier nation.

ADDITIONAL RESOURCES

For additional information on oral health, web-based oral health resources are given in Table 28.13.

Table 28.13. Web-Based Oral Health Resources

Organization	Website
American Academy of Pediatrics (AAP)	http://www.aap.org/healthtopics/oralhealth.cfm *AAP's statement on high incidence of caries in children*

American Association of Community Dental Programs (AACDP)	http://www.aacdp.com/
	Available publications:
	    Seal America: The Prevention Invention
	    A Guide for Developing and Enhancing Community Oral Health Programs
	    A Model Framework for Community Oral Health Programs Based Upon the Ten
	        Essential Public Health Services

American Association of Public Health Dentistry (AAPHD)	http://www.aaphd.org/ *Provides a focus for meeting the challenges to improve oral health*
American Board of Public Health Dentistry (ABPHD)	http://www.aaphd.org/default.asp?page=ABDPHMenu.htm *Tools and information on board eligibility, honorary diplomat policy, and an annual report of continuing education (accessed through the AAPHD Web site)*
American Dental Association (ADA)	http://www.ada.org/goto/fluoride *Overview of fluoride and fluoridation information*

American Dental Education Association	http://www.adea.org/
	*Services the predoctoral, postdoctoral, and allied dental education community.
	    Provides advocacy, professional development, and a wealth of expert information
	    and resources*

Table 28.13. (*continued*)

Organization	Website
American Public Health Association (APHA)	http://www.apha-oh.org/ *Provides information and resolutions on dental and public health policies, programs, and practices*
Association of State and Territorial Dental Directors (ASTDD)	http://www.astdd.org/docs/ASTDDGuidelines_BestPracLinksMay2005rev7final6.29.2005.pdf Guidelines for State and Territorial Oral Health Programs
Local, County, Regional or State Health Department	Check your local listings *Local health authorities of the area*
Healthy People 2010	http://www.healthypeople.gov/ *Provides a framework and national prevention goals for the United States including a chapter on oral health*
The Mobile-Portable Dental Manual	http://www.Mobile-PortableDentalManual.com *Provides detailed information and links to resources on planning, financing, equipping, staffing, operating, and evaluating mobile and portable dental programs.*
National Association of County and City Health Officials	http://www.naccho.org/topics/infrastructure/operational_definition.cfm *Operational Definition of a Local Public Health Agency*
National Institute Dental and Craniofacial Research	http://www.nidcr.nih.gov/HealthInformation/SpecialCareResources/ *Health information and research on dental and craniofacial health*
National Maternal and Child Oral Health Resource	http://www.mchoralhealth.org *A Guide for Developing and Enhancing Community Oral Health Programs and a variety of information on various aspects of oral health*
The National Network for Oral Health Access (NNOHA)	http://www.nnoha.org *NNOHA is a nationwide network of dental providers who care for patients in Migrant, Homeless, and Community Health Centers.*
Safety Net Dental Clinic Manual	http://www.DentalClinicManual.com *Manual for designing and implementing a safety net dental clinic*
U.S. Centers for Disease Control and Prevention (CDC)	http://www.cdc.gov/oralhealth *Collection of tools to assist states to build oral health program capacity*

REVIEW QUESTIONS

1. Why are oral diseases considered a neglected epidemic in the United States and why is oral health important?
2. Why are oral diseases considered a public health problem in need of a public health solution?
3. Why are there oral health disparities for vulnerable or high-risk populations, and how can they be resolved?
4. What are the major differences between individual and community-based dental prevention measures?
5. How can the 10 essential public health services as they relate to oral health in *A Model Framework for Community Oral Health Programs* be implemented and what impact would they have?
6. What is community water fluoridation? Why is it considered the foundation for better oral health?

7. How can *Healthy People 2010*, the *Guide to Community Preventive Services*, and the U.S. Surgeon General's Report on Oral Health help improve oral health in a community?

8. What are the advantages and disadvantages of the five effective community prevention programs?

9. What are the advantages of the Alaska Dental Therapist model for improving access to dental services?

10. What is the role of a local or state health department for improving oral health?

REFERENCES

1. US Department of Health and Human Services. *Oral Health in America: A Report of the Surgeon General.* Rockville, MD: US Dept of Health and Human Services, National Institute of Dental and Craniofacial Research, National Institutes of Health; 2000.

2. Allukian M. The neglected epidemic and the Surgeon General's Report: a call to action for better oral health (editorial). *Am J Public Health.* 2000; 90(6):843–45.

3. Brunelle JA, Bhat M, Lipton JA. Prevalence and distribution of selected occlusal characteristics in the US population, 1988–1991. *J Dent Res.* 75(February 1996)(Special issue):706–13.

4. Bhat M. Periodontal health of 14–17-year-old U.S. school children. *J Public Health Dent.* Winter 1991;51(1):5–11.

5. Dye BA, Tan S, Smith V, Lewis BG, Barker LK, Thornton-Evans G, et al. Trends in oral health status: United States, 1988–1994 and 1999–2004. National Center for Health Statistics. *Vital Health Stat.* 2007;11(248).

6. Jemal A, Siegal R, Ward E, Murray T, Xu J, Thun MJ. Cancer statistics, 2007. *CA Cancer J Clin.* 2007;43–66.

7. Edmonds LD, James LM. Temporal trends in the prevalence of congenital malformations at birth based on the Birth Defects Monitoring Program, United States, 1979–1987. *MMWR.* 1993;39: 19–23.

8. US Department of Health and Human Services. *Healthy People 2010, With Understanding and Improving Health Objectives for Improving Health.*

2nd ed. Washington, DC: US Government Printing Office; 2000.

9. Allukian M, Kazmi I, Foulds SH, Horgan W. The unmet dental needs of the homeless in Boston. Presented at the 112th Annual Meeting of the American Public Health Association; November 13, 1984; Anaheim, California.

10. Kelly M, Bruerd B. The prevalence of nursing bottle decay among two Native American populations. *J Public Health Dent.* 1987;47:94–7.

11. Becker DB, Needleman HL, Kotelchuck M. Child abuse and dentistry: orofacial trauma and its recognition by dentists. *J Am Dent Assoc.* 1978; 97(1):24–8.

12. Flanders R. Orofacial injuries: prevalence and prevention in Illinois. *Ill Dent J.* May/June 1992: 211–16.

13. Bloom B, Gift HC, Jack SS. *Dental Services and Oral Health; United States, 1989. Vital Health Stat.* 1992;10:183.

14. *Healthy People 2000: National Health Promotion and Disease Prevention Objectives.* Washington, DC: US Public Health Service; 1990. PHS publication no. 91-50212.

15. Kaste LW, Marcus P, Monopoli M, Allukian M, Douglass CW. Oral health status of homebound elders in Boston. Paper presented at the 18th Annual Meeting of the American Association for Dental Research; March 15–18, 1989; San Francisco, California.

16. Mueller CD, Schur CL, Paramore C. Access to dental care in the United States. *J Am Dent Assoc.* 1998;129:429–37.

17. Jackson J. Nursing home fined $100,000 for death Pleasant Care Corp. in bankruptcy; facilities in process of being sold. *Argus-Courier* (Petaluma, CA), July 2007.

18. Otto M. For want of a dentist: Pr. George's Boy dies after bacteria from tooth spread to brain. *Washington Post*, February 2007.

19. Dasanayake AP. Poor periodontal health of the pregnant woman as a risk factor for low birth weight. *Ann Periodontol.* 1998;70:206–11.

20. Offenbacher S, Katz V, Fertik G, et al. Periodontal infection as a possible factor for preterm low birth weight. *Ann Periodontol.* 1995;67(suppl 10): 1103–13.

21. Davenport ES, Willias CE, Sterne JA, et al. The East London study of maternal chronic periodontal disease and preterm low birth weight

infants: study design and prevalence data. *Ann Periodontol*. 1998;70:213–21.

22. Beck JD, Offenbacher S, Williams R, Gibbs P, Garcia R. Periodontitis: a risk factor for coronary heart disease? *Ann Periodontol*. 1998;70:127–41.

23. Genco RJ. Periodontal disease and risk for myocardial infarction and cardiovascular disease. *Cardiovasc Rev Rep*. 1998;19:34–40.

24. Slavkin HC. Does the mouth put the heart at risk? *J Am Dent Assoc*. 1999;130:109–13.

25. Jeffcoat MK, Geurs NC, Reddy MS, Cliver SI, Goldenberg RL, Hauth JC. Periodontal infection and preterm birth. *J Am Dent Assoc*. July 2001; 132:875–80.

26. Hollister MC, Weintraub JA. The association of oral status and systemic health, quality of life, and economic productivity. *J Dent Educ*. 1993;57(12): 901–12.

27. Lipton JS, Ship JA, Larach-Robinson D. Estimated prevalence and distribution of reported orofacial pain in the United States. *J Am Dent Assoc*. 1993; 124(10):115–21.

28. Gift HC, Reisine ST, Larach DC. The social impact of dental problems and visits. *Am J Public Health*. 1992;82(12):1663–8.

29. Adams PF, Benson V. Current estimates from the National Health Interview Survey, 1991. *Vital Health Stat*. 1992;10(184):46–7,54.

30. Adams PF, Marano MA. 1995. *Current Estimates from the National Health Interview Survey, 1994. Vital and Health Statistics*. Hyattsville, MD: US Dept of Health and Human Services, National Center for Health Statistics. Series 10, no. 193.

31. Center for Medicare & Medicaid Services, Office of the Actuary, *National Health Expenditures Aggregate, per Capita Amounts, Percent Distribution, and Average Annual Percent Growth, by Source of Funds: Selected Calendar Years 1960–2005*. Available at: http://www.cms.hhs .gov/natioanlhealthexpenddata/downloads/tables .pdf. Accessed April 16, 2008.

32. Health Care Financing Administration, Office of Actuary. *National Health Expenditure Amounts and Average Change by Type of Expenditure: Selected Calendar Years 1980–2010*. Available at: http://www.hcfa.gov/stats/NHE-Proj/Proj.2000/ tables/t2.htm. Accessed June 14, 2001.

33. Centers for Medicare & Medicaid Services, Office of the Actuary. *National Health Expenditure Amounts, and Annual Percent Change by Type of Expenditure: Selected Calendar Years 1999–2015*. Available at: http://www.cms.hhs.gov/ NationalHealthExpendData/downloatds/ proj2005.pdf. Accessed February 2007.

34. Gehshan S, Wyatt M. *Improving Oral Health Care for Young Children*. National Academy for State Health Policy. Portland, ME: April 2007. Available at: http://www.nashp.org/Files/Improving_ Oral_Health.pdf.

35. National Institute of Dental Research. *Oral Health of United States Children. The National Survey of Dental Caries in U.S. School Children, 1986–1987*. Bethesda, MD: US Dept of Health and Human Services; 1989. DHHS publication NIH 89–2247.

36. Vargas CM. Unpublished estimates, Third National Health and Nutrition Examination Survey, 2000. Personal communication.

37. Joshi A, Douglass CW, Jette A, Feldman H. The distribution of root caries in community-dwelling elders in New England. *J Public Health Dent*. Winter 1994:15–23.

38. Winn DM, et al. Coronal and root caries in the dentition of adults in the United States, 1988–1991. *J Dent Res*. 1996;75:642–51. Special issue.

39. Kaste LM, Gift HC. Baby bottle feeding behavior in children ages 2–5. *J Dent Res*. 1994;33(2):580.

40. *Cancers of the Oral Cavity and Pharynx: A Statistics Review Monograph, 1973–1987*. Atlanta, GA: Centers for Disease Control and the National Institutes of Health; 1991.

41. Prout MN, Heeren TC, Barber CE, et al. Use of health services before the diagnosis of head and neck cancer among Boston residents. *Am J Prev Med*. 1990;6:77–83.

42. Palmer C. NCAA forbids tobacco usage. *ADA News*. 1994;25:4.

43. Dolan, Atchison K Huynh, TR. Access to Dental Care Among Older Adults in the United States. *J Dent Educ*. 2005;69(9):961–74.

44. Brown, E., Jr. *Children Dental Visits and Expenses, United States, 2003*. Statistical Brief #117. March 2006. Agency for Healthcare Research and Quality, Rockville, MD. http://meps.ahrq.gov/papers/ st117.pdf.

45. Institute of Medicine, Committee for the Study of the Future of Public Health. *The Future of Public Health*. Washington, DC: National Academy Press; 1988.

46. Executive summary: application for continued recognition of dental public health as a dental specialty. *J Public Health Dent*. 1986;46(1): 35–7.

47. Rozier RG. Competency objectives for dental public health. *J Public Health Dent*. 1990;50(5): 338–44.

48. Dental public health competencies. *J Public Health Dept*. 1998;58(suppl 1):121–22.

49. Tomar SL. An assessment of the dental public health infrastructure in the United Sates. *J Public Health Dent*. 2006;66(1):5–16.

50. American Dental Association. *Report of the ADA-Recognized Dental Specialty Certifying Boards*. Council on Dental Education and Licensure. Chicago, IL. April 2007.

51. American Association for Community Dental Programs. *A Model Framework For Community Oral Health Programs: Based Upon The Ten Essential Public Health Services*. August 2005. Available at: http://www.aacdp.com/Docs/ Framework.pdf.

52. American Association for Community Dental Programs. *Guide for developing and enhancing community oral health programs*. (2006) Available at: http://www.aacdp.com/Docs/CommunityGuide .pdf.

53. Burt B. Proceedings of the workshop: cost effectiveness of caries prevention in dental public health. *J Public Health Dent*. 1989;49:5. Special issue.

54. Centers for Disease Control and Prevention. Recommendations for using fluoride to prevent and control dental caries in the United States. *MMWR*. 2001;50:1–42.

55. Wagener DK, Nourjah P, Horowitz A. *Trends in Childhood Use of Dental Care Products Containing Fluoride: U.S. 1983–1989*. Hyattsville, MD: National Center for Health Statistics; 1992. Advance data from Vital and Health Statistics no. 219.

56. *Review of Fluoride: Benefits and Risks*. Washington, DC: US Public Health Service; February 1991.

57. American Dental Association. Caries diagnosis and risk assessment. A review of preventive strategies and management. *J Am Dent Assoc*. 1995; 126(suppl).

58. Kaminsky LS, Mahoney MC, Leach JF, Melius JM, Miller MJ. Fluoride: benefits and risk of exposure. *Crit Rev Oral Biol Med*. 1990;1(4):261.

59. National Research Council. *Health Effects of Ingested Fluoride*. Washington, DC: National Academy Press; 1993.

60. Institute of Medicine Food and Nutrition Board. *Dietary Reference Intakes: Calcium, Phosphorus, Magnesium, Vitamin D and Fluoride*. Washington, DC: National Academy Press; 1997.

61. Centers for Disease Control and Prevention. Public health focus: fluoridation of community water systems. *MMWR*. 1992;2(41):372–381.

62. Griffins S, Jones K, Tomar S. An economic evaluation of community water fluoridation. *J Public Health Dept*. 2001;61:38–86.

63. Centers for Disease Control. *Water Fluoridation: A Manual for Engineers and Technicians*. Atlanta, GA: US Public Health Service; 1986:19.

64. Griffin SO, Jones,K. Cost-effectiveness of community water fluoridation. Fluorides & Oral Health Symposium: Symposium Proceedings. *Kuwait Foundation*, Dec 2006;123–26.

65. Centers for Disease Control and Prevention. Fluoridation of drinking water to prevent dental caries. *MMWR*. 1999;48:933–40.

66. Centers for Disease Control and Prevention. Populations receiving optimally fluoridated public drinking water—US, 1992–2006. *MMWR*. 2008; 57(27):737–741.

67. Center for Disease Control and Prevention Populations receiving optimally fluoridated drinking water-United States, 2000, *MMWR*. 51(07): 144–47, 2002.

68. San Antonio Water System. Fluoridation Q&A. http://www.saws.org/our_water/fluoride.shtml.

69. Allukian M, Ackerman J, Steinhurst J. Factors that influence the attitudes of first-term Massachusetts legislators toward fluoridation. *J Am Dent Assoc*. 1981;104(4):494.

70. Griffin SO, Gooch BF, Lockwood SA, Tomar SL. Quantifying the diffused benefit from water fluoridation in the United States. *Community Dent Oral Epidemiol*. 2001;29:120–129.

71. Cohen LA, Horowitz AM. Community-based sealant programs in the United States: results of a survey. *J Public Health Dent*. Fall 1993;53:4.

72. American Dental Association. *2000 Survey of Legal Provisions for Delegating Intraoral Functions to Chairside Assistants and Dental Hygienists*. Survey Center; June 2001.

73. American Dental Association. *2004 Survey of Legal Provisions for Delegation Intraoral*

Functions to Chairside Assistants and Dental Hygienists. Survey Center; June 2005.

74. Impact of targeted, school-based dental sealant programs in reducing racial and economic disparities in sealant prevalence among school children—Ohio, United States, 1998–1999. *MMWR.* 2001; 50(34):736–38.

75. US Preventive Services Task Force Report. *Guide to Clinical Preventive Services.* 2nd ed. Baltimore, MD: Williams and Wilkins; 1996.

76. Centers for Disease Control and Prevention. Proceedings from the National Strategic Planning Conference for the Prevention and Control of Oral and Pharyngeal Cancer, August 7–9, 1996, Atlanta. Bethesda, MD: 1997.

77. Centers for Disease Control and Prevention. Presenting and Controlling Oral and Pharyngeal Cancer. Recommendations from a National Strategic Planning Conference. *MMWR.* 1998; 47(RR 1–14):1–12.

78. Flanders R. Mouthguards and sports injuries. *Ill Dent J.* Jan/Feb 1993:13–16.

79. Missouri Dental Association. Child abuse update, 1994. Reprinted from the *Missouri Dent J.* 1994; 1–101.

80. National Cancer Institute. *How to Help Your Patients Stop Using Tobacco: Manual for the Oral Health Team.* Washington, DC: National Institutes of Health; 1991. PHS publication no. 91–3191.

81. Allukian M. Effective community prevention program. In: Depoala DP, Cheney JG, eds. *Handbook of Preventive Dentistry.* Littleton, MA: Publishing Services Group Inc; 1979.

82. Horowitz AM. Community-oriented preventive dentistry programs that work. *Health Values.* 1984;8(1):121–129.

83. Allukian M. Community oral health programs. In: Clark JW, ed. *Clinical Dentistry, II.* Philadelphia, PA: Harper & Row; 1987.

84. Association of State and Territorial Dental Directors. *Public Health Core Functions: Strategies for Addressing the Oral Health of the Nation.* March 1994. Discussion paper.

85. Association of State and Territorial Dental Directors. *Building Infrastructure and Capacity in State and Territorial Oral Health Programs, April 2000.*

86. Allukian M Jr. Horowitz AM. Effective community prevention programs for oral diseases. In: Gluck G, Morganstein W, eds. Jong's *Community Dental*

Health. 5th ed. St. Louis, MO: Mosby Press; 2002:237–76.

87. Isman RE. Integrating primary oral health care into primary care. *J Dent Educ.* 1993;47(12): 846–52.

88. Oral Health Coordinating Committee, Public Health Service. Toward improving the oral health of Americans: An overview of oral health status, resources, and care delivery. *Public Health Rep.* 1993;108(6):657–72.

89. Mouradian WE, Wehr E, Crall JJ. Disparities in children's oral health and access to dental care. *J Am Med Assoc.* 2000;284:2625–31.

90. Bolden AJ, Henry JL, Allukian M. Implications of access, utilization and need for oral health care by low income groups and minorities on the dental delivery system. *J Dent Educ.* 1993; 57(12): 888–900.

91. Shortage Designation Branch Office of Workforce Evaluation and Quality Assurance Bureau of Health Professions, HRSA. *Selected Statistics on Health Professional Shortage Areas.* As of March 31, 2007.

92. American Dental Education Association. *Official Guide to Dental Schools. Applying to Dental Schools.* Washington, DC, 2007.

93. American Dental Association, Health Policy Resources Center. *2006 American Dental Association Dental Workforce Model: 2004–2025.* Chicago: American Dental Association Health Policy Resources Center; 2006.

94. US Department of Health and Human Services. *Health Personnel in the United States, Eighth Report to Congress.* Allied Health, 1991. Washington, DC: HRSA/Bureau of Health Professions; September 1992.

95. Valachovic RW, Weaver RG, Sinkford JC, Haden NK. Trends in dentistry and dental education. *J Dent Educ.* June 2001:539–61.

96. American Dental Association, Survey Center. 2005 Survey of Dental Practice: Income from the Private Practice of Dentistry, January 2007.

97. U.S. Department of Labor, Bureau of Labor Statistics. *Occupational Employment Statistics, May 2005.* http://www.dol.gov. Accessed April 2007.

98. Professional Practice Environment of Dental Hygienists in the Fifty States and the District of Columbia, 2001. National Center for Health Workforce Analysis. Bureau of Health

Professions. Health Resources and Services Administration. April 2004.

99. *Comptroller General: Increased Use of Expanded Function Dental Auxiliaries Would Benefit Consumers, Dentists and Taxpayers. Report to the Congress.* Washington, DC: General Accounting Office; March 7, 1980. Publication HRD-80-51.

100. Governor Doyle announces plan to expand dental access for kids, families—$12 million dedicated to comprehensive dental care across the state. *The Dunn County News.* Milwaukee. Available at: http://www.dunnconnect.com/articles/2007/04/02/variety/variety03.txt. Accessed April 2, 2007.

101. American Dental Hygienists' Association. The latest legislative news in oral health from coast to coast: bills Relating to Dental Hygiene Sent to the Governor. Stateline is prepared by the ADHA Division of Governmental Affairs. Available at: http://www.adha.org/governmental_affairs/stateline.htm. Accessed July 1, 2006–June 1, 2007.

102. American Dental Hygiene Association. *Dental Hygiene Legislative Activity 1993 to 2006.* http://www.adha.org. Accessed October 10, 2006.

103. American Dental Hygiene Association. ADHA's Response to ADA Study: The Economic Impact of Unsupervised Dental Hygiene Practice and its Impact on Access to Care in the State of Colorado. ADHA. News. Available at: http://www.adha.org/news/archives/2005/012805-study.htm.

104. American Dental Hygiene Association. *States Which Directly Reimburse Dental Hygienists for Services under the Medicaid Program.* ADHA. Government Affairs: Hot Topics. Available at: http://www.adha.org/governmental_affairs/index.html.

105. American Public Health Association. *Support for the Alaska Dental Health Aide Therapist and Other Innovative Programs for Underserved Populations.* Policy Number 20064. November 8, 2006. http://www.apha.org/advocacy/policy/policysearch/default.htm?id=1328. Accessed April 2007.

106. *Alaska Dental Society v. Alaska Native Tribal Health Consortium*, No. 3AN-06-04797CI. In the Superior Court for the State of Alaska, Third Judicial District at Anchorage. Alaska Super. Ct. filed Jan. 31, 2006.

107. Alaska Dental Society, Inc. (full-page ad) Governor Murowski 2nd class care for Alaska Natives deserves a ferocious reaction! *Juneau Empire.* May 26, 2005:C7.

108. Liang JN, Orgur JD. *Restrictions on Dental Auxiliaries; An Economic Policy Analysis.* Washington, DC: General Accounting Office; March 7, 1980. Publication HRD-80-51.

109. American Dental Education Association. Washington, D.C. Dr. Richard Weaver. Personal Communication, August 2, 2007.

110. Health Resources and Services Administration (HRSA) Bureau of Health Professions. Factbook, *United States Health Workforce Personnel.* Rockville, MD: HRSA/Bureau of Health Professions; 1999.

111. Corbin SB, Mecklenburg RE. The future of dental public health report: preparing dental public health to meet the challenges and opportunities of the 21st century. *J Public Health Dent.* 1994; 54(2):80–91.

CHAPTER 29

The Public Health Laboratory

Ronald L. Cada, DrPH and Ralph Timperi, MPH

LEARNING OBJECTIVES

Upon completion of this chapter, the reader will be able to:

1. Summarize the history and reasons for emergence of public health laboratories.

2. Describe and discuss the core functions of public health laboratories.

3. Discriminate the role of public health laboratories with regard to other governmental laboratories and the private sector.

4. Explain the roles and functions of public health laboratories in surveillance and response to infectious and environmental disease control and prevention.

5. Discuss the role of the National Laboratory Training Network in public health.

6. Describe and discuss the effects of technology on current public health laboratory practices, on diagnostic testing, and on the future trends in laboratory science, for example:

   a. Biomonitoring for environmental diseases

   b. Pandemic influenza diagnosis and tracking for emergency preparedness

   c. Point-of-care (done at the site of treatment) and other simple test kits (rapid HIV test) for diagnostic testing

7. Explain the role of the United States public health laboratory in the international arena, and how global assistance may be provided; explain the role of surveillance and research in global public health.

KEY TERMS

Core Laboratory Responsibilities

Clinical Laboratory Improvement Amendments Act of 1988 (CLIA '88)

False Positive and False Negative Test Results

Proficiency Testing

Quality Assurance

Public health laboratories have contributed significantly to the capacity of health departments to carry out their essential services in support of community health. Developed out of a recognition of the opportunities for prevention of infectious diseases after the bacteriological discoveries of the late nineteenth century such as by Koch of the tubercle bacillus, they have grown to encompass additional roles in environmental heath, newborn screening, and emergency response. In addition to providing disease surveillance testing, public health laboratories have often provided diagnostic testing for patients enrolled in public health programs and hospital settings. Many state laboratories also play a significant role in the assurance of laboratory testing quality in community clinical laboratories through inspection and education services.

This chapter provides an overview of **core laboratory responsibilities** (services all public health laboratories should have available in house or through contract) and offers a vision for the future. We anticipate that acceleration of new technology development and changes in health care systems will result in significant changes in testing services and functions of public health laboratories. A growing need for assurance of the quality of community laboratory services will require the public health laboratory to increase its capacity to operate in this arena. Enhanced communication, information management, and analytic skills will be necessary if public health laboratories are to continue to be viable and effective entities to assure competent public health services.

HISTORICAL ROLE OF THE PUBLIC HEALTH LABORATORY

In many disease control circumstances, laboratory investigation provides objective data to underpin public health decision making. Decisions to treat individual patients, provide access to a program for HIV/AIDS patients, sanction a company found to be polluting a water supply, identify and prosecute a drunk driver, close a contaminated public water supply, or identify/evaluate a terrorist-related biological/chemical event—among other possible examples—all are based on laboratory information. Laboratory results are essential components in the search for solutions to public health problems.

Beginnings

Public health laboratory services grew as a core function of community health during the 1890s. Laboratories were integral in tracking the outbreaks of enteric and respiratory infections that periodically exploded among populations crowding into urban centers at that time. The unique responsibility of public health laboratories was to assist with the task of community health assessment through the scientific identification and measurement of disease incidence and prevalence in susceptible populations. As the relationship among host, agent, and environment was identified for specific disease agents, public health laboratories contributed to disease prevention by using community environmental monitoring to estimate disease risk. The need for more adequate characterization and quantification of environmental hazards will continue to challenge the capabilities of public health laboratories.[1]

Shift in Emphasis to Personal Health Care

More recently, since the passage of Medicare and Medicaid legislation, public health departments have become more involved in the delivery of personal health care services. In many local public health agencies, laboratories were merged or integrated with publicly owned hospital labs. The unique community assessment role of public health laboratories often disappeared as the tests they performed became indistinguishable from those of acute care hospitals and private clinical laboratories. As increasing resources were needed to support growing public health clinic and hospital workloads, priorities were adjusted, often resulting in a change in emphasis from epidemic surveillance and environmental monitoring efforts to clinical testing services for individual patients supported by health insurance reimbursements.

For uninsured or indigent patients whose costs are not covered by third-party payers, the public health laboratory often provided the service whether or not payment was available. With increasing demands for patient-based clinical testing using a greater proportion of limited public funding, the mission of public health laboratories to provide infectious disease surveillance, epidemic investigations, and environmental risk factor analysis has clearly suffered.

Public health laboratories, especially at the state and local level, often find themselves in the position of providing services in areas considered unprofitable by commercial testing facilities. In addition, many of these services involve diseases or disorders that are reportable to the state, adding the extra cost of providing governmental reports in a manner different from the usual clinical result report. For example, the state requires identifiers and locations that are not usually provided in clinical laboratory reports to the attending health care practitioner. Testing for the potential of rabies transmission by examination of animal tissue, for instance, has remained in the community health laboratory, both because it is a form of environmental disease monitoring and because this labor-intensive analysis has not been automated and would not be profitable in commercial test environments. Another example is the use of enteric pathogen serotyping and DNA typing as a surveillance mechanism for tracking disease outbreaks. This activity is essential for understanding the distribution of these organisms in population groups, but it is not helpful in individual patient interventions. As a result, these and similar tests are ignored by the clinician's commercial testing facilities.

CORE FUNCTIONS OF PUBLIC HEALTH LABORATORIES

It should be readily apparent from the preceding historical discussion that public laboratories have taken a direction decidedly different from that of private testing facilities. Although there are many similarities in technology between the public and private testing sectors, the utility of the information is different. Whereas the private sector's main responsibility is to identify disease in an individual for treatment of that individual, the public laboratory's purpose is to prevent disease by identifying disease in a group so that causation can be determined and disease control efforts can begin. Public health laboratories may be expected to test not only individuals but also the environment in which they exist, such as water, air, or food, which might be a source of infection. Public laboratories are expected to set a high priority in situational testing, that is, to give preference to testing community sources of infection rather than individuals in queue as specimens are received. These emergency response events have become the *raisons d'etre* of the public health laboratory in that they work in concert with first responders to an outbreak in determining causation. Many recent outbreaks of enteric organisms in foodstuffs and water sources are easily identified by the reader. Food quarantine and drinking water diversion have become a common event in recent years due to the ability of public laboratories to quickly identify and track disease outbreaks.

Two other major roles differentiate the public laboratory from clinical and environmental testing sites: **quality assurance** (a system of activities and monitoring intended to provide the most accurate test result possible) oversight and data sharing. In many disease outbreaks of regional or national (even international) importance, many public and private laboratories provide data toward understanding the dynamics of how the disease spread.

Providing adequate, timely, and comparable data is imperative to rapid diagnosis and disease control efforts. To use data provided by many vendors requires that the quality of each be assured and comparable to the others. This assurance has been a major role of public sector laboratories since the years of WWI when the Department of the Army attempted to standardize blood testing for syphilis as part of its disease control efforts of military personnel. Over the succeeding generations, this peer evaluation has developed into the concept of Quality Management by the definition of minimum standards for test performance. These standards address the quality of personnel, equipment, supplies, environment for testing, and data handling.

Despite the lack of credible empirical evidence that modern laboratory services constituted a threat to public health,[9] a federal law requiring licensing of all clinical laboratories was enacted in 1988. Primarily intended to bring clinical laboratory testing in physicians' offices under regulatory oversight, the **Clinical Laboratory Improvement Amendments Act of 1988 (CLIA '88)** (a federal licensure of laboratories that perform testing on human specimens) brought an estimated 135,000 previously unregulated testing sites under a complex system of federal licensure.[10] This highly contentious law classifies tests based upon their technical complexity as well as the risk to patients of incorrect results.

A major reason that federal regulations have prompted concern by public health officials and their laboratories is because personnel standards under CLIA '88 are based, to a great extent, on previous federal requirements designed for clinical laboratories in hospitals and independent commercial settings.[11] Some public health laboratory leaders believe it is essential to develop standards that recognize the unique nature of public health laboratory testing.[12]

Although some standardization is clearly accomplished by regulation at both the state and federal levels, it is also achieved through the use of voluntary or consensus guidelines. The Clinical Laboratory Standards Institute (CLSI), for example, is a consortium of representatives of laboratorian professional organizations, government, and industry that has a well-defined process to identify procedures in need of standardization and then to draft, review, and promulgate voluntary practice standards.[16]

Accurate data are not useful if not transmitted quickly and in a format understandable to the receiver and translatable with other testing methods. In recent years, state and federal standards organizations have attempted to develop and implement standards and mechanisms for laboratories to transmit adequate data to agencies charged with preventing or lessening effects of disease spread. The process has been slow because state and regional laboratories can only develop as allowed by their parent organizations and professional support.

Impact of New Technologies

A growing number of laboratory tests are now available for use outside the laboratory environment by nonlaboratory users. Rapidly developing technologies promise an ever-increasing list of procedures intended to be performed in locations where patients live and work, rather than by individuals specifically trained in laboratory processes working in closely controlled institutional environments. More and more laboratory tests can now be done at the patient's bedside, at nursing stations, in shopping malls, in physicians' offices, or at remote clinics and environmental sites. Patient self-testing or home testing for blood glucose and pregnancy are examples of over-the-counter test kit technologies readily available with or without a physician's order. The list of home-use tests will grow as individuals request more control over their personal health, and manufacturers respond to this market demand. The extent to which these testing methodologies can be safely and effectively used and interpreted by personnel without extensive laboratory training is a current topic of considerable debate.[2] Scant attention has been given to the need for changes in education (pre-service and continuing) to assure proficiency in a workforce where testing is moving out of the laboratory as manufacturers gain approval of waived tests that are viewed mistakenly as simple because they are rapid and involve few steps. As testing moves out of a laboratory environment, test results are produced in an environment of less robust quality assurance, and the frequency of undetected errors is likely to increase. **False positive and false negative test results** (those showing disease where there is none, and showing negative results in a disease state) can have significant adverse effects on patient outcomes causing unnecessary treatment and stigma in the former case, for example, and delayed effective treatment in the latter. In some cases, testing errors can cause broad societal adverse effects such as economic disruption in global markets due to a false positive test result and failure to avert a widespread outbreak due to a false negative test result.

In their traditional role, public health laboratories will need to take the initiative to assess the effects of the trend to make diagnostic testing available to home users as well as nonlaboratory health care professionals and propose effective strategies to assure the quality of these testing systems and protection of the public's health. As technology changes the field of diagnostic testing, public health laboratories will be challenged to change to accommodate the new practices but not fail to provide the leadership to maintain their essential functions in disease surveillance and quality assurance.

The Reference Laboratory and Improvement Activities

Since their inception, public health laboratories have collected specimens for testing when an issue of public health importance was at stake.[3] These specimens come from a variety of sources, including other laboratories.[4] Over time, public health laboratories have become *referral laboratories* for a number of investigations having community health implications.

As their expertise improved, some public laboratories developed strategies beyond the passive reference role and began activities to systematically improve the quality of testing in other laboratories. These activities were buttressed by early surveys of medical testing laboratories, which indicated that

test results were often below minimally acceptable levels.[5,6] Concerns were raised that poor results were so widespread as to constitute a serious threat to the public health. Comprehensive efforts to externally monitor laboratory quality were first introduced in military hospitals during World War II.[7] They were followed by similar efforts in private hospital laboratories in the late 1940s.[6] This external quality-control activity run by many state health departments is now a major component of laboratory accreditation and regulatory programs.[8]

Government Contributions

The recent evolution of practice guidelines for HIV/AIDS testing services provides an example of how federal agencies, such as the Centers for Disease Control and Prevention (CDC), and public health laboratories have worked to standardize and improve testing services for HIV antibody and T lymphocyte immunophenotyping. Public health laboratory officials at CDC and at state and local public health laboratories as well as test kit manufacturers recognized the need to evaluate performance, develop a consensus, and establish guidelines for HIV testing. After a number of ad hoc meetings of experts, the Association of State and Territorial Public Health Laboratory Directors (ASTPHLD) formed a human retrovirus testing committee to oversee this process.[13] Manufacturers, laboratory scientists, and pathologists from commercial and hospital laboratories contributed to the formulation of practice guidelines. The CDC provided "official" sanction to many of the practice recommendations by publishing them in supplements to the *Morbidity and Mortality Weekly Report (MMWR)*.[14]

In the mid-1980s, as the testing requirements to support response to the HIV epidemic exploded onto the public health scene, CDC reorganized its efforts in laboratory training and other improvement activities such as **proficiency testing** (in the laboratory scenario, specimens unknown to the tested but known to the tester). Most of these new efforts were focused on HIV/AIDS and related testing. The existing centralized, government-run training model was replaced by programs run through a National Laboratory Training Network (NLTN).[15] Seven regional Area Laboratory Training Alliances (ALTAs) were developed to serve as clearinghouses to assess, facilitate, and evaluate training activities. These centers work through training coordinators in state government laboratories. In early 2000, the CDC, in partnership with the Association of Public Health Laboratories, announced the reorganization of the network into a more specialized and centralized model. The increased role of more specialized laboratories, which currently use the most highly developed technology, will be to enable the network to more effectively transfer new technologies through distance-learning initiatives and the latest conferencing capabilities. In addition, the NLTN began the process of recovering costs of providing training through the application of training fees to individual students. This was instituted with the hope that the continued viability of the network would be assured.

BIOLOGICAL AND CHEMICAL TERRORISM PREPAREDNESS

In 2001, federal and state officials formally recognized the potential for infectious organisms to be used as terrorism agents. An interagency funding, training, and service initiative entitled the "Public Health Emergency Preparedness Cooperative Agreement" was used to renovate and expand laboratory space, technology, and staff to respond to potential terrorist events.[16] Designed to provide advanced-level testing for biologic agents, this Laboratory Response Network (LRN) integrated more than 150 federal, state, local, veterinary, military, environmental, food testing, and international laboratories in the screening, identification, and characterization of clinical and environmental specimens for response activities. In 2003, the LRN was expanded to include chemical warfare and radiological contaminants. Each laboratory in the system has been categorized as having a specified level

of performance scored on environmental safety, capability, and capacity in processing suspect material. Funding for continued development of this laboratory network has been inconsistent, and the political will at the national and state level to provide the major increases in resources to develop and sustain a strong public health laboratory network appears to be lacking. Technology and facilities for biological agents are familiar to public laboratories, testing for dangerous chemical agents has required many states to update their facilities or construct new laboratories to meet the safety requirements for handling unknown specimens and samples that may contain multiple hazards. Further gains in the laboratory network capabilities may await the next major unexpected disaster in which the laboratory responds well but insufficiently to meet demands of the crisis.

PUBLIC HEALTH LABORATORIES TODAY AND IN THE FUTURE

In 1988, the Institute of Medicine (IOM) delineated assessment, policy development, and assurance as the core functions of public health.[17] As the profession further refines the characteristics of these core functions, it is increasingly clear that public health laboratories have much to contribute to the accomplishment of each. Information obtained from laboratories is important in assessing risks to community health, establishing priorities for public policy making, and ensuring the availability and reliability of laboratory tests for decisions related to individual patient diagnosis and treatment.

Current Status

Not surprisingly, the roles, responsibilities, and priorities of a given public health laboratory today correlate closely with the mission of its parent agency. The public health agency that is a leader in disease control and environmental protection, for example, will likely support a laboratory program that provides leadership in information services for those areas. However, if the parent public health agency is heavily involved in providing direct medical services, its laboratory will likely have as its priority the provision of clinical laboratory testing. Community health programs would no doubt be enhanced by the separation of clinical laboratory responsibilities from those more traditionally associated with public health agencies, but such a separation would likely be impractical and unrealistic as well as inefficient in some jurisdictions within the present system. The formation of regionalized management care organizations and other reform measures promised to make health care, including diagnostic testing, available to the enrollee, but the net effect has often been to scatter testing within and among institutions, corporations, and the public. Tests that were traditionally performed in reference or specialized laboratories are now done at the bedside; those previously performed in local medical laboratories are now completed by individuals in their homes. Space age technology in medical testing is available and expanding at an increasing rate. The fragmentation of the public health system over the past several decades is mirrored in public health laboratories today. A number of traditional public health laboratory functions have been transferred from public health agencies to other agencies and institutions. For example, while the study of the distribution of *Salmonella* infections in the United States population is the responsibility of the CDC, the monitoring of water supplies, one of the vehicles of transmission for these organisms, is the purview of the Environmental Protection Agency (EPA). Similarly, the monitoring of food supplies, the most common vehicle for *Salmonella* outbreaks, is the responsibility of the Food and Drug Administration (FDA). At the state level, these responsibilities are often distributed widely to such entities as state departments of agriculture, consumer protection, and natural resources. Until these activities are unified or coordinated effectively, efficiency and effectiveness will not be maximized. As a lead agency for public health policy

development in the United States, the CDC will have among its most important tasks the provision of leadership and assistance to states and selected local laboratories in ensuring a public health laboratory system that is truly functional.

Public Health Laboratories of the Future

The existence and future direction of laboratory testing in support of public health is not just a challenge for public health laboratories. As described previously, laboratory information is essential to the existence of a scientific base for public health services. In a review of public health laboratory infrastructure, Walter Dowdle, retired deputy director of CDC, expressed concern over a lack of resources in public health and concluded that public health laboratories have generally not fared well during recent cutbacks. However, he also observed that a number of state laboratories had continued to thrive even in this environment.[18]

To thrive in changing times, public health agencies need to evaluate their capabilities and be willing to adjust to new realities, including adjusting their laboratory services. A public/private planning venture[19] involving public health laboratory directors, public health leaders, and laboratorians from the private sector assessed present public health laboratory structure and services and recommended changes to respond to national trends. Sadly, many of the needed capabilities envisioned in this planning document and espoused as core functions of public health are currently not available or are poorly developed in many public health agencies. These include monitoring of nutritional status and systematic assessment of environmental contaminants, among other capabilities.

Beginning in the mid-1970s, state public health laboratories began gathering annual service and effort data to document the range and capacity of services formed in this group of laboratories.[20] These data showed a tripling of laboratory budgets and a shift in service volume from disease tracking to metabolic testing over the 15-year period that these reports were generated. The belief that infectious diseases had been controlled and the search for chronic disease causes contributed to the changes in service direction. The decision in many states to outsource their laboratory testing resulted in the expansion of laboratory improvement and regulatory activities by many states, which also included laboratory training for private laboratories needing quality improvement of their services.

A laboratory-related objective within *Health People 2010*[21] reads: Increase the proportion of tribal, state, and local health agencies that provide or assure comprehensive laboratory services to support essential public health services. In 2004, the Association of Public Health Laboratories (APHL) revived and revised its survey of state public health laboratories to measure compliance with these objectives.[22] The questions were designed to reflect the attainment of Objective 23-13 by asking whether the laboratory provided or assured services within the 11 essential subobjectives proposed (see Table 29.1). Participants were graded as meeting each subobjective if they responded affirmatively to 70 percent or more of the service questions. As noted in the table, the respondents needed to answer 16 of the 22 indicator questions to meet the subobjective for disease prevention, control, and

surveillance. This was the first year these questions were asked and intended to give a baseline of laboratory services performance. These data showed a wide range of capabilities in meeting national needs for public health laboratory testing as summarized in Figure 29.1. This chart lists not only the percentage participants meeting the objective but also the national target value chosen by the Committee developing the survey. For example, better than 90 percent of the respondents provided adequate disease control testing in 2004 (target 98% by 2010), and two-thirds presently served as referral and specialized testing laboratories (target 80% by 2010). However, less than 5 percent provided testing in food safety, and one-quarter met the minimum capability to contribute information to an emergency response event, accidental or terrorist-related. Policy development and emergency response are recent additions to the essential services expected of public health laboratories, and food safety is routinely a part of the mission of agencies other than public health. This online survey of 56 state and territorial laboratories will be repeated at 2-year intervals and expanded to local public health and other governmental public health laboratories as they are able to do so.

Table 29.1. Indicators for Subobjectives of *Healthy People 2010* Objective 23-13

Subobjective		Number of indicators	70% passing score
23-13a	Disease Prevention, Control, and Surveillance	22	16
23-13b	Integrated Data Management	5	4
23-13c	Reference & Specialized Testing	8	6
23-13d	Environmental Health and Protection	12	9
23-13e	Food Safety	9	7
23-13f	Laboratory Improvement and Regulation	2	2
23-13g	Policy Development	3	3
23-13h	Emergency Response	12	9
23-13i	Public Health–Related Research	4	3
23-13j	Training and Education	6	5
23-13k	Partnerships and Communication	6	5

SOURCE: Delmar Cengage Learning.

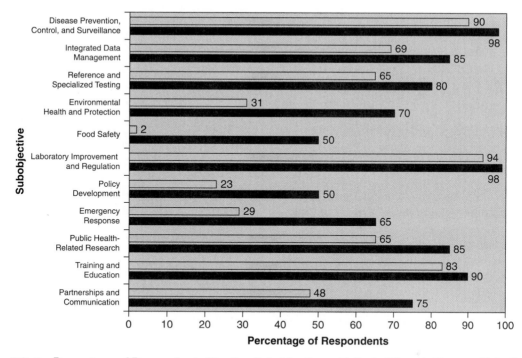

Figure 29.1. Percentage of Respondents Meeting Subobjective with End of Decade Targets. Light Gray Indicates Percentage of Respondents Meeting Subobjective; Black, End of Decade Targets

SOURCE: Delmar Cengage Learning.

The recent activity in completing the genome project has engendered a new paradigm of testing that public health agencies are pressed to consider. The tests being developed for identifying genetic disease, or the probability to develop disease, is an issue with which agencies and public health laboratories are ill-equipped to deal. Although state laboratories have been testing newborns for a variety of "inborn errors of metabolism" (e.g., phenylketonuria, hypothyroidism, and galactosemia), and evaluating hemoglobin for the presence of sickle cell disease and carrier states, genetic testing of individuals or the understanding of the results of these tests is not widely available in public health or health care sectors.[23,24] Public health laboratories are struggling to realize that they will be asked to take a leadership role in defining which tests should be used and how to evaluate their quality. The current status of many laboratories is that they

have minimal equipment, personnel, and training required for developing future tests. In many cases, these same laboratories will be asked to provide population testing as well as assure quality testing in other laboratories.

A major addition to the mission of public health laboratories was inserted when it was recognized that individuals, groups, and governments were attempting to infect and contaminate the community by the deliberate preparation and distribution of dangerous materials. Although the testing regimens for individual agents are available in most reference laboratories, artificially produced mixtures of biological, chemical, radiological, and explosive materials added a dimension to laboratory testing quite unknown and frightening to most laboratory employees. Training in handling these potentially lethal combinations proceeds at a rapid rate but is still a source of consternation for those handling and processing the test material. Few health care professionals are prepared to process patients, clinical material, or autopsy candidates at present.

The Impact of Health Care Reform

Under current conditions and predicting most probable health care reform scenarios, significant clinical and epidemiological laboratory roles remain the purview of state and local health departments. In an improved system, laboratory services should be universally available in a timely manner to the individual patient and the community. The experience of private-sector commercial laboratories may provide excellent models in this respect. These laboratories have connected networks of local, regional, and national testing facilities linked by electronic and courier networks. A rational system of public health laboratory services would share many characteristics of these private-sector systems.

Given the demand for high-quality, cost-effective services, it is clear that many smaller local agencies may not choose to maintain full-service laboratories. Even very large local departments may find it more effective to pool their resources with the state or other local health agencies. In some instances, sharing services with public or private hospital laboratories may be reasonable, as long as the information is available to public decision makers for assessment. The test of the utility of such mergers and reorganizations should be the continued ability to provide information in support of health programs, not short-term cost savings and political correctness.

Many expected that an evolved system of health care delivery would free public health departments from the responsibility for personal health care services. Under such a scenario, the public health laboratory could have returned to its primary purpose of protecting and promoting the public health through population-based programs.[25] The American Public Health Association (APHA) developed a vision of public health services in a reformed United States health care system.[26] Unfortunately, the envisioned health care reform did not occur.

Thus, it appears that the average public health laboratory will retain significant responsibility for providing clinical laboratory services to a large, medically underserved population.

A Vision of the Future Public Health Laboratory

What should the "typical" public health agency laboratory look like in the future? Although there will never be an archetypal laboratory, we anticipate that future public health laboratories will be different from public health laboratories supported today. It is likely they will have the characteristics discussed next.

Highly Integrated

The future public health laboratory will be integrated with intrastate clinical laboratories and an interstate public health laboratory network. Information standards and technologies and transportation systems will allow efficient integration.

Connected to Personal Health Care Information Systems

The electronic information highways envisioned under health care reform will funnel selected laboratory test results to the local, state, and federal health agencies. Public health laboratorians/epidemiologists will monitor communicable disease in the community, converting data into useful assessment information. On a routine basis, supplemental data will be collected from personal health care providers or special studies and will be integrated with routine, organized community surveys. The federal government has been challenged to develop and transport to local governments this electronic disease reporting system, which promises to link information across public and private laboratories, agency programs, and the federal government. This initiative, although improving the quality and speed of data acquisition, will not arrive without an expense to the system that may be greater than the present costs of collecting partial data.

Involved in Health-Related Environmental Testing

Food and water testing as well as other environmental testing will be expanded and directed more to health risk measurement. Testing will often depend on remote sensing systems with information passing to the health and environmental authorities for analysis and interpretation. Food monitoring will obtain real-time input from laboratories in food processing facilities to monitor changes in the endemic distribution of organisms and the emergence of potential community pathogens or toxins. Recent initiatives by the federal government to stimulate public health laboratories to develop capabilities in biomonitoring promise to link environmental contaminants with disease states or precursors to disease. These capabilities have not been available previously except in narrow research projects involving small groups of heavily contaminated individuals. This area of testing is tailor-made for the public laboratory sector because many provide both medical and environmental testing at the present.

Committed to Quality Assessment

Local, state, and federal laboratories will be positioned to assist personal health care providers and various professional organizations in monitoring and improving laboratory performance. Reference specimens of interest will be processed as needed for disease monitoring by the public health testing system. Feedback to personal health care laboratories will provide an opportunity to ensure the quality of testing services in the private sector.

Devoted to Laboratory Improvement

Most regulation of personal health care and environmental laboratories will have been replaced by a system of practice guidelines and peer review through professional accreditation agencies. Local or regional public health laboratories will monitor proficiency and patient-testing outcomes with an emphasis on feedback and focused interventions, using practice sanctions as a last resort. Information on testing problems will be used to design training and other intervention strategies. Local or regional organizations will coordinate delivery of training through traditional and innovative distance-based learning methods. Affiliations with local community colleges, universities, laboratory training programs, and schools of public health will enhance available public- and private-sector resources. The model of quality assurance in laboratory testing developed in the United States and adopted in components of the International Standards Organization (ISO) is fostering progress in quality management in private and public laboratories. Public health laboratories at the federal, state, and local levels are involved in working with international colleagues in instituting policies and procedures that monitor and improve quality, and 15 state public health laboratories were directly involved in collaborative efforts to support quality systems in international projects.

Dedicated to Providing a Safety Net of Bottom-Line Assurance Testing

Some orphan tests that are too specialized for managed care plans will find a home in the public health system if there is a consensus on public benefits and cost-effectiveness of such testing. In some instances, local health agencies, because of their expertise in managing selected diseases (e.g., HIV, TB), will contract with the managed care plans to provide personal health care services. Laboratories will provide or arrange for needed support services for diagnosis and treatment as well as monitoring of these diseases and conditions.

Committed to Rapid Response and Research

In some jurisdictions, resources will be allocated to improve assessment methods. Research and development sections will seek improvements in operations as well as basic and applied assessment testing. These centers may be affiliated with universities or research institutes. In addition, United States public health laboratories will be an important resource in strengthening international laboratory capacity for early detection and effective response to global disease threats such as SARS and pandemic influenza in collaboration with the United States CDC and the WHO Center for Surveillance and Response.

SUMMARY

Individual public health laboratories are rapidly changing although a national consensus on a vision for the future of these critical organizations is not yet in focus. As infectious diseases of global significance continue to present risks from natural and deliberate sources, and challenges and demands on these institutions become more complex and critical, laboratory directors and managers are judged on their scientific knowledge and their ability to perform and supervise skilled analyses. As technology and competition change the laboratory industry, laboratory leaders must become competent system and information managers.

The challenge is to participate in the development of effective reporting systems that produce standardized information for disease reporting. The ability to understand the decision-making needs of clients and the programs they serve, the menu of available tests, and the test procurement options available from the industry is now an essential skill for laboratory services managers. This transition to "testing-and-information" managers will require a radical shift of thinking for many laboratory directors. Laboratory directors who view their role as one of providing a service rather than providing information for public health decision making will continue to play a minor role in their organizations. The capacity to balance and manage issues of turnaround time, cost of testing, analytic quality, and legal issues will be the benchmark of the effective laboratory information manager and director of the future.

REVIEW QUESTIONS

1. What are the core functions of public health laboratories?
2. What is the role of United States public health laboratories in global disease control efforts?
3. What is the purpose of the Clinical Laboratory Improvement Amendments Act of 1988?
4. How do public health laboratories differ from clinical laboratories?
5. How has the Public Health Emergency Preparedness Cooperative Agreement changed the United States public health laboratory system?
6. What is the major change predicted to occur in the public health laboratory system?

REFERENCES

1. Burke TA. Understanding environmental risk: The role of the laboratory in epidemiology and policy setting. *Clin Chem*. 1992;38:1519–1522.
2. Ferris DG, Fischer PM. Elementary school students' performance with two ELISA test systems. *JAMA*. 1992;268:766–770.
3. Inhorn SL, ed. *Quality Assurance Practices for Health Laboratories*. Washington, DC: American Public Health Association; 1978.
4. Valdiserri RO. Temples of the future: An historical overview of the laboratory's role in public health practice. *Annu Rev Public Health*. 1993;14: 635–648.
5. Schaeffer M, ed. *Federal Legislation and the Clinical Laboratory*. Boston, MA: GK Hall Medical Publishers; 1981.
6. Belk WP, Sunderman FW. A survey of the accuracy of chemical analysis in clinical laboratories. *Am J Clin Pathol*. 1947;17:853–861.
7. Shuey HE, Cabel J. Standards of performance in clinical laboratory diagnosis. *Bull US Army Medical Dept*. 1949;9:799–815.
8. *Clinical Laboratory Improvement Amendments of 1988; Final Rule*. Washington, DC: Dept of Health and Human Services, Health Care Financing Administration; February 28, 1992. Federal Register 57;40:7002–7288.

9. Kenney ML. Quality assurance in changing times: Proposals for reform and research in the clinical laboratory field. *Clin Chem.* 1987;33:728–736.

10. Clinical Laboratory Improvement Act of 1967. Washington, DC: US Dept of Health, Education, and Welfare; 1967. Code of Federal Regulations Title 42, Part 74.

11. Sweet CE. Effect of CLIA-88 on public health laboratories. *Clin Microbiol Newsletter.* 1993;15: 60–62.

12. Hausler WJ. Commentary by a state public health laboratory director. Paper presented at Session 1090 of the 121st Annual Meeting of the American Public Health Association: San Francisco, CA; October 25, 1993.

13. *Committee on Retrovirus Testing: Second Consensus Conference on Human Retrovirus Testing.* Washington, DC: Association of State and Territorial Public Health Laboratory Directors; 1987.

14. Centers for Disease Control and Prevention. Interpretation and use of the Western blot assay for serodiagnosis of human immunodeficiency virus type 1 infections. *MMWR.* 1989;38:1–7.

15. Gore MJ. Keeping up with changing times: How the National Laboratory Training Network helps. *Clin Lab Sci.* 1993;6:268–271.

16. APHL: Public Health Laboratories issues in Brief: State Public Health Laboratory Bioterrorism Capacity. Available at: http://www.aphl.org/programs/emergency_preparedness/Pages/default.aspx. Accessed May 2007.

17. Institute of Medicine, Committee for the Study of the Future of Public Health. *The Future of Public Health.* Washington, DC: National Academy Press; 1988.

18. Dowdle WR. The future of the public health laboratory. *Annu Rev Public Health.* 1993;14: 649–664.

19. Counts JM. LIFT 2000: Laboratory initiatives for the year 2000. *Clin Chem.* 1992;38: 1517–1518.

20. USDHEW. 1977. Consolidated Annual Report on State and Territorial Public Health Laboratories. Fiscal Year 1976. HEW Pub. No. (CDC) 77-811. Atlanta, GA; 30333.

21. U.S. Department of Health and Human Services. *Health People 2010.* Conference edition, in two volumes. Washington, DC: US Department of Health and Human Services; 2000.

22. Inhorn SL, Wilcke BW, Downes FP, Adjanor OO, Cada RL, Ford JR. A Comprehensive Laboratory Services survey of State Public Health Laboratories. *J. Public Health Management Practice.* 2006; 12;6:514–521.

23. Leonard DGB. The future of molecular genetic testing. *Clin Chem.* 1999;45:726–731.

24. Holtzman NA. Promoting safe and effective genetic tests in the United States: Work of the Task Force on Genetic Testing. *Clin Chem.* 1999; 45:732–738.

25. Lee PR, Toomey KE. Epidemiology in public health in the era of health care reform. *Public Health Rep.* 1994;109:1–3.

26. American Public Health Association. APHA's vision: public health and a reformed health care system. *Nation's Health.* July 1993:9,11.

CHAPTER 30

Global Health

Alfredo E. Vergara, MS, PhD and Sten H. Vermund, MD, PhD

LEARNING OBJECTIVES

Upon completion of this chapter, the reader will be able to:

1. Recognize the major health problems affecting populations around the globe and their relative importance.

2. Explain basic global and regional health indicators as well as the Millennium Development Goals.

3. Explain principal differences in health problems among low-, middle-, and high-income countries, and the significance of the epidemiologic transition from infectious to chronic diseases.

4. Describe at least two important features of the epidemiology of HIV/AIDS, malaria, tuberculosis, sexually transmitted infections, vaccine preventable diseases, diarrheal diseases, acute respiratory infections, and maternal, child, and reproductive health.

5. Define neglected tropical diseases and emerging infectious diseases, and describe their significance.

6. Describe key constraints in addressing global health problems.

7. Appreciate the chronic global inequities in health care financing and health manpower distribution.

8. Understand the concept of task shifting to accommodate such challenges as HIV care in rural areas, male circumcision to reduce the efficiency of HIV transmission, and primary care in rural areas.

KEY TERMS

Barefoot Doctor

Brain Drain

Demographic and Health Surveys

Disability Adjusted Life Years (DALYs)

Disinhibition

Drug Resistance

Emerging Infectious Diseases

Epidemic

Epidemiological Transition

Family Planning

Female Genital Mutilation

Global Health

Hygiene

International Health

Mother-to-Child Transmission

Multidrug-Resistant TB (MDR-TB)

Multiple Indicator Cluster Surveys

Neglected Tropical Diseases (NTDs)

Pandemic

Severe Acute Respiratory Syndrome (SARS)

Stunting

Syndromic Detection and Management

Task Shifting

Tropical Medicine

Voluntary Counseling and Testing (VCT) for HIV

At the beginning of the twentieth century, the terms **hygiene** and **tropical medicine** were highlighted approaches to health problems in developing countries, characterized at the time by concerns of empire-building, colonization, and economic exploitation. The term *public health* was in vogue by the mid-twentieth century as a broader, generic term that highlighted preventive strategies to environmental, occupational, dietary, lifestyle, infectious, and other risks that might be avoided or mediated. By the 1960s, organizations such as the Rockefeller Foundation began to use the term *geographic medicine*, acknowledging that diseases requiring special expertise in control and prevention can occur in diverse zones, even if they have high hygienic standards (West Nile virus in New York City is a recent example) or are not in the tropics per se (e.g., trichinellosis among Inuit persons in the sub-Arctic). Paradoxically, the Rockefeller Foundation supported the creation of schools of public health administratively *apart* from medical schools and later supported divisions of geographic medicine on the express condition that they be located *within* medical schools. Later in the twentieth century, the word "medicine" gave way (again) to "health," acknowledging that prevention of disease by maintenance of health must be highlighted as a principal priority, and that health encompassed a broader swath of issues than those covered by the medical paradigm. **International health** departments or divisions arose both in schools of public health and medicine, and nursing schools developed international health certificate programs. Veterinarians, pharmacists, dentists, optometrists, and many other health professions began to highlight those aspects of their professions that needed special consideration in developing country settings.

As we write in 2007, the term **global health** is in fashion, and for good reason. For example, rural health approaches in Appalachia, the Mississippi Delta, remote Alaska, or Native American reservations might apply to Africa, Asia, or Latin America, or vice versa. Global health recognizes the lure of the city for health care workers and the logistical challenges in both industrialized and developing country rural venues; incentives applied in one setting may have analogies in the other. If a "buddy system" helps a recovering alcoholic avoid drinking in Norway or New Zealand, maybe a buddy system will help an AIDS patient remember daily medications in Nigeria or Nepal. Acknowledging that exigencies of a global economy and travel can bring a passenger incubating an infectious disease from nearly any part of the world to any other venue in one to two days, in contrast to the months required a century ago on a clipper ship, the concept of global health has emerged to highlight our similarities as well as our differences. Global health also acknowledges that many nations are neither rich nor poor but are middle income (Table 30.1). Many of these nations have reduced mortality rates from infectious diseases but have seen rates rise for chronic diseases related to diet, exercise, smoking, lifestyle, and aging. Hence, global health applies to all of us and highlights the need to parse problems as to their unique or similar characteristics across the often artificial and arbitrary political borders that history has bequeathed us.

Table 30.1. The Diversity of Global Economies (Nations or Territories) as Represented by the World Bank (WB) and United Nations (UN) Economic Classifications by Income Group, as of July 2007

Key: HIPC: heavily indebted poor countries (WB)
       LDC: least developed countries (UN)
       OECD: Organization for Economic Co-operation and Development of the European Monetary Union
       Rep.:   Republic

Economy	World Bank-Defined Income Group	Economy	World Bank-Defined Income Group
Afghanistan	Low income: HIPC; LDC	Chad	Low income: HIPC; LDC
Albania	Lower middle income	Channel Islands	High income: non-OECD
Algeria	Lower middle income	Chile	Upper middle income
American Samoa	Upper middle income	China	Lower middle income
Andorra	High income: non-OECD	Colombia	Lower middle income
Angola	Lower middle income: LDC	Comoros	Low income: HIPC; LDC
Antigua and Barbuda	High income: non-OECD	Congo, Democratic Republic	Low income: HIPC; LDC
Argentina	Upper middle income	Congo, Republic of the	Lower middle income: HIPC
Armenia	Lower middle income	Costa Rica	Upper middle income
Aruba	High income: non-OECD	Côte d'Ivoire	Low income: HIPC
Australia	High income: OECD	Croatia	Upper middle income
Austria	High income: OECD	Cuba	Lower middle income
Azerbaijan	Lower middle income	Cyprus	High income: non-OECD
Bahamas, The	High income: non-OECD	Czech Republic	High income: OECD
Bahrain	High income: non-OECD	Denmark	High income: OECD
Bangladesh	Low income: LDC	Djibouti	Lower middle income: LDC
Barbados	High income: non-OECD	Dominica	Upper middle income
Belarus	Lower middle income	Dominican Republic	Lower middle income
Belgium	High income: OECD	Ecuador	Lower middle income
Belize	Upper middle income	Egypt, Arab Republic of	Lower middle income
Benin	Low income: HIPC; LDC	El Salvador	Lower middle income
Bermuda	High income: non-OECD	Equatorial Guinea	Upper middle income: LDC
Bhutan	Lower middle income: LDC	Eritrea	Low income: HIPC; LDC
Bolivia	Lower middle income: HIPC	Estonia	High income: non-OECD
Bosnia and Herzegovina	Lower middle income	Ethiopia	Low income: HIPC; LDC
Botswana	Upper middle income	Faeroe Islands	High income: non-OECD
Brazil	Upper middle income	Fiji	Lower middle income
Brunei Darussalam	High income: non-OECD	Finland	High income: OECD
Bulgaria	Upper middle income	France	High income: OECD
Burkina Faso	Low income: HIPC; LDC	French Polynesia	High income: non-OECD
Burundi	Low income: HIPC; LDC	Gabon	Upper middle income
Cambodia	Low income: LDC	Gambia, The	Low income: HIPC; LDC
Cameroon	Lower middle income: HIPC	Georgia	Lower middle income
Canada	High income: OECD	Germany	High income: OECD
Cape Verde	Lower middle income: LDC	Ghana	Low income: HIPC
Cayman Islands	High income: non-OECD	Greece	High income: OECD
Central African Republic	Low income: HIPC; LDC	Greenland	High income: non-OECD

Table 30.1. (*continued*)

Economy	World Bank-Defined Income Group	Economy	World Bank-Defined Income Group
Grenada	Upper middle income	Malawi	Low income: HIPC; LDC
Guam	High income: non-OECD	Malaysia	Upper middle income
Guatemala	Lower middle income	Maldives	Lower middle income: LDC
Guinea	Low income: HIPC; LDC	Mali	Low income: HIPC; LDC
Guinea-Bissau	Low income: HIPC; LDC	Malta	High income: non-OECD
Guyana	Lower middle income: HIPC	Marshall Islands	Lower middle income
Haiti	Low income: HIPC; LDC	Mauritania	Low income: HIPC; LDC
Honduras	Lower middle income: HIPC	Mauritius	Upper middle income
Hong Kong, China	High income: non-OECD	Mayotte	Upper middle income
Hungary	Upper middle income	Mexico	Upper middle income
Iceland	High income: OECD	Micronesia, Federated States of	Lower middle income
India	Low income		
Indonesia	Lower middle income	Moldova	Lower middle income
Iran, Islamic Republic of	Lower middle income	Monaco	High income: non-OECD
Iraq	Lower middle income	Mongolia	Low income
Ireland	High income: OECD	Montenegro	Upper middle income
Isle of Man	High income: non-OECD	Morocco	Lower middle income
Israel	High income: non-OECD	Mozambique	Low income: HIPC; LDC
Italy	High income: OECD	Myanmar	Low income: LDC
Jamaica	Lower middle income	Namibia	Lower middle income
Japan	High income: OECD	Nepal	Low income: HIPC; LDC
Jordan	Lower middle income	Netherlands	High income: OECD
Kazakhstan	Upper middle income	Netherlands Antilles	High income: non-OECD
Kenya	Low income	New Caledonia	High income: non-OECD
Kiribati	Lower middle income: LDC	New Zealand	High income: OECD
Korea, Democratic Republic of	Low income	Nicaragua	Lower middle income: HIPC
Korea, Republic of	High income: OECD	Niger	Low income: HIPC; LDC
Kuwait	High income: non-OECD	Nigeria	Low income
Kyrgyz Republic	Low income: HIPC	Northern Mariana Islands	Upper middle income
Lao People's Democratic Rep.	Low income: LDC	Norway	High income: OECD
Latvia	Upper middle income	Oman	Upper middle income
Lebanon	Upper middle income	Pakistan	Low income
Lesotho	Lower middle income: LDC	Palau	Upper middle income
Liberia	Low income: HIPC; LDC	Panama	Upper middle income
Libya	Upper middle income	Papua New Guinea	Low income
Liechtenstein	High income: non-OECD	Paraguay	Lower middle income
Lithuania	Upper middle income	Peru	Lower middle income
Luxembourg	High income: OECD	Philippines	Lower middle income
Macao, China	High income: non-OECD	Poland	Upper middle income
Macedonia, Former Yugoslav Rep.	Lower middle income	Portugal	High income: OECD
		Puerto Rico	High income: non-OECD
Madagascar	Low income: HIPC; LDC	Qatar	High income: non-OECD

(*continued*)

Table 30.1. (*continued*)

Economy	World Bank-Defined Income Group	Economy	World Bank-Defined Income Group
Romania	Upper middle income	Syrian Arab Republic	Lower middle income
Russian Federation	Upper middle income	Tajikistan	Low income
Rwanda	Low income: HIPC; LDC	Tanzania	Low income: HIPC; LDC
Samoa	Lower middle income: LDC	Thailand	Lower middle income
San Marino	High income: non-OECD	Timor-Leste	Low income: LDC
São Tomé and Principe	Low income: HIPC; LDC	Togo	Low income: HIPC; LDC
Saudi Arabia	High income: non-OECD	Tonga	Lower middle income
Senegal	Low income: HIPC; LDC	Trinidad and Tobago	High income: non-OECD
Serbia	Upper middle income	Tunisia	Lower middle income
Seychelles	Upper middle income	Turkey	Upper middle income
Sierra Leone	Low income: HIPC; LDC	Turkmenistan	Lower middle income
Singapore	High income: non-OECD	Tuvalu	Not listed by World Bank; LDC
Slovak Republic	Upper middle income	Uganda	Low income: HIPC; LDC
Slovenia	High income: non-OECD	Ukraine	Lower middle income
Solomon Islands	Low income: LDC	United Arab Emirates	High income: non-OECD
Somalia	Low income: HIPC; LDC	United Kingdom	High income: OECD
South Africa	Upper middle income	United States	High income: OECD
Spain	High income: OECD	Uruguay	Upper middle income
Sri Lanka	Lower middle income	Uzbekistan	Low income
St. Kitts and Nevis	Upper middle income	Vanuatu	Lower middle income: LDC
St. Lucia	Upper middle income	Venezuela, Rep. Bolivariana de	Upper middle income
St. Vincent and the Grenadines	Upper middle income	Vietnam	Low income
Sudan	Low income: HIPC; LDC	Virgin Islands (U.S.)	High income: non-OECD
Suriname	Lower middle income	West Bank and Gaza	Lower middle income
Swaziland	Lower middle income	Yemen, Republic of	Low income: LDC
Sweden	High income: OECD	Zambia	Low income: LDC
Switzerland	High income: OECD	Zimbabwe	Low income

NOTES: Four principal classifications are used by the World Bank: Low, lower middle, upper middle, and high-income economies. Among high-income countries, European Monetary Union (OECD) members are highlighted. The World Bank further classifies 41 low-income countries as "heavily indebted poor countries (HIPC)." In an independent evaluation of economic development, the United Nations has a special category of "least developed countries (LDC)" based on three criteria:

1. Three-year average estimate of the gross national income (GNI) per capita (under $750 for inclusion, above $900 for graduation)
2. Human resource weakness based on a Human Assets Index (HAI) with four indicators: (a) nutrition; (b) health; (c) education; and (d) adult literacy
3. Economic vulnerability, based on a Economic Vulnerability Index (EVI) with six indicators: (a) instability of agricultural production; (b) instability of exports of goods and services; (c) economic importance of nontraditional activities (share of manufacturing and modern services in gross domestic product); (d) merchandise export concentration; and (e) handicap of economic smallness (as measured through the population in logarithm); and (f) percentage of population displaced by natural disasters.

SOURCE: Adapted from World Bank. The World Bank Data and Statistics: Country Classification, 2008.

WORLD POPULATION AND HEALTH

Of the factors affecting health, population density is an important but neglected aspect. Population density is closely tied to food and nutrition, water and sanitation, environmental contamination, access to health services, and general socio-economic well being. All of these factors have a direct link to the health of individuals and populations. In fact, much historical evidence describes the collapse of early societies after reaching a particular population size that could not be supported by the particular environment where they lived. Often the point at which collapse began, or the speed at which it developed depended on the richness or depletion of natural resources and on the ability of that society to interact positively (trade, mutual support, and exchange of goods and services) as opposed to negatively (war, isolation, and destructive competition for resources). Modern societies that are in a similar crisis include Bangladesh and Haiti where the local population may be too large for the land and resources available. Megacities, including Mexico City, Sao Paolo, Lagos, Nairobi, Mumbai, Shanghai, and many others, have far outstripped their infrastructures and face serious and chronic health and environmental challenges. Even Los Angeles, Phoenix, Las Vegas, and elsewhere in the arid southwest United States may encounter an analogous, if qualitatively different crisis if its population rise continues unabated, outstripping water and energy resources.

Today's global society has prompted the development of interactions among cities, countries, ethnic groups, and other natural groupings of people that are much closer, frequent, complex, and varied, among very different groups of people. Migration of people, resources, and information have become much easier, and as a result, disease agents turn up in populations or places where they were not living before, or they cause disease at rates higher than before. Tropical diseases turn up in regions with temperate climates transported by a host (or even a hitchhiking mosquito vector) who travel faster than the incubation period, resulting, for example, in malaria cases in London or Tokyo or New York. Environmental pollution and waste is exported for economic reasons or produced more rapidly and at greater levels, creating, for example, the unhealthy air quality of many megacities and beyond around the world. Lifestyles that may be detrimental to our health are enhanced via mass media, telecommunications, and transportation, such as increasing high-risk sexual activity associated with alcohol consumption in commercial transport corridors.

Our global ability to eradicate or control certain disease **epidemics** is hindered by the resource limitations. Less wealthy countries have poorer infrastructures (roads, hospitals, schools, communication systems), human resource pools limited in numbers or specialized capacity, and few financial resources to compensate for those deficiencies. Such nations are at a disadvantage in their abilities to implement strategies to control or eradicate disease. Examples include the difficulties in controlling the HIV **pandemic** in sub-Saharan Africa or including more costly vaccines for *Haemophilus influenzae* type B and pneumococcus in childhood vaccine schedules in low- and middle-income countries.

Wealth and density of populations do not predict health in a perfect correlation, however. There are rich countries that do not distribute their wealth equitably and underinvest in their health sectors. Among the globe's most dramatic examples is the small, oil-rich, medium-to-low population density nation of Equatorial Guinea that continues to languish on the United Nations list of Least Developed Countries despite its upper-middle income classification by the World Bank (refer to Table 30.1). Life expectancy in this small central African nation is only 42.3 years, and its infant mortality rate is 123/1000 live births in the context of one of the highest gross domestic products in the region.[2] HIV does not explain this, as Equatorial Guinea has an HIV rate of 3.2 percent in persons aged 15–49 years, far lower than other sub-Saharan countries whose trends toward worsening health indices are being driven by HIV. A second example of a "disconnect" is the difficulty in eradicating polio from northern India and northern Nigeria, while even more resourced-limited settings have accomplished regional elimination of transmission. Suboptimal progress in polio eradication has not been due to resource limitations but rather to regional rumor mongering that Christians (in Kano State, Nigeria) and Hindus (in Uttar Pradesh State, India) are trying to harm Muslim infants with the vaccine.

A third example of inconsistent correlation of crowding and wealth with health status is that of Western Europe. In a positive model of planning and resource distribution, the European democracies have coped with the serious potential consequences of overcrowding through urban planning, mass transportation, social safety nets, and maintenance of high public health standards.

In addition to the more traditional effects of poverty on health, some interesting transitions are reflected in global statistics. Even though overall childhood mortality has improved over the past 10 years, gaps within countries remain high and continue to be major sources of inequality; children of the poorest and least-educated parents have the highest mortality rates regardless of what nation is being studied. "Transitions" from previously dominant infectious to more prevalent chronic diseases are notable in middle-income countries but are also beginning to be seen in many parts of lower-income countries.[3]

MEASURES OF GLOBAL BURDEN OF DISEASE AND INDICATORS OF PROGRESS

The Global Burden of Disease Project (GBDP) began in 1990, commissioned by the World Bank to provide a comprehensive assessment of disease burden (from a list of more than 100 diseases and injuries) and risk factors (a list of 10 selected risk factors).[4] GBDP used time-based measures of premature mortality (Years of Life Lost [YLL]) and disability (Years of Life lived with Disability [YLD], weighted by disability type). The sum of the two measures is known as **Disability Adjusted Life Years (DALYs),** designed to describe disease burden far more comprehensively than crude or adjusted death rates can. Death rates from the GBDP in children and adults around the world are shown in Figures 30.1 and 30.2, respectively.[5]

In 2005, a World Health Organization (WHO) group estimated that 73 percent of the 10.6 million child (<5 years of age) annual deaths worldwide were from 1 of 6 causes: pneumonia, diarrhea, malaria, neonatal sepsis, preterm delivery, and asphyxia at birth.[6] Infant mortality rates (IMRs) are ≤5.0/1000 live births in 20 of 27 countries with available 2005 estimates (3 missing) in the Organization for Economic Co-operation and Development, a 30-nation list of the European Community and such other nations as Australia, Canada, Japan, and the United States.[7] Among 221 countries and territories listed in *The World Fact Book*, IMRs vary enormously (Table 30.2).[8] Oil-rich Angola is not even considered a low-income country by the World Bank (refer to Table 30.1), yet it has the worst estimated IMR in the world in 2007; more than 60 Angolan infants under age 1 die for every infant who dies in Hong Kong or Singapore (Table 30.2). In low-income countries, malaria, diarrheal diseases, respiratory infections, and other infectious and parasitic diseases account for about 80 percent of all child deaths. In sub-Saharan Africa, the single most important cause of death for children is likely malaria, and the malaria-specific death rate may have risen since 1990. Overall, among middle- and low-income countries, significant reductions in childhood mortality have been observed in Latin America, Middle East, North Africa, and South Asia comparing 1990 to 2001, but comparably little progress has been made in sub-Saharan Africa and in the East Asia and the Pacific region.

In 2001, almost half the estimated disease burden in low- and middle-income countries was from noncommunicable diseases, having increased in sub-Saharan Africa and the low- and middle-income countries of Europe and Central Asia between 1990 and 2001.[5] Ischemic heart disease and stroke were the leading causes of death, constituting about 20 percent of all deaths in high-income, middle-, and

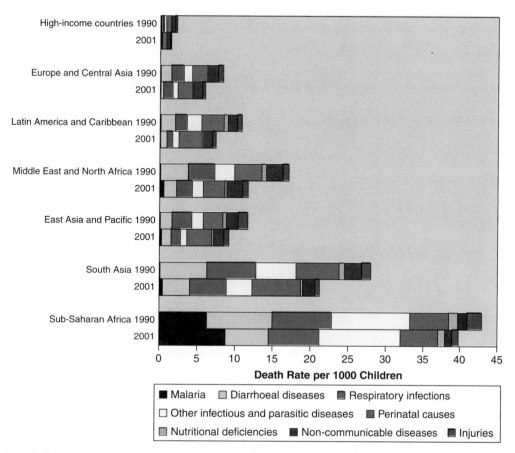

Figure 30.1. Death Rates by Disease Group and Region in 1990 and 2001 for Children Aged 0–4 Years

Cause-specific death rates for 1990 estimated from Murray and Lopez might not be completely comparable to those for 2001 because of changes in data availability and methods, plus some approximations in mapping 1990 estimates to the 2001 regions East Asia and Pacific, South Asia, and Europe and Central Asia. For all geographical regions, high-income countries excluded and shown as single group at top of graph. The geographical regions therefore refer to low-and-middle-income countries only. Reprinted with permission from Elsevier.

SOURCE: Reprinted from Nat Med, Lopez AD, Murray CC, The global burden of disease, 4:1241–3, © 1998, with permission from Elsevier.

low-income countries. In low- and middle-income countries, 5 of the 10 leading causes of death continue to be infectious in origin: respiratory infections, HIV/AIDS, diarrheal diseases, tuberculosis, and malaria. Excluding HIV/AIDS, 97 percent of deaths from communicable diseases, maternal and perinatal conditions, or nutritional deficiencies, occurred in low- and middle-income countries. Among adolescents and adults 15–59 years old, the distinctions in death rates are notable for different

country income levels and world regions. In high-income countries, death rates are almost entirely due to cardiovascular disease, cancer, other non-communicable diseases, and injuries. In many middle-income countries, notably much of eastern Europe, Central Asia, Latin America, the Caribbean, the Middle East, and North Africa, death rates from infectious diseases, maternal and perinatal conditions, or nutritional deficiencies represent no more than 20 percent of total mortality. The brunt of

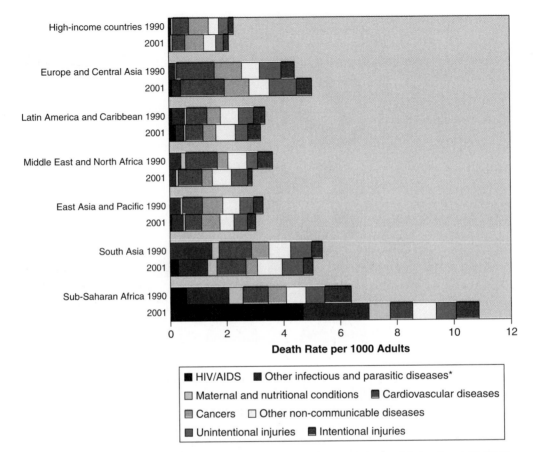

Figure 30.2. Death Rates by Disease Group and Region in 1990 and 2001 for Adults Aged 15–59 Years

*Includes respiratory infections. Cause-specific death rates for 1990 estimated from Murray and Lopez might not be completely comparable to those for 2001 because of changes in data availability and methods, plus some approximations in mapping 1990 estimates to the 2001 regions East Asia and Pacific, South Asia, and Europe and Central Asia. For all geographical regions, high-income countries excluded and shown as single group at top of graph. The geographical regions therefore refer to low-and-middle-income countries only. Reprinted with permission from Elsevier.

SOURCE: Reprinted from Nat Med, Lopez AD, Murray CC, The global burden of disease, 4:1241–3, © 1998, with permission from Elsevier.

mortality is due to chronic diseases and injuries. In dramatic contrast, in most low-income countries, most notably most of sub-Saharan Africa and parts of south/southeast Asia, >70 percent of mortality is due to infectious diseases, maternal and perinatal conditions, and nutrition deficiencies. Sub-Saharan Africa is further beleaguered with an unprecedented historic event, namely the HIV/AIDS epidemic. HIV/AIDS has reversed the gains in mortality

reduction and increased life expectancy of the past 40–50 years in high prevalence areas of southern Africa. Sub-Saharan Africa as a whole experienced a 9-fold rise in AIDS-specific mortality rates from 1990 to 2001.[5]

The role of clean water and sanitation, food and nutrition, education and literacy, and quality health services on individual and population health outcomes has been obvious to health workers, public

Table 30.2. Of 221 Countries and Territories, the 10 Highest and the 10 Lowest Infant Mortality Rate (IMR, Deaths in Children <1 Year of Age per 1000 Live Births) Estimates from 2007, *The World Fact Book*, Central Intelligence Agency

Country	IMR
Highest 10 IMR nations (9 Africa, 1 Asia)	
Angola	184.4
Sierra Leone	158.3
Afghanistan	157.4
Liberia	149.7
Niger	116.8
Somalia	113.1
Mozambique	109.9
Mali	105.7
Guinea-Bissau	103.5
Chad	102.1
Lowest 10 IMR nations (7 Europe, 3 Asia)	
Czech Republic	3.9
Malta	3.8
Norway	3.6
Finland	3.5
France	3.4
Iceland	3.3
Hong Kong	2.9
Japan	2.8
Sweden	2.8
Singapore	2.3

SOURCE: CIA. Rank Order-Infant Mortality Rate CIA Factbook.Washington DC: CIA; 2007.

health authorities, and governments for much of the twentieth century. However, in spite of decades of joint efforts from wealthy and poor nations, in concert with the UN and other international organizations, progress in the improvement of all these factors on health status and economic development was very slow for dozens of countries around the globe. At the UN Millennium Summit in September 2000, all 189 member countries signed a Millennium Declaration that outlined a new approach, committing governments and intergovernmental institutions to focused international cooperation

on eight Millennium Development Goals (MDGs). This commitment was a rare quantitative commitment by the international community in that all UN member states agreed to the MDGs as a joint framework for action to improve the human condition. Timetables are in place for achieving goals on measurable indicators within multiple mutually reinforcing development goals.[9]

The following sectors are measured to judge progress toward achieving MDGs: Economy, Education, Environment, Health, Information and Communication, Nutrition, and Women. The eight goals themselves are the following:

1. Eradicate extreme poverty and hunger.
2. Achieve universal primary education.
3. Promote gender equality and empower women.
4. Reduce child mortality.
5. Improve maternal health.
6. Combat HIV/AIDS, malaria, and other diseases.
7. Ensure environmental sustainability.
8. Develop a global partnership for development.

The many "measurable indicators" or targets being measured for health are to be achieved by 2015 for each goal and can be reviewed online.[10] The MDGs are a diverse set of indicators, some qualitative and others quantitative. Some focus on inputs, and some on outcomes. Some have measurable targets, though others do not. In addition, some targets are defined relative to unknown starting points, most focus on national averages rather than minimum standards for groups or regions, and some goals still need to be mapped into indicators that can be monitored. Although the MDGs do not cover all the health issues relevant to populations around the globe, they nonetheless address issues that affect a significant portion of the populations in developing countries and have helped galvanize interest in truly making a difference. MDG goals to prevent women from dying during childbirth, to protect young children from ill health and death, and to tackle the major communicable diseases, in particular HIV/AIDS and malaria, seek to use currently available knowledge and technology to scale up programs that we can and should implement.

DISEASES OF MAJOR IMPACT IN LOW- AND MIDDLE-INCOME COUNTRIES

Global health is a vast topic. This chapter can only provide an introduction. Given the continuing failure in disease control and prevention, it is an important part of global health to understand key elements of such diseases and their control strategies.

HIV/AIDS

The term "acquired immunodeficiency syndrome" (AIDS) was adopted by the CDC in 1982 after a rapidly growing epidemic of unusual symptoms and diseases was uncovered in 1981 among men who had sex with men and among injecting drug users. Soon thereafter, children of parents with risk factors and recipients of blood or blood products were also reported with AIDS, the disease was documented in the Caribbean and in Africa, and Europeans noted the same syndrome, notable for its high case fatality rates and characteristic links to sex, injected drugs, and blood or needle exposure. A human retrovirus was discovered in 1983 by the Pasteur Institute and was soon linked clearly to AIDS by investigators at the United States National Institutes for Health (NIH). By 1986, it was named human immunodeficiency virus (HIV) to avoid nomenclature confusion. For three decades, the number of cases around the world has been increasing rapidly, even exponentially, after introduction into vulnerable populations. This global rise in incidence continues even as death rates in western nations have fallen due to highly active antiretroviral therapies based on drugs licensed since 1987.[11-13] Benefits of antiretroviral therapy

are now reaching low-income country nations, albeit slowly, through such initiatives as the Global Fund to Fight AIDS, Tuberculosis, and Malaria and the President's Emergency Plan for AIDS Relief.[13-15] The global epidemic, termed a pandemic given its spread across continents, has resulted in the creation of thousands of local, regional, national, and international organizations to combat its spread and facilitate its care and treatment, among them UNAIDS.

An estimated 39 million (33 million–46 million) people worldwide were living with HIV in 2005, and an estimated 4.1 million became newly infected with HIV that year. UNAIDS and WHO further estimated that 2.8 million lost their lives to HIV disease in 2005. Although slightly more than one-tenth of the world's population lives in sub-Saharan Africa, it is home to 63 percent (24.5 million) of all people living with HIV.[16] In sub-Saharan Africa, the epidemics are "generalized," defined as having prevalence >1 percent; the main mode of transmission is heterosexual sexual contact. The epidemic in Africa is highly diverse and is especially severe in southern Africa. The prevalence rates of HIV infection in southernmost African countries range between 15 and 38 percent. Only the plague in fourteenth century Europe and pandemic influenza in the twentieth century rival HIV for single-organism devastation; both these were self-limiting, while HIV is a chronic infection such that many transmissions can occur, over many years, prior to the death of the index case. In fact, stable prevalence and incidence suggests that HIV is now endemic in much of the world and is in epidemic expansion only in some regions.

After sub-Saharan Africa, the Caribbean has the second highest prevalence rate for HIV infection with an estimated adult prevalence rate of 3–4 percent in the most afflicted nation, Haiti, and the exception of Cuba with an estimated adult prevalence of 0.1 percent.[17] By the end of 2005, UNAIDS estimated that 8.3 million people were living with HIV in Asia, at least two-thirds of whom lived in India. HIV prevalence has been declining in four states in India, Cambodia, and Thailand, likely due to successes in prevention. However, HIV prevalence is increasing in China, Indonesia, Papua New Guinea, and Vietnam, among others. The sudden and steep rise in HIV seroincidence among injection drug users (IDUs) in Pakistan stimulated an entire issue of the *Journal of Pakistan Medical Association* to be devoted to HIV/AIDS in 2006.[18] Ukraine and the Russian Federation have the worst AIDS epidemics in all of Europe, attributable largely to IDU and subsequent sexual spread. Increased transmission is noted among men who have sex with men (MSM), particularly those from minority populations and younger ages, in the United States and some countries in Europe, with evidence of largely hidden epidemics among MSMs in Latin America and Asia.[19]

As of 2005, 92 percent of HIV-infected persons lived in developing nations, up from an estimated 84 percent of the total in 1991. The epidemics in Western Europe and North America have stabilized since the late 1980s, with approximately the same number of new infections as deaths from AIDS each year until falling death rates were noted in the late 1990s due to highly active antiretroviral therapy. Now, industrialized countries have rising prevalence rates in the face of relatively stable incidence, due to longer life spans of persons on therapy. In contrast, incidence rates continue to remain high or rise in many middle- and low-income countries; as drug treatment is expanded, the numbers of people living with HIV will rise both as a consequence of incident infections and the life-prolonging effects of antiretroviral therapy.[20] Successes of "abstinence, be faithful, condom (ABC)" programs in Uganda and Thailand have resulted in a substantial reduction in incidence in both nations, a success not yet replicated at the national level elsewhere.[21,22] The pediatric HIV epidemic has been reduced massively in high-income countries through the use of **voluntary counseling and testing (VCT)** among pregnant women and antiretroviral prophylaxis for HIV-infected women and their newborns.[23] However, coverage is too low in developing countries, and **mother-to-child transmission** of HIV continues at high rates.[24,25]

The major route of HIV transmission worldwide is heterosexual sex, with special concern for sex workers, although risk factors for transmission vary within and across populations. In many regions of the world, men who have sex with men (MSM) and injection drug users (IDU) account for significant proportions of infections. Even in the United States, thought of as a relatively low-prevalence nation, HIV continues as a major public health problem due to a relatively constant HIV incidence of about 45,000 cases/year, a rising number of persons living with HIV/AIDS (>1 million), inability of all persons to access testing or care, and high HIV/AIDS prevalence among MSM and IDU.[26] IDU incidence rates have fallen markedly, likely due to clean needle and syringe exchange programs instituted through community activism in the face of a continuing federal government funding ban.[27–31]

Women represent almost half (48%) of all adults living with HIV/AIDS globally. By the end of 2005, 17.5 million women worldwide were infected with HIV according to the WHO estimates. The proportion of AIDS cases in women in 2005 was more than three times that in 1988. In sub-Saharan Africa, women represent more than half (59%) of all adults living with HIV/AIDS, and, on average, 3 adolescent women are infected for every adolescent man. In the Caribbean, young women are more than twice as likely to be infected with HIV compared to young men in countries such as Haiti, Guyana, and Jamaica, where heterosexual transmission is driving the epidemic.[32] Women are particularly vulnerable to heterosexual transmission of HIV due to biological risk related to mucosal exposure to infected seminal fluids, cervical ectopy, genital inflammation and ulcers, and other factors, not all of which are understood fully. Gender inequalities in sexual decision making, social status, and economic empowerment can increase women's vulnerability to HIV and even diminish access to prevention and care services. Sexual violence may also increase women's risk; young women are biologically more susceptible to HIV infection than men.[33]

Under-five child mortality rates have risen at historically unprecedented rates in sub-Saharan Africa due to HIV/AIDS (Figure 30.3). HIV-related demands have stretched the capacity of existing

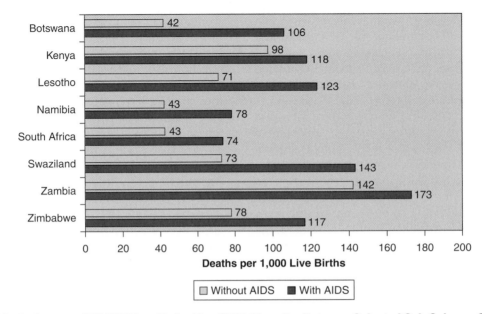

Figure 30.3. Impact of HIV/AIDS on Under-Five Child Mortality Rates on Selected Sub-Saharan Countries, 2002–2005, from UNAIDS Estimates

SOURCE: UNAIDS. Report on the global AIDS epidemic. Geneva: UNAIDS; 2006.

programs in antenatal care, oral rehydration, safe water, and immunization programs. As a result of increased adult mortality, the number of children orphaned by AIDS has increased steadily.[34,35] Exclusive breastfeeding is recommended for infants whose mothers do not have clean water and replacement feeding access; research is in progress to see whether prophylactic antiretroviral therapy may protect breastfeeding infants from HIV infection.

A review of HIV prevention and HIV research is beyond this chapter's scope, but the reader is referred to recent publications cited here. Vaccine and microbicide clinical trials have been disappointing to date, and neither modality is expected to be relevant for HIV prevention in the immediate future.[36–39] Although condom effectiveness is high, the intravaginal diaphragm did not protect women any better than condoms did in a Zimbabwe trial.[40–42] Male circumcision has proven to reduce HIV incidence by about 50 percent, although global expansion of circumcision services has been minimal since the first positive trial was published

in 2005.[43–45] The clinical trials confirmed earlier epidemiological observations and corrected for potential confounding factors such as religion and sexual practices.[46]

Prevention programs for sexual transmission are rooted in "ABC" programs, whether for MSM or heterosexuals, though the difficulty is in their implementation, uptake, and adherence. Abstinence-only programs have not demonstrated efficacy in richer countries and have not been reviewed systematically in developing countries.[47] Prevention of noninjection illicit drug use and alcohol abuse could improve success of ABC programs as well as having myriad other benefits. Opiate agonist-based treatment and needle exchange programs target IDU. Contingency management and "12-step" programs are among the approaches that can help reduce drug and alcohol-mediated sexual risk, although research is inconclusive to date.[48,49]

Global efforts to control HIV/AIDS depend on VCT for HIV as an essential entry point for risk-reduction education, perinatal transmission prevention, and appropriate care and treatment for infected persons.[50,51] As successful provision of antiretroviral medications and maternal/nursing adherence can prevent mother-to-child HIV transmission, VCT and referral to care and treatment with risk-reduction counseling can reduce transmission risk to sexual partners.[52] Expansion of antiretroviral therapy is expected to reduce the infectiousness of HIV-infected persons as plasma load correlates with genital viral load, albeit imperfectly. Lower plasma viral load is associated with lower HIV transmission.[53,54] However, **disinhibition** (sometimes termed "risk compensation") may result in paradoxical increased community risks, as when an HIV-infected person on therapy reduces condom use or increases the number of sexual partners [55,56] In other words, it is not yet established whether expanded treatment of HIV-infected persons will reduce or increase community HIV transmission due to reduced infectiousness or increased life expectancy and sexual risk taking, respectively. This underscores the importance of risk-reduction counseling among HIV-infected persons who are in care and may be on antiretroviral treatment.

As attention has been paid to the global HIV epidemic, the obvious shortage of qualified health care workers to cope with the magnitude of the clinical and public health need is apparent. **Task shifting** refers to less qualified health staff taking on the traditional duties of higher trained staff in an effort to cope with this workforce shortage. Practical training substitutes for formal medical training and workers take on the duties of unavailable physicians, nurses, pharmacists, and laboratory technicians, among others. Less optimistic predictions have been made as to the likely success of task shifting for antiretroviral therapy (ART) in Africa.[57,58] Nonetheless, the idea that physicians and nurses can be provided to every rural community needing primary care is fanciful; an emphasis on task shifting is prudent to provide broader care to rural populations. Task shifting must be accompanied by reform in drug availability and distribution, public health and clinical infrastructure investments, and appropriate training and upgrading of rural working conditions in the health sector.

Malaria

An estimated 350–500 million clinical malaria episodes occur annually around the globe, most caused by infection with *Plasmodium falciparum* and *P. vivax*.[59] About 60 percent of the cases of malaria worldwide, 75 percent of global falciparum malaria cases, and >80 percent of malaria deaths occur in sub-Saharan Africa. *P. falciparum* causes the vast majority of infections and deaths in this region, including about 18 percent of deaths in children under 5 years of age.[59] In high-transmission endemic settings in sub-Saharan Africa, 12 children per 1000 can die as a result of malaria infection each year.[60] Falciparum malaria cases account for 1–2 million deaths per year (some estimates are even higher) and is a contributor to much morbidity and mortality in conjunction with other diseases and nutritional status, especially among children in resource-poor countries.[61] In such settings, poor nutrition, repeated infections, and socioeconomic factors create a vicious cycle that can have adverse health effects continuing across generations. For example, premature children are at risk of early death or may survive and experience poor growth and development, which may result in **stunting** and being underweight during adolescence. This places young women at risk of, in turn, delivering premature or low birth weight children. Under-nutrition and repeated infections contribute to this cycle by reducing overall well-being, such as anemia and micronutrient deficiencies, with subsequent poor pregnancy outcomes.[62] Malaria results in about 400,000 pregnant women developing moderate to severe anemia as a result of malaria infection each year.[63]

Patterns of malaria transmission and disease vary markedly between regions and even within individual countries. This diversity results from variations between malaria parasites and mosquito vectors, ecological conditions that affect malaria transmission and socioeconomic factors, such as poverty and access to effective health care and prevention services. Public health strategies for malaria prevention and control include early diagnosis and effective treatment (including artemisinin-based combination therapies for falciparum malaria and intermittent preventive treatment for pregnant women); use of insecticide-treated bednets; appropriate treatment with indoor residual spraying of insecticides, larvicides, and other environmental control of mosquitoes; and strengthening of surveillance and reporting systems.[64] The use of these strategies depends on the epidemiological setting (endemic areas, unstable areas of outbreaks, strength of the health system) and requires strong components of public health education. Asia has experienced a resurgence of vivax and falciparum malaria during the past 20 years, particularly in areas where conflict and complex emergencies have debilitated health systems. Vivax malaria resurged in Central Asia and Trans-Caucasia, and falciparum malaria re-emerged in Tajikistan during the 1990s.[59] Southeast Asia has the highest rate of **drug resistance** in the world for malaria.[59] Since 1998, when routine monitoring of drug resistance was established, countries have stepped up prevention and control through insecticide-treated bednets, indoor residual spraying, larvicide use, and improved surveillance; substantial success has been observed in reducing incidence and epidemics.[65] In the Americas, roughly two thirds of malaria cases are due to *P. vivax*, about 18 percent to *P. falciparum*, and the remainder to *P. malariae*; infection rates have remained relatively stable in endemic countries since the early 1990s. The rise of *P. falciparum* drug resistance has spurred a change in treatment regimes to artemisinin-based combination therapies, but chloroquine remains the treatment of choice for *P. vivax* and other species.[59]

In highly endemic African countries, malaria accounts for 25–35 percent of all outpatient visits, 20–45 percent of hospital admissions and 15–35 percent of hospital deaths, imposing a great burden on already fragile health care systems. Evidence suggests that persons infected with HIV should receive continuous malaria prevention and prompt treatment both to help persons not receiving HIV care and to avoid undercutting successes from new care and treatment initiatives where they are being scaled up.[66] Malaria contributes synergistically with HIV/AIDS to morbidity and mortality in areas where both infections are highly prevalent, such as in Africa south of the Sahara. In addition to providing immediate health benefits, prevention and treatment of malaria may lessen transient increases in HIV viral load during malaria episodes and thus help limit the progression and transmission of HIV.[67,68]

In 1998, partly in response to concerns about re-emergence and development of drug resistance, the WHO launched the Roll Back Malaria (RBM) Partnership. This partnership has grown substantially since its creation and now involves in addition to UN agencies, affected and donor countries, the private sector, NGOs, philanthropic, research, and academic institutions. One of its goals is to cut malaria mortality in half by 2010; increasing funding from donors was pledged in 2007 at the Group of 8 (G8) summit through the Global Fund to Fight AIDS, Tuberculosis, and Malaria. Provision of insecticide-impregnated bednets will be a vital component of any strategy, given the nocturnal biting patterns of anopheline mosquitoes.[69]

Acute and Chronic Diarrheal Diseases

About 2 million people die as a result of diarrheal diseases each year in the world.[69,70] Most of these are children under 5 years of age ("under-fives"), but an increasing number of immunocompromised persons such as those infected with HIV have emerged in the death statistics over time. The majority of diarrheal disease episodes improve without antimicrobial medications, given adequate rehydration therapy and adequate baseline nutritional status. However, diarrhea results in substantial mortality and morbidity in places where water is poor quality, undernutrition is prevalent, and oral rehydration access is limited.[71] Major pathogenic organisms involved in diarrheal disease around the world include bacteria, viruses, and parasites. Prevalent bacterial species include *Campylobacter*, *Shigella*, *Salmonella*, *Vibrio*, and *E. coli*. Enteroviruses include rotaviruses, Norwalk-like caliciviruses, astroviruses, and adenoviruses. Parasitic etiologies include *Giardia lamblia*, *Entamoeba histolytica*, *Cryptosporidium spp.*, and *Cyclospora cayetanensis*.[72] Differences in pathogenicity are marked with rotaviruses and *Shigella* having the highest indices of pathogenicity.[73] It is estimated that 94 percent (CI 84–98%) of the diarrheal disease burden in developing countries is due to preventable environmental factors such as water quality and that over 1 billion people around the world do not have access to improved water sources.[70,74]

Very simple practices such as frequent hand washing with soap, boiling water, and adequate water storage containers have been proven to reduce transmission of microorganisms that cause diarrhea.[75] But even these practices are difficult to implement in very low resource settings and generally require effective community and health care worker education effort. Recently, efforts have moved in the direction of providing simple technologies for water treatment at the point of use—the household—for disinfection and also to improve the taste and appearance of water, factors that have been found to affect the adoption of disinfection technologies.[70,76,77]

Breastfeeding newborn children is another practice that, in addition to strengthening the infant's immune system, protects it by reducing contact with potentially contaminated food or water.[75] Restricting breastfeeding of an HIV-infected mother to reduce mother-to-child transmission of HIV in sub-Saharan Africa is not advisable unless she has resources for safe replacement feeding; diarrheal and respiratory disease and infant mortality rise in the nonbreastfeeding infant even in enhanced circumstances.[78] An outbreak of diarrheal disease caused by flooding in Botswana in 2005 identified the highest mortality in HIV-infected, nonbreastfeeding infants, suggesting the complexity of policy in sub-Saharan Africa that does not encourage breastfeeding.[79] Diarrheal disease mortality, particularly in children, is also exacerbated by nutrition deficiencies that are more prevalent in developing countries. Zinc supplementation has been shown to reduce the rates and severity of diarrhea[80–82] and

pneumonia,[83,84] as well as reduce mortality rates in children under five years of age.[84–86] One study suggested that vitamin A and zinc were synergistic and superior to zinc alone for diarrheal disease risk reduction.[87] Although the impact on infant mortality is less clear from epidemiologic data, there is enough consensus to recommend zinc for treatment of diarrhea, as well as support appropriate dietary zinc intake and study potential zinc supplement interventions that could have an impact on mortality and health outcomes including low birth weight children.[85] Since vitamin A in appropriate, that is, not too high, doses is recommended for a number of other conditions, vitamin A and zinc supplementation should be routine for infants and children in developing countries.

Diarrheal disease treatment and vaccine development are beyond the scope of this chapter. The backbone of primary prevention is provision of clean water and appropriate disposal of human and animal waste. However, prevention of serious disease is achieved with prompt provision of oral rehydration with WHO/UNICEF-recommended 90 mmol/L of sodium and 111 mmol/L glucose concentrations.[88] This innovation has lead to a decline in global mortality in children due to diarrhea such that acute respiratory infection is now the number one cause of death in under-fives, due to the decline in diarrhea-related mortality secondary to oral rehydration programs. Vaccines are not widely available in developing countries for diarrheal diseases, although measles vaccine has reduced measles-related diarrhea markedly. Two new rotavirus vaccines are now licensed in various parts of the world after many trials in >110,000 children showed high efficacy without increased intussusception rates. RotaTeq™ (Merck & Co., Inc., USA) is a live, oral pentavalent vaccine that contains 5 live reassortant rotaviruses. The first dose is recommended at 6–12 weeks of age and a 3-dose series is needed. Rotarix™ (GlaxoSmithKline Biologicals, Belgium) is a 2-dose oral live attenuated viral vaccine that is given with the first dose after 6 weeks of age and the second at least 4 weeks later and ideally before 15 weeks of age.

Tuberculosis

Tuberculosis (TB) is a contagious disease that spreads via respiratory droplets. More than 2 billion persons globally (as many as 1 in 3) are infected with TB bacilli. Only people whose lesions leak into lung alveoli are infectious to others. Most TB-infected persons are not infectious. However, when infectious, an individual increases infection risk to others through casual respiratory routes, for example, coughing, sneezing, talking, or spitting. Although a person can be infected by inhalation of just a few organisms, risk is dose-related. Left untreated, the WHO estimates that each person with active TB disease will infect on average between 10–15 people in a year.[89] The WHO also estimates that a person is newly infected with TB bacilli every second. Only 5–10 percent of people who are infected with TB bacilli will get sick and be infectious during their lifetime; the human immune system walls off bacilli, which can then live in a quiescent state. Antibiotics for TB act on a replicating bacterium, so drugs must be administered for months to ensure cure.[90] TB is a respiratory-borne bacterium that is more rarely transmitted through the gastrointestinal route. The organism can invade a variety of organs and cavities; extra-pulmonary TB is more difficult to diagnose, typically, than pulmonary disease. The principal cause is *Mycobacterium tuberculosis*, though related mycobacterial pathogens (*M. bovis*, *M. kansasii*, and others) may cause disease variants. Although the populous South-East Asia Region accounted for 34 percent of incident cases estimated by the WHO in 2005, the estimated incidence rate in sub-Saharan Africa is nearly twice that of the South-East Asia Region, at nearly 350 cases per 100,000 population (Table 30.3). An estimated 1.6 million deaths occurred from TB in 2005.

Although TB medicines have only been available since the mid-twentieth century, strains that are resistant to at least one anti-TB drug have been documented in every country surveyed. **Multidrug-resistant TB** (MDR-TB) refers to organisms that are resistant to at least two of the best, first-line anti-TB drugs, isoniazid and rifampin. Extensively drug resistant TB (XDR-TB) is a less common type of MDR-TB, defined as TB that is resistant to isoniazid and rifampin, plus resistant to a fluoroquinolone

Table 30.3. **Estimated Global Tuberculosis Incidence, Prevalence, and Mortality in 2005**

| WHO region | Incidence of TB | | | | Prevalence of TB | | TB Mortality | |
| | All forms | | Smear-positive* | | | | | |
	No. in (1000s) (% of total)	per 100,000 pop	No. in (1000s)	per 100,000 pop	No. in (1000s)	per 100,000 pop	No. in (1000s)	per 100,000 pop
Africa	2529 (29)	343	1088	147	3773	511	544	74
The Americas	352 (4)	39	157	18	448	50	49	5.5
Eastern Mediterranean	565 (6)	104	253	47	881	163	112	21
Europe	445 (5)	50	199	23	525	60	66	7.4
South-East Asia	2993 (34)	181	1339	81	4809	290	512	31
Western Pacific	1927 (22)	110	866	49	3616	206	295	17
Global	**8811 (100)**	**136**	**3902**	**60**	**14052**	**217**	**1 577**	**24**

*Smear-positive cases are those confirmed by smear microscopy and are the most infectious cases.

SOURCE: WHO. Global Tuberculosis Control 2008: Surveillance, Planning, and Financing. Geneva: WHO; 2008.

NOTE: Pop indicates population.

and at least one of three injectable second-line drugs, that is, amikacin, kanamycin, or capreomycin.[92] Drug-resistant TB is caused by inconsistent or partial treatment, when patients do not take all their medicines regularly for the required period because they start to feel better, because physicians and health workers prescribe the wrong treatment regimens, or because the drug supply is unreliable.[93–95] Rates of MDR-TB are high in some countries, especially in the former Soviet Union, and threaten TB control efforts globally. MDR-TB is treatable with extended chemotherapy for up to two years with more costly second-line anti-TB drugs. Adverse drug reactions are more severe with second-line drugs, but these reactions can be managed with adequate health care.[96] Much can be done if global resources and expertise are mobilized.[97]

The WHO's Stop TB Strategy was launched in 2006 as a follow-up to the directly observed therapy-short course (DOTS) strategy promulgated since 1995. In just over a decade, >22 million patients have been treated via DOTS. The six components of the Stop TB Strategy are the following:

1. Pursuing high-quality DOTS expansion and enhancement
2. Addressing TB/HIV, MDR-TB and other challenges
3. Contributing to health system strengthening
4. Engaging all care providers
5. Empowering people with TB, and communities
6. Enabling and promoting research

By 2004, 183 countries (including the 22 high-burden countries that account for 80% of all cases) were implementing DOTS in varying degrees of success.

The WHO estimates that up to 50 percent of TB patients in sub-Saharan Africa are also HIV infected.[89] The foremost cause of death due to HIV in developing countries is TB, responsible for at least 13 percent, and perhaps ≥30 percent of all.[98] HIV-induced immunosuppression is a principal contributor to TB reactivation; about one-quarter of HIV cases in a Cambodian study in 2004–2005 had active TB.[99] Furthermore the problem is growing despite the antiretroviral therapy (ART) "roll-out" in developing countries for at least four reasons. First, there is a substantial lag in ART availability versus the clinical need. Second, the ongoing high incidence of HIV continually generates a cadre of newly at-risk persons. Third, the aging of already HIV-infected persons increases the risk of *M. tuberculosis* reactivation due to advancing immunosuppression. Fourth, there remain serious program limitations that inhibit application of what we already know how to do in control and prevention of both HIV and TB, for example, primary prophylaxis and directly observed therapy-short course (DOTS) approaches.[100] Fortunately, cost-effectiveness analyses support TB investments, and this has helped galvanize increased global funding.[101–106] Nonetheless, HIV and TB can be managed successfully because the principles for care do not differ substantially with co-infection, depending on appropriate diagnostics, drug availability, and infrastructure for long-term follow-up and drug distribution with community and family support.[107]

Acute Respiratory Infections

UNICEF estimates that pneumonias kill more children than HIV/AIDS, malaria, and measles combined, probably more than one in four child deaths when neonatal pneumonias are included (Figure 30.4). Pneumonia also contributes to substantial morbidity, as with diarrheal diseases and malaria, with >150 million episodes of pneumonia in children under 5 in developing countries. Only 5 percent of these cases occur in under-fives in industrialized countries. From 11–20 million children with pneumonia are hospitalized; South Asia and Sub-Saharan Africa account for over half of the total global pneumonia episodes in this age group. Most of this mortality is completely preventable.[108]

Acute respiratory infection (ARI) represents both upper- (e.g., throat, nasal passages, epiglottis) and lower airways (e.g., below the epiglottis). Lower ARIs include common and potentially severe lung infections such as pneumonia that compromise

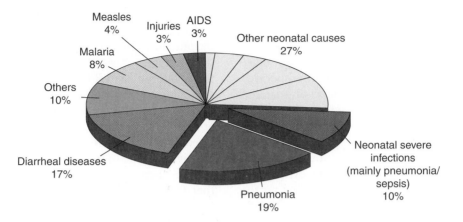

Figure 30.4. Global Distribution of Cause-Specific Mortality Among Children Under Age Five Years
SOURCE: WHO. Routine EPI Activities, 2007.

oxygenation. Syndromic management of pneumonia relies on identifying children with fever, cough, rapid breathing rates, and lower chest wall retraction during inhalation. Chest x-rays and microbiology laboratory availability are limited severely in most developing countries. National household surveys estimate pneumonia incidence rates based on maternal responses regarding whether children have experienced cough and fast or difficult breathing in the two weeks prior to the survey, as in **Demographic and Health Surveys** and **Multiple Indicator Cluster Surveys**.

Key prevention strategies include immunizing children against such common causes of pneumonia as measles, pneumococcus, and *H. influenzae* type B. The latter two are conjugate vaccines for pediatric use and are comparatively costly. New initiatives from the Bill & Melinda Gates foundation are trying to reduce the fiscal barriers, much as the Rotary Club International bought poliovirus vaccine for the global eradication campaign, enabling reinvestment of vaccine expenditures into infrastructure. Nutritional status is vital in helping a child weather respiratory illness, as with diarrheal diseases. Breastfeeding advocacy helps with both immunological and macronutrient status, whereas such supplements as zinc and vitamin A help build anti-infective capacities at both mucosal and systemic

levels. Environmental improvements can help children, particularly reducing indoor air pollution from tobacco or other types of smoking or cooking. HIV co-infection exacerbates incidence and severity of pneumonias, as it does with diarrhea and malaria.[109]

Excellent **syndromic detection and management** of pneumonia at a primary care level convenient to villages and neighborhoods can drop morbidity and mortality markedly, as is the case with diarrhea, malaria, and other scourges of poverty.[110] Timely treatment with a 5–10 day course of appropriate antibiotics is usually adequate because bacterial pneumonias are overrepresented in severe disease. Hence, health worker training is essential, as is a consistent and adequate supply of antibiotics suitable for childhood pneumonias. Physicians and nurses need not be the ones providing this care; basic training of community health workers can result in declines in pneumonia mortality when they are taught to diagnose and treat uncomplicated pneumonias with antibiotics, referring severe pneumonia patients to health facilities. "Lady Health Workers" manage ARIs in Pakistan, for example.[111] The now-defunct **"barefoot doctor"** system in China was a harbinger of the "task shifting" revolution in primary care; the Chinese rural primary care system resulted, with public health work and improved nutrition, in the rapid rise in life expectancy among the Chinese in the latter twentieth century.[112]

Mother and Child and Reproductive Health

In Chapter 26 in this book, mother and child health (MCH) issues are presented in detail, as are reproductive health and **family planning** issues. However, no chapter on global health can neglect to mention these pillars of prevention. Our presentations of acute respiratory infections, diarrhea, malaria, HIV, and vaccine-preventable diseases touch on key elements of child health. Nutritional management emphasizing breastfeeding, growth monitoring with simple prospective growth charts, injury prevention and counseling, and vaccination are among the preventive backbones of child health. Child health is inextricably tied to maternal health, especially in the first year of life. Good antenatal care, birthing practices, and post-partum care will start the infant on a healthy path. Breastfeeding is the most vital component of post-birth care, and any efforts to undermine this nutritional and immunological boon have proven disastrous. We discuss under-fives care in many other parts of this chapter. In an effort to reduce maternal–infant HIV transmission, UNAIDS, UNICEF, and the WHO have suggested implementation of a package with six components that one might generalize to benefiting mothers and infants, regardless of HIV risk per se.[113] These components of integrated mother and child care include the following:

1. Expansion and strengthening of family planning education and services, as well as HIV prevention activities

2. Early access to quality antenatal care from trained health-care workers

3. Voluntary counseling and HIV testing for women and their partners

4. Provision of antiretroviral medication to prevent HIV transmission from HIV-infected women to their babies

5. Improved care during labor, delivery, and the postpartum period

6. Counseling for HIV-positive women on infant feeding choices, making replacement feeding available when needed, and supporting women in all their feeding practices

Women's health in general, and during pregnancy in particular, may be neglected, in comparison to attention paid to children.[114] Pregnancy is a common and esteemed state for most women globally. Social and marital rejection and a loss of self-esteem are the unfortunate consequences of infertility in many societies. When pregnancy occurs, inadequate obstetric care for women who are often stunted from undernutrition results in maternal mortality ratios of >900 deaths per 100,000 live births in sub-Saharan Africa in contrast to rates <20 deaths per 100,000 live births in industrialized countries.[81] Consequences of dystocia (pelvic obstruction during childbirth) result from prolonged pressure of the fetal head in the pelvic canal and can be severe for those women who survive.[115] Vaginal fistulas are an all-too-common consequence of necrosis of the bladder wall from the prolonged pressure of a baby's head in the obstructed birth canal; fistulas result in chronic dribbling of urine through the vagina and chronic urinary tract infections, making women in many traditional societies pariahs in their own communities. Proper antenatal care and pregnancy management can prevent fistulas, but until this primary care function is upgraded, the global community needs to provide fistula care for women.[116] Access to cesarean section, when needed, can reduce maternal and infant mortality and morbidity and has been proven feasible even in rural settings.[117]

Female genital mutilation, especially the extreme "pharaonic infibulation" form, is designed to remove female sexual pleasure through removal of the clitoris and more. Its continuation has been steeped in strongly favorable social or religious traditions in the Sahel region and elsewhere.[118] Consequences include both immediate complications of hemorrhage, pain, fractures, increased risk of HIV transmission, infection, and shock, while later complications include keloid scars, dyspareunia (pain with intercourse), infection, ulcers, fistulas, and pregnancy complications; psychological problems from sexual dysfunction, loss of trust, and depression are reported.[119]

Family planning is an essential component of reproductive health services. Experience in resource-limited nations indicates that women must control their fertility if they are to maximize educational and health benefits to their wanted children. "Unmet need" refers to the circumstance when a woman wishes not to have more children but does not have access to family planning; unmet need is highly prevalent in such high fertility nations as Pakistan, indicating public health failures globally.[120] Oral contraception, depot hormone injections, diaphragms, intrauterine devices (IUDs), and tubal ligation have the advantage of being controlled by women themselves. Vasectomy, male condoms, and even female condoms require male cooperation and assent. Millennium Development Goals are being assessed, in part, on demographic, fertility, women's health, and child health goals.[121]

A neglected component of prevention of mother-to-child HIV prevention is facilitation of family planning for HIV-infected women who want it, to avoid having an unwanted child who may be HIV-infected.[122] Prevention of perinatal HIV transmission should be built on three elements: (1) primary prevention of HIV in women, (2) prevention of mother-to-child transmission of HIV with antiretroviral prophylaxis, and (3) strengthening of family planning services among HIV-infected women to prevent unplanned pregnancies.[122] Practitioner attitudes toward contraception can facilitate or impede women's access.[123]

Sexually Transmitted Infections

Sexually transmitted infections (STI) manifest with reproductive complications, liver disease (as with hepatitis B), immunologic collapse (as with HIV disease), and cancer (as with HPV). STI are more common in developing countries than where public health infrastructures are comparatively advanced.[124] HIV has been discussed earlier in the chapter. Infertility, ectopic pregnancy, facilitation of HIV

infection, and serious morbidity and even mortality can result from unrecognized, unremediated sexually transmitted infections. Adolescents are of particular concern for both biological and behavioral reasons.[125] Curable bacterial and parasitic infections include *Treponema pallidum* (syphilis), *Chlamydia trachomatis, Neisseria gonorrhoeae,* and *Trichomonas vaginalis.* All can be recognized syndromically to some degree, which is how diagnosis is made in the absence of laboratory testing capabilities.[126] Syphilis is often asymptomatic, but a simple serologic screen, such as the rapid plasma reagin test, is practical even in resource-limited settings that do not have microscopy or microbiology capabilities.[127] Contact tracing is an essential component of successful control programs globally, but such efforts are rare in developing countries.[128] Complications of curable STIs, sometimes complemented by consequences of past dystocia or genital mutilation/cutting, include high rates of infertility, ectopic pregnancy, and social rejection. Social rejection, in turn, drives some destitute and desperate women into sex work as has been noted with HIV stigma, exacerbating their health risks and social isolation. Although alleviation of poverty and female sexual exploitation would be most helpful, there are still many strategies for risk reduction that can prevent STIs even for women continuing sex work.[129] Sociodemographic factors that increase demand for sex work are also important drivers of STI/HIV via sex work.[130] Female or male sex work is an important multiplier for STI transmission, as are high sexual mixing rates (high rates of partner exchange, especially when multiple partners are concurrent and linked in sexual networks).[131–133]

Hepatitis B is almost completely preventable with vaccination, and global rates are declining slowly with the advent of universal infant vaccination.[134] Human papillomavirus (HPV) causes genital squamous carcinomas, including cancer of the cervix, vulva, vagina, penis, and anus. Cervical cancer is typically the number one or two cancer killer of women in developing countries, yet it is preventable with Pap smear screening. Given Pap smear logistical difficulties, visual inspection with acetic acid is proving promising, so-called "see and treat" approaches using liquid nitrogen cryosurgery or Loop Electrosurgical Excision Procedure (LEEP).[135,136] Although HPV vaccine is now available, both products' oncogenic coverage is for types 16 and 18; their relevance, due to type-specific immune responses and very high cost is uncertain.[137]

Herpes simplex virus type 2 is a chronic, incurable virus that flares up periodically and causes genital ulcers likely to facilitate HIV transmission.[138–140,8] A large clinical trial, the HIV Prevention Trials Network 039 protocol will be completed in 2008 to see if suppression of HSV-2 with acyclovir can reduce HIV acquisition.[141] A partner trial supported by the Bill & Melinda Gates foundation will look at HIV-1 and HSV-2 co-infected persons to see if HSV-2 suppression will reduce HIV-1 transmission to partners.

Male circumcision is likely to reduce sexually transmitted infections in general, as highlighted earlier vis-à-vis HIV.[46] Douching is another remediable risk factor for STI acquisition.[142–144] Both circumcision of men and education to discourage vaginal douching and insertion of nontherapeutic intravaginal substances might be expected to reduce STI rates.

Vaccine Preventable Diseases

Vaccines may be from live attenuated (weakened) strains or from a wide variety of killed or manufactured products. Increasingly common are genetically engineered subunit protein fragments that mimic the viral coat or bacterial wall of an organism, serving as an epitope to stimulate a vigorous immune response. Advances in conjugate vaccines have enabled linkage of a polysaccharide antigen to a chemical moiety that stimulates a vigorous immune response, especially in children under age two whose immune systems are immature.[145]

In developing countries, the WHO Expanded Program on Immunizations may include Bacille Calmette-Guérin (BCG) for tuberculosis, measles, poliovirus, diphtheria, pertussis (whooping cough), and tetanus (the latter also for women of child-bearing age); an example of a "bare-bones" program in Ethiopia is found in Table 30.4. (Vaccines in this schedule are provided free of charge. The plan calls for the routine immunization schedule to be completed before age one year.) In contrast, the current United States schedule is an impressive array of vaccines that protect against polio, diphtheria, pertussis, tetanus, *H. influenzae* type B, pneumococcus, varicella (chicken pox), hepatitis B, rotavirus, influenza, measles, mumps, rubella, and others for selected high risk populations (Table 30.5). These may include meningococcus, hepatitis A, human papillomavirus, and herpes simplex virus type 2 for girls in early adolescence, and others for persons with immunosuppression, pregnancy, or age-related risk.[146–149] Vaccine policies and successes are challenged by cost-effectiveness considerations and are constrained by poverty, poor education, program underfunding, anti-vaccine propaganda, and political considerations.[150–153]

Some diseases are theoretically eradicable with vaccines, as was done for smallpox.[154,155] Poliovirus has proven more difficult than anticipated, but nonetheless eradication is predicted as there are no animal or long-term environmental reservoirs, and human-to-human transmission chains are being reduced radically.[156] Many challenges in disease control for vaccine-preventable diseases are programmatic, community-education-related, or political and fiscal.[157]

Some observers state, with good rationale, that the vaccines against "easy diseases" have already been developed. When the human immune response clears the virus, correlating well with virus-specific antibody levels, for example, then the vaccinologists know what goal to seek. If the human being rarely, inefficiently, or inconsistently clears the agent and does so without a clear correlate of protective immunity, then our vaccine development goal is more elusive, as with many of the STI, HIV, and hepatitis C. Nonetheless, progress is being made against agents that just a decade ago were thought to have formidable obstacles.[160–163]

Neglected Tropical Diseases

Some diseases are considered **neglected tropical diseases (NTDs)** by the WHO, and as such merit

Table 30.4. The Routine Childhood Immunization Schedule in Ethiopia Comprises Six Vaccine Preventable Diseases: Measles, Diphtheria, Pertussis, Tetanus, Polio, and Tuberculosis

Vaccine*	Diseases	Age
BCG	Tuberculosis	At birth
DPT	Diphteria, Pertussis, Tetanus	6, 10, 14 weeks
OPV	Polio	At birth, 6, 10, 14 weeks
Measles	Measles	9 months

Schedule for tetanus toxoid administration in women of childbearing age to protect their unborn babies from tetanus.

Dose**	Time for Administration	Duration of Protection
TT1	At first contact	No protection
TT2	4 weeks after TT1	3 years
TT3	≥6 months after TT2	5 years
TT4	≥1 year after TT3	10 years
TT5	≥1 year after TT4	30 years?

*BCG = Bacille Calmette-Guérin; DPT = diphtheria-pertussis-tetanus; OPV = oral polio vaccine

**TT = tetanus toxoid

SOURCE: Modified from WHO. Routine EPI Activities, 2007.

special consideration. The list includes such conditions as Buruli ulcer (*Mycobacterium ulcerans*), cholera, cysticercosis, dracunculiasis (guinea-worm); food-borne trematodes such as fascioliasis, hydatidosis, leishmaniasis, leprosy, lymphatic filariasis, onchocerciasis, schistosomiasis, soil-transmitted helminthiasis, trachoma, trypanosomiasis; and arboviral diseases such as dengue.[164] At least 1 billion persons are infected with one or more of these diseases worldwide.[165] Diseases can be rapidly fatal (e.g., hemorrhagic fever viruses, cholera) or can result in chronic morbidity (e.g., dracunculiasis, hookworm). Disfigurement from leprosy or leishmaniasis can carry social stigmatization and even abandonment by family. For helminthic infections, low-cost and effective drugs can be used to reduce worm burden and pathology. Water and sanitation programs can reduce incidence further. Good drugs for leprosy, yaws, pinta, and trachoma have helped reduce global prevalence considerably.

Other NTDs depend on systematic case finding and management at an early stage to prevent advanced morbidity or mortality, including Buruli ulcer, Chagas disease, diarrheal diseases such as cholera, African trypanosomiasis, and leishmaniasis. Vector control can reduce dengue or Chagas disease incidence and disease burden. Unfortunately, simple diagnostic tools and safe and effective treatment regimens are not available for many NTDs, complicating control efforts. The Guinea-worm Eradication Programme was begun in the early 1980s when an estimated 3.5 million people in 20 endemic countries were infected with the disease. By 2005, ≈10,000 cases were reported in 9 endemic countries, and global eradication may be a reality by 2010.[166] The Onchocerciasis Control Programme in west Africa and Latin America has resulted in >25 million hectares of previously uninhabitable land being made available for cultivation and habitation thanks to onchocerciasis control.[167] The WHO has a Department of Control of

Table 30.5. Centers for Disease Control and Prevention Immunization Schedule Recommendations for 2006–2007, United States

Vaccine ▼ Age ▶	Birth	1 month	2 months	4 months	6 months	12 months	15 months	18 months	19–23 months	2–3 years	4–6 years
Hepatitis B[1]	HepB	HepB	see footnote1		HepB					HepB Series	
Rotavirus[2]			Rota	Rota	Rota						
Diphtheria, Tetanus, Pertussis[3]			DTaP	DTaP	DTaP		DTaP				DTaP
Haemophilus influenzae type b[4]			Hib	Hib	Hib[4]	Hib		Hib			
Pneumococcal[5]			PCV	PCV	PCV	PCV				PCV PPV	
Inactivated Poliovirus			IPV	IPV		IPV					IPV
Influenza[6]						Influenza (Yearly)					
Measles, Mumps, Rubella[7]						MMR					MMR
Varicella[8]						Varicella					Varicella
Hepatitis A[9]						HepA (2 doses)				HepA Series	
Meningococcal[10]											MPSV4

□ Range of recommended ages   ■ Catch-up immunization   ■ Certain high-risk groups

Vaccine ▼ Age ▶	Birth	1 month	2 months	4 months	6 months	12 months	15 months	18 months	19–23 months	2–3 years	4–6 years
Hepatitis B[1]	HepB	HepB	see footnote1		HepB						
Rotavirus[2]			Rota	Rota	Rota						
Diphtheria, Tetanus, Pertussis[3]			DTaP	DTaP	DTaP	see footnote3	DTaP				DTaP
Haemophilus influenzae type b[4]			Hib	Hib	Hib[4]	Hib					
Pneumococcal[5]			PCV	PCV	PCV	PCV				PPV	
Inactivated Poliovirus			IPV	IPV		IPV					IPV
Influenza[6]						Influenza (Yearly)					
Measles, Mumps, Rubella[7]						MMR					MMR
Varicella[8]						Varicella					Varicella
Hepatitis A[9]						HepA (2 doses)				HepA Series	
Meningococcal[10]											MCV4

□ Range of recommended ages   ■ Certain high-risk groups

Footnotes are omitted.

SOURCE: CDC. 2008 Child & Adolescent Immunization Schedules, 2008.

Neglected Tropical Diseases that supports member states and partners to improve global efforts against NTDs, including orphan drug programs for diseases of little economic interest to the pharmaceutical industry.[168] Efforts are being made to tackle these diseases as a whole, rather than through unintegrated vertical programs. This includes integrating with better funded HIV, TB, and malaria programs.[169]

Emerging Infectious Diseases

From successes such as smallpox eradication and diminishing infectious disease mortality in industrialized nations before the HIV/AIDS epidemic, a popular misconception emerged among health professionals and policy makers in industrialized nations that infectious diseases had been largely conquered and chronic diseases were the principal new frontier.[170]

Only a highly ethnocentric point of view that would ignore the developing world, combined with a naive optimism that no new pathogens would emerge or reemerge would confuse the rise in chronic diseases (true) with a conclusion that infectious diseases were defeated (false). The HIV/AIDS and global avian influenza pandemics have squashed this view. The first pandemic of the twenty-first century occurred when >8,400 cases and >800 deaths from **severe acute respiratory syndrome (SARS)** were reported in 32 countries within 5 months, resulting in a global control and research effort. Subsequently, the SARS coronavirus remains quiescent in human populations, but there are continuing fears of a bird virus making the genetic leap into human populations, resulting in a future pandemic from influenza type A from the H5N1 avian influenza circulating in Asia. The United States witnessed the largest encephalitis epidemic in its history from June 10 to December 31, 2002, due to West Nile virus.[171] This time period also saw the emergence of the first inhalational anthrax cases in the United States from an intentional act of bioterrorism that remains of mysterious origin.[172]

TB and malaria drug resistance are examples of how major killers can evolve so that treatment and global control becomes more difficult with the emergence of drug-resistant strains. By 2005, the global distribution of dengue viruses had become comparable to malaria, with 2.5 billion people living in areas at risk for epidemic transmission. Among the factors that contribute to **emerging infectious diseases** and reemerging infectious diseases are the following:

- Demographic factors, including population growth, migration, housing density, and distribution of population within a region
- Social and behavioral changes such as the increased use of child care, liberalized sexual behavior, outdoor recreational pursuits, alcohol and drug use, patterns and styles of the transportation of goods, and widespread business and leisure travel
- Advances in health care technology, including modern chemotherapies, styles and institutions of health care delivery, iatrogenic immunosuppression, health care-associated antibiosis and antisepsis with consequent selective pressure and development of drug resistance, and invasive catheter techniques that introduce foreign objects either through natural orifices or parenteral routes
- Changes in the treatment and handling of foodstuff, including mass production of nearly all food products, water processing, and use of adjunct agricultural practices such as antibiotics in animal feed
- Climatologic changes and environmental alterations such as those associated with the El Niño ocean current centered off the coast of Peru, global warming, natural disasters such as volcanic eruptions, deforestation, and land use development (including dams, farming, irrigation, and mining) with attendant expansion of vector–reservoir–human contacts
- Microbial evolution, including natural variation, mutation, and cross-species zoonotic transmission
- War and natural disasters with the consequent breakdown of public health measures, including disease control activities, with or without economic collapse

- Deliberate release of microorganisms as a component of war or terrorism as with the 2001 intentional release of *Bacillus anthracis* through the United States mail in 2001

The relationships between social or behavioral phenomena and the risk of emerging pathogens are complex, and only interdisciplinary approaches will succeed in comprehensive prevention and control.[173] These factors have been more finely subdivided by a subsequent IOM report. These include microbial adaptation and change, human susceptibility to infection, climate and weather, changing ecosystems, human demographics and behavior, economic development and land use, international travel and commerce, technology and industry, breakdown of public health measures, poverty and social inequality, war and famine, lack of political will, and intent to harm. These can result in the emergence of an infectious disease via interactions of (1) the causal agent, (2) the human host, and (3) the social and biological environment, often mediated through an animal reservoir and an insect vector. Host characteristics include biological and genetic predictors of susceptibility and infectiousness, often mediated by the complex behavioral, social, economic, political, religious, and technological features of a host environment. Environmental influences increase or diminish the degree to which an infectious agent and vulnerable humans come into contact or the likelihood with which humans become infected with the given agent. For example, higher temperature and humidity are obvious influences on insect vectors of disease and also are associated with wearing loose, light clothing that facilitates insect biting. Environmental pollution that changes vector breeding patterns, natural disasters, water use patterns, human waste and garbage sanitation, and social conditions that influence behavior all are critical contributors to disease incidence. The all-important political response that can temper or exacerbate disease is a variable often overlooked except in extremes of war or famine.[174,175] It is a misconception that natural balance between the infectious agent, the host, and the environment results in stability by keeping emerging diseases in check. Rather, recurrent epidemics and plagues, along with high endemic rates of many infectious diseases, are dynamic and evolving contributors to human history that continue into contemporary times.

Chronic Diseases and Global Constraints to Improving Public Health

Historically, communicable diseases and adverse reproductive outcomes have been associated with poverty. Poor water quality, lack of sanitation infrastructure and resulting poor hygiene, crowding, lack of education, poor access to adequate health care, and nutrition deficiencies are all far more common among the economically deprived. In contrast, non-communicable diseases or conditions have been associated with sedentary lifestyles, dietary factors, chemical exposures, accidents, and other factors associated with industrialized or high income country settings.[176] As population growth, urbanization, and population density increase, conditions previously encountered in "developed" urban areas begin to occur in rapidly urbanizing areas of low- and middle-income countries. Good examples can be found in the trends observed in Latin American countries during the past few decades. In the latter three decades of the twentieth century, the mortality rates related to chronic diseases and injury in Latin American countries have increased markedly. A comparative study of four countries (Guatemala, Mexico, Chile, and Uruguay) provided insight in the context of different stages of this epidemiologic transition; mortality from chronic disease and injury increased 30 percent from the 1970s to the 1990s. At the same time, reductions in communicable disease mortality were observed, and the proportion of the population that lived in urban settings increased in all four countries.[177] Increased life expectancy and changing patterns of morbidity can be correlated with population growth, urbanization, infrastructure, and economic improvements.[178]

Although some of the effects of the **epidemiological transition** are beneficial, reducing communicable disease and adverse reproductive outcome burdens, others are deleterious, namely the increases in chronic disease and injury mortality and morbidity. These transitions create new epidemiologic patterns demarcating disease along poverty lines that are very similar in high- and low-income countries. For example, wealthy persons in Asia and Africa confront diseases of overnutrition and hypertension today, much as if they lived in North America. Globalization, the epidemiologic transition, and shifts in the patterns of production and consumption at the family and community levels are at the core of some of the complex global and local changes observed in disease patterns.[176,179]

The effects of these forces are illustrated by the global obesity epidemic. In the recent past in developing countries, undernutrition was the principal dietary problem. More recently, obesity rates around the world have increased substantially in both industrialized and developing countries.[180–184] Changes in obesity incidence relate to lower levels of physical activity and "westernization" of diets that are linked to globalization and urbanization, including increased consumption in low dietary quality; processed, high energy food that is available at lower cost;[185] reduction of incentives and rising costs of traditional dietary sources;[186] and reduction of physical activity due typically to increased use of motorized vehicles.[187,188] Obesity is one of the most important health risk factors in the modern world and has been clearly established as an important contributor to cardiovascular disease, diabetes, and certain cancers. In 1993, the worldwide prevalence of diabetes was estimated to be 5.1 percent in adults (20–79 years of age), and the number of adults suffering with diabetes was estimated at 194 million, a figure expected to increase to 332 million by 2025.[189]

Changing disease patterns are noted in the increase and changing mix in injury-related disability and death. A large proportion of unintentional injuries involve road and pedestrian traffic crashes, poisonings, and other injuries related to modernization and urbanization. Nonaccidental injuries from firearms, homicide, or suicide are more common in urban settings. At the same time, burn injuries, common in rural settings with open fire cooking, tend to be less common in urbanized settings and electrified kitchens. Chronic diseases and injury contribute to mortality, but they also contribute greatly to morbidity and disability resulting in added physical, social, and economic burdens that pose particularly difficult challenges to people living in low- and middle-income countries. Rehabilitation-related challenges are often neglected in developing countries.

HEALTH CARE WORKFORCE CRISES

Health leaders from the Joint Learning Initiative estimated in 2004 that 4 million more health workers were then required to improve health status globally, and that sub-Saharan countries in particular needed at least 1 million additional health workers.[190] They further state that "nearly all countries are challenged by worker shortage, skill mix imbalance, maldistribution, negative work environment, and a weak knowledge base." In many resource-constrained countries or regions, the status of human resources in health services is very dire. Health workers are few, concentrated in major urban areas, poorly paid in the public sector, and have little economic mobility, a circumstance that clashes with their high social status as health workers. Public-sector workers are often under tremendous work-related stress with high patient volumes, poor quality of care due to very short contact time with each patient, and poor conditions due to a lack of equipment, needed materials, protective devices, and medicines. Some health workers are not well trained, having learned in institutions with few teachers, outmoded curricula, substandard libraries, poor mentoring and supervision, and suboptimal work-based learning situations.

As a consequence of low salaries, poor working conditions, and low morale, health workers are being drained from the poorest environments to the less poor environments, leaving the most resource-constrained areas in worse conditions than before. Given imbalances of remuneration around the globe, a very poor country such as Mozambique or Zambia lose health care workers to South Africa, which in turn loses them to Australia, the United Kingdom, or the United States This **brain drain** comes without compensation, as the poorer countries are functionally paying for health care workers for richer countries. In sub-Saharan Africa, the impact of the HIV pandemic and other diseases results in high health care worker mortality so that they cannot train enough new workers fast enough to even replace those who are lost to HIV/AIDS and the brain drain.

Solutions include improving working conditions, recruitment, and retention strategies, such as public sector salaries in poorer countries. Lack of financial resources poses very difficult barriers to salary increases in poor countries. In many cases, salary increases have to be subsidized from international aid, and efforts to step up training of health staff, preferably locally, have to be increased. In some countries, an international medical "force" has been implemented as a stop-gap measure. For example, in Mozambique, Russian, Chilean, Cuban, and Indian physicians have been working to supplement local health cadres under collaboration agreements with their respective countries. Cuba has demonstrated to be particularly successful in helping other poor countries supplement human resources for health as well as contribute to the training of health workers from countries around the globe. Currently, Cuba boasts of having 28,000 health professionals practicing in 68 countries and of having trained 30,000 health professionals from other poor nations.[191] In addition, in 2005, President Fidel Castro announced that Cuba will join with Venezuela to provide scholarships and training for 100,000 new physicians from poor populations in developing countries over the next 10 years. Volunteers in the workforce have been suggested as a solution, but this tends to work in discrete settings and may not be a long-term, sustainable solution.

RESEARCH AND THE FUTURE OF GLOBAL HEALTH

At the World Economic Forum in 2003, Bill Gates announced the Grand Challenges in Global Health (GCGH) Initiative, and a grant to the Foundation for the National Institutes of Health to lead the efforts. This initiative seeks to promote high-level research in key specific areas related to diseases that disproportionately affect developing nations, with the goal of producing innovations that will have a high global impact, high degree of feasibility, and can potentially remove critical barriers to improving health. The scientific board, with input widely requested from scientists around the world, put together a list of 14 areas of challenges, including vaccine development and delivery, vector control, medication and delivery system design, infectious disease therapies, nutritional interventions, and measurement of health and economic status. All addressed requirements of particular relevance to developing countries such as simplicity and low cost. The Bill & Melinda Gates foundation to date has contributed US$436.6 million to this endeavor in partnership with resources from the Wellcome Trust (UK) and the Canadian Institutes of Health Research.[192] Forty-three grants were awarded to scientists around the world who were selected from thousands of applicants. Grants include research on vaccines that do not require refrigeration or needles for delivery and can be administered soon after birth, innovative ways to control insect populations that transmit diseases such as malaria through interference with mosquitoes' olfactory system, drug discovery to cure latent infections (those that are dormant and do not produce physiologic symptoms), design of diagnostic systems that can detect multiple pathogens or conditions in a simple and low-cost fashion at the primary care level, design of information systems that can help measure population health status, and incorporation of an optimal and full range of nutrients in one staple food [192]. Applied, goal-directed research is intended to complement the historic basic science focus of the National Institutes of Health (NIH, United States), the world's largest research support organization, or the Howard Hughes Medical Institute, the world's largest foundation before the Bill & Melinda Gates foundation was created. The new NIH strategy called the NIH Roadmap, however, suggests a shift in some of the NIH research toward goal-directed investments.[193]

Focused global health activities have played a major role in bringing awareness and raising and making funds available for global health problems, but most have focused primarily on program implementation. A good example is the Stop TB Partnership.[194] Such initiatives often conduct outcomes and implementation research to seek the most efficient "real world" approaches to disease control, given what we know to be efficacious. In 1996, The Joint United Nations Programme on HIV/AIDS (UNAIDS) became operational as a multi-UN agency. UNAIDS has been a cornerstone of the global response to the epidemic, contributing to the creation of National AIDS Councils and national plans to combat HIV in nearly all UN member nations. It liaisons with organizations devoted to the coordination of efforts to fight the epidemic across multiple societal sectors, including governmental agencies and ministries. To marshal global improvements in health infrastructures, The Global Fund to Fight AIDS, Tuberculosis and Malaria was launched with UN co-sponsorship in 2002.[195] The Global Fund is a multinational initiative that provides financing from donor nations and technical support for programs to fight these interacting scourges. National proposals are vetted by an in-country multisector committee and selected by an international panel of experts based on merit and feasibility.[196]

In 2003, the United States President Bush launched PEPFAR, or the President's Emergency Plan for AIDS Relief, borne out of global concerns about the rapidly growing pandemic of HIV/AIDS particularly in sub-Saharan Africa and Asia. The 5-year plan has spent >$18 billion over 5 years, and its second phase 2008–2012 has recently been discussed for approval by the United States Senate

for more than $50 billion. This is the largest global health investment ever made to combat an epidemic, supporting bilateral programs through the CDC, the United States Agency for International Development, and other federal agencies, as well as supporting The Global Fund.[197] PEPFAR started by emphasizing 15 focus countries, 13 in sub-Saharan Africa, plus Haiti and Vietnam, and scaling up care and treatment activities. As of September 2007, PEPFAR funds and partners had supported ARV treatment for 1.45 million people, care for more than 2.7 million orphans and vulnerable children, care for 6.6 million people living with HIV/AIDS, and reached more than 56 million people through community outreach programs for HIV prevention and care.[197]

Another initiative that contributed to increasing efforts toward fighting the HIV/AIDS epidemic was the WHO 3 by 5 Initiative. Through a series of trainings, meetings, and guidance, the WHO advocated increasing treatment access to 3 million people by the year 2005.[198] Although failing to meet its objective, the campaign helped raise international consciousness as to the emergency of high mortality. The Clinton HIV/AIDS Initiative, launched in 2004, has worked with governments of high- and low-income countries to facilitate funding for treatment access and to reduce the prices of ARV drugs and laboratory costs associated with treatment for HIV/AIDS.[199]

Other examples of single-focus global initiatives include the 1998 meeting of an ad hoc Committee on the Tuberculosis Epidemic. At their London meeting, they established the Stop TB Initiative, which led to a Global Plan to Stop TB and the creation of the Stop TB Partnership in 2001, led by the WHO.[194] Similarly, the Roll-Back Malaria Partnership, also led by the WHO, remains a galvanizing advocate (http://www.rbm.who.int). PolioPlus of Rotary International is an example of an ambitious public-private global partnership whose goal is to rid the globe of polio forever (http://www.rotary.org/en/SERVICEANDFELLOWSHIP/POLIO/Pages/ridefault.aspx).

Finally, a global health chapter is incomplete without mention of the foundations. For decades, the Rockefeller Foundation has spearheaded interest in tropical disease control and family planning; the Ford Foundation has focused on education and poverty alleviation; the Edna McConnell Clark Foundation has targeted schistosomiasis, onchocerciasis, and trachoma; the Ellison Medical Foundation for global infectious diseases (http://www .ellisonfoundation.org/index.jsp); and others have contributed money and expertise. The largest and most recent contributor is the Bill and Melinda Gates foundation, with historically unprecedented investments being made into global health and development. In their words, the Bill & Melinda Gates foundation is "guided by the belief that every life has equal value" and "works to reduce inequities and improve lives around the world. In developing countries, it focuses on improving health, reducing extreme poverty, and increasing access to technology in public libraries" (http:// www.gatesfoundation.org). Its fiscal disbursements are increasingly demanding partnership payments, a strategy sure to inspire new consortia that will tackle the globe's toughest health problems.

In spite of the tremendous contribution all of these-disease focused initiatives have made, one major criticism dampens their effectiveness: the potential destabilization of the very same local health service infrastructures the initiatives seek to support. Often these "vertical" programs tend to be implemented outside the normal channels of health services and public health systems, mainly because they attempt to bypass poorly working, inefficient, or corrupt systems. In doing so, the vertical program can become a temporary fix, ignoring or doing little to the much larger systemic problems. If we fail to address human capacity development, brain drain, procurement and distribution logistics, coordination, maintenance and repair, management and administration and finance, information systems and telecommunications, and research, we fail to address the real problems that plague health care and public health systems around the world. Addressing these underlying problems is the only way to ensure sustainability in our efforts.

There has been a renewal of commitment worldwide in global health. The work of many multilateral organizations, bilateral government programs, foundations, nongovernment and community organizations, but most of all, the intensive efforts of many of our colleagues struggling under extremely difficult conditions to provide health care to poor populations around the world, symbolizes the new spirit to tackle any health problem, no matter how daunting. This new energy can give hope in the face of stark challenges.

REVIEW QUESTIONS

1. What are the most common neglected tropical diseases (NTDs), and why are they considered neglected?
2. Name three of the most common diseases affecting low-income countries, and describe those diseases' major epidemiologic features.
3. What is *epidemiologic transition,* and how is it manifested in global health?
4. The term "task shifted" has been applied to health manpower in developing countries. Describe the meaning of the term and the rationale for the strategy.
5. What are the most common determinants of infectious diseases in low- and middle-income countries?
6. What are the most common determinants of chronic diseases in low- and middle-income countries?
7. What are the most salient features of the HIV/AIDS epidemic in sub-Saharan Africa?
8. What are the principal public health interventions used in successful malaria control?
9. What are the main public health interventions for tuberculosis? How do the health care service section and public health preventive sector interface for TB control?
10. What are emerging infectious diseases, and why are they important?
11. What are the most significant causes of mortality for children under five years, and what are some of the most important public health interventions to address the consequent mortality and morbidity?

REFERENCES

1. World Bank. The World Bank Data and Statistics: Country Classification, 2008.

2. World Bank. Equatorial Guinea Data Profile. Washington DC: World Bank; 2006.

3. WHO. World Health Statistics 2006. Geneva: WHO; 2006.

4. Lopez AD, Murray CC. The global burden of disease, 1990–2020. *Nat Med* 1998;4:1241–3.

5. Lopez AD, Mathers CD, Ezzati M, Jamison DT, Murray CJL. Global and regional burden of disease and risk factors, 2001: Systematic analysis of population health data. *Lancet.* 2006;367: 1747–1757.

6. Bryce J, Boschi-Pinto C, Shibuya K, Black RE. WHO estimates of the causes of death in children. *Lancet.* 2005;365:1147–1152.

7. OECD. OCED Health Data 2007, 2007.

8. CIA. Rank Order-Infant Mortality Rate CIA Factbook. Washington DC: CIA; 2007.

9. Annan KA. "We the People" The Role of the United Nations in the 21st Century Millennium Report of the Secretary-General of the United Nations. New York, 2000.

10. UN. Millennium Development Goal Indicators United Nations Millennium Development Goals New York: UN; 2000.

11. Vermund SH. Millions of life-years saved with potent antiretroviral drugs in the United States: A celebration, with challenges. *J Infect Dis.* 2006; 194:1–5.

12. Jones J, Taylor B, Wilkin T, Hammer S. Advances in antiretroviral therapy. The 14th Conference on Retroviruses and Opportunistic Infections. Columbia University Medical Center, New York: Top HIV Med; 2007.

13. Stringer JSA, Zulu I, Levy J, et al. Rapid scale-up of antiretroviral therapy at primary care sites in Zambia: Feasibility and early outcomes. *JAMA.* 2006;296:782–793.

14. Severe P, Leger P, Charles M, et al. Antiretroviral therapy in a thousand patients with AIDS in Haiti. *N Engl J Med.* 2005;353:2325–2334.

15. George E, Noel F, Bois G, et al. Antiretroviral therapy for HIV-1-infected children in Haiti. *J Infect Dis.* 2007;195:1411–1418.

16. UNAIDS. Report on the global AIDS epidemic. Geneva: UNAIDS; 2006.

17. UNAIDS. Epidemiological Fact Sheet: Cuba. Geneva: UNAIDS, WHO; 2006.

18. Vermund SH, White H, Shah SA, et al. HIV/AIDS in Pakistan: Has the explosion begun? *J Pak Med Assoc.* 2006;56:S1–2.

19. UNAIDS. The changing HIV/AIDS epidemic in Europe and Central Asia. Geneva: UNAIDS; 2004.

20. USAID. Coverage of selected services for HIV/AIDS prevention, care, and support in low and middle-income countries in 2003. Washington DC: USAID; 2004.

21. Stoneburner RL, Low-Beer D. Population-level HIV declines and behavioral risk avoidance in Uganda. *Science* 2004;304:714–718.

22. Nelson KE, Celentano DD, Eiumtrakol S, et al. Changes in sexual behavior and a decline in HIV infection among young men in Thailand. *N Engl J Med.* 1996;335:297–303.

23. CDC. Epidemiology of HIV/AIDS—United States, 1981–2005. *MMWR Morb Mortal Wkly Rep.* 2006:589–92.

24. Stringer JSA, Sinkala M, Maclean CC, et al. Effectiveness of a citywide program to prevent mother-to-child HIV transmission in Lusaka, Zambia. *AIDS.* 2005;19:1309–1315.

25. Reithinger R, Megazzini K, Durako SJ, Harris DR, Vermund SH. Monitoring and evaluation of programmes to prevent mother to child transmission of HIV in Africa. *BMJ.* 2007;334:1143–1146.

26. GHPWG. Access to HIV Prevention: Closing the Gap Global HIV Prevention Working Group, 2003.

27. Schoenbaum EE, Hartel DM, Gourevitch MN. Needle exchange use among a cohort of injecting drug users. *AIDS.* 1996;10:1729–34.

28. Jarlais DCD, Marmor M, Paone D, et al. HIV incidence among injecting drug users in New York City syringe-exchange programmes. *Lancet.* 1996; 348:987–991.

29. Monterroso ER, Hamburger ME, Vlahov D, et al. Prevention of HIV infection in street-recruited injection drug users. *JAIDS.* 2000;25:63–70.

30. Heimer R. Syringe exchange programs: Lowering the transmission of syringe-borne diseases and beyond. *Public Health Rep.* 1998;113;Suppl 1: 67–74.

31. Kaplan EH, Heimer R. HIV incidence among New Haven needle exchange participants: updated estimates from syringe tracking and testing data. *J Acquir Immune Defic Syndr Hum Retrovirol.* 1995;10:175–6.

32. UNAIDS. *Women and HIV/AIDS: Confronting the Crisis.* Geneva: UNAIDS; 2004.

33. Moench TR, Chipato T, Padian NS. Preventing disease by protecting the cervix: The unexplored promise of internal vaginal barrier devices. *AIDS.* 2001;15:1595–602.

34. Makumbi FE, Gray RH, Serwadda D, et al. The incidence and prevalence of orphanhood associated with parental HIV infection: A population-based study in Rakai, Uganda. *AIDS.* 2005;19: 1669–1676.

35. Floyd S, Crampin AC, Glynn JR, et al. The social and economic impact of parental HIV on children in northern Malawi: Retrospective population-based cohort study. *AIDS Care.* 2007;19:781–790.

36. Johnston MI, Fauci AS. An HIV vaccine—evolving concepts. *N Engl J Med.* 2007;356:2073–81.

37. Berkley SF, Koff WC. Scientific and policy challenges to development of an AIDS vaccine. *Lancet.* 2007;370:94–101.

38. Wakabi W. HIV microbicide trials halted. *CMAJ.* 2007;176:1569–70.

39. McGowan I. Microbicides: A new frontier in HIV prevention. *Biologicals.* 2006;34:241–255.

40. Winer RL, Hughes JP, Feng Q, et al. Condom use and the risk of genital human Papillomavirus infection in young women. *N Engl J Med.* 2006; 354:2645–2654.

41. Holmes KK, Levine R, Weaver M. Effectiveness of condoms in preventing sexually transmitted infections. *Bull World Health Organ.* 2004;82: 454–61.

42. Padian NS, van der Straten A, Ramjee G, et al. Diaphragm and lubricant gel for prevention of HIV acquisition in southern African women: A randomised controlled trial. *Lancet.* 2007;370: 251–261.

43. Gray RH, Kigozi G, Serwadda D, et al. Male circumcision for HIV prevention in men in Rakai, Uganda: A randomised trial. *Lancet.* 2007;369: 657–666.

44. Bailey RC, Moses S, Parker CB, et al. Male circumcision for HIV prevention in young men in Kisumu, Kenya: A randomised controlled trial. *Lancet.* 2007;369:643–656.

45. Auvert B, Taljaard D, Lagarde E, et al.. Randomized, controlled intervention trial of male circumcision for reduction of HIV infection risk: The ANRS 1265 Trial. *PLoS Med.* 2005;2:e298.

46. Weiss HA, Thomas SL, Munabi SK, Hayes RJ. Male circumcision and risk of syphilis, chancroid, and genital herpes: A systematic review and meta-analysis. *Sex Transm Infect.* 2006;82:101–110.

47. Underhill K, Montgomery P, Operario D. Sexual abstinence only programmes to prevent HIV infection in high income countries: systematic review. *BMJ.* 2007;335:248.

48. Shoptaw S, Klausner J, Reback C, et al. A public health response to the methamphetamine epidemic: The implementation of contingency management to treat methamphetamine dependence. *BMC Public Health.* 2006;6:214.

49. Bryant KJ. Expanding research on the role of alcohol consumption and related risks in the prevention and treatment of HIV_AIDS. *Substance Use and Misuse.* 2006;41:1465–1507.

50. Vermund SH, Wilson CM. Barriers to HIV testing-where next? *Lancet.* 2002;360:1186–1187.

51. Sweat M, Gregorich S, Sangiwa G, et al. Cost-effectiveness of voluntary HIV-1 counseling and testing in reducing sexual transmission of HIV-1 in Kenya and Tanzania. *Lancet.* 2000;356:113–121.

52. Cohen MS, Gay C, Kashuba AD, Blower S, Paxton L. Narrative review: antiretroviral therapy to prevent the sexual transmission of HIV-1. *Ann Intern Med.* 2007;146:591–601.

53. Fideli US, Allen SA, Musonda R, et al. Virologic and immunologic determinants of heterosexual transmission of human immunodeficiency virus type 1 in Africa. *AIDS Res Hum Retroviruses.* 2001;17:901–10.

54. Quinn TC, Wawer MJ, Sewankambo N, et al. The Rakai Project study G. viral load and heterosexual transmission of human immunodeficiency virus type 1. *N Engl J Med.* 2000;342:921–929.

55. DiClemente RJ, Funkhouser E, Wingood G, Fawal H, Holmberg SD, Vermund SH. Protease inhibitor combination therapy and decreased condom use among gay men. *South Med J.* 2002;95:421–5.

56. Cassell MM, Halperin DT, Shelton JD, Stanton D. Risk compensation: The Achilles' heel of innovations in HIV prevention? *BMJ.* 2006;332:605–607.

57. Bedelu M, Ford N, Hilderbrand K, Reuter H. Implementing antiretroviral therapy in rural communities: the Lusikisiki model of decentralized HIV/AIDS care. *J Infect Dis.* 2007;196 Suppl 3: S464–8.

58. Philips M, Zachariah R, Venis S. Task shifting for antiretroviral treatment delivery in sub-Saharan Africa: Not a panacea. *Lancet.* 2008;371:682–4.

59. WHO. *World Malaria Report.* Geneva: WHO; 2005.

60. Snow RW, Korenromp EL, Gouws E. Pediatric mortality in Africa: plasmodium falciparum

malaria as a cause or risk? *Am J Trop Med Hyg.* 2004;71:16–24.

61. Breman JG. The ears of the hippopotamus: Manifestations, determinants, and estimates of the malaria burden. *Am J Trop Med Hyg.* 2001;64: 1-c-11.

62. Steketee RW. Pregnancy, nutrition and parasitic diseases. *J Nutr.* 2003;133:1661S–1667S.

63. Guyatt HL, Brooker S, Kihamia CM, Hall A, Bundy DA. Evaluation of efficacy of school-based anthelmintic treatments against anaemia in children in the United Republic of Tanzania. *Bull World Health Organ.* 2001;79:695–703.

64. Breman JG, Alilio MS, Mills A. Conquering the intolerable burden of malaria: What's new, what's needed: A summary. *Am J Trop Med Hyg.* 2004; 71:1–15.

65. Na-Bangchang K, Congpuong K. Current malaria status and distribution of drug resistance in East and Southeast Asia with special focus to Thailand. *Tohoku J Exp Med.* 2007;211:99–113.

66. Whitworth JA, Hewitt KA. Effect of malaria on HIV-1 progression and transmission. *Lancet.* 2005; 365:196–7.

67. Hewitt KA, Steketee RB, Mwapasa VC, Whitworth JD, French NE. Interactions between HIV and malaria in nonpregnant adults: Evidence and implications. *AIDS.* 2006;20:1993–2004.

68. Ter Kuile FO, Parise ME, Verhoeff FH, et al. The burden of co-infection with Human Immunodeficiency Virus type 1 and malaria in pregnant women in sub-Saharan Africa. *Am J Trop Med Hyg.* 2004;71:41–54.

69. Miller JM, Korenromp EL, Nahlen BL, W. Steketee R. Estimating the number of insecticide-treated nets required by African households to reach continent-wide malaria coverage targets. *JAMA.* 2007; 297:2241–2250.

70. WHO. *Managing Water in the Home: Accelerated Health Gains from Improved Water Supply.* Geneva: WHO; 2002.

71. Lima AA, Guerrant RL. Strategies to reduce the devastating costs of early childhood diarrhea and its potential long-term impact: Imperatives that we can no longer afford to ignore. *Clin Infect Dis.* 2004;38:1552–4.

72. O'Ryan M, Prado V, Pickering LK. A millennium update on pediatric diarrheal illness in the developing world. *Semin Pediatr Infect Dis.* 2005;16: 125–36.

73. Levine MM. Enteric infections and the vaccines to counter them: Future directions. *Vaccine.* 2006; 24:3865–73.

74. Pruss-Ustun A, Corvalan C. How much disease burden can be prevented by environmental interventions? *Epidemiology.* 2007;18:167–78.

75. Feachem RG. Interventions for the control of diarrhoeal diseases among young children: Promotion of personal and domestic hygiene. *Bull World Health Organ.* 1984;62:467–76.

76. Clasen T, Garcia Parra G, Boisson S, Collin S. Household-based ceramic water filters for the prevention of diarrhea: A randomized, controlled trial of a pilot program in Colombia. *Am J Trop Med Hyg.* 2005;73:790–5.

77. Crump JA, Otieno PO, Slutsker L, et al. Household based treatment of drinking water with flocculant-disinfectant for preventing diarrhoea in areas with turbid source water in rural western Kenya: cluster randomised controlled trial. *BMJ.* 2005;331:478.

78. Mbori-Ngacha D, Nduati R, John G, et al. Morbidity and mortality in breastfed and formula-fed infants of HIV-1-infected women: A randomized clinical trial. *JAMA.* 2001;286:2413–2420.

79. Creek T, Arvelo W, Kim A, et al. Role of infant feeding and HIV in a severe outbreak of diarrhea and malnutrition among young children. Botswana 2006 14th Conference on Retroviruses and Opportunist Infections. Los Angeles, CA: CDC; 2007.

80. Bhutta ZA, Bird SM, Black RE, et al. Therapeutic effects of oral zinc in acute and persistent diarrhea in children in developing countries: Pooled analysis of randomized controlled trials. *Am J Clin Nutr.* 2000;72:1516–22.

81. AbouZahr C. Global burden of maternal death and disability. *British Medical Bulletin.* 2003;67:1–11.

82. Bhandari N, Bahl R, Taneja S, et al. Substantial reduction in severe diarrheal morbidity by daily zinc supplementation in young north Indian children. *Pediatrics.* 2002;109:e86.

83. Bhutta ZA, Black RE, Brown KH, et al. Prevention of diarrhea and pneumonia by zinc supplementation in children in developing countries: pooled analysis of randomized controlled trials. Zinc Investigators' Collaborative Group. *J Pediatr.* 1999;135:689–97.

84. Black RE, Sazawal S. Zinc and childhood infectious disease morbidity and mortality. *Br J Nutr.* 2001;85 Suppl 2:S125–9.

85. Bhatnagar S. Effects of zinc supplementation on child mortality. *Lancet.* 2007;369:885–6.

86. Sazawal S, Black RE, Ramsan M, et al. Effect of zinc supplementation on mortality in children aged 1–48 months: A community-based randomised placebo-controlled trial. *Lancet.* 2007; 369:927–34.

87. Rahman MM, Vermund SH, Wahed MA, Fuchs GJ, Baqui AH, Alvarez JO. Simultaneous zinc and vitamin A supplementation in Bangladeshi children: Randomised double blind controlled trial. *BMJ.* 2001;323:314–318.

88. Fuchs GJ. A better oral rehydration solution? An important step, but not a leap forward. *BMJ.* 2001;323:59–60.

89. WHO. WHO Mediacenter. Tuberculosis, 2008.

90. Frieden TR, Sterling TR, Munsiff SS, Watt CJ, Dye C. Tuberculosis. *Lancet.* 2003;362: 887–899.

91. WHO. Global Tuberculosis Control 2008: Surveillance, Planning, and Financing. Geneva: WHO; 2008.

92. Gandhi NR, Moll A, Sturm AW, et al. Extensively drug-resistant tuberculosis as a cause of death in patients co-infected with tuberculosis and HIV in a rural area of South Africa. *Lancet.* 2006;368: 1575–1580.

93. Shah NS, Wright A, Bai GH, et al. Worldwide emergence of extensively drug-resistant tuberculosis. *Emerg Infect Dis.* 2007;13:380–7.

94. CDC. Emergence of Mycobacterium tuberculosis with extensive resistance to second-line drugs—worldwide, 2000–2004. *MMWR Morb Mortal Wkly Rep.* 2006;55:301–5.

95. Pablos-Mendez A, Gowda DK, Frieden TR. Controlling multidrug-resistant tuberculosis and access to expensive drugs: A rational framework. *Bull World Health Organ.* 2002;80:489–95; discussion 495–500.

96. Padayatchi N, Friedland G. Managing multiple and extensively drug-resistant tuberculosis and HIV. *Expert Opin Pharmacother.* 2007;8: 1035–1037.

97. Dukes Hamilton C, Sterling TR, Blumberg HM, et al. Extensively drug-resistant tuberculosis: Are we learning from history or repeating it? *Clinical Infectious Disease.* 2007;45:338–342.

98. Zumla A, Malon P, Henderson J, Grange JM. Impact of HIV infection on tuberculosis. *Postgrad Med J.* 2000;76:259–268.

99. Corbett EL, Watt CJ, Walker N, et al. The growing burden of tuberculosis: Global trends and interactions with the HIV epidemic. *Arch Intern Med.* 2003;163:1009–1021.

100. Selwyn PA, Hartel D, Lewis VA, et al. A prospective study of the risk of tuberculosis among intravenous drug users with human immunodeficiency virus infection. *N Engl J Med.* 1989;320:545–50.

101. Tupasi TE, Gupta R, Quelapio MID, et al. Feasibility and cost-effectiveness of treating multidrug-resistant tuberculosis: A cohort study in the Philippines. *PLoS Med.* 2006;3:e352.

102. Floyd K, Arora VK, Murthy KJ, et al. Cost and cost-effectiveness of PPM-DOTS for tuberculosis control: Evidence from India. *Bull World Health Organ.* 2006;84:437–45.

103. Baltussen R, Floyd K, Dye C. Cost effectiveness analysis of strategies for tuberculosis control in developing countries. *BMJ.* 2005;331:1364-.

104. Islam MA, Wakai S, Ishikawa N, Chowdhury AM, Vaughan JP. Cost-effectiveness of community health workers in tuberculosis control in Bangladesh. *Bull World Health Organ.* 2002; 80:445–50.

105. Schwartzman K, Oxlade O, Barr RG, et al. Domestic returns from investment in the control of tuberculosis in other countries. *N Engl J Med.* 2005;353:1008–1020.

106. Harcourt C, Donovan B. The many faces of sex work. *Sex Transm Infect.* 2005;81:201–206.

107. Friedland G. Tuberculosis, Drug Resistance, and HIV/AIDS: A Triple Threat. *Curr Infect Dis Rep.* 2007;9:252–61.

108. Schuchat A, Dowell SF. Pneumonia in children in the developing world: New challenges, new solutions. *Seminars in Pediatric Infectious Diseases.* 2004;15:181–189.

109. Jeena P. The role of HIV infection in acute respiratory infections among children in sub-Saharan Africa. *Int J Tuberc Lung Dis.* 2005;9:708–15.

110. Cashat-Cruz M, Morales-Aguirre JJ, Mendoza-Azpiri M. Respiratory tract infections in children in developing countries. *Seminars in Pediatric Infectious Diseases* 2005;16:84–92.

111. Khan TA, Madni SA, Zaidi AK. Acute respiratory infections in Pakistan: Have we made any progress? *J Coll Physicians Surg Pak.* 2004;14:440–8.

112. Horn JS. Building a rural health service in the People's Republic of China. *Int J Health Serv.* 1972;2:377–83.

113. Goldenberg RL, Stringer JS, Sinkala M, Vermund SH. Perinatal HIV transmission: developing country considerations. *J Matern Fetal Neonatal Med.* 2002;12:149–58.

114. Rosenfield A, Maine D. Maternal mortality—a neglected tragedy. Where is the M in MCH? *Lancet.* 1985;2:83–5.

115. Neilson JP, Lavender T, Quenby S, Wray S. Obstructed labour: Reducing maternal death and disability during pregnancy. *Br Med Bull.* 2003; 67:191–204.

116. Wall LL. Obstetric vesicovaginal fistula as an international public-health problem. *Lancet.* 2006; 368:1201–9.

117. Kwawukume EY. Caesarean section in developing countries. *Best Practice & Research Clinical Obstetrics & Gynaecology.* 2001;15:165–178.

118. Jones SD, Ehiri J, Anyanwu E. Female genital mutilation in developing countries: an agenda for public health response. *European Journal of Obstetrics & Gynecology and Reproductive Biology.* 2004;116:144–151.

119. Dorkenoo E. Combating female genital mutilation: an agenda for the next decade. *World Health Stat Q.* 1996;49:142–7.

120. Pasha O, Fikree F, Vermund S. Determinants of unmet need for family planning in squatter settlements in Karachi, Pakistan. *Asia Pac Popul J.* 2001; 16:93–108.

121. Wirth ME, Balk D, Delamonica E, Storeygard A, Sacks E, Minujin A. Setting the stage for equity-sensitive monitoring of the maternal and child health Millennium Development Goals. *Bull World Health Organ.* 2006;84:519–27.

122. Stringer EM, Kaseba C, Levy J, et al. A randomized trial of the intrauterine contraceptive device vs. hormonal contraception in women who are infected with the human immunodeficiency virus. *American Journal of Obstetrics and Gynecology.* 2007;197:144.e1–144.e8.

123. Stringer E, Sinkala M, Kumwenda R, Chapman V, Mwale A, Vermund SH, Goldenberg RL, Stringer JSA. Personal risk perception, HIV knowledge and risk avoidance behavior, and their relationships to actual HIV Serostatus in an urban African obstetric population. *JAIDS.* 2004;35:60–66.

124. Low N, Broutet N, Adu-Sarkodie Y, Barton P, Hossain M, Hawkes S. Global control of sexually transmitted infections. *Lancet.* 2006;368: 2001–2016.

125. Bearinger LH, Sieving RE, Ferguson J, Sharma V. Global perspectives on the sexual and reproductive health of adolescents: Patterns, prevention, and potential. *Lancet.* 2007;369:1220–1231.

126. Peeling RW, Holmes KK, Mabey D, Ronald A. Rapid tests for sexually transmitted infections (STIs): the way forward. *Sex Transm Infect.* 2006; 82:v1–6.

127. Sangani P, Rutherford G, Wilkinson D. Population-based interventions for reducing sexually transmitted infections, including HIV infection. *Cochrane Database Syst Rev.* 2004:CD001220.

128. Trelle S, Shang A, Nartey L, Cassell JA, Low N. Improved effectiveness of partner notification for patients with sexually transmitted infections: systematic review. *BMJ.* 2007;334–354.

129. Rekart ML. Sex-work harm reduction. *Lancet.* 2005;366:2123–34.

130. Tucker JD, Henderson GE, Wang TF, et al. Surplus men, sex work, and the spread of HIV in China. *AIDS.* 2005;19:539–547.

131. Peto J. AIDS and promiscuity. *Lancet.* 1986;2:979.

132. Doherty IA, Padian NS, Marlow C, Aral SO. Determinants and consequences of sexual networks as they affect the spread of sexually transmitted infections. *J Infect Dis.* 2005;191 Suppl 1: S42–54.

133. Anderson RM, Garnett G. Mathematical models of the transmission and control of sexually transmitted diseases. *Sexually Transmitted Diseases.* 2000;27:636–643.

134. Shepard CW, Simard EP, Finelli L, Fiore AE, Bell BP. Hepatitis B virus infection: epidemiology and vaccination. *Epidemiologic Review.* 2006;28: 112–125.

135. Sankaranarayanan R, Esmy PO, Rajkumar R, et al. Effect of visual screening on cervical cancer incidence and mortality in Tamil Nadu, India: a cluster-randomised trial. *Lancet.* 2007;370: 398–406.

136. Parham GP, Sahasrabuddhe VV, Mwanahamuntu MH, et al. Prevalence and predictors of squamous intraepithelial lesions of the cervix in HIV-infected women in Lusaka, Zambia. *Gynecologic Oncology.* 2006;103:1017–1022.

137. Sahasrabuddhe VV, Mwanahamuntu MH, Vermund SH, Huh WK, Lyon MD, Stringer JS, Parham GP. Prevalence and distribution of HPV genotypes among HIV-infected women in Zambia. *Br J Cancer.* 2007;96:1480–3.

138. Paz-Bailey G, Ramaswamy M, Hawkes SJ, Geretti AM. Herpes simplex virus type 2: Epidemiology and management options in developing countries. *Sex Transm Infect.* 2007;83:16–22.

139. Tita ATN, Grobman WA, Rouse DJ. Antenatal herpes serologic screening: An appraisal of the evidence. *Obstetrics and Gynecology.* 2006;108:1247–1253.

140. Reynolds SJ, Quinn TC. Developments in STD/HIV interactions: The intertwining epidemics of HIV and HSV-2. *Infectious Disease Clinics of North America.* 2005;19:415–425.

141. Celum CL, Robinson NJ, Cohen MS. Potential effect of HIV type 1 antiretroviral and herpes simplex virus type 2 antiviral therapy on transmission and acquisition of HIV type 1 infection. *J Infect Dis.* 2005;191 Suppl 1:S107–14.

142. Martino JL, Vermund SH. Vaginal Douching: Evidence for Risks or Benefits to Women's Health. *Epidemiologic Review* 2002;24:109–124.

143. Grimley D, Oh MK, Desmond R, Hook EW, Vermund SH. An intervention to reduce vaginal douching among adolescent and young adult women: A randomized, controlled trial. *Sexually Transmitted Diseases.* 2005;32:752–758.

144. Tsai CS, Shepard BE, et al. Does douching increase risk for sexually transmitted infections? A prospective study in high-risk adolescents. *Am J Obstet Gynecol.* In press, 2008.

145. Crowe JE, Williams JV. Immunology of viral respiratory tract infection in infancy. *Paediatric Respiratory Reviews.* 2003;4:112–119.

146. Zimmerman RK, Middleton DB. Vaccines for persons at high risk, 2007. *J Fam Pract.* 2007;56:S38–46, C4–5.

147. Pancharoen C, Ananworanich J, Thisyakorn U. Immunization for persons infected with human immunodeficiency virus. *Curr HIV Res.* 2004;2:293–9.

148. Healy CMa, Baker CJab. Prospects for prevention of childhood infections by maternal immunization. *Current Opinion in Infectious Diseases.* 2006; 19:271–276.

149. Gall SA. Maternal immunization to protect the mother and neonate. *Expert Review of Vaccines.* 2005;4:813–818.

150. Obaro SK, Palmer A. Vaccines for children: policies, politics and poverty. *Vaccine.* 2003;21:1423–1431.

151. Pickering LK, Orenstein WA. Development of pediatric vaccine recommendations and policies. *Semin Pediatr Infect Dis.* 2002;13:148–54.

152. Kimmel SR, Burns IT, Wolfe RM, Zimmerman RK. Addressing immunization barriers, benefits, and risks. *J Fam Pract.* 2007;56:S61–9.

153. Brent RL. Risks and benefits of immunizing pregnant women: The risk of doing nothing. *Reproductive Toxicology.* 2006;21:383–389.

154. Hinman A. Eradication of vaccine-preventable diseases. *Annu Rev Public Health.* 1999;20:211–29.

155. Moss WJ, Griffin DE. Global measles elimination. *Nat Rev Micro.* 2006;4:900–908.

156. Aylward RB. Eradicating polio: Today's challenges and tomorrow's legacy. *Ann Trop Med Parasitol.* 2006;100:401–13.

157. Salmon DA, Smith PJ, Navar AM, et al. Measuring Immunization Coverage among Preschool Children: Past, Present, and Future Opportunities. *Epidemiologic Review.* 2006;28:27–40.

158. WHO. Routine EPI Activities, 2007.

159. CDC. 2008 Child & Adolescent Immunization Schedules, 2008.

160. Kieny MP, Girard MP. Human vaccine research and development: An overview. *Vaccine.* 2005; 23:5705–5707.

161. Letvin NL. Progress and obstacles in the development of an AIDS vaccine. *Nat Rev Immunol.* 2006; 6:930–939.

162. Elliott LN, Lloyd AR, Ziegler JB, Ffrench RA. Protective immunity against hepatitis C virus infection. *Immunol Cell Biol.* 2006;84:239–249.

163. Cullen PA, Cameron CE. Progress towards an effective syphilis vaccine: The past, present and future. *Expert Review of Vaccines.* 2006;5:67–80.

164. Hotez P, Ottesen E, Fenwick A, Molyneux D. The neglected tropical diseases: The ancient afflictions of stigma and poverty and the prospects for their control and elimination. *Adv Exp Med Biol.* 2006;582:23–33.

165. Engels D, Savioli L. Reconsidering the underestimated burden caused by neglected tropical diseases. *Trends in Parasitology.* 2006;22:363–366.

166. Ruiz-Tiben E, Hopkins DR, David HM. Dracunculiasis (Guinea Worm Disease) Eradication Advances in Parasitology. Academic Press; 2006:275–309.

167. Brady MA, Hooper PJ, Ottesen EA. Projected benefits from integrating NTD programs in sub-Saharan Africa. *Trends in Parasitology.* 2006;22:285–291.

168. Pecoul B. New drugs for neglected diseases: From pipeline to patients. *PLoS Med.* 2004;1:e6.

169. Hotez PJ, Molyneux DH, Fenwick A, Ottesen E, Ehrlich Sachs S, Sachs JD. Incorporating a rapid-impact package for neglected tropical diseases with programs for HIV/AIDS, tuberculosis, and malaria. *PLoS Med.* 2006;3:e102.

170. Fauci AS, Touchette NA, Folkers GK. Emerging infectious diseases: A 10-year perspective from the National Institute of Allergy and Infectious Diseases. *Emerg Infect Dis.* 2005;11:519–25.

171. US Department of Health and Human Services. Centers for Disease Control and Prevention Epidemic/Epizootic West Nile Virus in the United States: Guidelines for Surveillance, Prevention, and Control, 3rd Revision. Fort Collins, CO: US Department of Health and Human Services; 2003.

172. Jernigan JA, Stephens DS, Ashford DA, et al. Bioterrorism-related inhalational anthrax: The first 10 cases reported in the United States. *Emerg Infect Dis.* 2001;7:933–44.

173. Lederberg J, Shope R, Oaks Jr S. Emerging infection: Microbial threats to health in the United States. Washington, DC: National Academy Press; 1992.

174. Garfield RM, Frieden T, Vermund SH. Health-related outcomes of war in Nicaragua. *Am J Public Health.* 1987;77:615–8.

175. Roberts L, Lafta R, Garfield R, Khudhairi J, Burnham G. Mortality before and after the 2003 invasion of Iraq: Cluster sample survey. *Lancet.* 2004;364:1857–1864.

176. Waters WF. Globalization, socioeconomic restructuring, and community health. *J Community Health.* 2001;26:79–92.

177. Albala C, Vio F, Yanez M. Epidemiological transition in Latin America: a comparison of four countries. *Rev Med Chil.* 1997;125:719–27.

178. Omran AR. The epidemiologic transition: a theory of the epidemiology of population change. 1971. *Milbank Q.* 2005;83:731–57.

179. Waters WF. Globalization and local response to epidemiological overlap in 21st century Ecuador. *Global Health.* 2006;2:8.

180. Popkin BM, Doak CM. The obesity epidemic is a worldwide phenomenon. *Nutr Rev.* 1998;56:106–14.

181. Monteiro CA, Conde WL, Popkin BM. Is obesity replacing or adding to undernutrition? Evidence from different social classes in Brazil. *Public Health Nutr.* 2002;5:105–12.

182. Moreno LA, Sarria A, Popkin BM. The nutrition transition in Spain: A European Mediterranean country. *Eur J Clin Nutr.* 2002;56:992–1003.

183. Popkin BM. An overview on the nutrition transition and its health implications: the Bellagio meeting. *Public Health Nutr.* 2002;5:93–103.

184. Popkin BM, Gordon-Larsen P. The nutrition transition: worldwide obesity dynamics and their determinants. *Int J Obes Relat Metab Disord.* 2004;28 Suppl 3:S2–9.

185. Hawkes C. Uneven dietary development: linking the policies and processes of globalization with the nutrition transition, obesity and diet-related chronic diseases. *Global Health* 2006;2:4.

186. Cassels S. Overweight in the Pacific: Links between foreign dependence, global food trade, and obesity in the Federated States of Micronesia. *Global Health.* 2006;2:10.

187. Bell AC, Ge K, Popkin BM. The road to obesity or the path to prevention: motorized transportation and obesity in China. *Obes Res.* 2002;10:277–83.

188. Du S, Lu B, Zhai F, Popkin BM. A new stage of the nutrition transition in China. *Public Health Nutr.* 2002;5:169–74.

189. International Diabetes Federation. *Diabetes Atlas: The e-Atlas,* 2007.

190. Chen L, Evans T, Anand S, et al. Human resources for health: overcoming the crisis. *Lancet.* 2004;364:1984–90.

191. MEDCC. Medical Education Cooperation with Cuba, 2007.

192. GCGH. Grand Challenges in Global Health. Goals and Challenges: Overcoming Barriers to Good Health, 2007.

193. NIH. *NIH Road Map for Medical Research.* Washington DC, 2007.

194. Stop TB. Stop TB Partnership, 2007.

195. The AIDS Monitor. *Overview of the Global Fund to Fight AIDS, Tuberculosis and Malaria Center for Global Development,* 2007.

196. The Global Fund. The Global Fund to fight AIDS, Tuberculosis and Malaria, 2007.

197. PEPFAR. *President's Emergency Plan for AIDS Relief,* 2007.

198. WHO. *Treating 3 Million by 2005.* Geneva: WHO, 2005.

199. The William J Clinton Foundation. Clinton HIV/AIDS Initiative, 2007.

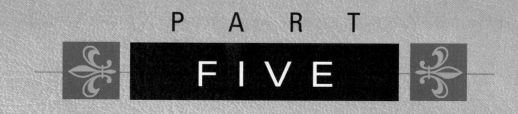

PART
FIVE

The Future of Public Health Practice

CHAPTER 31

The Future of Public Health

C. William Keck, MD, MPH and F. Douglas Scutchfield, MD

LEARNING OBJECTIVES

Upon completion of this chapter, the reader will be able to:

1. Describe the potential impact of preventive services on health status in the United States.
2. Discuss how changes in the illness care sector can affect public health practice.
3. Describe cultural, professional, and scientific elements that impact public health practice.
4. Describe attributes of local health departments that are key to their effectiveness.
5. List and discuss characteristics that will be found in the successful health departments of the future.

KEY TERMS

Accreditation
Bioterrorism
Certification
Clinical Preventive Services
Credentialing
Determinant
Disease Prevention
Genome
Global Warming
Health Disparities
Health Promotion
Health Status
Infrastructure
Institute of Medicine (IOM)
Life Expectancy
Lifestyle
Medical Care
Performance Standards
Premature Death
Social Justice
Surveillance

Significant gains in **health status** and **life expectancy** have occurred over the past 200 years in the United States as well as in most other industrialized nations. Many attribute those gains to advances in clinical medicine that tend to be dramatically and impressively chronicled in the electronic and print media. Indeed, our capacity to diagnose and treat illness has advanced rapidly. The reality remains, however, that most of the improvements in quality and length of life have come from measures aimed at protecting populations from environmental hazards and pursuing behaviors and activities that are known to be health promoting.[1] Health departments and other community agencies are responsible for developing the programs and relationships with individuals and neighborhoods that will continue to improve the health of citizens of this country.

In spite of this fact, the public health system has been largely ignored during the second half of the twentieth century. Resources were focused disproportionately on medical care while the public health system was allowed to atrophy compared to the growing need for its services. The two **Institute of Medicine (IOM)** reports often cited in this book, plus the tragedy of 9/11 and the subsequent anthrax episode, provided both a professional and public awakening to the need to reinvest in public health. Despite some positive steps, however, much remains to be done for public health practice to be in the best position to contribute what it can to the effort to improve health status. This chapter reviews the continuing potential for public health contributions to healthfulness, the relationships of public health to the medical care system, challenges facing the changing practice of public health, and likely characteristics of successful health departments of the future.

THE CONTRIBUTIONS OF PUBLIC HEALTH

Public health policies and actions have significantly improved the health status of the population of the United States. Their contribution is summarized in this section.

Public Health Measures and Previous Health Status Gains

Significant gains in population health status during the nineteenth and early twentieth centuries were based on activities ensuring the availability and safety of food and clean water, the adequate disposal of sewage, the provision of adequate and safe shelter with minimal crowding, and the adoption of personal behaviors that were health promoting. Due to these measures, substantial control of many communicable diseases was accomplished before the advent of vaccines and antibiotics. For example, tuberculosis deaths declined as a result of improved physical environments and better nutrition; the impact of fecally/orally transmitted pathogens declined with the separation of sewage and drinking water; and vector-borne conditions improved with vector habitat control.[2] These changes, combined with the discovery of vaccines and antibiotics, modified the major causes of death from infectious diseases at the turn of the previous century to chronic diseases, including heart disease, cancer, and stroke, currently. There has been a concomitant rapid gain of life expectancy from 48 years for men and 51 for women in 1900 to 75 and 80 years, respectively, in 2003.[3]

During the past four decades, there has been a growing emphasis on population-based prevention programs aimed at reducing risks for chronic disease. Programs aimed at reducing tobacco use, controlling blood pressure, diminishing obesity and dietary fat, reducing risks for occupational and home injury, and promoting use of seat belts and automobile air bags have contributed to a decline of 50 percent in stroke deaths, 40 percent in coronary heart disease deaths, and 25 percent in death rates for children.[2]

Potential for Further Gains in Health Status

The Centers for Disease Control and Prevention (CDC) reviewed the major causes of **premature death** in United States citizens.[4] Their findings confirmed that approximately 50 percent of premature mortality in this country is directly related to

Table 31.1. 10 Leading Causes of Death in the United States, 2003

Cause of Death	No. of Deaths
All Causes	2,448,288
Diseases of the Heart	685,089
Malignant Neoplasms	556,902
Cerbrovascular Diseases	157,689
Chronic Lower Respiratory Diseases	126,382
Unintentional Injuries	109,277
Diabetes Mellitus	74,219
Influenza and Pneumonia	65,163
Alzheimer's Disease	63,457
Nephritis, Nephrotic Syndrome, and Nephrosis	42,453
Septicemia	34,069

SOURCE: *Health, United States, 2006.* Available at: http://www.cdc.gov/nchs/data/hus/hus06.pdf.

Table 31.2. Leading Underlying Causes of Death in the United States, 2000

Cause of Death	No. of Deaths
Tobacco	435,000
Diet/Inactivity	400,000
Alcohol	85,000
Certain Infections	75,000
Toxic Agents	55,000
Motor Vehicles	43,000
Firearms	29,000
Sexual Behavior	20,000
Drug Use	17,000

SOURCE: Mokdad JM, Marks JS, Stroup DF, Gerberding JL. Actual causes of death in the United States, 2000. *JAMA.* 2004;291:1238–1245.

individual **lifestyle** and behavior, about 20 percent is related to environmental factors, an additional 20 percent is directly related to one's inherited genetic profile, and only about 10 percent is related to inadequate access to **medical care.** This means that fully 70 percent of the premature mortality suffered by the United States population will require population-based strategies in addition to medical care for effective control.

Traditional discussions of health status include a list of the major causes of death for the population of interest. That information is listed in Table 31.1 for the United States.

From a public health/preventive perspective, however, the real question is what underlying risk factors caused the fatal conditions listed in Table 31.1. The underlying causes of many of the premature deaths occurring in our population are listed in Table 31.2.

These factors, which are closely linked to the determinants of health discussed in Chapter 4, are at the root of the finding that 50 percent of premature mortality in the United States is due to factors related to lifestyle. These factors are the major causes of preventable conditions that carry a high cost in terms of morbidity, mortality, and dollars. Improving access to medical care is an important goal for those who lack access, but it alone will have little impact on diminishing the death and disability reflected in the disease figures just cited. AIDS will not be controlled by actions taken in physician's offices, low-birth-weight babies will not be prevented solely by the work of obstetricians, and heart disease will not continue to decline without extensive community outreach and education.

Human health is also directly related to the quality of the environment. Factors such as air pollution, food and water contaminants, radiation, toxic chemicals, wastes, disease vectors, safety hazards, and habitat alterations are at the root of the 20 percent excess mortality related to environmental issues in the United States. Long-term human health is dependent upon achieving ecological balance and maintaining health-promoting home, work, and leisure environments. Whereas we have a tendency to dwell on the negative aspects of environmental factors on health, we must also recognize that some aspects of our environment can enhance health. Frumpkin reviewed the positive features of our world that enhance health status. His findings suggest that the public health leader will need to acquire new skills, such as land-use planning, that were not previously thought necessary.[5]

The combination of ensuring access to medical care and paying attention to the **determinants** of health has been brought to national attention by the "100% Access, 0 Disparities" campaign proposed by the United States Department of Health and Human Service's Health Resources and Services Administration's Bureau of Primary Health Care in the mid-1990s.[6] This grassroots effort, which has evolved into a national movement called Communities Joined in Action,[7] challenges communities to reorganize and rationalize the distribution of health care locally, and to identify and confront the basic causes of **health disparities**. The latter will require that public health officials understand the impact of social and economic factors on health, and revamp their approach to disease control to address these causative factors.

PUBLIC HEALTH IN AN EVOLVING MEDICAL CARE SYSTEM

The United States continues to search for the "best" way to finance and deliver illness (medical) care. The nation's citizens are increasingly unhappy because the number of uninsured and underinsured continues to grow despite relative prosperity in the country overall. The insured are asked to carry more of the financial load through increased premiums, deductibles, and co-pays. Many can't find coverage for pre-existing conditions and face the potential of personal bankruptcy if severe illness occurs. Rising costs for health coverage are straining the traditional employer-based programs, and United States businesses offering health insurance are placed at a

financial disadvantage in competition with foreign companies in countries that enjoy government subsidized coverage, or where there is no expectation of coverage. Research continues to demonstrate that the quality of care given to the insured in the United States can often be substandard, and there is no question that the uninsured or underinsured population is less healthy than the population with "good" insurance.[8] Ominously, it is also clear that the nation is increasingly sedentary and overweight with the result that the prevalence of many associated chronic diseases is on the rise. The question is whether the sum total of these realities has reached sufficient mass to counterbalance well-funded constituencies that oppose change that would diminish their income or influence. Whether the result is continued "tinkering" with the system or a substantial reworking of it, the public health practitioner will be affected. This requires awareness of changes as they occur, at a minimum, or preferably, participation in the policy debates that are sure to continue in this area. The authors believe the United States medical care system is unsustainable in its current form, and major restructuring is desirable.

In many ways, the debate about health care reform is miscast. For the most part, the wrong question is being addressed. Attempts are made to seek better ways of providing and paying for illness care rather than to determine what should be done to create the healthiest population possible. With the courage and the foresight to frame the debate in these terms, it is readily apparent that improved health status depends on illness care reform *and* on public health reform.

For too long, those professionals who concentrate on the diagnosis and treatment of illness have been separated from those who concentrate on **health promotion**, **disease prevention**, and control of the environment. Instead of a seamless web of integrated services and activities focusing first on minimizing risks and then on early diagnosis and treatment of emerging disease, two separate systems have developed and evolved into two distinct cultures that are often at odds with one another. It is the responsibility of public health practitioners to help society understand the value of each approach and the need to integrate them into a quest for improving health status. As we noted in Chapter 3, the major professional organizations representing these two professions, the American Medical Association (AMA) and the American Public Health Association (APHA), have opened a dialogue around this issue and are encouraging discussions designed to bridge the gap between medical care and public health.[9,10] It is hard to believe that significant progress will be made, however, until health promotion and disease prevention are valued as much as illness diagnosis and therapy.

Obtaining medical care is very important for that segment of the population for whom access is denied or inappropriately restricted, of course. The approximately 10 percent of excess mortality in citizens of the United States that is related to inadequate access to medical care occurs principally in that group for whom access to care is limited by virtue of its cost. No illness is "deserved," and every member of society should have access to those interventions that have been developed to diagnose and treat disease and minimize suffering. It is also worth noting that significant contributions to disease prevention can be made in the context of a single patient's interaction with a physician or other health care provider. The activities described in the *Guide to Clinical Preventive Services*[11] are particularly recommended for their proven capacity to improve health and prevent disease and injury. It is also true that preventive care is underused for the almost 85 percent of the population that has access to primary care. A new report released recently by the Partnership for Prevention notes that the use of key preventive services by Americans remains low despite the evidence of the effectiveness of these services. The report states that increasing the use of just five preventive services (low dose aspirin for adults, advising smokers to quit, colorectal cancer screening, annual flu immunizations, and breast cancer screening) could save up to 100,000 lives annually.[12] Preventive and population-based services applied in both clinical and public health settings have the greatest potential to contribute to overall gains in health status.

THE CORE FUNCTIONS OF PUBLIC HEALTH

Population-based services are provided from a variety of sources in most communities. These sources include state and local health departments, community health agencies (e.g., family planning agencies, heart associations, kidney associations, cancer societies, mental health agencies, and drug abuse agencies, among others), hospitals, and schools, to name several. However, this chapter focuses on the local health department because it is only the local health department that has statutory responsibility for the health status of its constituent population. It is the health department, in most locations, that is ultimately responsible for the assurance that all citizens have access to the services they need in the community, no matter which groups or organizations ultimately deliver those services. This focus on the health needs of the entire community by an agency ultimately responsible to that community for its performance emphasizes the importance for health of "a governmental presence at the local level (AGPALL)."[13]

Institute of Medicine Reports

There exists wide variation in the size, sophistication, capacity, and roles of local health departments in the United States. In its 1988 report, *The Future of Public Health*, IOM's Committee for the Study of the Future of Public Health described widespread agreement across the country that "public health does things that benefit everybody," and that "public health prevents illness and educates the population."[14(p3)] However, it found little consensus on how those broad statements should be translated into action. Indeed, there is such great variability in resources, available services, and organizational arrangements "that contemporary public health is defined less by what public health professionals know how to do than by what the political system in a given area decides is appropriate or feasible."[14(p4)]

The committee concluded that "effective public health activities are essential to the health and well-being of the American people, now and in the future," but the variability across the country is so great that this essential system is currently in "disarray."[14(p6)]

In an effort to provide a set of directions for the discipline of public health that could attract the support of the whole society, the committee proposed a public health mission statement and a set of core functions. These are thoroughly reviewed in Chapter 3. In 2003, IOM completed a second report focused on the description of a framework for assuring the public's health in the future.[15] IOM's Committee on Assuring the Health of the Public in the 21st Century looked at health achievements and issues that undercut the potential for improvement in health status, the role of government in protecting and promoting public health, the importance of partnerships between governmental agencies and groups from other sectors of society, and trends that are likely to influence health in the coming decades. The report is highly recommended reading for those engaged in public health leadership and policy-making positions.

Unfortunately, the study committee found the conclusion of the 1988 IOM report that the governmental component of the nation's public health system was in disarray still valid 15 years later. To be sure, efforts have been made to improve the circumstances that led to that conclusion, but governmental public health agencies continue to suffer from under-funding, political neglect, and exclusion from forums where their expert advice and leadership are essential for an effective public health system.[15(p26)] These agencies continue to be saddled with deficiencies in the tools and other resources necessary to assure population health, and a secure future requires expansion of support for their resource needs and their inclusion in policy-making activities.

In addition, the IOM notes in the most recent report that the increasingly fragile health care sector threatens efforts to assure the health of the public. Particular problems noted include the growing number of uninsured and underinsured people in this country, the minimal coverage provided for preventive care by the Medicare program, the common lack of treatment options for people with mental health or substance abuse problems, inequality of care provided to racial and ethnic minorities compared to the white population, and the poor distribution of health care resources that limits the ability to address complex medical problems of an aging population or manage a large scale emergency.[15(pp27–28)] The IOM committee also noted the importance of broadening the segments of society responsible for, and involved in, activities likely to improve health status. In addition to elements of the public health and health care **infrastructure**, employers and businesses, the media, academia, and others are important players in a real public health "system" dedicated to creating the conditions necessary to assure the best possible health status.[15(p30)] All have a role to play in assuring the 10 essential services are delivered by the Local Public Health System (LPHS), tasks that can be monitored using the National Performance Standards (see Chapter 3). The committee described 6 areas of action and change that are central to the desire to create an effective intersectoral health system that can increase levels of health and longevity in the United States in the near future:

1. Adopt a population health approach that builds on evidence of the multiple determinants of health.

2. Strengthen the governmental public health infrastructure—the backbone of any public health system.

3. Create a new generation of partnerships to build consensus on health priorities and support community and individual health actions.

4. Develop appropriate systems of accountability at all levels to ensure that population health goals are met.

5. Assure that action is based on evidence.

6. Acknowledge communication as the key to forging partnerships, assuring accountability, and using evidence for decision making and action.[15(p33–34)]

We note in Chapter 3 that public health has been undergoing a philosophic renaissance during the past two decades. Significant problems remain, however, with the structure and funding of local public health services. These problems hinder the capacity of the system to provide the services required for our population to reach the maximum healthfulness our knowledge and technology make possible. The recommendations of the 2003 IOM committee recognize that future progress requires attention and action in the areas listed. Unfortunately, there is little evidence that major policy makers in the Congress or administration at the time of this writing perceive the nature of the problem in any detail, let alone share a commitment to lead the nation in a venture to improve health status. It is not likely that significant progress can be made until the nation commits itself to transforming the current illness care industry into a real health care system and actively engages those with the requisite expertise in such an undertaking.

PUBLIC HEALTH SYSTEM CHANGES

Although the basic organization and structure of local and state health departments has not evolved in a manner that matches the change that has occurred in public health thinking over the past several decades, there have been significant shifts in programmatic emphasis that have affected the public health system and raised questions about future trends. Chief among those, particularly in more recent years, have been the infusion of **bioterrorism** funds and the push away from the provision of direct medical services to individuals in health department settings.

Bioterrorism Funding

As noted in Chapter 3, the events of September 11, 2001, the anthrax attacks that came soon thereafter,

the SARS epidemic, and growing concern about avian influenza focused attention on the preparedness of the public health system (and others) to respond to natural and man-made events that threatened health on a grand scale. Public health professionals were not surprised by the verdict that readiness was deemed inadequate, at best. It was clear that the diverse practices of more than 3,000 local health departments, each of which had developed and evolved in a unique environment, did not constitute a "system" that could be easily coordinated to meet large national or regional threats. In addition, the public health workforce was small (inadequate) and lacked many of the competencies that an effective response to these emerging threats would require. Technology was limited to the degree that no comprehensive electronic surveillance and information system existed that crossed jurisdictional boundaries.[16]

America responded to these realities with relative speed. The Public Health Security and Bioterrorism Response Act of 2002 required national initiatives to develop countermeasures to catastrophes, infrastructure to handle mass casualties, and information systems linking relevant agencies, including health departments. The Homeland Security Act of 2002 was designed to improve the country's ability to prevent and respond to acts of terrorism. President Bush signed an Executive Order in April 2003 designating SARS a communicable disease for purposes of enacting control measures, if necessary. The CDC launched a website to inform the public about avian influenza. In addition, President Bush proposed substantial increases in funding to combat bioterrorism, and new attention was focused on strengthening the nation's public health infrastructure.

These initiatives fostered strong efforts to creatively improve preparedness capacity on the part of all agencies and institutions engaged in the effort, including state and local health departments. These efforts included increasing laboratory capabilities, strengthening disease **surveillance** and communication mechanisms, performing preparedness training, and conducting drills and exercises. These investments have clearly improved the capacity to deal with communicable disease outbreaks and other threats across the country.

Unfortunately, however, federal funds for other public health programs have been reduced during this period, and most states have experienced revenue shortfalls leading to public health budget reductions. The sum total of these realities is that health departments are faced with supporting ongoing public health service needs and the new preparedness initiatives with little additional funding.[17,18] The failure to address clearly how national protection activities should be organized and how government public health agencies should be configured to be maximally effective, however, leaves us with a situation where public expectations for the ability to respond almost certainly continue to exceed capacity. The need to reorganize and restructure governmental public health agencies and provide them with the resources necessary for them to meet their obligations is left for the future.

Shift Away from Direct Medical Services

The inadequacies of the medical care system(s) in the United States have driven much of nonenvironmental public health programming for decades. Health departments are often "courts of last resort" in their communities for populations who are unable to receive **clinical preventive services** or medical care through other means. Child health clinics, prenatal care services, family planning clinics, and so on, exist in local health departments to fill gaps in medical care. Public health leaders have sometimes bemoaned the fact that their resources would be better spent meeting health promotion and disease prevention objectives, but some have become financially dependent upon third-party payments for clinical services. Nonetheless, there has been a strong push from the federal government to "privatize" Medicaid and move clinical services into the private sector. This transition has largely occurred, and it has moved ahead in the absence of any clear policy initiatives to enhance the ability of health departments to meet national health status goals. As a matter of fact, there has never been a coherent and strong public policy agenda to improve population health in the United States.

An important issue facing leaders in both the medical care and public health sectors is the place of public health in a system when health care access issues are either solved or lessened, or where the provision of medical care services is made difficult for local health departments to accomplish. How does one re-educate the public to embrace and support a new version of public health activities when many continue to view public health's role to primarily be provision of health care to the poor? How does one meld public health with medicine more effectively in a culture that values treatment over prevention? How can one best introduce principles of population medicine into clinical practice?

If we prove unable to provide good answers to these questions in the near future, we are likely to experience a continuation of mission confusion with a poor coherence of approach. That will be characterized by a continuation of disproportionate funding going to medical care and by an expansion of orphan topics that become public health's responsibility alone by default (nutrition, aging, violence, drug abuse, built environment and urban sprawl, exercise, global warming, school health, etc.). We are left, therefore, with the large tasks of developing a national focus on populations as well as individuals, and better defining which population-centered programs work and which do not, so that appropriate population-based services can be defined and supported. In short, we will be in the business of determining who will fund, direct, control and evaluate public health services in the future. Local health departments must be prepared to understand and influence medical care policy change because of the impact such change has on public health programs. Questions about how best to organize and deliver health services are once more on the national agenda. The experience of attempted national health care reform in 1994 suggests we should remain a bit cynical about the likely outcome, but that should not dissuade us from full participation in the debate. It is an opportunity we should not allow to pass without our full engagement.

PUBLIC HEALTH IN RAPID EVOLUTION—NEW CHALLENGES

In addition to the internal and external forces described previously that are impacting the delivery of public health services, other cultural, professional, and scientific elements impacting our society are inevitably affecting the practice of public health.

Information, Informatics, and Communication

We live in a time of incredibly rapid change in our ability to communicate with each other. This age of electronic communication is characterized by continuous enhancement of the speed and sophistication with which large amounts of information can be created, processed, and distributed. The Internet provides a platform for extremely rapid access to huge amounts of information on almost any subject. It can be used for low-cost communication between individuals and groups who share common interests. Every state health department and almost every local health department is now connected to this medium that provides expanding opportunities to communicate with other agencies that have overlapping missions and interests, and to communicate directly with a large portion of the population for whom they have some responsibility. Increasingly sophisticated software allows for the development of electronic medical records, syndromic surveillance systems, new datasets, geographic information systems (GIS), sophisticated imaging and reporting, and on and on. As difficult as it is to keep up with this expansion of hardware and software, the effective public health agency will learn to take advantage of the opportunities that exist in this area to enhance its capacity to develop accurate information about communities, provide effective public health interventions and programs targeted at well described problems, and evaluate the effectiveness of interventions.

The advent of the electronic medical record provides a growing list of opportunities to use information about individuals from many sources to enhance the understanding of populations. There is a paradox inherent in this situation, however, because the potential for inappropriate use of information about individuals and their health problems has delayed the use of information that might impact individual privacy rights. Significant future energy will be spent on analyzing these competing interests and designing surveillance systems that can both inform public health practice and protect individuals.

Socioeconomic Determinants of Health

Chapter 4 provides a thorough review of the individual, environmental, and health care characteristics that affect individuals and populations. The impact of these characteristics on health status is reviewed in Chapter 4 and summarized to some degree at the beginning of this chapter. In an ideal world, the public health system would be able to turn most of its attention to amelioration of those factors (income, race, family structure, community resources, etc.) that can impact the social fabric in ways that are detrimental to health. In the less than ideal world in which we work, we have the challenge of moving in that direction in the absence of clear policy and funding prerogatives to do so.

To begin, public health will have to find its way to decision-making tables where it has been infrequently represented before. It can be argued that public health should be present whenever public policy decisions are made to assess the likely impact on population health, both positive and negative, of policy decisions. For example, the structure of the so-called built environment impacts health, so public health should be represented at forums where construction of housing, factories, parks, and roads is discussed. Programs that engage, or propose to engage, existing social networks should seek assistance in understanding the public health role in building human and social capital, and so on. The effective public health practitioner of the future will need to acquire knowledge and skills that will allow impact in these areas.

Building the Public Health Research Base

Given the lack of a real population focus in health policy and planning in the United States, it is not surprising that the bulk of health research dollars are spent in the area of disease diagnosis and treatment. This bias in investigative scholarship has left the field of public health lagging in understanding the structure, operation, and impact of public health programs and delivery systems. This, in turn, leaves public health policy makers and administrators with a thin portfolio for guidance in the establishment of effective public health interventions. Fortunately, concerted efforts are underway to systematically address public health research needs. The Community Preventive Services Guidelines process identifies community interventions where evidence related to their effectiveness is incomplete or absent, the Council on Linkages Between Academia and Public Health Practice has compiled a list of detailed public health systems research needs, the CDC's Office of Public Health Practice has developed a national agenda for public health systems research, and many of the profession's leading researchers, thinkers, and professional organizations are focusing new attention on improving the science base for public health practice. Academy Health, with funding from the Robert Wood Johnson Foundation, is engaged in a process with major public health research stakeholders of further refining and prioritizing a research agenda in preparation for a strong effort to attract new funding to this field.

Perhaps the best summary of the challenge that lies ahead was penned by Glen P. Mays, PhD, MPH in the Conclusion section of his white paper, "Understanding the Dimensions of Public Health Delivery Systems: Theory, Evidence, and Unanswered Questions," prepared for Academy Health in June, 2007:

> Addressing current and future research needs in public health will require more than a few rigorous and timely studies conducted on

high priority topics. A successful research enterprise on public health systems will require sustained commitments to building robust data resources that reflect the organizational, financial, and workforce characteristics of public health delivery systems at local, state, and national levels. Data elements that historically have been collected from multiple, episodic surveys of state and local public health agencies need to be standardized and routinely collected to support expanded research on systems. Additionally, public health agencies, professionals, and others involved in the delivery of public health services need to be engaged more directly in the conceptualization, design, and conduct of public health systems research studies. Such engagement will ensure that studies are asking the right questions, using the best data and measures, and capitalizing on opportunities for studying natural experiments that result from organizational and policy changes. Additionally, practitioner engagement—such as through practice-based research networks and participatory research designs—promises to reduce the cycle time required for disseminating and integrating new evidence into practice. If successful, expanded research on public health systems will strengthen the ability of governmental public health agencies and their private-sector partners to deliver services that protect and promote health. The result will be a continuously improving public health system that assures the conditions necessary for all Americans to enjoy healthier lives.

Assuring the involvement of practitioners is, as Dr. Mays notes, an important factor if research is to be useful. Since the 1988 IOM report lament about the major decoupling they found between academia and public health practice, much has been done to expand the connections between town and gown. Much remains to be done, however, and expanding and strengthening the linkages between them will be a required prerequisite for effectively completing public health services research and translating the results into effective patterns of practice. Both academic and practice settings will need to find or create expanded opportunities to develop working relationships that will facilitate the movement of students into practice settings for relevant learning experiences and will establish partnerships for service research. The academic health department is one approach to linking health departments and academic institutions that is gaining some traction.[19,20] One of the most attractive elements of this model is the involvement of practitioners in academic settings and vice versa, and the opportunities presented for training public health professionals in combined academic/practice venues. Practitioners and academics who link now will be in good position to take advantage of funding for service-related research likely to become available during the next decade.

Accreditation of Local Health Departments

As noted in Chapter 3, the **credentialing** of the public health workforce has already begun with the development of The National Board of Public Health Examiners and the administration of the first board examination for Master of Public Health graduates in 2008. The recent progress in the description of essential services a community must have in place to reach high levels of healthfulness, coupled with the development of **performance standards** for public health services at the national level and in many states, and the development by the National Association of County and City Health Officials (NACCHO) of an "Operational Definition of a Functional Local Health Department" in 2005[21] has set the stage for a process to measure agency capacity. A report commissioned by the Robert Wood Johnson Foundation in late 2004 noted that there was no real momentum for state health agency **certification**, but that there are many examples of innovative programming related to agency **accreditation** at the local level.[22] The importance of making local health departments accountable for their work across the country led to the establishment in October 2006 of a national

Public Health Accreditation Board (see http://www.exploringaccreditation.org). The board has implemented a voluntary national accreditation program. This is an example of "lap over" from the medical care system where concern about quality of service delivery has led to quality improvement activities, pay for performance, and so on, and effective health departments should begin to prepare themselves for new levels of accountability.

Population Shifts and Diversity

Health disparities among subpopulation groups in the United States have been well documented and have proved very difficult to resolve. To be sure, if access to care for all can be achieved, it will have some positive impact, but that alone will not cause health disparities to disappear. The evidence is growing that many of the roots of health disparities lie in the areas of social policy, economics, environment, and in our personal perceptions and prejudices,[23,24] and these are compounded by a constant influx of immigrants from around the world who bring with them their own unique cultural attributes, many of which affect their smooth integration into American society. The social environment, or our social health, should be as carefully monitored as the more traditional indicators of community health status.[25] The major difficulty in all of this is deciding the appropriate role for local health departments. Influencing social and economic policy making and confronting the realities of racism, sexism, and ageism are not simple tasks. They require broadly based partnerships at least, and at most a new paradigm of public health service delivery. It will be important for the public health community to become familiar with this new public health agenda item, to monitor the impact of new models of public health activity developing in some communities,[26] and to determine how best to influence social health in their own constituencies.

This suggests that there may well be a new set of skills that the public health practitioner will need. Practitioners might want to attend a planning and zoning committee meeting to provide input and suggestions for arranging the community to assure opportunities for exercise by providing parks and bike trails, for example. Additionally, one might ask whether the community offers enough opportunities for recreation and interaction of community members, and whether there are community centers where clubs and organizations can meet, parks where families and other groups can gather, bandstands, and so on.

Globalization

International health issues will become increasingly important for local public health. The most obvious issue is the repeated demonstration that many infectious diseases are not constrained by geopolitical boundaries. The reality that relatively large numbers of people travel to almost anywhere else in the world within the 24 hours of any given day creates the potential for any new or re-emerging infection to become a major public health problem in the United States at any time. This risk is compounded by the present day reality that both domestic and foreign enemies of the United States can choose to attack populations in this country with acts of violence against property (federal building bombing in Oklahoma, 9/11) or against people with toxic or infectious agents (anthrax) in an effort to create large numbers of casualties and population panic. As described previously, these activities have brought new awareness to the important role of public health in dealing with biological and chemical disasters, and resources directed to public health in recent years have improved response capacity for future disasters but also for more "routine" disease surveillance and outbreak control measures. Maintaining and improving preparedness will be a major public health practice issue for the foreseeable future.

The continuing degradation of the global physical environment has substantial implications for human health in all parts of the world, including the United States. Rain forest loss and desertification, species extinction, populations driven by poverty and hunger massing in so-called mega cities, **global warming**, and so on, will influence disease patterns around the globe. Persons anxious to escape poverty and conflict are migrating in large numbers to the so-called developed countries. In the United States, this results in a growing number and size of minority populations with a tendency to exacerbate the already unacceptable health disparities that exist between majority and minority groups in this country, despite special attention paid to this issue over the past decade or so. The need for cultural awareness and increased cross-cultural competency on the part of public health workers is both obvious and problematic. Bringing minority representatives into the public health workforce and minority students and faculty into academic institutions that train public health workers remains a priority that attains increasing urgency with the growing diversity of the United States population. The minimal success accomplished to date will need to be significantly enhanced if public health is to remain relevant to the needs of its constituents in the future.

The Human Genome

The deciphering of the human **genome** has been a remarkable scientific achievement. We now possess the master code for increased understanding of humans. The biologic and medical implications of this feat are increasingly apparent, and there is growing awareness of the ethical challenges inherent in that understanding. Little attention, so far, has been directed at the public health implications of being able to characterize human beings and their risk for disease in this manner, except for the wide practice of newborn genetic screening. Nevertheless, it is likely that human genomic understanding will produce new tools for the practice of public health, as well as significant challenges to the appropriateness of their use. The competencies that will be required of public health practitioners in this area have been delineated in a workshop sponsored by the CDC,[27(p70)] but few training programs and institutions have developed curriculum intended to assure that future public health graduates have a broad understanding of genomics and future use of the discipline in public health practice.

CAPACITY OF HEALTH DEPARTMENTS TO FULFILL CORE AND OTHER FUNCTIONS

Since the publication of the first IOM report dealing with the future of public health in 1988, there has been growing agreement in the public health community that the core functions and resulting 10 essential services of public health make sense. The profession has been busy defining the particulars of those services in the interim, as described earlier. The growing unity of thought about public health's core functions and essential services, however, begs the question of whether or not local and state health departments actually have the capacity to fulfill the core functions and the other tasks that may be required of them by their own communities. Indeed, available evidence suggests that there is great variability in capacity among the diverse agencies found at local and state levels.

Organizational Diversity

Chapter 10 in this book reviews the structure, governance, financing, and capacities of local health departments. The diversity that characterizes health departments is perhaps an indication of just how problematic it can be to provide public-sector services in a democracy. Competition for attention and resources among many interests in a system with multiple decision makers and policy makers makes it difficult to attain and sustain coherence and consistency of function.[14(p123)] In addition to the organizational variability of local public health agencies, there is also a great deal of programmatic variability that results from the deliberate delegation out of public health departments of a number of responsibilities previously considered to be in the purview of public health.

The 1988 IOM report noted that the coherence of public health activities is damaged by the administration of environmental health, mental health, and indigent care programs by separate agencies.[14(pp108–112)] This separation of responsibilities encourages the development of separate programs and fragmented data systems that impede integrated problem analysis and risk assessment. The result is diminished coherency in the efforts of government to provide service and a division of constituencies that might otherwise coalesce around a broad vision of the mission of public health.[14(pp123–124)]

Funding

In addition to the problems noted in the previous section, most local health departments must cope with inconsistent funding sources. Some local departments are comparatively well funded, but many face severe financial constraints and must rely heavily on sources of revenue that may very well result in inadequate and unstable funding. It has been clearly demonstrated, for example, that the performance of essential public health services in local health departments is directly associated with public health spending levels, even after controlling for system and community characteristics.[28] Where to find the needed resources will be a continuing challenge. The realization that the public health system is an integral part of preparedness has resulted in increased funding for that purpose with some positive spillover into more routine public health activities. At the same time, however, the period during which preparedness funding accelerated, also saw declines in federal support for other public health functions. Health departments need to be creative to find resources that can be applied to material needs for housing and equipment, and the solution of population health problems. Possible sources include private foundations, fees for service, hospital and other partnerships, research grants, and so on. With a wide diversity of funding sources, public health financial managers need to be more publicly accountable and develop management skills more akin to those found in the private sector.

Public Health Training in the Workforce

Most public health workers, including some public health leaders, have not had formal training in public health. The IOM report noted the need for well-trained public health professionals with "appropriate technical expertise, management and political skills, and a firm grounding in the commitment to the public good and **social justice** that gives public health its coherence as a professional calling."[14(p127)] The report further noted that public health leadership requires an appreciation of the role and nature of government. It also requires the capacity to continue to learn to stay current with the evolution of the discipline.

Chapter 17 contains a thorough review and analysis of the composition and current state of the public health workforce, including activities currently underway to address the problems described. The fragile nature of that workforce is highlighted from the perspective that growing shortages in competent professionals are predicted, and the authors note the importance of conducting rigorous inquiry into the nature of the workforce and its impact on health outcomes. They also note that health status in the future is dependent to a significant degree on the thoughtful deployment and nurturing of an evolving public health workforce.

An important component of public health training is integration of learning with practical experience. It is critical that public health students and workers receive training linked to practice by requiring practicum experiences in local health agencies for students; improving communication and collaboration among agencies and schools through such efforts as joint programs, research, and technical assistance, among others; making education and training programs more relevant to practice; and increasing the resources devoted to linking academia with practice.[29]

Until consistent, high-quality, easily accessible workforce development is available, on-the-job training will continue to be the major mechanism for integrating professionals into the public health workplace (see Chapter 10). There are, however, no formal standards for this kind of learning experience, so the presence of the values and skills required is inconstant at best in those who receive their training in public health in this manner.

Staff Size

An important indicator of the capacity of an agency's staff to fulfill the core functions of public health is the size of its staff. The large majority of health departments are small. NACCHO's *1990 National Profile of Local Health Departments*[30] revealed that 26 percent of local health departments in the United States at that time had 4 or fewer employees, and an additional 20 percent had between 5 and 9 employees. Information collected in 2001 showed that although local health departments, on average, employ 67 full-time staff, the median is 13. This would indicate a preponderance of very small departments.[31] More recent information from NACCHO reviewed in Chapter 10, Table 10.12, indicates that small local health departments serving small populations usually employ just a few occupations: typically, a director, nurses, environmental health specialists, and clerical staff. The larger departments, in contrast, are most likely to have significant numbers of staff with the public health or related training and resultant capacity to pursue assessment, policy development, and assurance functions as refined in the 10 essential services.

Technical Capacity

Technical capacity is closely linked to the issue of staffing, although it also includes the availability of equipment that might be required to provide for preventive health services, analysis of environmental health problems, laboratory services, and health education activities, among others. Few data exist regarding the distribution of equipment and facilities, but it is probably reasonable to assume that it follows the same distribution characteristics as the staff required to use it.

Accomplishment of the core functions and essential services relies heavily on the capacity of local health departments to collect, analyze, and use information. Information summarized in Chapter 10 indicates that approximately 80 percent of local health departments are now connected with the Internet, a clear improvement over the situation just five years ago. The current perception of public health leaders is that the larger, more sophisticated agencies are part of the "information superhighway," that the smallest agencies tend not to be involved with much data processing or information sharing, and that medium-sized agencies are improving their capacity to process information.

Leadership

The importance of leadership in public health and its characteristics are described in Chapter 18. There is no objective scale by which leadership can be measured, although most people seem to have a good notion of whether it is present or absent. Certainly, there are no formal efforts to measure the effectiveness of leadership in the public health world. There have been discussions of the nature of that leadership, however, with some praise mixed in with an apparent consensus that public health leadership is generally lacking.[14] That consensus has fueled efforts to provide leadership training opportunities at the national, state, and local levels as described in Chapter 18.

Although leadership is difficult to measure objectively, there are several questions to ask to assess whether a local health department is well led. For example, is the department respected in its community by both community leaders and citizens? Is the opinion of department leaders actively sought when the community faces public health problems? Does the department seek and maintain collaborative working arrangements with other community groups and agencies in such a manner that services to the public are provided efficiently and effectively? Is the department successful working within the political system? Are interactions with the medical community (physicians and hospitals) strong and productive? Is the department considered a source of innovative problem solving? Does the department exhibit a history of adequate and stable funding? Is the department involved in

teaching and research? There are many other questions that could be listed here as well. The sum total of impressions garnered from pursuing questions such as these leads to a judgment of the quality of leadership present in a particular local health department. Completion of the Performance Standards assessment by the LPHS (see Chapter 16) is a mechanism for addressing this question and holding local public health leadership accountable for their performance.

The quality and nature of public health leadership will be increasingly critical as practitioners struggle to bring some focus to the activities of all the disciplines and professions that impact the public's health. Health is the arena where social forces come together, and the growing awareness of the interrelationship of factors that influence health will continue to expand areas of involvement for health departments. Flexible and innovative public health leadership is essential for society to make decisions in all areas of human endeavor that are health promoting rather than health destroying.

THE EFFECTIVE HEALTH DEPARTMENT OF THE FUTURE

The public health system in the United States is in a state of significant flux. Some of the characteristics of this evolving system include shifts toward the provision of services based on demonstrated need and potential impact, modeled after the year 2010 objectives for the nation; multidisciplinary team-based approaches to problem solving; growing community involvement; closer linkages between prevention and treatment services; and closer linkages between practice and academia.

To be effective, public health agencies of the future must be aware of these continuing waves of change and exhibit the understanding and flexibility required to adapt activities to their environment so that public health services will be appropriately designed and effectively delivered. Also, to be effective, public health departments must be positioned as the health intelligence centers of their respective communities; that is, they must be the source of epidemiologically based thinking and analysis of their community's approach to dealing with health matters. They must be facilitators of strong and meaningful community participation in the assessment and prioritization of community health problems and issues. They must be major participants in public policy decision making, and they must both deliver and broker the delivery of services needed by their constituent populations. Finally, they must be focused on health outcomes as measures of the impact of interventions.

Accomplishing these tasks will require that health departments work from the strongest organizational base possible and that they hone and expand the capacities that are necessary to accomplish the core functions of public health and the other services assigned to them by their respective communities.

Many local health departments are too small and too resource-poor even to attempt to play the role now expected of them, let alone to be taken seriously as players by community decision makers. The findings of the 1988 and 2003 IOM reports and the description of local health departments contained in Chapter 10 demonstrate clearly that the old penchant for home rule has outlived its usefulness. To be effective, health departments must represent a constituency large enough that geographic boundaries of authority make sense to the citizenry, that funding is stable, and that the tax base is adequate to provide the local share of resources needed to ensure that at least the core functions of public health are accomplished.

Effective health departments require a governance structure that clearly delineates policy and administrative functions between the board of health (or other governing body) and the director of the department. Additionally, the primary concern of governance must be the description and solution of public health problems in the constituent community rather than the political correctness of the department's actions.

Those of today's public health leaders, who are reluctant to embrace community participation and adopt new ways of thinking and acting, may actually be significant barriers to the change that is required if every citizen is to be served by a strong and effective public health agency. Effective health departments will have leaders who exhibit commitment, charisma, and drive, and who embrace collective action, community empowerment, consumer advocacy, and egalitarianism.[32]

New technology is moving the nation into an information-rich future. Dealing appropriately with this reality requires computer equipment and analytical skills that provide access to the information available and allow for the correct interpretation of its meaning. Health departments must be able to analyze information about the world they find themselves in and determine the appropriate response to it. This means they must be connected to the information superhighway and be capable of recognizing information and trends that are relevant to the health of their constituents. Every department should have a high-speed connection to the Internet with e-mail capability. Departments must be able to collect and analyze information from their own communities, as well. They should be tracking the demographics of their communities and be thinking imaginatively about the potential use of home computers and interactive television in assessing community perceptions of health needs and priorities. These capacities are basic to future policy and program development and evaluation.

The effective health department will enable individual citizens to take responsibility for decision making related to the community's health as well as their own. Citizens will be involved both in setting the community's priorities for public health issue study and action and in assessing the impact of programs and services designed to improve community health. Effective citizen involvement will require a new level of cultural sensitivity and awareness, and a growing representation of minority groups among the public health workforce.

It is doubtful that any health department has the necessary resources available to carry out the community's full public health agenda. Thus, ensuring that all citizens receive the services they require for good health will require that public health departments build strong collaborative and cooperative linkages with other community health agencies and with the illness care system in the community. These collaborative arrangements will be with other health departments, other departments of local government, community health centers, school systems, and community agencies such as Planned Parenthood, the American Lung Association, the American Cancer Society, neighborhood block clubs, and environmental groups, to name just a few. Such collaboration is necessary for effective health promotion and disease prevention efforts to occur. Joint programming and service and referral arrangements with hospitals, managed care companies, group medical practices, individual physicians, and other providers of illness services are necessary to ensure that each citizen has access to a seamless web of services that promote health, prevent illness, diagnose disease early, and provide disease treatment that is efficient and effective.

Health departments should take the lead in assessing their community's capacity to deliver the 10 essential services by coordinating the use of the national performance standards. The partnerships inherent in such activities can also provide the base for responding to the threat of terrorism and for adjusting the local health care delivery system so that universal access to care can be realized, and social health can be monitored and deficiencies addressed.

Improvements in those activities and services intended to advance the public's health are strongly dependent upon increasing knowledge of the effectiveness of current or planned actions. They also depend upon the ability to bring well-trained professionals into the field of public health. The practice of, and the academic base for, public health have been allowed to become relatively isolated from one another. This reality has been recognized, and work is underway to link the two settings in a manner that will improve the level of training of local public health workers and increasingly focus research efforts on public health administration and service delivery concerns. If at all possible, the effective local health department will welcome stu-

dents and faculty from academic settings who have the potential to contribute to the understanding of local public health issues and strengthen the capacities of the local public health workforce. The health department should also be supportive of its current employees who want to pursue additional public health training and become adjunct or part-time faculty members. In addition, public health workers should be encouraged to join appropriate professional associations at the state and federal level (see appendix A). These groups can be very helpful in creating networking opportunities, keeping their members up-to-date on technical and organizational advancements, and representing member opinion in public policy-setting processes.

SUMMARY

This is an extraordinary time, and change is in the air. It is a time when no one is clearly in charge of the public health world. Consequently, there are remarkable opportunities for entrepreneurial efforts to reshape the public health system. It is a time for public health leaders to take responsibility for shaping the profession's collective destiny. If that leadership can be exerted so that the public health system can break out of old molds that are no longer functional, there is every reason to believe that public health workers will provide a valuable service to their communities and that it will be recognized as such. The most important element of that recognition, of course, will be steady, measurable gains in community health status.

REVIEW QUESTIONS

1. What potential exists for public health to continue to contribute to gains in health status in the United States?
2. What recommendations were made by the Institute of Medicine to increase levels of health and longevity in the United States in the near future?

3. List some of the new challenges confronting public health leaders.

4. List some of the traditional challenges faced by public health departments that will continue to be relevant in the future.

5. What are some of the key characteristics you think effective health departments of the future will illustrate?

REFERENCES

1. Bunker JP, Frazier HS, Mosteller F. Improving health: Measuring effects of medical care. *Milbank Q.* 1994;72(2):225–258.

2. *Health Care Reform and Public Health.* Washington, DC: Office of Disease Prevention and Health Promotion, US Public Health Service; 1993.

3. Health United States. *Chartbook on trends in the health of Americans.* Washington, DC: 2006; 60.

4. *Healthy People: The Surgeon General's Report on Health Promotion and Disease Prevention.* Washington, DC: US Dept of Health and Human Services, Public Health Service; 1979.

5. Frumpkin H. Beyond toxicity: Human health and the natural environment. *Am J Prev Med.* 2001; 20(3):234–240.

6. Buluran NL. The campaign for 100% access and zero health disparities. *Urban Health Update.* 1999;1(1):22–23.

7. Communities Joined in Action. Available at: http://www.cjaonline.net.

8. Institute of Medicine, Committee on the Consequences of Uninsurance. *Coverage Matters.* Washington, DC: National Academy Press; 2001.

9. Reiser SJ. Topics for our times: The medicine/public health initiative. *Am J Public Health.* 1997; 87(7):1098–1099.

10. Beitsch LM, Brooks RG, Glasser JH, Coble YD. The medicine and public health initiative: Ten years later. *AJPM.* 2005;29(2):149–153.

11. *Guide to Clinical Preventive Services.* 2nd ed. Baltimore, MD: Williams & Wilkins; 1996.

12. Partnership for Prevention. *Use of high-value preventive care and lives saved if used.* Available at: http://www.prevent.org/content/view/129/72/.

13. American Public Health Association, et al. *Model Standards: A Guide for Community Preventive Health Services.* 2nd ed. Washington, DC: American Public Health Association; 1985: 4.

14. Institute of Medicine, Committee for the Study of the Future of Public Health. *The Future of Public Health.* Washington, DC: National Academy Press; 1988.

15. Institute of Medicine, Committee on Assuring the Health of the Public in the 21st Century. *The Future of the Public's Health in the 21st Century.* Washington, DC: National Academy Press; 2003.

16. Shi L. *The relationship between public health system performance and social determinants of health, public policy, governance structure, and preparedness.* White paper prepared for Academy Health, June 2007.

17. New York Academy of Medicine. *Bioterrorism preparedness needs are draining funds from essential public health resources.* News and Publications. May 29, 2003. Available at: http://www.nyam.org/news/1143.html.

18. Robert Wood Johnson Foundation. *Health experts analyze the effects of increased federal funding on state bioterrorism preparedness.* Available at: http://www.rwjf.org/pr/product.jsp?id=16757.

19. Institute of Medicine. *Training Physicians for Public Health Careers.* Washington, DC: National Academy Press; 2007.

20. Keck CW. Lessons learned from an academic health department. *J Public Health Management Practice.* 2000;6(1):47–52.

21. National Association of County and City Health Officials. *Operational Definition of a Local Health Department.* Available at: http://www.naccho.org/topics/infrastructure/accreditation/OpDef.cfm.

22. Thielen L. *Exploring public health experience with standards and accreditation.* Available at: http://www.cdc.gov/nceh/ehs/EPHLI/Resources/Exploring_Public_Health.pdf.

23. Marmot M. Inequalities in health. *N Engl J Med.* 2001;345(2):134–135.

24. Miringoff M. *The Social Health of the Nation.* New York: Oxford University Press; 1999.

25. Schauffler HH, Scutchfield FD. Managed care and public health. *Am J Prev Med.* 1998;14(3): 240–241.

26. *Health Departments Take Action: A Compendium of State and Local Models Addressing Racial and*

Ethnic Disparities in Health. Washington, DC: Association of State and Territorial Health Officials; 2001.

27. CDC. *Genomics workforce competencies.* Available at: http://www.cdc.gov/genomics/training/competencies/comps.htm; 2001.

28. May GP, McHugh MC, Shim K, et al. *J Public Health Management Practice.* 2004;10(5):435–443.

29. Sorensen AA, Bialek RG. *The Public Health Faculty Agency Forum: Linking Graduate Education and Practice, Final Report.* Gainesville: University Press of Florida; 1993.

30. *National Profile of Local Health Departments.* Washington, DC: National Association of County Health Officials; 1990.

31. *Local Public Health Agency Infrastructure: A Chartbook.* Washington, DC: National Association of County and City Health Officials; 2001.

32. Lloyd P. Management competencies in health for all/new public settings. *J Health Admin Ed.* Spring 1994;12(2):187–207.

APPENDIX A

Major National Public Health Professional Associations

C. William Keck, MD, MPH and F. Douglas Scutchfield, MD

Two of the more difficult yet important challenges facing public health professionals are keeping up with developments at the state and national level that are relevant to their work and staying connected to a peer network of colleagues. Membership in professional associations can be very helpful in both these areas. Professional associations can be a mechanism for access to such useful items as relevant publications; technical and legislative updates, alerts, and summaries; issue analyses; trend forecasts; career opportunities; and policy development issues.

This appendix provides a list of some of the major national professional associations typically joined by public health workers. There are many other national organizations not listed here that might be of value to some in public health, and the reader is encouraged to search out and explore any group that might be professionally helpful or personally rewarding.

Public health professionals should also explore state-level professional associations in the state in which they work. Many of these associations provide the same benefits and opportunities at the state level that national associations provide at the national level. Indeed, many state associations are affiliated with national ones. Although there are

too many to list here, state associations deserve consideration and support.

American Association of Public Health Dentistry (AAPHD)

3085 Stevenson Drive
Suite 200
Springfield, IL 62703
Tel: 217-529-6941
Fax: 217-529-9120
Web: http://www.aaphd.org

American Association of Public Health Physicians (AAPHP)

3433 Kirchoff Road
Rolling Meadows, IL 60008-1842
Web: http://www.aaphp.org

American College of Preventive Medicine (ACPM)

1307 New York Avenue, NW
Suite 200
Washington, DC 20005
Tel: 202-466-2044
Fax: 202-466-2662
Web: http://www.acpm.org

America's Health Insurance
Plans (AHIP)

601 Pennsylvania Avenue, NW
South Building, Suite 500
Washington, DC 20004
Tel: 202-778-3200
Fax: 202-331-7487
Web: http://www.ahip.org

American Medical
Association (AMA)

515 N. State Street
Chicago, IL 60610
Tel: 800-621-8335
Web: http://www.ama-assn.org

American Nurses
Association (ANA)

8515 Georgia Avenue
Suite 400
Silver Spring, MD 20910
Tel: 301-628-5000
Fax: 301-628-5001
Web: http://www.ana.org

American Public Health
Association (APHA)

800 I Street NW
Washington, DC 20001-3710
Tel: 202-777-2742
Fax: 202-777-2534
Web: http://www.apha.org

Association of Schools of
Public Health (ASPH)

1101 15th Street NW
Suite 910
Washington, DC 20005
Tel: 202-296-1099
Fax: 202-296-1252
Web: http://www.asph.org

Association of State and Territorial
Health Officials (ASTHO)

2231 Crystal Drive
Suite 450
Arlington, VA 22202
Tel: 202-371-9090
Fax: 571-527-3189
Web: http://www.astho.org

Association for Prevention Teaching
and Research (APTR)

1001 Connecticut Avenue, NW
Suite 610
Washington, DC 20036
Tel: 202-463-0550
Fax: 202-463-0555
Web: http://www.atpm.org

Community Campus Partnerships
for Health (CCPH)

c/o Medical College of Wisconsin
Public and Community Health
Attn: Alicia Witten
8701 Watertown Plank Road
Milwaukee, WI 53226
Tel: 414-456-7404
Fax: 414-456-6431
Web: http://depts.washington.edu/ccph

National Association of County and
City Health Officials (NACCHO)

1100 17th Street NW
Second Floor
Washington, DC 20036
Tel: 202-783-5550
Fax: 202-783-1583
Web: http://www.naccho.org

National Association of Local
Boards of Health (NALBOH)

1840 E. Gypsy Lane Road
Bowling Green, OH 43402
Tel: 419-353-7714
Fax: 419-352-6278
Web: http://www.nalboh.org

*National Environmental Health
Association (NEHA)*

720 S. Colorado Boulevard
Suite 1000-N
Denver, CO 80246-1926
Tel: 303-756-9090
Fax: 303-691-9490
Web: http://www.neha.org

*Society for Public Health Education
(SOPHE)*

10 G Street, NE
Suite 605
Washington, DC 20002-4242
Tel: 202-408-9804
Fax: 202-408-9815
Web: http://www.sophe.org

APPENDIX B

What Is Evidence-Based Public Health?

Nancy A. Myers, RN, PhD

Public health practitioners are called upon to make decisions on a daily basis that will affect essential health services delivered to their communities or patients. In assessing options for action, many rely on their own experience or draw upon the experience of those around them. Others incorporate the opinions and advice of community members or other local experts. Some look beyond their own agencies or communities to find out how others have handled similar situations. These methods of gathering data about possible options for action may provide the practitioner with good ideas upon which to base his or her actions, but they are unlikely to yield the best available evidence upon which public health programs or policies should be based.

Evidence-based public health (EBPH) has been defined in several ways, but includes two key components. First and foremost, it is the development of public health programs and policies based on the *best available evidence* or information. Evidence can include epidemiologic data about the population(s) or condition(s) under consideration, as well as evaluations of program or policy interventions that have been tried by others. Evidence can be quantitative in nature (i.e., with outcomes reported in quantifiable or numeric units), or it can be obtained using qualitative study methods, including interviews or focus groups to gain individuals' insights into a particular issue. After the best

information or evidence to inform decision making has been located and assessed, EBPH practice includes another critical aspect: the incorporation of that evidence, and the lessons learned from it, with community- or patient-specific needs, values, and goals.[1,2]

Brownson et al.[1] have developed a framework for public health practice problem-solving. They include identifying and evaluating the scientific literature for evidence of what has been shown to work in other settings as a key part of the process. Their framework includes the following steps:

1. Develop an initial statement of the issue.
2. Quantify the issue.
3. Search the scientific literature and organize information.
4. Develop and prioritize program options.
5. Develop an action plan and implement interventions.
6. Evaluate the program or policy.
7. Re-tool, disseminate widely, or discontinue the program or policy.

Although all of these steps are critical to the process of locating, evaluating, using, and generating evidence in public health practice, the remainder of this appendix focuses on how to find and evaluate evidence (Step 3).

WHERE TO FIND EVIDENCE

After a problem or issue is identified for potential intervention, the public health practitioner should identify programs or policies that are currently in place or that have been implemented in the past that might present models to consider in designing their activities. If the issue being addressed is a fairly common one (e.g., obesity rates among school-age children), it is likely that programs or policies have been implemented and evaluated that can be assessed for their relevance to the specific community needs. If, however, the issue is fairly new, the practitioner may need to broaden the search to identify programs that have addressed similar issues. For example, there are few studies published to date that evaluate programs' or policies' success in increasing the rate of HPV vaccination among young adolescent girls. This doesn't mean that a practitioner can't rely on evidence of what has worked; the practitioner needs to identify similar issues for which there have been published evaluations. In the case of developing a program or policy related to HPV vaccination, one might consider looking for evaluations of efforts to improve rates of other newer vaccines that are recommended for children or adolescents, including the meningitis or hepatitis series. In addition, one might review the literature on how to approach education or programmatic efforts related to the prevention of sexually transmitted infections in the adolescent population to identify potential communication or cultural issues that should be taken into consideration when putting together an HPV prevention program.

A first step in finding evidence of what has or has not worked is a formal review of the existing published scientific literature to find journal articles, books, or manuscripts that may address the problem at hand. Several health databases can be accessed either on a personal- or an organization-based computer system, or through one's local public or university library, including (but not limited to) MEDLine, PubMed, CancerLit, PsycInfo,

and HealthSTAR. The National Library of Medicine (NLM) provides public access to MEDLine and PubMed, as well as the NLM catalog on its website (http://www.nlm.nih.gov).

Next, there are several resources for identifying past or current public health programs or policies that may provide evidence for future planning purposes. The Centers for Disease Control and Prevention's (CDC) website contains a section designed for public health professionals (http://www.cdc .gov/CDCForYou/health_professionals.html), with information on the latest programmatic or intervention recommendations. It also provides links to manuscripts or data on select public health issues.

Another excellent resource that is provided through the CDC is its *Guide to Community Preventive Services: Systematic Reviews and Evidence-Based Recommendations.* This publication, which is available free online (http://www.thecommunityguide .org) or for purchase in hard-copy format, provides a summary of the available evidence for community interventions for a variety of public health topics, such as oral health, physical activity, tobacco use, and injury prevention. It also gives evidence-based recommendations for practitioners to incorporate into their own program or policy planning. New topics are being added to the guide each year and are linked to the *Healthy People 2010* objectives.

Partners in Information Access for the Public Health Workforce (http://phpartners.org) is a collaboration among several public health organizations and the United States government; it provides a central access point for several public health resources for evidence-based practice that are available through the Internet. Links are also provided for educational resources for practitioners, and upcoming meetings and seminars.

The Cochrane Collaboration (http://www .cochrane.org/index.htm) is a subscription service that provides users with up-to-date systematic reviews of the evidence for individual clinical care as well as community or population-based interventions. It is published (either online, or in CD version) four times each year. Most medical libraries have access to this service.

Finally, many university or public health organization resources are available for no cost to public health practitioners. One example is the *Evidence-Based Practice for Public Health* website (http://library.umassmed.edu/ebpph/index.cfm), which includes links to descriptions of model programs or policies that have been successfully implemented and evaluated.

HOW TO ASSESS WHAT YOU FIND

Some of the resources listed previously provide a review of the applicability and strength of published evidence, as well as recommendations for incorporating best practices into future efforts. However, public health practitioners also need to review articles or manuscripts themselves to determine if the information provided about a program and its evaluation provides evidence that can be used in designing their own community-specific intervention. Although a full discussion of all of the elements of a program's design and evaluation that should be taken into consideration are beyond the scope of any single chapter or appendix, some basic questions to help guide the process of evaluating the evidence that has been published are discussed here.

Evaluating the description of a public health program or policy (as one would find in a journal article or other manuscript) should involve a careful assessment of how the intervention was designed and implemented, and how it was evaluated. First and foremost, practitioners should look for a clear and concise description of the problem or issue that is addressed, and the development of specific, measurable objectives that lay the foundation for evaluating the success (or lack of success) of an intervention. Do the authors present a review of the existing data to describe the health issue? Do they conduct and report on a thorough assessment of the literature (to show that their process of developing an intervention was based on existing

evidence for what works or does not work)? Are their objectives for improving the situation measurable; that is, do they quantify the change that they expect their intervention will bring? Are the objectives that have been defined consistent with the data about the issue; are they realistic or achievable? The foundation of any program or policy is the establishment of objectives that are based on what is known about the issue (or about issues that are similar in nature) and the population affected; this information should be clearly spelled out in an introduction or literature review.

In addition to assessing whether the authors present measurable objectives, one should assess whether or not the outcomes that they are defining and measuring are the best ones. Do the authors define summative outcome measures, which assess the actual change in attitudes, knowledge, behavior, or health status that they are hoping to affect? Many practitioners assume that if they conduct an intervention (e.g., a class on cancer prevention), then participants will be better off afterward (in this example, by having a better understanding of the topic and therefore adopting preventive behaviors or habits).

Do the authors identify formative outcome measures, which evaluate how well the program or policy was implemented (e.g., by defining operational objectives for implementation and then providing data on outcomes)? When a practitioner is considering duplicating some or all of an existing program or policy, having information about both types of outcomes is critical. All programs or policies should be evaluated on whether or not they actually effected a change in community members' health status; many studies report "success" as having implemented a program, without following through and measuring whether that program ultimately made a difference. For example, programs may report how many participants attended nutrition education sessions as a measure of success. Although this is an important formative measure (because it gives an indication of how well the program was designed, if it was advertised in a comprehensive way, and how accessible it was to potential participants), it doesn't provide the reviewer with the bottom line: did participants implement and sustain changes to their behavior that will lead to better health?

As stated earlier, a key aspect of EBPH is the incorporation of the best available evidence with the reality of one's own community needs, culture, and assets. In assessing the applicability of other program or policy interventions to the issue at hand, the practitioner should look for a complete description of the target population that was the focus of the program's interventions. Do the authors provide a description of their target audience in terms of socioeconomic status, race, ethnicity, literacy level, gender, age, and so on? Do they describe any community-specific attributes or concerns that were taken into consideration in designing their program? Were community members involved in defining the issue, developing the program, or evaluating its effectiveness; if so, what were their specific roles and what insight did they bring to the process? While a practitioner shouldn't discount a program that was carried out within the context of a community with a very different composition than his or her own target group, a successful program in one community may need substantial modification in another to translate that success.

As a side note, practitioners in the United States may not consider looking for data or program evaluations in the international public health literature, although it may be a more appropriate venue to search. If one is working within a very specific ethnic or immigrant community, it may be worthwhile to look for articles about successful programs tackling the same or similar issues in that ethnic or immigrant group's native country.

Public health issues are rarely caused by a single factor; they are multicausal in nature. Therefore, solutions to public health problems are generally complex and involve multiple approaches that can occur simultaneously. The best public health interventions, whether they are program-based or policy-oriented, are developed, implemented, and evaluated by multidisciplinary teams. A discussion of this teamwork in a program or policy report is helpful in identifying all of the perspectives that were taken into consideration, as well as illuminating what perspectives weren't (and perhaps should have been) included. This report and commentary

can assist the practitioner in determining which colleagues to include in the planning process.

A few key questions related to the design of the program or policy evaluation should be answered to determine how solid its findings are. The first helps to answer the question about whether the changes observed (either positive or negative) in the target audience were potentially attributable to the intervention that took place. People receive public health information from a variety of sources each day; television programs, radio advertisements, print media, and the web all provide important health messages to their consumer audiences. To determine if a change in program participants' outcomes (attitudes, knowledge, behaviors, or health assessment measures) has been influenced by the intervention that they received, data from a comparison group (which did not receive the intervention) should be presented. The comparison group should be as similar as possible (in demographic composition, location, culture, and potential exposure to outside sources of health information) to the group receiving the intervention. The same outcome measures (surveys of attitudes or knowledge, assessment of health risk behaviors, etc.) should be measured and reported for both groups. If there is a significant difference in outcomes between two groups that are similar with the exception of the intervention provided, the evidence for the efficacy of the intervention is stronger (than if there is not a comparison group).

One should also question whether the change in outcomes that occurred in the program participants was replicated in more than one group; this will also provide stronger evidence for an intervention's effectiveness. Practitioners should assess the evaluation process to determine if it included interventions and measurement of outcomes with more than one group of participants. Were results consistent across intervention groups? Were the same results achieved in groups that were heterogenous?

Another good practice when reviewing any article or manuscript is to compare whether the program's stated objectives or research questions were ultimately answered or addressed in the report of its evaluation. Did the authors report findings for all of the measures that they set out to use? Did they report on results for all of the objectives or questions that they began with? Did they provide an explanation for why or how their program or policy did (or did not) work that is reasonable?

Finally, a sound evaluation should conclude with a discussion of its limitations. No program, policy, or evaluation process is without flaws, some of which are known at the planning stage, and others do not become apparent until after implementation. This discussion should include what the program planners were not able to accomplish (and why), how they could have chosen to organize their program or evaluation (and why they did not), and what they believe subsequent programs or policies should include or do differently. This section often provides valuable insight for practitioners who are beginning their own program or policy planning process, so that they can avoid common pitfalls.

CHALLENGES TO EVIDENCE-BASED PRACTICE

Although the need for EBPH practice has been identified by virtually every national public health organization, practitioners working to adopt an evidence-based approach to their programmatic and policy activities are facing several challenges. Public health practitioners have been intervening with carefully planned and executed policies and programs to improve the health of their communities for decades. What is lacking, however, is the evidence of how these policies and programs have worked.

Although medical journals are filled each month with the reports of randomized control trials and other studies documenting the causes of and best treatments for disease in individual patients, public- or community-based intervention studies have not been conducted or published in great numbers. Public health evidence is sometimes difficult, if not impossible, to find. Complicating this lack of evidence overall is the reality of a phenomenon known as publication bias. Studies that are published in peer-reviewed journals generally demonstrate a positive impact of an intervention; that is, they demonstrate how well an intervention has worked. Negative findings—findings that document that an intervention didn't work—are much less likely to be published. Nonetheless, for a practitioner who is assessing what the evidence shows to be the best approach, knowing what *hasn't* worked and why is just as important as knowing what has been shown to be effective.

As referenced earlier, the causes of and solutions to community health problems are complex and multifaceted. Communities themselves can differ dramatically in their demographic makeup and culture, and in their level of available resources. It is unlikely that public health practitioners will find a best practice program or policy that can be duplicated "as is" in their own community; it is also unlikely that the evaluation of any single program includes many or all of the potential interventions that may be used to approach a particular issue. So, unlike a clinical researcher who can look to a few key articles that demonstrate the effectiveness of a single intervention on patient outcomes, a public health practitioner must integrate a wide array of information on potential solutions, from a variety of literatures. Public health as a science includes epidemiology, social/behavioral sciences, clinical sciences, allied health sciences, communication sciences, and education sciences. Becoming adept at referencing all of these potential fields' scientific literature can seem overwhelming; working with a reference librarian from a local college or university to learn how to become more adept at literature search techniques may help.

CONTRIBUTING TO THE FUTURE OF EVIDENCE-BASED PUBLIC HEALTH

Public health practitioners must become good consumers of scientific evidence and develop the skills to incorporate that evidence into their daily practice. Many organizations, schools, and programs have developed education modules to provide practitioners with some basic tools for EBPH.

For EBPH practice to become the norm, practitioners must also incorporate the routine, planned evaluation of programs and policies into their daily work. All practitioners should see themselves as generators of evidence, as well as consumers of evidence. One way to accomplish this is to look for academic partners who can assist in the development and implementation of sound program or policy evaluation, as well as provide support for the dissemination of findings via articles, manuscripts, or presentations. Although schools and programs of public health are natural partners in this endeavor, practitioners should also consider working with other academic departments that house graduate programs, including social/behavioral sciences,

allied health, and health education. Planning for the evaluation stage of a program or policy should be part of the earliest discussions; a sound evaluation plan should be in place before the intervention takes place, and may actually strengthen the intervention itself by raising new or different issues about how it will be operationalized.

REFERENCES

1. Brownson RC, Baker EA, Leet TL, Gillispie KN. *Evidence-Based Public Health*. New York: Oxford University Press; 2003.
2. Kohatsu ND, Robinson JG, Torner JC. Evidence-based public health: An evolving concept. *American Journal of Preventive Medicine.* 2004; 27(5):417–421.

APPENDIX C

Core Competencies for Public Health Practice

Diane Downing, RN, MSN

INTRODUCTION

Two important sets of public health core competencies are available to guide public health practice. In 2001, the Council on Linkages Between Academia and Public Health Practice released a list of core competencies for public health professionals. In 2006, the Association of Schools of Public Health (ASPH) developed a master's degree in public health (MPH) core competencies.

The core competencies developed by the Council on Linkages Between Academia and Public Health Practice represent 10 years of work on this subject by the Council and many other organizations and individuals in public health academic and practice settings. The Council compiled its work and cross-walked it with the 10 essential public health services to ensure the competencies help build the skills necessary for providing these essential services.

More than 1000 public health professionals reviewed the list during a public comment period. Feedback from reviewers led to this consensus set of core competencies for guiding public health

workforce development efforts. They represent a set of skills, knowledge, and attitudes necessary for the broad practice of public health divided into eight domains. This set of competencies applies to all public health workers in the job categories of front-line staff, senior-level staff, and supervisory and management staff. They serve as a starting point for curriculum development, public health workforce training needs assessment and performance measurement, and development of discipline specific competency sets. They also provide cross-cutting competencies that can be used by personnel systems to develop job descriptions for public health workers. The competencies can be found on the Web (http://www.train.org, click on Core Competencies) where they are also listed as they apply to the 10 essential public health services and as they apply to front-line staff, senior-level staff, and supervisory and management staff. The Council on Linkages is currently revisiting the competencies described previously and listed later in this appendix. The eight domains will be retained, although many of the competencies will be re-worded to both modernize them and improve their wording. When available, the revised competencies can be viewed at http://www.trainingfinder.org/competencies/list_nolevels.htm.

The ASPH master's degree in public health core competencies were developed in response to the challenges of twenty-first century public health practice, a proliferation of public health competency-based training, incorporation of competencies into accreditation criteria, and the move to develop a voluntary credentialing exam for MPH graduates. This set of core competencies reflects the work of 332 public health professionals from academia and public health practice. They include discipline-specific competencies for the five areas of knowledge offered in Council on Education for Public Health (CEPH) accredited programs and schools and a set of cross-cutting competencies divided into seven domains. The ASPH set of cross-cutting competencies present competencies all MPH students are expected to demonstrate upon graduation, irrespective of area of specialization or career trajectory. The ASPH set of core competencies serves as a resource guide for strengthening the quality and accountability of education offered in MPH schools and programs. The competencies can be found on the Web at http://www.asph.org/competency.

The domains and their associated competencies for both sets of core competencies are listed next.

COUNCIL ON LINKAGES BETWEEN ACADEMIA AND PUBLIC HEALTH PRACTICE CORE COMPETENCIES FOR PUBLIC HEALTH PRACTICE

Analytic/Assessment Skills

- Defines a problem.
- Determines appropriate uses and limitations of both quantitative and qualitative data.
- Selects and defines variables relevant to defined public health problems.
- Identifies relevant and appropriate data and information sources.
- Evaluates the integrity and comparability of data, and identifies gaps in data sources.
- Applies ethical principles to the collection, maintenance, use, and dissemination of data and information.
- Partners with communities to attach meaning to collected quantitative and qualitative data.
- Makes relevant inferences from quantitative and qualitative data.
- Obtains and interprets information regarding risks and benefits to the community.
- Applies data collection processes, information technology applications, and computer systems storage/retrieval strategies.
- Recognizes how the data illuminates ethical, political, scientific, economic, and overall public health issues.

Policy Development/Program Planning Skills

- Collects, summarizes, and interprets information relevant to an issue.
- States policy options, and writes clear and concise policy statements.
- Identifies, interprets, and implements public health laws, regulations, and policies related to specific programs.
- Articulates the health, fiscal, administrative, legal, social, and political implications of each policy option.
- States the feasibility and expected outcomes of each policy option.
- Utilizes current techniques in decision analysis and health planning.
- Decides on the appropriate course of action.
- Develops a plan to implement policy, including goals, outcome, and process objectives, and implementation steps.

- Translates policy into organizational plans, structures, and programs.
- Prepares and implements emergency response plans.
- Develops mechanisms to monitor and evaluate programs for their effectiveness and quality.

Communication Skills

- Communicates effectively both in writing and orally, or in other ways.
- Solicits input from individuals and organizations.
- Advocates for public health programs and resources.
- Leads and participates in groups to address specific issues.
- Uses the media, advanced technologies, and community networks to communicate information.
- Effectively presents accurate demographic, statistical, programmatic, and scientific information for professional and lay audiences.

Attitudes

- Listens to others in an unbiased manner, respects points of view of others, and promotes the expression of diverse opinions and perspectives.

Cultural Competency Skills

- Utilizes appropriate methods for interacting sensitively, effectively, and professionally with persons from diverse cultural, socioeconomic, educational, racial, ethnic, and professional backgrounds, and persons of all ages and lifestyle preferences.
- Identifies the role of cultural, social, and behavioral factors in determining the delivery of public health services.
- Develops and adapts approaches to problems that take into account cultural differences.

Attitudes

- Understands the dynamic forces contributing to cultural diversity.
- Understands the importance of a diverse public health workforce.

Community Dimensions of Practice Skills

- Establishes and maintains linkages with key stakeholders.
- Utilizes leadership, team building, negotiation, and conflict resolution skills to build community partnerships.
- Collaborates with community partners to promote the health of the population.
- Identifies how public and private organizations operate within a community.
- Accomplishes effective community engagements.
- Identifies community assets and available resources.
- Develops, implements, and evaluates a community public health assessment.
- Describes the role of government in the delivery of community health services.

Basic Public Health Sciences Skills

- Identifies the individual's and organization's responsibilities within the context of the essential public health services and core functions.
- Defines, assesses, and understands the health status of populations, determinants of health and illness, factors contributing to health promotion and disease prevention, and factors influencing the use of health services.
- Understands the historical development, structure, and interaction of public health and health care systems.
- Identifies and applies basic research methods used in public health.

- Applies the basic public health sciences, including behavioral and social sciences, biostatistics, epidemiology, environmental public health, and prevention of chronic and infectious diseases and injuries.
- Identifies and retrieves current relevant scientific evidence.
- Identifies the limitations of research and the importance of observations and interrelationships.

Attitudes

- Develops a lifelong commitment to rigorous critical thinking.

Financial Planning and Management Skills

- Develops and presents a budget.
- Manages programs within budget constraints.
- Applies budget processes.
- Develops strategies for determining budget priorities.
- Monitors program performance.
- Prepares proposals for funding from external sources.
- Applies basic human relations skills to the management of organizations, motivation of personnel, and resolution of conflicts.
- Manages information systems for collection, retrieval, and use of data for decision making.
- Negotiates and develops contracts and other documents for the provision of population-based services.
- Conducts cost-effectiveness, cost-benefit, and cost-utility analyses.

Leadership and Systems Thinking Skills

- Creates a culture of ethical standards within organizations and communities.
- Helps create key values and shared vision, and uses these principles to guide action.

- Identifies internal and external issues that may impact delivery of essential public health services (i.e., strategic planning).
- Facilitates collaboration with internal and external groups to ensure participation of key stakeholders.
- Promotes team and organizational learning.
- Contributes to development, implementation, and monitoring of organizational performance standards.
- Uses the legal and political system to effect change.
- Applies theory of organizational structures to professional practice.

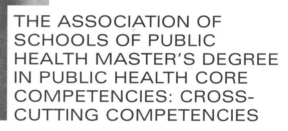

THE ASSOCIATION OF SCHOOLS OF PUBLIC HEALTH MASTER'S DEGREE IN PUBLIC HEALTH CORE COMPETENCIES: CROSS-CUTTING COMPETENCIES

Communication and Informatics

- Describe how the public health information infrastructure is used to collect, process, maintain, and disseminate data.
- Describe how societal, organizational, and individual factors influence and are influenced by public health communications.
- Discuss the influences of social, organizational, and individual factors on the use of information technology by end users.
- Apply theory and strategy-based communication principles across different settings and audiences.
- Apply legal and ethical principles to the use of information technology and resources in public health settings.

- Collaborate with communication and informatics specialists in the process of design, implementation, and evaluation of public health programs.

- Demonstrate effective written and oral skills for communicating with different audiences in the context of professional public health activities.

- Use information technology to access, evaluate, and interpret public health data.

- Use informatics methods and resources as strategic tools to promote public health.

- Use informatics and communication methods to advocate for community public health programs and policies.

Diversity and Culture

- Describe the roles of, history, power, privilege, and structural inequality in producing health disparities.

- Explain how professional ethics and practices relate to equity and accountability in diverse community settings.

- Explain why cultural competence alone cannot address health disparity.

- Discuss the importance and characteristics of a sustainable diverse public health workforce.

- Use the basic concepts and skills involved in culturally appropriate community engagement and empowerment with diverse communities.

- Apply the principles of community-based participatory research to improve health in diverse populations.

- Differentiate among availability, acceptability, and accessibility of health care across diverse populations.

- Differentiate among linguistic competence, cultural competency, and health literacy in public health practice.

- Cite examples of situations where consideration of culture-specific needs resulted in a more effective modification or adaptation of a health intervention.

- Develop public health programs and strategies responsive to the diverse cultural values and traditions of the communities being served.

Leadership

- Describe the attributes of leadership in public health.

- Describe alternative strategies for collaboration and partnership among organizations, focused on public health goals.

- Articulate an achievable mission, set of core values, and vision.

- Engage in dialogue and learning from others to advance public health goals.

- Demonstrate team building, negotiation, and conflict management skills.

- Demonstrate transparency, integrity, and honesty in all actions.

- Use collaborative methods for achieving organizational and community health goals.

- Apply social justice and human rights principles when addressing community needs.

- Develop strategies to motivate others for collaborative problem solving, decision making, and evaluation.

Public Health Biology

- Specify the role of the immune system in population health.

- Describe how behavior alters human biology.

- Identify the ethical, social, and legal issues implied by public health biology.

- Explain the biological and molecular basis of public health.

- Explain the role of biology in the ecological model of population-based health.

- Explain how genetics and genomics affect disease processes and public health policy and practice.

- Articulate how biological, chemical, and physical agents affect human health.

- Apply biological principles to development and implementation of disease prevention, control, or management programs.
- Apply evidence-based biological and molecular concepts to inform public health laws, policies, and regulations.
- Integrate general biological and molecular concepts into public health.

Professionalism

- Discuss sentinel events in the history and development of the public health profession and their relevance for practice in the field.
- Apply basic principles of ethical analysis (e.g., the Public Health Code of Ethics, human rights framework, other moral theories) to issues of public health practice and policy.
- Apply evidence-based principles and the scientific knowledge base to critical evaluation and decision making in public health.
- Apply the core functions of assessment, policy development, and assurance in the analysis of public health problems and their solutions.
- Promote high standards of personal and organizational integrity, compassion, honesty, and respect for all people.
- Analyze determinants of health and disease using an ecological framework.
- Analyze the potential impacts of legal and regulatory environments on the conduct of ethical public health research and practice.
- Distinguish between population and individual ethical considerations in relation to the benefits, costs, and burdens of public health programs.
- Embrace a definition of public health that captures the unique characteristics of the field (e.g., population-focused, community-oriented, prevention-motivated, and rooted in social justice) and how these contribute to professional practice.
- Appreciate the importance of working collaboratively with diverse communities and constituen-

cies (e.g., researchers, practitioners, agencies, and organizations).
- Value commitment to lifelong learning and professional service, including active participation in professional organizations.

Program Planning

- Describe how social, behavioral, environmental, and biological factors contribute to specific individual and community health outcomes.
- Describe the tasks necessary to assure that program implementation occurs as intended.
- Explain how the findings of a program evaluation can be used.
- Explain the contribution of logic models in program development, implementation, and evaluation.
- Differentiate among goals, measurable objectives, related activities, and expected outcomes for a public health program.
- Differentiate the purposes of formative, process, and outcome evaluation.
- Differentiate between qualitative and quantitative evaluation methods in relation to their strengths, limitations, and appropriate uses, and emphases on reliability and validity.
- Prepare a program budget with justification.
- In collaboration with others, prioritize individual, organizational, and community concerns and resources for public health programs.
- Assess evaluation reports in relation to their quality, utility, and impact on public health.

Systems Thinking

- Identify characteristics of a system.
- Identify unintended consequences produced by changes made to a public health system.
- Provide examples of feedback loops and "stocks and flows" within a public health system.

- Explain how systems (e.g., individuals, social networks, organizations, and communities) may be viewed as systems within systems in the analysis of public health problems.
- Explain how systems models can be tested and validated.
- Explain how the contexts of gender, race, poverty, history, migration, and culture are important in the design of interventions within public health systems.
- Illustrate how changes in public health systems (including input, processes, and output) can be measured.

- Analyze inter-relationships among systems that influence the quality of life of people in their communities.
- Analyze the effects of political, social, and economic policies on public health systems at the local, state, national, and international levels.
- Analyze the impact of global trends and interdependencies on public health problems and systems.
- Assess strengths and weaknesses of applying the systems approach to public health problems.

GLOSSARY

10 essential public health services A set of 10 activities that have been identified as defining elements of public health practice in promoting population health and preventing disease and disability. These activities were identified through the work of a consensus panel of experts convened by the U.S. Department of Health and Human Services.

45 CFR 46 Also known as the Common Rule, this legislation established the role of institutional review boards (IRBs) for research on human subjects. See also *common rule*.

abscess A localized collection of pus in a cavity formed by the disintegration of tissues.

absenteeism Health-related productivity loss measured by the number of missed workdays.

abuse a pattern of drug or alcohol use that leads to clinically significant impairment or distress as evidenced by failure to fulfill major obligations due to substance use, using the substance in a physically hazardous manner, recurrent legal problems, and/or continued use despite these recurrent problems.

academics Policy players who contribute to the development of policy options through theory and to the assessment of options through the application of methods supported by their disciplines; also commentators or "experts" who contribute to the debate over policy.

acceptability As applied to public health surveillance, the ability of the system to be adopted and used by those persons responsible.

accident An unscientific term applied to unintended events that may result in injury; the term has caused injuries to be considered by many to be unpredictable and therefore unpreventable.

accountability A means of assuring the quality and availability of public health services.

accounting The bookkeeping methods involved in making a financial record of business transactions and in the preparation of statements concerning the assets, liabilities, and operating results of a business, agency, or institution.

accreditation A process for external, reliable, and objective validation of agency performance against a specific set of standards, and some form of reward or recognition for agencies meeting those standards.

acid rain Atmospheric precipitation containing acids of sulfur and nitrogen from the combustion of fuels.

Acute Necrotizing Ulcerative Gingivitis (ANUG) An acute, inflammatory, painful process with ulceration of the interdental papillae; the tissues bleed easily, a pseudomembrane may be present, and an offensive mouth odor is usually associated with the necrosis.

advanced dental hygiene practitioner In 2004, the American Dental Hygienists Association initiated the advanced dental hygiene practitioner concept to help respond to national oral health needs. A Master's-level education that builds upon a foundation of dental hygiene education and includes basic restorative skills is required.

age adjustment A statistical process applied to rates of disease, death, injuries, or other health outcomes that allows communities with different age structures to be compared.

age standardized See *age adjustment*.

agenda The "list" of issues that are under active consideration for policy change or policy action. The agenda is limited by the scale and scope of the formal policy process, which is, in turn, restricted by time (the number of days in a legislative session, the election cycle), by the degree to which people can focus on a limited number of issues, and by the available resources that can be directed to a problem or issue (the budget or available income, resources, or staff).

agent factors Those entities necessary to cause disease in a susceptible host. An agent can be biological (a bacterium, parasite, or virus), physical (force in motor vehicle crashes), chemical (environmental toxins), or nutritional imbalance (e.g., rickets). Several characteristics of agents are important to consider: infectivity, the capacity to cause infection in a susceptible host; pathogenicity, the capacity to cause disease in a host; and virulence, the severity of disease that the agent causes in the host.

airborne transmission Airborne transmission involves the dissemination of microbial aerosols to a suitable portal of entry, usually the respiratory tract. Microbial aerosols are suspensions of particles in the air consisting partially or wholly of microorganisms. They may remain suspended in the air for long periods of time, some retaining and others losing infectivity or virulence.

Alaska Dental Therapist Native Alaskans in rural Alaska who were originally trained in two years at the University of Otago, New Zealand to drill, fill, and extract teeth. They are now trained in Alaska by the University of Washington. Alaska Dental Therapists are the only dental therapists permitted to practice in the United States at this time.

Alaska Native Tribal Health Consortium (ANTHC) The Alaska Native Tribal Health Consortium (ANTHC) is a nonprofit health organization based in Anchorage, Alaska, which provides health services to about 130,000 Alaska Natives and American Indians in Alaska. Established in 1997, ANTHC is owned and managed by Alaska Native tribal governments and their regional health organizations and is the sponsor of the Alaska Dental Therapist program.

alcohol A colorless liquid created by fermentation that is used in intoxicating beverages.

all-hazards plan Comprehensive emergency plans designed to provide a framework for preparing for and responding to the broadest range of events, disasters, and emergencies.

American Association for Community Dental Programs (AACDP) A nonprofit professional organization whose members include those who work in city, county, and community-based health programs with an interest in oral health issues, access to care, and serving the oral health needs of vulnerable populations at the community level.

American Association of Dental Research (AADR) A nonprofit professional organization with more than 4000 members who are primarily interested in dental research. Its mission is (1) to advance research and increase knowledge for the improvement of oral health; (2) to support and represent the oral health research community; and (3) to facilitate the communication and application of research findings.

American Association of Public Health Dentistry (AAPHD) A nonprofit professional organization whose members are primarily interested in public health and community health. Founded in 1937, the main purposes of this association are to promote effective efforts in disease prevention, health services, and delivery; to educate the public, health professionals, and decision makers; and to expand the knowledge base of dental public health competency and practice.

American Association of State and Territorial Dental Directors (ASTDD) A nonprofit professional organization whose members primarily include those who work for state and territorial government and are interested in oral health.

American Dental Association (ADA) A nonprofit professional organization that represents practicing dentists primarily and is dedicated to scientific and professional advancement. Founded in 1859, this is the world's largest and oldest national dental association.

American Dental Education Association (ADEA) A nonprofit professional organization representing individuals and institutions in dental education. ADEA addresses contemporary issues influencing education, research, and the delivery of oral health care for the improvement of public health.

American Legacy Foundation An independent tobacco control funding organization created by the Master Settlement Agreement between the states' attorneys general and the tobacco industry.

American Public Health Association (APHA) Founded in 1872, the APHA is the oldest and largest organization of public health professionals in the world. The APHA provides public health leadership and collaborates with partners to convene constituencies, champion prevention, promote evidence-based policy, and advocate for healthy people and healthy communities.

analytic epidemiology The aspect of epidemiology concerned with the search for health-related causes and effects. Uses comparison groups, which provide baseline data, to quantify the association between exposures and outcomes, and test hypotheses about causal relationships.

analytic horizon Time period during which the costs and benefits of health outcomes that occur as a result of the intervention are considered.

applied ethics Prescribed actions or policies in ethical situations commonly encountered in a particular profession.

applied research Examines the efficacy of new interventions in an effort to identify ever more powerful and less costly ways to prevent and control disease.

appropriations legislation Funding authority approved by Congress and signed by the President to expend a given amount of funds to carry out a federal program. The appropriations act specifies an amount of funding in each appropriation (fund) account of an agency.

aquifer A water-bearing permeable stratum of underground rock, gravel, or sand used for a water supply.

archetype A pattern seen over and over in many environments. There is power in the use of systems archetypes because they provide information and clarification for why things appear to be going right or not so right.

area warrant A general plan for inspection of buildings or other property that describes the area to be searched and the public health or safety purpose of the search. An area warrant may be issued by a health officer, fire marshal, or other public official with police powers.

asepsis The absence, or at least minimal presence of, pathogenic organisms achieved by thorough cleaning and hand washing.

assessment Each public health agency should regularly and systematically collect, assemble, analyze, and make available information on the health of the community, including statistics on health status, community health needs, and epidemiologic and other studies of health problems.

assurance Each public health agency should assure its constituents that services necessary to achieve agreed upon goals are provided, either by encouraging actions by other entities (private or public sector), by requiring such action through regulation, or by providing services directly.

attack rate A cumulative incidence rate used for particular groups observed for limited periods under special circumstances, such as during an epidemic. See also *rate*.

attributable fraction The amount of disease or injury that could be eliminated if a risk factor never occurred in a given population.

attributable risk The amount or proportion of incidence of disease or death (or risk of disease or death) in individuals exposed to a specific risk factor that can be attributed to exposure to that factor; the difference in the risk for unexposed versus exposed individuals.

audience Those who pay attention to what is written or said.

authorization legislation Legislation enacted by Congress that establishes or continues the legal operation of a federal program or agency, either indefinitely or for a specific period of time, or sanctions a particular type of obligation or expenditure within a program. Sometimes referred to as substantive legislation.

bacteriology A branch of microbiology dealing with identification, study, and cultivation of bacteria and with their applications in medicine, agriculture, industry, or biotechnology.

balancing loops A balancing loop attempts to move some current state (the way things are) to a desired state (goal or objective) though some action (whatever is done to reach the goal).

barefoot doctor Farmers who received minimal basic medical and paramedical training and worked in rural villages in the People's Republic of China providing primary health care to rural areas where urban-trained doctors would not settle. They promoted basic hygiene, preventive health care, and family planning and treated common illnesses. The name comes from southern farmers, who would often work barefoot in the rice paddies.

Behavioral Risk Factor Surveillance System (BRFSS) The world's largest telephone survey with 200,000 interviews conducted annually. Sponsored by the CDC, it has provided state-specific data on behavioral risk factors, such as tobacco use, for the past 20 years and is now operational in every state.

behavioral surveillance Plays a unique and important role in the field of chronic disease through its relevance to prevention and early intervention. Through behavioral risk factor surveillance, we can examine the relationship between risk behaviors at the population level and disease patterns in the population. It also provides appropriate and useful data to help us plan and evaluate health promotion and risk reduction programs.

Belmont Report A report on research ethics published in 1979 by the National Commission for the Protection of Human Subjects of Biomedical and Behavioral Research.

bias Systematic error in the design, conduct, or analysis of a study that results in a mistaken estimate of an exposure/disease relationship.

Biochemical Oxygen Deficit (BOD) Lowered dissolved oxygen in water, sometimes caused by decomposer organisms digesting raw sewage.

bioconcentrate Increase of contaminant content in organisms caused by high solubility of the contaminant in body tissue or ingestion of a large number of contaminated organisms that are lower in the food chain.

biodetection An extension of traditional and syndromic surveillance that uses environmental monitoring to identify the release of bioterrorism agents.

bioethics To some, this term is synonymous with ethics related to all living or health-related things. Most often, it is closely aligned more narrowly with medical ethics.

biological and chemical terrorism Illegal use or threatened use of force or violence using biological or chemical agents; typically with ideological and political motives and justifications.

bioremediation Cleanup of contaminants through ingestion by organisms.

biostatistics The application of statistics to biological and medical problems. This is one of the basic sciences of public health, applied in the analysis of vital and health statistics and in the use of statistical tests for associations, correlation, significance levels, and so on, in epidemiology, toxicology, environmental health sciences, and all other public health sciences.

bioterrorism Indiscriminate violent hostile acts against the general population that employs biological agents or toxic products to spread dangerous contagious disease.

brain drain An emigration of trained and talented individuals ("human capital") to other nations or jurisdictions, due to conflicts, lack of opportunity, health hazards where they are living, or other reasons. It parallels the term "capital flight," which refers to financial capital that is no longer invested in the country where its owner lived and earned it. Investment in higher education is lost when a trained individual leaves and does not return. Also, whatever social capital the individual has been a part of is reduced by his or her departure.

budgeting Preparing an itemized summary of estimated or intended expenditures for a given period along with proposals for financing them.

Building Related Illness (BRI) Identifiable and chronic adverse health effects from indoor pollution.

bureaucracies Management systems in which power derives from placement in office rather than from birthright or political connections.[1]

bureaucrats Individuals who work primarily in bureaucracies but may function outside of formal institutions as long as they adhere to a predictable pattern of action formed by enumerated rules and laws and in which they are able to rise in position.

capture-recapture methodology A well-accepted method in wildlife studies of estimating the size of a study population that makes use of overlapping, incomplete, but intersecting sets of data to derive reasonably accurate numerators and denominators for epidemiologic study, which has been adapted to epidemiology and surveillance of ill-defined human populations (sex workers, homeless, etc.). Most methods require multiple samples from a population and an ability to match cases, at least probabilistically. Typically, the method allows an estimate of the total number of cases, including those missed by the sampling methods.

case control study An analytic epidemiologic study in which the risk factors of people with a certain disease (cases) are compared with those of similar people without the disease (controls). Case-control studies are sometimes described as being retrospective because they are always performed looking back in time.

case definition Standard set of criteria for deciding whether, in an investigation or surveillance system, a person should be classified as having the disease or health condition under study. A case definition usually includes four components: clinical information about the disease; characteristics about the people who are affected; information about the location or place; and a specification of time during which the condition occurred.

categorical Pertaining to a specific disease, part of the body, or subset of the population.

categorical funding Funding provided to a public health agency for which expenditure is restricted to purposes and activities specified by the funding source.

causal loop diagram (CLD) A diagram used in systems thinking that aids in visualizing how interrelated variables affect one another.

cellulitis Inflammation of cellular or connective tissue.

certification Completion of education or other requirements to practice a profession.

chance A force assumed to cause events that cannot be foreseen or controlled; the unknown and unpredictable element in happenings that seems to have no assignable cause.

chi-square test A family of statistical tests used to determine whether two or more sets of data or populations differ significantly from one another based on comparing observed with expected distributions of the sets of data and calculating the statistical probability that the differences could be due to chance alone using the chi-square mathematical distribution.[1]

chloro-fluorocarbons (CFCs) Chemicals developed as propellants or insulation materials. Banned by the Montreal Protocol because they are believed to destroy stratospheric ozone, which can absorb some UV radiation that causes skin cancer and eye damage.

chronic diseases Persistent and lasting medical conditions that may be controlled rather than cured.

civil service system Those branches of public service that are not legislative, judicial, or military and in which employment is usually based on competitive examination.

cleft lip/cleft palate Fissures in the upper lip and palate caused by incomplete closing of the two sides of the face in the developing embryo.

Clinical Laboratory Improvement Amendments Act of 1988 (CLIA '88) A federal licensure of laboratories that perform testing on human specimens.

clinical preventive services Interventions used in clinical settings intended to promote good health and prevent disease and injury.

coaching Methods in which employers help employees solve some performance issue and develop abilities to do his or her job better.

coalition Unions of people and organizations working to influence outcomes on a specific problem.

cohort study An observational study in which a defined group of people (the cohort) is followed over time. Outcomes are compared in subsets of the cohort who were exposed or not exposed (or exposed at different levels) to an intervention or other factor of interest. Cohorts can be assembled in the present and followed into the future (a "concurrent cohort study"), or identified from past records and followed from that time up to the present (a "historical cohort study"). Because random allocation is not used, matching or statistical adjustment must be used to ensure that the comparison groups are as similar as possible.

color of state law When an individual acts with the legal power of the state or local government, either because he or she is a governmental employee or because the government supports the individual's actions.

command center Location established by the local or state Emergency Management Authority where the oversight of the emergency response is provided and the response from each of the numerous pertinent agencies is coordinated. Also called the Emergency Operations Center (EOC).

competency domains Areas of public health in which professionals have the ability and capability to perform.

common rule This legislation established the role of institutional review boards (IRBs) for research on human subjects. See also *45 CFR 46.*

communications The imparting or interchange of thoughts, opinions, or information by speech, writing, or signs; the sharing of information, arguments, and points of view.

community A group of people, for example, a neighborhood, village, or municipal or rural region, or a social group with a unifying common interest or trait, loosely organized into a recognizable unit.[1]

Community-Based Participatory Research (CBPR) A collaborative research approach that is designed to ensure and establish structures for participation by communities affected by the issue being studied, representatives of organizations, and researchers in all aspects of the research process to improve health and well-being through taking action, including social change.

community medicine The study of health and disease in a community that is considered an entity and the provision and evaluation of the health services of that community.

community mitigation Measures that might be instituted to decrease the spread of a highly contagious disease, such as pandemic influenza.

Community Oriented Primary Care (COPC) A variation of the primary care model in which major health problems of a defined population are identified and addressed through modifications in both primary care services and other appropriate community health programs.

community water fluoridation The adjustment of the fluoride level in a public water supply that is optimal for oral health. See *fluoridation* and *water fluoridation.*

competencies The skills, knowledge, and abilities necessary for the practice of public health.

conduction Transfer of heat by contact.

confidence interval The range within which the "true" value (e.g., size of effect of an intervention) is expected to lie with a given degree of certainty (e.g., 95% or 99%). For a 95 percent confidence interval, for repeated calculations of the interval for the same population, 95 percent of the intervals will be expected to contain the true population parameter. Confidence intervals represent the probability of random errors but not systematic errors (bias).

confidentiality Information, often of a private or sensitive nature, which a person has chosen to reveal but which is protected from being revealed to others. Confidential information should not be shared with anyone without consent except when there is a clear ethical justification (e.g., approval by a human subjects research review panel), or a legal requirement (e.g., regulations to protect children). Epidemiologic research use of identifiable data without consent requires showing importance of the research, minimal risk to those whose information is used, promise of benefit to society, and an obligation to maintain the confidentiality of the information.

confounding Occurs when a variable is a risk factor for an effect among nonexposed persons and is associated with the exposure of interest in the population from which the effect derives, without being affected by the exposure or the disease (without being an intermediate step in the causal pathway between the exposure and the effect).

continuing education A specific learning activity generally characterized by the issuance of a certificate or Continuing Education Units (CEU) to document attendance or completion of a course of instruction. Continuing education for core competencies helps the public health workforce maintain its current skills and develop new knowledge, skills, and abilities.

controlling The management activity that monitors and adjusts activities to achieve organizational goals.

convection Transfer of heat by transport of air or water currents.

core competencies A set of workforce skills, knowledge, and other attributes necessary for the effective practice of public health.

core functions (of public health) There are three core functions of public health as defined by the Institute of Medicine (IOM): assessment (of dental needs), policy development (for dental disease prevention and treatment), and assurance (of access to needed services).

core laboratory responsibilities Services all public health laboratories should have available in-house or through contract.

coronal tooth decay Tooth decay on the crown of the tooth.

coroner A public officer whose primary function is to investigate by inquest any death thought to be of other than natural causes. See also *medical examiners*.

cost analysis An economic evaluation technique that involves the systematic collection, categorization, and analysis of program costs.

cost-benefit analysis (CBA) A type of economic analysis in which all costs and benefits are converted into monetary (dollar) values and results are expressed as either the net present value or the benefits per dollars expended.

cost-effectiveness analysis (CEA) A type of economic evaluation in which all costs are related to a single, common effect. Results are usually stated as additional cost expended per additional health outcome achieved.

cost-utility analysis (CUA) A type of cost-effectiveness analysis in which benefits are expressed as the number of life years saved adjusted to account for loss of quality of life from morbidity of the health outcome or side effects from the intervention.

Council on Linkages An organization established in 1991 to bring representatives of the major public health professional organizations and federal agencies involved in public health together to address ways of increasing the linkages between public health academia and practice.

covert Unannounced release of a biologic agent that presents as illness in the community, and with contagious agents, has the potential for large-scale spread of disease before detection.

craniofacial anomalies Developmental irregularities of the skull and face, which may include cleft lip and cleft palate.

credentialing A mechanism, generally through testing, to certify competence of public health workers to practice their profession in a public health setting.

criminal justice The system of law enforcement, involving police, lawyers, courts, and corrections, used for all stages of criminal proceedings and punishment.

crisis leadership Requires that public health leaders become competent in a new set of skills necessary to work in a preparedness environment in addition to the skills needed to function in times of normalcy.

cumulative incidence rate Number of new cases or events occurring during a specified period of time divided by the population at risk. The population at risk includes people in the defined population at risk of the condition but condition-free at the beginning of the time period. See also *rate*.

deliberation The process of establishing intent and resolve, where a person or group explores different solutions before settling on a specific course of action.

demographic and health surveys The Demographic and Health Surveys (DHS) project has been initiated and funded by the U.S. Agency for International Development (USAID) to provide data and analysis on the population, health, and nutrition of women and children in developing countries. This is done through the implementation of standardized national population-based surveys.

denormalization A strategy developed in tobacco control campaigns to make smoking an unacceptable or undesirable behavior and to counter social norms that supported smoking in public places.

dental caries An infection and destructive process that results in decalcification of the enamel of teeth, which leads to destruction (cavities) of enamel and dentin and eventually the death of the tooth's nerve and blood supply, if not treated.

dental fluorosis Faint white markings on teeth due to excess fluoride intake while the teeth are developing. Usually considered a minor cosmetic problem.

Dental Health Management Organizations (HMOs) A corporation financed by insurance premiums whose member dentists and professional staff provide dental care within certain financial, geographic, and professional limits to enrolled volunteer members and their families.

Dental Health Professional Shortage Areas (DHPSA) A DHPSA is a federal designation reflecting a shortage of dental providers, in accordance with the federal guidelines. This designation may be established in urban or rural areas, population groups, or in medical or other public facilities. A geographic DHPSA includes the total population of all income levels that have less than 1 dentist per 5000 people, or less than 1 dentist per 4000 people in low-income populations.

dental insurance/benefit plan Dental insurance and benefit plans that help patients receive basic dental care at an affordable cost without causing harm to their financial position.

dental laboratory technicians Dental laboratory technicians make and repair prosthetic appliances such as dentures, bridges, and crowns, usually based on a prescription from a dentist.

dental personnel The various types of dental personnel are dentists, dental hygienists, Alaska dental therapists, dental assistants, and dental laboratory technicians.

dental provider Any one person or group who provides dental services such as dentists and dental hygienists. Some states such as Alaska allow for dental therapists.

dental public health Dental public health is the science and art of preventing and controlling dental diseases and promoting dental health through organized community efforts. It is the form of dental practice that serves the community as a patient rather than the individual.

dental sealant A thin plastic and protective coating that is applied to the biting surfaces of the back teeth, usually the first and second permanent molars. The sealant protects the tooth from getting a cavity by shielding against bacteria and plaque.

dentures An artificial substitute for missing natural teeth and adjacent tissues, usually made from plastic.

denturist A member of the oral health care team, usually a laboratory technician, who provides an oral health examination, takes impressions of the surrounding oral tissues, and constructs and delivers removable oral prosthesis (dentures and partial dentures) directly to the patient. Very few states have laws allowing denturists.

dependence A pattern of drug or alcohol use that leads to clinically significant impairment or distress as evidenced by the development of tolerance, withdrawal, taking larger amounts of the substance, inability to cut down, spending a great deal of time obtaining the substance, missing important activities, and/or continued use despite knowledge of the problem.

descriptive epidemiology The study of the amount and distribution of a disease in a specified population by person, place, and time.

determinant Any factor, whether event, characteristic, or other definable entity, that brings about change in a health condition or in other defined characteristics.

direct cost Medical and nonmedical costs identified and estimated for the cost of an intervention.

direct transmission Direct transmission may occur as a result of touching, biting, kissing, or sexual intercourse, or through direct projections (droplet spread) of droplet spray onto the conjunctiva or onto the mucous membranes of the eye, nose or mouth during sneezing, coughing, spitting, singing, or talking (usually limited to a distance of about 1 meter or less).

disability-adjusted life year (DALY) A key disease measurement that accounts for premature mortality, loss of quality of life, and social values for allocating resources to health programs.

Disaster Medical Assistance Teams Trained and equipped medical personnel who can be quickly mobilized to provide emergency medical care at the site of an emergency.

Disaster Mortuary Operational Response Teams (DMORT) Trained and equipped personnel who can recover, identify, and process deceased victims of a disaster.

Disaster Portable Morgue Unit Team Helps the DMORTs by setting up and running mortuary operations.

disasters Natural or man-made hazards that result in ecologic disruptions, or emergencies, of a severity and magnitude resulting in deaths, injuries, illness, and/or property damage that cannot be effectively managed by the application of routine procedures or resources and that result in a call for outside assistance.

discounting A method for converting the value of future costs and benefits accrued due to an intervention to an equivalent value today (present value) to account for time preference (i.e., $1 today is worth more than $1 a year from now).

disciplines Defined forms of training involving mastery of a specific body of knowledge and skills.

disease prevention The deferral or elimination of specific illnesses and conditions by one or more interventions of proven efficacy.

disease registry A dataset or a collection of specific data elements of a defined population, usually with a specific illness or risk factor (cancer, diabetes, birth defects, etc.). Information collected on individuals may include demographic data, risk factors, genetics, and other information relevant to monitoring health events or outcomes.

disinhibition A process, of whatever etiology, which results in an individual having a reduced capacity to edit or manage their immediate impulsive response to a situation.

disparities In reference to health, disparities refers to inequality in health status and health care experienced by individuals with different social characteristics. Chief among these are disparities experienced by patients with different racial or ethnic characteristics as well as those who differ in terms of education, income, and other measures of socioeconomic status.

distribution In epidemiology, the frequency and pattern of health-related characteristics and events in a population. In statistics, the observed or theoretical frequency of values of a variable.

drug resistance The reduction in effectiveness of a drug in curing a disease or improving a patient's symptoms. When the drug is not intended to kill or inhibit a pathogen, then the term is equivalent to dosage failure or drug tolerance. More commonly, the term is used in the context of diseases caused by pathogens.

drugs Any article, other than food, intended to affect the structure or any function of the body of humans or other animals.

Early Childhood Caries (ECC) Previously referred to as Baby Bottle Tooth Decay (BBTD), ECC is a disease that causes severe and rapid decay of baby teeth and is often due to improper baby bottle feeding such as putting the baby to sleep with milk or soda in a bottle. Occurring between the ages of six months and six years of age, it usually begins with the upper anterior teeth.

Early Periodic Screening Diagnosis and Treatment (EPSDT) Program The child dental health component of Medicaid that is required by federal law and is designed to improve the oral health of low-income children by financing appropriate and necessary dental services.

ecological leadership Professionals who are committed to the development of their leadership skills and competencies throughout their professional careers. These leaders are strongly committed to the appropriate application of these skills to their communities' changing health priorities.

ecological models Provide a framework for targeting system and structural changes within the environment and make it possible to tease out and assess how variations affect individual and community change.

economic evaluation The use of applied analytic techniques to identify, measure, value, and compare the costs and outcomes of alternative interventions.

economic inequality A difference in relative income experienced by a population, at either a national or local level. The term is related to the socioeconomic gradient, the steepness of which may be associated with disparities in health status.

effectiveness The improvement in health outcome that a prevention strategy can produce in typical community-based settings.

efficacy The improvement in health outcome that a prevention strategy can produce in expert hands under ideal circumstances.

efficiency A measure of the relationship between inputs and outputs in a prevention strategy. Efficiency goes beyond effectiveness of a prevention strategy by attempting to identify the maximum health output achievable for a set amount of resources.

elites Individuals usually identified by some group characteristic who have heavy influence over political and policy decisions. Their status may be conferred by their relative wealth, position, or role.

emergency management The organization of a response to disasters through multiple jurisdictions, agencies, and authorities.

Emergency Management Assistance Compact (EMAC) Mutual aid agreement for sharing resources and manpower among all states in the United States.

Emergency Management Authority (EMA) The governmental agency responsible for coordinating the use of all state assets during an emergency or disaster. Also called an Office of Emergency Preparedness (OEP).

Emergency Support Functions (ESF) Annexes within the National Response Framework that guide the response and delineate the roles and responsibilities of participating federal agencies during a disaster.

Emergency System for the Advance Registration of Health Professions Volunteers (ESAR-VHP) System for states to register, credential, and privilege health professional volunteers to provide a supplemental workforce during an emergency.

emerging infectious diseases New infections resulting from changes or evolution of existing organisms, known infections spreading to new geographic areas or populations, previously unrecognized infections appearing in areas undergoing ecologic transformation, and old infections reemerging as a result of antimicrobial resistance in known agents or breakdowns in public health measures.

employee recruitment, retention The process of attracting qualified candidates to agency employment and maintaining their employment with the agency.

enabling legislation Legislation enacted by Congress that gives appropriate government officials and agencies the authority to implement specified activities or enforce specified provisions of the law.

endodontics A recognized specialty of dentistry that deals with the tooth's pulp (nerve and blood supply) and the tissues surrounding the root of a tooth.

energy Kinetic energy (the energy of motion) is the agent of most injuries, such as lacerations and concussions; other injuries such as burns result from thermal, electrical, or chemical energy or ionizing radiation, and some result from interference with energy exchanges such as oxygen use (e.g., drowning) and thermal regulation (freezing).

enumeration A process of identifying the number and types of workers in a specific industry or professional domain. In public health, enumeration is being used to identify the numbers, demographics, and skills and training of workers currently employed in public health activities.

environmental factors The conditions or influences that are not part of either the agent or the host but that influence their interaction. A wide variety of factors, including physical, climatologic, biologic, social, and economic conditions, can come into play.

epidemic A classification of a disease that appears as new cases in a given human population, during a given period, at a rate that substantially exceeds what is "expected," based on recent experience (the number of new cases in the population during a specified period of time is called the "incidence rate"). The disease may or may not be contagious.

epidemic diseases Diseases affecting many persons at the same time and usually spreading from person to person in a locality where the disease is not usually prevalent.

epidemic period A time period when the number of cases of disease reported is greater than expected.

epidemiological transition Refers to a change in the pattern of disease in a country away from infectious diseases toward degenerative diseases.

epidemiology The study of the distribution and determinants of health-related states or events in specified populations and the application of the study to the control of health problems.

ESF 8 The Public Health and Medical Services Annex that covers public health emergencies and is overseen by the Department of Health and Human Services. Responsibilities include assessing the need for assistance on a number of issues such as surveillance, deployment of supplemental medical care personnel, worker health and safety, and patient care.

ethical standards Documents prepared by members of a public health discipline or representative professional society (e.g., American College of Epidemiology or the Public Health Leadership Society) containing core values, duties (obligations), and virtues of the profession, sometimes in the form of general principles. Distinguished from guidelines for good scientific practices and from rules of professional etiquette, ethics guidelines are consensus documents, providing a foundation for discussion of issues arising in practice such as minimizing risks and protecting the welfare of research participants, maintaining public trust, protecting confidentiality and privacy, and obligations to communities.

evaluation A process that attempts to determine as systematically and objectively as possible the relevance, effectiveness, and impact of activities in the light of their objectives.

event An occurrence that may result in injury. (Events are what many people would refer to as accidents.)

Expanded Function Dental Auxiliaries (EFDA) Dental assistants and hygienists who perform more intra-oral procedures than those usually taught in most schools such as drilling and filling teeth. EFDAs increase the dentist's productivity.

false positive and false negative test results Those showing disease where there is none, and showing negative results in a disease state, respectively.

family planning The deliberate effort by women and couples to determine the number of conceptions the woman will have and the timing of those conceptions.

federal regulation A rule or order issued by a federal executive-branch department or administrative agency, generally under authority granted by statute, which enforces or amplifies laws enacted by the legislature and has the force of law.

Federally Qualified Health Center (FQHCs) Health Centers that meet the criteria for and receive federal funding for the services they provide under Section 330 of the Public Health Services Act.

female genital mutilation (FGM) Procedures that intentionally alter or injure female genital organs for nonmedical reasons. It is practiced worldwide, with an estimated 100 to 140 million girls and women currently living with the consequences of FGM.

financial management Comprehensive management of an agency's funds, including budgeting, accounting, grants and contracts management, identifying funding sources, understanding policy issues underlying agency finance, and reporting on these and related matters.

first responder Term used to describe the first medically trained responder(s) to arrive on the scene of an emergency (i.e., police, fire, EMS, and emergency management agencies).

Fisher Exact Test A statistical test used when a sample size is too small to use chi-square analysis. As with chi-square, a comparison between expected and observed results is made to determine if the results vary significantly from what would be expected by chance.

fixed costs Costs that do not vary with volume or level of activity.

fluoridation The addition of fluorides to the public water supply to reduce the incidence of tooth decay.

fluoride A naturally occurring compound that is a component of minerals in rocks and soil, resulting in all water supplies naturally containing some fluoride. The fluoride ion is from the element fluorine, a gas that never occurs in nature in its free state.

food-borne illness A group of diseases caused by contamination of food and water by disease-causing agents, typically pathogenic organisms and their toxins.[1]

formative research The first step taken to identify and define the key problems that affect the target population (also known as needs assessment). This step is critical to achieving a comprehensive understanding of the target population and to provide data to inform the development of an intervention or program.

free radical An atom or group of atoms that has at least one unpaired electron and is therefore unstable and highly reactive.[2]

genome All of the genes existing in the DNA of an individual member of any existing species.[1]

gingivitis A milder and reversible form of periodontal disease that only affects the gums. Gingivitis may lead to more serious, destructive forms of periodontal disease called periodontitis.

global health Field at the intersection of several disciplines—epidemiology, economics, demography, and sociology—that is concerned with international health issues. The term global health, as opposed to international health, implies consideration of the health needs of the people of the whole planet above the concerns of particular nations.

Global Youth Tobacco Survey (GYTS) This outgrowth of the U.S. Youth Tobacco Survey in 1998, under World Health Organization auspices in 1999, became a true global system of in-depth and comparable tobacco surveillance, with city and regional, state, national, and international data available for comparison and analysis.

global warming The gradual rise of global mean surface temperature secondary to the accumulation of greenhouse gases, principally carbon dioxide, in the lower atmosphere. The major causes of increasing greenhouse gases are human activities (combustion of fossil fuels, deforestation, etc.).[2]

governance Where the ultimate authority for, or control of, agency activities resides.

Government Accounting Standards Board (GASB) Entity responsible for standards of financial accounting and reporting for state and local governmental entities.

government agency Organizations such as health departments within the executive branch of a government created and empowered by specific legislation (enabling statutes).

governmental functions Functions that are only done by government, or which are part of governmental policy making.

Great People Individuals who, by force of their personalities and being "in the right place at the right time" are able to effect great changes or influence many people. They are the "natural" or accidental leaders who transform the world or a major sector of the polity or society.

greenhouse gases Gasses in the lower atmosphere that permit the passage of solar radiation from the sun to the earth's surface but impede the escape back into space of long wavelength infrared radiation causing the earth's surface to increase in temperature as their concentration rises. Gasses implicated in this process include carbon dioxide, methane, oxides of sulfur and nitrogen, and chlorofluorocarbons (CFCs).[1]

Guide to Community Preventive Services Recommendations by an expert committee for population-based prevention activities.

habeas corpus Literally, "bring me the body." A petition to the court requesting the release of an individual who claims to be unjustly or illegally confined. The traditional remedy for a person who claims to have been improperly quarantined is to seek *habeas corpus*.

hazard vulnerability analysis (HVA) An analysis of the probability and severity of a variety of emergency events that might occur in a locality that could impact the health and safety of a community.

Head Start A federally funded, income-eligible, direct-service program providing comprehensive child and family development services for families with children from birth to age five. Head Start assists families with job skill development, employment search, and family counseling. Head Start focuses on health, mental health, child development, and early education services, as well as dental prevention.

health (World Health Organization definition) A complete state of physical, mental, and social well-being and not merely the absence of disease or infirmity. Societies that approach this ideal state will do so by appropriately balancing services for the diagnosis and treatment of illness with services that promote health and prevent disease.

health disparities Differing levels of health indicators that are observed among segments of a population, discernible in the size of the health gap between the highest and lowest segment of the population.

health educator Health educators are professionals who design, conduct, and evaluate activities to promote wellness and healthy lifestyles. Health educators teach individuals and communities about behaviors that encourage healthy living to prevent diseases and other problems.

Health Insurance Portability and Accountability Act (HIPAA) An Act adopted by the U.S. Congress in 1996 to ensure health insurance coverage after leaving an employer and also to provide standards for facilitating electronic transactions related to health care. HIPAA included administrative simplification provisions that required national standards for electronic health-care transactions. The HIPAA Privacy Rule provides the first national standards for protecting the privacy of health information. The Privacy Rule regulates how certain entities, called covered entities, use and disclose certain individually identifiable health information, called protected health information.

health officer The state or local government official vested with the power to enforce public health laws.

health policy Formal statements or procedures within institutions (notably government) that define priorities and the parameters for action.

health problem Any factor that prevents a state of complete physical, mental, and social well-being; not limited to disease or infirmity.

health promotion The policies and processes that enable people to increase control over and improve their health. These address the needs of the population as a whole in the context of their daily lives, rather than focusing on people at risk for specific diseases, and are directed toward action on the determinants or causes of health. Health promotion is action-oriented and based on public policies, for instance, provision of facilities such as bicycle pathways, recreational parks to encourage healthy behavior, and public meeting places to encourage social interaction; and deterring health-harming behavior by promoting smoke-free zones.

health protection A useful term to describe important activities of public health departments, specifically in food hygiene, water purification, environmental sanitation, drug safety, and other activities in which the emphasis is on actions that can be taken to eliminate as far as possible the risk of adverse consequences for health attributable to environmental hazards, unsafe or impure food and water, drugs, and so on.

health service All services performed, provided, or arranged to promote, improve, conserve, or restore the mental or physical well-being of communities. These services include but are not limited to the management of health services resources, such as manpower, monies, and facilities; preventive and curative health measures; emergency response; medical supply, equipment, and maintenance thereof; and medical intelligence services.

health status The degree to which a person or defined group can fulfill usually expected roles and functions physically, mentally, emotionally, and socially.

Healthy People 2010 A statement of national health objectives designed to identify the most significant preventable threats to health and to establish national goals by the year 2010 to reduce these threats. It can be used by states, communities, professional organizations, and others to guide them in developing programs to improve health.

history The branch of knowledge dealing with past events; the field of research producing a continuous narrative and a systematic analysis of past events of importance to the human race.

Hospital Incident Command System (HICS) The incident command system that defines the roles and responsibilities of hospital providers and employees during an emergency.

host factors Characteristic of the person, or in a more generic definition, the organism, that is susceptible to the effect of the agent. The status of the host is quite important and is generally classifiable as susceptible, immune, or infected. Finally, and also quite important, is that the host's response to exposure can vary widely, from showing no effect to manifesting subclinical disease, atypical symptoms, straightforward illness, or severe illness.

human resources The field of personnel recruitment and management.

human rights A philosophical and political view that every human being has equal dignity and worth and

thus must be ensured certain resources necessary for life and protection against certain harms.

hygiene Refers to practices associated with ensuring good health and cleanliness.

"iceberg" or "pyramid" The relationship between mortality and morbidity (or different degrees of severity) is referred to as the "pyramid of injury"; the actual ratio between each of the levels of that pyramid varies depending on the specific injury or the specific injury mechanism because some injuries are more lethal than others.

incidence A measure of the frequency with which an event, such as a new case of illness, occurs in a population over a period of time. For an incidence rate, the denominator is the population at risk; the numerator is the number of new cases occurring during a given time period.

incipient carious lesion Beginning dental caries or tooth decay; noncavitated.

Incident Action Plan (IAP) Objectives and strategies usually established by the incident commander and planning section for responding to events during an emergency.

Incident Command System (ICS) The standard management structure used in disaster response across the United States.

incident commander The individual responsible for the management of the emergency response and operations when using the Incident Command System at the scene of an emergency.

Incremental Cost-Effectiveness Ratio (ICER) The ratio of difference in net costs and net benefits between one scenario and another.

indemnity plan Indemnity policyholders pay for their medical or dental care as they go and are reimbursed by their health care provider either in full or partially.

independent practice Includes various forms of unsupervised dental practice or less restrictive practice. Usually used in regard to dental hygienists working independently from a dentist.

indirect cost Productivity losses identified and estimated for the cost of patients' participation in an intervention.

indirect transmission Transmission of infection from an infected person to a susceptible one in the absence of direct contact. Indirect transmission may be vehicle-borne (air, water, food, etc.) or vector-borne (mosquito, tick, flea, etc.). See also *vehicle-borne transmission* and *vector-borne transmission*.

industrial hygiene The discipline of anticipating, recognizing, evaluating, and controlling health hazards in the working environment with the objective of protecting workers' health and well-being and safeguarding the community at large.

infant mortality Deaths in the first year of life per 1000 live births.

informatics Encompasses the many and varied aspects of managing, using, and sharing information to promote decision making in assessment, priority setting, quality and effectiveness of work activities, and evaluation. Informatics draws from computer science, information technology, engineering, social and cognitive psychology, library science, and administration because all influence the processing and use of information.

information bias Bias that occurs during data collection; the three main types of information bias are misclassification bias (e.g., due to interviewer or recall), ecological fallacy (bias produced when analyses realized in an ecological [group level] analysis are used to make inferences at the individual level), and regression to the mean (phenomenon that a variable that shows an extreme value on its first assessment will tend to be closer to the center of its distribution on a later measurement).

informed consent Ensuring voluntary participation in research on human subjects. Potential study participants must be informed of all the likely risks and benefits of the research before they consent to participate.

infrastructure The assets that support an economy, such as roads, bridges, power supplies, water supplies, and public health services; these are typically owned and managed by local or central government. The investment in these assets is made with the intention that dividends will accrue through increased productivity, improved living conditions, and greater prosperity.

injuries Bodily damage related to acute exposure to some form of energy (kinetic, potential, or other) in amounts and at rates that exceed the individual's tolerance threshold.

injury prevention or control Intervention(s) aimed at preventing the initial event or blocking progression of the injury-producing process.

Institute of Medicine (IOM) A nonprofit membership organization, established by the U.S. National Academy of Sciences in 1970, which identifies, studies, and reports on medically relevant issues and problems, including many in the field of public health.

institutional review board (IRB) An officially sanctioned group that reviews and monitors ethical aspects of research.

intangible cost Costs associated with emotional anxiety and fear and with physical pain and suffering.

international health Also called *geographic medicine* or *global health*, this field of health care usually has a public health emphasis across regional or national boundaries.

interoperability The ability of information systems to operate in conjunction with each other encompassing communication protocols, hardware, software, application, and data compatibility layers.

inter-rater reliability The degree of correspondence among multiple observations that are collected on the same subject by two or more independent observers/raters.

intervention Efforts taken to reduce or stop drug or alcohol use after initiation of use.

job action sheets Documents that describe the duties and responsibilities for each function within the Incident Command System (ICS).

job description A formal description of a position title, qualifications, major duties, assessment criteria, and related matters.

key informants People who represent a specific community and are able to provide "expert" information about specific experiences, beliefs, and attitudes that are common to that community.

Laboratory Response Network (LRN) A network of laboratories organized into a three-level system to process biological or chemical specimens during an emergency.

leadership Leadership is creativity in action. It is the ability to see the present in terms of the future while maintaining respect for the past. Leadership is based on respect for history and the knowledge that true growth builds on existing strengths.

leadership development A key factor in organizational effectiveness and infrastructure development and refers to any activity that enhances the quality of leadership within an individual or organization.

Leading Health Indicators (LHI) Primary public health concerns in the United States that were chosen based on their ability to motivate action, the availability of data to measure their progress, and their relevance as broad public health issues.

leverage points A place in a system where pressure can be applied. In systems thinking, leverage points are where the smallest efforts can make the biggest differences.

liberal traditions The notion that all individuals have equal political rights and responsibilities was not realized until late in the twentieth century with passage of the civil rights acts. The primacy of the individual has now come to be recognized as the fundamental characteristic of the U.S. political system but stands at odds with the collective problems that public health copes with. There is a constant and dynamic tension between the rights of the individual and protections for the population in public health.

life expectancy The average number of years a person of specific age and sex is expected to live if current trends in mortality rates prevail in the future.

lifestyle The behavioral patterns, customs, and habits of persons or groups, generally considered in the context of consequences for health.

local health department An administrative or service unit of local or state government concerned with health and carrying some responsibility for the health of a jurisdiction smaller than the state.

Local Public Health System (LPHS) The consortium of agencies, institutions, and individuals whose work and activities impact community health status.

malocclusion A condition in which the upper and lower teeth do not fit together properly. Commonly known as crooked teeth, an overbite is a common example of a malocclusion.

managed care A form of fiscal management of medical services used by health maintenance organizations and other health care organizations to allocate referral and treatment services.

managerial accounting The process of identifying, measuring, analyzing, interpreting, and communicating information in pursuit of an organization's goals.

Master Settlement Agreement (MSA) An agreement between the states' attorneys general and the tobacco companies for the latter to pay the states billions of dollars a year and to voluntarily change some of their marketing behavior in consideration of the costs to states for medical care of those who contracted tobacco-related diseases. In exchange, the states relinquished their claims for reimbursement and agreed not to bring suit in the future.

Maternal and Child Health (MCH) Block Grant The Maternal and Child Health Block Grants are from the federal government with the purpose of improving the health of mothers, children, and their families. They are a major source of financial support for all state health departments.

maternal deaths A death is defined as maternal if it occurs during pregnancy or delivery or shortly after delivery, as a result of complications of the pregnancy or delivery.

maternal mortality Maternal deaths per 100,000 live births.

maternal mortality review (MMR) committees Highly effective in reducing maternal mortality during the middle third of the twentieth century through application of this methodology. Each maternal death was examined for whether it could have been prevented, and if so, how it could have been prevented.

Maximum Contaminant Level (MCL) The maximum concentration of a chemical that is allowed in public drinking water according to standards set by the U.S. Environmental Protection Agency for drinking water quality.[2]

MCH Block Grant See *Maternal and Child Health (MCH) Block Grant.*

measurement error The deviation of a measurement from its true value, expressed in absolute or relative form.

measurement noise Variation in values obtained for a measure due to random or systematic disturbances that interfere with measurement.

measurement sensitivity A performance measure's ability to detect true differences in performance across organizations and/or true changes in performance over time.

measurement specificity A performance measure's ability to distinguish performance levels from other phenomena that independently influence health.

media A term that refers to a very large sector of communication that is often associated with television and newspapers but involves a much wider scope. The popular media, which depends on viewership, subscriptions, and advertising revenue, can become influential due to its coverage (or lack of coverage) of events and the degree to which it editorializes on the events or issues.

Medicaid A governmental health insurance program for eligible low-income individuals and families, who normally meet a set of categorical health-need requirements, with a goal of providing medical and other health care services to help maintain health status and self-sufficiency.

Medicaid Managed Care Services paid for by Medicaid that are provided through health maintenance organizations.

medical care Care of sickness or injury provided by any qualified professional person in a health-related institution, clinic, or comparable setting.

medical ethics Ethics applied to interactions between clinicians and patients. Common concerns include the autonomy of the patient and the obligation of the clinician to not knowingly harm the patient.

medical examiner A public officer whose primary function is to investigate by inquest any death thought to be of other than natural causes. Most medical examiners are licensed physicians or forensic pathologists and are generally appointed (rather than elected). They may have jurisdiction over a county, district, or entire state. See also *coroner*.

Medical Reserve Corps (MRC) Federal group that recruits and deploys health care personnel as volunteers during emergencies.

medically underserved area A geographically contiguous area in which residents have a shortage of personal health services.

Medicare A federally funded and administered health insurance program for older Americans and those who are disabled. Individuals contribute to Medicare during their working years just as they do to social security.

medicine/public health initiative An attempt to bridge the gap between medicine and public health in a manner that promotes stronger working relationships between the two disciplines.

mentoring Teaching, supporting, encouraging, counseling, and acting as a friend to an individual.

merit system The system of appointing and promoting civil service personnel on the basis of merit rather than on political affiliation or loyalty.

meta-leadership Working across organizations to exert leadership beyond the borders of one's day to day sphere of responsibility.

mission A statement of the overall purpose of an organization that describes what it does, for whom it does it, and the benefit.

mitigate the hazard To correct the conditions or cease the activity that creates a hazard or public nuisance

mitigation Phase in comprehensive emergency management where actions are taken to reduce the harmful effects of a disaster such as those that may prevent further loss of life, disease, disability, or injury.

mobilization The act of assembling and making both troops and supplies ready for war; the organization or adaptation (of industries, transportation facilities, etc.) for service to the government in time of war.

Model Framework for Community Oral Health Program Provides guidance to public health agency leaders and policy makers who want to develop oral health programs and services at the local or community level.

models Representations of physical structures or processes and the interactions among these structures and processes that are meant more to describe and logically link phenomena together than to imply broader meanings underlying them.

Monitoring the Future (MTF) Study Conducted by the University of Michigan with support from the National Institute of Drug Abuse (NIDA), MTF has been in operation since 1976, tracking the use of tobacco and other substances among high school seniors. In the early 1990s, MTF added eighth and tenth grade samples to its school-based surveys.

morally defensible decision A decision with ethical implications that was determined by a fair process and took into account ethically important factors relevant to the situation.

morbidity The absence of health or physical or psychological well-being.

mortality The number of individuals within a defined population who die during a specific period.

mortality surveillance The systematic and ongoing collection of data on the causes of death for individuals.

mother-to-child transmission Also known as vertical transmission, mother-to-child transmission refers to transmission of an infection, such as HIV, hepatitis B, or hepatitis C, from mother to child during the perinatal period, the period immediately before, during, and after birth, including the period of breastfeeding.

MPH core competencies The skills, knowledge, and other attributes that should be evident in graduates with a generalist Master of Public Health (MPH) degree.

multidisciplinary teams Work groups composed of or combining several usually separate fields of expertise.

multidrug-resistant TB (MDR-TB) TB that is resistant at least to isoniazid (INH) and rifampicin (RMP), which are the first line of treatment drugs. Isolates that are multiply-resistant to any other combination of anti-TB drugs but not to INH and RMP are not classed as MDR-TB. MDR-TB can develop in the course of the treatment of fully sensitive TB and is in part the result of patients missing doses or failing to complete a course of treatment.

Multiple Indicator Cluster Surveys A survey program developed by the United Nations Children's Fund to provide internationally comparable, statistically rigorous data on the situation of children and women.

mutual aid Agreements made with surrounding jurisdictions for the provision of aid during an emergency.

natality Birth in a defined population over a period of time.

National Disaster Medical System (NDMS) A federally coordinated system that supplements the medical response capability of state and local authorities when dealing with the medical impacts of major disasters. Through NDMS, the government is able to deploy critical assets during an emergency. NDMS has several components.

National Health and Nutrition Examination Surveys (NHANES) The NHANES collects a combination of survey data and physical measures from blood samples to estimate national probabilities of exposure to risk factors and levels of health in the population.

National Health Interview Survey (NHIS) NHIS is the oldest and most continuous system, apart from tobacco sales, for monitoring tobacco use, and other critical health behaviors and conditions.

National Health Service Corps Founded in 1972 and part of the U.S. Department of Health and Human Services, the National Health Service Corps helps medically underserved communities recruit and retain primary care clinicians, including dental, mental, and behavioral health professionals, to serve in their community.

National Incident Management System (NIMS) A system, based on the Incident Command System (ICS), which is used for the management of emergencies. The NIMS standards, promulgated by the Department of Homeland Security, provide guidance for coordinating all levels of governmental response across the country.

National Network for Oral Health Access (NNOHA) A nonprofit organization made up primarily of dental providers and administrators who care for patients in migrant, homeless, and community health centers.

National Notifiable Diseases Surveillance System A surveillance system in the United States dating back to 1878, when Congress authorized the U.S. Marine Hospital Service (the forerunner of the Public Health Service) to collect morbidity reports regarding cholera, smallpox, plague, and yellow fever from U.S. consuls overseas.

National Nurse Response Team Provides supplemental nursing care during an emergency; can assist in Point of Distribution (POD) operations.

National Pharmacy Response Teams Assists in large-scale Point of Distribution (POD) operations and other activities requiring pharmacists.

National Response Framework (NRF) A federal guideline for operations during an emergency.

National Survey on Drug Use and Health (NSDUH) The NSDUH, recently expanded both in sample size and in depth of tobacco questions, as well as having improved computer methodology to obtain valid measures of illicit drug use and private information during interviews in the home, provides valuable information on the incidence of initiation of illicit drugs and on smoking, as well as the number of new smokers in a given year, and most recently, cigarette brand preference among adolescents.

needs assessment The determination of the needs of a community, population, or patient.

neglected epidemic An epidemic that affects large numbers of people but is not addressed or responded to by society.

neglected tropical diseases (NTDs) A group of tropical infections that are especially endemic in low-income populations in developing regions of Africa, Asia, and the Americas. Different groups define the set of diseases differently. Together, they cause an estimated 500,000 to 1 million deaths annually and cause a global disease burden equivalent to that of HIV-AIDS.

neonatal mortality Neonatal deaths per 1000 live births.

neonates Babies younger than 28 days.

net present value (NPV) The future stream of benefits and costs converted into equivalent values today.[2]

New Zealand Dental Therapist Training Program Originally begun in 1921 in New Zealand, this is a two-year training program for high school graduates to provide basic preventive and restorative dental care, including drilling, filling and extraction of teeth. In 2006, the curriculum for dental therapists and dental hygiene merged into a three-year academic program.

nicotine addiction The habituation and dependency on frequent doses of nicotine, usually from tobacco products, which develops as a result of the use of tobacco.

observational study A study in which nature is allowed to take its course. Changes or differences in one characteristic (e.g., whether or not people received the intervention of interest) are studied in relation to changes or differences in other(s) (e.g., whether or not they died), without the intervention of the investigator. There is a greater risk of selection bias than in experimental studies.

odds ratio The ratio of the odds of an event in the experimental (intervention) group to the odds of an event in the control group.

official capacity The actions that a government official takes that are part of his or her official duties and for which the governmental employer can be legally liable.

ONPRIME model A model that emphasizes the importance of seven process substeps (Organization, Needs/Resources Assessment, Priority Setting, Research, Interventions, Monitoring, and Evaluation).

operational planning Translating elements of a strategic plan into terms consistent with the way the subject agency functions; tactical planning.

oral and pharyngeal cancer Cancer that occurs in the mouth and/or pharynx.

oral contraceptives The most popular form of nonpermanent birth control.

oral diseases Diseases and infections that occur in the mouth such as gum diseases, dental caries, and oral and pharyngeal cancer.

Oral Health Section (APHA) Part of the American Public Health Association that works to promote oral health. The Section is made up primarily of oral health professionals and has sponsored many resolutions and educational programs on dental public health policies, programs, and practices.

organizational structure The relationships among elements of an organization, typically depicted in chart form.

orofacial injuries Injuries that occur to the mouth or jaw from physical activities or the external environment.

orthodontic treatment Dental treatment that focuses on the development, prevention, and correction of irregularities of the teeth, bite, and jaw.

outbreak investigation Outbreak investigation involves seven major steps:

1. Confirm whether there truly is an epidemic.
2. Identify the illness involved.
3. Enumerate all cases and characterize them according to time, place, and person.
4. Confirm the diagnosis.
5. Formulate a hypothesis about the cause of the epidemic and the means of transmission, and test that hypothesis.

6. Take control measures to end the epidemic.

7. Prepare and disseminate a report about the epidemic.

outcome evaluation The assessment of a program's or intervention's impact on the primary study outcome.

outcome indicators Measures that characterize the quality or performance of an enterprise based on the results obtained by consumers of the goods or services produced by the enterprise. For health-related programs and providers, these indicators may include measures of health status, satisfaction, quality of life, and economic impact.

overt Announced releases of biological or chemical agents.

P value The probability (ranging from zero to one) that the results observed in a study (or results more extreme) could have occurred by chance.

pandemic An epidemic of infectious disease that spreads through human populations across a large region (e.g., a continent), or even worldwide.

pandemic influenza The emergence of a novel strain of influenza, capable of causing significant morbidity and mortality because people have no immunity against the unique viral strains, accompanied by worldwide spread.

***parens patria* power** The power of the state to act as parent to protect an individual for the individual's own good. This is different from police power, in that the individual is protected because of the state's interest in not having to bear the burden of injured citizens. Motorcycle helmet laws are enacted under *parens patria*.

partnerships A relationship among individuals and groups that is characterized by mutual cooperation and responsibility.

pathognomonic Characteristic or indicative of a disease, denoting especially one or more typical symptoms that distinguish it from other diseases.

patronage The term is often used to describe the corrupt use of state resources to advance the interests of groups, families, ethnicities, or races in exchange for electoral support.

performance benchmark A quantitative assessment of performance that is used as a comparison point for evaluating the performance of public health programs or organizations. A benchmark may be based on the observed performance of one or more leading organizations or based on a percentile of all relevant organizations.

performance management The practice of using performance measures on an ongoing basis to improve the operation of a program, organization, or delivery system.

performance measures Criteria, often determined in advance by an expert committee, that are used to assess the performance of individuals, agencies, or institutions.

performance standard A statement of the expectations or requirements for carrying out a specific public health activity to reach a goal or objective. Performance standards may be based on professional consensus or empirical evidence about the actions necessary for goal attainment.

periodontal disease Periodontal disease is an infection of the tissues that support the teeth and is classified according to the severity of the disease. The two major stages are gingivitis and periodontitis.

periodontitis A severe form of periodontal disease where the tissues around a tooth, including the ligament and bone that holds the tooth in place is infected. Periodontitis can lead to bone loss and an eventual loss of teeth.

person-time rate A measure of the incidence rate of an event, for example, a disease or death, in a population at risk over an observed period of time that directly incorporates time into the denominator.

personal capacity Actions taken by a government official that are outside of his or her official duties and for which the individual can be held personally liable.

personal identifier An identifying data element associated with an individual, including the individual's name, social security number, any identifying particular assigned to the individual (fingerprint, voiceprint, photograph), or any other identifying number, symbol, unique retriever, or coding device that is assigned to or directly correlates with the individual.

personnel management Management of individuals working within a specified organization.

Plan-Do-Study-Act (PDSA) A quality improvement cycle developed by Shewhart that supports small-scale experimentation and the development of an evidence base in advance of broader action.

plume The trail of smoke, vapor, or other material emanating from a source, such as a smelter stack, and carried by prevailing winds in a particular direction.[1]

point-of-care Done at the site of treatment.

Point of Distribution sites (PODs) Sites where the well public comes to receive preventive medical interventions.

point source A single identifiable person or place and time that is the origin of an epidemic or pollutant.[1]

police power The power of the state to protect the health, safety, morals, and general welfare of the people. The police power is the power to restrict the liberty of individuals to protect other individuals. Communicable disease laws are enacted under the police power.

policy "All the rules" that guide behavior or people and institutions. These can be customs or they can be very specific procedure manuals or regulatory guidance based on general laws or statutes.

policy development Each public health agency should serve the public interest in the development of comprehensive public health policies by promoting use of the scientific knowledge base in decision making about public health and by leading in developing public health policy.

policy entrepreneurs Individuals who promote a specific policy solution that may or may not address a specific and matching problem. They are found in the wider policy field as well as in the specifics of public health.

political action committee A group organized to promote its members' views on selected policy issues, usually through raising money that is contributed to the campaign funds of candidates for elective office who support the group's position.

politics The process that decides who gets what, when, and how. Politics operates at many levels and in many places and institutions. Politics are invoked when there are things to be distributed or taken away from people and institutions.

population-based approach An approach that targets a population as the subject instead of the individual.

positive predictive value The probability that individuals with a positive test result have the disease the test is designed to detect.

poverty A state of deprivation of those things that determine the quality of life, including food, clothing, shelter, and feeling in control of one's own choices.

Preferred Provider Organizations (PPOs) A managed care organization of dentists, medical doctors, hospitals, and other health care providers who have an agreement with an insurer or a third-party administrator to provide health care at reduced rates to the insurer's or administrator's clients.

premature death Deaths that occur a considerable but undefined number of years before average life expectancy is achieved.

preparedness Phase in comprehensive emergency management where officials or the public plan a response to potential disasters.

presidential disaster declaration When the President determines that federal aid, including manpower and services, medicine and medical supplies, food and other consumables, and financial assistance, is required by states in response to a disaster.

preterm deliveries Deliveries at less than 37 weeks' gestation.

prevalence The number of people in a population with the disease at any given time.

prevalence odds ratio See *odds ratio*.

prevented fraction The amount of a health problem that actually has been prevented by a prevention strategy in the real world.

prevention Policies and actions to eliminate a disease or minimize its effect; to reduce the incidence and/or prevalence of disease, disability, and premature death; to reduce the prevalence of disease precursors and risk factors in the population; and, if none of this is feasible, to retard the progress of incurable disease.

prevention effectiveness The systematic assessment of the impact of prevention policies, programs, and practices on health outcomes.

preventive medicine The specialized branch of clinical medical practice devoted to promoting health and preventing disease and premature disability.

primary care Basic or general health care focused on the point at which a patient ideally first seeks assistance from the health care system.

Primary Care Health Professional Shortage Areas (HPSAs) Areas where there are fewer than 1 full-time equivalent primary care physician for each group of 3500 residents.

primary health care Social concept defined as essential health care that should be made available to everyone.

primary medical care See *primary health care.*

primary prevention Preventing a disease before it occurs. The most effective way to improve health and control costs.

primary teeth The baby teeth, usually 20 in number. Also known as deciduous teeth. The baby teeth are replaced by the adult teeth (permanent teeth), usually 32 in number.

privacy What a person claims as protected from scrutiny by others unless the person chooses to reveal it. Respect for privacy means that a person should not normally be expected to reveal personal information, conditions, or behavior unless he or she chooses to reveal it. Violation of privacy requires ethical justification, for example, in cases where it is argued such violations protect others from greater harm.

procedural due process The insurance of fundamental fairness in the legal procedure used. A physician who has his or her hospital privileges terminated has a right to a hearing before an impartial party to ensure the fairness of the termination proceeding.

process evaluation The assessment of the immediate impact of the program, program implementation, and quality control procedures (also known as intervention fidelity).

process indicators Measures that characterize the quality or performance of an enterprise based on the methods and procedures used by the enterprise and the services and activities produced by the enterprise. For health-related programs and providers, these indicators often show the degree of adherence to professional standards and evidence-based guidelines in delivering health services.

profession An occupation that requires specialized education or training that is often available only in a college or university and is usually assessed by a sequence of examinations.

professional A person in a skilled occupation requiring formal training or education; a person who is an expert in his or her work.

proficiency testing In the laboratory scenario, specimens unknown to the tested but known to the tester.

program evaluation A systematic way to improve and account for public health actions that involves procedures that are useful, feasible, ethical, and accurate. Program evaluation should go hand-in-hand with program delivery to determine whether a given program is actually achieving the intended outcomes.

program intervention A long-term, often multifaceted sequence of actions or events to respond to identified problems in a particular community.

prophylaxis A professional cleaning of the teeth with instruments to remove plaque, calculus (mineralized plaque), and stains to help prevent dental disease.

proprietary functions Activities that are not unique to government but are commonly done by private businesses.

prostheses An artificial substitute for a missing body part or missing teeth, such as dentures.

prosthodontics Prosthetic dentistry; the dental art and science pertaining to the restoration and maintenance of oral function by the replacement of missing teeth and adjacent structures by artificial devices or prostheses.

public health An organized activity of society to promote, protect, improve, and, when necessary, restore the health of individuals, specified groups, or the entire population. It is a combination of sciences, skills, and values that function through collective societal activities and involve programs, services, and institutions aimed at protecting and improving the health of all the people.

public health competencies Represent a set of skills, knowledge, and attitudes necessary for the broad practice of public health. They may be used in assessing training needs, training development, hiring, or performance evaluation.

public health dentist Dentists who are trained in public health and are concerned with the oral health needs of entire communities, or populations; they usually design, evaluate, and administer population-based prevention and dental care programs.

public health emergency Both natural and man-made events that have the potential to overwhelm routine public health capabilities due to their scale, timing, or unpredictability.

public health ethics Ethics applied to interactions between a public health agency and the population it serves. Common concerns are the interdependence of individuals and the tensions between the rights of individuals and the good of the community.

public health informatics The systematic application of information and computer science and technology to public health practice, research, and learning.

public health practice The planning, implementation, and evaluation of policies and programs to benefit the health of a particular population. The gathering of data for this purpose is often contrasted with research.

public health sentinel Health care workers who may identify an epidemic in an early stage through individual patients.

public health system The constellation of governmental and nongovernmental organizations that contribute to the performance of essential public health services for a defined community or population.

public nuisance An activity or condition of property that is hazardous or offensive to the community.

public policy A plan or course of action developed by public bodies or figures and intended to determine or influence decisions, actions, and other matters.

public-private alliances Collaboration between public and private organizations, which may include business, governmental, community, and academic partners, working toward a common goal.

quality-adjusted life years (QALYs) A measure standardized to one-year periods, which combines levels of health (measured in terms of their impact upon quality of life) with their duration.

quality assurance A system of activities and monitoring intended to provide the most accurate test result possible.

quarantine A strict isolation imposed to prevent the spread of disease; the word comes from the Italian (seventeenth century) language *quarantena*, meaning a 40-day period.

radiology The use of radiation (such as x-rays) or other imaging technologies (such as ultrasound and magnetic resonance imaging) to diagnose or treat disease.

radon A radioactive element that is a decay product of radium and uranium. It is occasionally an environmental health problem associated with childhood leukemia, adult lung cancer, and other malignancies in localities with high naturally occurring levels.[1]

randomized controlled trial An experimental approach in which subjects from a sample are randomly assigned to either a treatment or nontreatment group. The results are assessed by comparing outcomes in the treatment and control groups.

rate An expression of the frequency with which an event occurs in a defined population.

recovery Phase of a disaster where actions are taken (e.g., repairing infrastructure, damaged buildings, and critical facilities) to return a community to normal or the "new normal."

recurrent tooth decay Tooth decay that comes back after it has been treated.

redundancies Use of multiple methods to communicate in anticipation that one or more communication systems may fail.

referendum The principle or practice of referring measures proposed or passed by a legislative body to the vote of the electorate for approval or rejection.

reinforcing loops Loops in which an action produces a result that influences more of the same action thus resulting in growth or decline.

relative risk A comparison of the risk of some health-related event such as disease or death in two groups.

reliability A measure's ability to produce a consistent reflection of performance each time it is used.

remineralization The process of restoring mineral ions to the tooth structure, usually accomplished with fluoride.

replacement The number of children needed to replace the current generation.

reportable disease or injury A disease or injury that must be reported to an appropriate government authority regardless of issues of privacy or patient consent. Usually, infectious diseases must be reported to the health department, and intentional injuries must be reported to law enforcement.

representativeness The degree to which the characteristics of a sample correspond to those of the original population or reference population.

research The application of systematic methods to discover, interpret, and advance human knowledge of our world and the universe.

response Phase in comprehensive emergency management where relief is followed by recovery, including reconstruction of the community. Emergency relief activities include saving lives, providing first aid, restoring emergency communications and transportation systems, and providing immediate care and basic needs to survivors, such as food and clothing or medical and emotional care.

risk The probability that an event will occur, for example, that an individual will become ill or die within a stated period of time or age.

risk-adjustment A statistical method of rescoring performance measures to exclude the influence of factors deemed to be outside the control of the organizations being measured.

risk ratio See *relative risk*.

root planing The dental procedure by which the surfaces of the roots are made smooth with dental instruments by the removal of residual calculus and diseased cementum.

root surface tooth decay Tooth decay that occurs on the root surface of teeth.

sanitarians Persons knowledgeable about sanitary sciences. Persons technically trained to detect environmental risks to health due to such causes as deficiencies in sanitation, ventilation, and so on.

sanitation The development and application of measures to promote or improve health through environmental engineering, for example, provision of clean water supplies and the disposal of solid waste.

scaling The basic procedure by which calculus is removed from the surfaces of the teeth with dental instruments. Scaling is divided into supramarginal and submarginal scaling depending on the location of the calculus in relation to the gingival margin.

School Dietary Fluoride Supplement Programs A school-based program that ensures all children have access to fluoride by prescribing dietary fluoride supplements that are taken daily in school.

school fluoridation Similar to community water fluoridation, except the public school water system is fluoridated. See also *fluoridation*.

School Fluoride Rinse Program School Rinse Programs are not as effective as community water fluoridation but are effective in communities that are not fluoridated. Children rinse their mouths with a fluoride solution once a week for one minute in the classroom and then spit out the fluoride. The benefit to teeth from a fluoride rinse program is topical because the fluoride solution strengthens the outer layer of tooth enamel, and the fluoride is not swallowed.

school sealant program Provides sealants to vulnerable populations less likely to receive private dental care, such as children eligible for free or reduced-cost lunch programs, using portable dental equipment or a fixed facility within the school setting. See also *dental sealant*.

scientists Related to academics but restricted to those practitioners who adhere to a scientific process that calls for observation measurement and an attempt at objective reporting.

scope of practice The legal definition of the services that a health professional can or cannot do on patients.

seasonal influenza Common but frequently serious viral disease.

secondary attack rate A measure of the frequency of new cases of a disease among the contacts of known cases.

secondary prevention Treating or controlling a disease after it occurs, such as replacing an amalgam restoration.

second-hand smoke The exposure to the smoke emitted by the burning of another person's cigarette, either directly from the burning cigarette or indirectly from the exhaled smoke.

sectors Way in which the emergency management field organizes its activities; includes fire, police, and emergency medical services (EMS). Public health and health care organizations are part of the health sector.

secular trend A long-term movement or change in frequency, usually upward or downward.

security The protection of data from unauthorized (accidental or intentional) modification, destruction, or disclosure.

selection bias The error introduced when the study population does not represent the target population.

self-efficacy The confidence that a person has in his or her belief to achieve a specific desired behavior or state of cognition.

sensitivity The proportion of individuals with the target condition in a population who are correctly identified by a screening test. Also known as true positive rate. The ability of a surveillance system to detect epidemics and other changes in disease occurrence.

sensitivity analysis The process of changing the values of some parameters, variables, or model structures in a meaningful way to examine the robustness of the results.

sentinel Clinical laboratories that may identify an epidemic in an early stage through individual patient test results.

sentinel surveillance A surveillance system in which a pre-arranged sample of reporting sources agrees to report all cases of one or more notifiable conditions.

sepsis A blood stream infection.

servant leadership An individual who is committed to serving the public.

severe acute respiratory syndrome (SARS) A viral respiratory illness caused by a coronavirus, called SARS-associated coronavirus (SARS-CoV). SARS was first reported in Asia in February 2003. Over the next few months, the illness spread to more than two dozen countries in North America, South America, Europe, and Asia before the SARS global outbreak of 2003 was contained. According to the World Health Organization (WHO), a total of 8098 people worldwide became sick with SARS during the 2003 outbreak. Of these, 774 died. In the United States, only 8 people had laboratory evidence of SARS-CoV infection. All of these people had traveled to other parts of the world where SARS was present.

sexually transmitted diseases (STDs) More than two dozen diseases with a variety of causal agents that are transmitted from person to person by direct contact. These pathogens reside in the genital tract and/or blood and other body fluids and are transmitted principally through sexual activities.

sick building syndrome (SBS) A combination of symptoms or illnesses associated with poor indoor air quality in a place of work or residence. Poor indoor air quality may result from problems with heating, ventilation or air conditioning systems, outgassing of building materials such as volatile organic compounds, and toxic molds.

Siracusa Principles A set of four principles, established at a meeting in Siracusa Italy, regarding internationally recognized limitations on human rights.

smog An atmospheric mixture of smoke and fog often consisting of human generated air pollutants that can be harmful to living things.

smoke-free areas Settings in which smoking has been banned by "clean-air laws," most of which have been passed by local or state legislation.

smoothing techniques A class of statistical methods used to reduce irregularities (random fluctuations) in time series data. They provide a clearer view of the true underlying behavior of the series. See also *time series*.

social class A hierarchy within society or culture that differentiates the power of individuals based on their occupation, education, income, wealth, property, ancestry, or religion.

social determinants of health The economic and social conditions under which people live that largely determine their health status.

social justice The distribution of advantages and disadvantages within society. Public health leaders often justify actions through a social justice perspective, which includes the philosophy of equal health for all regardless of ability to pay.

social marketing The application of common marketing techniques and concepts to achieve a specific behavioral outcome (done for social good rather than financial gain).

social medicine The field of social medicine seeks to understand how social and economic conditions impact health and disease and to foster conditions in which this understanding can lead to a healthier society.

social norms The perceived prevalence of a behavior in a population, taken by individuals to mean that the behavior is acceptable and even expected by others.

soft tissue lesions Lesions in the mouth that occur on the soft tissue, that is, cheeks, gums, tongue, and lips.

sovereign immunity The common law doctrine that no one may sue the government (king).

span of control The number of people/subordinates that can be effectively managed by one manager.

Incident Command System (ICS) organizes tasks and functions into manageable components that ensure span of control.

span of impact The reach or penetration of an intervention in a population, measured by numbers of eligible people affected or percentage of targeted segments exposed to and influenced by the intervention.

special interests In the development of the American polity, the presence of factions or political interest groups was anticipated early in the development of the republic. The original concern was that the "mischief" that would be caused by factions would result in one single faction overcoming others and creating a centralized monarchy-in-all-but-name. The American political system was designed to thwart this tendency by creating separation of powers and a complex system where control was difficult, and sweeping changes were delayed if not completely deterred. At the same time, the system allows for the establishment of groups who can petition government and influence the policy process. This easy entry into the political stream and the constitutional freedoms of assembly and free speech have given the United States a very vibrant system of interest groups, who, in the minds of many political scientists, form the basis for our democratic discourse. Public health has its own interest group structures in the form of associations and organizations that petition government and attempt to sway elections, legislative votes, and executive discretion.

spit (smokeless) tobacco Includes snuff and chewing tobacco; not a safe alternative to smoking. Smokeless tobacco is as addictive as smoking and can cause cancer of the gum, cheek, lip, mouth, tongue, and throat.

Stafford Act Robert T. Stafford Disaster Relief and Emergency Assistance Act, signed into law November 23, 1988; amended the Disaster Relief Act of 1974, PL 93-288. This act constitutes the statutory authority for most federal disaster response activities.

Standardized Mortality/Morbidity Ratio (SMR) A widely used method of reporting death or disease, which adjusts for differences in age and sex across regions. It is a measure of premature mortality. Instead of giving an adjusted rate, the SMR gives a ratio that is a direct comparison with a standard (e.g., the entire country). It is also known as the Adjusted Mortality Ratio (AMR).

State Children's Health Insurance Program (SCHIP) A federal program to cover individuals who have incomes too high to qualify for medical assistance (Medicaid) but cannot obtain private insurance. All states participate, but some do not cover dental services.

statisticians Scientists trained in the science and art of collecting, summarizing, and analyzing data that are subject to random variation. Statistics is also applied to the data themselves and to summarizations of the data.

stillbirth Death in the womb of a fetus of at least 20 weeks gestation.

Strategic National Stockpile (SNS) Federal source of medicine and medical supplies, used to supplement local provisions during public health emergencies.

strategic planning Activity that seeks to define the organization and its future through systematic analysis.

stratosphere The atmospheric layer extending from about 7 to 12 miles above the earth's surface.

structural indicators Measures that characterize the quality or performance of an enterprise based on the resources used within that enterprise, including physical, human, financial, intellectual, and technological resources.

study perspective The viewpoint of the bearers of the costs and benefits of an intervention (e.g., society, government, health care providers, businesses, or patients).

stunting Reduced growth rate in human development that is a primary manifestation of malnutrition in early childhood, including malnutrition during fetal development brought on by the malnourished mother. Once established, stunting and its effects typically become permanent. Stunted children may never regain the height lost as a result of stunting, and most children will never gain the corresponding body weight. It also may lead to premature death later in life because vital organs never fully developed during childhood.

substantive due process The insurance of fundamental fairness in the result reached.

Surgeon General's Report Reviews of science and practice on specific health topics, issued periodically from the federal office of the Surgeon General of the

U.S. Department of Health and Human Services, the first of which was in 1964 on the harmful health effects of tobacco.

surveillance The systematic and routine collection of data to help identify and monitor health risks over time.

super-agency A single, large organization constructed of multiple agencies formerly operating independently. The term has also been used to refer to an organization given new and extraordinary powers or authority.

SWOT analysis Analysis of an organization's strengths, weaknesses, opportunities, and threats.

syndemic perspective Suggests that many community partners may need to work together to solve a problem because it may affect many of these partners in complex, interactive ways.

syndromic detection and management The approach of treating STI/RTI symptoms and signs based on the organisms most commonly responsible for each syndrome. Many sexually transmitted infections and reproductive tract infections (STIs/RTIs) can be identified and treated on the basis of characteristic symptoms and signs. Symptoms and signs can be grouped together into syndromes—upper respiratory infection, gastroenteritis, and vaginal discharge are examples of common syndromes. It is often difficult to know exactly what organism is causing the syndrome, however, and treatment may need to cover several possible infections.

syndromic surveillance Relatively new systems for conducting surveillance that rely on recognizing patterns of symptoms or behavior (e.g., buying anti-flu medications, absenteeism among large groups of people) rather than on diagnoses of specific diseases among individuals.

systemic fluoride Becomes part of the teeth while they are growing through the bloodstream by ingestion. Systemic fluoride can be derived from a food source, water source, or dietary supplements (pill, tablet, lozenge, drop).

systems model of leadership Defines effective leadership as a synthesis of wisdom, creativity, and intelligence. Public health leaders need creativity to generate ideas, analytic intelligence to evaluate those ideas, practical intelligence to implement the ideas and persuade others of their worth, and wisdom to balance the interests of all stakeholders and to ensure that the actions of the leaders contribute to the common good.

systems thinking A way of viewing systems from a broad perspective that includes seeing overall structures, patterns, and cycles in systems, rather than seeing only specific events in the system.

Task Force on Community Preventive Services A U.S. national panel of public health experts appointed by the director of the Centers for Disease Control and Prevention (CDC) to review the scientific literature on efficacy and effectiveness of public health interventions and to recommend their use in practice or further research on the basis of the strength of evidence.

task shifting This term has been applied to assigning tasks in clinical medicine to nurses or medical technicians that have traditionally been performed by physicians or other specialists. Task shifting has been used as a strategy to cope with the lack of health care personnel in low- and middle-income countries or in rural areas.

telemedicine The application of telecommunications technologies (e.g., telephone, video, and Internet technologies) to deliver a health intervention or to assist health personnel when the provider and the recipient are separated by distance.

temporomandibular dysfunction (TMD) Dysfunction of the temporomandibular joint. May result in headaches, jaw pain, and neck pain.

Ten Essential Public Health Services Provides a fundamental framework by describing the public health activities that should be undertaken by public health professionals in all communities. The Core Public Health Functions Steering Committee developed the framework for the Essential Services in 1994. This Steering Committee included representatives from U.S. Public Health Service agencies and other major public health organizations.

tertiary prevention Limiting a disability as a result of disease or rehabilitating an individual with a disability, such as providing dentures for those who have lost all their teeth.

The Joint Commission The organization that accredits health care organizations.

The law of the few (agent) The presence of certain types of people called Connectors, Mavens, and Salesmen.

The power of context (environment) Influences how quickly the innovation will spread.

The stickiness factor (host) The "contagiousness" of the message and the ability of the message to gain adherents.

theories Principles devised to explain a group of facts or phenomena, especially one that has been repeatedly tested or is widely accepted and can be used to make predictions about social and physical events.

time frame The period of time over which the costs of a policy, program, or intervention are tracked.

timeliness The lag between various points in the surveillance process (e.g., onset, symptoms, diagnosis, verification, report). Refers to how quickly the data can enable interventions to be put into place.

time series A sequence of observations that are ordered in time (or space). If observations are made on some phenomenon throughout time, it is most sensible to display the data in the order in which they arose, particularly because successive observations will probably be dependent.

tipping point In epidemiology, it is that moment in an epidemic when a virus reaches critical mass. Used in a sociological context, it is when what is unexpected or rare becomes reality.

topical fluorides A fluoride liquid or gel placed on teeth to help prevent caries.

toxic mold Molds that produce mytotoxins. While mold spores are nearly everywhere, large quantities of certain types of molds can create a health hazard potentially causing respiratory problems and other illnesses. Exposure to high levels of mycotoxins, produced by harmful molds, has been known to lead to neurological problems and sometimes death.

traditional thinking Linear thinking, where "A" leads to "B," which leads to "C," in a causal chain.

transactional leadership The transactional leadership style developed by Bass is based on the hypothesis that followers are motivated through a system of rewards and punishment.

transformational leadership A leader who examines and searches for the needs and motives of others. The three major activities of the public health transformational leader are (1) engaging in the development of mission, (2) visioning, and (3) monitoring and facilitating the process of change.

translation Putting proven public health interventions into practice.

treatment The use of behavioral and/or pharmacological methods to manage drug or alcohol abuse or dependence.

trench mouth A progressive painful infection of the mouth and throat with ulceration, swelling, and sloughing of dead tissue from the mouth and throat due to the spread of infection from the gums. See also *Acute Necrotizing Ulcerative Gingivitis (ANUG)*.

tropical medicine The branch of medicine that deals with health problems that occur uniquely, are more widespread, or prove more difficult to control in tropical and subtropical regions.

tuberculosis A bacterial disease caused by *Mycobacterium tuberculosis*.

Turning Point Initiative A foundation-funded effort to link public health agencies and their partners to other sectors of the community to better affect the underlying social causes of poor health and quality of life.

two-by-two table A table created to categorize observations according to two attributes (e.g., exposure and illness) and facilitate statistical calculations.

tyranny of the majority A liability or danger of utilitarianism in which a minority in the population suffers from a decision to benefit the majority.

umbrella agency A type of state-health agency with an overarching organizational structure consisting of two or more governmental functions, such as public health and social service programs or environmental quality, with a single appointed director who reports to the chief elected official such as a mayor, county commissioner, or governor.

Universal Declaration of Human Rights A United Nations statement of the minimum protection and benefits due to each human being, drafted in 1948.

U.S. Surgeon General's Report on Oral Health This report describes the oral health crisis in the United States, the relationship between oral health and general health, how oral disease is prevented, and the needs and opportunities to enhance oral health.

utilitarianism The philosophical view that the right thing to do is that which provides the greatest good to the greatest number of people.

vaccines Vaccines are suspensions of live (usually attenuated) or killed microorganisms (bacteria or viruses) or fractions thereof administered to induce immunity and prevent infectious disease or its sequelae.

vaccine efficacy (VE) A simple formula exists to determine vaccine efficacy (VE). VE = (ARU − ARV)/ ARU × 100 where ARU is the attack rate of disease in unvaccinated individuals, and ARV is the attack rate in vaccinated individuals.

validity A measure's ability to produce an accurate reflection of the intended aspect of performance.

values clarification Values are the general beliefs that set the foundation for how an organization will operate. Teams must clarify what is important and how the group will operate.

variable costs Costs that change with the level of organizational output or activity.

vector-borne transmission Vector-borne transmission may be mechanical or biological. Mechanical vector-borne transmission includes simple mechanical carriage by a crawling or flying insect through soiling of its feet or proboscis, or by passage of organisms through its gastrointestinal tract. This does not require multiplication or development of the organism. With biological vector-borne transmission, propagation (multiplication), cyclic development, or a combination of these is required before the arthropod can transit the infective form of the agent to humans.

vehicles (or vectors) Typically transfer energy to the host, resulting in injuries. *Vehicles* are the inanimate objects that transmit the energy (e.g., cars, matches, guns), whereas *vectors* are the plants, animals, or persons that transmit the energy (e.g., biting animals, poisonous snakes, human fists).

vehicle-borne transmission Vehicle-borne transmission may occur as a result of contaminated inanimate materials or objects (fomites) such as toys, handkerchiefs, cooking or eating utensils, water, food, milk, and blood. The agent may or may not have multiplied or developed in or on the vehicle before being transmitted.

Veterinary Medical Assistance Teams Provide veterinary services during emergencies.

vision A picture of the "preferred future"; a statement that describes how the future will look if the organization achieves its ultimate aims.

vital events See *vital statistics*.

vital records Document the registration of vital life events. These events are registered, and documents are stored and managed by state or local registrars as directed by law. Records may include birth certificates, marriage licenses, divorce documents, death certificates, and fetal death.

vital statistics Refers to the systematic tabulation of vital records creating statistics concerning important events in human life such as births, deaths, marriages, and migrations.

Voluntary Counseling and Testing (VCT) for HIV Usually involves two counseling sessions: one prior to taking the test known as "pre-test counseling" and one following the HIV test when the results are given, often referred to as "post-test counseling." Counseling focuses on the infection (HIV), the disease (AIDS), the test, and positive behavior change.

voluntary health organizations An industry comprised of establishments engaged in raising funds for health-related research, health education, and patient services.

vulnerable individuals People who are particularly susceptible to research abuses related to constrained possibilities for informed consent. Minors, pregnant women (or fetuses), and prisoners are most commonly considered vulnerable.

vulnerable populations Groups of people who are at a higher risk of disease than the general population, such as the elderly, the homeless, and low-income children.

warning or forecasting The monitoring of events to look for indicators that signify when and where a disaster might occur and what the magnitude might be.

water fluoridation The adjustment of the fluoride level in a public water supply that is optimal for oral health; also called community water fluoridation and fluoridation.

waterborne illness Disease caused by communicable pathogens of viral, bacterial, protozoan and helminthic origin, or chemical toxins that are transmitted by water.[1]

wetland Open water habitat as found in coastal tidal zones, inland marshes, and waterlogged land adjacent to lakes and rivers.[1]

window of opportunity These are relatively brief periods in policy cycles that allow for substantial change. They occur when a problem meets with an applicable solution and when there is a strong enough majority in a legislative body, sufficient public support, and available resources to enact a new or transformative policy. They can also occur when a focusing event such as a terrorist attack, a hurricane, or a handgun tragedy displaces other issues and forces decision makers to act.

Women, Infants, and Children (WIC) Supplemental food program for women, infants, and children administered by the U.S. Department of Agriculture and each state.

workforce The population employed in a specified occupation.

Years of Potential Life Lost (YPLL) A measure of the impact of premature mortality on a population, calculated as the sum of the differences between some predetermined minimum or desired life span and the age of death for individuals who died earlier than that predetermined age.

Youth Risk Behavior Survey (YRBS) The YRBS is conducted by the states, like the BRFSS, with the technical assistance and coordination of the Centers for Disease Control and Prevention (CDC), since 1990, providing national estimates and state-specific estimates in alternating years.

Youth Tobacco Survey (YTS) In contrast to the NSDUH, MTF, and YRBS (which are all multiple risk factor surveillance systems) covers just tobacco use. The YTS was developed in response to requests from those state health departments that received early settlements from tobacco industry litigation. The YTS began in Florida, Texas, and Mississippi in 1998, providing valuable data for program planning and evaluation purposes, and is currently being used in 45 states.

zoonosis A disease that is transmissible from animals to humans; usually a disease that also causes disease in animals.[1]

REFERENCES

1. Last JM. *A Dictionary of Public Health*. New York: Oxford University Press; 2007.
2. Breslow L. *Encyclopedia of Public Health*. New York: Macmillan Reference USA; 2002.

INDEX